Across Volume 5

• Physiology • Biochemistry

Eighth Edition

Saumya Shukla
DNB Radiodiagnosis
Assistant Professor
Nizam's Institute of Medical Sciences
Hyderabad, India

Anurag Shukla
MS MCh (Orth), UK

Siddharth Dixit
DO, DNB (Ophthalmology)
Glaucoma Consultant, L V Prasad Eye Institute,
Hyderabad, India

Khushi Shukla

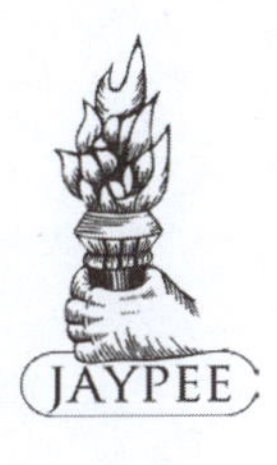

JAYPEE The Health Sciences Publisher
New Delhi | London | Panama

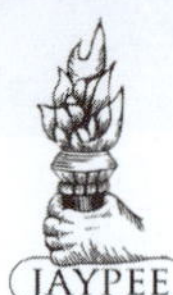

Jaypee Brothers Medical Publishers (P) Ltd

Headquarters
Jaypee Brothers Medical Publishers (P) Ltd.
4838/24, Ansari Road, Daryaganj
New Delhi 110 002, India
Phone: +91-11-43574357
Fax: +91-11-43574314
E-mail: jaypee@jaypeebrothers.com

Overseas Offices
J.P. Medical Ltd.
83, Victoria Street, London
SW1H 0HW (UK)
Phone: +44-20 3170 8910
Fax: +44(0)20 3008 6180
E-mail: info@jpmedpub.com

Jaypee-Highlights Medical Publishers Inc.
City of Knowledge, Bld. 235, 2nd Floor, Clayton
Panama City, Panama
Phone: +1 507-301-0496
Fax: +1 507-301-0499
E-mail: cservice@jphmedical.com

Jaypee Brothers Medical Publishers (P) Ltd.
17/1-B, Babar Road, Block-B, Shaymali
Mohammadpur, Dhaka-1207, Bangladesh
Mobile: +08801912003485
E-mail: jaypeedhaka@gmail.com

Jaypee Brothers Medical Publishers (P) Ltd.
Bhotahity, Kathmandu, Nepal
Phone: +977-9741283608
E-mail: kathmandu@jaypeebrothers.com

Website: www.jaypeebrothers.com
Website: www.jaypeedigital.com

Across Volume 5

Seventh Edition: 2015
Eighth Edition: 2017
ISBN: 978-93-5270-140-7
Printed at Sanat Printers

Contents

PHYSIOLOGY

MCQs with Answers and Explanations

Chapter -1 CENTRAL NERVOUS SYSTEM

QUESTIONS

Higher Function

1. Attention and concentration is mediated by:
A. Hypothalamus (AIIMS 14) ☐
B. Frontal lobe ☐
C. Parietal lobe ☐
D. Basal ganglia ☐

2. Human brain is more intelligent than monkey's brain due to: (PGI 03)
A. Larger brain ☐
B. Increased convulations ☐
C. Increased brain area compared to body surface area ☐
D. More blood supply ☐

3. True about function of brain are *all except:* (AI 06)
A. Sensitive to hypoxia ☐
B. Dependent on glucose ☐
C. Uses fatty acids in starvation ☐
D. Does not store energy ☐

4. Sematosensory area I largest representation is for-
A. Arm (NBE P 13) ☐
B. Leg ☐
C. Back ☐
D. Head ☐

5. Ablation of the 'somatosensory area I' of the cerebral cortex leads to:
(NBE P 15,14,13; AIIMS 14; AI 02)
A. Total loss of pain sensation ☐
B. Total loss of touch sensation ☐
C. Loss of tactile localization but not of two point discrimination ☐
D. Loss of tactile localization and two point discrimination ☐

6. The inability to perceive the texture & shape an object occurs in lesion of: (AIIMS 06)
A. Lateral spino-thalamic tract ☐
B. Nucleus gracils ☐
C. Spino reticular tract ☐
D. Nucleus cuneatus/tractus cuneatus ☐

7. Pt. is able to recognize person by name but not by face. Lesion is in......- (NBE P 13)
A. Post parietal region ☐
B. Occipital ☐
C. Frontal lobe ☐
D. Temporal lobe ☐

Emotions & Memory

8. The nucleus involved in Papez circuit is:
A. Pulvinar (AI 07) ☐
B. Intralaminar ☐
C. VPL nucleus ☐
D. Anterior nucleus of Thalamus ☐

9. Window of limbic system (Assam 04, WB –03)
A. Hypothalmus ☐
B. Amygdala ☐
C. Hippocampus ☐
D. Thalmus ☐

10. Functions of limbic system : (PGI 06)
A. Emotion ☐
B. Memory ☐
C. Higher function ☐
D. Planned motor activity ☐

11. Structure of brain involved in emotion :
A. Neocortex (PGI 04) ☐
B. Limbic system ☐
C. Thalamus ☐
D. Hippocampus ☐
E. Basal ganglia ☐

12. Self stimulation could be induced experimentally most effectively from which part of the brain OR Area of brain responsible for self stimulation reward on induction (i.e. reward centre) is?
A. Periaqueductal area (AI 12; AIIMS 14) ☐
B. Medial forebrain bundle ☐
C. Periventricular region of hypothalamus ☐
D. Mesencephalon ☐

13. Which of the following statements about 'Sham Range' is Not true: (AI 12)
A. Caused by Hypothalamic stimulation ☐
B. Abolished by Decortication ☐
C. Pathological Rage Reaction ☐
D. Association with sympathetic stimulation ☐

14. Which of the following nucleus of Hypothalamus is most closely related to sexual activity in males
A. Preoptic nucleus (AI 12) ☐
B. Supraoptic nucleus ☐
C. Lateral hypothalamic nuclei ☐
D. Posterior hypothalamic nuclei ☐

15. The mechanism of learning and memory, include all except: (AI 07)
A. Changes in level of neurotransmitter at synapse ☐
B. Increasing protein synthesis ☐
C. Recruitment by multiplication of neurons ☐
D. Spatial Reorganization of synapse ☐

16. The processing of short term memory to long term memory is done in OR Unable to consolidate long term memory indicate damage to OR Consolidation of long term memory occur in:
A. Prefrontal cortex (NBE P 15, 14, 13) ☐
B. Hippocampus (AIIMS 14,12; AI 07) ☐
C. Neocortex ☐
D. Amygdala ☐

17. All are true statement regarding memory except
- A. Structural changes occur in synapses during the development of long-term memory ☐
- B. Short term memory last as long as the person continues to think *(PGI 11)* ☐
- C. The site for storage of long term memory is in temporal lobe ☐
- D. Bilateral loss of hippocampal function leads to loss of the ability to encode events of the recent past in long term memory ☐
- E. Intermediate memory results from temporary change in synapse ☐

18. Associative learning- *(NBE P 13)*
- A. Associated with consciousness ☐
- B. Includes skills and habits ☐
- C. Relation of one stimulus to another ☐
- D. Facilitation of recognition of words ☐

19. Striatum damage affects priming- *(NBE P 13, 15)*
- A. Procedural memory ☐
- B. Short term memory ☐
- C. Long term memory ☐
- D. Explicit memory ☐

Sleep

20. Key regulators of sleep are located in
- A. Hypothalamus *(AI 09, AIIMS 12)* ☐
- B. Thalamus ☐
- C. Putamen ☐
- D. Limbic cortex ☐

21. Which of the following is likely to happen to the 'Sleep-wake cycle' if all environment/external cues are removed: *(AIIMS 12, AI12)*
- A. Will remain unchanged at 24 hrs ☐
- B. Will be prolonged to greater than 24 hrs cycle length ☐
- C. Will be shortened to less than 24 hours cycle length ☐
- D. Will become irregular/does not continue ☐

22. Which of the following nucleus controls the circadian rhythm? OR Diurnal variation of ACTH depends on- *(NBE P 15, 13; AIIMS 08, 13,15)*
- A. Supraoptic nucleus ☐
- B. Paraventricular nucleus ☐
- C. Suprachiasmatic nucleus ☐
- D. Premamillary nucleus ☐

Cereberal Dominance

23. Left lobe is responsible for *(AIIMS 12)*
- A. Appreciation of Music ☐
- B. Spatial orientation ☐
- C. Visual Stimuli Processing ☐
- D. Written and Spoken Language ☐

24. Agnosia is caused by lesion of- *(NBE P 13)*
- A. Representative hemisphere, left ☐
- B. Categorial hemisphere, left ☐
- C. Representative hemisphere, right ☐
- D. Categorial hemisphere, right ☐

25. Neurophysiological defects present in right lobe involvement are A/E *(AIIMS 09)*
- A. Visuospatial defect ☐
- B. Anosognosa ☐
- C. Dyscalculia ☐
- D. Dysgraphia ☐

Aphasia

26. Broca's area is present in- *(NBE P 13)*
- A. Superior temporal gyrus ☐
- B. Precentral gyrus ☐
- C. Post central gyrus ☐
- D. Inferior frontal gyrus ☐

27. Broca's area is concerned with: *(AI 07)*
- A. Word formation ☐
- B. Comprehension ☐
- C. Repetition ☐
- D. Reading ☐

28. Motor aphasia refers to defect in: *(AIIMS 08)*
- A. Peripheral speech apparatus ☐
- B. Verbal expression ☐
- C. Auditory comprehension ☐
- D. Verbal comprehension ☐

Hearing & Vision

29. Endolymph in ear equivalent to- *(NBE P 13)*
- A. ICF ☐
- B. Lymph ☐
- C. CSF ☐
- D. Blood ☐

30. Inner hair cells depolarises due to- *(NBE P 13)*
- A. K+ influx ☐
- B. Na+ influx ☐
- C. K+efflux ☐
- D. Voltage gated ca channels ☐

31. Semicircular canals are stimulated by- *(NBE P 13)*
- A. Gravity ☐
- B. Linear acceleration ☐
- C. Rotation ☐
- D. Sound ☐

32. Endo-cochlear potential is: *(AIIMS 16)*
- A. +45 mV ☐
- B. –45mV ☐
- C. –60mV ☐
- D. +85 mV ☐

33. Where do the peripheral processes of spiral ganglion end? *(AIIMS 16)*

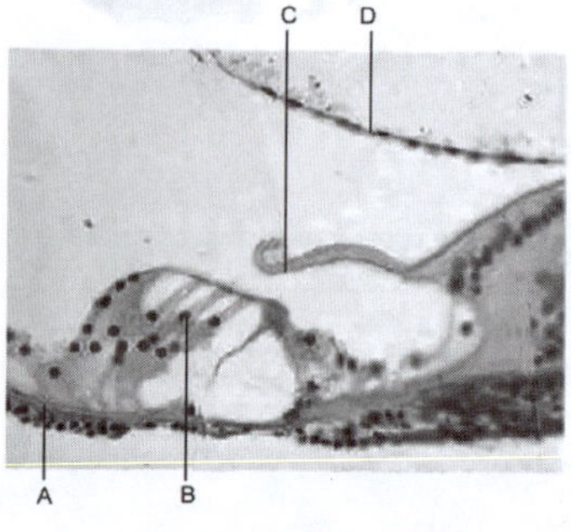

A. C
B. D
C. B
D. A

34. **True stereopsis is perceived due to the following:**
A. Overlay of contours (AIIMS 06)
B. Motion parallax
C. Bi- nasal disparity
D. Linear perspective

35. **The fibers from the contralateral nasal hemiretina project to the following layers of the lateral geniculate nucleus:**
A. Layers 2, 3 & 5. (AI 05)
B. Layers 1, 2 & 6.
C. Layers 1, 4 & 6.
D. Layers 4, 5 & 6.

36. **Most afferent fibers from the lateral geniculate nucleus terminate in the primary visual cortex is:**
A. Layer 1 (AI 06)
B. Layer 2 & 3
C. Layer 4
D. Layer 5 & 6

37. **The parvocellular pathway, from the lateral geniculate nucleus to the visual cortex, carries signals for the detection of:** (AI 06)
A. Movement, depth and flicker
B. Color vision, shape and fine details
C. Temporal frequency
D. Luminance contrast

38. **The parvocellular pathway from lateral geniculate nucleus to visual cortex is most sensitive for the stimulus of:** (AI 05)
A. Color contrast.
B. Luminance contrast.
C. Temporal frequency.
D. Saccadic eye movements.

39. **The blobs of the visual cortex are associated with:**
A. Ocular dominance (AI 06)
B. Orientation
C. Color processing
D. Saccadic eye movements

40. **Retinal cells which secrete acytyl choline-**
A. Bipolar cells (NBE P 13)
B. Ganglion cells
C. Amacrine cells
D. H cells

41. **Which is the first order neuron in optic pathway:**
A. Bipolar cells (NBE P 13)
B. Ganglionic cells
C. Cells of lateral geniculate body
D. Astrocytes

42. **Second order neuron-** (NBE P 13)
A. Optic nerve
B. MGB
C. LGB
D. Layer of retina

43. **Relative colour and luminosity of photoreceptive input under changing light conditions are regulated and maintained by:** (AIIMS 03)
A. Muller cells
B. Amacrine cells
C. Ganglion cells
D. Retinal astrocytes

44. **During the dark phase of visual cycle, which form of vitamin A combines with opsin to make Rhodopsin:** (AIIMS 04)
A. All trans-Retinaldehyde
B. All trans-Retinol
C. 11-cis-Retinaldehyde
D. 11-cis-Retinol

45. **Initiation of visual impulse is associated with**
A. Condensation of opsin with vitamin A aldehyde (AI 09)
B. Photoisomerization and hydrolysis of visual purple
C. ↓ NADP
D. ↓ NAD

46. **Photoreceptors on exposure to dark release-**
A. Acetyl choline (NBE P 13)
B. Glutamate
C. Adrenaline
D. Epinephrine

47. **Transducin is required for-** (NBE P 13)
A. Small
B. Hearing
C. Small
D. Vision

48. **Rods and cones differ in all, Except:**
A. Signal transduction (AIIMS 09)
B. Light sensitivity
C. Wavelength
D. Acuity

Color Vision, Taste & Olfaction

49. **For color vision, which is true?** (AIIMS 09)
A. Independent of wavelength of light
B. Depends on intensity discrimination
C. Involves opponent color cells
D. Minimum at fixation point

50. **Visible range of electromagnetic spectrum of human eye** (PGI 04)
A. 370 – 740 nm
B. 740 – 1140 nm
C. 200 – 340 nm
D. 200 – 370 nm
E. 370 – 770 nm

51. **Which of the following are Chemoreceptors-**
A. Rods (NBE P 13)
B. Cones
C. Taste buds
D. Muscle spindle

52. Salty taste is due to- *(NBE P 13)*
A. Ca^{+2} channels
B. Na^{+} channels
C. G-protein
D. H^{+} Channels

53. The receptors/buds responsible for carrying bitter taste sensation are situated- *(NBE P 13)*
A. At the tip of the tongue
B. Just behing the tip
C. At the sides
D. At the posterior aspect

54. Which is incorrectly matched- *(NBE P 13)*
A. Eyes-rods& cones
B. Olfaction-hair cells
C. Tongue-Na channels
D. Carotid body-chemoreceptor

Equilibrium & Basal Ganglia

55. Static equilibrium is due to- *(NBE P 13)*
A. Macula
B. Cupula
C. End organ of corti
D. Cristae ampulla

56. Nucleus of basal ganglia are:*(PGI 04,13; NBEP 14, 13)*
A. Dentate
B. Thalamus
C. Caudate nucleus / Putamen/ GP
D. Red nucleus

57. The efferent fiber bundle of the substantia nigra transmits dopamine to one of the following areas:
A. Thalamus *(AIIMS 04)*
B. Corpus striatum
C. Tegmentum of pons
D. Tectum of midbrain

58. The highest density of glutamate receptors in basal ganglia are found in *(AI 12)*
A. Substantia nigra
B. Globus pallidus interna
C. Globus pallidus externa
D. Putamen

59. Which of the following basal ganglia nucleus is primarily glutaminergic *(AI 12)*
A. Putamen
B. Subthalamic Nucleus
C. Globus pallidus
D. Substantial Nigra

60. Which of the following acts as the major neurotransmitter in substantia nigra (nigrostriatal pathway): *(NBE P 14, 13)*
A. Dopamine *(AIIMS 07, 14)*
B. Noradrenaline
C. Acetylcholine
D. Serotonin

61. Functions of basal ganglia *include*: *(PGI 02)*
A. Gross motor
B. Skilled movements
C. Emotions
D. Maintenance of equilibrium
E. Coordination of movements

62. Which of the following clearly states the role of basal ganglia in motor function:
A. Planning *(NBE P 13; PGI 05, 13,14)*
B. Skilled function
C. Coordinate function
D. Balance & Coarse movements

63. True about spinocerebellar tract is:
A. Equilibrium *(AIIMS 09, 10)*
B. Smoothens and coordinates movement
C. Learning induced by change in vestibulocular reflex
D. Planning and programming

64. Lesion of Globus pallidus causes- *(NBE P 13)*
A. Chorea
B. Ballismus
C. Athetosis
D. Akinesia

65. Disease of Basal ganglia dysfunction are all except-
A. Alziemer's disease *(NBE P 13)*
B. Parkinsonism
C. Chorea.
D. Athetosis

Blood Brain Barrier

66. Which of the following is not permeable through the Blood Brain Barrier: *(AIIMS 10)*
A. Water
B. Lipophilic drugs
C. Gas
D. Proteins

67. "Blood brain barrier" is present at all of the following sites except: *(AIIMS 14, 12; AI 2K)*
A. Hebenular nucleus
B. Subfornical organ
C. Cerebellum
D. Pontine nucleus

68. Circumentricular organ is- *(NBE P 13)*
A. Anterior pituitary
B. Posterior pituitary
C. Pineal gland
D. None

69. Vomiting centre- *(NBE P 13)*
A. Area postrema
B. Suprachiasmatic
C. Medial nuclei
D. Lateral nuclei

70. Vomiting centre is situated in the- *(NBE P 13)*
A. Hypothalamus
B. Amygdala
C. Rons
D. Medulla

Cerebellum, Posture & Decortication

71. **Flocculo nodular lobe has direct connection with :**
    A. Red nucleus *(AI 08)*
    B. Inferior olivary nucleus
    C. Vestibular nucleus
    D. Dentate nucleus
72. **Vestibulocerebellar tract terminates in the... of cerebellum-** *(JIPMER 04)*
    A. Flocculus
    B. Lingula
    C. Nodulus
    D. Uvula
    E. All of the above
73. **Cerebellar connection to other parts of the brain is projected through which cell OR Output from the cerebellum is solely from::** *(AI 04)*
    A. Golgi cells
    B. Basket cells
    C. Purkinje cells
    D. Oligodendrocytes
74. **Purkinje cells from the cerebellum end in OR Purkinje fibres are inhibitory for:** *(NBE P 14, 13)*
    A. Extrapyramidal system *(Jipmer 05)*
    B. Cranial nerve nuclei
    C. Deep Cerebellar nuclei
    D. Cerebral cortex
75. **All are true about cerebellum except** *(AI 04; PGI 05)*
    A. It has 3 layers, 4 nucleus & 5 cells
    B. Climbing fibres are afferent inputs
    C. Mossy fibres inhibit Purkinje cells
    D. Climbing fibres excite Purkinje cells
76. **Which is a cerebellar nucleus-** *(NBE P 13)*
    A. Caudate
    B. Subthalamic
    C. Globus pallidus
    D. Dentate
77. **Cells present in Cerebellar cortex are all except.**
    A. Purkinje *(AIIMS 08)*
    B. Bipolar
    C. Granule
    D. Golgi
78. **True about cerebellum :** *(PGI 04)*
    A. Cerebral cortex have mostly inhibitory effects
    B. Co-ordination
    C. Planning of motor movements
    D. Decreased tone
    E. Excitatory effect from deep nuclei
79. **Which one of the following clearly states the role of cerebellum in motor performance:** *(AIIMS 04)*
    A. Planning and programming of movement
    B. Convert abstract thought into voluntary action
    C. Initiation of skilled voluntary action
    D. Smoothens and coordinates ongoing movements
80. **Lesions of the lateral cerebellum cause all of the following, Except:** *(NBE P 15, 13, 14; AI 10; AIIMS 10)*
    A. Incoordination
    B. Intention tremor/Dymetria
    C. Resting tremor
    D. Ataxia/Hypotonia
81. **Which of the following does not carry proprioceptive impulses?** *(NBE P 13)*
    A. Olivo cerebellar tract
    B. Tecto cerebellar tract
    C. Spino cerebellar tract
    D. Cuneo cerebellar tract
82. **Destruction of anterior cerebellum in a decerebrate animal leads to-** *(NBE P 13)*
    A. No effect on rigidity
    B. Increased flexor muscle tone
    C. Increased rigidity via alpha motor neurouns
    D. Decrease in rigidity
83. **True about spinocerebellar tract is-** *(NBE P 13)*
    A. Equilibrium
    B. Smoothens and coordinates movement
    C. Learining induced by change in vestibulocular reflex
    D. Planning and programming
84. **Vestibulo ocular reflex is concerned with-**
    A. Archicerebellum *(NBE P 13)*
    B. Flocculonodular lobe
    C. Neocerbellum
    D. Occipital lobe
85. **Setting posture before planned movement-**
    A. Premotor cortex *(NBE P 13)*
    B. Motor cortex
    C. Frontal
    D. Supplementary motor cortex
86. **The maintenance of posture in a normal adult human being depends upon:** *(AI 06)*
    A. Integrity of reflex arc
    B. Muscle power
    C. Type of muscle fibers
    D. Joint movements in physiological range
87. **Posture is maintained by-** *(NBE P 13)*
    A. Crosse extensor reflex
    B. Stretch reflex
    C. Golgi tendon refkex
    D. None
88. **In decorticate animal which reflex is lost?** *(NBE P 13)*
    A. Hoping and placing reflex
    B. Tonic neck reflex
    C. Tonic labyrinthine reflex
    D. Stretch reflex
89. **Postural reflex with integrating center in spine-**
    A. Righting reflex *(NBE P 13)*
    B. Tonic labyrinthine reflex
    C. Righting reflex
    D. Crossed extensor reflex
90. **All of the following are true about Kluver-Buey syndrome except:** *(NBE P 13)*
    A. Hypersexuality
    B. Hyperactivity
    C. Hypermetamorphosis
    D. Placidity

Appetite

91. The principal polypeptide that increase food intake are all except- *(NBE P 13)*
A. Neuropeptide Y
B. Leptin
C. Orexin A
D. Ghrelin

92. Appetite is stimulated by all of the following peptides, Except: *(AI 09, AIIMS 10)*
A. Agouti – Related Peptide (AGRP)
B. Melanocyte Stimulating hormone (MSH)
C. Melanin Concentrating Hormone (MCH)
D. Neuropeptide Y

93. Which hormone is secreted from stomach that control intake of food and stimulate growth:
A. Orexin *(NBE P 15, 13; AIIMS 10)*
B. Insulin like growth hormone
C. Cholecystokinin
D. Ghrelin

94. Regarding Gherlin which of false- *(NBE P 13)*
A. Secreted from oxyntic cells
B. Increases fat deposition
C. Stimulates appetite
D. Secretion increased in anorexia

95. The cell bodies of orexinergic neurons are present in: *(AI 06)*
A. Locus ceruleus
B. Dorsal raphe
C. Lateral hypothalamic area
D. Hippocampus

Neurotransmitter

96. Which is not a peptide neurotransmitters-
A. Enkephalin *(NBE P 13)*
B. Substance P
C. Endorphin
D. Serotonin

97. All are true about neuropeptide Y except:
A. Consist of 36 amino acids *(AIIMS 10)*
B. Decreases thermogenesis
C. Decreased in starvation
D. Same effect like melanocorticotropin

98. Substance P is increased in response to pain in periphery by which of the following?
A. Mast cells *(AIIMS 09)*
B. Endothelium
C. Plasma
D. Nerve terminals

99. The main excitatory neurotransmitter in the CNS is
A. Glycine *(PGI 04, AI 04)*
B. Acetylcholine
C. Aspartate
D. Glutamate

100. The inhibitory neurotransmitter in CNS neurons is
A. Glutamate *(AIIMS 04)*
B. Aspartate
C. Gamma-amino butyric acid
D. Taurine

101. The hyperkinetic features of the Huntington's disease are due to the loss of: *(AI 06)*
A. Nigrostriatal dopaminergic system
B. Intrastriatal cholinergic system
C. GABA-ergic and cholinergic system
D. Intrastriatal GABA-ergic and cholinergic syste

Thalamus & Thirst Control

102. Pain and temperature in thalamus is controlled by nucleus- *(NBE P 13)*
A. VPM
B. VPL
C. Anterior
D. Posterior

103. Location of osmoreceptor is OR Injection of hypertonic saline in which region of hypothalamus produces intense thirst: *(AIIMS 07, 02)*
A. Posterior region
B. Paraventricular
C. Preoptic nucleus of anterior hypothalamus
D. Supraoptic

104. Drinking can be induced by: *(AIIMS 04)*
A. Electrical stimulation of the posterior hypothalamus
B. Osmotic stimulation of supraoptic nucleus
C. Lesions in the paraventicular nucleus
D. Neuronal lesion of the preoptic nucleus

105. Vasopressin induced thirst is through- *(NBE P 13)*
A. Subfornicial nuclei
B. Posterior hypothalamus osmoreceptors
C. Pretectal nucleus

Temperature Regulation

106. Temperature at which regulating mechanism does not work- *(NBE P 13)*
A. 40°C
B. 35°C
C. 30°C
D. 25°C

107. Hyperthermia- *(NBE P 13)*
A. Temperature>41.5
B. >40 with autonomic dysfunctuion
C. No change in hypothalamic thermostat
D. One which normalizes with antipyretic

108. Function of preptic nucleus of hypothalamus-
A. Temperature regulation *(NBE P 13)*
B. Thirst
C. GI stimulation
D. Satiety centre

109. Lesion of preoptic nucleus of hypothalamus causes-
A. Hyperphagia *(NBE P 13)*
B. Hyperdypsia
C. Hyperthermia
D. Hyperglycemia

110. Which of the following nucleus controls the circadian rhythm? *(NBE P 13)*
A. Supraoptic nucleus
B. Paraventricular nucleus
C. Suprachiasmatic nucleus
D. Premamillary nucleus

111. Vasopressin is secreted by- *(NBE P 13)*
A. Supraoptic
B. Preoptic
C. Paraventricular
D. Posterior nucleus

112. A/E is under the control of hypothalamus:
A. Increases heart rate with exercise
B. Food intake *(AIIMS 05, AI 07)*
C. Pituitary hormone (hypophyseal) regulation
D. Temperature regulation

113. Sweating a result of exertion is mediated through OR During acclimitisation, decreased sweating is due to down regulation of: *(NBE P 14, 13)*
A. Adrenal hormones *(PGI 15,13,09)*
B. Sympathetic cholinergic
C. Sympathetic adrenergic (ACh)
D. Parasympathetic cholinergic (NA)

114. Heat loss from the body depends mostly on:
A. Thermoregulatory center *(AI 2K)*
B. Warming of air during inspiration
C. On the environmental temperature
D. Radiation and evaporation

115. Main mechanism in thermoregulation-heat loss is-
A. Radiation *(NBE P 13)*
B. Evaporation
C. Conduction
D. Convection

116. The first physiological response to high environmental temperature is: *(AI 05)*
A. Sweating.
B. Vasodilatation.
C. Decreased heat production.
D. Non-shivering thermogenesis.

117. Under physiological conditions heat acclimatization is accomplished A/E. *(AIIMS 08)*
A. Decreased Renal Blood Flow
B. Increased urine sodium
C. Increased aldosterone secretion
D. Excessive sweating

118. The physiological effect in unacclimatised person suddenly exposed to cold is: *(AIIMS 01)*
A. Tachycardia
B. Shift of blood from shell to core
C. Non shivering thermogenesis
D. Hypertension

119. Nonshivering thermogenesis in adults is due to
A. Thyroid hormone *(AI 02)*
B. Brown fat between the shoulders
C. Noradrenaline
D. Muscle metabolism

120. Endogenous non-shivering thermogens are secreted by all except : *(AI 03)*
A. Liver
B. Spleen
C. Heart
D. Small intestine

121. Non-shivering thermogenesis is mediated by:
A. α_1 receptor. *(NBE P 15,13; PGI 03, 14, 13)*
B. β_2 receptor
C. β_3 adrenergic receptor & UCP1
D. UCP-2

122. All the following can occur in a neonate for heat production except: *(AIIMS 12)*
A. Shivering
B. Breakdown of brown fat with adrenaline secretion
C. Universal flexion like a fetus
D. Cutaneous vasoconstriction

123. The hormone associated with cold adaption is:
A. Growth hormone *(AIIMS 03)*
B. Thyroxine
C. Insulin.
D. Melanocyte Stimulating Hormone.

124. True regarding animals that are chronically exposed to cold? *(AIIMS 11)*
A. Increased sympathetic stimulation
B. Increased vagal action
C. Increased insulin levels in blood
D. Decrease blood supply to adipose tissue

125. A 10 degree decrease in temperature causes decrease in cerebral metabolic rate by: *(AIIMS 02)*
A. 10%
B. 30%
C. 50%
D. 70%

126. In human being, the least useful physiological response to low environmental temperature is:
A. Shivering *(AI 06)*
B. Vasoconstriction
C. Release of thyroxine
D. Piloerection

127. Which of the following site doesn't contain brown adipose tissues? *(AIIMS 15)*
A. Scapula
B. Subcutaneous tissue
C. Around blood vessel
D. Around adrenal cortex

128. Adrenergic beta-receptors having lipolysis property in fat cells is: *(AIIMS 15)*
A. Alpha-1
B. Alpha-2
C. Beta-1
D. Beta-3

129. Adverse effects of hypothermia are all except:
A. Cardiac arrhythmias *(AIIMS11)*
B. Renal failure
C. Decreased peripheral resistance
D. Reversible coagulopathy

Cells of CNS

130. Features of Neuroglia cells include *all except:*
- A. Protoplasmic astrocytes are found in grey matter *(NBE P 15, 13; AI 08)* ☐
- B. Oligodendrocytes are derived from ectoderm and form myelin ☐
- C. Microglia are mesodermal in origin ☐
- D. Central neuroglial cells are derived from Schwann Cells ☐

131. Function of microglia in CNS: *(NBE P 15; PGI 03)*
- A. Phagocytosis (like macrophage) ☐
- B. Myeline synthesis ☐
- C. Fibrosis ☐

Nerve Regeneration

132. A politician is shot in the back at level of D8 vertebral body. Immediately after the shot he loses all the sensation below the level of transaction. He is put on treatment. No recovery is noted even after proper treatment. All of the following are the possible reasons for his non recovery, except:
- A. Glial scar formation *(AIIMS 12)* ☐
- B. Absence of growth factors ☐
- C. Lack of myelin inhibiting substance ☐
- D. Absence of endoneural tube ☐

Cerebrospinal Fluid (CSF)

133. About CSF following statement (s) true is A/E: *(NBE P 15,13;PGI 08)*
- A. Specific gravity is 1.003–1.0008 ☐
- B. CSF/plasma glucose ratio is 0.6 to 0.8 (2/3) ☐
- C. CSF volume is 150ml, daily production is 550ml/day & pH is 7.33 ☐
- D. CSF/plasma protein ratio is 0.3 ☐

134. CSF pressure (lumbar) - *(AIIMS 2K)*
- A. 70 - 180 mm CSF ☐
- B. 50 - 100 mm CSF ☐
- C. > 200 mm CSF ☐
- D. 150 - 200 mm CSF ☐

135. CSF does not pass through - *(AI 09)*
- A. Ventricles ☐
- B. Venous sinuses ☐
- C. Epidural spaces ☐
- D. Subarachnoid space ☐

136. CSF is principally secreted by - *(NBE P 15,13)*
- A. Choroid plexus *(AIIMS 14)* ☐
- B. Arachnoid granulation ☐
- C. Floor of fourth ventricle ☐
- D. Periaqueductal grey ☐

137. The normal adult CSF pressure is:
- A. 1-2 mm Hg *(AIIMS 03)* ☐
- B. 6-12 mm Hg ☐
- C. 15-30 mm Hg ☐
- D. 730 mm Hg ☐

138. Low CSF protein may be seen in all of the following conditions, Except: *(AI 10)*
- A. Recurrent Lumbar Puncture ☐
- B. Hypothyroidism ☐
- C. Pseudotumor cerebri ☐
- D. Infants ☐

139. Regarding CSF all the following statements are true except *(AIIMS 07)*
- A. Its pH is less than blood ☐
- B. No neutrophils present normally ☐
- C. Formed by arachnoid villi ☐
- D. Persistent leakage can cause headache ☐

140. CSF pressure is mainly regulated by:
- A. Rate of CSF formation *(AIIMS 12,11, 08)* ☐
- B. Rate of CSF absorption ☐
- C. Cerebral blood flow ☐
- D. Venous pressure ☐

141. True about cerebrospinal fluid: *(PGI 12)*
- A. Produced by choroid plexus ☐
- B. Travels from subarachnoid space to third ventricle ☐
- C. Absorbed by arachnoid villi ☐
- D. Flow from spinal cord to brain ☐

142. Concentration of potassium in children's CSF is:
- A. 3 mEq/L *(PGI 12)* ☐
- B. 5 mEq/L ☐
- C. 10 mEq/L ☐
- D. 15 mEq/L ☐
- E. 20 mEq/L ☐

143. Enzymes found in CSF: *(AIIMS 12)*
- A. ALP+ CK-MB ☐
- B. CK+ LDH ☐
- C. Deaminase and peroxidase ☐
- D. GGT+ALP ☐

Intracranial Tension & Transection

144. All are seen in cerebral herniation, except:
- A. Neck stiffness *(AIIMS 01)* ☐
- B. Loss of consciousness ☐
- C. Pupil dilatation ☐
- D. Autonomic disturbances ☐

145. Increase in intracranial pressure is NOT associated with: *(AIIMS 14,08,02; NBE P 15, 14)*
- A. Deterioration of consciousness ☐
- B. Tachycardia ☐
- C. Respiratory depression ☐
- D. Increase in BP ☐

146. Increased BP & decreased heart rate is seen in-
- A. Hemorrhage *(NBE P 13)* ☐
- B. High altitude ☐
- C. Raised intracranial pressure ☐
- D. Anemia ☐

147. In an encephala isole preparation, the transections is done at: *(AIIMS 14)*
- A. First cervical spinal segment ☐
- B. Level of medulla ☐
- C. Midpontine level ☐
- D. Midcollicular level ☐

EEG

148. What are the EEG waves recored for parietooccipital rgion with subject awake & eye closed- *(NBE P 13)*
A. Alpha waves
B. Beta waves
C. Delta waves
D. Theta waves

149. True about EEG (Buerger) alpha (α) wave is:
A. Frequency is 8-13 /sec. *(PGI 2K)*
B. Voltage is 50 microvolts usually
C. Seen in awake patients at rest with eyes closed and mind wandering
D. These are Buerger (EEG) curves seen in hippocampus.
E. Found in emotional stress.

150. True about EEG (Buerger) β wave is /are *(PGI 01)*
A. Frequency is 13-30 per second
B. Frequency is < 13 per second
C. Predominant activity in REM sleep
D. Predominant activity in NRFM sleep

151. Beta waveforms in electroencephalogram designate which of the following states of the patient:
A. Deep Anaesthesia *(AIIMS 05)*
B. Surgical Anaesthesia
C. Light Anaesthesia, eyes closed, relaxed
D. Awake/alert state

152. Delta waves are seen in : *(AI 07)*
A. Deep sleep
B. REM sleep
C. Awake state
D. Stage I NREM sleep

153. EEG rhythm having lowest frequency is-
A. Alpha *(DNB 14, AI 04)*
B. Beta
C. Delta
D. Theta

154. Slow wave sleep associated with: *(PGI 06)*
A. Dreams
B. Cardiac arrhythmia
C. Penile intumescence
D. Delta activity

155. The EEG recorded shown below is normally recordable during which stage of sleep? *(AIIMS 15,14,03)*

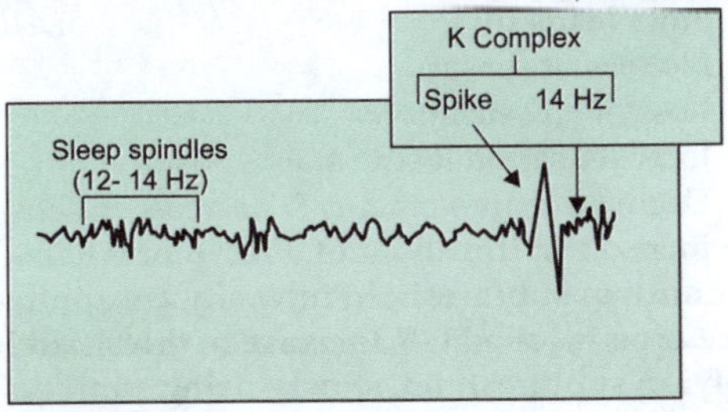

A. Stage I
B. Stage II
C. Stage III
D. Stage IV

156. In the given image, wave B represents: *(AIIMS 15)*

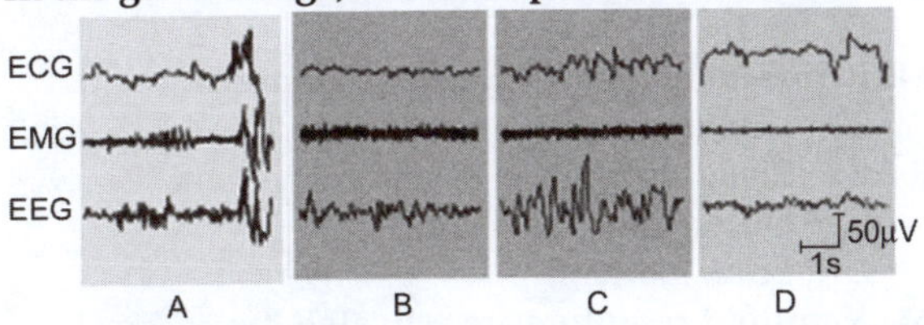

A. REM
B. NREM
C. Quiet wakefulness
D. Awake

157. About paradoxical sleep. True is: *(AIIMS 07)*
A. Prominent beta waves
B. Prominent alpha waves
C. Also known as NREM sleep.
D. Low amplitude, mixed frequency waves.

158. Nightmare is seen in : *(AI 04)*
A. REM sleep
B. Stage II NREM sleep
C. Stage IV NREM sleep
D. Stage I NREM sleep

159. Which one of the following phenomena is closely associated with slow wave sleep:
A. Dreaming *(AIIMS 04)*
B. Atonia
C. Sleep walking
D. Irregular heart rate

160. The normal adult human electroencephalogram (EEG): *(AIIMS 04)*
A. Will not show high frequency waves during Stage 3 sleep
B. Shows alpha rhythm when a person is awake but inattentive
C. Has lower frequency waves during mental activity
D. Is predominated by large amplitude waves during REM sleep

161. Polysomnography contains all of the following tests except: *(AIIMS 16)*
A. Electroencephalography
B. Pulse oximetry
C. Electrooculography
D. Arterial pCO_2 measurement

Pain / Analgesia & Receptors

162. Free nerve endings carrying nociceptive fibers are seen in: *(AIIMS 14)*
A. Intestine
B. Spleen
C. Liver
D. Mesentery

163. Nerve ending sensitive to noxious stimuli are present in all except: *(PGI 09)*
A. Stomach
B. Intestine
C. Mesentry

D. Liver ☐
E. Brain ☐

164. Pain-sensitive intracranial structure is:
A. Piamater *(NBE P 15,13; PGI 15; AI 06)* ☐
B. Pial vessels ☐
C. Duramater ☐
D. Brain matter ☐

165. Vanilloid receptors are activated by:
A. Pain *(AIIMS 06)* ☐
B. Vibration ☐
C. Touch ☐
D. Pressure ☐

166. Perception of normal sensory stimuli as painful is called *(AIIMS 08)*
A. Hyperalgesia ☐
B. Allodynia ☐
C. Hyperpathia ☐
D. Causalgia ☐

167. Repetitive stimulation increases pain sensation, The probable cause is:
A. Hyper-sensitization *(AIIMS 09)* ☐
B. Decreased reflex time ☐
C. Increase in threshold of pain ☐
D. Decreased receptor area ☐

168. True about Visceral pain: *(PGI 11)*
A. It is poorly localized ☐
B. Resembles "fast pain" produced by noxious stimulation of the skin ☐
C. Mediated by B fibers in the dorsal roots of the spinal nerves ☐
D. Causes relaxation of nearby skeletal muscles ☐
E. Shows relatively rapid adaptation ☐

169. Ascending pain pathway is inhibited in dorsal midbrain by encephalin and: *(PGI 10)*
A. 5-HT (serotonin) ☐
B. Noradrenaline ☐
C. Substance P ☐
D. Glutamate ☐
E. Adenosine ☐

170. Hot water bottle relieves pain of abdominal spasm by: *(AI 10)*
A. Simulation of adrenergic fibers ☐
B. Stimulation of cholinergic fibers ☐
C. Inhibition of cold receptors ☐
D. Inhibition of heat receptors ☐

171. Mechanism of analgesia is by: *(PGI 05)*
A. Nociceptin stimulation ☐
B. Nocistatin stimulation ☐
C. O.L.R.I ☐
D. Anadamide receptors ☐
E. Nicotinic & cholinergic receptors ☐

172. Transcutaneous Electrical Nerve Stimulation (TENS) is based on: *(AIIMS 13)*
A. Central pain ☐
B. Referred pain ☐
C. Gate controlled theory of pain ☐
D. Allodynia ☐

173. Massage and the application of liniments to painful areas in the body relieves pain due to: *(AIIMS 04)*
A. Stimulation of endogenous analgesic system ☐
B. Release of endorphins by the first order neurons in the brain stem ☐
C. Release of glutamate and substance P in the spinal cord ☐
D. Inhibition by large myelinated afferent fibres ☐

174. Which of the following is effect of μ (mu) receptor of opioids: *(AIIMS 02)*
A. Sedation ☐
B. Dysphoria ☐
C. Miosis ☐
D. Bradycardia ☐

175. Na^+ & /or K^+ is /are involved in mechanism of action of which of the following receptor (s): *(PGI 09)*
A. GABAA receptor ☐
B. Nm receptor ☐
C. Nn receptor ☐
D. 5-HT3 receptor ☐
E. Dopamine ☐

176. All of the following are thermal modalities except:
A. Cold receptor *(PGI 05, 14,15)* ☐
B. Warm receptor ☐
C. Pain receptor ☐
D. Stretch receptor ☐
E. Pressure receptor ☐

177. Which of the following phrase adequately describes Pacinian corpuscles i.e. Pacinian corpuscles transmit which sensation:: *(AIIMS 04)*
A. A type of pain receptors ☐
B. Slowly adapting touch receptors ☐
C. Rapidly adapting touch receptors ☐
D. Located in the joints ☐

178. Meissener's corpuscle are for- *(NBE P 13)*
A. Touch ☐
B. Temperature ☐
C. Pressure ☐
D. Progrioception ☐

179. The mechanostretch receptors in joints and ligaments are: *(AIIMS 14)*
A. Fast adapting ☐
B. Slow adapting ☐
C. Non adapting ☐
D. Adapt differentially for different stresses ☐

180. During hip replacement, loss of joint and ligament receptors leads to: *(AIIMS 14)*
A. No loss of sensation ☐
B. Loss of all sensations ☐
C. Joint sensation lost in stable position ☐
D. Decrease in movements & decrease in sensation ☐

181. The increase in threshold of a receptor when a series of stimuli of subthreshold intensity are applied in succession is called OR Increase in threshold level on applying subthreshold, slowly rising stimulus is k/a:
A. Adaptation *(AIIMS 08, 06)* ☐
B. Accomodation ☐
C. Initiation ☐
D. Resistance ☐

Spinal Cord & Tracts

182. Kinesthetic sensation is: *(AI 04)*
- A. Transmitted by the β-type of sensory nerve ☐
- B. Located in Merkl's disc ☐
- C. Transmitted by Meissner's corpuscles ☐
- D. Means abnormal perception of sensation ☐

183. Pyramids are formed by- *(NBE P 13)*
- A. Arcuate nucleus ☐
- B. Vestibular nuclei ☐
- C. Interstitial cells of cajal ☐
- D. Lateral corticospinal tract ☐

184. UMN includes: *(PGI 02)*
- A. Pyramidal cells ☐
- B. Peripheral nerves ☐
- C. Anterior horn cells ☐
- D. Glial Cells ☐
- E. Schwann cells ☐

185. True about lateral corticospinal tract:
- A. Crossed *(PGI 06)* ☐
- B. Uncrossed ☐
- C. Stops in midthoracic region ☐
- D. Crossed at midspinal level ☐
- E. Only 20% crossed ☐

186. Cortcospinal tract lesion leads to: *(PGI 10)*
- A. Spaticity ☐
- B. Extensor plantar response ☐
- C. Cogwheel rigidity ☐
- D. Resting tremors ☐
- E. Exaggerated tendon reflexes ☐

187. Features of pyramidal tract lesion are all except
- A. Clasp knife rigidity *(AI 08)* ☐
- B. Involuntary movements ☐
- C. Positive Babiniski sign ☐
- D. Exaggerated reflexes & increased tone ☐

188. Following are the features of corticospinal involvement except: *(AI 03)*
- A. Cog-wheel rigidity ☐
- B. Spasticity ☐
- C. Planter extensor response ☐
- D. Exaggerated deep tendon reflexes. ☐

189. Amyotrophic lateral sclerosis involves: *(AI 03)*
- A. Upper motor neuron and lower motor neuron both ☐
- B. Posterior column only ☐
- C. Lower motor neuron only ☐
- D. Raphae nucleus ☐

190. True about medial lemniscus system; *(PGI 12)*
- A. Formed from fasciculus gracilis and fasciculus cuneatus ☐
- B. Carries discriminative touch and proprioception ☐
- C. Convey pain and temperature ☐
- D. Joins spinothalamic tract ☐
- E. Decussate at lower medulla ☐

191. Posterior column lesion which of the following is not affected: *(AIIMS 15,14; PGI 08, 14, 15)*
- A. Vibration & Proprioception ☐
- B. Temperature / Crude Sense & Pain ☐
- C. Fine touch ☐
- D. Position sense ☐

192. Concious proprioception is carried by: *(NBE P 14)*
- A. Dorsal column fibres *(AI 03)* ☐
- B. Anterior spinothalamic tract ☐
- C. Lateral spinothalamic tract ☐
- D. Vestibular tract ☐

193. Which of the following sensation are transmitted by the Dorsal Tract/ Posterior column: *(AIIMS 15)*
- A. Fine touch, Propioception *(NBE P 15,14)* ☐
- B. Pain *(PGI 14)* ☐
- C. Temperature ☐
- D. All of the above ☐

194. Which of the following tracts is concerned with pain & temperature *(NBE P 15,13; AI 08; AIIMS 14)*
- A. Pyramidal tract ☐
- B. Anterior spinothalmic tract ☐
- C. Lateral spinothalmic tract ☐
- D. Dorsal spinocerebellar tract ☐

195. A lesion of ventrolateral part of spinal cord will lead to loss (below the level of lesion) of: *(AI 03)*
- A. Pain sensation on the ipsilateral side ☐
- B. Proprioception on the contralateral side ☐
- C. Pain sensation on the contralateral side ☐
- D. Propriception on the ipsilateral side ☐

196. An anterolateral (ventrolateral) corodotomy relieving pain in right leg is effective because it interrupts the: *(NBE P 14,13)*
- A. Left dorsal column *(AI 12, AIIMS 14, 05)* ☐
- B. Left ventral spinothalmic tract ☐
- C. Left lateral spinothalmic tract ☐
- D. Right lateral spinothalmic tract ☐

197. All are true about brown sequard syndrome
- A. Ipsilateral loss of joint sensation *(PGI 09)* ☐
- B. Contralateral loss of joint sensation ☐
- C. Ipsilateral loss of pain & temperature ☐
- D. Segmental sign are bilateral ☐
- E. Contralateral loss of vibration ☐

198. All are seen in Brown – Sequard syndrome except
- A. I/L Pyrimidal tract features *(AIIMS 11)* ☐
- B. C/L Dorsal column ☐
- C. C/L Spinothalamic tract ☐
- D. I/L Plantar extensor ☐

199. Unlikely to be involved in lesion of anterior spinal artery is: *(PGI 09, 15)*
- A. Pain and temp ☐
- B. Vibration and proprioception ☐
- C. Pyramidal tract ☐
- D. Sphincters ☐

Reflexes

200. Salivation by dog seen when food is given along with ringing of bell is : *(AIIMS 05)*
- A. Conditioned reflex ☐

B. Reinforcement
C. Habituation
D. Innate reflex

201. Decrease reflex response after repetitive stimulation- *(NBE P 13)*
A. Summation
B. Fatigue
C. Irradiation
D. Occlusion

202. A/E are true properties of spinal cord reflex :
A. Memory *(AIIMS 04)*
B. Summation
C. Delay
D. Fatigue

203. The first reflex response to appear as spinal shock wears off in humans is: *(AI 06, NBE P 13)*
A. Tympanic reflex
B. Withdrawal reflex / Bulbocavernous
C. Neck righting reflex
D. Labyrinthine reflex

Sensory Reception

204. The distance by which two touch stimull must be separated to be perceived as two separate stimull is greastes at- *(NBE P 13)*
A. The lips
B. The palm of the hand
C. The back of scapula
D. The dorsum of the hand

205. If a single spinal nerve is cut, the area of tactile loss is always greater than the area of loss of painful sensations, because: *(AIIMS 04)*
A. Tactile information is carried by myelinated fast conducting fibres
B. Tactile receptors adapt quickly
C. Degree of overlap of fibres carrying tactile sensation is much less
D. In the primary sensory cortex tactile sensation is represented on a larger area

Autonomic Nervous System

206. Parasympathetic supply is from- *(NBE P 13)*
A. C234
B. T234
C. L234
D. S234

207. True regarding autonomic system is: *(AIIMS 08, 06)*
A. High centre of integration is medulla oblongata
B. Conduction autonomic fibres is same as in somatic motor fibres.
C. Preganglionic parasympathetic fibres are more lengthy.
D. Ratio of preganglionic and post ganglionic fibres is 20:1

208. Post ganglionic fibers are longer in? *(NBE P 13)*
A. Para sympathetic system
B. Sympathetic system
C. Both have same length
D. It is variable

209. All are effects of sympathetic stimulation, EXCEPT
A. Increased conduction velocity *(NBE P 13)*
B. Increased heart rate *(AIIMS 03, 14)*
C. Increased refractory period
D. Increased contractility of heart

210. During Flight or Fight reaction, which of the following is responsible for increase in local blood flow: *(AI 02)*
A. Sympathetic system mediated Cholinergic release
B. Local hormones
C. Para-sympathetic cholinergic
D. Endocrine factors only

211. α - adrenoreceptor stimulation effects are :
A. Vasoconstriction *(PGI 04)*
B. Vasodilatation
C. Broncho constriction
D. Alveolar bronchoconstriction
E. Bronchodilatation

212. Not a direct effect of Ach- *(NBE P 13)*
A. Decrease BP
B. Increase contraction of heart
C. Decrease heart rate
D. Decrease conduction

213. Sympathetic stimulation increases blood flow to all except: *(AIIMS 13)*
A. Skin
B. Coronary circulation
C. Cerebral
D. Renal

214. Catecholamines- *(NBE P 13)*
A. Decrease gut contraction
B. Bronchoconstriction
C. Decrease plasma glucose
D. Inhibit lipoysis

215. Epinephrine reduces insulin by – *(NBE P 13)*
A. Alpha action predominantly
B. Beta action predominantly
C. Alpha and beta
D. Muscarinic receptors

216. All is/are true about ANS except: *(AIIMS 09)*
A. Ciliary, otic, submandibular and pterygopalatine ganglia contain postganglionic parasympathetic neurons
B. Celiac and superior & inferior mesenteric ganglia contain post ganglionic sympathetic neurons
C. Acetyl choline is neurotransmitter for both pre & post ganglionic synapses in parasympathetic division as well as preganglionic sympathetic neurons.
D. NE is the NT of all postganglionic sympathetic neurons including merocrine sweat glands.

217. Nerve fibres innervating sweat glands release the following at their endings- *(NBE P 13)*
A. Noradrenaline ☐
B. Acetycholine ☐
C. Doparmine ☐
D. Histamine ☐

218. Simulation of post ganglion sympathetic neurons leads to: *(PGI 02)*
A. Fast EPSP ☐
B. Slow EPSP ☐
C. Fast IPSP ☐
D. Slow IPSP ☐
E. Very slow EPSP ☐

219. Slow IPSP in autonomic is generated by: *(PGI 05)*
A. Nicotinic cholinergic ☐
B. Muscarinic cholinergic ☐
C. Dopamine ☐
D. GnRH ☐
E. Adrenaline ☐

220. Tyramine acts by *(AIIMS 03)*
A. Inhibit acetylcholinesterase ☐
B. Stimulate α_1 receptor ☐
C. Release norepinephrine ☐
D. Stimulate β receptor ☐

221. True about Galvanic Skin Response: *(PGI 09)*
A. Indicator of thermal sweating ☐
B. ↑ by sweating because of sweat has electrolytes ☐
C. Fall when sympathetic activity is high ☐
D. Fall is associated with yogic practice ☐

ANSWERS AND EXPLANATIONS:

Higher Function

1. **B i.e. Frontal lobe** *[Ref: Ganong 24/e p. 294]*

Frontal lobe is the largest lobe. It is responsible for **attention, concentration**[Q], **personality**, behaviour, planning, **judgement**, motivation, organization and **word choice (expressive language)**[Q].

2. **A i.e. Larger brain** *[Ref: Ganong 22/e P-272]*

Human brain is more intelligent than monkey's brain d/t larger brain, greater size of association area and higher brain/body weight ratio[Q].

3. **C i.e. Use fatty acid in starvation** *[Ref: NMS biochemistry 3/e P-516, Lippincotts 2/e P- 294, 188, Ganong 22/e P-283]*

Brain uses ketone bodies (not fatty acid) in starvation[Q].

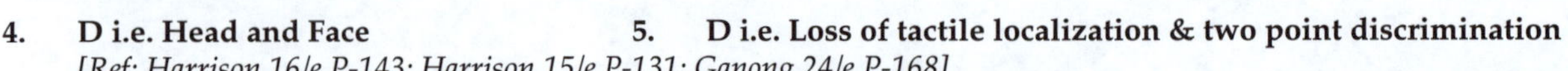

4. **D i.e. Head and Face** 5. **D i.e. Loss of tactile localization & two point discrimination**

[Ref: Harrison 16/e P-143; Harrison 15/e P-131; Ganong 24/e P-168]

- **Largest representation in somatosensory area I (post central gyrus)** is for **hand (thumb especially)** and **face** (esp **mouth** parts concerned with speech i.e. **lips, tongue** etc)[Q]. **Trunk & back** has **very small representation.**
- ***Ablation of somatosensory area I (SI) of cerebral cortex leads to loss of tactile localization and two point discrimination***[Q].

6. **D i.e. Nucleus cuneatus** *[Ref: Ganong 22/e P-147;Textbook of Human neuroanatomy I.B Singh 6/e P 12]*

The **middle part of cuneate nucleus, the pars rotunds** which receives impulses from ***digits, palm, dorsum of hand & forearm is specific for stereognosis***[Q].

Stereognosis

Stereognosis is determination of texture & size of an obect, is function of cerebral cortex.
The sensory information of stereognosis to brain is carried by ***posterior column***[Q]. Which includes *tractus gracilis* & *tractus cuneatus.*

Tractus gracilis	**Tractus cuneatus**
brings sensation from lumbar & sacral *segments to nucleus gracilis* (less specific for stereognoses)	brings sensation from *cervical & thoracic segments* to nucleus cuneatus.

[Mn: "Gracilis for lower segment & cuneatus for upper segment – G comes after C"]

7. **D i.e. Temporal lobe** *[Ref: Ganong 23/ep 298]*

Right inferior temporal lobe (in right handed person) **stores visual inputs (representation) of objects especially faces**. So lesion in this area causes **prosopagnosia i.e. inability to recognize familiar faces**[Q]. However, they **can recognize people from their voice or names.** They can also show autonomic responses (anxiety) on seeing familiar faces (but not on seeing unfamiliar faces).

Emotions

8. **D i.e. Anterior nucleus of thalmus**

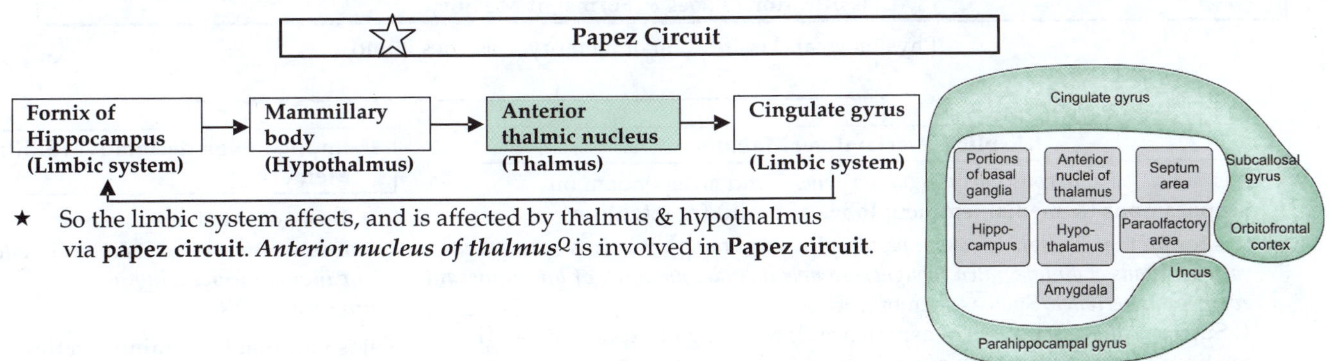

★ So the limbic system affects, and is affected by thalmus & hypothalmus via **papez circuit**. *Anterior nucleus of thalmus*[Q] is involved in **Papez circuit**.

9. B i.e. Amygdala

10. A i.e. Emotion B i.e., Memory C i.e., Higher function

11. B i.e. Limbic system; D i.e. Hippocampus

12. B i.e. Medial forebrain bundle

13. B i.e. Abolished by Decortication

14. A i.e.Preoptic nucleus

[Ref: Ganong's 24/e p 309; Guyton 12/e p 717; Gallagher & Nelson 2/e p 348; Chaudhary 6/e p 354]

- *Amygdala is the window through which limbic system sees the place of person in the world*[Q].
- **Reward center** (ie area of brain responsible for self stimulation reward on induction) includes *medial forebrain bundle*[Q], especially in **lateral** and *ventro medial nuclei of hypothalamus*[Q].
- The *hypothalamus and limbic system*[Q] are responsible for *instinctual behaviour & emotions.* **Limbic system** is responsible for emotions *(emotional behavior & motivational drives) and memory (higher functions)*[Q].
- **Sham (false) rage is an outburst of pathological (inappropriate, uncontrolled & violent) anger & fear in decorticate animals** on mild peripheral stimulation. It can be caused by **stimulation of punishment center of hypothalamus** and presents with *features of sympathetic stimulation*[Q].
- *Preoptic nucleus (MPOA) of hypothalamus*[Q] is most closely related **to sexcual activity in males.**

15. C i.e. Recruitment by multiplication of neurons

16. B i.e. Hippocampus

17. C i.e. The site for storage of long term memory is in temporal lobe *[Ref: Ganong 24/e p 283-90; Guyton 12/e p705-708;Berne & Levy 6/e p210-14;Harrison 16/e p-2394; Journal of Neuroscience vol.16, no-10 p. 3189-98]*

- **Mechanism of learning and long term memory** include **gene activation leading to ↑protein synthesis & spatial reorganization (restructuring) of synapse** changing their sensitivity by **increasing the number of transmitter vesicles / vesicle release sites / level of neurotransmitter at synapse / presynaptic terminals** as well as changes in dendritic spine that permit transmission of stronger signals. **Change in number of neuron & their connectivity** is significant in initial week / month / years of life but this *recruitment of neurons is from already existing pool (not by multiplication) mainly*[Q]
- **Hippocampus (in medial temporal lobe)** is the site where *short term memory is processed and converted into long term memory*[Q]. While the encoding process for short term explicit memory involves hippocampus, *long term memories are stored in various parts of neocortex*[Q]. **Hippocampus causes consolidation of long term memory**[Q].
- **Short term memory** lasts as long *as the person continues to think.* **Intermediate memory** results from **temporary changes in synapses**, whereas **structural changes** occur in synapses during development of **long term memory.**

18. C i.e. Relation of one stimulus to another

19. A i.e. Procedural memory

Classification (Types & Forms) of Memory

Physiological classification of memory, classifies it into

I. Explicit (Declarative) Memory

- It is *associated with consciousness (or awareness)* and is dependent on **hippocampus (& medial temporal lobes of brain) for retention**
- It is for ***factual knowledge*** *about people, places and things.* It involves *memory of various details of an integrated thought, example includes* ***memory of an important event or experience.*** Such as memory of 1) Surroundings, 2) Causes of experience, 3) Meaning of experience, 4) Time relationship and 5) Memory of one's deductions that were left in the person's mind.
- Explicit memories that are required initially during activities like learning bicycle riding can become implicit once the task is thoroughly learned.
- Explicit memory can be divided into

Semantic (Fact) Memory

- For facts like words, rules & language
- May be short to long term
- *Inferolateral temporal lobe* is also involved (along with **hippocampus**)

Episodic (Event) Memory

- For *event and experiences*
- May be short to long term
- *Anterior thalamic nuclei,* ***prefrontal cortex & medial temporal lobe*** is also involved

II. Implicit (Non declarative /Skill) Memory

- It **does not involve awareness (consciousness)** and its retention ***does not involve processing in hippocampus***[Q]
- It is important for **training reflexive motor or perceptual skills** *such as all skills developed for hitting a tennis / cricket ball*, including automatic memories to (1) sight the ball, (2) calculate the speed of ball & positioning of bat, (3) deduce rapidly the motions of body to hit the ball- all these activated instantly based on previous learning of game – and then moving on to next stroke while forgetting the details of previous stroke.
- It can be of 4 types

Priming

Recognition of **words or objects** by prior exposure to them is dependent on **neocortex**

Procedural Memory

Includes **habits & skills**, which after acquisition, become **unconscious and automatic**. Procedural memory is processed in **striatum (part of basal ganglia)**[Q]

Associative Learning

It involves **classical & operant conditioning in which relationship between one stimulus and another is learnt**[Q]**.** It is dependent on **amygdala** for **emotional responses** and **cerebellum for motor (skeletal musculature) responses**

Non-associative ie Learning

It involves **habituation & sensitization** and is dependent on various **reflex pathways**

Sleep

20. A i.e. Hypothalamus

Ref: Harrison's 17th/e p.172-73; Textbook of Physiology Gabriel C Ezeilo 472-80; Guyton 11th/e p. 740-41; Ganong 23rd/e p. 236-39

Hypothalmic ventro lateral preoptic (VLPO) neurons play a ***key executive role in sleep regulation***[Q].

21. B i.e. Will be prolonged to greater than 24 hours cycle length >> A i.e. Will remain unchanged at 24 hrs

22. C i.e. Suprachiasmatic nucleus *[Ref:Ganong 24/e p.278-79; Best & Taylor 13/e p.869-70,657,1205; Berne & Levy 6/e p.207-8, 655]*

- In the liver circadian rhythm is influenced by pattern of food intake, but ***in almost all other cells the circadian rhythm is entertained by paired suprachiasmatic nuclei***[Q].
- **Endogenous (built in or self sustained) circadian periodicity of sleep wake cycle** is about **25 hours** (i.e. slightly greater than 24 hours). It is **entrained (adjusted or synchronized) by external (environmental) cues (or Zeitgebers = time givers)** mainly the **day-night** (or **light-dark) cycle** to attain 24 hour periodicity. Therefore, if **all external or environmental cues (Zeitgebers) are removed or in a constant environment**, the **sleep wake cycle becomes free running** and slightly drifts away from 24 hour cycle to become **> 24 (to 25) cycle**.

Cerebral Dominance

23. D i.e. Written and Spoken Language

24. C i.e. Representative hemisphere, right

25. C i.e. Dyscalculia *[Ref: Berne & Levy 6/e p 213-208; Ganong 24/e p 291-294; Guyton 12/e p 701-704]*

- **Categorical (dominant) hemisphere (ie left lobe** in most cases) is responsible for **sequential – analytic processes** such as **language (understanding language, verbal memory, motor speech, written & spoken language)** and **mathematical ability**. Therefore lesions of left (dominant) side produce **aphasias (receptive & expressive), dyslexia and dyscalculia.**
- **Representational (non dominant mostly right) hemisphere** is responsible **for visuo-spatial orientation & musical (art) awareness.** Its lesion causes **anosognosia and dysgraphia**.

Aphasia

26. D i.e. Inferior frontal gyrus

[Ref: Fuller 2nd/10; Harrison 16/e P-146, 147; Ganong 22/e P-274-275]

27. A i.e. Word formation

28. B i.e. Verbal expression

Broca's (nonfluent/motor'/ expressive) aphasia is caused by lesion in ***inferior frontal gyrus***Q. It is ***a disorder of word finding (formation)*** resulting in ***inadequate verbal expression*** Q.

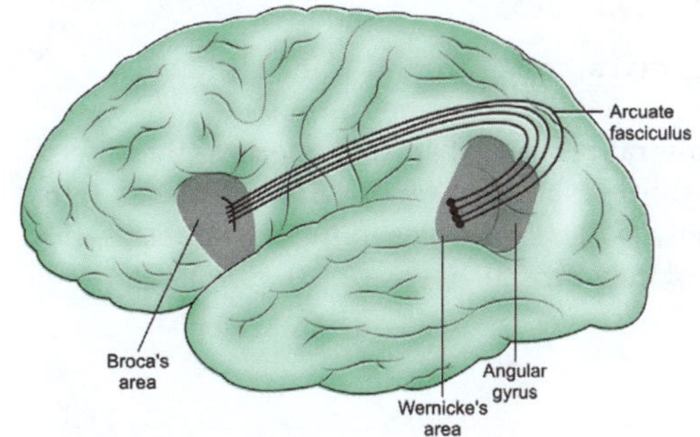

Hearing & Vision

29. A i.e. ICF

Perilymph
Rich in Na^+ & resembles ECF (& CSF)Q
- **Communicates with CSF** via aqueduct of cochlea - Fills space between bony & membranous labyrinth i.e. **scale vestibule & tympani**

Endo lymph
Rich in K^+ and resembles ICFQ
- Secreted by **stria vascularis** (of cochlea) and **dark cells** (of utricle & ampulatted ends of SCCs) - Fills **membranous labyrinth** including **sale media** (cochlear duct)

30. A i.e. K+ influx

31. C i.e. Rotation *[Ref: Ganong 24/ep 202-205]*

Inner Hair cells (in auditory pathway) **depolarize due to influx of K^+ ion (>>>>) and Ca^{++}**Q

Hair cells (HCs) Sensory Receptors of Ear

- **HCs (6 Patches) are mechanoreceptors**, which signal

Hearing	In organ of Corti
Horizontal accelerationQ	**In Utricle**Q
Verticle accelerationQ	**In Saccule**
Rotational accelerationQ	**(A patch) in all 3 SCCs**Q

- **Base of HCs** is in contact with afferent neuron and supporting cells (surmounted by **otolith membrane** embded with **calcium carbonate crystals or otoliths).**
- **Apical end of HCs** have **30-150 rod shaped processes (hairs or stereocilia). Kinocilium** (not found in cochlea) is **largest non motile, true** hair process with clubbed end. It has 1 central and 9 circumferential pairs of microtubules. All stereocilia are of same height *(along perpendicular axis) but along an axis towards kinocilium they increase in height progressively*
- Tips of adjacent stereocilia are connected *by tip links controlling opening of mechanosensitive* ***cation transduction channel*** *in taller stereocilia.*

- **Movement of shorter stereocilia towards taller stereocilia (i.e. deflection of stereocilium towards kinocilium) cause opening (or increased open time) of transduction channel resulting in influx of K+ (Most abundant endolymph cation)Q and Ca^{++}(In lesser amount). This produces depolarization of hair cells.** RMP of hair cells is -60 mV and it is decreased to-50 mv.
- Depolarization of HCs cause **opening of voltage gated (not transduction) Ca^{++} channels** at their **base** allowing more Ca^{++} **influx** resulting in **release of NT-glutamate**. Finally **voltage sensitive K+ channels** at base cause **K+ efflux restoring Resting membrane potential (RMP).**
- But a/t recent text, **myosin based molecular motor** in taller cilia **moves the transduction channel towards base and so releasing tension in tip link**. This **closes Ca^{++} channel** and restores resting state.
- **Movement of stereocilia away from kinocilium causes closure of transduction channel and hyper polarizationQ**

32. D i.e. +85 mV *[Ref: Guyton 11/ep 657]*

Endocochlear potential is **positive (+) 80 to 100 mVQ** voltage seen in cochlear endolymphatic space (i.e. b/w endolymph & perilymph) with positive inside scala media and negative outside. It is generated by **continuous secretion of K^+ ions into scale media by stria vascularis.**

33. A i.e. C *[Ref: Ganong 24/e p 208]*

- Sensory neurons that arborize around hair cells have their cell bodies located in **spiral ganglion**
- **90-95% of peripheral process of spiral ganglion** (these sensory neurons) **innervate inner hair cellQ** (i.e. C in diagram) and only **5-10%** innervates more numerous outer hair cells (B in diagram).

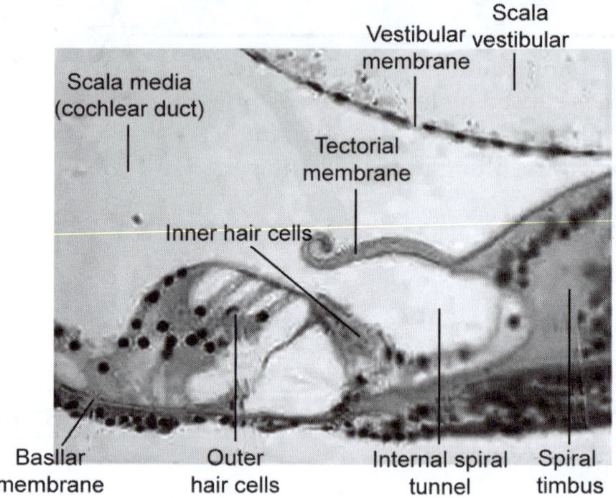

34. C i.e. Binasal disparity *[Ref: Ganong 22/e P-167- 68]*

True stereospsis is perceived due to binasal disparityQ.

35. C i.e. Layers 1,4,6 **36. C i.e. Layer 4** **37. B i.e. Colour vision, shape, fine details**
38. A i.e. Color contrast **39. C i.e. Colour processing** *[Ref: Neuroanatomy by I.B.S 6/e P-233; Ganong 22/e P-160- 61]*

- **Fibres from contralateral nasal hemiretina** project to the ***layers (laminae) 1,4 and 6 of lateral geniculate bodyQ.***
- **Most afferent fibers from the lateral geniculate body terminate in the primary visual cortex layer 4Q.**
- The **parvocellular pathway from** layers 3 to 6 of **lateral geniculate nucleus** to the visual cortex, **carries signals for color vision (contrast), texture, shape and fine detailQ.**
- ***Blobs are arranged in a mosaic in visual cortex and are concerned with colour vision.***

40. C i.e. Amacrine cells **41. A i.e. Bipolar cells** **42. A i.e. Optic nerve** *[Ref: Guyton 12 ep-617: Ganong 24/ep 179-92]*

Visual Pathway	
Sensory (Photo) Receptors	**Rods & cones**
1st Order Neuron	**Bipolar cell axonQ** (in retina)
2nd Order Neuron	**Ganglionic cell axonQ** (form optic disc-**nerve-chiasma-tract)Q**
3rd Order Neuron	**LGB nerve cell axons** (form optic radiation)

- **Amacrine cells** secrete 5 inhibitory neurotransmitters **AChQ**, GABA, Glycine, Dopamine & Indolamine.
- Only **ganglionic cell** in retina produce **propagating action potential** (always depolarizing). All other cells develop graded local potential which is decremental, non propogative & does not follow all or none law.
- **Photoreceptors (rods & cones) release glutamate at their synapse with bipolar cells (in dark)Q**

43. **B i.e. Amacrine cells** *[Ref: Guyton 11th/e p. 635-637]*

Amacrine cells serve important function of ***increasing visual acuity by modulating photoreceptive signals, serving to adjust or maintain the relative colour & luminosity inputs under changing light conditions***Q. So ***amacrine cells regulate and maintain relative color luminosity of photoreceptive input under changing light conditions*** Q.

44. **C i.e. 11-Cis – Retinalaldehyde** *[Ref: Lippincott 2/e P 332; Ganong 22/e P-158, Chaudhuri 5/e P-506]*

In the dark phase – ***11-Cis- retinal***Q exists combined with opsin. **In the light phase** – 11 trans – retinal exist combined with opsin.

45. **B i.e. Photoisomerization and hydrolysis of visual purple** *[Ref: Harrison- 409; Lippincott's 4th/e p. 381- 84; Garner & Klintworth pathology of ocular disease 3/e pg- 1066-67; Robbin's 7/ed pg- 451]*

Initiation of visual cycle is associated with ***condensation of opsin with vitamin A aldehyde (11-cis retinaldehyde)***Q whereas, **initiation of visual (nerve) impulse** is associated with *photochemical isomerization & hydrolysis (bleaching) of visual purple (rhodopsin)* resulting in release of all trans retinal & opsin.

46. **B i.e. Glutamate** 47. **D i.e. Vision** 48. **A i.e. Signal transduction**
[Ref: Ganong 23rd/e p. 190-92; Neuroscience: Mark, Bear, Barry 3/e p. 296; CNS Per Broda 3/e p. 188; Guyton 11th/e p. 626-31, 636]

- **Both rods cones release glutamate at their synapses with bipolar cells and remain in depolarized state (-40 mv membrane potential) in dark**Q. So **photo transduction is a unique type of sensory transmission** that is associated with decreased neurotransmitter **(glutamate) release** from photoreceptors in light. Unlike other receptors, the photoreceptors (rods and cones) & bipolar cells are **hyperpolarized (instead of depolarized) and *do not produce action potential***Q. **Instead they produce hyperpolarizing local graded potential**Q
- ***Process of phototransduction (response to light) in rods and cones is virtually the same***Q. And the sequence of events are:

Incident light → structural change in retinene 1 of photopigment → conformational change of photopigment opsin → **activation of transducin (Gt1) in rods / Gt2 in cones**Q → activation of photodiesterase →↓ **intracellular C-GMP→ closure of Na^+ channels →↓ intracellular Na^+ → hyperpolarization → dcreased release of synaptic transmitter (glutamate)**Q → **response in bipolar cells.**

Color Vision & Taste

49. **C i.e. Involves opponent color cells** *[Ref: Ganong 23rd/e p. 195-98; Gabriel C Ezeilo p. 441, 449-50; 439, Guyton 11th/e p.638-32]*

Colour vision involves opponent color coding cone cellsQ.

50. **A i.e. 370-740 nm** *[Ref: Guyton 10/e P- 643]*

The **visible** range is ***350nm-600nm***Q

51. **C i.e. Taste buds** 52. **B i.e. Na^+ channels** 53. **D i.e. At the posterior aspect** *[Ref: Ganong 24/ep 223-24]*

(R) Receptors (On★)	Substance	R-Type
Salty Anterior half of tongueQ ★	Sodium chloride	**Ligand gated (ionotropic) channels: Amiloride sensitive sodium (Na^+) selective epithelial channels (ENaC)**Q
Sour Edges of tongueQ ★	HCL	Ligand gated (ionotropic) channel: **ENaC permitting entry of proton (H^+ ions)**Q; H^+ can also block *K+ sensitive channels*; **HCN** (hyper polarization-activated cyclic nucleotide gated cation channel)
Sweet Tip of tongueQ ★	Glucose etc	**GPCR (metabotropic) receptors: T1R3 (Sac locus) family of G protein coupled receptors (GPCR) coupling to G protein Gustducin**
Bitter Back of tongueQ ★	Poisons	**GPCR (T2R family)** interact with **gustducin** e.g. strychnine; some are membrane permeabe & K^+ channel blockers
Unami	L-glutamate	**Metabotropic glutamate Receptors (M-Glu R4)**

54. **B i.e. Olfaction-hair cells**

Olfactory receptors are unique as receptor cell itself (not hair cell)[Q] is neuron.

Equilibrium & Basal Ganglia

55. **A i.e. Macula** *[Ref: Ganong 23/e p. 206]*

Macula (Otolith Organ = Stretch receptors) in Utricle & Saccule	**Maintain Static equilibrium i.e. head position in reference to gravity[Q]**
Cristae at ampullated ends of **Semicircular Canals**	Respond to **angular (rotational) acceleration & deacceleration[Q].**

56. **C i.e. Caudate nucleus /Putamen/GP**
57. **B i.e. Corpus striatum**
58. **D i.e. Putamen**
59. **B i.e. Subthalamic Nucleus**

[Ref: Ganong's 24/e p 136-142, 243-45; Guyton 12/e p 689-94; Best & Taylor 13/e p 1194-95; Berne & Levy 6/e p 188-193]

- **Basal ganglia** consists of – *caudate nucleus[Q], putamen, globus pallidus, subthalmic nucleus, and substantia nigra[Q].* **Striatum** (term derived from the **striated appearance** of these nuclei) refers to the **caudate nucleus and putamen**. Whereas the combination of **putamen and globus pallidus** is often referred to as **lentiform nucleus**
- **Efferent fiber bundle of substantia nigra (pars compacta) transmit dopaminergic fibers to corpus striatum / striatum (dopaminergic nigro striatal projection).**
- **Subthalamic nucleus** (a diencephalic grey matter part of basal ganglia) is the only nucleus of basal ganglia that actually **produce excitatory neurotransmitter glutamate**. Subthalamic nucleus receives inhibitory (GABA - nergic) imput from globus pallidus external segment (GPe) and has excitatory (glutaminergic) projections to both GPe and GPi (globus pallidus internal segment). Subthalamic nucleus plays an important role in stimulation of **indirect SNpc-GPi** (substantia nigra – pars compacta – globus pallidus internal segment) **pathway**.
- Although the majority of striatal neurons are **GABA nergic medium spiny neurons**, the **highest density of glutamate receptors** in basal ganglia is found ***in corpus striatum (putamen + caudate nucleus)[Q]***, which receives 2 main inputs (both of which are excitatory glutaminergic) **from cerebral cortex (cortico striatal pathway)** and **from intralaminar nuclei of thalamus (thalamostriatal pathway).**

60. **A i.e. Dopamine** *[Ref. Ganong 22/e P-213]*

Dopamine is the ***major neurotransmitter in substantia nigra[Q] (nigrostriatal pathway)[Q].***

61. **B i.e. Skilled movement** *[Ref: Ganong 23/e p. 242-57; Guyton 11th/e p. 700]*
62. **A i.e. Planning**
63. **B i.e. Smoothens and coordinates movement**

Basal ganglia is concerned with **planning and organizing voluntary (skilled) movements[Q]** whereas, **spinocerebellum (spinocerebellar tract) smoothen & coordinates movements[Q]**

Functions of

Basal ganglia	Cerebellum	Limbic system
- **Planning and programming of movements[Q]** - **Subconscious execution of learned pattern of movement[Q]** - Cognitive control of sequence of motor pattern.	- Concerned with **equilibrium[Q]** - **Co- ordination of motor function[Q]**	- Olfaction - Autonomic responses (along with hypothalamus) - Emotion of rage, fear and motivation

- **Gross motor function[Q]** → by cortico motro area
- **Sensory relay station[Q]** → Thalamus
- **Short term memory[Q]** → Hippocampus

64. **C i.e. Athetosis**
65. **A i.e. Alziemer's disease**

Disorder	**Basal Ganglia (Part) involved**
Parkinson's Disease	**Dopaminergic neurons in Substantia nigra pars compacta[Q]** (most severely affecting **putamen**)
Athetosis	**Globus pallidus[Q] >>> Subthalmic nucleus**
Ballismus	**Subthalmic nuclei[Q]**
Huntington Chorea	**Striatum (Caudate nucleus >> Putamen)**

Dysfunction in any of three biochemical pathways of basal ganglia [i.e. (1) **nigrostriatal dopaminergic system, (2) intrastriatal cholinergic system** and (3) **GABA ergic system]** may result in two type of motor disorders i.e.

1. **Hypokinetic disorders** like **akinesia & bradykinesia.**
2. **Hyperkinetic** disorders like **athetosis, ballismus, chorea, cog-wheel rigidity & resting tremors**Q

Blood Brain Barrier (BBB)

66. D i.e. Proteins *[Ref: Ganong 23/e p-572-74; Guyton 11/e p-766]*

Blood-CSF Barrier & Blood-Brain Barriers are **highly permeable to water, CO_2 (carbondioxide), O_2 (oxygen)$_2$, and most lipid soluble (lipophilic) substances such as free forms of steroid hormones, alcohol and anesthetics**Q; slightly permeable to electrolytes like Na^+ (sodium), K^+ (potassium) and Cl^- (chloride); and almost **totally impermeable** to plasma proteins, protein bound forms of steroid hormones, protein antibodies and most non lipid soluble large organic molecules (i.e. impermeable to, in general, **all proteins and polypeptides)**Q. It slows penetration of some smaller molecules like urea.

BBB is Formed by
- **Tight junction of the endothelial cells**Q - **Foot process of the astrocytes around the capillaries** Q (astrocytes send processes to blood vessels where they induce capillaries)

67. B i.e. Subfornical organ **68. B i.e. Posterior pituitary** **69. A i.e. Area postrema** **70. D i.e. Medulla**
[Ref: Ganong 23/e P-573-74; MTx]

- **Circumventricular organs without bloor brain barrier** includes **Median eminence of hypothalamus, Subfornical organ (SFO),** Organum Vasculosum of lamina Terminalis (OVLT, supraoptic crest), **Area postrema (chemoreceptor trigger zone = CTZ = Vomiting Center)**Q, **Posterior pituitary**Q (Neurohypolysis).
- **Medulla** contains **centers for swallowing, vomiting, coughing, sneezing & VMC** (vasomotor center).

Cerebellum, Posture & Decortication

71. C i.e. Vestibular nucleus **72. A i.e. Flocculus; C i.e. Nodulus** **73. C i.e. Purkinje cells**
74. C i.e. Cerebellar nuclei **75. C i.e. Mossy fibres inhibit Purkinje cells** **76. D i.e. Dentate**
77. B i.e. Bipolar **78. A i.e.Cerebral cortex; B i.e.Co-ordination; D i.e. Decreased tone; E i.e. Excitatory effect**
79. D i.e. Smoothens and coordinates ongoing movement **80. C i.e. Resting tremor**
Ref: Ganong 23/e p. 255-58; Guyton 12 SAE 699-709; Gray's 40/e p. 300; Snell's NA 8/e p. 223-225; IBS NA 6/e p.158]

- **Flocculonodular lobe** constitutes the vestibulo- cerebellum. **Output from flocculonodular lobe goes directly to the brainstem**Q **(vestibular nucleus),** bypassing the deep cerebellar nuclei and is **concerned with maintenance of equlibrium**Q.
- **Cerebellar connection to other parts of the brain is projected through (or output from the cerebellum is solely from) purkinje cells**Q. Purkinje cells are amongst the biggest neurons in the body. Their axons are the **only output from the cerebellar cortex from where they are projected to deep cerebellar nuclei**Q.
- **Efferents arising from cerebellar cortex (purkinje fibers) end in deep cerebellar nuclei & have inhibitory effects**Q. Whereas **output arising in deep cerebellar nuclei is always excitatory**Q and project to centre outside the cerebellum to brainstem & thalamus.
- **The afferent input to the cerebellum is excitatory and comes through – Climbing fibers and Mossy fibers.**

Cerebellum has **4 deep nuclei**: - **d**entate, **e**mboliform, **f**astigial & **g**loboseQ (Mn: 'DEFG').

Cerebellar cortex contains 5 types of neuron cells Mn: **"Go Park & Basket Granular starts"**

GO **Park &** **Basket** **Granular** **Stars**	**Golgi** cells **Purkinje** cells **Basket** cells **Granule** cells **Stell**ate cells

- ***Cerebellum** smoothens & coordinates ongoing movement* in motor performance this is the reason why lesion of cerebellum causes *1)* ***Ataxia*** (lack of coordination of movement) 2) ***Asynergia*** (lack of coordination b/w different group of muscles), 3) ***Astasia*** (Unsteady voluntary movement) 4) ***Dysdiadochokinesia*** **= Rebound Phenomenon** (Inability to do rapid alternate successive movement).

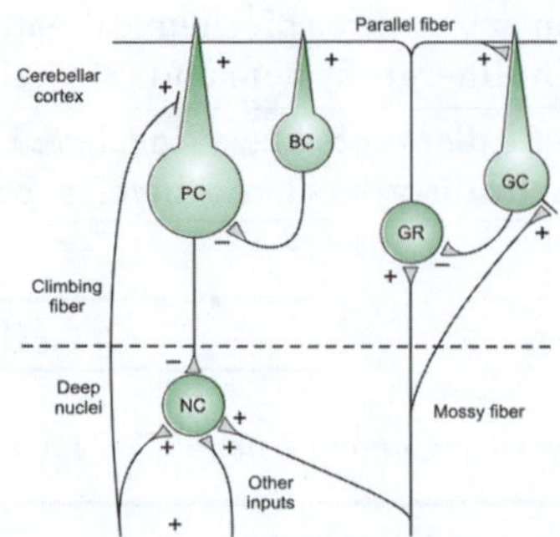

Diagram of neural connections in the cerebellum. Plus (+) and minus (-) sign indicate whether endings are excitory or inhibitory. BC basket cell; GC, Golgi cell; GR, granule cell; NC, cell in deep nucleus; PC, Purkinje cell. Note that PCs and BCs are inhibitory. The connections of the stellate cells, which are not shown, are similar to those of the basket cells, except that they end for the most part on Purkije cell dendrites.

- **Cerebellar lesions** are associated with **unsteady-drunken gait, slurred-scanning speech, dissection-decomposition of movement** (i.e. b/o difficulty in performing action that involve simultaneous movement at more than one joint patient dissect such motion & carry them out one joint at a time). **Slurred-scanning speech, hypotonic, dysmetria (Past pointing) & intentional tremors**Q whereas, **resting tremors** occur in **lesions of basal ganglia**Q.

81. **B i.e. Tecto cerebellar tract**

Spino/Olivo/Cuneo-Cerebellar (Mnz SOCC) tracts carry proprioceptive impulses whereas tecto cerebellar tract carry auditory & visual impulses.

Afferent Tracts	Transmits
Vestibulo-cerebellar	Vestibular impulses from labyrinths, direct and via ***vestibular nuclei***Q
Dorsal /Ventral spinocerebellar	**Proprioceptive** and exteroceptive impulses from body
Cuneo cerebellar	**Proprioceptive** impulses, especially from head and neck
Tectocerebellar	**Auditory and visual impulses** via inferior and superior colliculi
Pontocerebellar	Impulses from motor and other parts of cerebral cortex via pontine nuclei
Olivocerebellar	**Proprioceptive**Q input from whole body via relay in inferior olive

82. **C i.e. Increased rigidity via alpha motor neurouns** *[Ref: Ganong 24/e p. 241-43]*

Mid-Collicular Decerebration

- **Complete transaction of brain stem (i.e. lesion) between superior & inferior colliculi** permits brain stem pathways to function independent **from all inputs from cortex** (corticospinal & corticobulbar tracts) **and red nucleus** (rubrospinal tract) mainly to distal muscles of Extremities
- Inhibitory & excitatory **reticulospinal pathway to postural extensor muscles remain intact leading to hyperactivity & rigidity in extensor muscles of all 4 extremities**Q
- Reticulospinal tract activates **γ motor neurons,** which indirectly (via Ia spindle afferent activity) activate **α motor neurons** (k/a **Gamma loop). Sections of dorsal root eliminate** extensor rigidity by breaking this **myotactic stretch reflex**. It is seen in **uncal herniation** d/t large cerebral tumor or hemorrhage.

Decorticate Rigidity

- **Decortication (i.e. removal of cerebral cortex)** produces
  - **Flexion of upper extremities** at elbow (d/t rubrospinal excitation) &
  - **Extensor hyperactivity in lower** limbs (cause similar to midcollicular decerebration)
- It is seen in **hemiplegia d/t internal capsular bleed.**

Decerebellate Rigidity

- **Extensor muscle hyperactivity is exaggerated by removing anterior lobe of cerebellum in decerebrate animals (decerebellate rigidity)**Q d/t elimination of cortical inhibition of cerebellar fastigial nucleus
- This shows that decerebrate rigidity also l/t **direct activation of α motor neurons**Q **(independent of gamma loop)**Q**. So subsequent dorsal root cut does not reverses rigidity**Q

83. **B i.e. Smoothens and coordinates movement**

84. **B i.e. Flocculonodular lobe**

Functional Division of Cerebellum (3 parts)

1. Vestibulo-cerebellum

- Phylogenetically the *oldest*[Q] *part of cerebellum*
- Includes *flocculus & nodule in the vermis so also k/a Flocculonodular lobe*[Q]
- **Concerned with *equilibrium, gait*** & learning induced changes in ***VOR* (Vestibulo-Ocular Reflex)**
- Output passes directly to brainstem

2. Spinocerebellum

- Includes rest of *vermis & adjacent medial portion of hemispheres*[Q]
- Receives propioceptive infut from all body & motor plan from motor cortex. By comparing both it ***smoothens & coordinates movements*** that are ongoing
- Output through *Emboliform, Fastigial or Globose nuclei* to brainstem

3. Neocerebellum/Cerebro-cerebellum

- Phylogenetically the *newest*[Q] part of cerebellum
- Includes *lateral portion of cerebellar hemisphere*[Q]
- Interact with motor cortex in *planning & programming movements*[Q]
- Output through ***Dentate nucleus***[Q] to *ventrolateral nucleus of thalamus*

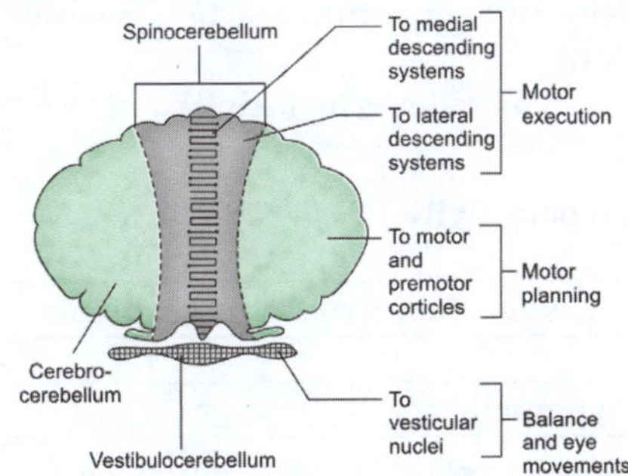

85. **A i.e. Premotor cortex**

Control of Posture & Movements

Part	Function
Cortical Association Areas	***Commands for Voluntary movements originate***[Q]
Basal ganglia & neocerebellum (lateral portion of cerebellum) & cortex	Are part of a feedback circuit to premotor & motor cortex that is concerned with ***planning & organizing voluntary movement***[Q]
Supplementary motor area	Involved primarily in *programming motor sequences*. Lesions l/t awkwardness in performing complex activities & difficulty with bimanual co - ordination
Premotor Cortex	**Concerned with *setting posture at the start of a planned movement* and with getting individual ready to perform**[Q]
Somatosensory area (Posterior parietal cortex)	Lesion causes *inability to execute learned sequences of movements* as eating with knife & fork. Neurons in *area 5* is concerned with *aiming hand toward an object* & manipulating it, where as area 7 is concerned with *hand- eye co-ordination.*
Spinocerebellum (medial & intermediate portion of cerebellum)	Movements is ***smoothened & co- ordinated***[Q]
Cortico spinal & Cortico-bulbar system	Primary pathway for the ***initiation of skilled voluntary movements***[Q].
Rubrospinal, Reticulo-spinal, Tecto-spinal & Vestibulo spinal tracts	Are main brainstem pathways concerned with *posture & co- ordination*

86. **A i.e. Integrity of Reflex arc:** *[Ref: Ganong 22/e P-206; Chaudhari 7/ep 602]*

87. **B i.e. Stretch reflex**

- *'Postural Reflexes not only maintain the body in an upright balanced position but also provide the constant adjustments necessary to maintain a stable postural background for voluntary activity'- Ganong 22nd/207*
- ***Integrity of the postural reflex arc is therefore the single best answer of choice.***
- **Posture is maintained by altering postural (stretch) reflexes**[Q]**.** In any posture some muscles are contracted & others are relaxed. For example in erect posture **antigravity muscle (extensors) of neck, spine, hip & knee have high tone.**

88. **A i.e. Hoping and placing reflex** *[Ref: Ganong 24/e p 240-41 & Internet]*

89. **D i.e. Crossed extensor reflex**

In decorticate animals, Postural reflex integrated in cerebral cortex i.e. **long loop stretch reflex & hopping-placing reflexes are lost**[Q]

Integrating Center	Postural Reflexes
Cerebral cortex	**Long Loop Stretch reflex, Hopping & placing reflex**[Q]
Mid Brain	**Rightining reflex**
Medulla oblongata	**Tonic Neck & Labyrinthine reflexes**[Q]
Spinal cord	Muscle tone, Positive supporting reaction & **crossed extensor reflexes**[Q]

Postural Reflexes

- Optical rightning reflex, placing reactions & hopping reactions are integrated in cerebral cortex
  - Labyrinthine / Neck / Body on head / Body on body – **rightining reflexes** are integrated in **midbrain**
  - **Tonic** neck reflex, tonic **labyrinthine reflexes & streth reflex** are integrated in medulla.
  - **Negative** supporting reaction, **positive supporting (magnet) reaction and stretch reflexes**[Q] are integrated in **spinal cord**
- Antigravity reflexes in medulla and locomotor reflex in midbrain & thalamus

90. B i.e. Hyperactivity *[Ref: MTx]*

Kluver-Bucy Syndrome i.e. Bilateral ablation of Amygdale (anterior temporal lobe) Clinical Presentation

1. Hyperorality

Tendency to place everything in mouth

2. Hypersexuality

Strong sex drive so much so that it attempts to copulate even with wrong (immature, wrong sex, different species) anmials & inanimate objects.

3. Hypermetamorphosis

4. Placidity (Tameness or Docility)

Opposite of hyperactivity

Other Features include

- Loss of fear, extreme curosity, forgets rapidly
- Visual agnosia, altered dietary habits (d/t hyperorality)
- Depression, apathy, agitation & **anxiety**
- Sensory-motor-memory deficit.

Appetite

91. B i.e. Leptin **92. B i.e. Melanocyte Stimulating hormone (MSH)** **93. D i.e. Ghrelin**
94. B i.e. Increases fat deposition **95. C i.e. Lateral Hypothalamic Area**
[Ref: Harrison's 17th/ed pg-255, 464; Guyton 11/e p. 867-70, 923-24; Handbook of obesity 2/ed pg-302; Ganong 23/e 384, 448, 237]

- **MSH reduce apetite whereas MCH increase it**[Q]. **MSH** (α-melanocyte stimulating hormone) and **CART** (cocaine & amphetamine regulated transcript) releasing **POMC** (pro-opio-melano-cortin) neurons are **anorexigenic /anti-orexigenic** (i.e. produce satiety & decrease appetite). Whereas, **AGRP** (agouti-related-peptide) and **NPY** (neuropeptide Y) releasing neurons of arcuate nuclei of hypothalamus are **orexigenic** (i.e. increase appetite & cause obesity).
- **Ghrelin**, is released by **oxyntic cells of stomach**[Q], especially **during fasting** (in **anorexia)** and **stimulates appetite**[Q] **(orexigenic)**. It is also produced in **hypothalamus & stimulates growth hormone (GH) secretion & activity**[Q]**. CCK, Peptide YY/PYY** (secreted from entire gitract but especially from ileum & colon), **glucagon like peptide** (secreted by intestines d/t presence of food) and **insulin** (produced in response to GLP) are gastrointestinal hormonal factors, which suppress feeding i.e. cause satiety (**anorexigenic**). Whereas, **ghrelin** another gastrointestinal hormone produced mainly by **stomach** is orexigenic (i.e. increase appetite).
- **'Orexins are synthesized in neurons located in the lateral hypothalamus'. And neurons that produce orexigenic substances NPY & AGRP have their cell bodies in arcuate nuclei and project to paraventricular nuclei of hypothalamus.**

Regulation of Food Intake

- Hypothalmus contains hunger (feeding) and satiety centers. The **lateral nuclei of hypothalamus** serve as a **feeding (hunger) center** and **ventromedial nuclei of hypothalamus** serve as the **satiety center**. Stimulation of feeding center & /or destruction of satiety center cause *voracious appetite (hyperphagia) & obesity*. Whereas, destruction of feeding center & /or stimulation of satiety center cause *anorexia (complete satiety* /lack of desire for food) & progressive *inanition (weight loss*).
- Lesions of **paraventricular nuclei** of hypothalamus cause *excessive eating* and lesions of **dorsomedial nuclei** usually depress eating behaviour.
- **Arcuate nuclei of hypothalamus**, are the sites where *multiple hormones released from gastrointestinal tract and adiose tissue converge to regulate food intake & energy expenditure*. It has 2 types of neurons.

POMC / CART - (anorexigenic) Neurons	AGRP/NPY (orexigenic) - Neurons
Propiomelanocortin (POMC) neurons produce **α-MSH** (α-melanocyte stimulating hormone) and **CART** (cocaine and amphetamine regulated transcript), *decreasing food intake (anorexigenic) and increasing energy expenditure.*	These neurons produce **orexigenic** substances ***neuropeptide Y (NPY)*** & **agouti related protein (AGRP)**, increasing food intake & reducing energy expenditure.

α- MSH released by POMC neurons stimulate **melanocortin receptor (MCR)**, esp. MCR-3 & (MCR-4) present in neurons of **paraventricular nuclei (PVN)** of hypothalamus, which then activate neuronal pathways that project to **nucleus tractus solitarius (NTS)**, thereby increasing sympathetic activity & energy expenditure. So defective signaling of melanocortin pathway & /or mutations of MCR-4 are a/w obesity. Whereas excessive activation of melanocortin system reduces appetite. (eg anorexia a/w cancers & infections.)

- **AGRP** is a natural **antagonist of MCR-3 & MCR-4** and so **increases appetite & obesity by inhibiting the stimulatory effects of α-MSH on MCR receptors.**
- When energy stores of body are low, orexigenic neurons release NPY to stimulate appetite.

Insulin, leptin and CCK hormones inhibit AGRP- NPY neurons and stimulate POMC-CART neurons, thereby reducing food intake	**Gherlin** hormone secreted from **stomach** (mainly) activates **AGRP-NPY** neurons & stimulate food ntake.

Appetite Stimulatory Peptides (Orexigenic)

These peptides increase appetite/ food intake and obesity

AOrB	**Orexin A & Orexin B**
Why Neuro	**Neuro**peptide Y (NPY)
MCH	**M**elanin **C**oncentrating **H**ormone (**MCH**)
Gala	**Gala**nin (GAL) **Gala**nin like peptie (GALP) **G**hrelin
a Gout patient	**Agouti** Related **P**eptide (Ag RP) **A**minoacids (glutamate & α amino butyric acid)
Ended Or	**End**orphin B **Or**exin A or B
Released His Gonadal	**Gona**dotropin **Releasing H**ormone
Growth	**Growth** Hormone **Releasing** Hormone (GHRH) Cortisol

Mn – **"A or B why Neuro MCH Big (Gala) Gout patient Ended Or Released His Gonadal Growth"**

Satiety Causing Peptides (Antiorexigenic)

These peptides decrease food intake and inaniation

A MS	**α MS**H (Melanocyte stimulating Hormone)
Gastro	**Gastro**intestinal peptides such as - Glucagon - Glucagons like peptide (GLP) - Insulin - Cholecystokinin (CCK) - Somatostatin - Peptide YY (PYY) - GRP
CR (Chief Resident)	• **CART** (Cocaine / Amphetamine Regulated Transcript) • **CR**H (Corticotropin **R**eleasing Hormone) • **CGRP** (**C**alcitonin Gene **R**elated peptide)
Slept On tense Bomb	**S**erotonin, **Leptin** **O**xytocin, Norepinephrine Neuro **tensin** **Bomb**esin

Mn – **" A MS Gastro Chief Resident (CR) Slept On Tense Bomb"**

Variety of **Cytokines** can induce **cachexia** (**anorexia** + other inflammatory responses)

- Tumor necrosis factor (TNF)
- Interleukin 6 (IL6)
- Inteleukin 1 (IL1)
- Interferon (IFN)
- Ciliary netrotrophic factor (CNTF)
- Leukemia inhibitory factor (LIF)

Neurotransmitter

96. D i.e. Serotonin

Large Molecule NTs	Small Molecule Neurotransmitters
Neuropeptides e.g. Enkephalins, β-Endorphins, Substance PQ & Hypothalamic releasing hormone	1. **Amino acids** e.g. Aspartate, Glutamate, Glycine, GABA 2. **Amines e.g. Serotonine**Q, Dopamine, Epinephrine, Nor epinephrine **3. Acetylcholine**

97. C i.e. Decreased in starvation *[Ref: Guyton 11/e 868-70, 563-64, 874, 956-57; Gaong 23/e p 145, 379; 22/e p-114, 96, 351, 224, 238-39, 230, 602; Harrison 17/e p-464; Martin obesity surgery p-52; Sembulingm 5/e p 273]*

Neuropeptide Y (NPY) is a ***36 aminoacid***Q polypeptide, which **increases during starvation** (Martin-52)/ **and feeding** (Ganong 22/e p 238) ***to increase the food intake and reduce energy expenditure*** *(i.e.* basal /resting metabolic rate, adaptive **thermogenesis**, thermic effect of exercise and energy cost of metabolizing and storing food). NP-Y decreases during satiety.

NPY & MCH (melanin concentrating hormone) increase appetite whereas, **MSH (α-metanocyte stimulating hormone)** *decrease appetite. NPY decrease the firing of POMC neurons, thereby* ***decreasing the activity of melanocortin (i.e. MSH secreting) pathway.*** (So the option D has some mistake).

98. D i.e. Nerve terminals *[Ref: Ganong 23rd/e p. 143, 175, 448; Gabriel C Ezeilo p. 146, 248, 251, 427; MTx]*

- The synaptic neurotransmitter released by **primary afferent nerve fibers** in dorsal horn grey matter (substentia gelatinosa) subserving fast mild pain is **glutamate** and the transmitter subserving slow severe pain is **substance P.**
- **Substance P** is involved in **pain transmission, neuroendocrinal regulation, axon reflex and peristalsis (intestinal)**Q.

99. D i.e. Glutamate **100. C i.e. Gamma- amino butyric acid** *[Ref: Ganong 22/e P-107, 109]*

- **Glutamate** is the ***main excitatory transmitter in brain & spinal cord***Q, responsible for 75% excitatory transmission in brain.
- **GABA** is the ***major inhibitory mediator in brain***Q.

Neurotransmitters of CNS

Excitatory amino acid	Inhibitory amino acid
- *Glutamate*Q - *Aspartate*Q	- Gama amino butyric acid ***(GABA)***Q - ***Glycine***Q

101. C i.e. GABA-ergic and cholinergic system *[Ref: Ganong 22/e P-215]*

'In Huntington's disease, a loss of the intrastriatal GABA ergic and cholinergic neurons occurs'.

The loss of GABA ergic pathway to the external pallidum releases inhibition, permitting the hyperkinetic features of the disease to develop. *Degeneration of Nigrostriatal dopaminergic system causes Parkinson's disease*Q.

Thirst Control

102. B i.e. VPL *[Ref: Ganong 24/ep 169-170]*

- **Ventro-lateral Spinothalmic tract (from nociceptors & thermo-receptors) carrying pain and temperature synapse in VPL (Ventral-posterior-lateral) nucleus**. Some fibers also project to **centrolateral nucleus of thalamus** (through **spinoreticular pathway).** Thalamic pain syndrome is chronic pain on contralateral side of body during recovery from thalamic infarct.
- **Dorsal column** carrying **touch, vibration & proprioception** synapse in **gracilis & cuneate nuclei.** 2nd order neuron **(medial lemniscus)** cross midline and end in contralateral **VPL.**

103. C i.e. Preoptic nucleus of anterior hypothalamus *[Ref: Ganong 22/e P- 244-245,615; Harrison 16/e P- 2097-2097]*

104. B i.e. Osmotic stimulation of supraoptic nucleus (most probably)

105. A i.e. Subfornicial nuclei

Drinking or **thirst can be induced** by **hypertonic (hyper osmotic) stimulation of osmoreceptors located in thirst center (or preoptic nucleus of anterior hypothalamus)**Q mainly, or **by Osmoitic stimulation of supraoptic nucleus**Q (which is although mainly responsible for increased ADH secretion)

↑ **Osmolality** (Hypertonicity)	↓ **ECF volume (Hypovolemia)**
Osmoreceptors (Anterior hypothalamus)Q **Stimulation of thirst centers located in preoptic nucleus**	Via rennin- Angiotensin system • **Angiotensin II action** - **Subfornical organ**Q in diencephalons - Organum vasculosum of lamina terminalis (OVLT) / **Supraoptic crest**Q • **Baroreceptors**Q **in** - heart & - blood vessel

Thirst

Temperature Regulation

106. D i.e. 25°C

Zone of thermo neutrality i.e. zone of least thermoregulatory effort is narrow range of ambient temperature (25 to 27°C)Q in which normal body temperature can be maintained by physical (not regulatory) mechanism.

107. C i.e. No change in hypothalamic thermostat *[Ref: Harrison 17/e p. 118]*

Hyperthermia is uncontrolled increase in body temperature that exceeds body's ability to lose heat d/t failed thermoregulatory mechanism, unlike fever; there is no change in hypothalamic thermostat (thermoregulatory) settings, so antipyretics are not effectiveQ**.**

108. A i.e. Temperature regulation

109. C i.e. Hyperthermia

110. C i.e. Suprachiasmatic nucleus

111. A i.e. Supraoptic *[Ref: Gygton 12/ep 716]*

Hypothalamus Part	Function
Anterior hypothalamic (Pre-optic area)	**Temperature regulation (thermostatic detection & control center of body temperature)**Q
- **Anterior hypothalamus**	- Responds to **heat** so lesion l/t **hyperthermia**
- **Posterior hypothalamus (Shivering center)**	- Responds to **cold** so lesion l/t **hypothermia**
Supraoptic Crest/OVLT in anterior hypothalamus	**Osmoreceptors (regulating Vasopressin/ADH secretion)**
Preoptic nucleusQ (Ganong)/ **Lateral superior hypothalamus** (Guyton)	**Thirst center**
Lateral Hypothalamus	**Feeding center**
Ventromedial Nucleus	**Satiety center**
Suprachiasmatic NucleusQ	**Circadian rhythm**Q

Hypothalamic part	Hormone Released
Supraoptic (SO) Nuclei	**Vasopressin/ADH**Q (some by PV nuclei)
Para ventricular (PV) nuclei	**Oxytocin** (also by SO), TRH, CRH
Periventricular Nuclei esp. Arcuate Nucleus	**Somatostatin**, GnRH
Preoptic area	GnRH
Dorsal & Posterior hypothalamus	Catecholamine's

112. A i.e. Increases heart rate with exercise *[Ref: Ganong 22/e P- 228, 610]*

Increase in heart rate with exercise is under medullary control.Q

113. B i.e. Sympathetic cholinergic (ACh) **114. C i.e. On the environmental temperature** **115. A i.e. Radiation**
116. B i.e. Vasodilatation **117. B i.e. Increased urine sodium** **118. B i.e. Shift of blood from shell to core**
119. C i.e. Noradrenalin **120. B i.e. Spleen** **121. C i.e. β_3 receptor & UCP –1**
122. A i.e. Shivering **123. B i.e. Thyroxine** **124. A i.e. Increased sympathetic stimulation**
125. D i.e. 70% **126. D i.e. Piloerection**

[Ref: Ganong 24/e p 316-19; Levy & Berne 6/e p 664, 228; Best & Taylor 13/e p 1168, 287; Guyton 12/e p 865-867-77; Lee 12/e p 292]

- **Sweat glands** are innervated by **sympathetic postganglionic cholinergic fibres.**Q Stimulation of sympathetic system result in sweating. The major thermoregulatory responses to high environmental temperature include **cutaneous vasodilatation & sweating. Cutaneous vasodilatation is first physiological response.**Q & prerequisite for sweating to occur.
- **Heat acclimatization** (ie person exposed to hot weather for 1 to 6 weeks) results in **excessive sweat production, increased secretion of aldosterone, decrease in sodium chloride (salt) concentration in sweat and urine**Q and decreased renal blood flow.
- **Heat loss from body depends mostly on the environmental temperature**Q**. Heat is lost from the body when environmental temperature falls below the body temperature.**Q
- **Modes of heat lost from skin in a nude person (at normal room temperature)** include **radiation (60%)**Q**, Conduction** (to air =15% & direct conduction to solid objects e.g. chair= 3%) and **evaporation** (sweating =**22%**)Q. Conduction of heat from body to air is self limited unless air **currents (convection)** continually moves air away from skin.
- **Cutaneous vasoconstriction shifts the blood from shell to core and decrease heat loss**Q in person suddenly exposed to cold.
- **With each fall of 1°C, metabolism is reduced by 6.7%**Q**. So in 10°C fall it will decrease by 67% (~70%)**Q
- In heat acclimatization there is decrease in urine sodium.
- **Endogenous non sievering thermogens** are secreted by liver, intestine and muscles (eg cardiac) but **not by spleen. Nonshivering thermogenesis** is seen in brown fat, which is abundant in infants & is mediated by **UCP –1 (Uncoupler protein) and β_3- adrenergic receptors**Q. Stimulating the sympathetic nervous system, with liberation of nor epinephrine and epinephrine, increases the metabolic rate of many tissues of the body. These hormones **stimulate glycogenolysis in liver, muscle other tissue and increase cellular activity, (thermogenesis)** Q.
- **Neonates cannot produce heat by shivering**Q. However, neonates can assume universal flexion posture like fetus (to decrease surface area) & cutaneous vasoconstriction to decrease heat loss as well as non shivering thermogenesis (ie breakdown of brown fat with adrenaline secretion) for heat production.
- **Thyroxine** is the **hormone associated with long term cold adaptation**Q**.**
- **Skin vasoconstriction, sympathetic stimulation , increased thyroxine output shivering, non exercise activity thermogenesis** or **NEAT** (increased energy expenditure in form of small, fidgety movements; also responsible for slower weight gain), **non shivering thermogenesis** (important in neonates with brown fat), **voluntary behavioural responses** such as **universal flexion** or **curling up in a ball posture** = more important in animals and neonates), **piloerection (horripilation = goose pimples)** and **shunt vessels** (counter current exchange of blood from artery to deep venae comitantes) are physiological **responses to low body temperature (cold).**
- **Piloerection, shunt vessels and curling up are important in animals but not in humans as a physiological response to cold**Q

127. B i.e. Subcutaneous tissue **128. D i.e. Beta-3**

Non Shivering Thermogenesis

- Is a cold induced increase in oxygen consumption to generate heat and is mediated by *sympathetic nervous system.*
- Depends directly on the availability of brown fat and is a common feature in *neonates.*
- The magnitude of this type of thermogenesis in adult human ***being, who has virtually no brown fat, is less than 15%.***Q

Sites	Mechanism
• **Sites of brown adipose tissue deposition** - **between the shoulder blades** - **around the neck** - **behind the sternum** - **along the great vessels in thorax & abdomen** - **around the kidney & adrenal gland**Q (Brown adipose tissue is found **only in neonates** – Samson wright) • Norephinephrine stimulates glycogenolysis ***in liver, muscle***Q & other tissue. • Thyroxine • ***Intestine***Q	Brown fat contains **large number of mitochondria and many small globules of fat** instead of one large fat globule. In brown fat cells the process of **oxidative phosphrylation in mitochondria is mainly uncoupled** ie on sympathetic stimulation, mitochondria **produce large amount of heat but almost no ATP,** therefore almost all the released energy in oxidative phosphorylation becomes heat. **Sympathetic Stimulation & Release of Epinephrine and Norepinephrine** **β_3 adrenergic receptor mediated Direct action on muscle & liver cells** - **Increased glycogenolysis, lipolysis & fatty acid oxidation**Q - Increased BMR and heat production Indirect action in cells of **brown fat** with large no of mitochondria **UCP-1 mediated uncoupling of oxidative phosphorylation producing large amounts of heat but no ATP**

129. C i.e. Decreased peripheral resistance *[Ref Harrison 18/e p 166-167]*

Hypothermia may lead to **cardiac arrhythmias, reversible coagulopathy, increased pulmonary> systemic vascular resistance, decreased cardiac output and renal blood flow, renal failure** (in severe), cold induced diuresis (in mild cases) increased haematocrit (2% for each 1°C drop), dehydration, areflexia, **maladaptive** behavior, **leftward shift of oxyhemoglobin dissociation curve**, and decreased bowel motality and secondary dilation.

Cells of CNS

130. D i.e. Central neuroglial cells are derived from schwann cells *[Ref: Ganong 23/e P-80-82]*

131. A i.e. Phagocytosis *[Ref: Ganong 22/e P- 63]*

Schwann cells form myelin around axons ***in the peripheral nervous system***Q. They are not found in central nervous system. In **CNS myelination** is done by ***oligodendrocyte***Q.

Function of CNS Neuroglia

Microglia	**Oligodendrogliocytes**	**Astrocytes**
PhagocytosisQ	*Myelin formation*Q	***Blood brain barrier***Q

Origin of Neuroglial Cells
Three types are seen in CNS

Ectodermal originQ

Arise from cells of the neural tube (Ependymal cells or Neuroepithelial cell)

AstrocytesQ.

- Send proceses to blood where they induce capillaries to form the tight junction that *form the blood-brain barrier*Q. Two types:

i) ***Fibrous astrocytes*** – Found ***in white matter***Q & Rich in intermediate filament

ii) ***Protoplasmic astrocytes*** – found in ***gray matter***Q – Have granular cytoplasm

- They produce substances that are ***trophic to neuron***Q

OligodendrocytesQ

- ***Form myelin in CNS***Q
- Unlike Schwann cells which form myelin between two nodes of ranvier on *single neuron* (in PNS) oligodendrocytes form myelin on *many neighbouring axons.*

Mesodermal originQ

- These do not develop from cells of neural tube
- They probably come *from the bone marrow* and enter the nervous system from circulating *blood vessels.*

MicrogliaQ **(Macrophage of CNS)**

Scavanger cells resembling ***tissue macrophage***Q***and are responsible for phagocytosis***Q**.** These **small sized** glial cells are of **mesodermal origin** & derived from **circulating monocytes**. Example includes **Gitter, Rod & Siderophage cells.**

Nerve Regeneration

132. C i.e. Lack of myelin inhibiting substance *[Ref: Ganong 24/e p. 93-95; Guyton 12 SAE p. 75-76; Berne 6/e p. 63]*

Factors responsible for non recovery (non-regeneration) of CNS neurons (i.e. neurons in brain & spinal cord) include absence of growth promoting factors/ Schwann cells/ neurilemma = endoneural tube or Henle's sheath and presence of myelin associated inhibitors of regenerationQ (i.e. Nogo, MAG= myelin associated glycoprotein, OM gp = oligodendrocyte myelin glycoprotein & transmembrane semaphorin 4D)/ **glial scar formation**Q **/ astrocytic proliferation/ microglial activation**/inflammation & invasion of immure cells .

Cerebro Spinal Fluid (CSF)

133. D i.e. CSF/plasma protein ratio is 0.3
134. A i.e. 70-180 mm CSF
135. C i.e. Epidural space
136. A i.e. Choroid plexus
137. B i.e. 6 – 12 mmHg
138. B i.e. Hypothyroidism
139. C i.e. Formed by arachnoid villi
140. B i.e. Rate of CSF absorption

[Ref: Guyton 11/e p. 763-67; Ganong 23rd/e p. 571-72; Ganong 22/e p. 612-14; Shinde & Chatterjea 7/e p. 676; Harrison 17/e Appendix table 6; Wallach 8/e p 315; MTx]

- CSF is principally secreted by **choroid plexus**Q; it does not pass through epidural spaces. **Cerebro spinal fluid (CSF) pressure** is mainly **regulated by rate of CSF absorption by arachnoidal villi**Q. The **normal pressure in CSF** when one is lying in horizontal position averages **10mmHg or 130 mm of water**Q**. Although this may range from 65-195 milliliters of water.**
- **Rate of CSF formation** is **550ml/day (2.3ml/hr or 0.38ml/min)**Q; it s **specific gravity** is **1.006-1.007**Q, **pH 7.33**Q (i.e. < plasma pH 7.4) and **CSF/Plasma glucose ratio** is **~0.66**Q **(CSF sugar is 2/3 of plasma sugar). CSF/Plasma protein ratio is 0.003**Q.
- **Hyperthyroidism** cause **decreased** whereas, **hypothyroidism/myxoedema** is associated with **increased CSF protein.**

141. A i.e. Produced by choroid plexus; C i.e. Absorbed by arachnoid villi
142. A i.e. 3 mEq/L *[Ref: Adam's 10/e p. 16-20]*

CSF is produced by choroid plexus, flow from 3rd ventricle to subarachnoid space and brain to spinal cord and is absorbed by arachnoid villQ**. Concentration of K^+ in CSF is 3 mEq/L in children & adults**Q**.**

143. B i.e. CK+ LDH *[Ref: Adam's 10/e p. 17-18; Henray's Clinical DM/LM 22/e p. 630]*

Enzymes found in CSF include **creatine kinase (CK) BB, lactate dehydrogenase (LDH), adenosine deaminase, enolase, neopterin, lysozyme** and alpha fetoprotein.

Intracranial Tension & Transection

144. A i.e. Neck stiffness *[Ref: Harrison 16/e P-1626; Fuller 2nd/e P-199, 200]*

Neck stiffness is seen in those condition in which the meninges are irritated e.g. meningitis ***not in cerebral herniation***Q.

145. B i.e. Tachycardia *[Ref: Ganong 22/e P- 609]*
146. C i.e. Raised intracranial pressure

- When intracranial pressure is elevated to more than 33 mmHg over a short period, cerebral blood is significantly reduced l/t deterioration of consciousness. The resultant ischemia stimulates the vasomotor area & **systemic blood pressure rises.**Q
- Stimulation of vagal outflow produces **bradycardia & respiration is slowed**Q. The blood pressure rise helps to maintain the cerebral blood flow **(Cushing reflex)**Q**.**

147. A i.e. First cervical spinal segment

Encephale Isole (Line A) Transection	An animal with **caudal medulla or post medullary (i.e. at 1st cervical spine segment of spinal cord) transection.** It remains alert, has sleep wake cycles, normal pupillary reactions & EEG and its **respiration is maintained artificially.**
Cerveau Isole (Line B) Transection	**Mesencephalon transection** separating forebrain from more caudal structures at mid point of colliculi. **Animal breathes spontaneously** but is unresponsive, with abnormal pupils (usually dilated) and a continuous sleep pattern in EEG.

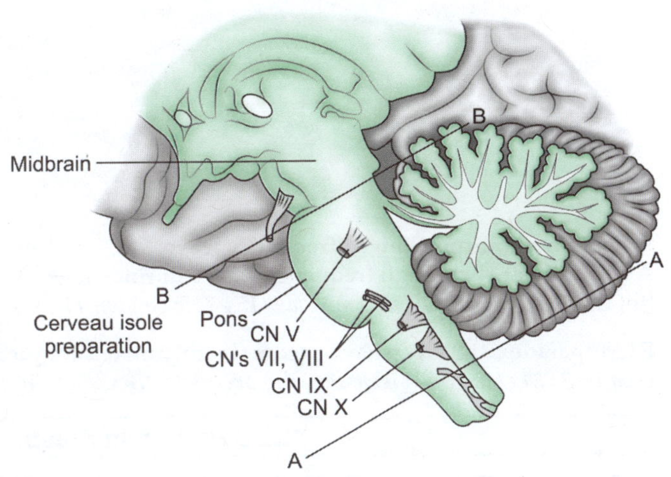

EEG

148. A i.e. Alpha waves *[Ref: Ganong 24/e p. 274; Guyton 11/e p. 764]*
149. A i.e. Frequency is 8-13 /sec.; B i.e. Voltage is 50 microvolts usually; C i.e. Predominant activity in REM sleep
150. A i.e. Frequency is 13-30 per second; C i.e. Predominant activity in REM sleep
151. D i.e. Awake /alert state
152. A i.e. Deep sleep
153. C i.e. Delta
154. D i.e. Delta activity
155. B i.e. Stage II
156. B i.e. NREM (stage 2) see diagram

- **Alpha (α) EEG or Berger's rhythm** has frequency of **8-13 Hz,** voltage of **50 micro volts usually** and is seen in **parietooccipital region** of **awake patient at rest with eyes closed, and mind wandering**Q.
- **Theta waves** are seen in **hippocampus**Q and during **emotional stress.**
- **β waves** have **>14 H z frequency**Q are seen in **awake alert patient at rest with eyes open and in REM (paradoxical) sleep**Q.
- **Lowest frequency (3-5 Hz) delta waves** are seen in stage **III/IV NREM deep sleep (or slow wave sleep)**Q.
- **Sleep spindles & K- complexes are found in stage 2 NREM sleep.**

Various EEG Patterns [Mnemonic: "BAT Dance"]

——— Order in which **frequency decreases & amplitude increases** ⟶

	Beta (β) Wave	Alpha (α) Wave	Theta Wave	Delta Wave
Recorded from/seen in	- **From parietal & frontal**Q region during specific activation of these parts of brain - Seen in **drowsiness & children & patients awake, at rest with eyes open**Q	- Recorded from **parieto occipital region**Q. - Seen in almost all normal adults when they are awake and in quiet resting state of cerebration - **Seen in awake patient at rest**Q with mind wandering and **eyes closed**Q	- Seen in **hippocampus**Q - **In parietal and temporal regions of normal children**Q & drowsiness, emotional stress in adults especially disappointment and frustration	Seen in **very deep NREM sleep**Q & **infant**Q, serious organic brain disease, in subcortical transactions separating the ceberal cortex from thalamus.
Frequency	**> 14Hz**Q	**8-13 Hz**Q	- 4 – 7 Hz	- **3-5 Hz (min)**Q
Amplitude	**Low amplitude**Q	- **High amplitude**Q	- **High amplitude**Q	- **Large amplitude(Max)**Q
Voltage		- 50 micro volts (usually) to 100	-	- **2 to 4 times greater than most other types**

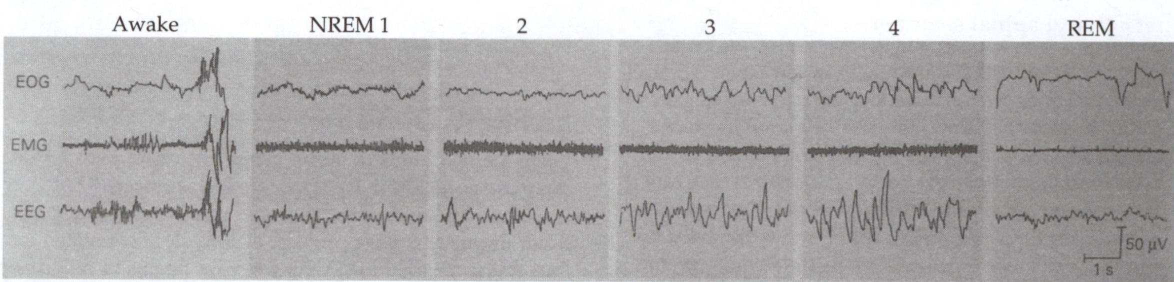

157. D i.e. Low amplitude, mixed frequency wave. **158. A i.e. REM sleep** **159. C i.e. Sleep walking**

160. A i.e. Will not show high frequency waves during stage –3 sleep; B i.e. Shows alpha rhythm when a person is awake but inattentive. *[Ref: Harrison 16/e P-154-155; Guyton 11/e p 741-743; 10/e P-692; Ganong 22/e p.193-198; Ahuja 5/e P-140, 148]*

REM (paradoxical) sleep have **predominantly mixed frequency low amplitude waves** (β like activity). ***Nightmare is seen in REM sleep and sleep walking occurs in NREM sleep***[Q].

*EEG Pattern In Sleep

Non Rapid Eye Movement (NREM) Sleep /Slow wave sleep / *Orthodox sleep*[Q] *70-80%* of total sleep	Rapid Eye Movement (REM) Sleep *Paradoxical sleep*[Q] *20-30%* of total sleep
Stage I: (dozing): First & lighest stage of sleep. - Predominatly **theta wave**[Q] is seen. **Stage II**: (Unequivocal) – Characterized by - **Sleep spindles**[Q] - **K- complex (easily evoked)** [Q] **Stage III**: (deep sleep transition) - **δ (delta) wave first appear**[Q] - K- **complex** (with strong stimuli only) **Stage IV:** (Cerebral sleep) - **Predominant δ (delta) activity**[Q].	- Light phase of sleep, **but arousal is difficult**[Q]. - **Mixed frequency, low amplitude**[Q] waves on EEG, predominantly **β-like activity**[Q]. - Also known as **Desynchronized**[Q] or paradoxical sleep (because EEG is rapid) - A – wave sleep - Active sleep
It is called **dreamless sleep** but **dreams do occur**[Q], which are mostly **not registered in memory**[Q]. Imagery may be reported but lack vividness & detail	Dreaming is seen. Recall of vivid dream imagery > 80%. Dreams are associated with **more bodily muscle activity**[Q].
-ve	Increased autonomic activity, presence of penile erection & bursts of eye movements and muscle tone decreased.
Regular respiration, ↓ BP, ↓ HR	Irregular respiration, variable BP & HR, arrhythmia present
Sleep disorder during NREM IV 1. Sleep walking **(Somnambulism)**[Q] 2. Sleep talking **(Somniloquy)**[Q] 3. **Night terror**[Q] (Pavor nocturnus) 4. **Bruxism**[Q] (tooth grinding) 5. **Nocturnal enuresis**[Q] (bed wetting)	**Sleep disorder of REM** 1. **Night mares**[Q] 2. **Narcolepsy**[Q]: The hallmark of this disorder being decreased sleep latency 3. **Nocturnal penile trumescene**[Q]

Normal EEG

- ***Alpha wave*** is most striking component & reflects the *synchronized brain activity.*
- The alpha wave wax & wave spontaneously & are slowed down with sleep, disappears during deep sleep & *are suppressed completely with eye opening or attention directed to some specific mental activity* eg light stimulation and are replaced by β waves.
- **Alpha block**: When eyes is opened the alpha rhythm is replaced by alpha block (a fast irregular low voltage activity)
- **Desynchronization**: When alpha pattern is replaced by another wave pattern during sensory stimulation/ mental concentration, it is called dysynchronization. This is also called *alerting or arousal* response.

★ **NREM / Slow wave sleep** is called *dreamless sleep* but ***dreams do occur***[Q].
- *NREM dreams* are ***not registered***[Q] in the memory.
- *REM dreams* are associated with ***more bodily muscle activity***[Q].

161. D i.e. Arterial pCO_2 measurement *[Ref: Ganong 24/ep 276]*

- **Polysomnography (PSG) (noninvasive) procedure** includes EEG (brain), EOG (eye), EMG (muscle) & ECG (heart) monitoring.
- **Arterial $PaCO_2$ measurement is an invasive procedure.**

Pain and Analgesia

162. D i.e. Mesentery

- **Pain receptors (i.e. nerve endings sensitive to noxious stumuli) are absent in liver parenchyma, lung alveoli, brain parenchyma, arachnoidmater, piamater, pial veins, & choroids plexus**Q.So these are **pain insensitive organs/structures.**
- Free **nerve endings carrying nociceptive fibers are seen in mesentery**Q.

Pain Sensitive/Insensitive Viscera

- **Pain receptors (nociceptors)** are **free nerve endings**Q widely distributed in superficial layers of skin and certain internal tissues, such as periosteum, arterial walls, joint surfaces and falx and tentorium in the cranial vault. Most other deep tissues are only sparsely supplied with pain endings.
- **Visceral pain** originating **in thoracic and abdominal cavities** is transmitted through **small type C pain fibers and so can only be of chronic aching- suffering type of pain**. Stumuli which cause true visceral pain are – **ischemia, chemical damage, spasm of smooth muscle of hollow viscus (eg gut, gall bladder, bile duct, ureter etc), over distention of a hollow viscus and stretching of the connective tissue**Q surrounding or within the viscus.
- **Insensitive viscera** – Few viscera like **parenchyma of liver and alveoli of lungs**Q are almost completely insensitive to pain of anytype. Yet the liver capsule, bile ducts, parietal pleura and bronchi are very sensitive to pain.
- Intracranial structures insensitive to pain are – **brain parenchyma, ventricular ependyma, duramater over convexity of skull, piamater, pial veins, arachnoidmater and choroids plexus**Q. Whearas, scalp, aponeurotica, **duramater around venous sinuses & vessels, falx & tentorium cerebri**, cranial venous sinuses with afferent veins, arteries at the base of brain and arteries of duramater including middle meningeal artery, proximal large pial arteries and 2, 3, 5, 7, 9, 10 cranial nerves are **pain sensitive**.
- Due to a **relative deficiency of A δ nerve fibers in deep structures** there is only a little rapid, bright pain. Instead deep & **visceral pain are poorly localized, nauseating, a/w autonomic symptoms like sweating and changes in blood pressure and may initiate reflex contraction of nearby skeletal muscle (i.e. reflex spasm or guarding)**. Ischemic muscle pain like angina pectoralis occurs d/t accumulation of a chemical agent **Lewis's P factor** (whose identity is not settled but it could be **K^+**). Visceral pain often radiates to other somatic structure that developed from same embryonic segment or dermatome – (**dermatomal rule**). This occurs d/t convergence of somatic and visceral pain fibers on same 2nd order neurons in lamina I-VIII of dorsal horn that project to the thalamus & then to somatosensory cortex (**convergence – projection theory**). Somatic nociceptive fibers normally donot activate the second order neurons but prolonged visceral pain facilitate somatic fiber endings – Causing stimulation of 2nd order neuron, and ofcourse brain cannot determine the source of stimulus is viscera or area of referral.
- Viscera have **no proprioceptors** and few temperature, touch and pain receptors (sparsely distributed than in somatic structures), Afferent fibers from viscera reach CNS via **sympathetic pathway** (from structures b/w the pain lines i.e. lower esophagus to distal colon, lungs, diaphragm, hepatobiliary system, Kidney, ureter, bladder, uterus & fallopian tubes etc) and **parasympathetic** pathway (from structures above thoracic & below pelvic pain line i.e. larynx, trachea, cervix & upper vagina, bladder triagnone, prostate, urethra, testicle, upper food pipe & rectum etc). Their cell bodies are located in dorsal roots & homologous cranial nerve ganglia. (esp facial, glossopharyngeal, vagus nerves, thoracic, upper lumbar & sacral roots).

163. D, E i.e. Liver, Brain
164. C i.e.Duramater
165. A i.e. Pain
166. B i.e. Allodynia
167. A i.e. Hyper – sensitization
168. A i.e. It is poorly localized

- **Vanilloid receptors – VR1** are activated not only by **pain causing agents capsaicin**Q but also by **protons & temperatures above 43°C**Q.
- **Perception of normal innocuous sensory stumuli (eg touch) as painful**Q is known as **allodynia** or **different pain**; whereas **hyperalgesia** is a **hypesensitization of pain receptors**Q, thus lowering their threshold and causing **exaggerated response on minor pain producing stumili**Q.
- **Visceral pain** (of thoracic & abdominal cavities) is transmitted through **small type C fibers** and so can only be of **chronic aching- suffering type showing slow adaptation**Q. Due to relative **deficiency of Aδ nerve fibers** in deep (visceral) structures there is **only very little rapid, bright, fast pain**. Visceral pain is **poorly localized**Q (often referred & radiating), nauseating & a/w autonomous symptoms and **spasm (reflex contraction of nearby skeletal muscle)**Q

169. A > > B i.e. 5-HT (serotonin) > > Noradrenaline **170. A i.e. Simulation of adrenergic fibers**
[Ref: Guyton 11/e 59, 564, 602-3; Ganong 23/167-179, 150-143, 262-267; Harrison 17/83]

Ascending pain pathway is **inhibited in dorsal midbrain** by ***enkephalins and serotonin (5HT)***[Q]. (Guyton). **Serotonergic & Noradrenergic neurons in brain stem activate opioid (enkephalin) interneurons and suppress the activity of spinothalamic projection neurons.** (Ganong p- 178- fig 11.5)

171. B i.e. Nocistatin stimulation; D i.e. Anandamide receptor; E i.e. Nicotinic & Cholinergic receptors
172. C i.e. Gate controlled theory of pain **173. D i.e. Inhibition by large myelinated afferent fibres**
[Ref: Ganong 23/e 262-267, 179 Q-2; Guyton 11/e 59]

- **Analgesia** is produced by **nocistatin stimulation** (ie inhibition of pain receptors), **nicotinic-cholinergic (α^4 & β^2) agonism** and **anandamide- cannabinoid agonism.**
- **TENS (i.e. trans cutaneous electrical nerve stimulation), Massage and application of liniments or hot bottles** to painful areas in the body relieves pain due to **gate control mechanism** i.e. **simultaneous stimulation of large myelinated Aβ fibers**[Q] from non painful tactile sensation block/close/inhibit the gate to painful stimuli.

174. C i.e. Miosis > A i.e. Sedation *[Ref: Ganong 23/e p. 144; KDT 5/e P-428]*

Miosis is produced by **μ (mu) opioid receptor** and **sedation** is produced by **μ and κ (kappa) opioid receptors.**

175. B, C, D, E i.e. Nm receptor, Nn receptor, 5-HT3 receptor, Dopamine *[Ref: Ganong 23/e 133; 141-42; KDT 6/e p-48, 96, 163, 415; Guyton 11/e p-561]*

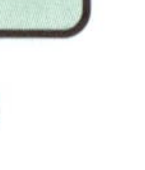

Na⁺ and/or **K⁺** are involved in **nicotinic cholinergic (Nn & Nm) receptor, serotonin (5HT) receptor, dopamine (D_2) receptor, norepinephrine (α_1 & α_2) receptor, glutamate and $GABA_B$ receptors but not in $GABA_A$ and glycine receptors.**

176. A i.e. Cold receptor B i.e. Warm receptor C i.e. Pain receptor *[Ref: Ganong 23/e p. 167-168; Guyton 11/e p. 607-8]*

Cold, warmth (heat) and pain receptors are **thermal receptors.**

177. C i.e. Rapidly adapting touch receptors *[Ref: Ganong 23/e p. 150-49; Guyton 11/e p. 576-574; 585-86]*
178. A i.e. Touch **179. B i.e. Slow adapting**

Pacinion Corpuscles are ***rapidly adapting touch receptors***[Q]. It responds only to *transient touch*, not to sustained pressure because the corpuscle *rapidly adapts and dissipates* the pressure.

*Tactile / Touch Receptors

(Touch receptors are most numerous in the skin of fingers & lips & scarce in the skin of trunk)

Rapidly adapting

- Detect change in stimulus strength and are also known as *'Rate receptors', 'Movement receptors' or phasic receptors.*
- They adapt rapidly so cannot be used to transmit a continuous signal because these receptors are stimulated only when the stimulus strength changes.
- **Examples :** Light touch is rapidly adapting *(otherwise it would be distracting)* [Mnemonic: **"My hair pack"**]

1) **Meissener corpuscle** – An elongated encapsulated nerve ending, **detects touch**[Q].
2) **Hair end organ** – detects touch
3) **Pacinian corpuscle**[Q] – detects **deep pressure & vibration**

★ *Pressure is maintained touch.*

Slowly adapting receptors

- They are also known as ***'tonic receptors'***
- They continue to transmit impulses to the brain as long as stimulus is present. Examples include

1) **Muscle Spindle Input (from stretch receptors in joint & ligaments) maintaining posture & Nociceptor input** are slowly adapting [Mn- **"Free Rough Disc"**]
2) **Free nerve endings** – found every where in the skin can detect touch & pressure.
3) **Ruffini's ending** – Detects touch and pressure
4) **Merckel's disc** – are expanded tip tactile receptors which detect touch, and are found in areas that contain large numbers of Meissner's corpuscles. These are often grouped together in **Iggo dome receptor** which projects upwards.

180. A i.e. No loss of sensation *[Ref: Ganong 23/e p. 158; Campbell 11/e p. 2348]*

During joint replacement (hip, knee etc) there is no loss of sensation[Q] despite loss of joint & ligament receptors.

181. B i.e. Accomodation *[Ref: Ganong 22/e P- 56, 124; Guyton 11/e p. 575- 76, 668, 608, 599, 568 –69, Sembulingam 4/e p. 695, 720, 892, 702; www.lib.mcg.edu/edu/eshuphysio/program/section1/1ch4/s1ch4-65.htm]*

☆ ***Increase in threshold level** (of a receptor) **on applying series of subthreshold slowly rising stimulus in succession** is called **accomodation**[Q].*

Spinal Cord & Tracts

182. A i.e. Transmitted by the β - type of sensory nerve *[Ref: Ganong 23/e p. 89; Guyton 11/e p. 594-95]*

☆ **Kinesthetic** sensation is ability to perceive the extent, direction or rate of movements. i.e. *perception of touch and pressure* and is therefore transmitted ***by Aβ type of fibers***[Q].

183. D i.e. Lateral corticospinal tract **184. A i.e. Pyramidal cells** **185. A i.e. Crossed**
186. A, B, E i.e. Spaticity, Extensor plantar response, Exaggerated tendon reflexes
187. B i.e. Involuntary movements **188. A i.e. Cog-Wheel rigidity**
[Ref: Chaudhuri 5/e P- 525-29; Ganong 22/e P- 192-204, 253; Hutchinson's 20/e p 268; Guyton 11/e p. 687- 89; Harrison 17/e p 147]

☆
- **Upper motor neurons (UMN)** consists of **pyramidal (corticospinal) tract**[Q] (pyramidal cells & their neurons). **80% of corticospinal tract fibers cross in lower medulla to form lateral corticospinal tract**[Q].
- **Pyramidal (Corticospinal) tract lesion** leads to ***increased muscle tone, spasticity (or clasp knife rigidity), clonus, exaggerated deep tendon reflexes and extensor plantar reflex (i.e. positive Babinski sign)***[Q].
- **Involuntary movements** (i.e. **athetosis, ballism** and **chorea**), **tremor at rest** and ***cogwheel (lead-pipe) rigidity***[Q] are hyperkinetic whereas, akinesia, and bradykinesia are hypokinetic features of ***extrapyramidal system (EPS) like basal ganglia lesion or disease*** **(eg Parkinson disease). Wing beating tremor or asterixis, dysarthria**, unsteady gait, and rigidity occur in hepato lenticular degeneration (Wilson's disease) involving **putamen of lenticular nucleus.**

189. A i.e. Upper motor neuron and lower motor neuron both.

☆ **Amyotrophic lateral sclerosis** [ALS] is the most common form of progeressive motor neuron disease. *It involves* both ***upper motor neuron (UMN) & lower motor neuron (LMN)***[Q].

190. A i.e. Formed from fasciculus gracilis...; B i.e. Carries discriminative touch...; E i.e. Decussate at lower medulla
191. B i.e. Temperature, Crude sense *[Ref: Ganong 24/e p. 167-169; Guyton 12/SAE p. 693-94]*
192. A i.e. Dorsal column fibers **193. A i.e. Fine touch & Propioception** **194. C i.e. Lateral spinothalmic tract**

☆
- **Dorsal column medial lemniscus pathway** is formed from ***fasciculus gracilis and fasciculus cuneatus*** (1st order, sensory neurons). The 2nd order neurons ***(medial lemniscus) cross the midline (decussate) at lower medulla***[Q]**.** It carries ***fine & discriminative touch, proprioception and joint position sense.***
- **Posterior (dorsal) column-medial lemniscal system** carries **fine touch, vibration, joint position and proprioception (conscious proprioception)**[Q]**.**

Somatic – Sensory Pathways

Dorsal Column-Medial Lemniscal System (Pathway)

Fibers mediating fine touch & proprioception **ascend ipsilaterally** in the dorsal column of the spinal cord to medulla, where they synapse in **gracilus & cuneate nuclei**. The first order neurons in dorsal columns are k/a **fasciculus gracilis** and **fasciculus cuneatus**. The **second order neurons** from the gracile & cuneate nuclei **cross the midline (decussate) at lower medulla**[Q] and ascend in the **medial lemniscus** to end in **contralateral** VPL (ventral posterior lateral) nucleus etc in **thalamus** (sensory relay area called **ventrobasal complex**).
Additional fibers from *sensory nuclei of trigeminal nerve* (subserving same functions from head) join medial leminiscus. **Third order neurons** project from VB complex to *somatosensory area I (post central gyrus of cerebral cortex) mainly* and also to SSA II (lateral parietal cortex).

Antero Lateral Spinothalamic Tract

Anterior (Ventral) Spinothalamic Tract	Lateral Spinothalamic Tract
- *Crude touch*[Q] - *Crude pressure*[Q] (capable only of crude localizing ability on the surface of body)	- *Pain*[Q] (pin prick) - **Temperature** /Thermal sensation (both warm & cold) - **Itch, Tickle**

★ Sexual sensations also travel in anterolateral system.

- ***Fine (light) touch***[Q] (requiring a high degree of localization of stimulus or requiring transmission of fine gradations of intensity)
- ***Fine (light) pressure***[Q]
- **Two point discrimination (discriminative touch,** tactile discrimination or **discrete localization)**
- Phasic sensations such as **vibration (pallesthesia)**
- Sensations that signal *movement against the skin*
- ***Joint-position sense***[Q]
- ***Proprioception***[Q] (**static position sense** i.e. conscious perception of orientation of different parts of body with respect to one another; and **rate of movement sense /kinesthesia or dynamic proprioception**).

195. C i.e. Pain sensation on the contralateral side **196. C i.e. Left lateral spinothalamic tract**

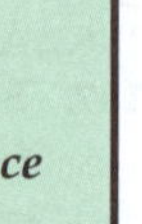

- A **lesion of antero (ventro) lateral part of spinal cord** (i.e. **anterolateral ascending spinothalamic tract**) will lead to *loss of pain, temperature (& ± crude touch)*[Q] below the level of lesion beginning 1-2 /2-6 segments below.
- **Antero (ventro-) lateral cordotomy** is effective in relieving pain because it cuts /interrupts ***lateral (not anterior) spinothalanic tract carrying pain (& temperature) from the opposite side of body***[Q]. This is the reason why, ***to produce relief of pain in right leg the contralateral (i.e. left) lateral spinothalamic tract is cut or interrupted***[Q].

197. A i.e. Ipsilateral loss of joint sensation **198. B i.e. C/L Dorsal column**

[Ref: Ganong 23/e p. 177; Guyton 11/ep 606; Harrison 17/ep- 2589; Chaudhari 5/e p 592-93; Fuller p-153, 165]

Brown Sequard Syndrome, a functional hemisection of cord results in **ipsilateral loss of dorsal column – medial lemniscus** (i.e. discriminative touch, vibration, proprioception, kinesthetic and position sensations, discrete localization) and **corticospinal-pyramidal-motor tract** (i.e. weakness and spasticity) modalities and **contralateral** loss of **spinothalamic** (i.e. pain, temperature) modalities.

199. B i.e. Vibration and Proprioception *[Ref: Harrison 16/e P-2440]*

In anterior spinal artery syndrome all spinal cord function (motor, sensory and autonomic) are lost below the level of lesion with the striking exception of ***retained vibration and position sense***[Q].[As posterior column is supplied by posterior spinal artery]

Reflexes

200. D i.e. Innate reflex *[Ref: Ganong 22/e P-267, 268]*

- Salivation by dog on seeing food- i***nnate reflex* (unconditioned reflex)**[Q].
- Salivation by dog on ringing the bell only (without food) is **conditioned reflex** [Q].

201. B i.e. Fatigue **202. A i.e. Memory** *[Ref: Chaudhuri 5/e P- 477; Ganong 24/e p. 286]*

Properties of spinal cord reflex includes summation, delay and fatigue but not memory[Q] as memory is strictly a function of brain (stored in neocortex, amygdala & corpus striatum) **not seen in spinal reflexes**.

Properties of Spinal Cord Reflex

Delay[Q]

- Between the application of stimulus & starting of the response there is a time – interval.
- Most of the delay occurs at the synapse **(central delay)**. But is may also be **peripheral delay** (in afferent or efferent limb).

Fatigue[Q]

- When a **nerve is repetatively stimulated at a rapid rate,** flexor response appears within a few millisecond because of spinal reflex. Then in the next few seconds **the reflex begins to** decrease b/o fatigue **of synaptic transmission**[Q]**.**

Summation[Q]: Two types

a) **Temporal summation** – A single subthreshold stimulus fails to produce a response two (or more) subthreshold stimuli, applied *in quick succession*, can evoke a response.

b) **Spatial summation** – Two subthreshold stimuli, *applied simultaneously* but at different spots, can evoke a response.

Irradiation

Stimulus intensity	Reflex contraction
Low	Few (flexor) muscle
Strong	Large no. of fibers (withdrawl)

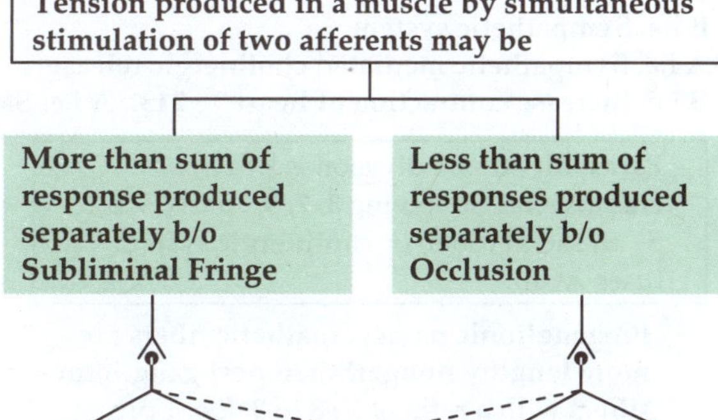

- In **Occlusion,** Fiber 1,2,3 are excited by Nerve A stimulation and Fiber 3, 4, 5 are stimulated by Nerve B. So there is less response on simultaneous stimulation.
- In **Subliminal Fringe,** Fiber 3 is excited when both A & B are stimulated only

Adaptations

Repeated application of stimuli may cause response intensity to

Decreased (i.e. Habituation)	**Increase (i.e. Sensitization)**
If stimuli is **non—injurious**	If stimuli is **injurious**

203. B i.e. Withdrawal Reflex/ Bulbocavernous *[Ref: Ganong 24/e P-235]*

Transaction of spinal cord in all vertebrates is followed by **spinal shock,** in which all spinal reflexes are profoundly depressed. **The first reflex response to appear as spinal shock wears off in human is the Bulbocavernous > Cremastric > Babinski > Withdrawl reflex**[Q] (ie a slight contraction of leg flexors and adductors in response to a noxious stimulus.

Sensory Reception

204. C i.e. The back of scapula *[Ref: Ganong 24/e 162]*

Tactile acuity (indicated by 2 point discrimination threshold or minimum distance at which 2 points touched simultaneously are perceived separate) measured by **two point threshold test. It is dependent on number of touch receptors (TR).**

↓ TR are most abundant on **finger tips** so two point discrimination distance is **2mm**[Q]

↓ TR is least and so TPD distance is **>65mm** on **back (of scapula)**[Q]

205. C i.e. Degree of overlap of fibres carrying tactile sensation is much less. *[Ref: Adam's Neurology 10/e 153-159]*

Following *injury to a cutaneous nerve*, the area of *sensory loss is always less* than its anatomic distribution because of overlap from adjacent nerve. But ***area of sensory loss for touch > pain***[Q]***. The area of tactile loss, is greater than that of pain***[Q] ***because*** in **tactile fibers** there is **much less degree of overlap** of fibers and theres is **lack of collateralization (ie rapid collateral regeneration)**[Q]. Whereas, in pain fibers there is greater overlap and rapid collateral regeneration.

Autonomic Nervous System

206. D i.e. S234
207. C i.e. Preganglionic parasympathetic fibres are more lengthy
208. B i.e. Sympathetic system
209. C i.e. Increased refractory period
210. A i.e. Sympathetic mediated cholinergic release
211. A i.e. Vasoconstriction
212. B i.e. Increase contraction of heart
213. A i.e. Skin *[Ref: Ganong 24/e p. 256-58; BRS 5/e p. 276-265; Guyton 12/SAE p. 608]*

- **Parasympathetic** division is k/a **craniosacral** (involving **3, 7, 9, 10 CN & S_2, S_3, S_4** sacral roots) or **cholinergic system** (uses ACh).

- **Preganglionic parasympathetic fibers are more lengthy (longer) than post ganglionic fibers** with a ratio of **1 : 8 to 9** (i.e. 1 pre ganglionic fiber diverges to 8 to 9 post ganglonic fibers). Whereas, **postganglionic fibers are longer in sympathetic system**Q.
- **Flight or fight reaction** is caused by ***sympathetic system mediated cholinergic release***Q. Sympathetic stimulation causes increased heart rate, conduction velocily and contractility but ***decreased refractory period***Q.
- **Vasoconstriction** is **α_1 adrenergic stimulation** response whereas **vasodilation and bronchodilation** are **β_2 adrenergic** stimulation responses.

- **Sympathetic stimulation** cause **vasoconstriction** and so **decreases blood flow in skin and splanchnic vessles**Q

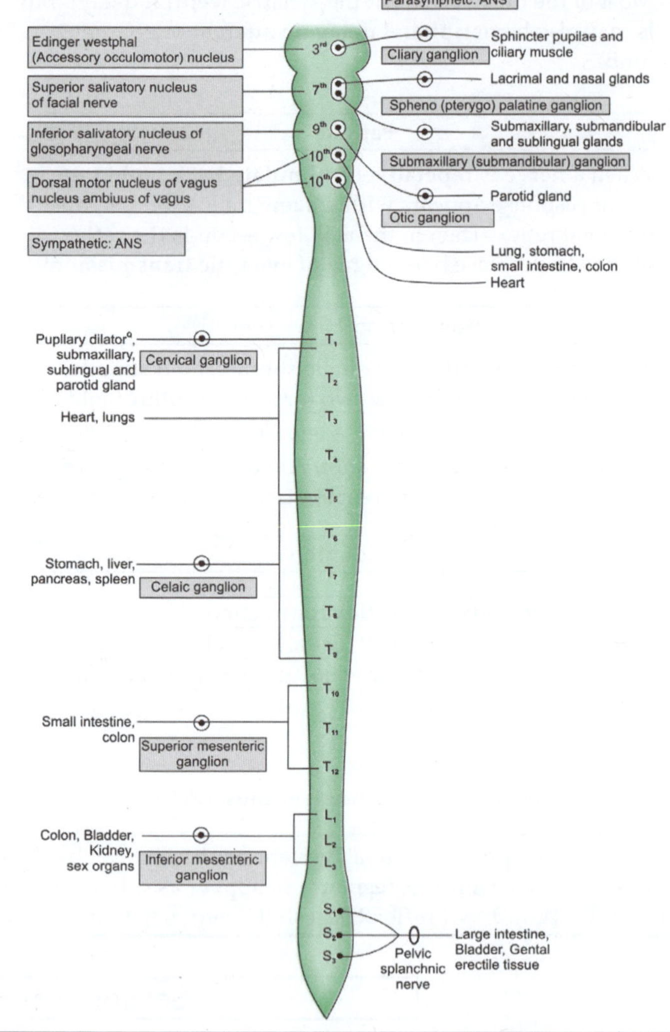

Heart/Skin	Parsympathetic (Cholinergic/ Ach) Response	Sympathetic (Adrenergic)	
		Response	Receptor
S-A node	**Decrease in heart rate, vagal arrest**Q	Increase in heart rate	β_1
Atria & ventricles	**Decrease in contractility and (usually) increase in conduction velocity**Q	Increase in contractility and conduction velocity	β_1, β_2
A-V node, His-Purkinje System	**Decrease in conduction velocity**Q	Increase in conduction velocity	β_1
Arterioles (vascular smooth muscles)			
- **Skin, splanchnic vessels**	-	**Contracts**	α_1
- **Skeletal muscle vessels**	-	Dilation/Contracts	β_2M/α_1
Systemic veins	-	Dilation/Contracts	$\beta_2/\alpha_1,\alpha_2$
Sweat glands	**Generalized secretions**Q	Slight localized secretion in thermoregulation & stress (apocrine)	M
Pilomotor Muscles	-	Contraction	$\alpha1$

214. A i.e. Decrease gut contraction *[Ref: MTx Autonomic System]*

Effector organ	Parsympathetic (Cholinergic) Response	Sympathetic (Adrenergic)	
		Receptor	Response
GIT (Stomach & Intestine) Motility & tone Sphincters Walls Secretion	 Increases **(Gut contraction)**[Q] Relaxation Contrtacts **Stimulation**[Q]	 α_1, α_2, β_2 (β_1 in S. intestine) α_1 - α_2	 **Decrease (usually)**[Q] Contraction Relax Inhibition
Gallbladder and ducts	Contraction	β_2	Relaxation
Urinary bladder			
Detrusor	Contraction	β_2	Relaxation usually
Trigone and sphincter	Relaxation	α_1	Contraction
Uterus (Motality & tone)	-	Increases, Contraction (pregnant) Relaxation (pregnant & non pregnant)	α_1 β_2
Male sex organs (Penis & seminal vesicle)	**Erection**	α_1	**Ejaculation**
Spleen capsule	-	Contraction/Relaxation	α_1/β_2
Adrenal medulla	-	-	**NE & Epinephrine secretion**
Liver	-	α_1, β_2	**Glycogenolysis, gluconeogenesis**
Pancreas			
Acini	Increased secretions	α	Decreased secretion
Islets		α_2	**Decreased insulin** and **glucagon secretion**[Q], **increase plasma glucose (mostly)**
		β_2	Increased insulin and glucagons secretion
Salivary glands	**Profuse, watery secretion**	α_1	**Thick, viscous secretion**
		β	Amylase secretion
Lacrimal & naso pharyngeal glands	**Secretion**	-	-
Adipose tissue	-	β_3	**Lipolysis**[Q]
Juxtaglomerular cells	-	β_1	**Increased rennin secretion**
Pineal gland	-	β	**Increased melatonin synthesis and secretion**
Eye Radial muscle of iris (dilator pupillae) Sphincter muscle of iris (pupillae) Ciliary muscle	 - - - **Contraction (miosis)**[Q] Contraction for near vision (accomodation)	 α_1 - - - β_2	 Mydriasis - - - Relaxation for far vision
Lungs: Bronchial muscle	**Contraction**[Q]	β_2	**Relaxation**[Q]

215. A i.e. Alpha action predominantly

Sympathetic (adrenergic) system decreases secretion of insulin & glucagon by α_2 receptor action[Q] (and **increases it by β_2 receptor action) on β cells (for insulin) or α cells (for glucagon).**

α- Actions	Adrenergic	β- Action
- *Vaso constriction*[Q] l/t ↑ BP (α_1)	**Arterioles & veins**	- *Vasodilation*[Q] l/t ↓BP (β_2)
- Arrhythmia at high dose, otherwise little effect (α_1)	**Heart**	- Cardiac stimulation (β_1) l/t ↑HR, force & conduction velocity
- ---------	**Lung**	- ***Bronchodilation***[Q] (β_2)
- ***Mydriasis***[Q] d/t contraction of radialis muscle (α_1) & decreased aqueous secretion	**Eye**	- No effect on iris & ciliar muscles. Enhanced aqueous secretion
- Intestinal relaxation, contraction of sphincters	**Intestine**	- Intestinal relaxation (β_2)
- Trigone contraction	**Bladder**	- Detrusor relaxation
- Contraction	**Uterus**	- Relaxation (β_2)
- Contraction	**Spleenic capsule**	- Relaxation (β_2)
- Contraction	**Pilomotor & Nictitating membrane**	-
- Transmission facilitated (↑ACH release)	**Neuromuscular**	- Active state prolonged in fast contracting muscle, abbreviated in slow contracting muscle tremor (β_2)
- Ejaculation	**Male sex organ**	- Ptylin secretion
- K^+ & water secretion (α_1)	**Salivary Gland**	- Liver glycogenolysis[Q] (β_2) → hyperlactacidemia
- Liver glycogenolysis (±)	**Metabolism**	- Muscle – glycogenolysis[Q] (β_2) → hyperlactacidemia - Fat- *lipolysis*[Q] (β_3) →↑ FFA, ***Calorigenesis***[Q]
- **Insulin secretion inhibited (α_2)[Q]**	**Pancreas**	- **Increase insulin (mild) & glucagon secretion (β_2)[Q]**
	Kidney	- Renin release

216. D i.e. NE is the NT of all postganglionic sympathetic neurons including merocrine sweat glands

217. B i.e. Acetycholine

- Ciliary, Otic, Submandibular and pTerygopalatine ganglia contain postganglionic parasympathetic neurons (Mn = "**COST**" = Parasympathetic ganglia).
- Celiac and superior & inferior mesenteric ganglia contain post ganglionic sympathetic neurons. (Mn=**Seal (Celiary) Mess** = Sympathetic ganglia).
- **Acetyl choline is neurotransmitter for both pre & post ganglionic synapses in parasympathetic division as well as preganglionic sympathetic neurons**[Q]**.**
- **Nor epinephrine** is the ***neurotransmitter of post ganglionic neurons, with the exception of merocrine (eccrine) sweat glands***[Q] and **some blood vessels that receive cholinergic sympathetic innervations**[Q]. However, **apocrine sweat glands of axilla** and most blood vessels are innervated by **post ganglionic sympathetic adrenergic fibers.**
- **Riley-Day syndrome** (familial dysautonomia l/t abnormal sweating & BP instability), ***Horner syndrome (interrupted sympathetic innervations to face)***[Q], peptic ulcer disease (d/t increased parasympathetic tone), Raynauds disease (? increased sympathetic activity), botulism and Hirschsprung disease are possible diseases resulting from ANS dysfunction.

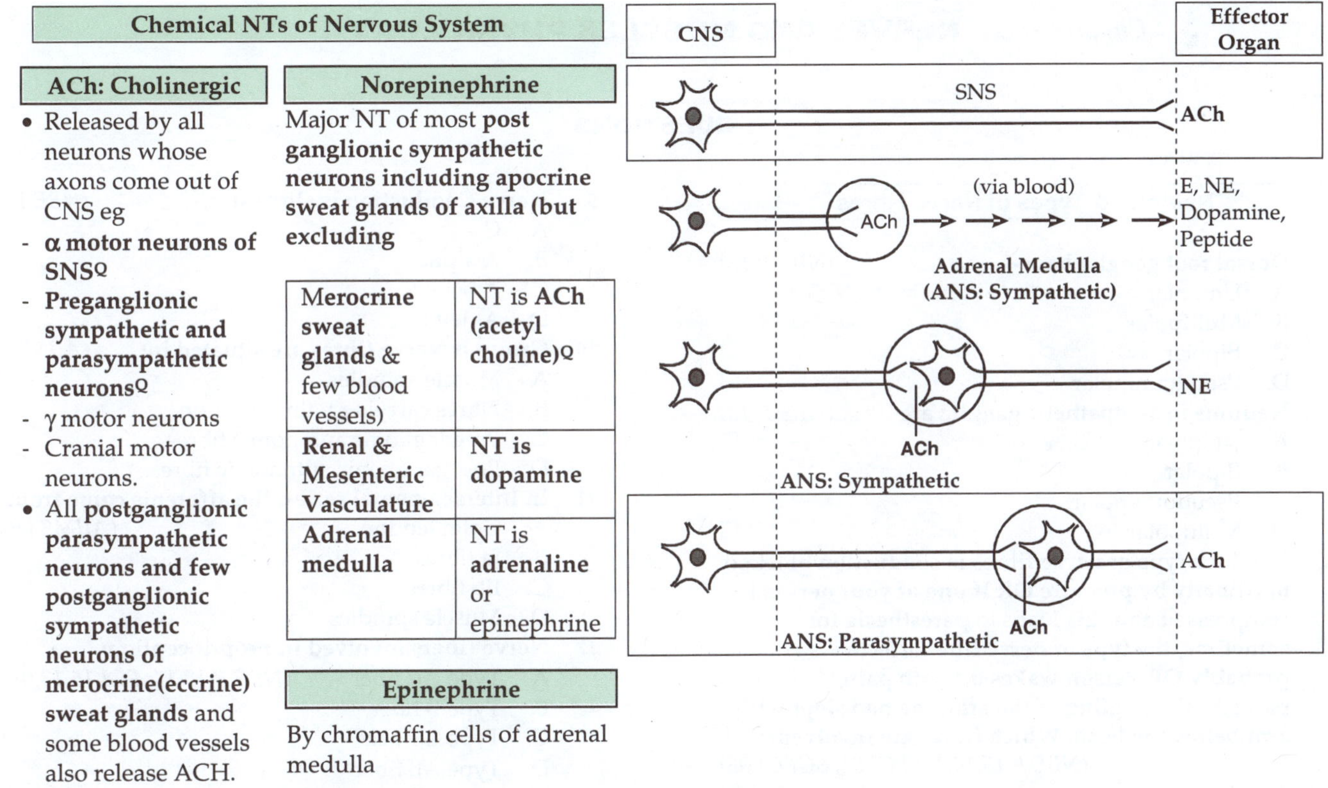

Chemical NTs of Nervous System

ACh: Cholinergic

- Released by all neurons whose axons come out of CNS eg
  - **α motor neurons of SNS**[Q]
  - **Preganglionic sympathetic and parasympathetic neurons**[Q]
  - γ motor neurons
  - Cranial motor neurons.
- All **postganglionic parasympathetic neurons and few postganglionic sympathetic neurons of merocrine(eccrine) sweat glands** and some blood vessels also release ACH.

Norepinephrine

Major NT of most **post ganglionic sympathetic neurons including apocrine sweat glands of axilla (but excluding**

Merocrine sweat glands & few blood vessels)	NT is **ACh (acetyl choline)**[Q]
Renal & Mesenteric Vasculature	**NT is dopamine**
Adrenal medulla	NT is **adrenaline** or epinephrine

Epinephrine

By chromaffin cells of adrenal medulla

218. A i.e. Fast EPSP, B i.e. Slow EPSP, D i.e. Slow IPSP

219. C i.e. Dopamine *[Ref: Ganong 24/e P- 121-24]*

- **Stimulation of post ganglionic sympathetic neurons leads to fast EPSP, slow EPSP, late slow EPSP and slow IPSP**[Q]**.**
- **Slow IPSP is generated by dopamine**[Q]**.**

220. C i.e. Release norepinephrine *[Ref: Ganong 22/e P-230]*

Tyramine, ephedrine & amphetamine (TEA) augment autonomic activity by ***releasing norepinephrine***[Q] from endings of post-ganglionic neurons.

221. A, B, D i.e. Indicator of thermal sweating, ↑ by sweating because of sweat has electrolytes, Fall is associated with yogic

Galvanic skin response is an indicator of thermal sweating[Q]**. GSR is increased by sweating (as in high sympathetic activity) because sweat has electrolytes, and falls in relaxed states like during yoag**[Q]**.**

Chapter -2 NERVES AND MUSCLES PHYSIOLOGY

QUESTIONS

Neurons & Types of Nerve Fibres

1. **Dorsal root ganglia have-** *(NBE P 13)*
   A. Unipolar ☐
   B. Multipolar ☐
   C. Bipolar ☐
   D. Pseudounipolar ☐
2. **Neurons in sympathetic ganglia are-** *(NBE P 13)*
   A. Unipolar ☐
   B. Bipolar ☐
   C. Pseudounipolar ☐
   D. Multipolar ☐
3. **In which type of nerve fibres is conduction blocked maximally by pressure OR If one of your nerves is compressed and this leads to paresthesia for sometime, the type of nerve fiber affected is probably OR Person wakes up with pain, parasthesia, tingling of the arms, he had slept with arm below the head. Which fibres are involved?:** *(NBE P 15,14,13; PGI 01, SGPGI 06)*
   A. Aa ☐
   B. Ab ☐
   C. Ag ☐
   D. C ☐
4. **A man slept with head over forearm, next morning he complains of tingling, numbness over forearm. It is caused by-** *(NBE P 13)*
   A. Sensitivity to hypoxia is A>B>C ☐
   B. Sensitivity to pressure is A>B>C ☐
   C. Sensitivity to hypoxia is C>B>A ☐
   D. Sensitivity to pressure is B>A>C ☐
5. **True about Nerve fibre 'C' is** *(TN 08, AP 01, UP 02)*
   A. Most susceptible to Hypoxia *(BHU 03)* ☐
   B. Unmyelinated ☐
   C. Preganglionic autonomic ☐
   D. Not for temp. & pain senses ☐
6. **Nociception from abdomen is transmitted by-**
   A. A gamma *(NBE P 13)* ☐
   B. Aα ☐
   C. C fibres ☐
   D. B ☐
7. **Burning pain is carried by which type of fibres-**
   A. A alpha *(NBE P 13)* ☐
   B. A delta ☐
   C. A beta ☐
   D. C ☐
8. **Maximum conduction occurs in which fibres**
   A. B-fibres *(UP 09, Bihar 03, Delhi 04)* ☐
   B. Aa fibre ☐
   C. Sympathetic fibre ☐
   D. C-fibre ☐
9. **Nerve Conduction is slowest in-** *(NBE P 13)*
   A. C ☐
   B. A alpha ☐
   C. A beta ☐
   D. A delta ☐
10. **Group B Nerve fibres are situated in:** *(AIIMS 02)*
    A. Muscle spindles ☐
    B. Fibres carrying pain sensation ☐
    C. Preganglionic autonomic fibres ☐
    D. Post ganglionic autonomic fibres. ☐
11. **In Intersegmental reflex, the afferents come from:**
    A. Golgi tendon *(AIIMS 09)* ☐
    B. Ia fibres ☐
    C. IIb fibres ☐
    D. Muscle spindles ☐
12. **Nerve fibers involved in proprioception:**
    A. Type Aα fiber *(NBE P 15,14; PGI 15,13,08)* ☐
    B. Type B fiber ☐
    C. Type C fiber ☐
    D. Type Aβ fiber ☐
13. **Most sensitive nerve fiber to hypoxia-** *(NBE P 13)*
    A. A ☐
    B. B ☐
    C. C ☐
    D. All are equally sensitive ☐
14. **Group A nerve fibers most susceptible to:**
    A. Pressure *(AIIMS 05)* ☐
    B. Hypoxia ☐
    C. Local anesthetics ☐
    D. Temperature ☐
15. **The afferent fibers which are most sensitive to local anesthetic belong to Group OR Post ganglionic sympathetic fibres are:** *(AIIMS 04; NBE P 15,13)*
    A. A ☐
    B. B ☐
    C. C ☐
    D. D ☐
16. **The correct order of susceptibility of the different types of nerve fibres to local anesthetics is:**
    A. B > C > A *(AIIMS 08)* ☐
    B. A > B > C ☐
    C. C > A > B ☐
    D. C > B > A ☐
17. **A gamma nerve diameter is-** *(NBE P 13)*
    A. 13-20 ☐
    B. 4-13 ☐
    C. 3-6 ☐
    D. 0.2-1.0 ☐
18. **Thickening of axon leads to-** *(NBE P 13)*
    A. Increased speed of conduction ☐
    B. Decreased speed of conduction ☐

C. Increased absolute refractory period
D. Unmyelination

19. Increased velocity of conduction in a nerve is favored by: *(PGI 08)*
A. Increased capacitance
B. Decreased capacitance
C. Increased resistance
D. Decreased resistance
E. Increased velocity

20. Which of the following is an amineneuro-transmitter *(AIIMS 03)*
A. Acetylcholine
B. GABA
C. Glutamate
D. Epinephrine

Muscle Spindle

21. Which of the following is true regarding alpha and gamma motor neurons during initiation of voluntary movements? *(AIIMS 15)*
A. Alpha motor neurons are activated first followed by gamma motor neurons
B. Gamma motor neurons are activated first followed by alpha motor neurons
C. Both are activated together
D. Only alpha motor neurons get activated

22. The intrafusal fibers of the striated skeletal muscles are innervated by one of the following type of motor neurons. Choose the correct answer: *(AIIMS 04)*
A. Alpha
B. Beta
C. Gamma
D. Delta

23. You are testing knee jerk reflex in a patient. The afferents in deep tendon reflexes are carried by:
A. Dynamic intrafusal fibers *(AIIMS 14)*
B. Golgi tendon organ
C. Nuclear bag and static chain fibers
D. Both Golgi tendon and muscle spindle

24. Lowest most level of integration of stretch reflex is at
A. Cerebral cortex
B. Medulla
C. Lower medulla
D. Spinal cord

25. What is true regarding the gamma efferent neuron?
A. An 'A' group *(Jipmer 05)*
B. Motor neuron with a smaller diameter than that of alpha efferent neurons
C. Innervates intrafusal fibres
D. Innervates muscle fibres that stretch annulospiral endings
E. All of the above

26. Muscle spindle is - *(AI 2K)*
A. Receptor for a variety of multisynaptic reflexes
B. Receptor for myotatic or stretch receptor reflex
C. Occurs only in antigravity extensor muscles
D. Excited by both stretch and contraction of the muscles in which it is located.

27. Find faulty statement regarding muscle spindle *(SGPGI-02, Jipmer-01, UP-04, Bihar 05)*
A. Central zone has no active & myosin
B. Peripheral zone has no actin & myosin
C. Type 1 nuclear bag fibers has low myosin ATP ase activity
D. Type 2 nuclear bag fiber has has high level of myosin ATPase activity

28. Contractile part of intrafusal fiber
A. Ends *(WB-01, Assam-03)*
B. Center *(SGPGI 09, UP-03)*
C. Both
D. None

29. Find false statement regarding sensory endings
A. Flower spray is secondary *(Jhar-04, Jipmer 08)*
B. Primary ending is annulospiral
C. Primary ending conduct Ia fibers
D. Annulospiral wrap the ends

30. Central wraping is done by *(PGI 08, DNB 12)*
A. Flower spray endings
B. Annulospiral ending
C. Golgitendon
D. Type II fiber

31. Dynamic response is due to
A. Primary ending *(AMU-04, WB-03, UP-06)*
B. Secondary ending
C. Tertiary ending
D. All

32. True is all except regarding intrafusal fibers *(UP-01)*
A. Nuclear chain fibers are shorter & thinner
B. Nuclear bag fibers are lesser *(PGI 06, WB 09)*
C. Primary endings excited by bag fibers only
D. Secondary endings excited by chain fibers only

33. Group II sensory fibers are attached to
A. Annulospiral ending *(AIIMS 04)*
B. Flower spray ending
C. Golgi tendon
D. Pacinian corpsucle

34. Plate endings are feature of *(PGI 14,12, SGPGI-03)*
A. Nuclear chain fibers *(NBE P 14, 13; UP 05)*
B. Nuclear bag fibers
C. Extrafusal
D. Golgi tendon

35. Leksell efferents go to *(Bihar 03, MP 04)*
A. Interneurons
B. Golgi bottle cells
C. Golgi tendon organ
D. Spindle

36. Nuclear bag fibres are related to: *(AIIMS 14)*
A. Force
B. Length
C. Tone
D. Length and velocity

37. Muscle spindle (stretch reflex) detects:
A. Tension *(AIIMS 09,15,13; NBE P 15,14)*
B. Length
C. Proprioception
D. Stretch Length

Golgi Tendon

38. In stretch reflex, the stimulus is- *(NBE P 13)*
A. Change in muscle length
B. Change in muscle tension
C. Pain in muscle
D. Cessation of blood supply

39. Golgi tendon organs detect *(AIIMS 08,15,13,14)*
A. Static muscle length *(NBE P 15,14,13)*
B. Dynamic muscle length
C. Muscle tension
D. Muscle action

40. Regarding Golgi tendon organ true is *(AIIMS 11, 06)*
A. Senses dynamic length of muscle
B. Involved in reciprocal innervation
C. α-motor neuron stimulation
D. Senses muscle tension

41. True statement about golgi tendon organ is
A. High threshold *(PGI 08, WB-03, KA-05)*
B. Dynamic response only
C. Detects length change
D. 3-25 muscle fibers.

42. Number of golgi tendon organs per 100 muscle fibres- *(NBE P 13)*
A. 1-20
B. 200-400
C. 50-60
D. 80-100

43. Golgi tendon organ true is A/E *(Jipmer 04, TN 05)*
A. Static & dynamic response *(Assam-06)*
B. Activated by both stretch and contraction of muscle
C. Responsible for stretch reflex
D. Transmit to Ib fibers.

44. Tendon organ , correct is A/E *(Raj 05)*
A. Ramified nobby nerve endings
B. Regulates tension *(SGPGI 06, Andhra 04)*
C. Weak stretch activates inverse stretch reflex
D. Myelinated Ib fibers

45. Autogenic inhibition is function of *(PGI 02)*
A. Intrafusal fiber *(AIIMS-03, UP 05)*
B. Extrafusal fiber
C. Golgi tendon organ
D. Muscle spindle

46. Crossed extensor reflex is a - *(AIIMS 02, JIPMER 09)*
A. Withdrawal reflex
B. Postural reflex
C. Monosynaptic reflex
D. Sympathetic

Nerve Injury

47. Most susceptible tissue to hypoxia-
A. Muscle *(NBE P 15,14; AIIMS 15,13)*
B. Neurons
C. Hepatocytes
D. Myocytes

48. Neuronal degeneration is seen in all of the following *except* OR Best prognosis in nerve injury: *(AI 05; NBE P 15,14)*
A. Crush nerve injury & Neurotemesis
B. Axontemesis
C. Senescence.
D. Neuropraxia.

49. Axonotmesis includes discontinuity in: *(NBE P 14)*
A. Perineurium *(PGI 06)*
B. Epineurium
C. Endoneurium
D. Axon & Myelin sheath

50. Motor march is seen in- *(NBE P 13)*
A. Axontemesis
B. Neurotemesis
C. Neuropraxia
D. Nerve regeneration

51. Difference between neuropraxia and neuronotomesis is: *(PGI 10)*
A. EMG finding
B. Sensory loss
C. Motor loss
D. Nerve conduction studies in distal fragment
E. Axon integrity

52. First change observed in distal part, of a cut nerve is: *(AI 04; AIIMS 02)*
A. Axonal degeneration f/b myelin degeneration
B. Chromatolysis
C. Degeneration of neurilema
D. Schawn cells proliferation & Sprouting

Nerve Conduction & N.M. Junction

53. If a supramaximal stimulus is applied to an excitable tissue like a nerve or a muscle and it elicits a response, then the tissue is said to be in:
A. Absolute refractory period *(NBE P 13)*
B. Relative refractory period
C. Latent period
D. After-depolarization

54. If a supramaximal stimulus is applied to an excitable tissue like a nerve or a muscle and it elicits a response, then the tissue is said to be in:
A. Absolute refractory period *(NBE P 13)*
B. Relative refractory period *(AIIMS 14)*
C. Latent period
D. After-depolarization

55. Action potential is generated in excitable cells. These cells are: *(PGI 11)*
A. Nerves

B. Muscle
C. Glands
D. Contractile tissue
E. Neuroglial cells

56. "Nerve terminals release chemicals was discovered by: *(PGI 10)*
A. Dale
B. Withering
C. Domagk
D. Langley
E. Loewi

57. Na+ channel concentration is highest at- *(NBE P 13)*
A. Dendrites
B. Soma
C. Axon hillock
D. Axon

58. True regarding Na+ ion- *(NBE P 13)*
A. Responsible for Donnan effect
B. Responsible for Resting membrane potential
C. Responsible for Depolarization
D. Does not help other ions in transport

59. Initiation of nerve impulse occurs at the axon hillock because : *(AI 04, 02)*
A. It has a lower threshold than the rest of axon
B. It is unmyelinated
C. Neurotransmitter release occurs here
D. None of the above

60. Nerve depolarization is due to- *(NBE P 13)*
A. Opening of sodium channels
B. Opening of chloride channels
C. Opening of potassium channels
D. Opening of calcium channels

61. Which is TRUE regarding nerve conduction:
A. All or none phenomenon *(AIIMS 04)*
B. Conduction independent of amplitude
C. Propagated action potential is generated in dendrites
D. Faster in unmyelinated fibres

62. Action potential is: *(Raj 09, AMU 04, MAHE 02)*
A. Decremental phenomenon
B. Doesn't obey all or none phenomenon
C. K+ goes from ECF to ICF
D. Threshold stimulus is required

63. Which ion causes repolarization – *(NBE P 13)*
A. Magnesium
B. Calcium
C. Potassium
D. Sodium

64. Resting membrane potential of neuron is close to the isoelectrical (equilibrium) potential of -
A. Na *(NBE P 14; (AIIMS 08)*
B. CI
C. K+
D. Mg ++

65. Most diffusable ion in excitable tissue is :
A. Na^+ *(AI 08)*
B. K^+
C. PO_4^{--}
D. Cl^-

66. Excitable tissue at rest is least permeable to:
A. Na^+ *(AI 06, AIIMS 13)*
B. K^+
C. Ca^{++}
D. Cl^-

67. Resting membrane potential in nerve fibre
A. Is equal to the potential of ventricular muscle fibre *(UP 2K, SGPGI 04)*
B. Can be measured by surface electrodes
C. Increases as extra cellular K+ increases
D. Depends upon K+ equilibrium

68. A travelling nerve impulse does not depolarize the area immediately behind it, because : *(AIIMS 02)*
A. It is hyperpolarized
B. It is refractory
C. It is not self propagating
D. The condition is always orthodromic

69. True about nerve impulse is: *(AIIMS 94)*
A. Travels in one direction along axon
B. If current is increased too slow nerve respond fast
C. Travels in one direction at synapse
D. Travels with the speed of electric current

70. Unidirectional flow of a nerve impulse is at:
A. Synapse *(AI 06)*
B. Axon
C. Dendrites
D. All of the above

71. Orthodromic conduction is
(AMU 04, SGPGI 04;(NBE P 15,14,13; AIIMS 14)
A. An axon can conduct impulse in one direction only
B. An axon can conduct impulse in both direction
C. The jumping of depolarization from node to node
D. The point at which a runaway spike potential

72. Synaptic conduction is mostly orthodromic because:
A. Dendrites cannot be depolarized *(AI 03)*
B. Once repolarized, an area cannot be depolarized
C. The strength of antidromic impulse is less
D. Chemical mediator is localised only in the presynaptic terminal.

73. Function of Dendrites: *(PGI 03, 12)*
A. It generates the action potential
B. Wave activity in E.E.G.
C. $\downarrow_{ed}$ Retrograde firing
D. $\uparrow_{ed}$ Retrograde firing
E. Involved in memory

74. In a neuron, graded electrogenesis occurs at-
A. Soma-dendritic zone *(NBE P 13)*
B. Initial segment
C. Axon
D. Nerve ending

75. Most permeable to pure phospholipid bi layer is-
A. Oxygen *(NBE P 13)*

B. Na ☐
C. Cl ☐
D. Water ☐

76. True about Nissl granule: *(PGI 10, 14)*
A. Involves in RNA synthesis ☐
B. Present in axon ☐
C. Present in dendrite ☐
D. Involves in protein synthesis ☐
E. Structurally they are endoplasmic reticulum ☐

77. Node of Ranvier is seen in- *(NBE P 13)*
A. Cell body ☐
B. Dendrites ☐
C. Axons ☐
D. Terminal butons ☐

78. Which of the following statements is true for excitatory postsynaptic potentials (EPSP): *(AI 03)*
A. Are self propagating ☐
B. Show all or none response ☐
C. Are proportional to the amount of transmitter released by the presynaptic neuron ☐
D. Are inhibitory at presynaptic terminal ☐

79. Simulation of post ganglion sympathetic neurons leads to: *(PGI 02)*
A. Fast EPSP ☐
B. Slow EPSP ☐
C. Fast IPSP ☐
D. Slow IPSP ☐
E. Very slow EPSP ☐

80. Equal strength stimulus of which type is least likely to produce a nerve stimulation: *(AIIMS 02)* 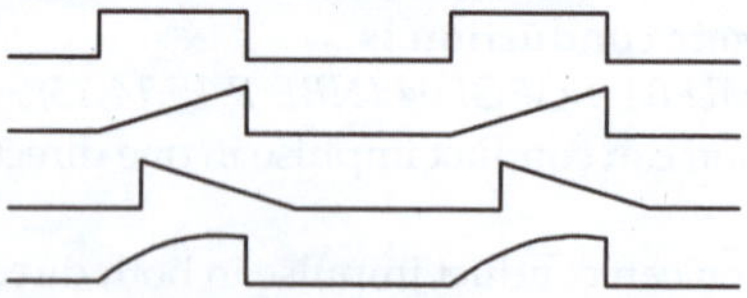
A. ☐
B. ☐
C. ☐
D. ☐

81. Which of the following statements is true about presynaptic inhibition? *(AIIMS 08)*
A. It results due to failure of the action potential to reach the synapse. ☐
B. It occurs due to hyperpolarisation of presynaptic membrane. ☐
C. It occurs due to inhibition of release of neurotransmitter from presynaptic terminal. ☐
D. It occurs due to blockade of neurotransmitter receptors ☐

82. Regarding presynaptic inhibition which of the following combination is true: *(AIIMS 01)*
a) Affected by axo-axonic transmission.
b) Not affected by pharmacologic agent
c) Prolonged by anaesthetic agents
d) Not prolonged by strychnine.
e) Inhibited by picrotoxin
f) It will increase EPSP
A. a, c and f are true. ☐
B. a, d, e are true. ☐
C. d, c and b are true. ☐
D. a, d and b are true. ☐

83. TRUE about Renshaw cell inhibition is:
A. Add on collateral sensation *(AIIMS 2K)* ☐
B. Increases by local anaesthetics. ☐
C. Has memory for spinal cord. ☐
D. Inhibition of feedback propogation. ☐

84. Renshaw inhibition- *(NBE P 13)*
A. Feedback facilitation ☐
B. Feedforward inhibhition ☐
C. Feedforward facilitation ☐
D. Feedback inhibhition ☐

85. Presynaptic facilitation is caused by- *(NBE P 13)*
A. Prolonged opening of calcium channels ☐
B. Prolonged opening of chloride channels ☐
C. Prolonged opening of sodium channels ☐
D. Prolonged closure of potassium channels ☐

86. Synaptic potentials can be recorded by: *(AIIMS 05)*
A. Patch clamp technique ☐
B. Voltage clamp technique ☐
C. Microelectrode ☐
D. EEG ☐

87. Type principle that is the spinal cord dorsal roots are sensory and the ventral roots are motor is known as– *(NBE P 13)*
A. Laplace's law ☐
B. Bell-Magendle's law ☐
C. Frank Starling's law ☐
D. Weber-Fechner's law ☐

88. Phantom limb sensations are best described by:
A. Weber Fechner law *(AIIMS 05)* ☐
B. Power law ☐
C. Bell-Magendie law ☐
D. Law of projection ☐

89. Weber Fechner law is related with : *(AI 03)*
A. Amplitude ☐
B. Surface area ☐
C. Number of sensory fibre involvement ☐
D. Stimulus discrimination ☐

90. Weber fechner law is: *(AIIMS 08)*
A. Magnitude of stimulus strength perceived is approximately proportionate to the log of the intensity of stimulus strength ☐
B. Magnitude of stimulus strength perceived is directly proportional to the intensity of stimulus strength ☐
C. Threshold of receptor is directly proportional to stimulus strength ☐
D. Threshold of receptor is inversely proportional to stimulus strength ☐

91. Intensity of sensory stimulation is directly related to: *(AIIMS 02)*
A. Duration of action potential (AP) ☐
B. Frequency of AP ☐
C. Amplitude of AP ☐
D. All of the above. ☐

92. Spontaneous release of acetylcholine at the neuro-muscular junction produces: *(AI 05)*

A. Miniature end-plate potential ☐
B. Action potential ☐
C. Post-tetanic potential ☐
D. Resting membrane potential ☐

Neuromuscular Junction

93. A short duration high frequency stimulation with 5 Hz of perforating substance pathway in hippocampus leads to: *(AIIMS 14)*
A. Long term potentiation ☐
B. Post tetanic potentiation ☐
C. Long term depression ☐
D. Habituation ☐

94. Release of synaptic vesicles from the presynaptic terminals is inhibited by? *(AIIMS 13)*
A. Preventing depolarization of nerve terminal ☐
B. Inhibition of conduction of nerve implse ☐
C. Prevention of Ca^{2+} influx ☐
D. Prevention of Na^{+} influx ☐

95. Contraction of muscle can be caused by- *(NBE P 13)*
A. Release of noradrenaline ☐
B. Release of acetylcholine ☐
C. Release of serotonin ☐
D. Release of histamine ☐

96. Which of the following events happens when a nerve impulse arrives at the Neuromuscular Junction: *(AI 12)*
A. Release of Calcium from the Sarcoplasmic Reticulum ☐
B. Acetylcholine binds to receptors on the postsynaptic sarcolemmal membrane ☐
C. Initiation of formation of cross bridges to allow muscle contraction ☐
D. Efflux of calcium through synaptic vesicles into the synaptic cleft ☐

97. Skeletal muscle contraction ends when- *(NBE P 13)*
A. Ions move out of cytoplasm ☐
B. Ach is absorbed from the NMJ ☐
C. Closure and indrawing of receptors ☐
D. Decreased calcium outside reticulum ☐

98. Myasthenia gravis is a disorder of: *(AI 05)*
A. Motor neuron ☐
B. Neuromuscular junction ☐
C. Peripheral nerve ☐
D. Spinal cord ☐

Muscle Contraction

99. Sarcomere extends between- *(NBE P 13)*
A. A band & I band ☐
B. Two Z lines ☐
C. Two I bands ☐
D. None ☐

100. In the following electron micrograph of the sarcomere, correctly identify the area labeled as "E".

A. band *(AIIMS 16)* ☐
B. I-band ☐
C. M-band ☐
D. H-zone ☐

101. Thin filament consists of all except- *(NBE P 13)*
A. Actin ☐
B. Troponin ☐
C. Myosin ☐
D. Tropomyosin ☐

102. Which of the following is not a Sarcolemmal Proteins? *(AI 08)*
A. Sarcoglycan ☐
B. Dystrophin ☐
C. Dystroglycan ☐
D. Perlecan ☐

103. Myosin filament has a fixed length of- *(NBE P 13)*
A. 0.16nm ☐
B. 1.6 microm ☐
C. 16nm ☐
D. .6mm ☐

104. The band which disappears on muscular contraction is *(AIIMS 14, PGI 15)*
A. A ☐
B. H ☐
C. I ☐
D. M or CM ☐

105. In Muscle contraction all are true except
A. A bond remains unchanged *[PGI 14,03]* ☐
B. H zone disappears ☐
C. I band becomes wider ☐
D. Two Z lines come closer ☐

106. Which protein prevents contraction by covering binding sites on actin and myosin : *(AI 08, NBE P 14)*
A. Troponin ☐
B. Calmodulin ☐
C. Thymosin ☐
D. Tropomyosin ☐

107. Tropomyosin: *(AI 02)*
A. Helps in the fusion of actin and myosin ☐
B. Covers myosin & prevents attachments of actin & myosin ☐
C. Slides over myosin ☐
D. Causes Ca^{2+} release ☐

108. The site where myosin heads bind to actin in skeletal muscles are covered by OR Actin's active site are covered by: *(AI 08; NBE P 15,13; AIIMS 15)*
A. Tropomyosin ☐
B. Troponin ☐
C. Calcium ☐
D. None of the above ☐

109. All of the following are true about excitation contraction coupling except: *(AIIMS 13)*
A. Accetylcholine is released at the nerve terminal
B. Calcium is pumped back into the sacroplasmic reticulum during relaxation
C. Calcium is released from sacroplasmic reticulum during contraction
D. Calcium binds to tropomyosin to initiate muscle contraction

110. Which of the following triggers muscle contraction
A. Ca binding tropomyosin *(AIIMS 15,13; AI 08)*
B. Ca binding troponin C
C. ATP breakdown
D. Ca binding troponin I

111. Type I muscle fibers are- *(NBE P 13)*
A. Red
B. Anerobic
C. Large
D. Glycolytic

112. Features of slow twinching muscle is/are *(PGI 11)*
A. Contain large amounts of myoglubin
B. Composed of smaller fibers
C. Contain larger amount of glycolytic enzyme
D. White in colour
E. It has high ATPase activity

113. The properties of fast twitch muscle are: *(PGI 11,13)*
A. Extensive sarcoplasmic reticulum
B. Extensive blood supply
C. Large glycolytic pathway
D. Abundant mitochondria
E. Made up of large so of small fibers with some long fibre muscles

114. Fast fatigue fibres are recruited during walking:
A. In the beginning *(AIIMS 14)*
B. In the end
C. Throughout the walking process
D. When small neurons are excited

115. True for smooth muscle contraction is A/E *(PGI 09)*
A. Latch bridge are less cycle less ATP bridges
B. Dephosphorylation causes definite relaxation
C. LC phosphatase is essential for binding
D. Slow & prolonged contractile response independent of nerve supply
E. Length tension relationship does not exist

116. Increase in cytosolic calcium from intracellular storage, during smooth muscle contraction is/are due to: *(PGI 08)*
A. CAMP
B. CGMP
C. CCMP
D. IP3- DAG
E. Ca $^{2+}$ channel

117. Action of calmodulin is: *(PGI 02)*
A. Ca^{2+} dependent
B. Through calmodulin dependent kinases
C. Through CAMP dependent kinases
D. Through CGMP dependent kinases

118. The difference between skeletal an smooth muscle contraction and relaxation is/are:
A. Troponin (+ve) *(NBE P 15,13;PGI 06)*
B. Myosin light chain kinase
C. Ca^{2+}
D. Actin & Myosin

119. True regarding excitation contraction coupling in smooth muscles is : *(AIIMS 02)*
A. Presence of troponin is essential
B. Sustained contraction occurs with high calcium concentration
C. Phosphorylation of actin is required for contraction
D. Presence of cellular calcium is essential to cause muscle contraction

120. The force of muscle contraction can be increased by all of the following except : *(AI 04)*
A. Increasing the frequency of activation of motor units
B. Increasing the number of motor units activated
C. Increasing the amplitude of action potentials in the motor neurons
D. Recruiting larger motor units

121. Twitch of a single motor unit is called : *(AI 06)*
A. Myoclonic-jerk
B. Fasciculation
C. Tremor
D. Chorea

122. Tetanic contraction is due to accumulation of –
A. Na^{+} *(NBE P 13)*
B. Ca^{+2}
C. K^{+}
D. Cl^{-}

123. There is mutation of gene coding for the ryanodine receptors in malignant hyperthermia. Which of the following statements best explains the increased heat production in malignant hyperthermia?
A. Increased muscle metabolism by excess of Ca ions *(AIIMS 05)*
B. Thermic effect of blood
C. Increased sympathetic discharge
D. Mitochondria thermogenesis

124. When the tension in a muscle fibre is maximum, its length is called as- *(NBE P 13)*
A. Equlibrium length
B. Optimum length
C. Initial length
D. None

125. Considering the latent period of a muscle twitch to be 10 ms, contraction time 40 ms and relaxation time 50 ms, what will be the tetanizing frequency for this muscle? *(AIIMS 15)*
A. 25 Hz
B. 50 Hz
C. 100 Hz
D. 75 Hz

ANSWERS AND EXPLANATIONS:

Neurons & Types of Nerve Fibres

1. **D i.e. Pseudounipolar**

2. **D i.e. Multipolar** *[Ref: BRS Anatomy p 18]*

Unipolar Neurons	Pseudounipolar N	Bipolar N	Multipolar Neuron
Invertebrates	**Dorsal root ganglion[Q]**	**Bipolar cells (retina)**	**Purkinje** (cerebellar) cells **pyramidal cells** of hyppocampus, **sympathetic ganglion & chain, motor neuron** Mn="PMS"

3. **B i.e. Ab** 4. **B i.e. i.e. Sensitivity to pressure is A>B>C** 5. **B i.e. Unmyelinated** 6. **C i.e. C fibres**
7. **D i.e. C** 8. **B i.e. Aa fibre** 9. **A i.e. C** 10. **C i.e. Preganglionic autonomic fibres**
11. **D i.e. Muscle spindle** 12. **A i.e. Aα fibers** 13. **B i.e. B** 14. **A i.e. Pressure**
15. **C i.e. 'C'** 16. **D i.e. C > B > A** 17. **C i.e. 3-6** *[Ref: Ganong 24/e p. 92-94; Berbe 6/e p. 77; Guyton 12 SAE p. 73]*

- *A (Aα, Aβ, Aγ, Aδ) and B* fibers are *myelinated* but *C fibers are unmyelinated.*
- **Fiber diameter and hence conduction velocity** in decreasing order is *A (Aα> Aβ> Aγ) > B > C.*
- Relative **decreasing order of susceptibility of nerve fibers to conduction block** produced by various agents is: **pressure (ABC = A > B > C); hypoxia (BAC = B > A > C);** and **local anesthetics (CBA = C > B > A).** That means **A fibers are most susceptible to pressure, B to hypoxia and C to LA.**
- **Pressure on a nerve** (eg Saturday night or Sunday morning palsy) can cause loss of conduction in **large diameter motor (Aα), touch and pressure (Aβ) fibers[Q]** while pain sensation (Aδ) remains relatively intact.
- **Type Aα fibers** are involved in **proprioception[Q]**; group **B** are *preganglionic autonomic[Q]* and **group C** are **post ganglionic autonomic** (sympathetic) & dorsal root fibers[Q]. **Visceral pain (nociception) e.g. from abdomen is carried by c fibers[Q].**
- **Thermo receptors** for cold are **A delta (Aδ) fibers for hot (heat/warmth/burn)** are on C **fibers[Q]. Visceral pain (nociception) eg from abdomen is carried by C fibers.**

- **Thermoreceptors** for cold are **A delta (Aδ) fibers** and for **hot (heat/warmth/burn)** are on **C fibers[Q].**

Mammalian Nerve Fibers: Types & Function

Numerical (N) & Erlanger – Gasser (EG) Fiber Type Classification of Sensory Neurons

N Type	EG Type	Origin	Function	Myelinated	Fiber Dia meter (μm)	Velocity (m/s)	Spike Duration (ms)	Absolute Refractory period
Ia	A α	*Annulospiral ending of muscle spindle[Q]* **(primary muscle spindle receptor a/w extrafusal muscle fiber)**	**Proprioception, somatic motor**	**Yes**	12-20	70-120		
Ib	A α	*Golgi-tendon organ[Q]*						
II	A β	- *Flower spray ending of muscle spindle[Q] (Secondary muscle spindle receptor)* - Fibers from most cutaneous **mechano receptor** (i.e. **discrete cutaneous tactile,** receptor)	**Touch, pressure,** motor	**Yes**	5-12	30-70	0. 4-0.5	0.4-1

III	**A δ**	Nociceptors of **neospinothalamic tract, cold thermoreceptor,** free nerve endings of crude touch & pressure (skin mechanoreceptors)	**Pricking pain, cold (temperature), crude touch**	**Thin**	2-5	12-30		
IV	**C (dorsal root)**	**Nociceptors** of **paleospinothalamic tract, warmth** receptor	**Slow pain, temperature (hot),** crude touch, itch & tickle	**Unmyeli-nated**	0.4-1.2	0.5-2	2	2

Classification of Motor Fibers (Neurons)

Motor type	**EG type**							
α	**A α**	*Annulospiral ending of muscle spindle*[Q] **(primary receptor a/w extrafusal muscle fiber)**	**Proprioception, somatic motor**	**Yes**	12-20	70-120		
γ	**A γ**	Associated with **intrafusal muscle fiber**	**Motor to muscle spindle**	**Yes**	**3-6**[Q]	15-30		

Classification of Autonomic (Motor) Neurons

Preganglionic	**B**	***Preganglionic autonomic***[Q]	**Yes**	***<3***	***3-15***	***1.2***	***1.2***
Post ganglionic	**C**	***Postganglionic sympathetic***[Q]	**No**	0.3-1.3	0.7-2.3	2	2

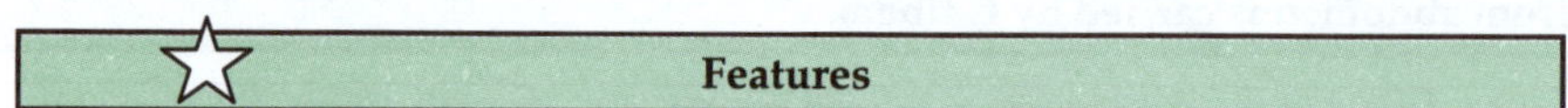
Features

- Greater the diameter of a given nerve fibre, ***greater is the speed of conduction***[Q]. **Diameter** & hence the **velocity of conduction** in decreasing order is

Aα > Aβ > Aγ > Aδ > B > C

- Large axons are primarily concerned with:
  - Proprioceptive sensation
  - Somatic motor function
  - Conscious touch & pressure
- Small axons are primarily concerned with
  - Pain
  - Temperature
  - Autonomic function
- Refractory period & spike duration
  Minimum – Aα
  Maximum – C fibres

Relative susceptibility of mammalian A, B and C nerve fibres to conduction block produced by various agents:

Suscepti-bility to	**Most Susceptible**	**Inter-mediate**	**Least Susceptible**
Hypoxia	B	A	C
Pressure	A	B	C
Local anesthetics	C	B	A

- Touch is carried by – AB, Aδ
- Pain by – **Aδ**, **C** fibres **[PA DC]**
- **A (A_α, A_β, A_γ, A_δ) and B** fibers are **myelinated** but **C fibers are unmyelinated.**

18. A i.e. Increased speed of conduction

19. A & D i.e. Increased capacitance & decreased resistance

[Ref: Gabriel C Ezeilo p. 33; Mathews- cellular physiology of nerve and muscle 4/ed pg-50; Ganong 23rd/e p.89-83]

Velocity of conduction in a nerve is increased by ***myelination, increase in diameter (thick nerve) and capacitance and decrease in resistance***[Q].

Factors Affecting Nerve Conduction Velocity

Fiber Diameter

Ability of an action potential to spread is proportional to amount of cytosol.

- **Small diameter** fibers **have less cytosol (& more membrane)** which means **less capacitance** (and **more resistance**) causing **slower** conduction velocity
- **Large diameter** fiber offers **lesser resistance and higher capacitance** through its **thick axoplasmic core** and so the conduction velocity is **faster.**

Degree of Myelination

- Nerve conduction velocity is directly proportional to *degree of myelination*
- Degree of myelination and so the conduction velocity decrease from A (α β γ δ) to B to C (eg Aα fibers are heavily myelinated where C fibers are unmyelinated)

20. D i.e. Epinephrine *[Ref: Ganong 24/e p. 136-53; Berne 6/e p. 95-103]*

Histamine, epinephrine, norepinephrine, serotonin and dopamine are **biogenic mono-amine neurotransmitters. (Mn" HENS do are monoamine NTs").**

Muscle Spindle

21. C i.e. Both are activated together

22. C i.e. Gamma *[Ref: Ganong 24/ep 232, Guyton 13/ep 694]*

- **The main motor** supply **of intrafusal fibres is Y (gamma) neurons.**Q Y motor neuron exclusively supply intrafusal fibresQ. Intrafusal fibres are also supplied by β fibres. β fibres also supply the extrafusal fibres [**β** for both]. **The main motor supply of extrafusal fibres are α neurons.**

- **During initiation of voluntary movements**, in response to descending excitatory inputs to spinal motor circuits i.e. whenever signals are transmitted from motor cortex etc, **both gamma (γ) and alpha (α) motor neurons are stimulated simultaneously. This co activation effect of α and γ neurons causes simultaneous contraction of both extrafusal skeletal muscle fibers and intrafusal muscle spindle fibers**Q

23. A i.e. Dynamic intrafusal fibers

Afferent in deep tendon reflex (eg knee jerk) is carried by **dynamic intrafusal fibers (nuclear bag fibers type 1)**Q.

24. D i.e. Spinal cord
25. E i.e. All
26. B i.e. Receptor for stretch receptor reflex
27. B i.e. Peripheral zone has no action & myosin
28. A i.e. Ends
29. D i.e. Annulospiral wrap the ends
30. B i.e. Anulospiral ending
31. A i.e. Primary ending
32. C i.e. Primary endings excited by bag fibers only
33. B i.e. Flower spray ending
34. B i.e. Nuclear bag fibers
35. D i.e. Spindle
36. D i.e. Length and velocity
37. B i.e. Length *[Ref: Guyton 12/SAE p.686,770-72; Ganong 24/e p. 229-33]*

Golgi tendon organ function as a transducer in feedback circuit that regulate *muscle force (or tension)*Q in a fashion analogus to the **muscle spindle (dynamic nuclear bag fibers)** feed back circuit that regulates ***muscle length and velocity***Q. Mn – "T for T & L for L"

Muscle Spindle

Each muscle spindle is 3-10mm long structure consisting of 3 elements (1) tiny **intrafusal muscle fibers =ifmf** (3-12 in number) with *contractile polar ends and noncontractile center;* (2) large diameter myelinated **type Ia and II afferent nerves** originating in *the central portion of* ifmf and (3) small diameter myelinated **γ motor efferent nerves** supplying the *polar contractile region of ifmf*. Muscle spindle is a sense organ which sends information about **muscle length**Q and **rate of change of length** (i.e. **speed of movement**Q. Because the change in muscle length is associated with **change in joint angle,** therefore muscle spindle also provide information on **joint position (proprioception**). Muscle spindle acts through **monosynaptic muscle stretch (myotatic) reflex**Q.

Intrafusal Muscle Fibers (IFMF)

- ***Central (mid) part of fibers has few or no actin & myosin filaments, so the ends of intrafusal fibers are contractile whereas central portions are not***[Q]. It's central portion functions as sensory receptor.
- IFMFs **lie parallel to** regular contractile units of muscle ie *extrafusal fibers* attached to its tendons. But it *does not contribute to the overall contractile force of muscle.* Two types of intrafusal fibers are

Nuclear bag fibers

- Several nuclei are *congregated in expanded central bag*. Typically 2 (1-3) bag fibers occurs per spindle.
- There are 2 subtypes of nuclear bag fibers: static and dynamic. ***Nuclear bag fiber 1 with low level of myosin ATPase activity and nuclear bag fiber 2 with high level of myosin ATPase activity***[Q].

Nuclear chain fibers

- ***Shorter & thinner***[Q] (about half) as compared to bag fibers and lacks a definite bag. Nuclei are arranged in a chain throughout receptor area.
- 3-9 fibers per spindle

Afferent (Sensory) Nerve Endings

- Central sensory receptor portion of muscle spindle is stimulated by stretching of midportion either by lengthening of whole muscle or even by contraction of end portion of intrafusal fibers.
- Two type of **sensory nerve endings are**

Group Ia: Primary (Annulospiral) Endings

- Are terminations of rapidly conducting (70-120 m/s) 17μ diameter ***group Ia afferent fibers***[Q]***. It wraps (encircles) the central position of nuclear bag (dynamic and static) & nuclear chain fibers***[Q].
- So **annulospiral endings are innervated (excited) by both nuclear bag (dynamic & static) and nuclear chain fibers**.
- Ia fibers are very sensitive to **velocity (speed) of change in muscle length** during stretch **(dynamic response).**
- When the length of spindle receptor increases suddenly (i.e., **dynamic response to rate of change of receptor length),** ***only primary endings are stimulated***[Q]

Group II: Secondary (Flower spray) Endings

- Are terminations of ***group II sensory fibers***[Q] (8μ diameter)
- May encircle fiber but usually it spreads like *branches on a bush*.
- ***Located near the ends but only on nuclear chain fibers***[Q] ***&static nuclear bag fibers. These do not innervate dynamic nuclear bag fibers***[Q]***.***
- ***There are upto 8 group II secondary endings in each muscle spindle.***
- Static response **d/t slow stretching of muscle spindle stimulate** ***both primary & secondary ending***[Q]

Efferent (Motor) Nerves

- **Main motor supply of muscle spindle** is through 3-6μ diameter ***gamma motor neuron (type A- γ motor fibers)***[Q]. Because of their characteristic smaller size they are called **γefferent of LeKell or small motor nerve system**. It has 2 histological types of motor end plates.

Gamma-Dynamic (γ-d)	Gamma-Static (γ-S)
Plate endings on **nuclear bag dynamic fibers**	Trail network endings on **nuclear chain fibers and static nuclear bag fibers**

- **Alpha motor neurons** (type **Aα-fibers**) are other type of anterior motor neuron of 14μdiameter mainly supplying *extrafusal fibers* and causing contraction of muscle fibers.
- So the muscle can be made to contract by stimulation of *α motor neuron* (innervating extrafusal fiber) or *γmotor neuron* (indirectly via stretch reflex). Intrafusal fibers are less strong & lesser in number to cause muscle contraction. However, their contraction by γ neuron deforms annulspiral endings & initiate stretch reflex.

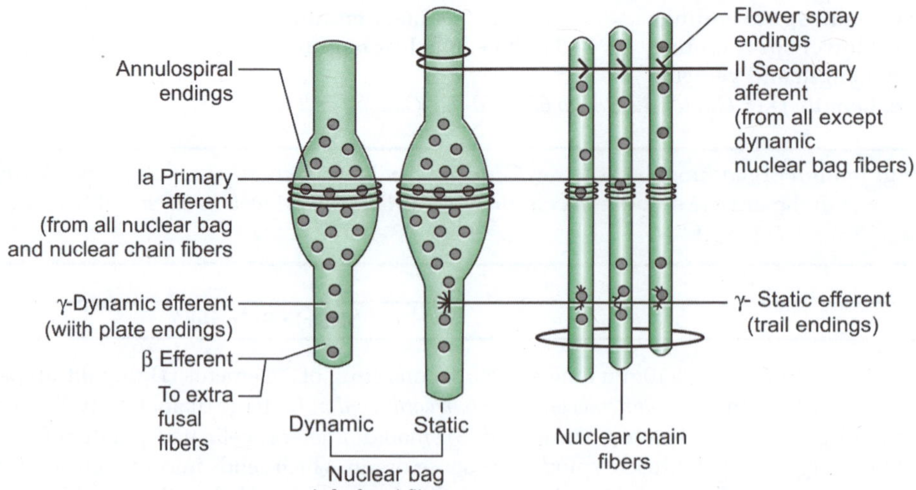

Mammalian Muscle Spindle: Afferents & Efferents

Golgi Tendon

38. **A i.e. Change in muscle length**
39. **C i.e. Muscle tension**
40. **D i.e. Senses muscle tension**
41. **D i.e. 3-25 muscle fibers.**
42. **A i.e. 1-20**
43. **C i.e. Responsible for stretch reflex**
44. **C i.e. Weak stretch activates reflex**
45. **C i.e. Golgi tendon organ**

[Ref: Ganong 24/e p. 230-233; Guyton 12/SAE p. 770-74; Oxford physiology 3/e p.254]

- **Muscle spindle** (responsible for **stretch reflex**) located in muscle belly send information about **muscle length** and **rate (speed** or **velocity) of change of length**. Whereas **golgi tedon organs** located in muscle tendons transmit information about **muscle tendon tension or rate of change of tension[Q].**
- Golgi tendon organ has **low threshold** and **strong stretch is required to produce relaxation** (i.e. **inverse stretch reflex** or **autogenic protective inhibitory negative feedback lengthening reaction).**
- **Golgi tendon (or ramified net like knobby nerve endings)** are both **activated by passive stretch and active contraction of muscle[Q]** and has both **dynamic as well as static response.**
- Each goligi tendon is attached to **3-25 muscle fibers.**

46. **A i.e. Withdrawal reflex** *[Ref: Guyton & Hall 11/e p.681 – 82; Ganong 22/e p.135]*

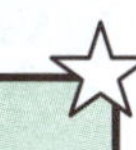

Crossed extensor reflex is withdrawl reflex[Q].

Nerve Injury

47. **B i.e. Neurons**

Hypoxic Susceptibility of Cells

Type	**High susceptibility**	Intermediate	**Low susceptibility**
Damage time	3-5 minutes	20-120 minutes	**Hours**
Cells	**Neurons (nerve cell)[Q]**	**Myocardium (Myocyte), Hepatocyte, Renal epithelial cell**	Fibroblast, epidermis, **skeletal muscle**

48. **D i.e. Neuropraxia**
49. **D i.e. Axon & Myelin Sheath**
50. **A i.e. Axontemesis**
51. **A, D, E i.e. EMG finding, Nerve conduction studies.., Axon integrity**
52. **A i.e. Axonal degeneration**

[Ref: Guyton 12/SAE p. 74-76; Samson Wright 13/e p. 288; Chaudhari 5/e p. 46; Apley's 8/e P-231; Sembulingam 4/e p. 687; CSDT 11/e p. 128, 913; Maheshwari 3/e p. 50-51]

- **Neuropraxia** refers to physiological disruption of conduction only, no structural changes or degeneration occur. **Neuronal degeneration is seen in[Q]** - Crush nerve injury, Fetal development, Senescence.
- **No neuronal degeneration (anatomical disruption or axonal disintegrity) is seen in neuroprexia. Axontemesis** includes **discontinuity in axons and myelin sheaths[Q]**. Whereas, in **neurontemesis** there is **complete discontinuation** of nerve (ie axon with myelin sheath & neural tube or perineurium, epineurium & endoneurium).
- Type of nerve injury can be differentiated by **EMG** & **nerve conduction studies.**
- **1st change** occurring in distal part of cut nerve is **axonal degeneration followed by** (2nd change) **myelin degeneration[Q].**

Seddon's Classification of Nerve Injury

Features	**Neuropraxia**	**Axontemesis**	**Neurontemesis**
Pathology	- No anatomical disruption - Both axon & sheath intact - Physiological disruption of conduction only	**Axons & myelin sheath disrupted but endoneural perineurium and epineurium sheath (neural tube) is intact[Q]**	- Complete division of nerve - Axon & neural tube (i.e. perineurium, epineurium, & endoneural sheath) both are divided.
Degeneration	**No degeneration [Q]**	Degeneration present proximal + distal (Wallerian)	Degeneration present proximal + Distal (Wallerian)
Neuroma	No	In continuity	**End or side neuroma**
Tinel's sign[Q] / Motor march	Absent	**Advancing (present)[Q]**	Static
Prognosis	- Excellent - Recovery is complete usually **with in 6 weeks**	- Good /fair /poor - Occurs as regenerating axons grow into intact sheath	Poor

- **Electrodiagnostic studies** (like **nerve conduction study & EMG**) are used to **distinguish between partial & complete lesion**[Q] **and to establish a baseline for monitoring subsequent functional recovery**[Q]. However, these are not helpful until 2-3 weeks after an acute injury.
- If a muscle lose its nerve supply (d/t nerve injury), **EMG** shows **denervation potential** at 3rd week; which exludes neuropraxia but however does not differentiate between axontmesis and neurontemesis.
- All types of injuries may cause sensory, motor or both loss depending on type of nerve damaged.

★ Each **axon** is covered by **myelin sheath** (in myelinated nerve only) &/or **neurilemma (Schwann sheath)**. Each *nerve fiber* (containing many axons) is covered by **endoneurium**. Each *fasciculus* (containing many nerve fibres) is covered by **perineurium**. And each nerve (containing mamy fasciculus) is covered by **epineurium**.

Nerve Conduction & N.M. Junction

53. B i.e. Relative refractory period **54. B i.e. Relative refractory period**
55. A i.e. Nerves; B i.e. Muscle; C i.e. Glands; D i.e. Contractile tissue
[Ref: Ganong 24/e p. 88; Guyton 12/e p. 64-65, 666; Chaudhary 6/e p. 17; Best & Taylor 13/e p.155-62]

Action potential develops in excitable cells such as **nerves (neurons), muscle (skeletal, smooth and cardiac),** and other **contractile tissues** such as **few glands**[Q]. Glial cells such as neuroglial cells do not generate action potential.

Refractory Period (RP)

Absolute RP	Relative RP
- It correspond to period from time the firing level is reached until repolarization is 1/3rd complete - **No stimulus no matter how strong, will excite the nerve.**	- **From the end of absolute R.P to start of after depolarization.** - **In this period only very strong stimulus can cause excitation**[Q]

56. E i.e. Loewi

Otto Loewi ***discovered that nerve terminals or synapse release chemicals***. In his most famous experiment, Loewi took fluid from one frog heart (**vagus stoff** or later found to be **acetylcholine**) and applied it to another, slowing the second heart and showing that synaptic signaling used chemical messengers.

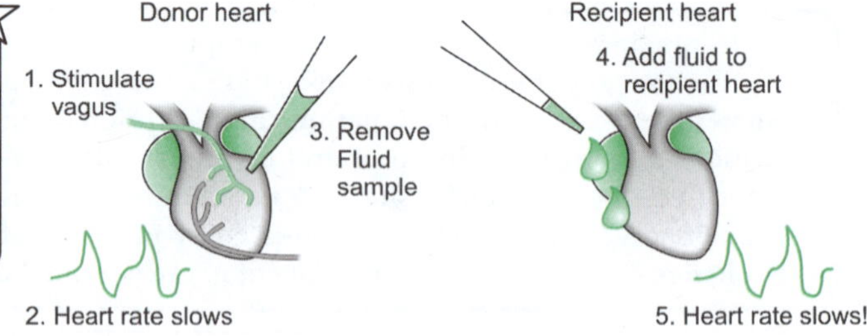

Otto Loewi's Experiment

57. C i.e. Axon hillock **58. C i.e. Responsible for Depolarization** **59. A i.e. It has lower threshold than rest of axon**
60. A i.e. Opening of sodium channels **61. A i.e. All or none phenomenon** **62. D i.e. Threshold stimulus is required**
63. C i.e. Potassium **64. C i.e. K^+** **65. B i.e. K^+ potassium ion is most diffusible ion.**
66. A i.e. Na^+ **67. D i.e. Depends on potassium ion equilibrium** **68. B i.e. It is refractory**
69. C i.e. Travels in one direction at synapse **70. A i.e. Synapse** **71. A i.e. An Axon can conduct impulse in ...**
72. D i.e. Chemical mediator is located only in the presynaptic terminal
[Ref: Ganong 24/e p. 86-92; Guyton 12/SAE p. 71-73; Berne 6/e p. 65-76; Chaudhari 5/e p. 469-70]

- **Initiation of nerve impulse (depolarization) occurs at axon hillock** because **it has lower threshold for excitation than the rest of axon (neuron)**Q mainly because of **greater concentration of voltage gated Na+ channels.**
- **Development of AP (i.e. depolarization spike) occurs d/t Na^+ influx (from opening of Na^+ channels)**Q and **rapid return of membrane towards resting membrane potential/RMP (i.e. repolarization)** is d/t closing of Na^+ Channels and **opening of K^+ channel**Q.
- **Development of action potential** (or nerve conduction) is an **"all or none phenomenon"**Q ie neither AP occurs below threshold intensity nor does the further increase in intensity of stimulus produces increase in AP.
- **Because of more open K^+ channels and greater membrane permeability to K^+**(in comparison to Na^+) **at rest, the resting membrane potential in neurons** is usually about **-70 mV,** which is **close to equilibrium (isoelectric) potential for K^+**Q - Summary of Ganong 24/e p. 88
- **Order of permeability in excitable tissue at rest: $K^+ > Cl^- > Na^+$**Q
- **The nerve impulse is self propagating**Q due to circular current flow and succive electronic depolarization to the firing level of membrane ahead of action potential.
- **Once initiated moving impulse does not depolarize the area behind it to the firing level, because this area is refractory**Q**.**
- **Axons** can conduct nerve impulses **in either direction**Q **(anti-dromic conduction)** unlike **synapses,** which **permit conduction of nerve impulses in one direction (orthodromic) only because the neurotransmitter substance responsible for conduction is present in vesicles of presynaptic neurons only**Q**. The post synaptic neuron does not contain any neurotransmitter**Q. It has protein molecules embedded in it which serve as receptor for the neurotransmitter.
- **Orthodromic conduction means conduction in one direction only, from one neuron called the presynaptic neuron to another neuron called the postsynaptic neuron**Q**.**

PRESYNAPTIC NEURON (SYNAPTIC KNOB)	⟶ SYNAPTIC CLEFT ⟶	POST SYNAPTIC NEURON
- Neurotransmitter vesicles		*- NO neurotransmitter vesicles* - Receptors present for them.

- **Electrical synapses can transmit signals in either direction.**Q

73. **B i.e. Wave activity in EEG (C) ↓ed retrograde firing (E) Involved in memory**
[Ref: Ganong 24/e P-125-26, 84-85; Guyton 12/SAE P-671-72, 676; Berne 6/e p. 53-54]

Functions of dendrites are learning & long term potentiation of memory, decreased retrograde firing and production of ware activity in EEGQ**.**

74. **B i.e. Initial segment**
75. **A i.e. Oxygen**
76. **C, D, E i.e. Present in dendrite; Involves in protein synthesis; Structurally they are endoplasmic reticulum**
77. **C i.e. Axons**

- From **Cell body (Soma)** of neuron arises 5-7 **Dendrites and Axon Hillock (initial thick segment of axon=Nerve impulse generator)**Q**. Nodes of Ranvier are periodic gaps in myelin sheath of axons**Q**.**
- Dendrites & soma are receptor zone. **Axon hillock is nerve impulse generator (graded electro genesis),** Axon is transmitter and nerve terminal is **neurotransmitter (NT) release zone.**

- **Nissl body (or granule) / tigroid body is large rough endoplasmic reticulum (i.e. containing ribosomes), seen in soma (or perikaryon , or cyton, or cell body, the bulbous end of a neuron, containing the cell nucleus)**Q **and dendrites**Q**, of neurons but not in axon or axon hillock**Q**. They are the site of protein synthesis**Q involved in for production of neurotransmitters such acetylcholine.

78. **C i.e. Are proportional to the amount of transmitter released by the presynaptic neuron**
[Ref: Ganong 24/e P-122-23, 161, 259; Berne 6/e p. 85, 89-90, 158, 222]

Excitatory post synaptic potential (EPSP) or **generator (receptor) potential** (which is EPSP in Pacinian corpuscles) is a **nonpropagating localized depolarizing potential, the magnitude of which is proportional to the intensity of stimulus (i.e. the amount of transmitters released by the pre synaptic neurons)**Q. So EPSP or GP(RP) are **graded potentials** rather than "all or none" action potential.

79. A i.e. Fast EPSP, B i.e. Slow EPSP, D i.e. Slow IPSP

The response produced in post ganglionic sympathetic neurons by stimulation of their preganglionic innervations generates rapid depolarization ***(Fast EPSP)***[Q], ***slow EPSP***[Q], a ***late slow (prolonged) EPSP***[Q], *and* ***prolonged inhibitory post synaptic potential (slow IPSP)***[Q].

80. B i.e. *[Ref: Ganong 24/e p. 90-91; Berne 6/e p. 65-67; Chaudhary 2/e p. 19]*

Only the ***current or stimulus which rises to its peak intensity rapidly causes the action potential to develop***[Q]. The **current which rises to its peak very slowly (as in graph B) does not produce AP**, although, at peak level, its strength may be adequate. This is called **accommodation**, & occurs because the **activation or opening up of Na^+ channels do not develop with slowly rising current strength**. In graphs A & C the rise to peak is rapid; where as the rise to peak is faster in D and slowest in B.

81. C i.e. It occurs due to inhibition of release of neurotransmitter from presynaptic terminal.
82. B i.e. a, d, e
83. D i.e. Inhibition of feedback propogation
84. D i.e. Feedback inhibhition
85. A i.e. Prolonged opening of calcium channels
[Ref: Ganong 24/e p134-36; Gabriel C Ezeilo p. 45-46; Guyton 11th/e p. 567-66; Sembulingum 3/e P- 642; Chaudhuri 5/e P- 472, 473]

- **Indirect preynaptic inhibition** occurs **due to decrease or inhibition of release of excitatory neurotransmitter from pre synaptic terminal**[Q] **(because of GABA mediated increased Cl- influx, increased K+ outflux, decreased size of action potential, decreased Ca++ entery, decreased NT release causing decrease in EPSP).** Whereas **direct reciprocal postsynaptic inhibition** occurs d/t release of inhibitory neurotransmitter (glycine / GABA) on post synaptic membrane producing **hyperpolarization & IPSP**.
- **Pricrotoxin (not LA) inhibits or antagonizes presynaptic inhibition whereas strychnine antagonizes postsynaptic inhibition**[Q]**.**
- **Presynaptic facilitation is caused by prolonged opening of Ca^{++} channels**[Q] **and early closing of K+ channels**[Q]**.**
- **Renshaw cell inhibition** is **negative feedback inhibition or inhibition of feedback propogation**[Q]**.**

86. C i.e. Microelectrode *[Ref: Ganong 24/e P-87-91]*

By electrical, chemical or mechanical stimulus, two types of physio chemical disturbances are produced in nerves- 1) **Local, non propagated potential – synaptic, electrotonic or generator potential,** 2) **Propogated disturbance – action potential (nerve impulse)**. The electric events in neurons are rapid being measured in millisecond (ms) and the potential changes are small, measured in millivolts (mv). The electrical activity can be measured by (i) ***Microelectrode***[Q] with tip diameter of less than 1 micron (ii) Electronic amplifier (iii) Cathode ray oscilloscope

87. B i.e. Bell-Magendle's law
88. D i.e. Law of projection
89. D i.e. Stimulus discrimation
90. A i.e. Magnitude of stimulus strength perceived is approximately proportionate to the log of the intensity of stimulus strength *[Ref: Ganong 23rd/e p. 152-54; 22/ed pg-126; Guyton 11th/e p. 594-96; Gabriel C Ezeilo p. 452]*
91. B i.e. Frequency of AP

Weber Fechner law	"Magnitude of sensation felt is proportionate to the log of intensity of the stimulus". So **stimulus strength discrimination (gradation)** is dependent on **frequency of AP**[Q], number of receptors activated and amount of receptor potential.
Bell Magentic law	In the spinal cord – **d**orsal roots are **s**ensory and **v**entral roots are **m**otor **[DS VM]**
Law of projection	Describe ***phantom limb sensation***[Q]

92. A i.e. Miniature end plate potential *[Ref: Ganong 22/e P-117]*

Small quanta (packets) of *acetylcholine (Ach) are released* randomly from the nerve cell membrane at rest, each producing a minute depolarizing spike called a ***miniature end- plate potential.***[Q]

Neuromuscular Junction

93. A i.e. Long term potentiation

Synaptic Plasticity and Learning

1. Post tetanic Potentiation (PTP)

- Production of enhanced post synaptic potentiation in **response to brief tetanizing train of stimuli in pre synaptic neuron** (which causes **Ca^{++} to accumulate in presynaptic neuron)**
- Lasts upto **60 seconds.**

2. Long term Potentiation (LTP)

- Like post tetanic potentiation but is **much more prolonged and can last for days**[Q]**.**
- Unlike PTP it is initiated by increase in intracellular Ca^{++} in postsynaptic (rather than presynaptic) neuron.
- Studied maximally in **hippocampus (perforating substance pathway)**[Q]**.**

3. Long Term Depression

- LTD is **opposite to LTP** characterized by decreased synaptic strength.
- It is produced by **slower stimulation of presynaptic neurons** and a/w smaller rise in intracellular Ca^{++} than LTP. It is d/t **dephosphorylation of AMPA receptors.**
- In cerebellum, LTD of climbing fibers causes decrease firing of parallel fibers
- First noted in **hippocampus** but occurs throughout brain.

4. Habituation

5. Sensitizationz

94. C i.e. Prevention of Ca^{2+} influx

95. B i.e. Release of acetylcholine

96. B i.e. Acetylcholine binds to receptors on the postsynaptic sarcolemmal membrane
[Ref: Ganong 24/e p 115, 104, 127-29; Guyton 12/e p 84-88; Berne & Levy 6/e p 234, Best & Taylor 13/e p 80-81]

- **Action potential** conducted along the nerve fiber **enhances the endocytic release of ACh (acetyl choline) from vesicles (packets) into the neuromuscular cleft by enhancing the permeability of presynaptic membrane to Ca^{++} ions (l/t Ca^{++} influx not efflux through voltage gated channels).**
- Sequence of events when a nerve impulse arrives at neuromuscular junction is: **Calcium influx in presynaptic neural membrane though voltage gated Ca^{++} channels → Exocytosis of ACh from synaptic vesicles into synaptic cleft → ACh binds to Nm receptors on post synaptic sarcolemmal membrane** which are ligand gated Na^{+} channels **→ Na^{+} influx; development of EPP & current sink** → AP conducted in both directions and enter muscle fiber via T-tubules **→ Ca^{++} released (efflux) from sarcoplasmic reticulum** (ryanodine receptor channels) in response to voltage change sensed by DHPR on T tubules → Binding of Ca^{++} to troponin C, uncovering myosin binding sites of actin l/t **formation of cross linkage (bridging) that allows muscle contraction.**
- ***Release of synaptic vesicles from presynaptic terminals is inhibited by prevention of calcium influx***[Q]; examples include **Lambert-Eaton syndrome (LEMS)** & use of **aminoglycoside** antibiotics. (Although preventing depolarization/ conduction/ Na^{+} influx can also prevent NM transmission but the best answer is prevention of Ca^{++} influx because of above examples)**. LEMS**, usually a/w cancer has **autoimmune damage of neuromuscular voltage gated Ca^{++} channels decreasing Ca^{++} influx** and acetylcholine release resulting in muscle weakness**. Aminoglycosides** can also impair Ca^{++} channel function. Whereas **aminopyridines** used in treatment of LEMS facilitate ACH release (so improve muscle strength) by blocking presynaptic K^{+} channels and activating voltage gated Ca^{++} channels.

97. D i.e. Decreased calcium outside reticulum *[Ref: Mtx of NMJ transmission & muscle contraction]*

ACh degradation at NMJ by ACh Esterase prevents continued muscle reexcitation (contraction)[Q]**, whereas pumping back of Ca^{++} from sarcoplasm into sarcoplasmic reticulum by ATP dependent pump (resulting in decreased Ca^{++} outside reticulum) ends skeletal muscle contraction (i.e. causes relaxation).**

98. B i.e. Neuromuscular junction *[Ref: Harrison 16/e P- 2518]*

Myasthenia gravis is a ***neuromuscular disorder***[Q] characterized by weakness and fatiguability of skeletal muscle. The underlying defect is a decrease in the number of available nicotinic Ach receptor at the *Neuromuscular junction* due to an ***antibody mediated autoimmune attack.***[Q]

Muscle Contraction

99. B i.e. Two Z lines

100. B i.e. I-band

Skeletal Muscle: Myofibrils

I ,Z

I (Light) Band –

It is formed by thin filament mainly actin.

The **light (Isotropic)** I band is divided into two by Z line.

Z Line –

each myofibril is divided into number of compartments by z-line.

A H M

A (Dark) Band-

In this band myosin & action filaments overlap

- This band is **dark** because of overlapping and presence of myosin.

H Zone –

This is a narrow lighter area at the middle of A band

There is no actin in this zone.

M Line-

A transverse line seen in the middle H zone

★ So in Q of AIIMS 2016, A = A Band, B = Actin Filament, C = Sacromere width, D = H zone and **E = Isotropic (Light) I Band**[Q].

Skeletal muscle in relaxed state

|← **Sacromere** →|

Z line M line Z line

Actin

Myosin

Myosin

H zone

I band A band

Sarcomere is the **portion of myofibril in between two adjacent Z lines. It is the *structural and functional unit of skeletal muscle***[Q].

Sarcomere = ½ I band + one full A band + ½ I band

101. C i.e. Myosin

Skeletal Muscle Morphology

- A muscle consist of large number of muscle fibers and each *muscle fibres* contains large number of *myofibrils*. Each myofibril contains two types of filament:
  - **Actin (active, thin)** [Q]
  - **Myosin (M for mota, thick)** [Q]
- Myosin & actin can become connected with each other by cross bridges. *Top of cross bridge is called myosin head &* it has sites for attachment for *actin and ATP*.
- Each myosin filament is surrounded by six actin filaments.

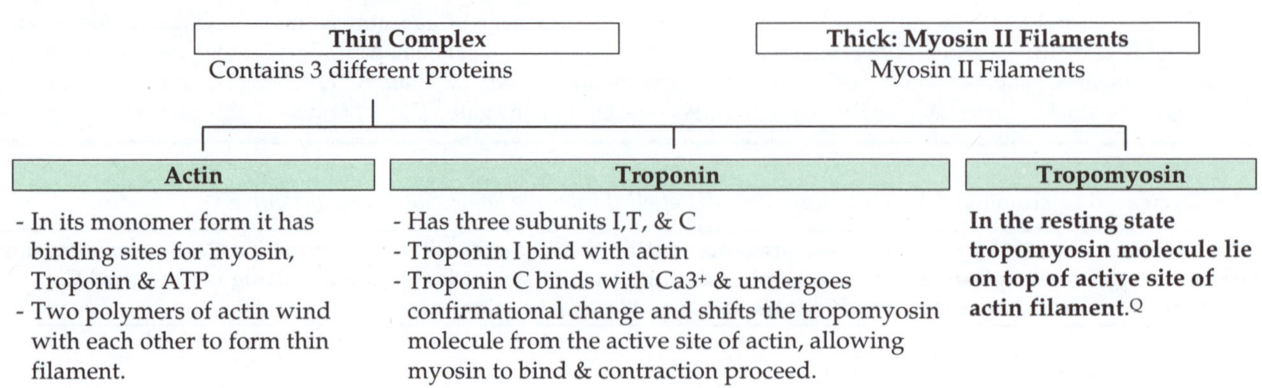

102. D i.e. Perlecan *[Ref: Ganong 22/e p. 68; Guyton 11/e p. 72, 90; Harrison 17/e p. 2683-84]*

Caplin, dystrophin, dysferlin, dystroglycan, sacroglycan, caveoli & integrins are sacrolemmal proteinsQ. Where as **perlecan** is a large multidomain proteoglycan, which is **synthesized by both vascular endothelium and smooth muscle cells and deposited in extra cellular matrix**Q.

103. B i.e. 1.6 microm

Myosin filament has a fixed (uniform) length of 1.5 micronsQ.

104. B i.e. H
105. C i.e. I band becomes wider
106. D i.e. Tropomyosin
107. B i.e. Covers myosin and prevents attachment of actin and myosin
108. A i.e. Tropomyosin
109. D i.e. Calcium binds to tropomyosin to initiate muscle contraction
110. B i.e. Calcium binding troponin C
[Ref: Ganong 24/e P- 97-104; Chaudhuri 5/e P- 428-30; Sembulingum 3/e P-127]

- In each sarcomere, during muscle contraction - **H zone disappears (greatly narrowed), I band is reduced (narrowed) and A band remains unchanged**Q.
- **Tropomyosin protein prevents muscle contraction** by **covering the active sites of actin where myosin head binds to actin**Q and thus preventing attachment of both.
- **Calcium (Ca^{++}) binding to troponin C (not tropomyosin) initiates or triggers muscle contraction**Q.
- **During excitation-contraction coupling, ACh (acetylcholine) is released at the nerve terminal. Calcium is pumped back into the sacroplasmic reticulum during relaxation. Calcium is released from sacroplasmic reticulum during contraction**

111. A i.e. Red
112. A i.e. Contain large amounts of myoglubin; B i.e. Composed of smaller fibers
113. A i.e. Extensive sarcoplasmic reticulum; C i.e. Large glycolytic pathway
[Ref: Berne & Levy 6/e p 243-44; Guyton 12/e p 79, 1036; Ganong 24/e p 106-107]

- **Fast twitch (type II) fibers have larger (more) diameter, number, sarcoplasmic reticulum, SERCA1, glycolytic pathway & myosin ATPase activity. Type II A are red oxidative-glycolytic whereas, II B are white glycolytic.**
- **Slow twitch red glycolytic**Q **(type I)** fibers have **smaller (lesser) diameter, number, force / velocity of contraction & fatigability**; glycolysis, SR, SERCA1 and ATPase activity but their **mitochondrial content, capillary density, myoglobin (responsible for red color)** and **oxidative (aerobic) capacity are higher**.

114. B i.e. In the end *[Ref: Ganong 24/e p. 107; Guyton 12/e p. 1036]*

According to **'Size Principle' for recruitment of motor units** during muscle contraction, a general scheme followed during a specific muscle action is

(1) Initial recruitment of S (slow) muscle unit to produce **controlled contraction.** Eg. during **standing.**

↓

(2) Followed by recruitment of FR (Fast Resistant to fatigue) units, resulting in more powerful response over a short period of time. Eg during initiation of walking.

↓

(3) Lastly (in the end) FF (Fast Fatiguable) units are recruited for most demanding tasks eg **running, jumping.**

Classification of Fiber Types in Skeletal Muscles

Feature	Type I: Slow Oxidative (SO) Red	Type IIA: Fast Oxidative Glycolytic (FOG) Red	Type IIB: Fast Glycolytic (FG) White
Color	**Red** (d/t myoglobin)	**Red** (d/t myoglobin)	**White**
Speed of contraction (time to develop peak tension)	**Slow twitch**	**Fast twitch**	**Fast twitch**
Myosin ATPase activity (rate)	**Slow**	**Fast**	**Fast**
Oxidative capacity, activity of enzymes of oxidative phosphorylation, generation of aerobic energy, mitochondrial content,myoglobin, number (density) of capillaries	**High**	Very high (a/t Berne): but oxidative capacity is moderate a/t Ganong	**Low**

Glycolytic capacity & activity of glycolytic enzymes	**Moderate**	High	**High**
Fatigability	Low (slow) b/o dependence of oxidative phosphorylation	-	High (rapid) b/o dependence on glycolytic pathway
Used for	More **sustaind activity**, for **endurance** eg maintaince of posture, marathon, swimming	-	**Occasionally & for brief periods** eg jumping , sprinters
Associated motor unit type	**Slow (s)**	**Fast resistant to fatigue (FR)**	**Fast fatigable (FF)**
Number of fibers; **Fiber diameter; Force & velocity of contraction & Fatigability**	**Lesser (smaller, lower)**		**Higher (larger)**
Diffusion distance (diameter)	Moderate	Small	**Large**
Innervating nerve cell diameter & conduction velocity Excitability of nerve	Smaller (fast) High		Larger (very fast) Low
Sarcoplasmic reticulum content; Calcium pumping capacity of SR; SERCA 1 activity and Calcium reuptake into SR	**Moderate**	**High**	**High**
Relaxation time	Slower		Quicker (d/t SERCA1)
Begin to develop tension at	Lower Ca++ concentration		Higher Ca++ conc.
Low affinity Ca++ binding sites in troponin C	1		2
Deliver	Prolonged strength of contraction for minutes to hours ie **endurance**		Extreme amount of power for few seconds to a minute
Example muscles **Sports activity**	Soleus muscle Marathon, swimming		Lateral rectus > gastrocnemius Sprinter, jumping

115. B & C i.e. Dephosphorylation causes definite relaxation & LC phosphatase is essential for binding

116. D & E i.e. IP3- DAG & Ca^{2+} channel *Ref: Guyton 11th/e p. 90, 98-99; Gabriel C Ezeilo P.56-57; Ganong 23rd/e p. 110-12, 125*

- During **smooth muscle contraction** increase in cytosolic calcium is due to influx through ***voltage or ligand gated plasma membrane Ca^{++} channels***Q and release of Ca^{++} from sarcoplasmic reticulum activated by ***IP3 receptor calcium channels***Q.
- **In smooth muscles,** *length tension relationship does not exist* & and **contraction** (slow & prolonged) and **relaxation are independent of nerve supply**Q**. Myosin light chain (MLC) phosphyrylation by MLC kinase (not phosphatese) is essential**Q for its actin-binding. However **MLC dephosphorylation by MLC phosphatese** ***does not necessarily l/t relaxation***Q**. Latch bridges** are **less (attachment- detachment) cycle, less ATP requiring bridge,** which maintain prolonged contractions without much expenditure of energy.

117. A i.e. Ca^{2+} dependent; B i.e. Through calmodulin dependent kinase *[Ref: Ganong 24/e P- 56-58; Chaudhuri 5/e P-455]*

Calmodulin is a ***calcium (dependent) binding protein which acts through calmodulin dependent protein kinases***Q like Ca^{++}/ calmodulin kinase I, II, III; MLC kinase and phosphorylase kinase.

118. A i.e. Troponin (+ve) **119. D i.e. Presence of cellular calcium essential to cause muscle contraction.**

In smooth muscles troponin is not required for contractionQ**. Presence of intracellular Ca^{2+} is required for the contraction of all the three types of muscles –smooth, skeletal & cardiac**Q**.**

Excitation – Contraction Coupling

In Smooth muscle
AP causes release of stored Ca^{2+}→**Ca^{2+} binds to calmodulin**Q → activates calmodulin dependent myosin light chain kinase → phosphorylates myosin. **Phosphorylation of myosin is essential for contraction.**Q

In Cardia /Skeletal muscle
Ca^{2+} ions initiate the process of contraction by binding with troponin CQ → uncover myosin binding sites on actin → actin gets attached to myosin → contraction

★ **Sustained contraction**:- is produced **d/t latch bridge mechanism.**Q By which myosin cross bridges remains attached to actin for some time after cytoplasmic Ca^{2+} concentration falls.

Skeleton Muscles	Smooth Muscles
Contain Actin (A), Myosin (M), Tropomyosin (TM) & **troponin**	Contain A, M, Tm **but lack troponin**[Q]
RMP > (-90mv), chronaxie is longer, contraction is phasic & EPP present	**RMP < (-50 mv),** tonic sustained contraction and **EPP absent**
Automaticity (A), Rythmicity (R), & Cross striations (C) absent & has single nucleus	RAC and multiple nucleus present

120. C i.e. Increasing the amplitude of action potential in the motor neurons.

Action potential follows an all or none law. If sufficient amplitude is reached to produces a response, increasing the amplitude further will not have any effect on the function to follow.

121. B i.e. Fasciculation

Fasciculation	is visible or palpable *twitch* within a single muscle ***due to spontaneous discharge of one motor unit.***[Q] [Each single motor neuron & the muscle fibres it innervates constitute a motor unit]
Fibrillation	Fine, irregular contraction of individual fibers, they are not visible grossly.
Tremor	Rhythmic abnormal involuntary movement.
Chorea	Rapid, jerky, semipurposive irregular movement more commonly occurring in the distal part.

122. B i.e. Ca^{+2}

123. A i.e. Increased muscle metabolism by excess of Ca^{2+} ions. *[Ref: Harrison 16/e P-105,390; Goodman & Gilman's 10/e P-204]*

In malignant hyperthermia (d/t mutation in gene coding **ryanodine receptor)** increased heat production is produced **by increased muscle metabolism by uncontrolled (excess) release of Ca^{++} ions from sarcoplasmic reticulum**[Q]**.**

124. B i.e. Optimum length

Initial length	**Length at relaxed state**
Optimal length	**Length at which tension in muscle i.e. force generated by muscle is maximal**[Q]**.**

125. A i.e. 25 Hz *[Ref: Ganong 24/e p. 104]*

- **Tetany** means **continuous contraction of muscle (fibre) without latency & relaxation (i.e. no latent period & relaxation time)**[Q]**.**
- So **tetanizing frequency** (i.e. the frequency at which muscles can contract) **depends only on contraction time of muscle (i.e. twitch duration)** and not on latency period & relaxation time.
- Because twitch (contraction) duration = 40 miliseconds = 0.04 seconds
  So tetanizing frequency = 1/0.04 = **25 Hz**[Q]

Chapter: 3 RESPIRATORY SYSTEM

QUESTIONS

Transport of Gases

1. **Defference in the amount of O_2 inspired and CO_2 expired-** *(NBE P 13)*
   A. 20ml/min
   B. 50ml/min
   C. 75 ml/min
   D. 100 ml/min
2. **Largest fraction of CO_2 is present in blood as or CO_2 is primarily transported in the arterial blood as**
   A. Dissolved CO_2. *(AIIMS 03, AI 05)*
   B. Carbonic Acid.
   C. Carbamino-hemoglobin.
   D. Bicarbonate
3. **Haldane effect-** *(NBE P 13)*
   A. Effect of 2,3-BPG
   B. Dissociation of CO_2 on oxygenation
   C. Dissociation of O_2 on addition of CO_2
   D. Chloride shift
4. **Venous blood with high hematocrit is seen in-**
   A. RBC high chloride. *(NBE P 13)*
   B. Plasma high Na
   C. Plasma high HCO_3
   D. RBC high K
5. **Normal diffusion of CO_2 at rest-** *(NBE P 13)*
   A. 20-25ml/min
   B. 50-100ml/min
   C. 100-200ml/min
   D. 300-400ml/min
6. **Which of the following does not occur as the blood passes through systemic capillaries?** *(AIIMS 07)*
   A. Increased protein content
   B. Shift of Hemoglobin dissociation curve to left
   C. Increased hematocrit
   D. Decreased pH
7. **Hemoglobin unlike myoglobin shows:** *(PGI 02)*
   A. Sigmoid curve of oxygen dissociation
   B. Positive cooperativity
   C. Hills coefficient of one
   D. None of above
8. **The normal value of P_{50} on the oxyhaemoglobin dissociation curve in an adult is:** *(AIIMS 04)*
   A. 1.8 kPa
   B. 2.7 kPa
   C. 3.6 kPa
   D. 4.5 kPa
9. **One intern calculated the concentration of O_2 in blood as 0.0025 ml/ml of blood. Considering atmospheric pressure as 760mmHg, how much approx. O_2 tension could have been in the blood?** *(AI 04)*
   A. 40mmHg
   B. 60mmHg
   C. 80mmHg
   D. 100mmHg
10. **Gas used to measure diffusion in lung:**
    A. CO *(AIIMS 10)*
    B. NO
    C. CO_2
    D. Nitrogen
11. **CO_2 diffuse more easily than O_2 because:**
    A. Less dense *(AIIMS 10)*
    B. More soluble in plasma
    C. Less molecular weight of CO_2
    D. Less pCO_2 in the alveoli
12. **Carbon monoxide transfer factor is increased in:**
    A. Anaemia *(NBE P 14; AIIMS 16, 14; PGI 13,15)*
    B. L→R shunt & Polycythemia
    C. R→L shunt
    D. Pulmonary embolism
13. **Arterial blood O_2 in ml of O_2 per dL:** *(PGI 01)*
    A. 12.1
    B. 19.8
    C. 15.6
    D. 27.8
14. **The Normal value of PO_2 in healthy man is :**
    A. 45 mm Hg *(AIIMS 2K)*
    B. 110 mm Hg
    C. 80 mm Hg
    D. 60 mm Hg
15. **Amount of dissolved oxygen transported in 100 ml of plasma in a subject breathing 100% oxygen at 4 ATA (Atmospheric pressure) will be:** *(AI 12)*
    A. 9 ml
    B. 6 ml
    C. 3 ml
    D. 0.3 ml
16. **The additional amount of oxygen transported in 100 ml of blood in a subject breathing 100% oxygen under hyperbaric conditions of 4 ATA compared to normobaric conditions (1ATA) will be:** *(AI 12)*
    A. 9 ml
    B. 6 ml
    C. 3 ml
    D. 0.3 ml
17. **Percentage of O_2 carried in chemical combination**
    A. 97% *(PGI 04)*
    B. 3%
    C. 66%
    D. 33%
18. **Arterial carbon dioxide level** *(PGI 04)*
    A. 40 mm Hg
    B. 37 mm Hg

C. 45 mm Hg ☐
D. 60 mm Hg ☐
E. 42 mm Hg ☐

19. O_2 delivery to tissues depends on all/except:
A. Cardiac output *(AIIMS 07)* ☐
B. Type of fluid administered ☐
C. Hemoglobin concentration ☐
D. Affinity of hemoglobin for O_2 ☐

20. The fraction of inspired air in mouth-to-mouth respiration is: *(AI 06, NBE P 13)*
A. 0.16 ☐
B. 0.19 ☐
C. 0.21 ☐
D. 0.26 ☐

21. Mouth-to-mouth respiration provides an oxygen concentration of: *(DNB 14, AI 04)*
A. 16% ☐
B. 20% ☐
C. 22% ☐
D. 24% ☐

22. Arterial blood gas of a 5 year old child done at sea level gives the following results: pH 7.41, PaO_2 100 mmHg, and $PaCO_2$ 40 mm Hg. The child is being ventilated with 80% oxygen. What is the (A-a) PO_2 *(AIIMS 05)*
A. 570.4 mm Hg ☐
B. 520.4 mm Hg ☐
C. 470.4 mm Hg ☐
D. 420.4 mm Hg ☐

23. What is charle's law- *(NBE P 13)*
A. PV=constant ☐
B. P/T=constant ☐
C. PV=nRT ☐
D. None ☐

24. In the following graph, the curve A represents the normal relationship between Alveolar ventilation and pCO2, when pO2 is 100 mm Hg. Of pH is changed from 7.4 to 7.3, where will the original curve shift? *(AIIMS 16)*

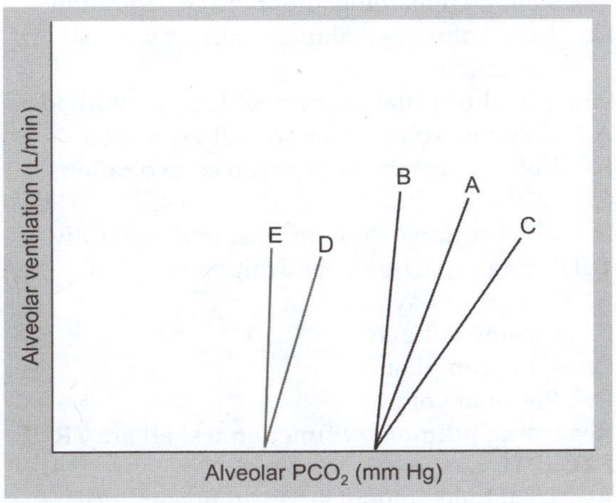

A. C ☐
B. A ☐
C. B ☐
D. D ☐

O_2 Dissociation Curve

25. The sigmoid nature of Hb-O_2 dissociation curve is because of : *(NBE P 14, 13; AI 09, AIIMS 11)*
A. Binding of one O_2 molecule increase the affinity for the next O_2 molecule. ☐
B. Alpha chain has more affinity for O_2 than beta chain ☐
C. Beta chain has more affinity for O_2 than alpha chain and Haemoglobin is acidic in nature ☐
D. Binding of one oxygen molecule decrease the affinity of binding other O_2 molecules ☐

26. Increased oxygen delivery to tissues in reponse to increased CO_2 is- *(NBE P 13)*
A. Bohr effect ☐
B. Haldane Effect ☐
C. Hamburger effect ☐
D. Chloride shift ☐

27. Bohr Effect is? *(NBE P 13)*
A. Facilitates oxygen transport ☐
B. Facilitates CO_2 transport ☐
C. Facilitates chloride transport ☐
D. None ☐

28. In anemia, the concentration of 2, 3-DPG is-
A. Decreased *(DNB 09)* ☐
B. Increased ☐
C. A or b ☐
D. Not changed ☐

29. Role of 2, 3 DPG in hemoglobin - *(AI 06)*
A. Unloading oxygen to tissues ☐
B. Increased affinity for oxygen ☐
C. Buffering capacity ☐
D. Osmotic fraglity ☐

30. An increase in the concentration of 2-3 Biphosphoglycerate (2, 3 DPG) may be seen in all of the following except. *(AI 09, NBE P 12)*
A. Anemia ☐
B. Hypoxia ☐
C. Inosine ☐
D. Hypoxanthine. ☐

31. In hyperventilation *(PGI 07)*
A. p50 and Hb affinity for O_2 increases ☐
B. p50 and Hb affinity for O_2 decreases ☐
C. p50 increases and O_2 affinity decreases ☐
D. p50 decreases and O_2 affinity increases ☐
E. no change ☐

32. Increase in P50 in oxygenation curve is due to decrease in- *(NBE P 13)*
A. PH ☐
B. Oxygen ☐
C. Temperature ☐
D. CO_2 ☐

33. Fetal hemoglobin has higher affinity for oxygen due to: *(AIIMS 09)*
A. Decreased 2, 3 DPG concentration ☐
B. Reduced pH ☐
C. Increased release of carbon dioxide ☐
D. Oxygen dissociation curve is shifted to right ☐

34. During exercise increase in O_2 delivery to muscles is because of all except : *(AI 2K, DNB 09)*
A. Oxygen dissociation curve shifts to left ☐
B. Increased stroke volume ☐
C. Increased extraction of oxygen from the blood ☐
D. Increased blood flow to muscles ☐

35. Oxygen dissociation curve shifts to right in all except:
A. Diabetic ketoacidosis *(AI 2K, DNB 11)* ☐
B. Blood transfusion ☐
C. High altitude ☐
D. Anaemia ☐

36. Which compound shifts the Oxygen dissociation curve to the right: *(NBE P 14,13; AI 04)*
A. 1, Phosphoglycerate ☐
B. 2, 3 DPG ☐
C. 1, 3 DPG ☐
D. Glyceraldehyde ☐

37. Oxygen dissociation curve shift to right in A/E:
A. Hypothermia/Fetal Hb ☐
B. Hypercarbia *(NBE P 15,14,13; PGI 14,13)* ☐
C. Anemia ☐
D. Sickle Hb ☐

38. O_2 dissociation curve is shifted to right in all except:
A. Hypercapnea / Hypercarbia ($\uparrow CO_2$) ☐
B. Rise in temperature *(AIIMS 08,14; NBE P 15,13)* ☐
C. Raised2, 3 DPG level ☐
D. Metabolic alkalosis (Decreased H^+ ion) ☐

39. The important feature of 2.3 Diposphoglycerate includes: *(AI 07)*
A. Higher concentration in adult blood ☐
B. Contribution to Bohr effect ☐
C. Increases affinity of O_2 to haemoglobin ☐
D. Associated with foetal blood to promote oxygenation. ☐

40. True about Hb dissociation curve is:
A. Acidosis shifts O_2 dissociation curve to right ☐
B. $\uparrow CO_2$ shifts the curve to left *(PGI 08,09)* ☐
C. Hypoxia shifts curve to left ☐
D. 2.3 DPG has no effect on curve ☐

41. All of the following factors influence hemoglobin dissociation curve, except: *(PGI 12, AIIMS 06)*
A. Chloride ion concentration ☐
B. CO_2 tension (pressure) ☐
C. Temperature ☐
D. 2-3 DPG levels ☐
E. Acidosis ☐

42. An increase in which of the following parameters will shift the O_2 dissociation curve to the left:
A. Temperature *(NBE P 14, AI 03)* ☐
B. Partial pressure of CO_2 ☐
C. 2,3 DPG concentration ☐
D. Oxygen affinity of hemoglobin ☐

43. Oxygen affinity is increased by all of the following *except:* *(NBE P 13, AI 05)*
A. Alkalosis ☐
B. Hypoxia ☐
C. Increased HbF ☐
D. Hypothermia ☐

44. O_2 delivery to tissue is decreased by A/E: *(NBE P 14)*
A. $\downarrow_{ed}$ Haemoglobin level *(PGI 03, 13)* ☐
B. $\downarrow_{ed}$ PaO_2 ☐
C. $\uparrow_{ed}$ pH. ☐
D. $\uparrow_{ed}$ HCO_3 & $\uparrow_{ed}$ Pa CO_2 ☐

45. The factor responsible for the left shift of Hb-O_2 dissociation curve is: *(AIIMS 14,15, 09)*
A. Increase in 2,3 DPG in RBC ☐
B. Fall in temperature ☐
C. Fall in pH ☐
D. Increase level of CO_2 in blood ☐

46. Which of the following statement (s) is /are true about Hb-O_2 dissociation curve: *(NBE P 15,13,14,13; PGI 12,08)*
A. Fetal Hb & hypothermia Shifts curve to Left ☐
B. Hyperthermia shifts curve to Left ☐
C. Hypercarbia shifts curve to Left ☐
D. Left shift cause more O2 release to tissue ☐

Lung Volume & Capacities

47. Tidal volume is calculated by: *(AI 06)*
A. Inspiratory capacity minus the inspiratory reserve volume ☐
B. Total lung capacity minus the reserve volume ☐
C. Functional residual capacity minus residual volume ☐
D. Vital capacity minus expiratory reserve volumes ☐

48. Volume of air taken in and given out during normal respiration is referred to as:
A. IRV *(NBE P 15, 13; PGI 02, 14, 13)* ☐
B. TV ☐
C. ERV ☐
D. VC ☐

49. Functional residual capacity is: *(AIIMS 03)*
A. Volume remaining after forced expiration ☐
B. Tidal volume + volume inspired forcefully ☐
C. Volume remaining after normal expiration ☐
D. Tidal volume + volume expired by forced expiration. ☐

50. Functional residual capacity of lung is defined as:
A. Volume expired after normal expiration ☐
B. Volume remaining after forced expiration ☐
C. ERV + RV *(PGI 07)* ☐
D. Tidal volume + volume inspired forcefully ☐

51. Total lung capacity depends upon : *(AI 08)*
A. Size of airway ☐
B. Closing volume ☐
C. Lung compliance ☐
D. Residual volume ☐

52. Regarding pulmonary function test all are TRUE, EXCEPT: *(AIIMS 09)*
A. Total lung volume increases in emphysema ☐
B. Compliance decreases in interstitial lung disease. ☐
C. Compliance is total lung distensibility ☐
D. FEV1 is forced expiratory rate at one minute ☐

53. Which of the following is used to measure the resistance to small airways OR Best denotes airway resistance *(NBE P 15,13; AIIMS 15,07)*
- A. Vital capacity ☐
- B. FEV_1 ☐
- C. Max. mid respiratory flow rates. ☐
- D. Closing volume ☐

54. Respiratory minute volume of lung is- *(NBE P 13)*
- A. 6L ☐
- B. 4L ☐
- C. 500mL ☐
- D. 125L ☐

55. Total alveolar ventilation volume (in L/min) is:
- A. 1.5 *(AI 10, NBE P 13)* ☐
- B. 3.5 ☐
- C. 4.2 ☐
- D. 5.0 ☐

56. Calculate the Alveolar ventillation per minute of a patient with respiratory rate 14/min, tidal vol. 500 ml with a vital capacity 7000 ml : *(AIIMS 01)*
- A. 4900 ml ☐
- B. 2000 ml ☐
- C. 7700 ml ☐
- D. 7000 ml ☐

57. In normal adult Vd/Vt ratio is: *(PGI 13, NBE P 13)*
- A. 20 ☐
- B. 0.35 ☐
- C. 40 ☐
- D. 50 ☐

58. Critical Closing volume is *(AIIMS 12)*
- A. Volume at the end of forceful expiration ☐
- B. Volume at the end of forceful inspiration ☐
- C. Volume remaining after Functional Residual Capacity is measured ☐
- D. Close to Residual Volume ☐

59. True about Hyaline membrane disease: *(AIIMS 10, NBE P 13)*
- A. FRC above the closing volume ☐
- B. FRC below the closing volume ☐
- C. FRC is equal to closing volume ☐
- D. FRC doesn't depend on closing volume ☐

60. Pulmonary function abnormalities in interstitial lung diseases include all of the following except:
- A. Reduced vital capacity *(AIIMS 05)* ☐
- B. Reduced FEV1/FVC ratio ☐
- C. Reduced diffusion capacity ☐
- D. Reduced total lung capacity ☐

61. Set of data which correctly defines restrictive lung disease is: *(AI 08, NBE P 13)*
- A. ↑FRC,↑ compliance of lung tissue ☐
- B. ↑FEV_1/FVC, ↓compliance of lung tissue ☐
- C. ↓FEV_1/FVC, ↓compliance of lung tissue ☐
- D. ↑TLC, RV is ↓ ☐

62. In upper air way obstruction all of the following changes are seen except : *(AI 09)*
- A. Decreased Maximum breathing capacity ☐
- B. RV decreased ☐
- C. Decreased FEV ☐
- D. Decreased vital capacity ☐

63. Pulmonary function changes seen in Emphysema are
- A. ↑TLC *(AI 06)* ☐
- B. ↓RV ☐
- C. ↑FEV_1 ☐
- D. ↑VC ☐

64. A person is having normal lung compliance and increased airway resistance. The most economical way of breathing for him: *(AIIMS 02)*
- A. Rapid & deep ☐
- B. Rapid & shallow ☐
- C. Slow & deep ☐
- D. Slow & sallow ☐

Test for Pulmonary Compliance

65. In body Plethysmography, a person is asked to expire against a closed glottis. Whiat will be the change in the pressure in the lung and the box *(AI 11)*
- A. Increase in both ☐
- B. Decrease in both ☐
- C. Increase in lung decrease in box ☐
- D. Decrease in lung increase in box ☐

66. Vital capacity is sum of- *(NBE P 13)*
- A. Inspiratory reserve volme, Tidal volume and Expiratory reserve volume ☐
- B. Tidal volume, Inspiratory reserve volume and Residual volume ☐
- C. Expiratory rerve volume, Inspiratory reserve volume and Residual volume ☐
- D. Residual volume, Inspiratory volume, and Expiratory volume. ☐

67. Spirometry measure (s): *(PGI 12)*
- A. Tidal volume ☐
- B. TLC ☐
- C. ERV ☐
- D. FRC ☐
- E. IRV ☐

68. Spirometry can demonstrate and measure all of the following except: *(NBE P 15,14,13; AI 10,03; AIIMS 15)*
- A. Tidal volume ☐
- B. Residual volume ☐
- C. Vital capacity ☐
- D. Inspiratory reserve capacity ☐

69. Routine spirometry can't estimate : *(PGI 08, 04)*
- A. FRC ☐
- B. VC ☐
- C. RV ☐
- D. ERV ☐
- E. FEV_1 ☐

70. Nitrogen washout method is used for estimating:
- A. Dead space volume *(PGI 04)* ☐
- B. Functional residual capacity ☐
- C. Tidal volume ☐
- D. Diffusion capacity ☐

71. Measurement of anatomic dead space is by- *(NBE P 13)*
A. O_2 breath test ☐
B. Helium dilution test ☐
C. N_2 breath test ☐
D. PCO_2 ☐

72. Regarding Dead space Volume in a normal individual- *(NBE P 13)*
A. Anatomical dead space>Physiological Dead space ☐
B. Anatomical dead space=Physiological Dead space ☐
C. Anatomical dead space>Physiological Dead space ☐
D. Anatomical dead space is not related to Physiological Dead space ☐

73. Which of the following methods is used for calculation of anatomical dead space? *(AIIMS 15)*
A. Xenon dilution technique ☐
B. Bohler's method ☐
C. Spirometry ☐
D. Single breath nitrogen test ☐

74. Examine the shape of the flow volume curve carefully. This flow volume loop indicates one of the following: *(AIIMS 04)*

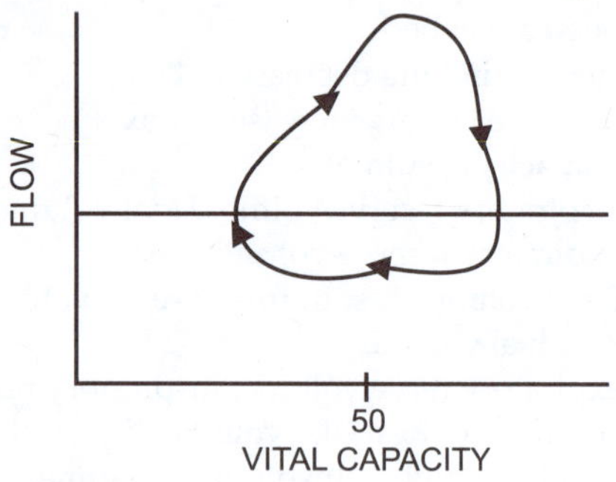

FLOW
50
VITAL CAPACITY

A. Normal ☐
B. Extrathoracic obstruction ☐
C. Intrathoracic obstruction ☐
D. Fixed large airway obstruction ☐

75. The given graph likely depicts which of the following disease? *(AIIMS 15)*
A. Bronchial asthma ☐
B. Emphysema ☐
C. Interstitial lung disease ☐
D. Normal study ☐

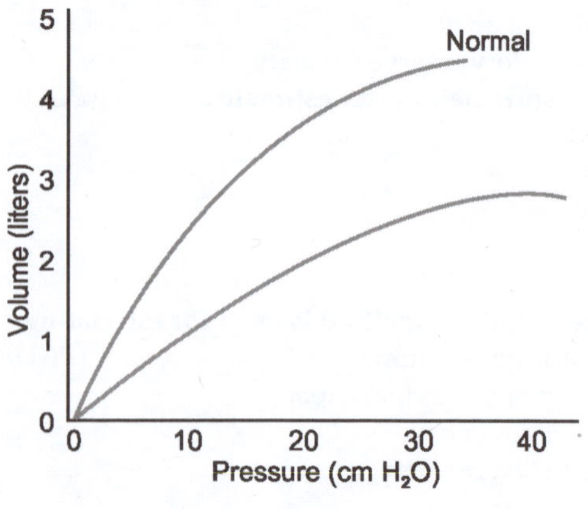

Normal
Volume (liters)
0 1 2 3 4 5
0 10 20 30 40
Pressure (cm H_2O)

Pressure During Breathing Cycle

76. Intrapleural pressure is- *(NBE P 13)*
A. Transpulmonary pressure+Alveolar pressure ☐
B. Transpulmonary pressure –Alveolar pressure ☐
C. Transmural pressure+Alveolar pressure ☐
D. Alveolar pressure-Transpulmonary pressure ☐

77. True about inspiration; the intrapleural pressure becomes: *(PGI 06)*
A. More – ve ☐
B. More +ve ☐
C. Same ☐
D. Initially positive, then negative ☐
E. No relation ☐

78. The intrapleural pressure is negative both during inspiration and expiration because: *(AIIMS 05)*
A. Intrapulmonary pressure is always negative ☐
B. Thoracic cage and lungs are elastic structure ☐
C. Transpulmonary pressure determines the negativity ☐
D. Surfactant prevents the lungs to collapse ☐

79. Normal Intrapleural Pressure is Negative because
A. The chestwall and lungs recoil in opposite directions *(AI 12)* ☐
B. The surfactant prevents pulmonary collapse ☐
C. Intrapulmonary Pressure is Negative ☐
D. Tranplmonary Pressure is Negative ☐

80. Negative Intrapleural pressure is maintained by: *(AIIMS 10; AI 12)*
A. Uniform distribution of surfactant over alveoli ☐
B. Cartilaginous rings in large airways ☐
C. Lymphatic drainage of pleural cavity ☐
D. Negative intraveolar pressure ☐

81. Increased airway resistance is/are caused by *(PGI 11)*
A. Forced expiration ☐
B. Dense air ☐
C. Low lung volume ☐
D. High lung volume ☐

82. More resistance in expiration is due to: *(AIIMS 03)*
A. Increased compression of airway ☐
B. Due to change from linear to turbulent flow ☐
C. Saturation with moisture ☐
D. Increased rate of flow during expiration ☐

83. Respiration stops in the last stage of expiration, in forced expiration b/c of: *(AIIMS 08)*
A. Respiratory muscle fatigue ☐
B. Collapse of alveoli ☐
C. Dynamic compression of airways ☐
D. Breaking effect of inspiratory muscles ☐

Expiration

84. True about normal expiration *(PGI 10)*
A. At the end of normal expiration air in lung is ERV ☐
B. At the end of normal expiration air in lung is ERV ☐
C. In expiration pleural pressure is equal to alveolar pressure ☐
D. Muscles that elevate the chest cage are classified as muscles of expiration ☐

Work Load of Breathing

85. Effort during normal respiration is done due to -
A. Lung elasticity (DNB 04, Delhi 13) ☐
B. Respiratory air passages ☐
C. Alveolar air spaces ☐
D. Creating negative pleural pressure ☐

86. Which of the following adaptations will be apt to increase the work capacity at high altitude: *(AI 07)*
A. Increasing workload, decreasing duration of exercise ☐
B. Increasing workload, increasing duration of exercise ☐
C. Decreasing workload, increasing duration of exercise ☐
D. Decreasing workload, decreasing duration of exercise ☐

87. When gases flow through an orifice which factor to least likely to effect turbulence- *(NBE P 13)*
A. Density of gas ☐
B. Viscosity of gas ☐
C. Pressure of gas ☐
D. Diameter of orifice ☐

Compliance

88. Specific lung compliance is decreased in all except
A. Pulmonary congestion *(AIIMS 15, AI 11)* ☐
B. Chronic bronchitis ☐
C. Pulmonary fibrosis ☐
D. Decreased surfactant ☐

89. Compliance of lung is measured by- *(NBE P 14,13)*
A. Elasticity ☐
B. Amount of air ☐
C. Blood flow ☐
D. Presence if fluid ☐

90. Compliance of lungs is- *(AIIMS 14; NBE P 13)*
A. 200ml/cm water ☐
B. 500ml/cm water ☐
C. 800 ml/cm water ☐
D. 1000 ml/cm water ☐

Ventilation & Perfusion

91. High Oxygen tension in alveoli is due to:
A. Right to left shunt *(AIIMS 04)* ☐
B. Ventilation perfusion mismatch ☐
C. Bronchial Asthma ☐
D. Inappropriate gas exchange ☐

92. PO_2 is maximum- *(NBE P 15,14,13)*
A. Base of lung ☐
B. Posterior lobe ☐
C. Apex of lung ☐
D. Middle lobe ☐

93. Ventilation perfusion ratio is maximum at :
A. Apex of lung *(NBE P 15,14; AI 10)* ☐
B. Base of lung ☐
C. Posterior lobe of lung ☐
D. Middle of the lung ☐

94. Ventilation perfusion ratio is least at- *(NBE P 15,13)*
A. Apex ☐
B. Middle lob ☐
C. Base ☐
D. None ☐

95. True statement regarding Pulmonary ventilation is
A. PaO_2 is maximum at the apex. *(AI 04)* ☐
B. V/Q is maximum at the base. ☐
C. Ventilation per unit lung volume is maximum at the apex ☐
D. Blood circulation is minimum at the base. ☐

96. Not a stimulus for pulmonary vasoconstriction:
A. Hypoxemia *(NBE P 15,13; AIIMS 04, 15)* ☐
B. Hypercapnia (Hypercarbia) ☐
C. PGI_2 ☐
D. Thromboxane A_2 ☐

Hypoxia

97. All of the following cause Hyperventilation *except:*
A. Decreased pH in CSF *(DNB 10)* ☐
B. Decreased plasma HCO_3 ☐
C. CO poisoning ☐
D. Increased adrenergic levels ☐

98. Arterial blood gas analysis in Carbon monoxide poisoning shows: *(AIIMS 07)*
A. PO_2 less, O_2 saturation normal ☐
B. PO_2 normal, O_2 saturation less with normal or slightly decreased PCO_2 ☐
C. PO_2 less, O_2 saturation normal ☐
D. PO_2 less, O_2 saturation decreased ☐

99. Which of the following variants of hypoxia does not stimulate peripheral chemoreceptors OR Oxygen therapy is least useful in: *(NBE P 15,14,13; AI 07)*
A. Hypoxic hypoxia *(AIIMS 14)* ☐
B. Anaemic hypoxia ☐
C. Stagnant hypoxia ☐
D. Histotoxic hypoxia ☐

100. Anemic hypoxia is due to : *(AI 06)*
A. $\downarrow PO_2$ in arterial blood ☐
B. $\uparrow PO_2$ in arterial blood ☐
C. $\uparrow PCO_2$ in arterial blood ☐
D. $\downarrow O_2$ content in arterial blood ☐

101. Which is the best parameter for analysis of Hypoxic hypoxia: *(AI 04)*
A. Arterial PO_2 ☐
B. Arterial PCO_2 ☐
C. Venous PO_2 ☐
D. A-V Difference ☐

102. Which of the following conditions leads to tissue hypoxia without alteration of oxygen content of blood? *(AIIMS 05)*
A. CO poisoning ☐
B. Met Hb ☐
C. Cyanide poisoning ☐
D. Respiratory acidosis ☐

103. Which combination of the following statements is correct with reference to hypoxia: *(AIIMS 04)*
a) When it is severe, causes stimulation of the sympathetic nervous system
b) It leads to the accumulation of hydrogen and lactate ions
c) It causes decrease in cerebral blood flow
d) If it is chronic, causes rightward shift of oxygen Hb curve
A. All of the above statements are correct
B. b & c
C. a,b & d
D. b,c & d

104. Tachycardia is caused by hypoxia due to:
A. Reflexly through peripheral chemoreceptors
B. Diffuse vasodilatation *(AIIMS 08)*
C. Through central chemoreceptor
D. Secondarily after by hyperventilation

105. The neurons may get irreversibly damaged if exposed to significant hypoxia for : *(AIIMS 02)*
A. 8 min
B. 2 min
C. 30 sec
D. 15 sec

106. Which of the following is most prone to hypoxic injury *(PGI 04)*
A. Thalamus
B. Hippocampus
C. Caudate nucleus
D. Cerebellum

107. Hypoxemia does not depend on:
A. $PaCO_2$ *(AIIMS 10)*
B. Altitude
C. Hb
D. FiO_2

Cyanosis

108. Condition where severe hypoxaemia occurs without cyanosis *(PGI 13,15; NBE P 15,13)*
A. CO poisoning & Anemia
B. High altitude
C. Interstitial lung disease
D. Pulmonary A. V. malformation

109. Cyanosis does not occur in severe anemia because:
A. Hypoxia stimulates erythropoietin production
B. Oxygen carrying capacity of available Hb is increased *(AI 09)*
C. Critical concentration of Hb required to produce cyanosis is reduced
D. Oxygen Hemoglobin curve shift to the right

110. Central cyanosis is seen if: *(PGI 01)*
A. Methemoglobin 0.5 gm/dl
B. O_2 saturation < 85%
C. O_2 saturation < 94%
D. Hb – 4 gm%

111. Central cyanosis not occurs when total Hb and reduced Hb level is respectively (in gm%): *(PGI 12)*
A. 10.9 & 4.1
B. 10.9 & 5.1
C. 10.9 & 6.1
D. 8.9 & 4.1
E. 8.9 & 6.1

112. Cyanosis in trauma is interpreted as:
A. Early sign of hypoxia *(AIIMS 10)*
B. Late sign of Hypoxia
C. Absence of cyanosis indicates adequate airway / ventilation
D. Absence of cyanosis indicates good tissue oxygenation

113. Concentration of methemoglobin to appears cyanosis
A. 5 gm/dl *(PGI 07)*
B. 2 gm/dl
C. 1.5 gm/dl
D. 12 gm/dl

114. Cause of methaemoglobinemia are all except :
A. Nitrites *(NBE P 13)*
B. Phenacetin
C. Sulfonamide
D. Phenytoin

115. Antidote for sodium nitrate poisoning is : *(NBE P 13)*
A. Methylene blue IV
B. Egg albumin
C. EDTA
D. Animal charcoal

116. Apnoea is defined as: *(PGI 03)*
A. Stoppage of heart beat
B. Cessation of respiration
C. Irregular respiration
D. RR

117. In which of the following a reduction in arterial oxygen tension occurs? *(AI 05)*
A. Anaemia.
B. CO poisoning.
C. Moderate exercise.
D. Hypoventilation.

CO, O_2 and CO_2 Toxicity

118. Which of the following statements about Carbon Monoxide poisoning is not true: *(AI 12)*
A. Carboxy haemoglobin (COHb) causes left shift of oxyhaemoglobin dissociation curve
B. Partial pressuresas low as 0.6 mm Hg can be lethal
C. Tissue toxicity plays an important role in clinical CO poisoning
D. Hyperbaric oxygen is used for treatment

119. Regarding carbon monoxide toxicity true are A/E
A. Cytochrome toxicity is lethal *(PGI 08)*
B. Treated by 5% CO_2
C. PO_2 is decreased
D. Shift HbO_2 dissociation cure to left
E. Gaseous vasodilator

120. Transport of Carbon monoxide (CO) is diffusion limited because: *(AIIMS 09)*
A. High affinity of CO for haemoglobin

B. Alveolar membrane is less permeable to CO ☐
C. CO crosses epithelial barrier slowly ☐
D. On exposure to air there is sudden increase in partial pressure ☐

121. Carbon monoxide poisoning is a type of- *(NBE P 13)*
A. Anemic hypoxia ☐
B. Histotoxic hypoxia ☐
C. Hypoxic hypoxia ☐
D. Stagnant hypoxia ☐

122. Hyperbaric oxygen is dangerous because it:
A. Decreases displacement of O_2 from kHb ☐
B. Decreases respiratory drive *(PGI 04)* ☐
C. Enzyme damage (☐
D. Is toxic to tissures ☐

123. Toxic effects of high oxygen tension include all of the following except: *(AI 07)*
A. Pulmonary edema ☐
B. Decreased cerebral blood flow ☐
C. Retinal damage ☐
D. CNS excitation and convulsion ☐

Smoking

124. Physiological response to smoking, are all, except:
A. Decreased HDL *(AIIMS 09)* ☐
B. Increased hematocrit ☐
C. Increased heart rate and increased catecholamine release ☐
D. Decreased carboxyhemoglobin ☐

Respiratory Failure

125. The gradient of alveolar arterial oxygen tension increases in A/E: *(AIIMS 08)*
A. Diffusion defect ☐
B. Right – Left shunt ☐
C. Hypoventilation ☐
D. Ventilation perfusion abnormality ☐

126. Alveolar hypoventilation is present in A/E:
A. Bulber poliomyelitis *(AIIMS 05)* ☐
B. COPD ☐
C. Kyphoscoliosis ☐
D. Lobar pneumonia ☐

127. CO_2 retention is seen in A/E: *(PGI 10, 01)*
A. Carbon monoxide poisoning/ High altitude ☐
B. Respiratory / Ventilatory failure ☐
C. Pulmonary edema ☐
D. Drowning ☐

128. Hypercarbia is characterized by: *(AIIMS 01)*
A. Miosis ☐
B. Cool extremities ☐
C. Bradycardia ☐
D. Hypertension ☐

Regulation Of Breathing

129. Pacemaker of respiration OR Spontaneous rhythmic respiration initiated in? *(AIIMS 10,14, 15)*
A. Dorsal nuclear group ☐
B. Apneustic centre ☐
C. Pnemotaxic centre ☐
D. Pre Botzinger complex ☐

130. If a cat apneustic center is destroyed along with cutting of vagi. Which of the following statement is correct regarding the breathing pattern seen in cat?
A. Prolonged inspiratory spasm *(PGI 05)* ☐
B. Prolonged expiratory spasm ☐
C. Slow and shallow respiration ☐
D. Animal will die ☐

131. Inspiratory depth is halted by- *(NBE P 13)*
A. Pneumotaxic centre ☐
B. Apneustic centre ☐
C. Inspiratory centre ☐
D. Expiratory centre ☐

132. Transection at mid pons level results in?
A. Hyperventilation *(AIIMS 09)* ☐
B. Apneusis ☐
C. Rapid and shallow breathing ☐
D. Hypoxia ☐

133. What will be the effect on respiration if a transmission is made between the pons & medulla
A. Apnoea *(AIIMS 04)* ☐
B. Irregular & gasping ☐
C. No effect ☐
D. Slow & deep ☐

134. CO_2 increases ventilation by acting mainly on receptors of- *(NBE P 13)*
A. Apneustic center ☐
B. Pneumotaxic center ☐
C. Ventral surface of medulla ☐
D. DRG ☐

135. True regarding respiratory center is *(AIIMS 03)*
A. Directly stimulated by fall in PaO_2 ☐
B. Inhibited during swallowing ☐
C. Connected with cardiac center ☐
D. Situated in midbrain ☐

136. Central Chemoreceptors are mot sensitive to following changes in blood: *(AI 09)*
A. $\uparrow PCO_2$ ☐
B. $\downarrow PCO_2$ ☐
C. $\uparrow H^+$ ☐
D. $\uparrow PO_2$ ☐

137. The primary direct stimulus for excitation of central chemoreceptors regulating ventilation is:
A. $\uparrow H^+$ *(AIIMS 11, AI 09)* ☐
B. $\uparrow CO_2$ ☐
C. $\uparrow O_2$ ☐
D. $\downarrow CO_2$ ☐

138. Most important stimulus to peripheral chemoreceptrs
A. PO_2 *(NBE P 13)* ☐
B. CO_2 ☐
C. pH ☐
D. HCO_3 ☐

139. Peripheral & central chemoreceptors may both contribute to increased ventilation that occurs as a result of decreased- *(NBE P 13)*
A. Arterial BP ☐
B. Arterial tension ☐
C. Arterial O_2 concentration ☐
D. H^+ ☐

140. Which of the following does NOT stimulate peripheral chemoreceptors: *(NBE P 15, 13; AI 05)*
A. Hypoxia
B. Hypocapnia
C. Acidosis
D. Low perfusion pressure

141. Administration of pure O_2 to hypoxic patients is dangerous because: *(PGI 09)*
A. Apnea occurs due to hypostimulation of peripheral chemoreceptors
B. Pulmonary edema
C. DPG
D. Convulsions

142. Tidal volume excessive load is prevented by activation of which of the following receptors:
A. J receptor *(AIIMS 11)*
B. Thoracic muscle spindle
C. Bronchial stretch receptors
D. Arterial baroreceptor

143. Herring Breuer reflex is an increase in- *(NBE P 13)*
A. Duration of inspiration
B. Duration of expiration
C. Depth of inspiration
D. Depth of expiration

144. "Inflation of lungs induces further inflation" is explained by:
A. Hering-Breuer inflation reflex *(AIIMS 03)*
B. Hering-Breuer deflation reflex
C. Head's paradoxical reflex
D. J-reflex

145. All of the following affect resting ventilation except
A. Stretch receptors *(AIIMS 10)*
B. J receptor
C. Oxygen
D. PCO_2

Surfactant

146. Surfactant production in lungs starts at:
A. 28 weeks *(AI 04,NBE P 14,13)*
B. 32 wks
C. 34 wks
D. 36 wks

147. Surfactant is produced by : *(NBE P 14,13; AI 04)*
A. Type II pneumocytes
B. Type I pneumocytes
C. Macrophages
D. Endothelial cells

148. Surfacant is made up of OR In human body, the action of surfactant is done by: *(NBE P 15; AIMS 13,06)*
A. Fibrin
B. Mucoprotein
C. Phospholipids & Proteins
D. Fibrinogen

149. Main part of surfactant is formed by- *(NBE P 15)*
A. Dipalmitoyl phosphatidyl choline
B. Phosphotidyl-inositol
C. Dipalmitoyl cephaline
D. Dipalmitoyl serine

150. Pulmonary surfactant *(PGI 08)*
A. Secreted from 26th weeks of gestation & maintain minimum alveolar integrity
B. In Hyaline membrane disease deficiency occurs
C. Theraputic application seen
D. Abundant secretion in bronchoalveolar carcinoma
E. It is mucin & secreted by pneumocyte 1

151. Stability of alveoli is maintained by?
A. Lung compliance *(AIIMS 09)*
B. Negative intrapleural pressure
C. Increase in alveolar surface area by the surfactant
D. Residual air in alveoli

152. Correct about action of surfactant? *(AIIMS 07)*
A. Binds O_2
B. Lubricates CO_2 flow
C. Make capillary surface hydrophilic
D. Breaks structure of water in alveoli

153. Alveoli are kept dry because of- *(NBE P 13)*
A. Surfactants
B. Glycoproteins
C. Buffers
D. Bohr's Effect

154. Hyaline membrane contains: *(NEET 12, AI 04)*
A. Albumin
B. Fibrin
C. Globulin
D. WBCs

Non Respiratory Functions of Lung

155. Which of the following is the best-known metabolic function of the lung: *(AIIMS 04)*
A. Inactivation of serotonin
B. Conversion of angiotensin-I to angiotensin-II
C. Inactivation of bradykinin
D. Metabolism of basic drugs by cytochrome P-450 system

156. An important non-respiratory function of Lungs:
A. Anion balance *(AI 10)*
B. Sodium balance
C. Potassium balance
D. Calcium balance

157. Which of the following is true for the pulmonary neuroendocrine cells? *(AIIMS 13)*
A. Contain catecholamines
B. Contain serotonin
C. Have only cholinergic nerve supply
D. Respond to a decrease in PO_2

158. True is all except about Acid-Base disorder
A. pH determined by P_{CO2} and HCO_3^- *(AIIMS 10)*
B. Respiratory acidosis is compensated by $\downarrow HCO_3^-$
C. Metabolic acidosis is compensated by $\downarrow P_{CO2}$
D. Buffering may be intra & extra cellular

159. Uncompensated metabolic acidosis shows- *(NBE P 13)*
A. Increased pH with increased HCO_3- ☐
B. Increased pH with Decreased HCO_3- ☐
C. Decreased pH with increased HCO_3- ☐
D. Decreased pH with Decreased HCO_3- ☐

High Altitude

160. During acclimatization to high altitude all of the following take place except: *(AI 04)*
A. Increase in minute ventilation ☐
B. Increase in the sensitivity of central chemoreceptors ☐
C. Increase in the sensitivity of carotid body to hypoxia ☐
D. Shift in the oxygen dissociation curve to the left ☐

161. A person goes to the mountains. When he reaches about 5000 ft. he develops dyspnea. Which of following correctly explains for the symptoms:
A. CNS depression *(AIIMS 2K)* ☐
B. CO_2 wash out. ☐
C. Increased work of breathing ☐
D. Increased blood flow to the pulmonary tissues ☐

162. A mountaineer ascents 18,000 feet in 2 days without supplemental oxygen. At the height of ascent the changes are: *(PGI 03)*
A. $\uparrow_{ed}$ Pa CO_2 ☐
B. $\downarrow_{ed}$ Barometric pressure ☐
C. $\downarrow_{ed}$ inspired O_2 ☐
D. $\downarrow_{ed}$ PaO_2 ☐
E. $\uparrow_{ed}$ PH ☐

163. Which of the following is seen in high attitude climbers:
A. Hyperventilation *(PGI 01)* ☐
B. Decreased $PaCO_2$ ☐
C. Pulmonary edema ☐
D. Hypertension ☐
E. Bradycardia ☐

164. A person unacclimatised develops pulmonary edema-
A. 19-21 days *(NBE P 13)* ☐
B. 2nd-3rd month ☐
C. 2-3 days ☐
D. 6-7 days ☐

165. In high altitude mountain sickness, feature of pulmonary edema is: *(PGI 06)*
A. Decreased pulmonary capillary permeability ☐
B. Increased pulmonary capillary pressure ☐
C. Normal left atrial pressure ☐
D. Increases left ventricular back pressure ☐

166. Compensating mechanisms involved in acclimatization to altitude : *(PGI 04)*
A. Hyperventilation ☐
B. Hypoventilation ☐
C. Respiratory depression ☐
D. Respiratory acidosis ☐
E. Respiratory alkalosis ☐

Decompression Sickness

167. In caissons disease pain in joint is because of-
A. Nitrogen bubble *(NBE P 14, 13)* ☐
B. Oxygen bubble ☐
C. Carbon monoxide ☐
D. Air in joint ☐

168. Caisson's disease *(NBE P 14,13; AIIMS 13)*
A. Gas embolism d/t N2 release from tissue ☐
B. Amniotic fluid embolism ☐
C. Tumor embolism ☐
D. Air embolism d/t CO_2 release from tissue. ☐

169. Decompression sickness is seen in: *(PGI 02)*
A. Diver ☐
B. Pilot ☐
C. Diver and pilot ☐
D. Diver, pilot and mountaineer ☐
E. Diver, pilot, mountaineer and astronauts ☐

170. Nitrogen narcosis is caused due to: *(AIIMS 11, 08)*
A. Nitrogen inhibits dismutase enzyme ☐
B. Increase production of nitrous oxide ☐
C. Increased solubility of nitrogen in nerve cell membrane ☐
D. Decrease in oxygen free radicals ☐

ANSWERS & EXPLANATIONS:

Transport of Gases

1. **B i.e. 50ml/min**

Amount of O_2 enters the body/min = *250 ml/min*Q. Amount of CO_2 excreted by lung/min = ***200 ml/min*Q *(288 L/day)*Q.So difference in amount of O_2 inspired & CO_2 expired is 50ml/minQ**. CO_2 is 20 times more soluble than O_2.

2. **D i.e. Bicarbonate** *[Ref: Ganong 24/e P-644-46; Sembulingum 3/e P-577,582; Chaudhuri5/e P-139]*
3. **B i.e. Dissociation of CO_2 on oxygenation**
4. **A i.e. RBC high chloride**

Transport of CO_2 in the form of bicarbonate ions accounts for approximately 70% of transported carbon dioxide from the tissues to lungs Q. So CO_2 is transported as plasma HCO_3^- > RBC>HCO_3^- >Carbamino compound > dissolved CO_2 Q

Transport of Carbon Dioxide

Carbon dioxide is transported in the blood as: *HCO_3^- (70%) > carbamino compounds (23%) > dissolved CO_2 (7%)*

Fate of CO_2 in Blood

In Plasma
- Dissolved
- Carbamino compound with plasma protein
- Hydration, H^+ buffered, HCO_3^- in plasma

In Red Blood Cells
- Dissolved
- Carbamino–Hb
- Hydration, H^+ buffered, 70% of HCO_3^- enters the plasma
- Cl^- shifts into Cells, mosm in cell increases

Haldane Effect/CDH (Christian, Douglas, Haldane) Effect

If the Hb is oxygenated, the CO_2 dissociation curve shifts to the right, that is, the blood begins to lose some CO_2 as it becomes oxygenated ***(Deoxygenated Hb binds more H^+ than oxyhemoglobin*Q**, binding of O_2 to Hb reduces its affinity for CO_2)

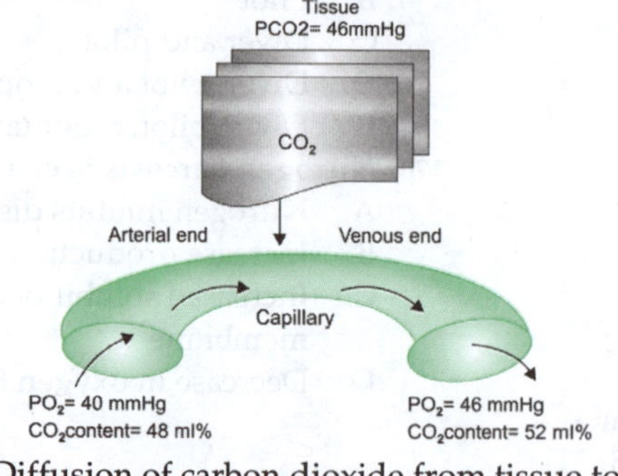

Diffusion of carbon dioxide from tissue to capillary

Chloride Shift/ Hamburger Phenomenon

- When the negatively charged (HCO_3^-) bicarbonate ions move out of red blood cell into the plasma, to maintain the electrolytic equilibrium the negatively charged chloride ions move into the Red blood Cells from plasma (In plasma plenty of sodium chloride is present).
- This process is mediated by *band 3 membrane protein*
- **Chloride shift occurs in: 1 secondQ**
- **Hematocrit of venous blood is: greater (by 3%)than that of arterial bloodQ**
- **PH of venous blood (7.36) is lower than that of arterial blood (7.40)Q**

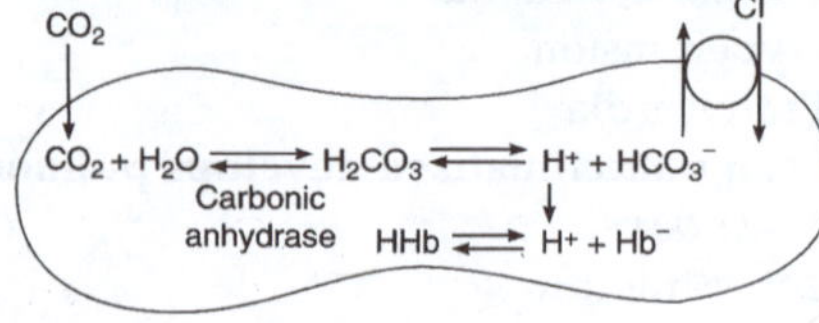

★ **For each CO_2 molecule added to RBC there is increase in one osmotically active particle in cell either HCO_3^- or Cl^-.** So RBC take up water & swell. For this reason plus a fact that some arterial fluid returns via lymphatics rather than the veins, the **hematocrit of venous blood is 3% greater than arterial bloodQ.**

5. **D i.e. 300-400ml/min**

- The normal diffusing capacity (D_L) for O_2 is about **25ml/min/mmHg**; and it increases to 2 to 3 times during exercise because of **recruitment and distension of pulmonary capillaries**. To convert D_{LCO} to D_{LO2}, the value obtained is multiplied by **1.23.**
- Both O_2 & CO_2 are highly soluble in lipids, therefore membrane barrier offers no hindrance to their diffusion; instead the **limitation is their diffusion through tissue water (plasma). CO_2 is 20 times more soluble in water than O_2** (Solubility of CO_2/O_2 in water=0.06/0.003= 20).
- This explains the fact **that although CO_2 has higher (but not very different) molecular weight than O_2, it diffuses nearly 20 times more rapidly across the alveolar capillary barrier than O_2Q**. So diffusion capacity of **~400-500 ml/minQ**.

6. **B i.e. Shift of hemoglobin dissociation curve to left** *[Ref: Ganong 24/e p. 641-47; Guyton 11/e p. 189, 508]*

In **systemic capillaries,** ***O_2 is released (i.e., O_2 dissociation curve shifted to right) and CO_2 is acquired***[Q] (CO_2 dissociation curve shifted to left). In systemic capillaries, there is **decrease** in ***pH***[Q] and **increase** in ***hematocrit, protein content, H+, Cl⁻, & HCO_3^- ion concentration***[Q].

7. **A i.e. Sigmoid curve of oxygen dissociation & B i.e. Positive co-operativity** *[Ref: Ganong 24/e 644; Sembulingum 3/581-82]*

Hemoglobin (unlike myoglobin) *shows* ***sigmoid curve of O_2 dissociation and positive co-operative binding***[Q].

Unlike Myoglobin, Hemoglobin shows:

- Tetrameric structure
- ***Can bind four O_2 molecule***[Q]
- ***Sigmoid saturation kinetics***[Q]
- **Co-operativity or co-operative binding kinetics:** property that permits it to bind a maximal quantity of O_2 at respiratory organs & to deliver a maximal quantity of O_2 at peripheral tissue. Here binding of Hb with O_2 facilitates binding of other O_2 molecules thus positive co-operativity.

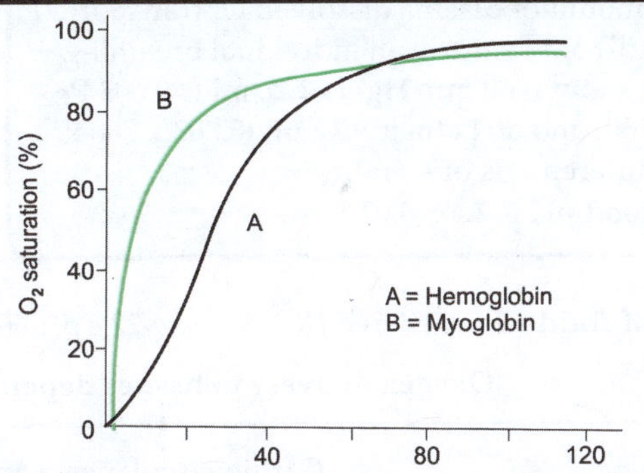

Dissociation curve of hemoglobin and myoglobin

8. **C i.e., 3.6 K Pa P_{50} is the PO_2 at which hemoglobin is half saturated with O_2.**

P_{50} is the PO_2 at which hemoglobin is half (50%) saturated with O_2[Q]***. The value of P_{50} is 25mm Hg(~ 3.6 Kpa***[Q]***)***

9. **C i.e. 80 mm Hg** *[Ref: Ganong 22/e P-667]*

PO_2 (mm Hg)		Dissolved O_2 (ml/dl)		% Saturation
10		0.03		13.5
20		0.06		35
30		0.09		57
40	Difference of	0.12	Table of 3	75
50	10	0.15		83.5
60		0.18		89
70		0.21		92.7
80		**0.24**[Q]		94.5
90		0.27		96.5
100		0.30		97.5

Given concentration of oxygen is in ml/ml and needs to be converted into ml/dl.

$$0.0025\ ml/ml = \frac{0.0025\ ml}{1/100\ dl}$$

(as 1 dl = 100 ml)

= 0.0025 x 100 ml/dl = 0.25 ml/dl.

From the table a value of dissolved oxygen of 0.25 ml/dl corresponds to 94.5% saturation of Hb and 80 mm Hg of PO_2.

10. **A i.e. CO** *[Ref: John West 8/e p 26-33; Michel Levitzky: Pulmonary physiology 6/e p 132; Ganong 23/e p 613;*
11. **B i.e. More soluble in plasma** *Guyton 11/e p 510-12; Gabriel p-190-91, 203; Berne and Levy 6/e p- 457-60]*

- **Carbon dioxide (CO_2) is 20 times more soluble in water (= plasma) than oxygen (O_2),** this is the reason why **CO_2 diffuses about 20 times more rapidly than does O_2 across the alveolar-capillary barrier** (although CO_2 has a higher but not very different molecular weight than O_2). Rate of diffusion α solubility/ $\sqrt{MW}$.
- Because the **transfer of carbon monoxide (CO)** across blood gas barrier of lung is **limited solely by diffusion,** and therefore ***CO is the gas of choice for measuring the diffusion properties of lung***[Q].

12. **B i.e. Polycythemia &. L→R shunt** *[Ref: John West 9/e p. 31-33; Guyton 12 SAE p. 352; Berne 6/e p. 459-60]*

Carbon monoxide transfer factor is increased in ***polycythemia and L→R shunt***[Q]; whereas, it is decreased in anemia, R→L shunt and pulmonary embolism.

13. **B i.e. 19.8** 14. **C i.e. 80 mm Hg** 15. **A i.e. 9 ml**
16. **B i.e. 6 ml** 17. **A i.e. 97%;** 18. **A i.e. 40 mmHg**

[Ref: Ganong 24/e p. 641-43; Guyton 12/e p. 485-99; John West 9/e p.78-84, 151-52; Chaudhuri5/e P-135; Sembulingum 3/e P--577]

- Arterial blood contains **19.8 ml O_2/dl** of which **19.5ml bound to Hb** and **0.29 ml dissolved in plasma**Q.
- **97%**Q of O_2 is transported in chemical combination with Hb and only 3% is transported in dissolved state in water of plasma & cells.
- **P_{CO_2} in arterial blood is 40mm Hg.**
- The total amount of plasma dissolved O_2 transported in 100ml (1dl) of plasma in an individual breathing 100% O_2 at **1 atm (760 mm Hg)** is **2.28 ml** (=0.003 P_{O_2} = 0.003 x 760) and at **4 atm** is **9.12 ml** (0.003 x 760 x 4). So the difference is of **~ 6ml.**
- **Arterial blood pH** is **7.4** ± 0.02

Feature	Arterial Blood	Venous Blood
P_{O_2} (Oxygen Tension)	95 (±5)mm Hg	40 (± 2)mm Hg
O_2 content (ml/dL or ml/100ml)	**19.8 ml/dl**Q (19.5 ml Hb bound & 0.29 ml plasma dissolved)	**15.22 ml/dl** (15.1 ml Hb bound and 0.12 ml plasma dissolved)
Hb saturation (%)	95 (± 2)%	75%
P_{CO_2} (CO_2 tension)	40 mmHg	46 mmHg
CO_2 content	49.02 ml/dl (46.4 Hb bound + 2.62 plasma dissolved)	52.68 ml/dl (49.7 Hb bound + 2.98 plasma dissolved)
N_2 content	0.98 (plasma dissolved)	0.98 (plasma dissolved)

19. B i.e. Type of fluid administered *[Ref: Ganong 22/e p. 666–69]*

Oxygen delivery to tissues depends on

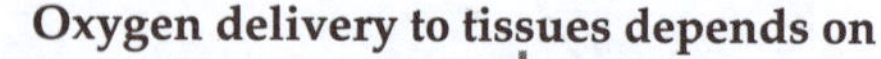

Lung
- Amount of O_2 entering the lungs **(ventilation)**
- Adequacy of pulmonary gas exchange **(diffusion)**

Cardiovascular system

Blood flow to tissue i.e.,
- ***Cardiac out put***Q
- ***Peripheral vascular resistance***Q i.e., degree of constriction of vascular bed in the tissue.

Blood

Capacity of blood to carry O_2, which depends on
- Amount of dissolved O_2 in plasma
- ***Amount of hemoglobin***Q
- ***Affinity of Hb for O_2***Q

Which is represented by O2 –Hb dissociation curve and ***depends on 2-3, BPG, pH and temperature***Q.

20. A i.e. 0.16

21. A i.e. 16% *[Ref: Sembulingum 3/e P- 574, 612]*

Mouth – to mouth respiration **provides 16% of O_2. In mouth- to – mouth respiration** the resuscitor takes a deep breath & exhales into the subject's mouth. It provides **16% (15.7%) of O_2 (amount of O_2 that is present in expired air).** So the fraction is **0.16**Q.

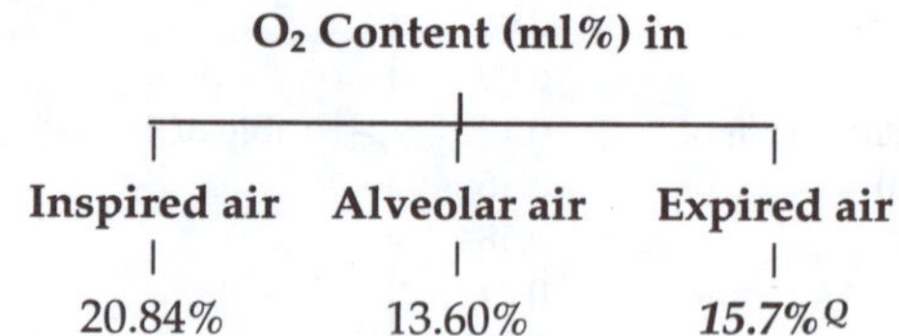

O_2 Content (ml%) in

Inspired air	Alveolar air	Expired air
20.84%	13.60%	*15.7%*Q

22. D i.e. 420. 4 mm Hg *[Ref: Chaudhuri 5/e P-141]*

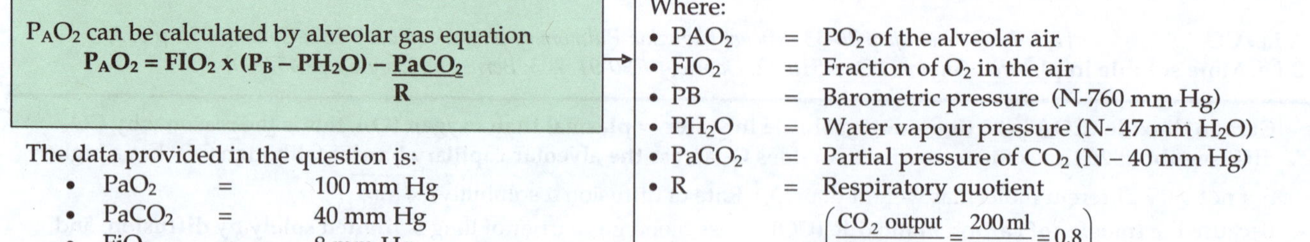

P_AO_2 can be calculated by alveolar gas equation

$$P_AO_2 = FIO_2 \times (P_B - PH_2O) - \frac{PaCO_2}{R}$$

Where:
- PAO_2 = PO_2 of the alveolar air
- FIO_2 = Fraction of O_2 in the air
- PB = Barometric pressure (N-760 mm Hg)
- PH_2O = Water vapour pressure (N- 47 mm H_2O)
- $PaCO_2$ = Partial pressure of CO_2 (N – 40 mm Hg)
- R = Respiratory quotient $\left(\frac{CO_2 \text{ output}}{O_2 \text{ uptake}} = \frac{200 \text{ ml}}{250 \text{ ml}} = 0.8\right)$

The data provided in the question is:
- PaO_2 = 100 mm Hg
- $PaCO_2$ = 40 mm Hg
- FiO_2 = 8 mm Hg

FiO_2 – Fraction of inspired Oxygen
At sea level (760 mm Hg pressure), the composition of air – O_2 = 20%; N_2 = 80%

So FiO_2 is $\frac{20}{100} = 0.2$

In this question, the child is being ventilated with 80% O_2

So FiO_2 is $\frac{80}{100} = 0.8$

Substituting these values

P_AO_2 = 0.8 x (760-47) – 40/0.8
= 520.4 mm Hg

Therefore $P_AO_2 - PaO_2$ = (520.4 mm Hg–100mm Hg)
= 420.4 mm Hg.

23. B i.e. P/T=constant

Charl's Law

At constant volume (V)

Pressure (P) ∝ Absolute temperature (T)

P/T = Constant

Boyle's law

At constant temperature

P ∝ 1/V or

PV= Constant

Gas equation

PV=nRT,

where R is gas constant and n is gram molecules of gas

Dalton's Partial Pressure Law

In a mixture of gas, **each gas exerts a pressure (k/a partial pressure) a/t its own concentration (as if it is present alone)**

Avogadro's Hypothesis

All gases at same temperature (T), pressure (P) & dryness contain same number of molecules. e.g. at STD (O°C, 760 mmHg, dry) a gram molecule of any gas occupies **22.4 liters**

24. D i.e. D *[Ref: Guyton 11/ep 519-20]*

- **In graph drawn between Alveolar ventilation & Alveolar PCO_2**
  - At same pH, **line tilts towards right with increase in PO_2** and viceversa
  - **With decrease in pH, the family of lines (curves) displace towards left**Q and viceversa.
- So curve of PO_2 100 will remain parallel **but shift towards left with decrease in pH**. This means original curve A (at PO_2 100 mm Hg) will become D at lower pH.

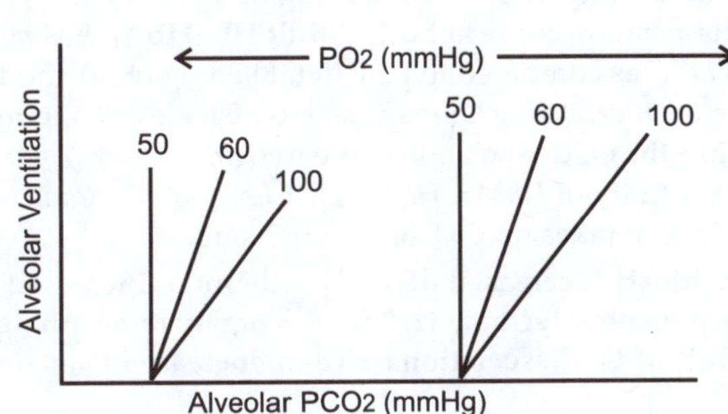

O_2 - Dissociation Curve

25. A i.e. Binding of one O_2 molecule increase affinity for the next O_2 molecule *[Ref:Ganong 23/ 609-11; Sembulingum 3/ 581-82]*

Oxygen – hemoglobin dissociation curve is sigmoid (or S) shaped because ***binding of one oxygen molecule to heme increases the affinity of second heme molecule for oxygen***Q an so on.

26. A i.e. Bohr effect

27. A i.e. Facilitates oxygen transport

- **Bohr effect: The presence of CO_2 (↓ pH) decreases the affinity of Hb for O_2, this enhances further release of O_2 to the tissue and the O_2 dissociation curve is shifted to right.** This is known as Bohr effect. ***So decrease in O_2 affinity of hemoglobin when pH of blood falls is called Bohr effect***Q. And it is caused by the fact that deoxygenated hemoglobin binds H+ more actively than does oxyhemoglobin. All the factors, which shift the O_2- dissociation curve to the right enhances the Bohr effect.
- ***Binding of O_2 to hemoglobin reduces its affinity for CO_2***Q or in other words CO_2 disociation curve shifts to right (i.e. blood begins to lose some CO_2 as it becomes oxygenated) is called **Haldane – Christian – Douglas effect.**

28. B i.e. Increased **29. A i.e. Unloading oxygen to tissues** **30. D i.e. Hypoxanthine**

[Ref: Ganong 23rd/e p. pg- 609-11; Lippincott Biochemistry 4th/e p. 31-32, 147, 294; Wintrobe's clinical hematology 12/ed pg-675]

While inosine increase / maintain 2, 3 – BPG content, hypoxanthine does notQ.

31. D i.e. p_{50} decreases & O_2 affinity increases **32. A i.e. PH** **33. A i.e. Decreased 2, 3 DPG concentration**
34. A i.e. Oxygen dissociation curve shifts to left **35. B i.e. Blood transfusion** **36. B i.e. 2,3, DPG**
37. A i.e. Hypthermia/HBF **38. D i.e. Matabolic alkalosis** **39. A i.e. Higher concentration are found in adult blood**
40. A i.e. Acidosis shifts O_2 dissociation curve to right. **41. A i.e. Chloride ion Concentration**
42. D i.e. Oxygen affinity of hemoglobin **43. B i.e. Hypoxia** **44. D i.e. ↑$PaCO_2$ & ↑ HCO_3^-**
45. B i.e. Fall in Temperature **46. A i.e. Fetal Hb & Hypothermia shifts curve to Left**

[Ref: Best & Taylor 13/e p 604-5; West respiratory physiology 9/e p 79-82; Egan's p 234; Ganong 24/e p 643-48; Berne & Levy 6/e p461-64; Nelson 17/e p 1603-2; Chattarjea 7/e p 149; Kumar & Clark 6/e p 430]

- **Alkalosis (increased pH), hypothermia (decreased temperature), hypocarbia (decreased p CO_2, and decreased 2, 3, DPG** cause **left shift of O_2 dissociation curve (ie decreased P_{50} = increased O_2 affinity = decreased tissue delivery of O_2)**
- **Hypocarbia due to hyperventilation shifts O_2 dissociation curve towards left i.e., P_{50} decreases & oxygen affinity increases**Q.
- O_2 saturation of maternal blood in placenta is so low that the fetus might suffer hypoxia damage if **fetal RBCs** did not have a **greater O_2 affinity than adult RBCs**. The cause of this greater O_2 affinity is *poor binding of 2, 3 – DPG by γpolypeptide chains that replace β chains in fetal Hb*Q. Because HbF binds less with 2, 3 DPG & so is able to bind O_2 more accounting for left shifted O_2 dissociation curve at birth. **Adult Hb (HbA_1)** has *more 2, 3 DPG* as compared to HbF (fetal hemoglobin) and it is *better at delivering O_2 to tissue*. **HbS** (sickle cell anemia) shift the O_2 dissociation curve to *right*.
- O_2 affinity of *HbM < HbA < Hb Chesapeake & Rainier*. Because Mb- O_2 disociation curve lies left of HbO_2 dissociation curve, it takes up O_2 from Hb in blood.
- **Acidosis (decreased pH), hyperthermia (increased temperature), hyper carbia (increased CO_2) & high levels of 2, 3, biphosphoglycerate (2, 3 BPG = organic phosphate) d/t exercise, high altitude or anemia (sickle cell Hb) cause right shift of O_2 dissociation curve (ie increased P_{50} = decreased O_2 affinity = increased tissue delivery of O_2)**

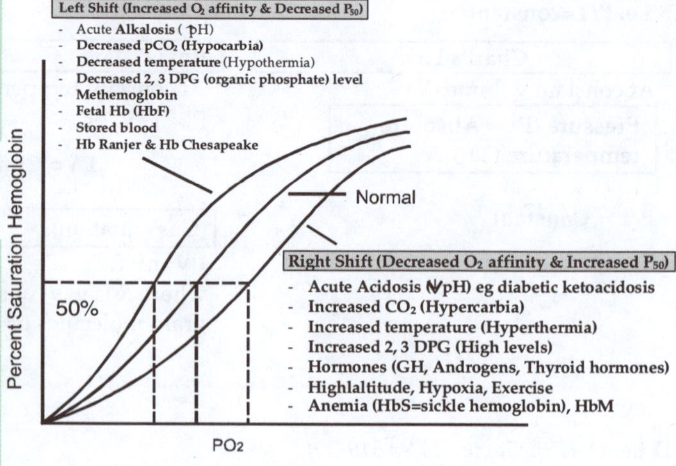

Factors Shifting O_2 Dissociation Curve

Towards **Left** ie **Increasing O_2 affinity to Hb and decreasing release = Decreased p50**	**Towards Right ie Decreasing O_2 affinity to hemoglobin and promoting release of O_2 in** tissue = **Increased p50**
- Acute **Alkalosis** (↑pH) - **Decreased pCO_2 (Hypocarbia)** - **Decreased temperature** (Hypothermia) - **Decreased 2, 3 DPG (organic phosphate) level** - **Methemoglobin** - **Fetal Hb (HbF)** - **Stored blood** - **Hb Ranier & Hb Chesapeake**	- **Acute Acidosis (↓pH) eg diabetic ketoacidosis** - **Increased CO_2 (Hypercarbia)** - **Increased temperature (Hyperthermia)** - **Increased 2, 3 DPG (High levels)** - **Hormones (GH, Androgens, Thyroid hormones)** - **High altitude, Hypoxia, Exercise** - **Anemia (HbS=sickle hemoglobin), HbM**

★Exercise: Oxygen dissociation Curve shifts to the right in exercising muscles. Stroke volume is increased during isotonic muscle exercise. Blood flow to muscles is increased.

2, 3 DPG

Is found in red blood cells. It is responsible for ***lowering the oxygen affinity of hemoglobin***Q, thus **allowing Hb to release oxygen (unloading)**Q more efficiently. It is

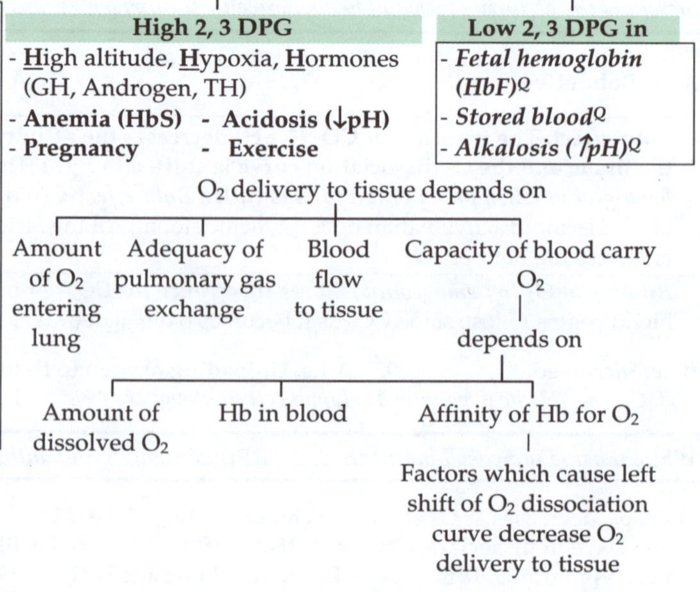

Lung Volume and Capacities

47. A i.e. Inspiratory Capacity minus Inspiratory Reserve volume
48. B i.e. TV
49. C i.e. Volume remaining after normal expiration
50. C i.e. ERV + RV
51. C i.e. Compliance of lung
52. D i.e. FEV_1 is forced expiratory rate at one minute
[Ref: Ganong 24/e P-629-31; Sembulingum 3/e P-561-62; Chaudhuri5/e P-154-155]

- *Volume of air taken in & given out during normal respiration is called as tidal volume (TV)*[Q]. **TV = IC - IRV**[Q].
- **Functional residual capacity (FRC)** *is volume remaining after normal (tidal) expiration*[Q]. **FRC = ERV + RV**[Q].
- **Total lung capacity (TLC)** depends on *lung compliance (distensibility)*[Q]. **Compliance decreases in interstitial lung diseases.**
- **FEV_1** or **timed vital capacity** is *fraction of VC expired (or forced expiratory volume) in 1 second*[Q].

53. C i.e. Max mid respiratory flow rates *[Ref: Harrison 16th/1498, 1500, Ganong 22/e P-651, Sembulingum 3/e P- 567, 570]*

Resistance to small air ways is **best measured by** *maximal mid expiratory flow rates (MMFR)* **followed by FEV_1.**[Q]
In early obstructive disease, which originates in the small airways FEV1/FVC may be normal but *FEF 25-75% - (Max mid expiratory flow rate)* may be depressed.

54. A i.e. 6L **55. C i.e. 4.2** **56. A i.e. 4900 ml** *[Ref: Ganong 24/e P-629-30; Sembulingum 3/e P- 567, 570]*

Alveolar ventilation (rest)	*4.2L/min.*[Q]
Total lung capacity	*4 – 6 lit.*[Q]
Respiratory minute volume (rest)	*6 L/min.*[Q]
Maximum voluntary ventilation	*125- 170 L/min.*[Q]
Timed vital capacity - In 1 sec (FeV_1)	*83%*[Q]
- In 3 sec	*97%*[Q]
Work of quiet breathing	*0.5 kg – m/min*[Q]
Maximum work of breathing	*10 kg- ml breath*

Alveolar ventilation = (TV – dead space volume) x RR
= (500 – 150 ml) x 14
= 4900 ml

★ Normally we consider dead space to be 150 ml. But also know that '*Dead space volume of a person is equal to twice his body weight* i.e. a person weighing 70 kg has a dead space volume of 140 ml.

57. B i.e. 0.35 *[Ref: Best & Taylors 12/e P-527]*

V_d = Dead space volume & V_t = Tidal Volume, so $V_d/V_t = \frac{150}{100} = 0.3$

Normal value of V_d/V_t in adults = ***0.2 - 0.35***[Q]

58. D i.e. Close to Residual volume
59. B i.e. FRC below the closing volume
[Ref: Ganong 24/e p 633-34; John West 9/e p 169-70; Nelson 18/e p 732-35; Cloherty 6/e p336; Rogers TPIC 3/e p 287-88; Berne & Levy 6/e p 431-434]

- **Closing volume (CV)** or critical CV is minimal volume of gas *necessary to prevent small airway collapse*. In young adults it is **10% of vital capacity (ie = 480 ML)** and becomes equal to **~ 40% of VC (ie = FRC) at the age of 65 years. In RDS (hyaline membrane disease), the FRC decreases below closing volume (FRC < CV)** indicating collapse of some alveolar segments during tidal breathing.
- Volume of air in lung at the end of (1) **force ful inspiration is TLC**; (2) **forceful expiration** is residual volume (RV) and ; (3) **normal tidal expiration** is FRC. RV is 1200mL and FRC is 2200 mL. Therefore normally closing volume is more close to RV than to FRC.

60. B i.e. Reduced FEV1/FVC ratio
61. B i.e.↑ FEV_1/FVC, ↓Compliance of lung tissue
62. B i.e. RV decreased
63. A i.e.↑ TLC *[Ref: Berne & Levy 6/e p. 443; Harrison 16/e P-1500]*

- **The hallmark of restrictive lung disease (eg interstitial lung disease) is decrease in lung volumes primarily TLC, RV and VC, decreased lung compliance (distensibility), reduced diffusion capacity but increased FEV_1/FVC ratio**[Q].
- **The hallmark of obstructive lung disease (eg emphysema)** are *increase in lung volumes RV & TLC*[Q] *(but not VC which is decreased)*[Q], **decrease in expiratory flow rates (FEF_{25-75}) & decrease in FEV_1/FVC**[Q].

64. C i.e. Slow and deep *[Ref: Harrison 16/e P-1549]*

As the lung deflates, the intrapleural pressure rises from negative to zero → this creates a situation when the bronchioles are no more stretched → bronchodilation ceases → bronchial narrowing → increased air flow resistance → drop of rate of airflow.

Slow and deep breathing is better[Q] than rapid and shallow breathing:
- Because of the dead space, rapid shallow breathing produces much less alveolar ventilation than slow deep breathing at the same respiratory minute volume. - Slow and deep breathing encounter less airway resistance.

Tests for Pulmonary Compliance

65. C i.e. Increase in lung decrease in box *[Ref:Berne 6/ 431-32;Sembulingam 5/ 665-66; Ganong 23/ 539; John West 8/ 14-16,165-66]*

Because of Boyle's law ($P_1V_1 = P_2V_2$), during **expiration** when **lung volume decreases, the pressure inside the lung increases** and **pressure inside** the air tight **box decreases** because the gas volume in box increases – **in body plethysmography** in which the subject sits in an air tight chamber.

66. A i.e. Inspiratory reserve volme, Tidal volume and Expiratory reserve volume
67. A, C, E i.e. Tidal volume, ERV, IRV
68. B i.e. Residual Volume
69. A i.e. FRC C i.e. RV
70. B i.e. Functional residual Capacity *[Ref: Guyton 12/e p 469-71, 517]*

- **Residual volume** is the amount of air left inside the lungs at the end of forced expiration. ***It cannot be measured by simple spirometer***[Q] *because the air in the residual volume of lungs cannot be expired into spirometer.* Because **spirometer cannot measure RV**, it can't be used to measure lung capacities requiring RV such as **functional residual capacity** (RFC = ERV + RV) and **total lung capacity** (TLC = VC + RV).
- **Spirometery** can **not** be used in a direct way to measure – ***Functional residual capacity (FRC), residual volume (RV) and total lung capacity (TLC)***[Q]. Helium dilution method is used to measure them.
- **Spirometry can measure tidal volume (TV), inspiratory reserve volume (IRV), inspiratory capacity (IC), expiratory reserve volume (ERV) and vital capacity (VC).**

Measurements of Lung Volumes

Spirometer[Q] (Computerized spirometer)	- **Helium dilution technique** - **Nitrogen washout[Q] method** - **Plethysmography**
- A spirometer records movements of lid, which moves upward when person inspires & downward when expires. - RV neither measured by volume of air expired (e.g. TV or VC), nor by air inspired (IRV). - Disadvantage – ***It cannot measure RV[Q], FRC[Q] and TLC.[Q]***	Used to measure **Residual volume (RV) and FRC[Q]**

VC = TV + IRV + ERV
= IC + ERV

FRC = ERV + RV

TLC = TV + IRV + ERV + RV
= VC + RV
= IC + FRC

71. C i.e. N_2 breath test **72. B ie. Anatomical dead space=Physiological dead space** **73. D ie. Single breath nitrogen test**

Measurement of Dead Space Volume

Anatomical Dead Space

Single Breath N_2 Method (Fowler's Method)

- After quiet expiration, subject takes a **single deep breath of pure (100%) O_2** and breathes it out slowly & steadily. **N_2 analysis in expired air is done**
- Pure O_2 fills dead space with 100% O_2 and it comes out first in expiration so **initial volume of air (during expiration) that is N_2 free gives anatomical dead space**[Q].
- **In healthy individuals, normally Anatomical dead space= Physiological dead space=150ml**[Q]

Physiological Dead Space (Volume)

Bohr's Method (Equation)

$$= \frac{TV\,(F_ACO_2 - F_ECO_2)}{F_ACO_2}$$

$$= \frac{T_V\,(P_aCO_2 - P_ECO_2}{P_aCO_2}$$

TV= tidal volume, $F_A\,CO_2$ & $F_E\,CO_2$= CO_2 Concentration in alveolar air (A) and expired air (E). **$PaCO_2$ & P_ECO_2** = Partial pressure of CO_2 in artery (a) & expired air (e)

★Since concentration of gas is α partial pressure ($F_{A/E}$= $P_{A/E}$) and alveolar Pco_2=arterial PCO_2 (So P_ACO_2= $PaCO_2$).

74. B i.e. Extrathoracic obstruction *[Ref: Morgan 3/e P-542]*

Pressure – Volume Curve

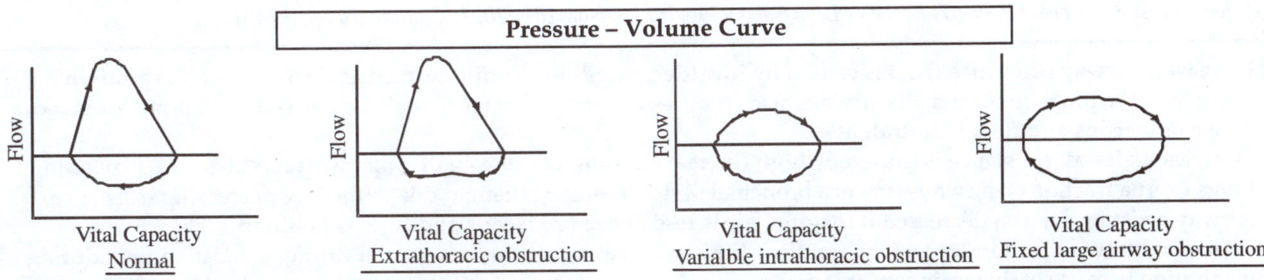

75. C i.e. Interstitial lung disease *[Ref: Ganong 24/e p. 63]*

Pressure Volume Curve

Compliance Decreased i.e. Curve Shifted to Downwards & Right	Compliance Increased i.e Curve Shifted to Upwards & Left
- **Pulmonary interstitial fibrosis**[Q] - **Interstitial lung disease**[Q] - Alveolar edema (prevents inflation of some alveoli) - ***Pulmonary congestion (increased pulmonary venous pressure)***[Q] - If lung remains unventilated for long period especially if lung volume is low - ***Decreased surfactant***[Q] (causing increased surface tension and alveolar atelectasis) - Deformities of thorax eg kyphosis, scoliosis - Paralysis of respiratory muscles - Pleural effusion pneumo/hydro/hemo-thorax	- **Emphysema**[Q] - **Normal aging lung** - **During an asthma attack**[Q]

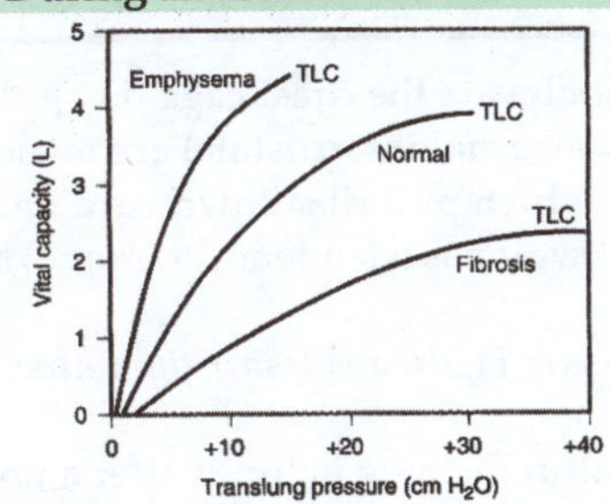

Pressure During Breathing Cycle

76. D i.e. Alveolar pressure-Transpulmonary pressure

77. A i.e. More – ve

78. B i.e. Thoracic cage and lungs are elastic structures.

79. A i.e. The chest wall and lungs recoil in opposite directions

80. C i.e. Lymphatic drainage of pleural cavity

[Ref: Guyton 11/e p. 489-90; Ganong 23/e p. 599; John West 8/e p 114-15; 110-11, Berne & Levy 6/e p-433-435; Chaudhari 5/e p 121]

The pressure difference between the air spaces (**alveolar pressure = P_A**) and pressure surrounding the lung (i.e. **pleural pressure = P_{Pl}**) is called **transmural pressure across lung or transpulmonary /trans lung pressure** (P_L) $P_L = P_A - P_{PL}$ The lung requires positive transpulmonary pressure (i.e. relatively more alveolar or lesser pleural pressure) to increase its volume and the lung volume increases with increasing P_L.

So, **Pleural (Intra Pleural) Pressure (P_{PL}) = Alveolar Pressure (P_A) – Trans Pulmonary/ Lung / Mural Pressure (i.e. P_L)**

- **Normal negative intrapleural pressure** is maintained by ***opposing elastic recoil forces of chest wall and lung***[Q] (ie the **expansile recoil tendency of chest wall and retractile recoil tendency of lung)** along with efficient drainage of excessive intrapleural fluid by **lymphatic pump** and **osmotic forces** across pleural **membrane maintaining a slight suction** and only a thin layer of serous fluid between parietal pleural surface of thoracic cavity and visceral pleural surface of lung.
- The basic cause of **negative pressure in most tissue spaces of body (including intrapleural cavity)** is ***lymphatic drainage (i.e. pumping of fluid from space by lymphatics)***[Q].
- **Intra pleural pressure is negative during the normal breathing cycle** (i.e. both ***during inspiration and expiration) because of elasticity of lung and chest wall***[Q].

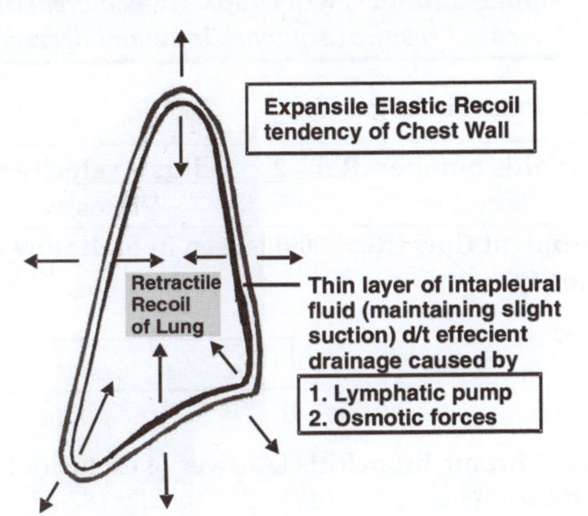

Negative Intrapleural Pressure

81. A, B, C i.e. Forced expiration, Dense air, Low lung volume

82. A i.e. Increased compression of airways

83. C i.e. Dynamic compression of airways

[Ref: John West 8/e p 114-17; 96-97; Berne & Levy 6/e p 439-41; Harrison 18th /2091; Chaudhary 6/e p 145]

- **Increased Airway resistance (R_{aw})** is caused by **low (decreased) lung volume such as during forced expiration**^Q because as the lungs compress, the airways also compress. Airway resistance is also increased **if inspired air is more dense or viscous and flow is turbulent**^Q
- **Decreased airway resistance** is caused by **high (increased) lung volume eg during inspiration** because expanding lungs exert a traction on airways (trachea bronchial system) causing them to dilate (thereby decreasing resistance). Airway resistance is also decreased if **inspired air is less dense or viscous and flow is laminar**^Q.
- **Expiatory flow** is **effort independent** and **flow limited.** Airway resistance is greater during exhalation than during inspiration because of **dynamic compression of airways**^Q which **stops last stage of forced expiration.**
- **Expiration** in quiet breathing is passive and requires no muscle activity. Lung recoil pulls the chest back and the airway pressure becomes slightly positive.

Expiration

84. B i.e. At the end of normal expiration air in lung is ERV *[Ref: Ganong 23/e 591-94; Berne & Levy 6/e p-425-35; Guyton 11/e 471-74; John West8/e p 114, 96-97; Gabriel p 178-184]*

- Muscles that **elevate the chest cage (i.e. pull the ribs upwards and farwards, thus increasing both AP and lateral diameters = external intercostals) are muscles of inspiration** whereas muscles that **depress the chest cage (i.e. internal intercostals which pull ribs downward and inwards, decreasing the thoracic volume)** are **muscles of expiration.**
- Elastic **chest wall** has a tendency to **move outward** which is balanced by **inward recoil of alveoli.** At **FRC** both are balanced
- ***Pleural pressure is always lesser than alveolar pressure***^Q, because it is a suction (slightly negative) pressure holding the lungs open
- Amount of air remaining in lungs after a normal tidal expiration is **functional residual capacity (FRC),** which is equal to the sum of residual volume (RV) and expiratory reserve volume (ERV). ERV is the amount of air that can be enhaled with maximal effort in excess of tidal expiration. RV is amount of air remaining in lungs after maximum expiration; which keeps alveoli inflated between breathes and mixes with fresh air on net inspiration **FRC = RV + ERV**.

Workload of Breathing

85. A i.e. Lung elasticity

86. D i.e., Decrease workload and decrease duration of exercise

[Ref: Guyton 11/e p. 539- 41; John West 8/e p. 98-100; Ganong 22/e p.657]

- **Efforts during respiration (inspiration) is done due to lung elasticity** i.e. to expand elastic lung.
- At high altitudes, **work capacity** ***is increased by acclimatization, increased rate of O_2 upake the body can achieve, decreased respiratory work load and decreased duration of exercise***^Q.

87. C i.e. Pressure of gas

$$\text{Reynolds number (Re)} = \frac{2 \times \text{radius} \times \text{velocity} \times \text{density}}{\text{Viscosity}} = \frac{2rvd}{\eta}$$

Turbulent flow (Re>2000) is seen in **high flow rates & large airways** and **laminar flow** is seen in **small airways & low velocity.**

Compliance

88. B i.e. Chronic bronchitis (Answer of exclusion)

89. A i.e. Elasticity

90. A i.e. 200ml/cm water

[Ref: Berne & Levy 6/e p 431-32; Gabriel p 182-83; John West 8/e p 99, 117; Guyton 11/e p 473-75; Ganong 23/e p 595-97]

- Unit of **compliance** (i.e. **stretchability** or **elasticity**) is mL (or liter) per cm H_2O. The compliance of normal human (both) lung is ***0.2L/cm H_2O (200 mL/Cm H_2O,)***[Q] which means every time the transpulmonary pressure increases 1 cm H_2O, the lung volume will expand 200 ml (0.2 L) after 10-20 seconds.
- **Specific lung compliance** is **decreased** in ***pulmonary fibrosis, pulmonary congestion and decreased surfactant***[Q].

Ventilation & Perfusion

91. B i.e. Ventilation – Perfusion mismatch *[Ref: Harrison 16/e pg 1503, 1504; Ganong 22/e pg 662,663]*

In **ventilation perfusion mismatch** the O_2 contained in the alveoli, *cannot be transmitted to arteries*. This leads to ***accumulation of O_2 in the alveoli***[Q], causing increased O_2 tension.

92. C i.e Apex of lung **93. A i.e. Apex of lung** **94. B i.e. Base** **95. A i.e. P_aO_2 is maximum at apex**
[Ref: Ganong 22/e P- 663,662, Sembulingum 3/e P- 572]

Ventilation Perfusion Ratio is maximum (3) at the Apex of lung[Q] and minimum (0.6) at base. PaO_2 is maximum at apex[Q]. Average V/P ratio for whole lung is 0.8[Q].

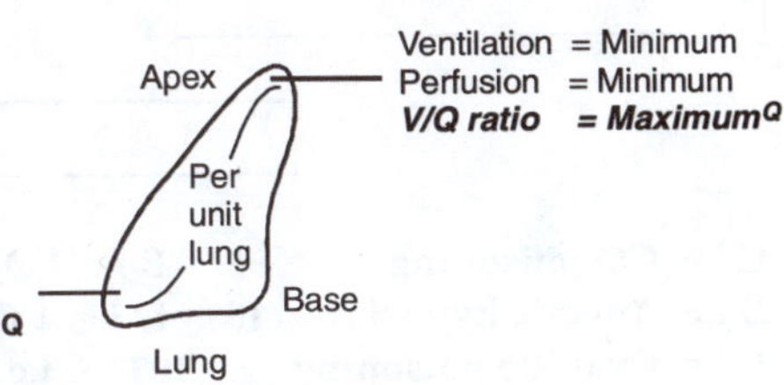

Ventilation/Perfusion Ratio

The ratio of pulmonary ventilation to pulmonary blood flow for the whole lung at rest is – 0.8 (4.2 L/min ventilation divided by 5.5 L/min pulmonary blood flow)[Q]

If the ventilation of an alveolus is reduced
- PO_2 falls because of less O_2 delivery - PCO_2 rises because less CO_2 is expired from alveolus,

If perfusion is reduced relative to ventilation:
- PO_2 rises in alveolus because less O_2 enters the blood - PCO_2 falls because less CO_2 is delivered.

- Ventilation as well as perfusion, in an upright position declines from the bases to the apices of the lung (in linear fashion). But the change in blood from apex to base is greater than the relative change in ventilation, therefore ***V/Q ratio is low at the base and high at the apex***[Q].
- In an upright position
  - Ventilation per unit lung volume is greatest at base
  - Perfusion per unit lung volume is greatest at base
  - ***P_aO_2 is maximum at apex***[Q].
- *High V- P ratio at the apex accounts for predilection of the tuberculosis for this area.*
- In patient with unilateral lung disease the patient is positioned such that the good lung is in dependent position. Arterial oxygenation is improved in this position due to effect of gravity on ventilation. (The situation in infants is opposite. i.e. infants do better with the diseased lung in the dependent position)

96. C i.e. PGI_2 *[Ref: Ganong 22/e P-663-664; KDT 5/e 158-160]*

The unique feature of **pulmonary vasculature** is that the **hypoxia tends to produce Vasconstriction** (where as *in other system it produces Vasodilation). **PGI_2 is uniformly vasodilator***[Q].

Substance Causing

Vasodilation (Nitric oxide mediated)		Vasoconstriction	
- α_2- adrenergic stimulation - β_2- adrenergic stimulation - **Prostacyclin (PGI_2)**Q - Histamine - Endothelium derived hyperpolarizing factor - Atrial **natriuretic** peptide - Vasopressin	Mn: **2-α, β, I** **2-Hi, Hy** **Na, Va**	- **α1** Adrenergic - ThromboxaneQ ($TX\text{-}A_2$) - **Angiotensin II** - LTC_4, LTD_4 - **Endothelin [ETA]**Q - ***Hypoxia***Q - ***Hypercapnia***Q	Mn: α_1 **A_2, A II** **CD_4** **E-A** **$\downarrow O_2$ $\uparrow CO_2$**

PGE_2 & PGF_2 α	Causes ***vasodilation in most but not all vascular beds. PGF_2 α causes vasoconstriction in many larger veins.***Q
PGI_2	Is *Uniformly Vasodilator.*
PG endoperoxidases (G_2 and H_2)	Are *inherently Vasoconstrictor, but* often produce vasodilatation or biphasic response.
TXA_2 & Leucotrienes (LTC_4 & LTD_4)	Consistently produces *vasoconstriction*

Hypoxia

97. C i.e. CO poisoning
98. B i.e. PO_2 normal O_2, saturation less with normal or slightly decreases PCO_2
99. B i.e. Anemic hypoxia
100. D i.e. ↓ O_2 content in arterial blood
101. A i.e. Arterial PO_2
102. C i.e. Cyanide poisoning
103. C i.e. a,b & d
104. B i.e. Diffuse vasodilation
105. A i.e. 8 min.
106. B i.e. Hippocampus
107. C i.e. Hb

[Ref: Berne & Levy 6/e p 454-65; John West 8/e p 57, 90, 134; Gabriel p 512-17; 69, 194; Ganong 23/e p 616-23; Guyton 11/e p 530-31; Harrison 17/e p 1591; Lee 12/e p 292.

- **Arterial hypoxemia** is defined as an **arterial P_{O2} (partial pressure of oxygen) less than 80 mmHg,** who is breathing room air at sea level. And because the partial pressure of a gas is determined by the soluble fraction of gas and not by the amount carried chemically bound to hemoglobin – the ***Hb does not determine P_{O2} and hypoxemia does not depend on Hb level***Q.
- In CO poisoning ***effective hemoglobin that can carry O_2 decreases***Q (because CO occupies Hb binding site) since ***P_{O2} or arterial blood O_2 remains normal***Q, *peripheral chemoreceptors are not stimulated* and hyperventilation is not seen.
- In hypoxia, with the reduction of PO_2 cerebral blood flow ***increases (d/t vaso dilatation)***Q to maintain O_2 delivery in the brain.
- The cerebral cortex can tolerate acute hypoxia for **5-10 min at 28°C**Q, *20 min at 20°C, and 50 min at 50°C.*
- **Hypoxic ischemia almost** invariably involve **hippocampus**. The hippocampal CA1 neurons are vulnerable to even brief episodes of hypoxic ischemia.

Cyanosis

108. A i.e. CO poisoning & Anemia
109. C i.e. Critical concentration of Hb required to produce cyanosis is reduced
110. B i.e. O_2 saturation < 85%
111. A, D i.e. 10.9 & 4.1; 8.9 & 4.1
112. B i.e. Late sign of Hypoxia *[Ref: Ganong 23/e 612; Harrison 17/e p 230-31; Guyton 11/ 531; John West 8/ 78; Wintrobe 6/e p. 194]*

- **The critical concentration of reduced hemoglobin** required to produce cynosis is **4** (Harrison) / **5** (wintrobe) *gram/ dl.* In ***severe anemia, the total concentration of hemoglobin may be < 4-5gm/ dl and so cynosis will not be manifested because the critical concentration can not be reached***Q.
- ***Cyanosis is a late sign of hypoxia***Q; so it is never advisible to wait for cyanosis to appear to diagnose hypoxia.
- **Cyanosis occurs when concentration of reduced hemoglobin is > 4-5 gm %** in capillary blood. Whereas when concentration of reduced Hb is less than 4/5 gm % (like 4.1) cyanosis would not occur.

113. C i.e. 1.5 g/dl **114. D i.e. Phenytoin** **115. A i.e. Methylene blue** *[Ref: Sembulingam 4/e p. 72 – 73]*

- **Concentration of methemoglobin** to cause cyanosis is **1.5 gm/dl**[Q].
- **Causes of methemoglobinemia** includes ***nitrites, sulfonamides and phenacetin not phenytoin***[Q]***. Antidote of Na-nitrate poisoning is methylene blue IV***[Q].

116. B i.e. Cessation of respiration

Apnea is cessation or stoppage of respiration[Q]

117. D i.e. Hypoventilation *[Ref: Chaudhuri5/e P-143]*

Arterial O_2 tension may be *reduced* either from a *defect in oxygenation* **(Type I failure)** or *Ventilation* **(type II failure)=hypoventilation.**

CO, O_2 and CO_2 Toxicity

118. C i.e. Tissue toxicity plays an important role .. **119. A & C i.e. Cytochrome toxicity is lethal & PO_2 is decreased**
120. A i.e. High affinity of CO for haemoglobin **121. A i.e. Anemic hypoxia**
Ref: Ganong 23rd/e p. 621, 564, 525; Guyton 12/e p. 501; 11th/e p. 509-12, 196, 492, 499

- ***Transport and toxicity of carbon monoxide (CO) is limited to its diffusing capacity because hemoglobin combines with this gas so rapidly***[Q] that its partial pressure never has time to build up and is essentially *zero* in blood. The affinity of Hb for CO is **210 greater** than its affinity for O_2. So the ***partial pressure as low as 0.6mmHg of CO may be lethal***[Q]***. CO is toxic to tissue cytochromes at level that is 1000 times of lethal dose. Therefore tissue toxicity plays no role in clinical CO poisoning***[Q]. It is treated by **hyperbaric pure oxygen and 5% CO_2.**
- ***Carbon monoxide (CO) poisoning shifts oxyhemoglobin dissocation curve towards left***[Q] (i.e. reduces amount of O_2 released in tissue). It **reduces the amount of Hb that can carry O_2** and causes **anemic hypoxia.**

122. D i.e. Is toxic to tissues **123. B i.e. Decreased cerebral flow**
[Ref : Sembulingum 3/e p. 595; Guyton 11/e p. 547; Chaudhari 5/e p. 148, 228; Goodman Gillman 11/e p. 393- 94]

Decreased cerebral blood flow due to cerebral vasoconstriction caused by high O_2 tension is its ***protective effect***[Q] (not toxic). Which protects brain from free radicle injury.

Smoking

124. D i.e. Decreased carboxyhemoglobin *[Ref: Harrison's 17/ed pg-2738; The risk of passive smoking: Roy J Shepherd p. 71; www.springerlink.com/content / a 74832479802343 K/]*

Smoking decreases HDL and increases RBC, hemotocrit, adrenaline, heart rate, catecholamines and carboxyhemogolobin[Q].

Respiratory Failure

125. C i.e Hypoventilation **126. D i.e Lobar Pneumonia.**
127. A i.e. Carbon monoxide poisoning/ High altitude *[Ref: Ganong 23/e p. 618-21; Harrison 17/e p. 1676; Guyton 11/e p. 531-32; API-Medicine 6/e p. 278; John West 8/e p. 85-87; Berne & Levy 6/e p. 465-66; 645-47, 447, 441; Gabriel p. 201-202]*

- **Type II respiratory failure**, which occurs d/t **hypoventilation (i.e. failure of ventilation)** is characterized by **hypoxemia with hypercapnia (CO_2) retention but normal (not increased) alveolar-arterial oxygen gradient (P_{AaO2})**
- **Hypercapnia (hypercarbia or CO_2 retention)** is defined as an **elevation in arterial partial pressure of carbon dioxide (P_{CO2})**. It characteristically occurs secondary to **inadequate alveolar ventilation (hypoventilation), in type II respiratory failure.**
- **Type II respiratory failure (or alveolar hypoventilation = alveolar ventilatory failure = hypercapnia = hypercarbia = CO_2 retention = respiratory acidosis)** or **normal P_{A-aO2}** is seen in reduced compliance of chest like ***kyphoscoliosis***Q, reduced lung compliance like ***pulmonary (alveolar) edema***Q, obstructive lung disease like ***COPD***Q, weakness of respiratory muscle (***like bulbar poliomyelitis***Q), bronchospasm and decreased central respiratory drive. Drowning may cause bronchospasm & pulmonary edema & so CO_2 retention.
- **Type I respiratory failure** results from **failure in exchange (diffusion)** of respiratory gases **at the alveolar-capillary junction** as a result of ***disease of lung parenchyma (like pneumonia), or vasculature (like right to left shunt), and ventilation-perfusion mismatch***Q. It is characterized by ***increased alveolar-arterial oxygen gradient (P_{A-aO2})*** Q, hypoxemia and normal or low P_{aCO2}.
- At high altitudes alveolar CO_2 decreases b/o hyperventilation.

128. D i.e. Hypertension *[Ref: Lee's 12/e P-42; Sembulingum 3/e P-595]*

Hypercarbia (hypercapnia) is characterized by ***hypertension, tachycardia, and mydriasis d/t sympathetic stimulation***Q. It also **increase intracranial tension.**

Regulation of Breathing

129. D i.e. Pre Botzinger complex **130. A i.e. Prolonged inspiratory spasm** **131. A i.e. Pneumotaxic centre**
[Ref:Ganong 23/e 626-27; Guyton 11/e p 514-16; John West 8/e p-124-26; Berne 6/e p 469-72; Gabriel p 197-99; MTx]

Spontaneous automatic rhythmic respiration is initiated by a small group of synaptically coupled **pacemaker cells** in the **pre-Biotzinger complex (Pre-BOTC)** situated on either side of medulla between **nucleus ambiguous and lateral reticular nucleus.**

Medullary Respiratory Centers (MRC)	**Pre Botzinger complex (Pre BOTC)**	**Pacemaker of respiration**Q **i.e. spontaneous automatic rhythmic respiration is initiated**Q
	Dorsal Respiratory Group (DRG)	Mainly cause **rhythmic inspiratory discharge**Q
	Ventral Respiratory group (VRG)	Mainly controls **forceful expiration**Q & some inspiration
Pontine Respiratory Centers (PRC)	**Pneumotaxic center (PC)**	**Halt (limit) inspiratory depth**Q by **fine tuning** respiratory rhythm **and switching** between inspiration & expiration
	Apneustic center (AC)	**Excites inspiration center (DRG) to prolong inspiration**

132. B i.e. Apneusis **133. B i.e. Irregular and gasping**
[Ref: Samson Wright 13/168; Ganong 23/ 626-27; Sembulingum 3/e P-585-587; NMS physiology 4/e P-253-57; Guyton 9/e P 525-26]

The main component of *respiratory control pattern generator* responsible for automatic respiration are located *in the medulla*. After transection of brain stem at inferior border of pons spontaneous respiration continues, albeit ***somewhat irregular and gasping***.Q Whereas, transection at mid (upper) pons leads to ***slow and deep breathing***Q (vagi intact) or ***apneustic breathing (or prolonged respiratory spasm)*** Q, when vagi are also cut.

Effects of transection of the brainstem at different levels on respiration. Note the additional effect of cutting the vagus (the Hering-Breuer inflation reflex).

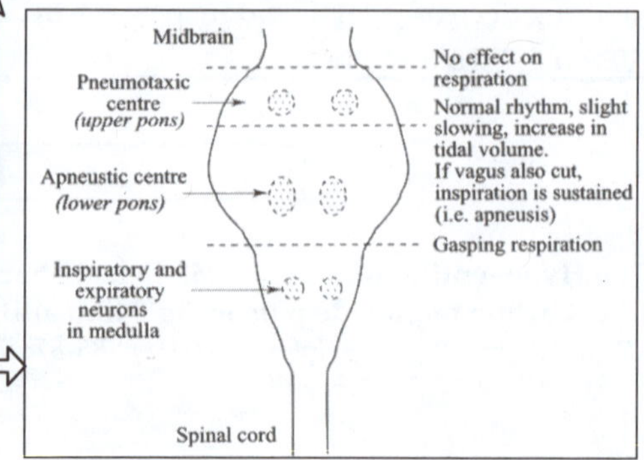

Effect of Lesion/ Transection

Above (rostral) pons	In Pons & medulla where autonomic centers are situated		Below medulla
	At upper or mid-pons	**At inferior border of pons & upper border of medulla**	
- Loss of voluntary control - *Respiration remains normal*	- **Pneumotaxis center** damage: respiration becomes ***slower &tidal volume greater (slow & deep)***Q ***but no change in rate or rhythm.*** - If **pneumotaxis center** is damaged **along with vagus** – this causes removal of inhibitory influence on Apneustic center and leads to ***prolonged respiratory spasm*** that resembles breath holding k/a ***Apneusis or Apneustic breathing*** Q i.e. breathing stops in deep inspiration which may be interrupted by occasional expiration. - If **only vegi** are cut ***depth of inspiraton is increased***Q	- *Spontaneous respiration* continues, although some what- ***irregular and gasping***Q (Ganong) - *Rhythmic respiration* persis but the pattern is ***less smooth***Q	Respiration stops

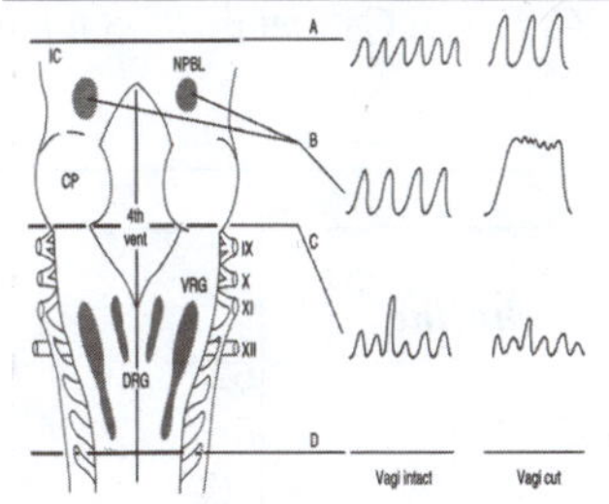

134. C i.e. Ventral surface of medulla **135. B i.e. Inhibited during swallowing** **136. A i.e. ↑PCO_2**
137. A i.e. ↑H^+ **138. A i.e. PO_2** **139. D i.e. H^+**
140. B i.e. Hypocapnia **141. A i.e. Apnea occurs due to hypostimulation of peripheral chemo receptor**
[Ref: John West 8/e p 126-31; Ganong 23/e p. 627-29; Guyton 11/e 517-18; Berne & Levy 6/e p 471-72; Gabriel p-200]

- **Respiratory center is inhibited during swallowing to prevent food aspiration**Q
- Reduction in partial pressure of oxygen is most potent stimulant for the peripheral chemoreceptor and send impulses to respiratory centers. If the O_2 dissolved in blood is high (as in hyperbaric O_2) the peripheral receptors will not be stimulated and **lack of respiratory drive leads to apnea.**Q
- **Central chemoreceptors (in ventral surface of medulla)**Q **are sensitive to dissolved CO_2 (P_{CO2}) in blood (but not to P_{O2}, H^+ concentration or pH of blood) and respond to pH (i.e. H^+ concentration) of CSF (i.e. ECF or interstitial fluid)**Q**. Therefore primary indirect stimulus for excitation of central chemoreceptor is increase in P_{CO2} in blood and primary direct (and more important) stimulus is increase in H^+ ion concentration (or decrease in pH) of CSF**Q**.**
- **Peripheral chemoreceptors (carotid & aortic bodies)** respond to **decrease in P_{O2} (most important stimulus) and pH (↑ H^+ ion concentration in blood)**Q **and increase in arterial P_{CO2}**Q**. Hypercapnia (↑CO_2) does not stimulate either peripheral or central chemoreceptors (only hypercapnia stimulate central receptors)**Q**.**
- If **the peripheral chemo receptor** is denervated the response to - (1) **Arterial hypoxemia (P_{O2}) and pH is completely abolished**Q**. (2) Hyper capnia (arterial P_{CO2}) is reduced by 30%.**

142. C i.e. Bronchial stretch receptors **143. B i.e. Duration of expiration** **144. C i.e Head's paradoxical reflex**
145. B i.e. J receptor*[Ref: Best&Taylor 13/653-649; Ganong 24/664-66; Gabriel p198-99; Berne&Levy 6/ 472-74; JohnWest 8/129-31;Guyton11/ 521-16]*

- **Tidal volume excessive load is prevented by** (or **lung maintains the tidal volume** by) activation of **slowly adapting pulmonary (or bronchial) stretch receptors**Q**.**
- **"Inflation of lungs induces further inflation"** due to elastic recoil of alveoli. With inflation of the lungs, there is augmentation of respiratory effort= **Head's paradoxical reflex.**
- Excessive inflation of lungs cause reflex inhibition of inflation **(& increase duration of expiration)**Q- this is **Hering Breuer inflation reflex** mediated by vagus. Conversely, excessive deflation of lungs cause reflex **inhibition of expiration (decrease duration)**– this is **Hering- Breuer deflation reflex.**
- Physiological role of **J (juxta-capilary/alveolar) reflex** is uncertain but it occurs in **pathological states such as pulmonary congestion, pulmonary edema**Q and embolism when the J recptors are stimulated by large lung hyper inflation, or intravascular chemicals like capsaicin, bradykinin & serotonin etc.
- **Slowly adapting pulmonary stretch receptors** are stimulated by lung inflation (not hyper inflation) - Ganong p 632 table 37.2. Hyper inflation (over stretching) of lungs stimulate stretch receptors and lead to Hering – Breuer inflation reflex. However, more recent work indicates HB reflex **may be important in new born babies but are largely inactive in adult human unless the tidal volume exceeds 1 liter** (John west) /1.5 liter (Guyton), as in exercise. So we can extract inference that, although stretch receptors get stimulated by (normal-quiet) inflation, the HBI reflex occurs only after lung hyper inflation.

Surfactant

146. A i.e. 28 Weeks **147. A i.e. Type II pneumocyte** **148. C i.e. Phospholipids**
149. A i.e. Dipalmitoyl phosphatidyl choline
150. A i.e. Secreted from 26th week..; B i.e. In hyaline membrane disease deficiency …; C i.e. Theraputic application is seen
151. C i.e. Increase in alveolar surface area by the surfactant **152. D i.e. Breaks structure of water in alveoli**
153. A i.e. Surfactants *[Ref: Mtx; Ganong 23/e 596-98; Guyton 11/e 474; Croftan Doughlas 5/e p 19-20, 41, 85; Gabriel p 181-83; John West 8/e p 99-104, 10; Berne & Levy 6/e p 426-27; Langman's 11/e p 204]*

Surfactant is produced by **type II pneumocytes after 20 weeks of gestational age**Q is a mixture of **phospholipids and protein.** It **maintains alveolar stability (integrity)** by **decreasing the surface tension in alveoli (i.e. increasing alveolar surface area by not dissolving uniformly in fluid linning the alveoli = breaking the structure of water in alveoli = keeping alveoli dry)**Q. It is **deficient in hyaline membrane disease where it is therapeutically used**Q. **Surfactant breaks structure of water in alveoli**Q.

Components	%
1. **Phospholipids** eg	77
- ***Dipalmitoyl phosphatidyl choline (DPPC)***Q	62
- Phosphatidyl glycerol (PG)	5
- Other **phospholipids**	10
2. Neutral lipids eg cholesterol and its ester	13
3. Protein: surfactant proteins (SP) like **SP-A, SP-B, SP-C, SP-D**	8
4. Carbohydrate 5. Fatty acid, Calcium	2

154. B i.e. Fibrin *[Ref: Ganong 23/e p.598; Gabriel p. 182; Langman 11/e p. 206Robbins 6/e P 472]*

Hyaline membranes are made up of **fibrinogen**Q and **fibrin**Q mixed with cell debris derived from necrotic type II pneumocytes. **In HMD, functional residual capacity (FRC) is below closing volume (CV)**Q.

Non Respiratory Functions of Lung

155. B i.e. Conversion of angiotensin – I to angiotension II.
156. B i.e. Sodium balance *[Ref: Ganong 23/e p 605-6; John West 8/e p 49-51; Berne & Levy 6/e p 477-83; Pulmonary physiology, Lange 6/e p 215-25; Lecture notes on human physiology 4/e p 400; Respiratory System: Devis & Moore (2003) p 28-29]*

- One of the **most important metabolic (non-respiratory) function of lungs** is **activation of** relatively physiologically inactive decapeptide **angiotensin I** to 50 times more potent (active) vasoconstrictor, pressure (↑BP), aldosterone stimulating octapeptid **angiotensin II** by extracellular ACE on the **surface of endothelial cells in pulmonary circulation.**
- As a part of renin – angiotensin-aldesterone system, lungs indirectly regulate sodium and water balance (and BP). However, lungs also ***directly affect Na+ balane***Q via **epithelial Na+ channels (E NaCs)**. Absorption of excess fluid from alveolar lumen and airways require active transepithelial transport of Na+ by ENaCs (mainly of alveolar type II and possibly type I cells.)

Prolonged immaturity of ENaCs in **IRDS or hyaline membrane disease** result in fluid accumulation and failure of gas exchange.	AR, **cystic fibrosis** disease is characterized by thick, tenacious and dehydrated airway secretions. In CF, mutations in **CFTR (cystic fibrosis trans membrane conductance regulator)**, which is a regulated **Cl⁻ channel**, causes decreased ability to secrete Cl⁻ and therefore **enhance Na+ and water absorption out of airway**. This reduces pericillary fluid and results in thick, sticky and inspissated mucous that cannot be cleared from the mucociliary clearance system l/t recurrent infections.

157. B i.e. Contain serotonin>>D i.e. Respond to a decrease in PO_2 *[Ref:Berne 6/e p.421-25; CRMR vol 4(2008) p. 174-186 PNEC system: Curtz et al]*

Pulmonary neuroendocrinal cell (PNEC) like Kultschitzky cells secrete biological amines including dopamine & **5-hydroxy tryptamine (serotonin).** These cells are more numerous in **fetus** (than adults), **have dual nerve supply** and are **cells of origin for bronchial carcinoid**.

158. B i.e. Respiratory acidosis is compensated by ↓ HCO_3 *[Ref: Ganong 23/e p. 629, 615, 681, 683; John West 8/e p. 84-87; Berne 6/e p – 647-49]*

Respiratory acidosis (↑P_{CO2}) is compensated by **↑HCO_3^-**Q, whereas **metabolic acidosis (↓HCO_3^-)** is compensated by **↓PCO_2**Q.

159. D i.e. Decreased pH with Decreased HCO_3.

Condition	Causes	pH	Primary alteration	Compensation	Defence Mechanism
Normal		7.40	HCO_3^- = 24.1 meq/L	Pco_2 = 40mmHg	
Respiratory Acidosis	- **Hypoventilation** eg emphysema - Breathing 7% CO_2	↓	P_{CO2}↑	HCO_3^-↑	ICF buffers ↑Renal NAE
Respiratory Alkalosis	- **Hyperventilation** - **High altitude**	↑	P_{CO2}↓	HCO_3^-↓	ICF buffers ↓Renal NAE
Metabolic Acidosis	- **Diabetic acidosis** - **Lactic acidosis** (hypoxia) - NH_4Cl ingestion	↓Q	HCO_3^-↓Q	P_{CO2}↓	ICF & ECF buffers Hyper ventilation (↓Pco_2) ↑Renal NAE
Metabolic Alkalosis	- Prolonged vomiting - $NaHCO_3$ ingestion	↑	HCO_3^-↑	Often none or P_{CO2}↑	ICF & ECF buffers Hypoventilation (↑Pco_2) ↓Renal NAE

High Altitude

160. D i.e. Shift of oxygen dissociation curve to the left **161. B i.e. CO_2 wash out**
162. B i.e. ↓ed Barometric pressure, (D) ↓ed PaO_2, (E) ↑ed pH
163. A i.e. Hyperventilation, (B) i.e. Decreased Pa CO_2 (C) pulmonary edema. **164. C i.e. 2-3 days**
165. B i.e. Increased pulmonary capillary pressure (C) i.e. Normal left atrial pressure
[Ref: Guyton 11/e p. 538-41; Ganong 22/e P-684– 686; Chaudhuri5/e P-141-142]

- **In unacclimatized persons mountain (high altitude) sickness i.e. pulmonary &/or cerebral edema develops 8-24 hours after climb and last for 4-8 days**Q.
- **High altitude climbers (at ↓ barometric pressure)** develop **↓PaO_2, increased sensitivity of central chemoreceptors (carotid body receptors) to hypoxia, hyperventilation (↑ed minute ventilation), CO_2 washout causing dyspnea, ↓$PaCO_2$ & ↑pH**Q.
- **Pulmonary edema** in climbers leads to **↑pulmonary capillary pressure & permeability and normal left atrial pressure**Q.

166. A i.e. Hyperventilation; E i.e. Respiratory alkalosis

Acclimatization to altitude occurs through ***respiratory alkalosis produced by the hyperventilation***Q, which shifts the O_2- Hb dissociation curve to left. However, ↑23DPG in RBC of climbers cause ***O_2 dissociation curve to shift right***Q.

Decompression Sickness

167. A i.e. Nitrogen bubble **168. A i.e. Gas embolism d/t N_2** **169. A i.e. Diver; B i.e. Pilot; C i.e. Divers and pilot**
[Ref: Robbins 8/e p 127; Best and Taylor 12/e p 594-95; Guyton 11/e 548-50, 178; Gabriel p 517-19; Sembulingam 5/e p 712-13]

- **Caisson's Disease** is ***nitrogen (N_2) gas embolism***[Q] seen in ***deep sea divers and aviators (pilots)***[Q] on sudden decompression.
- **Air embolim** occurs in **neuro-cranial surgery** and escape from submarines (i.e. person breathing compressed air from a tank). Because the veins in the skull are in non-collapsible chamber, so they cannot collapse and a **negative (suction) pressure develops in dural sinuses** (- 10 mmHg in saggital sinus in standing position). Therefore if dural sinus is opened during surgery, air can be sucked (causing **air embolism**) in venous system. Similarly when a person ascends (from deep sea in submarine) the gases in lung expand and sometimes rupture pulmonary blood vessel, forcing the gases (air) to enter the vessels and cause air embolism.

170. C i.e. Increased solubility of nitrogen in nerve cell membrane *[Ref: Guyton 11th/e p. 545- 46; Gabriel p. 518]*

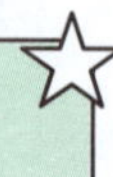

Nitrogen narcosis (toxicity) or raptures of death sets in at around 120 feet and below sea surface because at high tissue concentrations, N_2 behave as anesthetic gases and show **increased solubility in lipid (fatty) substances of neuronal membrane and makes them less excitable by altering ionic conductance**[Q].

Chapter -4 CARDIOVASCULAR SYSTEM

QUESTIONS

Electrical Activity of Heart

1. The following statements are true regarding the SA node except: *(AIIMS 05)*
- A. Is located at the right border of the ascending aorta
- B. It contains specialized nodal cardiac muscle
- C. It is supplied by the artial branches of the right coronary artery
- D. It initiates cardiac conduction

2. Prepotential in SA node is due to all EXCEPT? *(NBE P 13)*
- A. Ca^{2+} spark
- B. Fast sodium channels opening
- C. K^+
- D. Transient Ca chnnel opening

3. Hyperpolarizing cyclic nucleotide (HCN) gated channels have a role in: *(AIIMS 16)*
- A. Cardiac rhythm generation
- B. Generation of mitochondrial action potential
- C. Memory formation
- D. Myocardial muscle contraction

4. Inward flow of Na+ in heart leads to- *(NBE P 13)*
- A. Plateu phase
- B. Action potential
- C. Repolarization
- D. No change

5. Plateau phase of ventricular muscle is d/f opening of
- A. Na+ channel *(NBE P 14,13; PGI 15,12,11)*
- B. K+ channel
- C. Ca++ - Na+ channel
- D. Closure of K+ channel
- E. Closure of CL channel

6. S.A. node acts as a pacemaker of the heart because of the fact that it: *(NBE P 15, 13; AI 05)*
- A. Is capable of generating impulses spontaneously
- B. Has rich sympathetic innervations.
- C. Has poor cholinergic innervations.
- D. Generates impulses at the highest rate.

7. Highest conduction rate in m/s is observed in:
- A. SA node *(NBE P 15,14,13; PGI 05, AI 05)*
- B. AV node
- C. Bundle of His
- D. Purkinje system

8. Least conduction velocity is seen in OR Gatekeeper of the heart is: *(NBE P 15,14,13; PGI 08)*
- A. AV node
- B. Purkinje fibres
- C. Bundle of his
- D. Ventricular myocardial fibres

9. Which of the following is the order of activation after stimulation of Purkinji fibrs is : *(AIIMS 05)*
- A. Septum –> Endocardium –> Epicardium
- B. Endocrdium –> Septum –> Epicardium
- C. Epicardium –> Septum –> Endocardium
- D. Septum –> Epicardium –> Endocardium

10. Repolarization in isolated muscle piece fibre proceeds from: *(PGI 08)*
- A. Epicardium to endocardium
- B. Endocardium to epicardium
- C. Left to right
- D. Right to left

11. Preload leads to- *(NEB P 13)*
- A. Isovolulmetric relaxation
- B. Isovolumetric contraction
- C. Peripheral resistance
- D. Parasympathetic nervous system activation

12. During the cardiac cycle the opening of the aortic valve takes place at the : *(AI 04)*
- A. Beginning of systole
- B. End of isovolumetric contraction
- C. End of diastole
- D. End of diastasis

13. Of the following which one correlates with isovolumic contraction phase: *(AIIMS 08)*
- A. AV opening and aortic and pulmonary valve closure.
- B. AV closure and aortic & pulmonary valve opening.
- C. Both valves are closed
- D. Both valves are open

14. Isovolumic relaxation phase of the cardiac cycle ends with :
- A. Peak of 'C' waves *(AI 2K, NEET 13)*
- B. Opening of A.V. valve
- C. Closure of semilunar valve
- D. Beginning of 'T' wave.

15. Isometric relaxation is defined as- *(NBE P 13)*
- A. Relaxation of both atria
- B. Relaxation of both atria with all valves open
- C. Relaxation of LV with mitral & aortic valve closed

16. Einthovens law- *(NBE P 13)*
- A. I+III=II
- B. I+III=II
- C. I+II+III=0
- D. I+III=avL

17. Einthoven's triangle, what is the value of lead III when lead 1=2mv and Lead =I mv- *(NBE P 13)*
- A. 1
- B. 2
- C. 3
- D. 4

18. C' wave in JVP is due to *(AI 09)*
- A. Atrial contraction
- B. Atrial filling with tricuspid valves closed
- C. Rapid right ventricular filling
- D. Bulging of tricuspid valve into the right atrium

19. The feature of JVP in cardiac tamponade is: *(PGI 09)*
A. Prominent x descent with prominent 'y'descent ☐
B. Prominent x descent with absent 'y' descent ☐
C. Absent x descent with prominent 'y' descent ☐
D. Absent x descent with absent 'y' descent ☐

20. A wave in JVP is due to- *(NBE P 13)*
A. Atrial systole ☐
B. Atrial diastole ☐
C. Ventricular systole ☐
D. Ventricular diastole ☐

21. The left atrial 'v' wave is larger than 'a' wave in comparison to right atrium because: *(AIIMS 14)*
A. Left side is high pressure system ☐
B. Left atrium is more compliant ☐
C. Left atrium is compressed posteriorly by pulmonary veins ☐
D. Right atrial pressure is transmitted into the pulmonary circulation ☐

22. True statement about instantaneous means vector:
A. Equal & same as mean QRS vector *(PGI 11)* ☐
B. It is drawn through the centre of vector in a direction from base toward apex ☐
C. Summated vector of generated potential at particular instant cause by inflowing septal depolarization ☐
D. When a vector is exactly horizontal and directed toward the person's left side, the vector is said to extend in the direction of 0°. ☐

23. Ventricular contraction lasts for: *(PGI 11)*
A. Beginning of Q wave to end of S wave ☐
B. Beginning of Q wave to the end of T wave ☐
C. Beginning of P wave to end of T wave ☐
D. Beginning of R wave to the end of T wave, if Q wave is absent ☐
E. Beginning of P wave to the end of S wave ☐

24. QRS complex indicates : *(AI 08)*
A. Atrial repolarization ☐
B. Atrial depolarization ☐
C. Ventricular repolarization ☐
D. Ventricular depolarization ☐

25. P wave in absent in- *(NBE P 13)*
A. Atrial fibrillation ☐
B. CCF ☐
C. Atrial flutter ☐
D. PSVT ☐

26. Normal duration of PR interval- *(NBE P 13)*
A. 0.12-0.2sec ☐
B. 0.2-0.3sec ☐
C. 0.3-0.4sec ☐
D. 0.4-0.5sec ☐

27. Electromechanical Systole is best defined as the interval between *(AI 12)*
A. Q wave and S2 (Q-S2 Interval) ☐
B. Q wave and S1 (Q-S1 Interval) ☐
C. Q wave and beginning of T wave ☐
D. Q wave and R wave ☐

28. The ECG of a 40 year old male was recorded using standard bipolar limb leads. The sum of voltage of the three standard leads was found to be 5 millivolts. This indicates: *(AIIMS 05)*
A. A normal heart ☐
B. Right ventricular hypertrophy ☐
C. Left ventricular hypertrophy ☐
D. Increased cardiac muscle mass ☐

29. On increasing vagal tone following occurs in pacemaker- *(NBE P 13)*
A. Increased Na^+ increased slop ☐
B. Decreased Na^+ decreased slop ☐
C. Increased Na^+ decreased slop ☐
D. Decreased Na^+ increased slop ☐

30. Vagal stimulation of the heart causes: *(AIIMS 08)*
A. Increased heart rate ☐
B. Increased R – R interval in ECG ☐
C. Increased force of heart contraction ☐
D. Increased cardiac output ☐

31. Hypokalemia ECG changes all except- *(NBE P 13)*
A. Tall T waves ☐
B. Prolonged QRS interval ☐
C. Depressed ST segment ☐
D. Prominent U waves ☐

32. A cardiologist asks for measurement of electromechanical systole (QS_2) and left ventricular ejection time (LVET), and pre-ejection period (PEP). The cardiologist is informed by the technician that the carotid transducer is not functioning. Which of the following readings could not be obtained
A. QS_2 *(AIIMS 02)* ☐
B. QS_2 and LVET ☐
C. QS_2 and PEP ☐
D. LVET and PEP ☐

33. Duration of 2nd heart sound is – *(NBE P 13)*
A. 0.15sec ☐
B. 0.12sec ☐
C. 0.08sec ☐
D. 0.1sec ☐

34. 3rd heart sound is d/t- *(NBE P 13)*
A. Closure of av valve ☐
B. Closure of aortic valve ☐
C. Mid diastolic flow in the ventricle ☐
D. Atrial contraction ☐

35. Fourth heart sound is caused by- *(NBE P 13)*
A. Closure of AV valves ☐
B. Closure of semilunar valves ☐
C. Rapid ventricular filling ☐
D. Atrial contraction ☐

36. Which of the following is true about fourth heart sound 'S4': *(AI 07)*
A. Can be heard by the unaided ear ☐
B. Frequency is greater than 20 Hz ☐
C. Heard during ventricular filling phase ☐
D. Heard during ventricular ejection phase ☐

37. During cardiac imaging the phase of minimum motion of heart is: *(AI 10)*
A. Late systole ☐

B. Mid systole
C. Late diastole
D. Mid diastole

Heart as a Pump

38. Cardiac index in a normal person is
A. 2.1 *(NBE P 13, 14; TN 08, KA 07)*
B. 3.2
C. 4.6
D. 5.9

39. In a patient with cardiac output 5 liters/minute and body surface area 1.7 m² what will be the cardiac index *(PGI 04)*
A. 3 liter/min/m²
B. 4 liter/min/m²
C. 5 liter/min/m²
D. 2.5 liter/mkin/m²
E. 4.7 liter/min/m²

40. Amount of blood in heart- *(NBE P 13)*
A. 250-300ml
B. 500-600ml
C. 1-2 litre
D. 100-200ml

41. Ejection fraction is- *(NBE P 13)*
A. SV/EDV
B. EDV/SV
C. ESV/EDV
D. SV/EDV

42. What is the normal left ventricular ejection fraction? *(NBE P 13)*
A. 20%
B. 30%
C. 50%
D. 65%

43. Basal cardiac output in an adult in nearly:
A. 7.5 litre *(PGI 09)*
B. 5 litre
C. 12 litre
D. 10 litre

44. Cardiac output in L/min divided by heart rate equals:
A. Cardiac efficiency *(NBE P 15,13; AIIMS 14; AI 05)*
B. Mean stroke volume
C. Cardiac index
D. Mean arterial pressure

45. Cardiac index is defined as: *(PGI 06)*
A. Stroke volume M²/BSA
B. C.O.P. per unit body surface area
C. Syst press/M² BSA
D. End diastolic volume

46. The cardiac output can be determined by all except
A. Fick's principle *(PGI 09)*
B. V/Q ratio
C. Echocardiography
D. Thermodilution

47. Cardiac output decreases during: *(AI 12)*
A. High Environmental temperature
B. Anxiety and excitement
C. Eating
D. Standing from lying position

48. Cardiac output is increased in- *(NBE P 13)*
A. Sleep
B. Pregnancy
C. Sitting
D. Standing

49. Which scientific principle is the basis for Thermodilution method used in measurement of cardiac output by pulmonary catheter? *(AIIMS 12)*
A. Hagen-Poisseuille Principle
B. Stewart-Hamilton Principle
C. Bernoulli's Principle
D. Universal Gas Equation

50. Starlings law implies- *(NBE P 13)*
A. Increased VR-increased CO
B. Increased discharge-increased CO
C. Increased HR-increased CO
D. Increased BP-increased CO

51. Preload is increased by- *(NBE P 13)*
A. Increased blood volume
B. Increased total peripheral resistance
C. Standing
D. Sitting

52. End diastolic volume increases due to *(AIIMS 12)*
A. Increase in intrapericardial pressure
B. Decrease in ventricular compliance
C. Decrease in total blood volume
D. Increase in negative intrathoracic pressure

53. All of the following factors normally increase the length of the ventricular cardiac muscle fibers except:
A. Increased venous tone. *(AI 05)*
B. Increased total blood volume.
C. Increased negative intrathoracic pressure.
D. Lying-to-standing change in posture

54. Single most important factor in control of automatic contractility of heart is: *(AI 03)*
A. Myocordial wall thickness
B. Right atrial volume
C. SA node pacemaker potential
D. Sympathetic stimulation

55. Discharge from Baroreceptors causes inhibition of
A. Caudal Ventrolateral Medulla *(AI 12; NBE P 14)*
B. Rostral Ventrolateral Medulla
C. Nucleus ambiguous
D. Nucleus tractus solitarus

56. Which of the following statements about vasomotor centre (VMC) of medulla is true *(AIIMS 11, AI 09)*
A. Independent of corticohypothlamic inputs
B. Influenced by baroceptor signals but not by chemoreceptors
C. Acts along with the cardiovagal centre (CVC) to maintain Blood pressure.
D. Essentially Silent in sleep

57. Baroreceptor reflex, true is- *(NBE P 13)*
A. From aortic and carotid body
B. Causes arterial vasoconstriction when BP falls

C. Causes decrease in HR when BP increases
D. Causes increase in HR when BP increases

58. Baroreceptor stimulation produces: *(PGI 15,13,05)*
A. Decreased heart rate & BP
B. Increased heart rate & BP
C. Increased cardiac contractility
D. Decreased cardiac contractility

59. Clamping of the carotid arteries below the carotid sinus is likely to produce; *(AIIMS 12)*
A. Increase in discharge of carotid sinus afferent nerves
B. Decreased heart rate and blood pressure
C. Increase in vasomotor centre activity
D. Baroreceptor adaptation

60. Clamping of the carotid arteries below (proximal) the carotid sinus is likely to produce: *(AI 12)*
A. Increase in Blood pressure and increase in Heart Rate
B. Decrease in Blood pressure and decrease in Heart Rate
C. Increase in Blood pressure and decrease in Heart Rate
D. Decrease in Blood Pressure and increase in Heart Rate

61. Volume receptors are- *(NBE P 13)*
A. Affected by total cardiovascular output
B. Stimulated by atrial systole and diastole
C. Stimulated by left ventricular contraction
D. Stimulated by aortic pressure

62. A Patient with increased BP and decreased heart rate is likely to have: *(PGI 10,15)*
A. Increased ICT
B. Deep sea diving
C. Brain tumor
D. Head trauma

63. The triad of hypertension, bradycardia and irregular respiration is seen in: *(AIIMS 14)*
A. Cushing's reflex
B. Bezold-Zarisch reflex
C. Herring-Bruer reflex
D. Bainbridge's reflex

64. Which of the following statement is least correct: *(AI 08)*
A. Vagal stimulation decreases rate of contraction
B. Noradrenaline increases force of contraction
C. Denervated heart has more heart rate
D. During Exercise Systole is shortened more than diastole

65. TRUE regarding human heart *(AI 08)*
A. Conduction of impulse from endocardium to inwards
B. During exercise duration of systole is reduced more than diastole
C. HR increases with parasympathetic denervation
D. Vagal stimulation decreases force of contraction

66. Volume determining preload is: *(PGI 08)*
A. End diastolic volume of ventricles
B. Endo systolic volume
C. Volume of blood in aorta
D. Ventricular ejection volume

67. Sympathetic stimulation causes all of the following except : *(NBE P 14, AI 09)*
A. Increase in heart rate
B. Increase in blood pressure
C. Increase in total peripheral resistance
D. Increase in venous capacitance

68. Stroke volume is decreased in- *(NBE P 13)*
A. Lying down
B. Standing
C. Hypervolemia
D. Increased muscle tone

69. When a person changes position from standing to lying down position, following occurs: *(AIIMS 07)*
A. Heart rate increases and settles at a higher level
B. Venous return to the heart rises immediately
C. Cerebral blood flow becomes more than that in standing position and settles at a higher level
D. Decrease in blood flow to the lung apex

70. A shift of posture from supine to upright posture is associated with cardiovascular adjustments. Which of the following is NOT true in this context: *(AIIMS 03)*
A. Rise in central venous pressure.
B. Rise in heart rate.
C. Decrease in cardiac output.
D. Decrease in stroke volume.

71. When a normal person changes position from standing to lying down (supine), following change is seen: *(AIIMS 13, AI 09)*
A. Heart rate increases
B. Venous return to heart increases immediately
C. Cerebral blood flow increases
D. Blood flow at apices of lung decreases

72. In the given circuit, the inward flow pressure is 100mm Hg and the outward flow pressure is 10 mm Hg. Each of the parallel circuit has a resistance of 5 mm Hg/mL/min. Calculate the flow across the circuit: *(AIIMS 14)*

5mmHg/ml/min
5mmHg/ml/min
→ 100 mmHg A
5mmHg/ml/min
→ 100 mmHg B
5mmHg/ml/min
5mmHg/ml/min

A. 45 mL
B. 90 mL
C. 3.6 mL
D. 135 mL

Blood Pressure

73. Which of the following is true about measurement of blood pressure? *(AIIMS 14)*
A. Bladder in the blood pressure cuff should cover more than 80% of the arm area
B. The person should be comfortably sitting and blood pressure cuff should be at a higher level than the heart
C. Caffeine intake induces decrease in blood pressure
D. Blood pressure increases during sleep

74. The blood pressure measured by a sphygmomanometer: *(AI 08)*
A. Is lower than the intraarterial pressure
B. Is higher than the intraarterial pressure
C. Is same as the intraarterial pressure
D. Is the same with different cuff sizes

75. True about blood pressure measurement is all/except:
A. Cuff width should be 40% of arm circumference *(AIIMS 07)*
B. Diastolic blood pressure is indicated by fourth Korotkoff sound
C. Small cuff measures spuriously elevated Diastolic blood pressure
D. Monkenberg sclerosis causes pseudohypertension

76. True statement regarding arterial BP; *(PGI 13)*
A. Diurnal variation present
B. Low when taken with small cuff
C. Standing increases both SBP & DBP
D. Should be measured in both arms
E. Exercise increases both SBP & DBP

77. Windkessel effect is seen in- *(NBE P 13)*
A. Large elastic vessels
B. Capacitance vessels
C. Throughfare channels
D. Capillaries

78. During Diastole, the arterial pressure is maintained by *(AI 09)*
A. Elastic Recoil of aorta
B. Musculature of arteries
C. Constriction of capillaries
D. Contraction of left ventricle

79. Mean arterial pressure is : *(NBE P 14; AI 06)*
A. Systolic + (Diastolic BP)/2
B. Systolic + 1/3rd Pulse pressure
C. Diastolic + (Systolic BP)/2
D. Diastolic + 1/3rd Pulse pressure

80. Mean arterial pressure is calculated as:
A. (SBP + 2DBP)/3 *(NBE P 15; AIIMS 11, 06)*
B. (DBP + 2SBP)/3
C. (SBP + 3DBP)/2
D. (DBP + 3SBP)/2

81. Which of the following defines the pressure in the vascular system in the absence of blood flow? (Asked twice) *(AIIMS 15,14; NBE P 13)*
A. Pulse pressure
B. Critical closing pressure
C. Mean circulatory filling pressure
D. Perfusion pressure

82. Mean circulatory filling pressure is?
A. Difference between systemic and pulmonary arterial pressure *(AIIMS 15,13,08)*
B. Difference between central venous pressure and central arterial pressure
C. Mean atrial pressure
D. Arterial pressure taken at the point when heart stops beating

83. Venous return (VR) is given by formula - *(DNB 09)*
A. VR = (RVR – RAP)/ MFSP
B. VR = (MFSP – RVR)/RAP
C. VR = (MFSP – RAP)/RVR
D. None

84. Blood pressure is defined as the product of:
A. Systolic pressure × pulse *(NBE P 14,13; PGI 08)*
B. Diastolic pressure × pulse rate
C. Pulse pressure × pulse rate
D. Cardiac output × peripheral resistance

85. Spuriously high BP is seen in A/E : *(AIIMS 01)*
A. Auscultatory gap
B. Small cuff
C. Thick calcified vessels
D. Obesity

86. Which is true about measurement of BP with syphgnomonmeter versus intraarterial pressure measurements: *(AI 01)*
A. Less than intravascular pressure
B. More than intravascular pressure
C. Equal to intravascular pressure
D. Depends upon blood flow

87. In a study to measure BP, two students Rakesh and Arif conduct a study on a dog. Rakesh measures BP using a mercury sphygmomanometer on the right femoral artery and Arif measures using a pressure transducer and pulse tracing on the left femoral artery. The mean arterial pressure for both Rakesh and Arif is the same i.e. 100 mmHg. After 5 minutes of injection of adrenaline, Rakesh measures blood pressure 130 mmHg and Arif as 120 mmHg. The difference of 10 mmHg is explained by: *(AIIMS 02)*
A. Falsely high values at low pressure in pulse tracing
B. Falsely low values at high pressure in pulse tracings
C. Femoral artery is more sensitive to adrenaline on right side
D. Ventricular filling affects diastole period

88. As a part of space-research program, a physiologist was asked to investigate the effect of flight-induced stress on blood pressure. Accordingly, the blood pressure of the cosmonauts were to be measured twice: once before the take-off and once after the spacecraft entered the designated orbit around the earth. For a proper comparison, the preflight blood pressure should be recorded in: *(AI 03)*
A. The lying down position

B. The sitting position ☐
C. The standing position ☐
D. Any position, as long as the post-flight recording is made in the same position ☐

89. SI unit for measuring Blood Pressure is : *(AI 02)*
A. Torr ☐
B. mmHg ☐
C. kP_a ☐
D. Barr ☐

90. Pressure on carotid sinus cause: *(PGI 09, AI 10)*
A. Hyperapnea ☐
B. Reflex bradycardia ☐
C. Tachycardia ☐
D. Dyspnea ☐

91. Two students, Vineet and Kamlesh were asked to demonstrate in dogs the role of sinus nerve in hypovolemic shock. Vineet severed the sinus nerve when the mean blood pressure (MBP) was 85 mm Hg and Kamlesh cut the sinus nerve when the mean blood pressure was 60 mm Hg. On cutting the sinus nerve
A. Vineet recorded the increase in MBP but Kamlesh recorded a decrease in MBP ☐
B. Vineet recorded a decrease in MBP but Kamlesh recorded an increase in MBP ☐
C. Both recorded an increase in MBP *(AI 03)* ☐
D. Both recorded a decrease in MBP ☐

92. A pilot in Sukhoi aircraft is experiencing negative G. Which of the following physiological events will manifest in such situation? *(AIIMS 04, AI 06)*
A. The hydrostatic pressure in veins of lower limb increases ☐
B. The cardiac output decreases ☐
C. Black out occurs ☐
D. The cerebral arterial pressure rises ☐

93. Shape of the arterial pulse is influenced by:
A. Viscosity of blood *(AIIMS 06)* ☐
B. Velocity of blood ☐
C. Arterial wall expansion ☐
D. Cross sectional area of artery. ☐

94. A 0.5 litre blood loss in 30 minutes will lead to
A. Increase in HR, decrease in BP *(AI 01)* ☐
B. Slight increase in HR, normal BP ☐
C. Decrease in HR and BP ☐
D. Prominent increase in HR ☐

Cardiovascular Regulatory Mechanism

95. True regarding endothelin-1 are all except:
A. Bronchodilatation *(AIIMS 07)* ☐
B. Vasoconstriction ☐
C. Decreased GFR ☐
D. Has inotropic effect ☐

96. Nitric Oxide is produced in: *(PGI 14, 12, 08)*
A. Endothelium ☐
B. Plasma ☐
C. Platelets ☐
D. Serum ☐

97. All are vasodilators except- *(NBE P 13)*
A. Prostacyclin ☐
B. NO ☐
C. Bradykinin ☐
D. Endothelin ☐

98. Which is not synthesized by vascular endothelium- *(NBE P 13)*
A. Prostacyclin ☐
B. Angiotensin 2 ☐
C. Endothelin ☐
D. Heparin ☐

Circulation Through Special Regions

99. Normal interstitial pressure is- *(NBE P 13)*
A. 10 to 15 mmHg ☐
B. -5 to 0 mmHg ☐
C. 20 to 30 mmHg ☐
D. -10 to -20 mmHg ☐

100. Which of the following favours filtration at the arteriolar end of the capillary bed. *(AIIMS 06)*
A. Decrease in hydrostatic pressure of capillaries ☐
B. Increase in hydrostatic pressure of capillaries ☐
C. Increase in oncotic pressure of capillaries ☐
D. Decrease in oncotic pressure of interstitium ☐

101. Which of the following causes maximal cerebral vasodilation: *(AI 12)*
A. Hypercarbia ☐
B. Hypoxia ☐
C. Lactic Acidosis ☐
D. Exercise ☐

102. Cerebral blood flow is regulated by all except:
A. Blood pressure *(AIIMS 07, 08)* ☐
B. Arterial PCO_2 ☐
C. Potassium ions ☐
D. Cerebral metabolic rate ☐

103. The best method to access the adequacy of replacement of fluid a case of shock: *(AIIMS 2K)*
A. Decrease in thirst ☐
B. Increased PaO_2 ☐
C. Increase in urine output ☐
D. Blood pressure ☐

104. Which of the following is NOT correct regarding capillaries: *(AI 01)*
A. Greatest cross sectional area ☐
B. Contain 25% of blood ☐
C. Contains less blood than veins ☐
D. Have single layer of cells bounding the lumen ☐

105. Which of the following statements is true about capillaries : *(AI 06)*
A. Contain 5% of total blood volume ☐
B. Contain 10 % of total blood volume ☐
C. Velocity of blood flow is maximum ☐
D. Offer maximum resistance to blood flow ☐

106. All are true regarding capillaries *except:* *(NBE P 15,13; AI 04; AIIMS 13)*
A. Have large total cross-sectional area ☐
B. Contain larger quantity of blood than veins ☐

C. Site of gaseous exchange ☐
D. Lined by endothelium ☐

107. Which of the following statements about cutaneous shunt vessels is true: *(AIIMS 11, AI 09)*
A. Perform nutritive function ☐
B. Have role in thermoregulation ☐
C. Not under the control of autonomic nervous system ☐
D. These vessels are evenly distributed throughout the skin ☐

108. The velocity of blood is maximum in the: *(AIIMS 05)*
A. Large veins ☐
B. Small veins ☐
C. Venules ☐
D. Capillaries ☐

109. Maximum difference of BP occurs between: *(PGI 07)*
A. Descending Aorta & common iliac artery ☐
B. Femoral artery & femoral vein ☐
C. Arterial end & venous end ☐
D. Capillaries & venules ☐
E. Venules & vein ☐

110. Microcirculation consist of- *(NBE P 13)*
A. Capillaries ☐
B. Capillaries venules and arterioles ☐
C. Aorta ☐
D. Arteries and veins ☐

111. Arteriole is- *(NBE P 13)*
A. Conduction vessel ☐
B. Resistance vessel ☐
C. Exchange vessels ☐
D. Capacitance vessel ☐

112. Maximum reservoir of blood OR Hightest compliance is seen in which vessel - *(NBE P 13)*
A. Veins ☐
B. Aorta ☐
C. Heart ☐
D. Capillaries ☐

113. Gas exchange in tissues takes place at- *(NBE P 13)*
A. Artery ☐
B. Capillary ☐
C. Vein ☐
D. Venules ☐

114. All are true regarding circulation except *(PGI 09)*
A. Pulsatile flow affects gene transcription ☐
B. Transfused blood is mainly distributed in arteries ☐
C. Hematocrit markedly change peripheral resistance ☐
D. Increased viscosity increases mean blood pressure ☐
E. Non pulsatile flow is recommended ☐

115. Distribution of blood flow in mainly regulated by the: *(AI 05)*
A. Arteries. ☐
B. Arterioles. ☐
C. Capillaries. ☐
D. Venules ☐

116. What is the rise of blood flow if the radius of blood vessel is increased by 50%? *(AIIMS 15)*
A. 5 times ☐
B. 10 times ☐
C. 20 times ☐
D. 100 times ☐

117. True about shear stress on vessel: *(PGI 13)*
A. Parallel to the long axis of blood vessel ☐
B. Perpendicular to long axis of blood vessel ☐
C. Increases with increase in axial velocity of fluid ☐
D. Poiseuille-Hagen equation correlate flow with viscosity ☐
E. Depend upon viscosity ☐

118. Flow is laminar in small vessels because *(AI 11)*
A. Reynolds number is >2000 ☐
B. Total cross sectional area of small vessels is smaller ☐
C. Diameter of smaller vessels is less ☐
D. Effective velocity in small vessels is less ☐

119. Which of the following increases turbulence in blood flow *(AIIMS 06)*
A. Reynolds number less than 2000 ☐
B. Decreases in velocity of blood ☐
C. Decrease in density of blood ☐
D. Increase in diameter of blood vessel ☐

120. Which of these mediate the precapillary sphincter relaxation: *(AIIMS 08)*
A. Local hormones ☐
B. Sympathetic stimulations ☐
C. Catecholamines ☐
D. Capillary filling ☐

121. Coronary blood flow, true is- *(NBE P 13)*
A. 250ml/min ☐
B. Maximum during systole ☐
C. Adenosine decreases it ☐
D. More than skin ☐

122. Blood flow to skeletal muscles (ml/min)- *(NBE P 13)*
A. 100 ☐
B. 200 ☐
C. 400 ☐
D. 800 ☐

123. Brain blood supply- *(NBE P 13)*
A. 55ml/100 gm/min ☐
B. 400ml/100gm/min ☐
C. 100ml/100gm/min ☐
D. 200ml/100gm/min ☐

124. True about blood flow in various organs: *(PGI 13,09,02)*
A. Liver>Kidney>Brain > Heart ☐
B. Liver > Brain > Kidney > Heart ☐
C. Kidney > Brain > Heart > Liver ☐
D. Liver > Heart > Brain > Kidney ☐

125. The local control in blood flow is seen in A/E : *(AI 05, AIIMS 09)*
A. Skin ☐
B. Muscle ☐
C. Splanchnic vessels ☐
D. Cerebrum ☐

126. According to myogenic hypothesis of renal autoregulation, the afferent arterioles contract in response to stretch induced by: *(AIIMS 05)*
A. No release
B. Narodrenaline release
C. Opening of Ca^{2+} channels
D. Adenosine release

127. P.G. increasing the renal blood flow and causing renal vasodilation is/are: *(PGI 03)*
A. PGI_2
B. PGE_2
C. TXA_2
D. $PGF_{1\alpha}$
E. PGF_2

128. Regulation of coronary circulation is? *(NBE P 13)*
A. Autonomic
B. Autoregulatory
C. Hormonal
D. Sympathelic

129. Which one of the following is the correct statement regarding coronary food flow? *(AIIMS 06)*
A. Coronary blood flow is directly related to perfusion pressure and inversely related to resistance
B. Coronary blood flow is inversely related to perfusion pressure and inversely related to resistance
C. Coronary blood flow is directly related to perfusion pressure and also to resistance
D. Coronary blood flow is inversely related to both pressures and resistance

130. True about pulmonary circulation: *(PGI 03)*
A. It receives 30% of cardiac output
B. Hypoxia causes vasoconstriction
C. Blood volume in lung is 450 ml.
D. Pulmonary capillaries contain most of the blood volume in lung
E. It as low resistance

131. True regarding vascularity of lung is: *(AIIMS 02)*
A. Hypoxia causes vasodilation
B. Pulmonary resistance is half of the systemic vascular resistance
C. Perfusion is more in the apical lobe than in base
D. Distended pulmonary veins in the lower lobe

132. Pulmonary circulation differs from systemic circulation *(AIIMS 06, 08)*
A. Pulmonary vasodilation in hypoxia
B. Pulmonary vasoconstriction in hypoxia
C. Decreased blood volume during systole
D. Increased basal vasoconstrictor tone

133. Physiological dead space in lung is
A. Zone 1 *(Jipmer 06, UP08)*
B. Zone 2
C. Zone 3
D. Zone 4

134. True is all except about lung circulation
A. V/P ratio at rest is 0.8 *(PGI 09, WB05, KA03)*
B. In apex ventilation is less than at base
C. Decreased vital capacity in supine position
D. Most blood is in pulmonary capillaries

135. During heavy exercise the cardiac output (CO) increases upto five fold while pulmonary arterial pressure rises very little. This physiological ability of the pulmonary circulation is best explained by:
A. Increase in the number of open capillaries
B. Sympathetically mediated greater distensibility of pulmonary vessels *(AI 10)*
C. Large amount of smooth muscle in pulmonary arterioles
D. Smaller surface area of pulmonary circulation

136. Pulmonary micro-circulation differs from systemic circulation in having: *(AI 05)*
A. Resistance low, pulsatile flow high
B. Resistance low, capillary pressure low
C. Resistance high, pulsatile flow low
D. Resistance high, capillary pressure high

137. All of the following statements about bronchial circulation are true, Except: *(AI 10)*
A. Contribute 2% of systemic circulation
B. Contribute to gaseous exchange
C. Cause venous admixing of blood
D. Provide nutritive function to lung

138. Deoxigenated Blood is carried by all except:
A. Pulmonary Artery *(AI 11)*
B. Umbilical Vein
C. Right ventricle
D. Umbilical Art.

139. Max. blood supply to liver is by: *(PGI 2K)*
A. Portal Vein
B. Hepatic A
C. Splenic A
D. Mesenteric A

140. Wedged hepatic venous pressure represents pressure in: *(AIIMS 04)*
A. Main portal vein
B. Main hepatic vein
C. Sinusoids
D. Central vein radicles

141. Effectiveness of blood brain barrier is by:
A. Tight endothelial function *(AIIMS 2K)*
B. Microglial cell
C. Thick basement membrane
D. Tight arrangement of astrocyfes

142. Protein filtration across cerebral capillaries is limited by: *(AIIMS 05, 02)*
A. Fibrous tissue
B. Foot process of astrocytes
C. Low BP
D. High CSF pressure

143. Which of the following statements about myocardial oxygen demand is true: *(AI 09)*
A. Correlates with heart rate
B. Is directly proportional to external cardiac work
C. Is negligible when heart is at rest
D. Depends upon duration of systole

144. True regarding myocardial O_2 demand? *(AIIMS 11)*
A. Inversely related to heart rate
B. Has constant relation to external cardiac work
C. Directly proportional to duration of systole
D. Is negligible at rest

145. About Myocardial Oxygen Consumption true is:
A. Inverse relation with heart rate *(AIIMS 07)*
B. Inverse relation to mean systolic arterial pressure
C. Constant relation to external work done
D. Negligible in quiescent heart
E. Directly proportional to mean arterial pressure

146. Myocardial oxygen demand depend upon:
A. Preload *(PGI 09)*
B. Afterload
C. Intramyocardial tension
D. Myocardial muscle mass
E. Blood Hb concentration

147. Blood supply during exercise is increased in:
A. Cutaneous circulation *(AI 05)*
B. Hepato-splanchnic circulation
C. Renal circulation
D. Coronary circulation

148. Aerobic capacity is maximally increased by :
A. Regular 3 minute exercise *(AI 07)*
B. Spurts of exercise
C. Prolonged exercises
D. Sternous exercises

149. In a patient with a transplanted heart which of these are the reasons for increased cardiac output during exercise: *(PGI 02)*
A. Reinnervation of transplanted heart by vagus
B. Intrinsic mechanism
C. Epinephrine from medulla
D. Bainbridge reflex
E. Frank-Starling mechanism

150. Blood in splanchnic area during exercise is decreased due to : *(AI 07)*
A. Venoconstriction with decreased blood flow
B. Venodilation with decreased blood flow
C. Venodilation with increased blood flow
D. Venodilation with normal blood flow

151. The vasodilatation produced by carbon dioxide is maximum in one of the following: *(AI 05)*
A. Kidney.
B. Brain.
C. Liver.
D. Heart.

152. Patients having acute cardiac failure do not show oedema, because : *(AI 04)*
A. The plasma oncotic pressure is high
B. There is renal compensation
C. There is an increase in cardiac output
D. There is a fall in the systemic capillary hydrostatic pressure

153. The pressure-volume curve is shifted to the left in
A. Mitral regurgitation *(AIIMS 04)*
B. Aortic regurgitation
C. Mitral stenosis
D. Aortic stenosis

154. In the following diagram, left ventricular pressure is equal to diastolic blood pressure indicated by which point? *(AIIMS 15)*

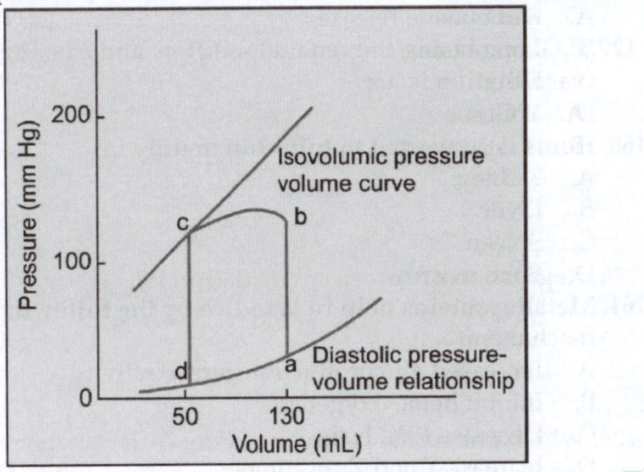

A. A
B. B
C. C
D. D

155. Calculate the ejection fraction from the given volume pressure curve: *(AIIMS 15)*

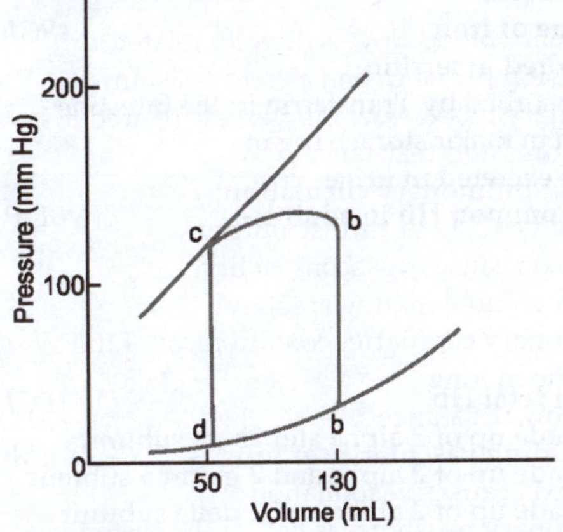

A. 40%
B. 50%
C. 55%
D. 60%

Circulating Body Fluid

156. Lymphocytes are produced in- *(NBE P 13)*
A. Lymph node
B. Thymus
C. Bone marrow
D. None

157. In Fetal life RBC are produced in all except-
A. Liver *(NBE P 13)*
B. Lymph node
C. Spleen
D. Bone marrow

158. Erythopoiesis in gestation age takes place in- *(NBE P 13)*
A. Yolk sac
B. Placenta
C. Amniotic sac
D. Chorion

159. Site of RBC formation in 20 year old healthy male is *(AI 07)*
A. Flat bones
B. Long bones
C. Liver
D. Yolk sac

160. Heme is converted to bilirubin mainly in: *(AI 05)*
A. Kidney.
B. Liver.
C. Spleen.
D. Bone marrow.

161. Metalloproteins help in jaundice by the following mechanism : *(AI 01)*
A. Increased glucoronyl transferase activity
B. Inhibit heme oxygenase
C. Decrease RBC lysis
D. Increase Y and Z receptors

162. Which of the following protein inhibits heme loss from plasma- *(NBE P 13)*
A. Ferritin
B. Hemopexin
C. Ceruloplasmin
D. Hmosiderin

163. What is true of iron: *(PGI 2K)*
A. It is stored in ferritin
B. It is absorbed by Transferrin in the intestine
C. Spleen in major storage organ
D. Fe^{++} is excreted in urine

164. 2nd Most Common Hb in adult is- *(NBE P 13)*
A. $\alpha2\beta$
B. $\alpha2\gamma2$
C. $\alpha2\delta2$
D. $\beta2\gamma2$

165. True about fetal Hb *(PGI 12)*
A. It is made up of 2 alpha and 2beta subunit
B. It is made up of 2 alpha and 2 gamma subunit
C. It is made up of 2 alpha and 2 delta subunit
D. It has high affinity for oxygen
E. It has low affinity for oxygen

166. The type of hemoglobin that has least affinity for 2,3-Diphosphoglycerate (2,3-DPG) or (2,3-BPG) is:
A. Hg A. *(AI 05)*
B. Hg F.
C. H B.
D. Hg A_2.

167. Embryonic hemoglobin is mainly composed of?
A. Alpha and gamma chains *(AIIMS 13)*
B. Alpha and beta chains
C. Zeta and epsilon chains
D. Alpha and delta chains

168. ADT test is for: *(PGI 08)*
A. Bence jounes protein
B. Fetabl Hb
C. Albumin
D. Myoglobin

169. The following image shows cell count in different squares of a Neubauer's chamber after charging with 20 times diluted blood. What is the total leukocyte count? *(AIIMS 16)*

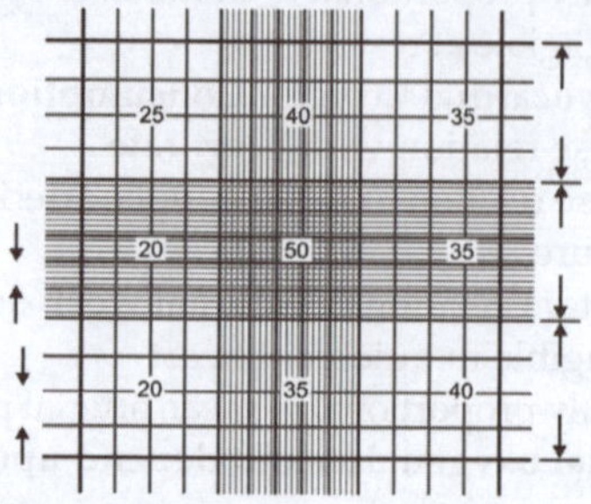

A. 6000 per cu mm
B. 2400 per cu mm
C. 3000 per cu mm
D. 14200 per cu mm

170. In this Leishman's stained blood smear, identify the cell which is raised markedly in worm infestations.

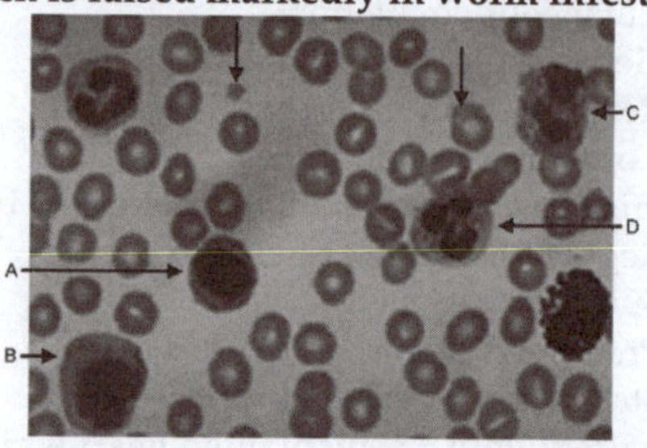

A. C *(AIIMS 16)*
B. B
C. D
D. A

171. Which of the following situations will lead to increased viscosity of blood: *(AIIMS 05)*
A. Fasting state
B. Hypoglycemia
C. Multiple myeloma
D. Amyloidogenesis

172. Albumin is important factor in maintaining osmotic pressure, has: *(AIIMS 08)*
A. Low molecular weight and high blood concentration
B. Low molecular weight and low blood concentration.
C. High molecular weight and low blood concentration.
D. High molecular weight and high blood concentration.

173. Thrombosthenin is a/an: *(AIIMS 07)*
A. Thrombosis preventing protein
B. Contractile protein
C. Coagulation protein
D. Protein for regulating platelets production

174. Central lymphoid organs are: *(PGI 03)*
A. Bone marrow
B. Lymph node
C. Thymus

D. Spleen ☐
E. Tonsil ☐

175. True about cytokines are all except: *(PGI 07)*
A. It is polypeptide ☐
B. Have autocrine and paracrine effects ☐
C. Involve in leukocytic movements ☐
D. It takes part in intrinsic enzymatic reaction ☐

176. Helper and cytotoxic cells belong to:
A. T cells *(PGI 07)* ☐
B. B cells ☐
C. Monocytes ☐
D. Macrophages ☐

177. Lysozymes are found in: *(PGI 05)*
A. Eukaryotes ☐
B. Prokaryotes ☐
C. Plants ☐
D. Bacteriophage ☐
E. Virus ☐

178. G-CSF and GMCSF in haematopoisis causes:
A. Leucocytosis *(AI 09, 06)* ☐
B. Erythrocytosis ☐
C. Leucopenia ☐
D. Thrombocytosis ☐

179. Macrophages release(s): *(PGI 12)*
A. IL-2 ☐
B. IL-6 ☐
C. IL-1 ☐
D. TNF-α ☐
E. Interferon ☐

180. Neutrophil secretes: *(PGI 02)*
A. Superoxide dismutase ☐
B. Myeloperoxidase ☐
C. Lysozymal enzyme ☐
D. Catalase ☐
E. Cathepsin G ☐

181. Which is/are true of NK cell: *(PGI 12)*
A. It is a large glanular lymphocyte ☐
B. Releases granzymes and perforins ☐
C. Depends on antibody for killing ☐
D. Depend on thymus for killing ☐
E. Can kill virus infected and cancer cells ☐

182. Absolute monocytosis is seen in: *(PGI 06)*
A. Infectious mononucleosis ☐
B. Kala-azar ☐
C. TB ☐
D. Brucellosis ☐

183. Source of TNF are *(PGI 04)*
A. Endothelium ☐
B. Neutrophil ☐
C. Macrophage ☐
D. Basophils ☐
E. B Cells ☐

184. Life span of neutrophils is: *(PGI 07)*
A. 6 hours ☐
B. 6 days ☐
C. 10 days ☐
D. 15 days ☐

185. Function of lymphatics *(PGI 02)*
A. Increases oncotic pressure ☐
B. Carries protein ☐
C. Immunocompetent cells ☐
D. Fat absorption ☐
E. Preventive role in infection ☐

Clotting & Anticlotting

186. All are vitamin K dependent clotting factors of hepatic origin except: *(PGI 15,13,09)*
A. II ☐
B. VII ☐
C. VIII ☐
D. X ☐

187. Not a vit. K dependent factor: *(NBE P 13, 15; PGI 08)*
A. II ☐
B. VII ☐
C. IX ☐
D. XII ☐

188. Activity of factor VIII procoagulant is deficient in:
A. Haemophilia *(PGI 08)* ☐
B. Von Willibrand's disease ☐
C. ITP ☐
D. Sickle cell anemia ☐

189. True about Haemophilia A are all *except* :
A. PTT increased *(AI 01)* ☐
B. PT increased ☐
C. Clotting time is increased. ☐
D. Serum levels of factor VIII are decreased. ☐

190. Which of the following is not involved in intrinsic pathway?
A. Factor XII *(AI 09, AIIMS 15,13)* ☐
B. Factor XI ☐
C. Factor IX ☐
D. Factor VII ☐

191. The substance that is present in both serum and plasma is:
A. Fibrinogen *(AI 07)* ☐
B. Factor VII ☐
C. Factor V ☐
D. Factor II ☐

192. Half life of factor VIII- *(NBE P 13)*
A. 2-4 ☐
B. 8-12 ☐
C. 6 minutes ☐
D. 60 days ☐

193. Which of the following helps in bridging the fibrin in a clot and stabilizes the clot OR The clot formed is not stable unless extensive cross-linking occurs. This extensive cross-linking of blood clot is done by?
A. Factor XIII *(AIIMS 15,14; AI 09)* ☐
B. Factor V ☐
C. Factor VIII ☐
D. Factor III ☐

194. Conversionof fibrinogen to fibrin is by- *(NBE P 13)*
A. Prothrombin ☐
B. Factor XIII ☐
C. Thrombin ☐
D. Kallikrein ☐

195. Which of the following coagulation factors causes cross linking and stabilization of clot *(AI 08)*

A. Factor XIII ☐
B. Thrombin ☐
C. Factor VIII ☐
D. Factor IX ☐

196. Which of the following anticoagulants prevent clotting of blood in the normal vascular system: *(AI 12)*

A. Antithrombin III ☐
B. Plasminogen ☐
C. Fibrinogen ☐
D. Heparin ☐

197. Thrombomodulin I is produced by all of the following EXCEPT *(AI 08)*

A. Splanchnic circulation ☐
B. Skin circulation ☐
C. Cerebral circulation ☐
D. Muscle circulation ☐

198. The blood within the vessels does not clot normally because: *(AI 08)*

A. Vitamin K antagonists are present in plasma ☐
B. Thrombin has a positive feedback on plasminogen. ☐
C. Sodium citrate in plasma chelates calcium ions ☐
D. Vascular endothelium is smooth and coated with glycocalyx ☐

199. Thrombin activity is inhibited by *(AI 08)*

A. Chymotrypsin ☐
B. Heparin cofactor II ☐
C. Alpha 2 antitrypsin ☐
D. Alpha 2 macroglobulin ☐

200. Thromboxane A2 causes- *(NBE P 13)*

A. Vasodilatation and platelet aggregartion ☐
B. Vasodilatation and anti platelet aggregatory ☐
C. Vasoconstriction and anti platelet aggregatory ☐
D. Vasoconstriction and platelet aggregartion ☐

201. During homeostasis, platelet affects the coagulation area: *(PGI 04)*

A. Platelet adhesion to exposed endothelium ☐
B. Clot retraction ☐
C. Activation of prothrombinase complex ☐
D. Vasoconstriction ☐
E. Conversion of fibrinogen to fibrin ☐

202. Although more than 400 blood groups have been identified, the ABO blood group system remains the most important in clinical medicine because:

A. It was the first blood group system to be discovered. *(AIIMS 03)* ☐
B. It has four different blood groups A,B,AB,O(H) ☐
C. ABO (H) antigens are present in most body tissues and fluids. ☐
D. ABO (H) antibodies are invariably present in plasma when persons RBC lacks the corresponding antigen. ☐

203. True about ABO blood group antigen: *(PGI 11)*

A. Found on RBC membrane ☐
B. Glycprotein in nature ☐
C. Highly immunogenic ☐
D. Autosomal recessive inheritance ☐

204. The genotype of a person with blood group 'A' should be:

A. OO *(AI 12)* ☐
B. BO ☐
C. AB ☐
D. AO ☐

205. Memory cell in immune system are long lived and escape apoptosis because of: *(PGI 09)*

A. Insulin like growth factor ☐
B. Fibroblast growth factor (FGF) ☐
C. Platelet derived growth factor ☐
D. Nerve growth factor ☐

206. Erythropoiesis is promoted by all of the following except: *(AIIMS 04)*

A. ACTH ☐
B. Thyroxine ☐
C. Oestrogen ☐
D. Prolactin ☐

207. What is not true for extrasystole in ventricle :

A. Falls to produce radial pulse *(AIIMS 09)* ☐
B. Hints at serious heart ailment ☐
C. Associated with abnormal QRS complex ☐
D. Tendency to be followed by a compensatory pause ☐

208. Reticulocytes are stained with: *(AIIMS 04)*

A. Methyl violet ☐
B. Brilliant cresyl blue ☐
C. Sudan Black ☐
D. Indigocarmine ☐

209. A procoagulant not normally circulating in the plasma is: *(AIIMS 03)*

A. Prothrombin ☐
B. Fibrinogen ☐
C. Antithemophilic factor ☐
D. Factor V ☐
E. None of the above ☐

210. Furasol DA is : *(AI 06)*

A. Free radical ☐
B. Artificial blood ☐
C. CO antagonist ☐
D. Used to increase O_2 delivery to tissue ☐

211. Which of the following is true regarding hydroxyl ethyl starch : *(AI 02)*

A. It is an anesthetic agent ☐
B. It is a plasma expander ☐
C. It is a crystalloid ☐
D. Used as a nutritional agent ☐

212. Hydroxyethyl starch is a *(AI 04)*

A. Vasodilator ☐
B. Inotrope ☐
C. Plasma expander ☐
D. Diuretic ☐

213. Ringer lactate contains all EXCEPT:

A. Chloride *(AIIMS 07)* ☐
B. Sodium ☐
C. Bicarbonate ☐
D. Potassium ☐

ANSWERS & EXPLANATIONS:

Electrical Activity of Heart

1. **A i.e. Is located at the right border of ascending aorta** *[Ref: Moore 4/e P-137; BDC 4/e Vol. I P-245-50]*

> **S.A node** is located at the ***junction of superior venacave with right atrium***Q just deep to the epicardium, near the superior end of sulcus terminalis and **AV node** is located in the *right postero-inferior region of interatrial septum* near the opening of coronary sinus.

2. **B i.e. Fast sodium channels opening** *[Ref: Ganong 24/ep 523]*

> **Prepotential or Pacemaker potential i.e. the action potential in SA & AV** nodes are ***d/t*** Ca^{++}***, with no contribution by*** Na^{+} ***influx***Q, so there is no sharp, rapid depolarizing spike before the plateau, as there in other parts. *Prepotentials are prominent only in SA & AV nodes*, **but latent pacemakers are present in other parts of conducting system. However, atrial & ventricular muscles do not have prepotentials**Q

Pacemaker (Pre) Potential

- The various parts of conducting system and myocardium are capable of spontaneous discharge. However ***SA node normally discharges most rapidly***Q, depolarization spreading from it to the other regions before they discharge. The SA node is there fore the **normal cardiac pacemaker**, its rate of discharge determining the rate at which the heart beats.
- Rhythmically discharging cells have a membrane potential, that after each impulse, declines to the firing level. Thus this **prepotential or pacemaker potential** triggers the next impulse.

Repolarization	At the peak of each impulse **IK (the K^{+} current, K^{+} efflux) by opening of K^{+} channels** begins &brings about repolarization
Depolarization (Start)	**IK then declines (K^{+} efflux decreases)**, the membrane begins to depolarize forming the *first part of prepotential*

Slow depolarization starts d/t opening of **Funny (F)/Hyper polarization (H) channels** (so called because of their **unusual/funny activation by hyper polarization and can pass both Na^{+} & K^{+}). As funny current (I_h) increases, depolarization begins forming first part of prepotential**

Depolarization (Late)	- The calcium current **(Ica)** d/t opening of **T (transient)** channels *completes the prepotential* and **Ica** d/t opening of **L (long lasting)** channels produce the impulse. - **Local Ca^{++} release *(Ca^{++} spark)* from sarcoplasmic reticulum occurs during prepotential**Q

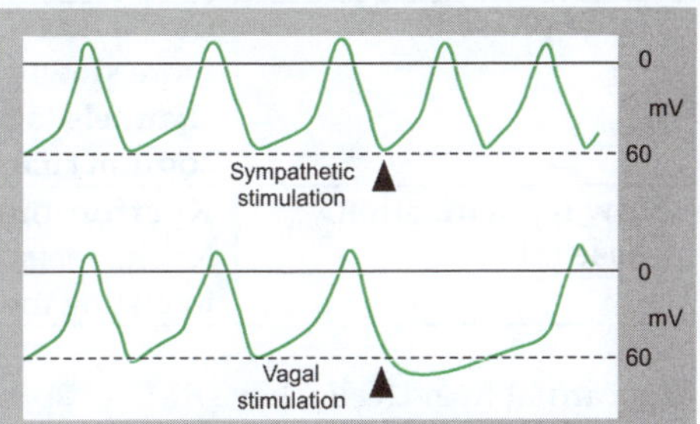

Effect of sympathetic (noradrenergic) and vagal (cholinergic) stimulation on the membrane potential of the SA node.

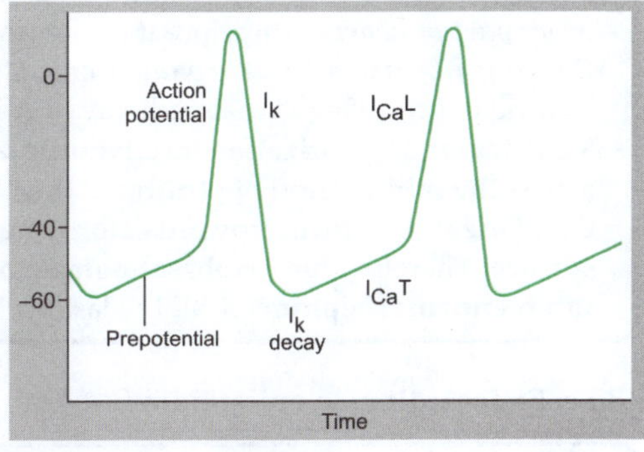

- When the *cholinergic (vagal)* fibers to nodal tissue are stimulated, the membrane becomes *hyperpolarized* and the *slope of prepotentials decreased*, because Ach acts on M_2 muscarinic receptors and *open K+ channels*. The resulting IKAch *counters the decay of IK*. In addition activation of M_2 receptors decreases C- AMP and *slows opening of Ca^{++} channels* resulting in decrease in firing rate.
- **Sympathetic stimulation** *increases* the *rate of spontaneous discharge* and makes the *membrane potential fall more rapidly* (d/t opening of *L channels*)
- Discharge frequency also increase with temperature rise (1/t tachycardia) and *digitalis* exerts effect like that of vagal stmulation particularly on the AV node.

3. **A i.e. Cardiac rhythm generation** *[Ref: Ganong 24/ep 523]*

- **Hyper polarization activated cyctic Nucleotide Gated (HCN) channels** also k/a **H channels or Funny (F) channels d/t unusual (funny) activation** (in hyper polarization phase), are nonselective cation channels found in plasma membranes of **heart & brain cells**. It is encoded by 4 genes HCN 1, 2, 3.

- It is also k/a **pacemaker channel** as it generates **rhythmic activity in SA/AV nodes** and neuronal rhythmicity in CNS. It produces **funny/hyperpolarizing current (I_F or I_h).**

4. **B i.e. Action potential**

5. **C i.e. Ca^{++}-Na^+ Channel** *[Ref: Ganong 24/e p – 522-23; Guyton 12/e p 115-117, 102-103]*

In **Cardiac (e.g. Ventricular) Muscle**

Phase	Is due to
Rapid depolarization phase or development of action potential (O)	**Na^+ influx** through **rapidly opening fast Na^+ channels** (Na^+ current, INa)
Initial rapid repolarization phase (1)	Inactivation of Na^+ channel
Platue phase (2)	Ca^{++} influx (Ca^{++}current, Ica) through more **slowly opening (slow) Ca^{++} channels** (also called **calcium-sodium channels)**
Slow repolarization phase (3)	**K^+ efflux** through multiple types of K^+ channels, allows the cell to return to resting membrane potential

Myocardial fibers (cells) have RMP of approximately **-90mv.**

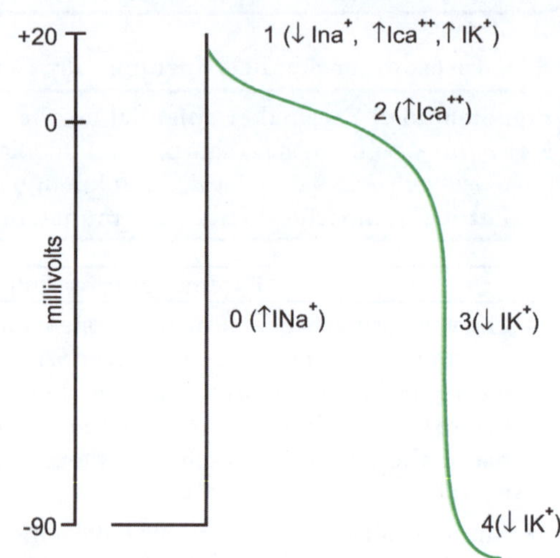

6. **D i.e. Generates impulses at the highest rate.**

7. **D i.e. Purkinje system**

8. **A i.e. AV node**
[Ref: Ganong 24/e p. 524; Berne & Levy 6/e p. 308]

9. **A i.e. Septum – Endocardium – Epicardium**

- ***Sinus node (located sub epicardially)***[Q] controls the beat of heart because ***its rate of discharge is greater than that of any other part of heart***[Q]. Therefore it is the *pacemaker of heart*.
- ***Purkinje fibers has fastest conduction***[Q]**. Conduction Rate in decreasing order: *Purkinje fibers*** [Q] > Bundle of His = Ventricular muscle = Atrial pathway> SA node > ***AV node***[Q].So **AV node is k/a "Gate keeper of heart".**
- **Ventricular depolarization (excitation)** starts from ***left side of interventricular septum***[Q] and moves first to the **right across the mid portion of septum**. It then travels **down the septum to the apex of heart**. From apex, the wave of depolarization **returns upwards along the ventricular walls to AV groove**, proceeding from **endocardial to epicardial surface**. Therefore, **posterobasal portion of the left ventricle, pulmonary conus** and **uppermost portion of interventicular septum** are all the last parts of heart to be depolorized (excited).

10. **B i.e. Endocardium to epicardium** *[Ref: Harrison 16/e P-1314; Best and Taylor's 12/e P 177, Guyton 8/27]*

Repolarization in isolated ventricular muscle fibre is from endocardium to epicardium[Q], whereas in whole heart the direction is from epicardium to endocardium.

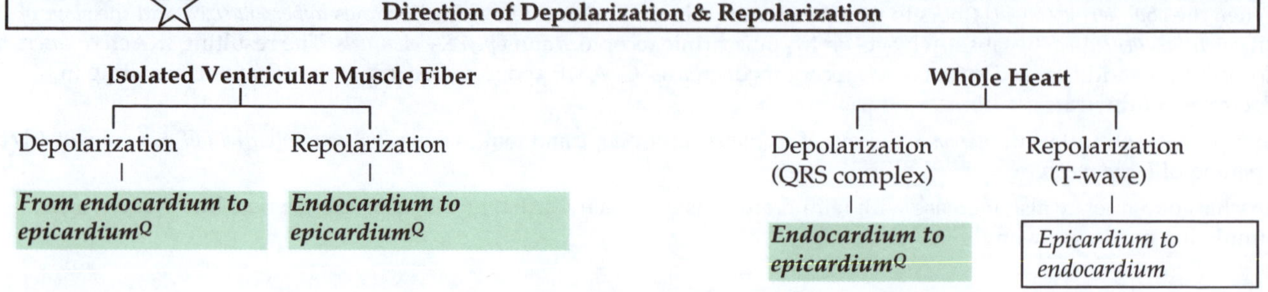

Normal Spread of Cardiac Excitation (Depolarization or Electrical Activity)

- **Depolarization begins in SA node** (located subepicardially) which is the **pacemaker of heart** as it ***generates impulses at the highest rate***[Q].
- The excitation (depolarization) spreads through **atria** to converge on **AVnode.** Because of slow conduction in **AV node**, there is a **AV node delay** of about **0.1s** before depolarization spreads to **ventricle**. This delay is ***shortened by sympathetic stimulation and lengthened by vagal stimulation.*** A marked loss of conduction is seen when there is *lack of I_{Na} in depolarization phase (O).*
- After AV node, the wave of excitation spreads **from top of septum in rapidly conducting Purkinje fibers to all parts of ventricle** in 0.08 – 0.1s.
- **Ventricular depolarization (excitation)** starts from ***left side of interventricular septum***[Q] and moves first to the **right across the mid portion of septum**. It then travels **down the septum to the apex of heart**. From apex, the wave of depolarization **returns upwards along the ventricular walls to AV groove**, proceeding from **endocardial to epicardial surface**. Therefore, **posterobasal portion of the left ventricle, pulmonary conus** and **uppermost portion of interventicular septum** are all the last parts of heart to be depolarized (excited).

Order of Depolarization of Septum

- Left → Mid → Right
- Upper → Lower → Upper most

Order of Depolarization (Activation) of Ventricular Muscle

- Endocardial surface of both ventricles are activated rapidly but the wave of **excitation spreads from endocardium** to epicardium at a slower velocity (0.3 – 0.4 m/sec)
- **Epicardial surface of right ventricle is depolarized (activated) earlier than left** because of its thinner wall.
- **Apical and central epicardial** regions of both ventricles are activated earlier than their respective basal regions.

Purkinje system inside the inter ventricular septum (excluding basal portion) is **depolarized first (along with papillary muscles)**

↓

Entire **endocardium** of ventricles

|

through **ventricular muscle**

↓

Epicardium

Conduction Rates (Speeds) in Cardiac Tissue*

Tissue	Conduction rate (m/s)	Relative value
S A node	0.05	***2nd least*** [Q]
Atrial pathway	1	
AV node	0.02 – 0.05	***Least*** [Q]
Bundle of His	1	
Purkinje system	4[Q]	***Highest***[Q]
Ventricular muscle	1	

- **Conduction Rate in decreasing order:** ***Purkinje fibers*** [Q] > Bundle of His=Ventricular muscle=Atrial pathway> SA node > ***AV node***[Q]

Rhythmicity of Heart

Tissue	Rate of impulse generation
SA node	70-80/minutes ***(Highest)***[Q]
AV node	40-60/minutes
Bundle of His	40/minutes
Purkinje system	24/minutes

- **Rate of impulse generation to decreasing order:**
- ***SA node***[Q] > AV node > Bundle of His > ***purkinje system***[Q]
- *AV node* and *purkinje fibres* are also capable of generating impulses spontaneously but SA node discharges most rapidly (70-80/min) & depolarizes the AV node and purkinje fibres before they can reach their own threshold for self excitation.

Order of Activation of Ventricular Muscle

First the Purkinje system inside the **septum**[Q]

↓

Entire ***Endocardium***[Q] of ventricle

↓ *through ventricular muscle*

Epicardium[Q]

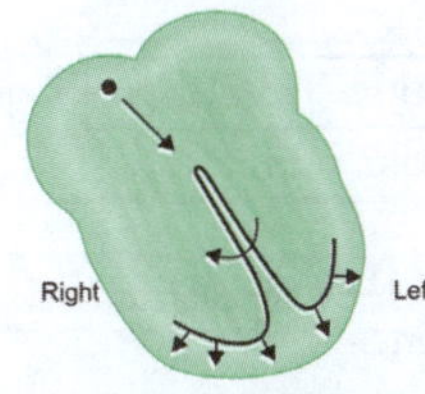

From SA node to AV node; Left to Right; Endo to Epi cardium[Q]

Normal Spread of Electrical Activity

- **Order of spread of cardiac excitation**
  SA node → Atrium → AV node →Bundle of His → Purkinje system →Ventricular muscles
- **Order of activation of ventricular muscle**
  - Depolarization starts at the ***left side of interventricular septum***[Q] → Moves first to the right across the *mid portion of septum* → Activation of *anteroseptal region of ventricular mayocardium (apex)* → Major portion of ventricular myocardium from ***endocardium to epicardium***[Q].
  - Last part to be depolarized are:

1-Posterobasal portion of left ventricle[Q] ***(epicardial region)***
2-Pulmonary Conus
3-Upper most (basal) portion of interventricular septum[Q]

11. B i.e. Isovolumetric contraction

Preload	Tension on muscle when it starts to contract. For heart it is usually end diastolic pressure when ventricles has filled
After load	Load against which muscle contracts. For heart it is pressure in aorta or resistance in circulation

12. B i.e. End of isovolumetric contraction

13. C i.e. Both value are closed

14. B i.e. Opening of A.V. value *[Ref: Ganong 24/e P- 540-45; Chaudhuri 5/e P- 176; Sembulingum 3/e P- 436]*

15. C i.e. Relaxation of LV with mitral & aortic valve closed

- **During isovolumic contraction phase both semilunar (=aortic & pulmonary) valves and AV (mitral & tricuspid) valves are closed**[Q]**. Opening of aortic & pulmonary valves** take place **at the end of isovolumetric contraction & or at the beginning of ventricular ejection**[Q].
- Similarly during **isovolumetric ventricular relaxation phase both AV and semilunar valves are closed. It ends with opening of AV valves**[Q], permitting the ventricles to fill.

Mechanical Events in Cardiac Cycle (= 0.80 sec)

Valves	**Ventricular systole=0.27 sec**		**Diastole = 0.53 sec**			
	Isovolumetric Ventricular Contraction = 0.05sec	**Ventricular Ejection = 0.22 sec**	**Proto-diastole 0.04 sec**	**Isovolumetric Ventricular Relaxation =0.08sec**	**Late Diastole VF**	**Atrial Systole VF**
AV (Bi/Tricuspid)	Closed	Closed	Closed	Closed	Open	Open
Aortic & Pulmonary	Closed	Open	Closed	Closed	Closed	Closed

Valvular event (valves)	Cardiac events	ECG	JVP (Jugular Venous Pressure curve)
Opening of AV valve[Q]	**End of isovolumic relaxation phase**[Q]	**End of T wave**[Q] (phase b/w T wave and new p wave)	**V-Y descent**[Q]
Closure of AV valve	-End of diastole - Beginning of isovolumic contraction	Later half of R wave	**End of 'x' descent**
Opening of semilunar valve	**End of isovolumic contraction**[Q]	ST segment	**Peak of 'C' wave**[Q]
Closure of semilunar valve	- Beginning of isovolumic relaxation phase - Beginning of diastole	Later half of T wave	

16. A i.e. I+III=II

Einthoven's Equilateral Triangle

- With the **heart in center** as moving dipole, it is formed by **two shoulder & pubis.**
- But electrodes are connected to **left arm (LA), right arm (RA)** and **left leg (LL)** for convenience.
- All 3 corners **always have O potentials** and so are k/a **indifferent electrode (central terminal of Wilson).**

17. A i.e. 1 *[Ref: Guyton 12/e p 125]*

Einthoven's Bipolar (Standard) Limb Leads between

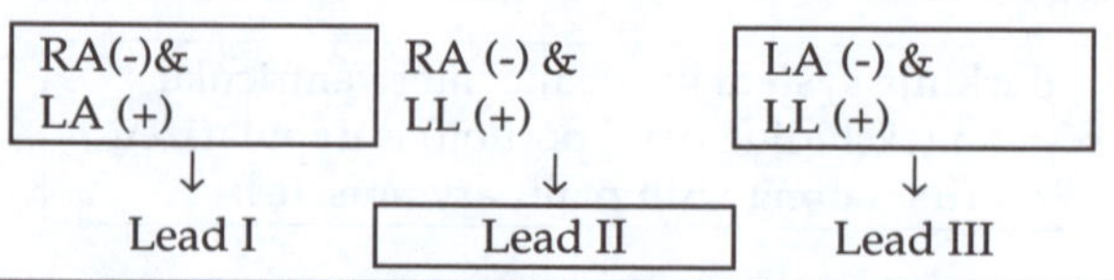

Einthoven's Law for Sum of Electrical Potential (Voltage) in Leads

I+III=II

18. **D i.e. Bulging of tricuspid valve into the right atrium** *[Ref: Harrison 16/e P- 1305,1306]*
19. **B i.e. Prominent X descent with absent 'Y' descent.**
20. **A i.e. Atrial systole**

- **'C 'wave** in JVP is due to **bulging of tricuspid (AV) valve into right atrium**[Q] during right ventricular isovolumetric contraction.
- JVP in **cardiac temponade** has **prominent x descent** with **absent Y descent**[Q].

☆ Jugular Venous Pattern (JVP)

a waves:	Due to distention produced by **right atrial contraction**[Q].
c waves:	Are positive waves produced by **bulging of tricuspid valve into right atrium during right ventricular**[Q] isovolumetric contraction.
v waves:	**Due to increasing volume of blood in the right atrium during ventricular systole when the tricuspid valve is closed.**[Q]
a – x descent:	Due both to atrial relaxation and to the downward displacement of the tricuspid valve during ventricular systole. **Accentuated in:** - Constrictive pericarditis - Cardiac temponade - Restrictive cardiomyopathy **Reduced with:** - Right ventricular dilatation **Reversed with:** - Tricuspid Regurgitation
v – y descent:	By the opening of the tricuspid valve and the subsequent rapid inflow of blood into the right ventricle. **Accentuated in:** - Tricuspid regurgitation - Constrictive pericarditis **Reduced with:** - Tricuspid stenosis - Right / Atrial Myxoma (Suggests obstruction to right ventricular filling)
y – a descent:	Due to continuous diastolic inflow of blood into great veins, right atrium and ventricle which are all in free communication during diastole.

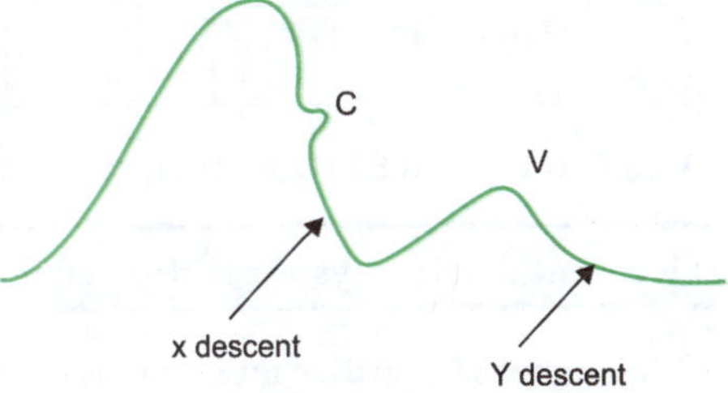

Features of JVP in:

Cardiac temponade	Constrictive pericarditis
- Prominent 'X' descent	- Prominent 'Y' descent
- Absent 'Y' descent	- Present 'X' descent

21. **A i.e. Left side is high pressure system** *[Ref: Braunwald 9/e p. 1110-12]*

In comparison to right atrium, the left atrial V wave is larger than a wave (in JVP) because lft side is high pressure system.

22. **A, B,C, D i.e. Instantaneous mean vector is equal & same as mean QRS vector; It is drawn through the centre of vector in a direction from base toward apex; Summated vector of generated potential at particular instant cause by inflowing septal depolarization; When a vector is exactly horizontal and directed toward the person's left side, the vector is said to extend in the direction of 0°.**
23. **B i.e. Beginning of Q wave to the end of T wave; D i.e. Beginning of R wave to the end of T wave, if Q wave is absent**
24. **D i.e. Ventricular depolarization** *[Ref: Ganong 24/e p 526-28; Guyton 12/e p. 129-137, 121-123; Harrison 18/e p. 1832; Berne 6/e p 310-11]*

QRS complex (wave) reflects ventricular depolarization [Q]
QT interval (or **period of electrical systole of ventricles**) is closely correlated with the **mean action potential duration of ventricular myocytes**. Contraction of ventricles lasts from the **beginning of Q wave** (or **R wave**, if Q wave is absent) **to the end of T wave**: an interval k/a QT interval.

25. **A i.e. Atrial fibrillation**
26. **A i.e. 0.12-0.2sec**

P wave (in ECG) indicate **atrial depolarization**. It is characteristically **absent in hyperkalemia (↑K^+), atrial fibrillation**[Q], **SA block, AV node rhythm, and ventricular tachycardia**[Q].

ECG

Intervals /Wave	Normal Duration (sec)		Events in the heart
	Average	Range	
P wave			**Atrial depolarization**Q
T wave			**Ventricular Repolarization**Q
PR (PQ) interval	0.18	**0.12-0.20**Q	**Atrio ventricular conduction** (from onset of atrial activation to onset of ventricular excitation)
QRS complex (wave)	***0.08*** Q	to 0.10	Ventricular depolarization (& atrial repolarization **is masked)**
QT (RT) interval	0.40	to 0.43	**Ventricular action potential or contraction**Q (Ventricular depolarization + Ventricular repolarization)
ST interval (QT minus QRS)	0.32		**Platue phase of ventricle action potential** (Ventricular repolarization)

27. **A i.e Q wave and S2 (Q-S2 Interval)** *[Ref: Ganong 24/e p 542-43; Katz 5/e p 340-42]*

Electromechanical systole is best defined y ***QS_2 interval***Q

28. **D i.e. Increased cardiac muscle mass** *[Ref: Ganong 22/e P- 550; Guyton 10/e P 127]*

When the sum of *voltages of all the QRS complexes of the three standard leads is greater* ***than 4 millivolts***, the ECG is considered as **high voltage electrocardiogram**. Most often due to ***increased cardiac muscle mass***Q.

The voltage in the three standard leads is measured from the *peak of R wave to the bottom of S wave* = 0.5 – 2.0 millivolts. *Highest voltage is* in lead II, *lowest* in lead III.

29. **B i.e. Decreased Na^+ decreased slop**
30. **B i.e. Increased R – R interval in ECG** *[Ref: Guyton 11th/e p. 113; Ganong 23rd/e p. 502-4; 494; Gabriel C Ezeilo p. 122, 124]*

- **SA node** (develops from right side of embryo) is supplied by **right vagus** and **AV node** (develops from left so) is supplied by **left vagus. Vagal or parasympathetic stimulation** of heart causes ***decreased*** **conduction (negative dromotropic), decreased force of contraction, cardiac out put, ejection fraction and heart rate**Q **(negative chronotropic) and increased R –R interval on ECG**Q**. It also increases refractory period.**

- **R R interval** is used to *define a cardiac cycle and determine heart rate from ECG.* A Heart beat occurs at every R wave, one small division represents 0.04 s & 1 minute is represented by 1500 (60/ 0.04) small divisions. So heart rate (HR) is

HR = Number of ' RR intervals in 1 minute (or 1500 small divisions)

$$HR = \frac{1500}{\text{Number of small division in one R R interval}}$$

So **increased R R interval** means ***decreased heart rate (bradycardia)***Q and decreased R R interval means increased heart rate (tachycardia)

- **Pacemaker (pre) Potential** is mainly d/t **Na^+ influx. Vagal stimulation decreases Na^+ influx and cause decrease in slope (=flattening) of pacemaker (pre) potential**Q. So time taken to reach threshold is increased & HR is decreased.
- **Sympathetic stimulation causes positive chronotropic (↑HR d/t increased slope of phase 4 of pacemaker potential), positive ionotropic (↑ contractility), positive dromotropic (↑ conduction velocity), positive bathmotropic** (increased automaticity) but **decreased refractory period**

31. **A i.e. Tall T waves** *[Ref: Harrison 17/ep 282]*

Prolonged PR interval, QRS widening & depressed/sagged ST segment is seen in, both hypo & hyperkalemia. So both are differentiated by

Hypokalemia
- **Prominent U wave (earliest)**Q
- **Flat & inverted T wave**Q **& Prolonged QT interval**

Hyperkalemia
- **Tall-tented (Narrow & peaked) T waves**
- **Sine wave configuration**
- **Ventricular systole**

32. **D i.e. LVET and PEP.** *[Ref: Ganong 22/e P- 568]*

> ***If carotid transducer is not functioning we would not be able to measure LVET and PEP***Q

33. **B i.e. 0.12sec** 34. **C i.e. Mid diastolic flow in the ventricle** 35. **C i.e. Rapid ventricular filling**
36. **C i.e. Heard during ventricular filling** *[Ref: Guyton 11/e p.269-70; Ganong 22/e p. 569; Harrison 16/e p. 1308]*

> - **3rd heart sound is d/t mid (middle third) diastolic flow (rapid filling) of ventricle**Q.
> - S4 is a **low pitched presystolic sound which can almost never be heard with a stethoscope (& ear) because of its weakness and very low frequency – usually ≤20 cycles/ second (H_z)**Q. It is caused by **in thrushing of blood into ventricles (ventricular filling**Q, which initiates vibration) **when the atria contracts**Q.

Feature	1st heart sound	2nd heart sound	3rd heat sound	4th heart sound *
Character	Low pitched (frequency) slightly prolonged "lub"	Shorter high pitched "dup"	Soft low pitched weak rumbling	Arterial heart sound
Duration	**0.14 (0.15)second**	**0.11 (0.12) sec**	0.1 sec	-
Frequency	25-45 Hz	50 Hz	-	***< 20 Hz***Q
Cause	Sudden closure of mitral & tricuspid valves	Closure of aortic & pulmonary valves	***Rapid ventricular filling***Q d/t inthrushing of blood from atria	***Ventricular filling***Q d/t atrial contraction causing inthrushing of blood
Timing	Start of ventricular systole	Just after end of ventricular systole	**Begining of middle third of diastole**Q	Immediately before 1st heart sound (presystolic)
Heard	S_1 & S_2 can be heard with stethoscope		***S_3 & S_4 can not be heard by stethoscope (ear)***Q. S_3 oftenly and S_4 sometimes can be recorded in phonocardiorgam	

37. **D i.e. Mid diastole** *[Ref: Braunwald (2002) p 227; MDCT : A practical approach (2006) p-213; MDCT: From protocol to practice (2008) p 213; CT of CVS (2007) p 110; Becker : Multislice CT 3/e p 197]*

> - **During cardiac imaging** (such as **MRI, CT, electron beam tomography), mid diastolic phase (or diastasis) of cardiac cycle is usually (but not always) associated with lowest (minimum) mean motion of heart.**Q
> - **Optimum phase** (i.e. with **minimum cardiac motion**) for cardiac and coronary vessel imaging is **mid-diastole (diastasis)** at low or intermediate heart rates; but is variable and may occur in **late systole** at **high heart rates.**

Heart As Pump

38. **B i.e. 3.2** 39. **A i.e. 3 liters / min /m²** *[Ref: Guyton 10/e P- 551]*

$$\textbf{Cardiac Index} = \frac{\textbf{Cardiac Output}}{\textbf{Body Surface Area}} = \frac{5}{1.7} = \textbf{3L / min /m}^2$$

40. **B i.e. 500-600ml**

Heart contains 12% of blood volume i.e. ~600mlQ **(of 5L).**

41. **A i.e. SV/EDV** 42. **D i.e. 65%** 43. **B i.e. 5 litre** 44. **B i.e. Mean stroke volume**
45. **B i.e. COP per unit body surface area** 46. **B i.e. V/Q ratio [Measures ventilation perfusion ratio]**

Cardiac output	*5L/min*Q	The output of the heart per unit time. It can be measured by **Fick's principle,** *thermodilution technique* and *Doppler echocardiography*Q.
Stroke volume	*70 ml*Q	**The amount of blood pumped out of each ventricle per beat. It is difference between end diastolic & end systolic ventricle volume (i.e. differences b/w volume of blood in left ventricle at the end of diastole i.e. 120 ml and at the end of systole i.e. 50 ml)** **Mean stroke volume**Q **= Cardiac output/Heart rate**

Ejection Fraction (EF)	**Percentage of stroke volume (SV) that is ejected by each stroke**[Q]. it is **valuable index of ventricular pump function**[Q] and decreases in failing heart $EF=\frac{\text{Stroke volume (SV)}}{\text{End diastolic ventricle volume (EDV)}}\times 100=\frac{70}{120}\times 100=60\%^{Q}$	
Cardiac Index	*3.2L/min/m²*[Q]	*Cardiac output/ body surface area*[Q]

47. D i.e. Standing from lying position

48. B i.e. Pregnancy

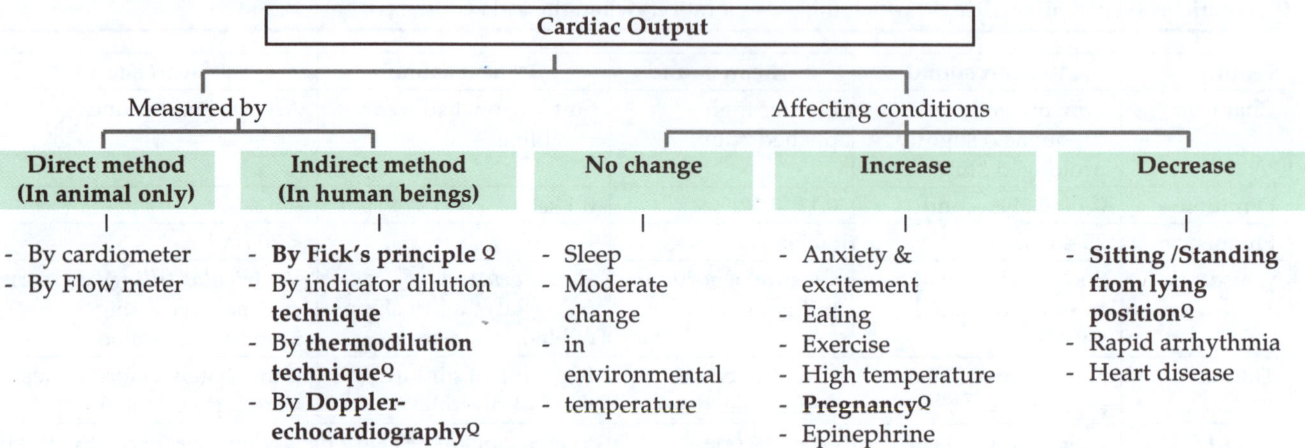

49. B i.e. Setwart-Hamilton Principle: *[Ref: Ganong 24/e p 545-46; Guyton 12/e p 240-41 & Net]*

Thermodilution (cold saline) method, a type of **indicator (dye / radioactive isotope) dilution method** measures cardiac output by pulmonary artery catheter using *Stewart – Hamilton principle*[Q].

50. A i.e. Increased VR-increased CO

51. A i.e. Increased blood volume

52. D i.e. Increase in negative intrathoracic pressure

53. D i.e. Lying to standing change in posture

[Ref: Ganong 24/e p. 540, 547; 23/e p. 515; 22/e p. 572; Guyton's 12 SAE p. 168, 207-11]

- When a person moves from a supine position to standing position volume of blood pools in the lower extremity because of high compliance of veins & venous return decreases. As a result of decreased venous return ***the length of ventricular cardiac muscle fibres is decreased***[Q] and so the cardiac output in accordance with **Frank-Sterling law**.
- ***Preload** or **end diastolic volume/pressure** or **venous return** or **length of ventricular cardiac muscle fiber increases due to increase in negative intrathoracic pressure***[Q], **increased total blood volume**[Q] and increased venous tone. Whereas **EDV decreases on standing**, increased intrapericardial pressure and decreased ventricular compliance.
- Increase in negative intrathoracic pressure (ie more expansion of thorax) would increase the pressure gradient and thus would increase the venous return to heart, thereby increasing preload or EDV.

Preload /Venous Return /End Diastolic Volume (EDV) or Pressure (EDP) / Length of Ventricular Cardiac Muscle Fiber

Preload is the degree of tension on the muscle which begins to contract. For cardiac contraction it is **end diastolic pressure (EDP)** of filled ventricles which inturn corresponds to ventricular filling (**end diastolic volume= EDV**) or **venous return** or **stretch/length of ventricular cardiac muscle fiber. According to Frank Starling law, force of cardiac contraction (so stroke volume & cardiac output) is proportional to muscle fiber length (preload). After load is the load against which the muscle exerts its contractile force. For heart it is pressure in aorta. Preload/EDV/EDP/VR/VCMF length is**

Increase by factors causing increased venous return	Decreased by factors causing decreased venous return
- **Increased total blood volume**Q - **Increased venous tone (or stiffness) or decreased venous compliance**Q - **Muscular activity or increased pumping action of skeletal muscle**Q - **Increased negative intrathoracic pressure** (ie more expanded chest) - Strong atrial contraction - Squatting	- **Increased venous compliance** - **Decreased ventricular compliance (ie increased ventricular stiffness)** due to MI, myopathy etc. - **Increased intrapericardial pressure** due to cardiac temponade, pericardial effusion, constrictive pericarditis or tumor - **Standing (from lying)**Q

54. **D i.e. Sympathetic stimulation** *[Ref: Ganong 24/e P- 547-50]*

Sympathetic stimulation is the single **most important factor in control of automatic myocardial cantractility**Q.

Catecholamines liberated by adrenergic (sympathetic) stimulation cause cardiac acceleration **(increased heart rate = + chronotropic action)** and increased strength of cardiac contraction **(increased myocardial contractility = + inotropic action).**

55. **B i.e. Rostral Ventrolateral Medulla** 56. **C i.e. Acts along with the cardiovagal centre (CVC) to maintain BP**
57. **C i.e. Causes decrease in HR when BP increases** 58. **A i.e. Decreased HR & BP; D i.e. Decreased cardiac contractility**

[Ref: Textbook of physiology: Gabriel C ezeilo (oxford) p- 142- 43, 385, 481; Guyton 11th/e p. 212-13, 210; Ganong 23/e P-556-59]

- **Vasomotor centre (VMC) controlling sympathetic outflow acts along with cardiovagal centre (CVC) controlling parasympathetic out flow to maintain blood pressure**Q.
- **Baroreceptors, chemoreceptors and corticohypothalmic inputs influence VMC**Q.
- **Baroreceptors** are **tonically active stretch receptors located in walls of aortic arch & carotid sinus (not body).** Discharge from baroreceptors cause **inhibition of C1 neurons of vasomotor center (VMC) situated in upper (rostral) half of ventrolateral mdulla**Q and **facilitation of cardiovagal centre (CVC) or nucleus ambiguous.**
- **Baroreceptors** are the stretch receptors in the walls of heart & blood vessels eg carotid sinus & aortic arch receptors, receptors in walls of atria at enterance of SVC, IVC & pulmonary veins and receptors in pulmonary circulation **(cardio-pulmonary receptors)**. These are stimulated by distension of the structure in which they are located l/t vagal innervation of heart and producing **vasodilation, venodilation, a drop in BP, bradycardia & decrease cardiac output (contractility)** Q.

Baroreceptor Discharge (+)

↓

Through NTS (Nucleus Tractus Solitaries) cause

Inhibition of (-) VMC=Vasomotor Center C1 Neurons in Upper/Rostral- Ventro-Lateral Medulla (RVLM)	**Facilitation (+) of CVC=Cardio Vagal Center or Nucleus Ambiguous**
Vasodilatation & ↓BPQ	**Bradycardia & Decreased Cardiac Output (Contractility)**

59. **C i.e. Increase in vasomotor centre activity**
60. **A i.e. Increase in Blood pressure and increase in Heart Rate:** *[Ref: Ganong 24/e p 589-93; Guyton 12/e p 206]*

- **Stretching of carotid sinus baroreceptors [d/t clamping of bilateral carotid arteries above (distal to) carotid sinus]** stimulate their firing which leads to **peripheral vasodilation decreased heart rate, decreased strength of contraction, decreased cardiac output and decreased blood pressure (BP) by excitation of vagal parasympathetic center.**

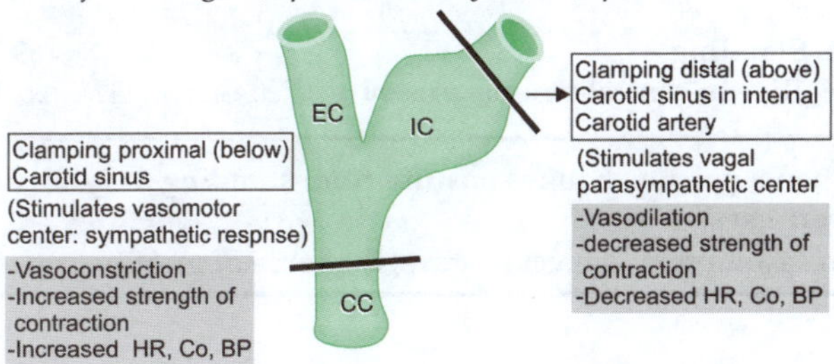

- **Clamping of carotid arteries proximal (below) the carotid sinus**, decreases pressure within the sinus reducing its discharge. This inturn **stimulates vasomotor center** in medulla and inhibits vagal parasympathetic center. This induces reciprocal compensatory response causing **peripheral vasoconstriction, increased heart rate, increased strength of contraction, increased cardiac output and increased blood pressure (BP)**. When bilateral vagatomy is also performed the *BP rise ≥300/200mmHg and is unstable.*
- **Bilateral destruction of visceral afferent nucleus ie nucleus tractus solitaries (NTS)**, which is the site of termination of baro receptor afferents, also causes a **marked (severe may be even fatal) hypertension.**

61. A i.e. Affected by total cardiovascular output

Volume (Low pressure) receptors are located in **walls of right and left atrium at the entrance of SVC and IVC** and **pulmonary veins** as well as in **pulmonary circulation**. In **low pressure part of circulation**, these are k/a **Cardiopulmonary receptors**. These are **stimulated by** ***distension or pressure rise in structure*** **(total cardiovascular output)**[Q]**.**

62. A, C, D i.e. Increased ICT, Brain tumor, Head trauma **63. A i.e. Cushing's reflex**

[Ganong 24/e 607; Guyton 11/e 213; Gabriel p 150-171; Berne & Levy 6/e p- 362]

Elevated intracranial pressure, as caused by **space occupying lesion like brain tumor or head trauma** with associated intracranial bleeding (eg epidural /subdural/cerebral- haemorrhage), results in **triad of irregular respiration,** ***increased systemic blood pressure (↑BP) and bradycardia***[Q] (rather than tachycardia), This response is called ***Cushing's reflex or phenomenon.***

64. D i.e. During exercise systole is shortened more than diastole *[Ref: Guyton 11/e p. 112-13; Ganong 22/e 603-05, 566-68*

65. C i.e. Heart rate increases with parasympathetic denervation *Chaudhauri 6/e p. 191, 202; KDT 6/e p. 478]*

The duration of systole is much more fixed than that of diastole and when the heart rate is increased (eg. in exercise), diastole is shortened to a much greater degree.[Q]

66. A i.e End diastolic volume of ventricles *[Ref: Ganong 22/e P- 572-573]*

According to frank-starling law, **the length of muscle fibers (extent of the pre-load) is proportionate to the end diastolic volume**[Q]

67. D i.e. Increase in venous capacitance

Effect of Sympathetic Stimulation On

Heart	Blood vessels
- Increase the **heart rate (+ve chronotropic action)** - Increases the strength of **cardiac contraction (+ve inotropic action)**[Q]	- Venoconstriction: ***decrease in venous capacitance***[Q] - ***Vasoconstriction: increased blood pressure***[Q] *& increased peripheral resistance*

Feature	Sympathetic (adrenergic) stimulation	Parasympathetic (cholinergic) stimulation
Heart rate (chronotropic)	**Increased**[Q]	**Decreased (main)**
Conduction	**Increased**[Q]	**Decreased**
Force of contraction (Ionotropic)	**Increased**[Q]	**Decreased (to a lesser extent)**

68. B i.e. Standing **69. B i.e. Venous return to heart rises immediately**

70. A i.e. Rise in central venous pressure *[Ref: Ganong 22/e p.630 – 31, 615-18, 662; Guyton 11/e p. 762]*

- **When a person changes posture from standing to lying down position, heart rate decreases and venous return to heart rises.**
- On assumption of erect posture, **the force of gravity opposes the return of blood (i.e.↓ in central venous pressure)**[Q]

Cardiovascular Feature	Effect on Standing	Supine (Lying down) Position	Standing (Upright) Position
Peripheral venous pooling	*300 –500 ml blood pools* in venous capacitance vessels of lower extremities		400 ml
Central blood pool	Same amount of *blood decreases*		400 ml
Central venous pressure	Decreases		3mm Hg
Arterial blood pressure	Sudden decrease followed by a relative gradual rise and settles at a lower level.		
Stroke volume	**Decrease by 40%**[Q]		40%
Cardiac output (& venous return)	***Decrease by 25%***[Q]		25%
Abdominal & limb flow	Decrease by 25%		25%
Heart rate	***Increase by 25***[Q]		25%
Total peripheral resistance	***Increase by 25%***[Q]		25%
Abdominal & limb resistance	Increase		
Small vein pressure	Increase by 10 mmHg		10 mmHg

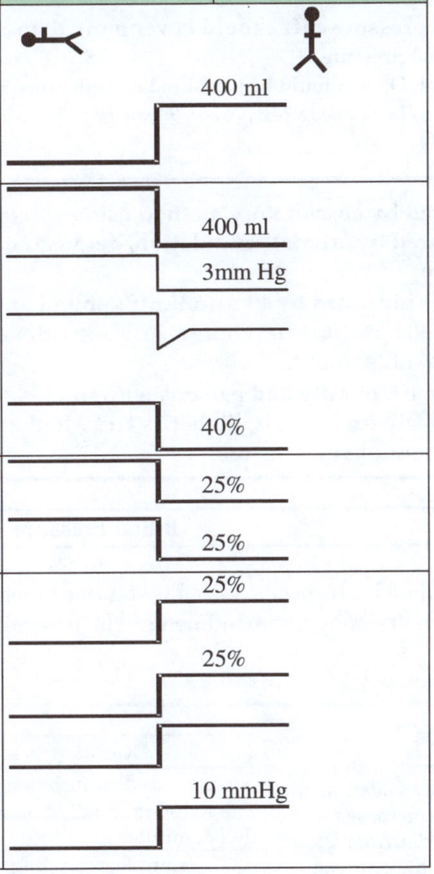

71. **B i.e. Venous return to heart increases immediately**

In standing posture, *300- 500ml of blood pools in venous capacitance vessels of lower extremities, which is immediately returned towards heart*[Q] on assuming lying down posture.

72. **B i.e. 90 mL** *[Ref: Ganong 24/e p. 573]*

Five (5) resistance of 5mm Hg/ml/min connected in parallel. So net resistance in circuit (circulation) according to Ohm's

Law would be $\frac{1}{R} = \frac{1}{R_1} + \frac{1}{R_2} + \frac{1}{R_3} + \frac{1}{R_4} + \frac{1}{R_5}$

$$= \frac{1}{5} + \frac{1}{5} + \frac{1}{5} + \frac{1}{5} + \frac{1}{5} = 1\,\text{mmHg/ml/min}$$

Now, $\text{Flow in any portion of vascular system} = \frac{\text{Effective Perfusion Pressure}}{\text{Net Resistance}}$

$$\text{Flow} = \frac{\text{Inward flow pressure} - \text{Outward flow pressure}}{\text{Net Resistance}} = \frac{100\text{-}10}{1} = 90\,\text{ml/min}$$

Blood Pressure

73. A i.e. Bladder in the blood pressure cuff should cover more than 80% of the arm area

74. B i.e. Is higher than intraarterial pressure

75. B i.e. Diastolic BP is indicated by 4th Kovotkoff's sound

76. A i.e. Diurnal variation present; D i.e. Should be measured in both arms; E i.e. Exercise increases both SBP & DBP

77. A i.e. Large elastic vessels *[Ref: Ganong 24/e p. 578-79; Jain 5/e p. 360-62; Snow Screening for disease (2004) p.135; Medicine for anesthesia 4/285; Guyton 11/p166-67,175-76]*

- **Blood pressure measured by auscultatory method using sphygmomanometer tends to be higher than true intra-arterial pressure measured by arterial cannulation, because some cuff pressure gets dissipated between the cuff and artery**[Q], in the soft tissue.
- **Systolic pressure is best indicated by 1st Korotkoff's sound and diastolic pressure in adults by 5th korotkoff's sound**[Q]. Where as diastolic pressure in children, in adults after exercise, hyperthyroidism & aortic insufficiency best correlates with 4th Korotkoff's sound.
- **Using relatively small cuff, obesity and persons with thick calcified & sclerotic vessels that are difficult to compress (eg in elderly, atherosclerosis, diabetics and Monkenberg's arteriosclerosis)**[Q] are the reasons of **spuriously high blood pressure (Pseudohypertension).**

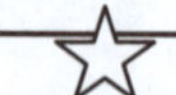

Blood Pressure

Auscultatory method described by *Nicolay Korotkoff* is standard method for BP measurement. It uses inflatable cuff (**Riva-Rocci-cuf**) attached to a mercury sphygmomanometer, which is **gold standard** but may be supplemented by aneroid sphygmomanometer.

Technique

- **Person should be comfortably seated, with back & arm supported, legs uncrossed & upper** ***arm at the level of right atrium***[Q].
- *Snugly wrapped cuff* should allow only *one finger* to be slipped b/w it & skin.
- The cuff is *rapidly inflated to 30 mm Hg* above the point at which radial pulse disappears. *Deflation* rate should be *2-3 mm/second.*
- Two readings should be at least 1 minute apart.
- ***BP should be measured in both arms***[Q] **to rule out diseases of blood vessels like Takayasu's disease.**

Appropriate Cuff size

- Ratio of width of compression cavity of cuff (bladder) to circumference of extremity is of critical importance. According to American Heart Association

Bladder **width** ***should be 40% of circumference or 1.2 times of diameter of extremity***[Q]	Bladder **length** should be ***80% of arm circumference***[Q]

Length to width ratio is 2 : 1

- If the person's limb measurement is on the borderline of two different cuff sizes the chance of error is *decreased if the larger of two cuff sizes is used.*
- So in obese and recording BP in thigh wider cuff size provide more accurate results.

Korotkoff's sound

- Are produced by turbulent flow in artery. The sound gradually become louder, then dull & muffled.

1.	Faint, clear, tapping sounds It indicates ***systolic BP***[Q]
2.	Murmur / swishing sounds
3.	More intense, crisper sounds
4.	Distinct abrupt muffle f sounds *Indicates diastolic BP in children, in adults after exercise, hyperthyroidism, & aortic insufficiency.*
5.	No sound ***Best correlates with diastolic BP in normal adults***[Q].

- It tends to give values for ***systolic pressure that are lower than true intra arterial pressure & diastolic values that are higher***[Q].

Diurnal variation

Diurnal variation of 5-10 mm Hg in systolic BP (SBP)[Q] with lowest values in early morning and peak values during afternoon is common. Night workers have reverse rhythm.

Changes in Exercise and Posture

Exercise increases both SBP and DBP[Q]***. On standing arterial BP decreases***[Q] (Ganong). On standing SBP decreases but DBP increases (AK Jain). DBP changes with body posture i.e. increases on standing, remains normal on sitting and decreases in lying posture (AK Jain).

Source of error

False High values are found in

- Thick overlying soft tissue causing more dissipation of pressure eg. obese
- **Hard sclerotic vessels with low compressibility** such as
  - Elderly
  - Atherosclerosis
  - Diabetics
  - ***Mokenberg's arteriosclerosis***[Q],
- **Retatively small size of cuff (bladder)** eg standard arm cuff used in thigh
- Too slow inflation rate l/t too high diastolic pressure

False low values are found in

- **Large (wide) cuff** eg standard arm cuff used in forearm.
- **Too fast Deflation rate** leads to too low systolic pressure.

Auscultatory gap

It is the interval of pressure where Korotkoff's sounds indicating true systolic pressure fade away and reappear at a lower pressure. The improper interpretation of this gap may l/t errors made in **falsely low recording of systolic BP.** It usually occurs at high pressures, when there is silence at pressures greater than systolic BP, except that the pulse can still be palpated.

78. A i.e. Elastic Recoil of aorta *[Ref: Ganong 23rd/e p. 507; 543- 47; 'Human Physiology ' by Muthayya 3rd / 342; Cardiovascular system at a glance 2nd / 9 Cardiovascular Physiology by Mohrman (2006) / 50]*

Windkessel (Elastic reservoir) effect is the ***recoiling of large elastic vessel wall of aorta and large arteries during diastole***Q that have been stretched during systole, which ***maintains continuous forward flow, and arterial pressure during diastole***Q.

79. B i.e. Systolic +1/3rd pulse pressure

80. A i.e. (SBP + 2DBP) /3 *[Ref: Chaudhuri 5/e P- 244]*

Mean arterial pressure (BP) = ***Diastolic BP + 1/3rd pulse pressure*** Q

= Diastolic BP +1/3rd (Systolic BP – Diastolic BP)

$$= DBP + \frac{SBP}{3} - \frac{DBP}{3} = \frac{SBP}{3} + DBP - \frac{DBP}{3} = \frac{SBP}{3} + \frac{2}{3}DBP = \frac{1}{3}(SBP + 2DBP)$$

Mean BP: It is the 'weighed' mean pressure of the blood. So like **BP it depends on cardiac output & peripheral resistance**Q. In a cardiac cycle, the systole lasts for 0.3sec and diastole for 0.5 sec. Therefore in a subject having a cardiac cycle of 0.8 sec, the mean BP cannot be taken as (systolic BP + diastolic BP)/2
Difference between systolic and diastolic pressure is k/a Pulse Pressure.

81. C i.e. Mean circulatory filling pressure

82. D i.e. Arterial pressure taken at the point when heart stops beating *[Ref: Guyton 11th/e p. 239- 40; Gabriel C Ezeilo p.158]*

Mean circulatory filling pressure (MCFP) is the *arterial pressure taken at the point when* heart *stops beating*Q. It is the equilibrium pressure reached throughout the cardiovascular system (i.e. everywhere in circulation = both systemic and pulmonary) when cardiac output (i.e. heart pumping) has stopped completely.Q

83. C i.e. VR = (MSFP-RAP)/RVR

84. D i.e. Peripheral resistance x cardiac output

85. A i.e. Auscultatory gap

86. B i.e. More than intravascular pressure

[Ref: Ganong 24/e P- 578-82, Chaudhuri 5/e P- 210; Bijlani 1/e P 189]

- **Venous return (VR) = (MSFP - RAP)/RVR;** whereas **blood pressure (BP) = cardiac output × peripheral resistance**Q.
- BP appears **spuriously (falsely) low** in **auscultatory gap**Q and falsely high in obesity, calcified thick vessels and small cuff.
- **Direct intraarterial method** measures accurate BP. Whereas **indirect sphygmomanometer method gives falsely high reading**Q.

87. B i.e. Falsely low values at high pressure in pulse tracing *[Ref Ganong 22/e P- 588- 589]*

Bernoulli's principle: In a tube or a blood vessel the total *energy (kinetic energy of flow+ potential energy) is constant*
When a *vessel is narrowed* (e.g. in adrenalin administration), the velocity of flow in the narrowed portion increases & so the kinetic energy (1/2 mv2). As the total energy is constant (Bernoulli's principle), potential energy decreases in narrowed segment.
Therefore when the velocity of flow is increased the *lateral pressure distending the wall* at the constriction *is decreased* and narrowing tends to maintain itself.
Pressure transducer measures arterial pressure directly, so it gives falsely low value after adrenaline injection (at high pressure)

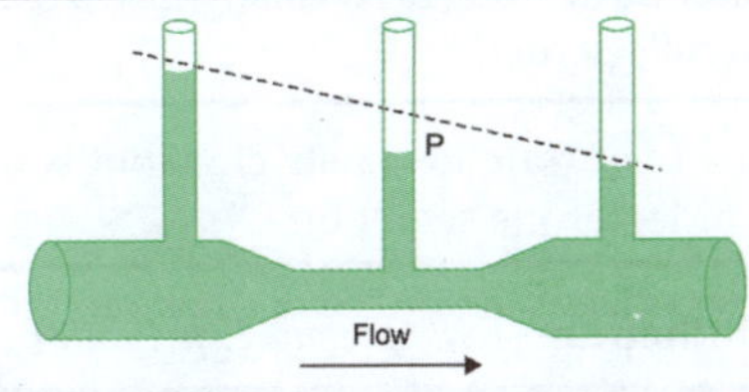

When fluid flows through the narrow portion of the tube, the kinetic energy of flow increases as the velocity increases, and the potential energy is reduced. Consequently, the measured pressure (P) is lower than it would have been at that point if the tube had been narrowed. The dashed line indicates what the pressure drop due to friction forces would have been if the tube had been of uniform diameter.

88. A i.e. The lying down position

For two values to be comparable (to remove any bias) we must remove as many confounding variables as possible.
The confounding variable in this question is gravity. Gravity is present on earth but is not present in space.
The *best position in which the effect of gravity is nullified is lying down.*

89. C i.e. KPa *[Ref: Taber's Medical Dictionary /2216]*

Pressure in SI unit is measured in pascal [Pa]. *Blood pressure in SI unit* is measured ***in KPa***[Q]

90. B i.e. Reflex bradycardia *[Ref: Ganong 24/e P-588-93; Wright 13/e p. 124-25]*

91. C i.e. Both recorded an increase in MBP

- Pressure on carotid sinus **or stimulation of baroreceptors** (usually by high BP) **decreases sympathetic and increases parasympathetic (vagal) activity.** ***So there is reflex bradycardia and decreased BP***[Q]**.**
- **Bilateral section of baroreceptor nerves (ie carotid sinus nerve & aortic depressor nerves) or bilateral lesions of NTS cause initial dramatic rise of BP**[Q]. However, mean BP returns to near control levels after a period of time, but *there are large fluctuations in BP during the course of day* and *the individual cannot adjust their BP in response to stimuli that cause abrupt changes in blood volume, cardiac output, or peripheral resistance, including exercise and postural changes.* Loss of baroreceptor reflex control cause **neurogenic hypertension** in long term.

92. D i.e. The cerebral arterial pressure rises: *[Ref: Ganong 22/e P-/632; Guyton 10/e p.500-501]*

'Negative 'g' causes increased cardiac output, a rise in cerebral arterial pressure, intense congestion of the head and neck vessels, ecchymosis around the eyes, severe throbbing head pain and eventually mental confusion (red out)'.

93. C i.e. Arterial wall expansion *[Ref: Ganong 22/e P- 568]*

The blood forced into the aorta during systole not only moves the blood in the vessels forward but also sets up a pressure wave that travel along the arteries. ***The pressure wave expends the arterial wall***[Q] *as it travels, and expansion is palpable as the pulse.*

94. B i.e. Slight increase in H.R, normal BP *[Ref: Harrison 16/e P-616, Bailey& love 23/e P275]*

Blood loss of upto 20% of blood volume are normally tolerated by redistribution of blood flow, mediated by vasospasm[Q]**.**

500ml blood accounts for about 10% of total blood volume (5 litres)

Blood loss	<15%	15-30%[Q]	30-40%	>40%
BP	No change	*No change*	Reduced	Markedly reduced
Heart rate	Slight Increase	*100-120 (slight)*	>120, weak	>120, thready
Respiratory rate	Normal	Increased	>20	20-30

Cardiovascular Regulatory Mechanism

95. A i.e. Bronchodilation *[Ref: Ganong 22/e p.599-600,446, Guyton & Hall 11/e p. 202,322, Harrison 16/e p. 1366, 1509, 213 , www.cvphysiology.com]*

Endothelin 1 is broncho constrictor (not bronchodilator) & vaso constrictor[Q] **(so ↓GFR)**[Q]. It is inotropic and stimulates ANP and aldosterone secretion.

96. A i.e. Endothelium *[Ref: Ganong 22/e P-598]*

97. D i.e. Endothelin

Nitric oxide is synthesized from arginine by the enzyme *NO synthetase* (NOS) *in endothelial cells*[Q]. It causes vasodilation.

Synthesis of NO/Endothelium Derived Relaxing Factor

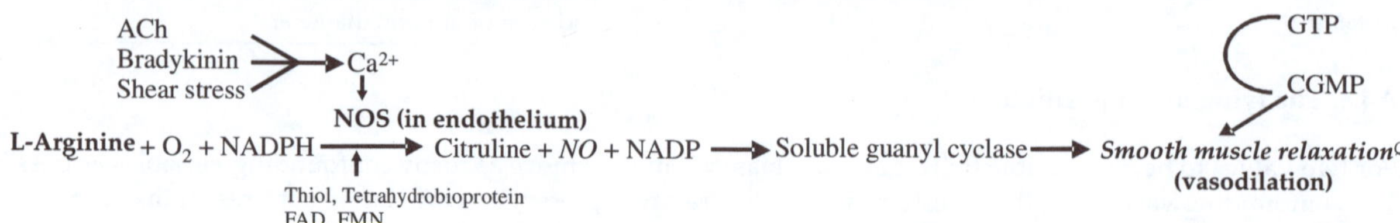

Factors Affecting the Caliber of Arteriole

Constriction		Dilatation
- Decreased local temperature - Autoregulation	**Local factors**	- Increased K^+, adenosine. - Increased CO_2 - Decreased O_2 - Decreased local pH - Decreased local temperature
- **Endothelin-1**[Q] - Platelet serotonin - **Thromboxane A_2**[Q]	**Endothelin products**	- **NO**[Q] - **Prostacyclin**[Q] - **Kinins**[Q] eg **Bradykinin**[Q]
- Epinephrin (except in skeletal muscle & liver) - Norepinephrin - AVP - Angiotensin II - Neuropeptide Y	**Circulating hormones**	- ***Epinephrin in skeletal muscle & liver***[Q] - ***Substance P***[Q] - ***Histamine***[Q] - ANP - VIP

Precapillary Sphincter Caliber

Precapillary sphincters are layer of smooth muscle fibres present just at the point where a capillary originates from a metarteriole.

- There is ***no innervation on precapillary sphincter.***[Q]
- Their *dilatation* or *constriction* (to control the blood flow) ***depends on local hormones.***[Q], circulating substance, end product of metabolism, hydrogen ions etc.
- *Catecholamines* causes *sphincter constriction.*

Effects of Prostaglandins

	Blood vessels	Platelets	Bronchi	Kidney	Uterus
PGE_2	Vasodilation	Variable effect	Dilatation	Vasodila-tation Renin release	Contraction Softening of cervix
$PFF_2\alpha$	Vasodilation	-	Constriction	-	Contraction Softening of cervix
PGI_2	Vasodilation	Antiaggre-gatory	Dilatation	Vasodilation Renin release	-
TXA_2	Vasocons-triction	Aggregation	Constriction	Vasocons-triction	-

98. B i.e. Angiotensin 2

Angiotensin converting enzyme/ACE (not angiotensin II) is synthesized in endothelium cells of lung capillaries (mainly)[Q]**.**

Endothelial Cell Function/Activity (By production of)

Anticoagulant- Antithrombotic

- **Prostacyclin (PGI_2), Heparin**[Q]**,**
- Protein S, Thrombomodulin, NO

Prothrombotic Activity

vW factor & Tissue factor

Vasoconstriction

ACE[Q] **& Endothelin**[Q]

Vasodilatation

Prostacycline, NO[Q]

Inflammation & Immunity

IL1 &6, HLA, VCAM-1, ICAM, E & P Selections

Cell growth stimulation

PDGF, CSF, FGF

Cell growth inhibitors

Heparin, TGFβ

Circulation Through Special Regions

99. B i.e. -5 to 0 mmHg

In most tissues, **interstitial pressure (i.e. interstitial fluid hydrostatic pressure) is normally sub atmospheric (or negative) ranging from-5 mm Hg to-1 mm Hg**[Q]**.**

100. B i.e. Increase in hydrostatic pressure of capillaries *[Ref: Ganong 22/e p. 592; Guyton & Hall 11/e p. 184-85]*

High capillary hydrostatic pressure & interstitial fluid colloid osmotic pressure tend to cause osmosis (filteration) of fluid outward through capillary membrane[Q]**.**

101. A i.e. Hypercarbia **102. A i.e. Blood pressure >> C i.e. Potassium ions**

[Ref: Ganong 22/e p.611- 19, 597; Lee's anesthesia 12/e p-441; Lange , anesthesia 4/e p- 615]

- **Cerebral blood flow** is insensitive to ***hormones, sympathetic nerve activity and virtually remain constant despite changes in arterial blood pressure***[Q].
- Cerebral circulation shares many features of coronary circulation. Both heart & bain have a high metabolic rate, extract & use large amount of O_2 & have limited ability to use anaerobic glycolysis for metbolism. Their vasculature have a limited ability to constrict in response to sympathetic nerve stimulation but an ***excellent ability to auto regulate blood flow at arterial blood pressure from 50-60 mmHg to 150- 160 mm Hg***[Q].
- **Potassium ion (K+) & lactate** cause vasodilation in *skeletal muscle*, whereas **adenoside** may cause vasodilation in *cardiac muscle* but not in skeletal muscle.
- ***Since ions (H^+, K^+, HCO_3^-), proteins, polypeptides and protein bound forms do not cross blood brain barrier as easily as water, CO_2, O_2 and lipid soluble substances, the ions have little effect on cerebral blood flow***[Q]. Cerebral blood flow, like other areas of body, is highly related to *metabolic rate of tissue*. Reaction of CBF to ***CO_2, H^+ and K^+***[Q] (i.e., chemicals released by increased brain activity) is a part of overall process of matching braines metabolic needs to its blood supply of nutrients & O_2.
- **Hypercarbia (↑CO_2 concentration in arterial blood)** is the ***most potent cerebral vasodilator***[Q] because of ease of permeability across BBB. CO_2 causes vasodilation by increasing the **H+ ion concentration in cerebral vessels.** However, H+ ions in blood do not cross BBB easily
- The 10-30% increase in blood flow in areas of brain excited by mental or visual activity and peripheral nerve stimulation, may be related to these three substances released from active nerve cells. ***Cerebral vasculature also dilates when the O_2 content of arterial blood is reduced but the vasodilatory effect is much less powerful than of elevated CO_2***[Q].

103. C i.e. Increase in urine output *[Ref: Shwartz 8/e P-132,133 CSDT Pg 217, Harrison 16/e P-1600–1617; Oxford Surgery P–120]*

Urine output is ***quantitative and relatively reliable indicator of organ perfusion***[Q]

The most reliable clinical guide in assessing hypovolumic shock is skin perfusion. (skin on the extremeties becomes pale, cool and moist).

As a general principle, measurements of *blood pressure and pulse are less reliable than change in urine output* in assessing the severity of shock.

B.P : Hypotension is not a reliable early sign of hypovolumea. In healthy patient blood volume must decrease by 30-40% before hypotension occur.

CVP: CVP measurement helps in distinguishing b/w Cardiogenesis shock and hypovolumic shock.

"A Central venous catheter can *give information about the relationship b/w intravascular volume & right ventricular function* but should not be used to assess either factor independently."

CVP is not a good indicator in septic shock because patient can develop pulmonary edema when it is in the normal range.

104. B i.e. Contains 25% of blood **105. A i.e. Contains 5% of blood volume**

106. B i.e. Contains larger quantities of blood than veins *[Ref: Ganong 23/e P-537-543]*

Vessel	Percentage of blood	Cross- sectional area $(cm)^2$
Aorta	2%	4.5
Artery	8%	20
Arteriole	1%	400
Capillary	5%[Q]	4500 ***(maximum)***[Q]
Venule	54% ***(maximum)***[Q]	18
Vein		
Vena cava		

- ***Maximum blood is contained in the veins (venous system)***[Q], while capillaries contain only 5% of blood volume.
- **Capillaries**
  - ***Maximum cross – sectional area***[Q] (1000 times of aorta)
  - **Minimum velocity** in circulation is seen in capillaries (Inverse relationship with cross- sectional area)
  - ***Are lined by single layer of endothelial cells.***[Q]

107. B i.e. Have role in thermoregulation

[Ref: An introduction to cardiovascular physiology – Levick, Butterworth, Heinemann 1995; 'Cardiovascular Physiology in Exercise & Sport' by Bell (2008) / 60, 61; Case Based Medical Physiology' by Bell (2005) / 115, Neuroimmunology of the skin (2008) / 24]

Cutaneous (anterior- venous anastomosis) shunt vessels play an important role in ***temperature thermoregulation***[Q].

108. A i.e. Large veins *[Ref: Ganong 22/e P- 584]*

The velocity of blood is inversely proportional to the total cross – sectional area at that point.

Order of Velocity of Blood	Order of Cross – Sectional Area:
Velocity is inversely proportional to total cross section area. So, velocity is highest in aorta, declines steadily in smaller vessels & lowest in capillaries. Velocity increases again as blood enters veins & is relatively high in vena cava but not so high as in aorta. ***Aorta > Vena cava***Q > Artery > Arteriole > ***Capillary (min)***Q	***Capillaries (max)***Q > Arteriole > Artery > Vena cava > Aorta ★ Mean velocity of blood in the aorta is = ***40 cm/sec***Q. Average normal **arm to tongue circulation time** is 15 seconds.

109. B i.e. Femoral artery and femoral vein *[Ref: Ganong 22/e p. 586 – 95 , 21/e p. 589]*

- **Blood pressure in decreasing order** ***is: Aorta > arteries > arterioles > capillaries > venule > vein > vena cava***Q.
- Blood pressure in aorta is 120/80 mmHg. It falls very slightly in the *large & medium sized arteries* becauswe their resistance to flow is small. But BP falls rapidly in **small arteries & arterioles*, which are the main site of peripheral resistance***Q against which the heart pumps. So these are referred to as **resistance vessels**. The mean pressure at the end of arteriole is *30-38 mmHg* and pulse pressure 5 mmHg. *Capillary pressure (BP) at arteriolar end* is *32 mmHg* with pulse pressure 5 mmHg and at *venous end* is *15 mmHg* with pulse pressure 0 mmHg. In capillary, blood velocity is 0.07 cm/s and transit time 1 – 2 seconds. The pressure in *venules* is *12-18mm Hg* which falls steadily in larger veins to about *5.5 mmHg* in great veins outside the thorax. The pressure in great veins at their entrance into right atrium in thorax (**central venous pressure**) averages *4.6 mm Hg*.
- Both **arterial pressure** and **peripheral venous pressure** are affected by gravity, in a way that it is increased ***0.77 mm Hg for each centimeter***Q below the right atrium and decreased by same amount for each centimeter above the right atrium
- **Windkessel (elastic reservoir) effect** is the recoiling of elastic vessel wall of aorta & large arteries during diastole that have been stretched during systole, which maintains continuous forward flow.

110. B i.e. Capillaries venules and arterioles **111. B i.e. Resistance vessel** **112. A i.e. Veins** **113. B i.e. Capillary**

114. B, C, & E i.e. Transfused blood is mainly distributed in arteries, Hematocrit markedly change peripheral resistance, & Non pulsatile flow is recommended *[Ref: Ganong 23rd/e p. 542- 47; Guyton 12/e p. 157]*

- A large amount of blood can be added to *veins* and therefore are called **capacitance vessels**. The ***small arteries and arterioles***Q are referred to as **resistance vessels** because they are the **principal site of peripheral resistance**. ***So increased radius of resistance vessel increases capillary blood flow***Q
- When extra blood is **transfused**, < 1% of it is distributed in arterial system (**High pressure system**) and *all the rest is found* in systemic veins, pulmonary circulation, & heart chamber other than left ventricle (**Low pressure system**)
- Resistance to blood flow is determined by *vascular hindrance (radius of blood vessels) and viscosity* of blood. The viscosity depends mostly on hematocrit (i.e.% volume of blood occupied by RBC) ***In large vessels, hematocrit increase causes appreciable increase in viscosity***Q ***and so increased mean blood pressure***Q. However , in vessels smaller than 100μm diameter (i.e. arteriole, capillaries & venules) – the ***viscosity change per unit change in hematocrit is much less than it is in large bore vessels***Q. d/t difference in nature of flow through smaller vessels. So the net change in viscosity (Poisenill- Hagen formula) per unit change in hematocrit is considerable smaller in vivo than in vitro. This is why ***hematocrit changes have relatively little effect on peripheral resistance***Q. Except when the changes are large.
- Mean velocity of blood flow in proximal aorta is *40 cm/s* (ranges from 120 cm/s during systole to negative at the time of transient back flow before the aortic valve closes in diastole) the flow is *phasic*. ***Pulsatile flow maintains optimal tissue function (by gene transcription)***Q. If an organ is perfused by a non pulsatile flow, inflammatory markers are produced, there is gradual rise in vascular resistance & ultimately tissue perfusion fails.

☆ Functional Classification of Vessel Wall

Vessel Type	Include	Feature
Elastic Arteries (Windkessel Vessels)Q	Aorta, Pulmonary artery & major branches	**Elastic recoil maintains continuous blood flow & diastolic arterial pressure**Q
Conduct (muscular) Arteries	Main arteries eg cerebral, coronary, popliteal , radial	Thicker muscle in tunica media
Resistance vessels	**Smallest terminal arteries & arterioles**Q	- Single layer of muscle in tunica media - Regulate local blood flow to match local demands
Arteriovenous anstomosis	**Shunt vessels**Q (dia 20-135) mm	- Connect arteriole to venule by passing capillaries - Present in skin & nasal mucosa **Regulate temperature**Q
Exchange vessels	**Capillaries**Q	- **Largest cross section area**Q - **Provide O2 and nutrition to tissues**Q
Capacitance (Compliance) vessels	**Veins**	- **Store large volumes of blood**Q
Capacitance V.	**Veins**Q	Store large amount of blood
Microcirculation	**Arteriole → Metarteriole → Precapillary sphincter → Capillary → Venule**Q	

115. B i.e. Arterioles *[Ref: Ganong 24/e p. 575; Chaudhuri 5/e P-198]*

116. A i.e. 5 times

Distribution of blood flow is mainly regulated by arteriolesQ, by alteration in their diameter. They can increase or decrease, the peripheral resistance to blood flow. Also called **precapillary resistance vessel** Q.

Arterioles are major site of resistance to blood flow, often termed as *seat of peripheral vascular resistance.*Q Small change in their caliber cause large change in total peripheral resistance & affect distribution of blood flow. **Poiseuille-Hagen Formula.**

$$R = \frac{8nL}{\pi r^4}$$

R = Resistance L= Length of the tube
r = radius of vessel η = viscosity

$$K = \frac{8nL}{\pi} = \text{constant}$$

$$F = \frac{P_A - P_B}{R}$$

F = Flow, $P_A - P_B$ = Pressure difference between two ends of tube

$$R \propto \frac{1}{r^4} \text{ and Flow (F)} \propto \text{radius } (r)^4$$

So, on **increasing radius 50% (i.e. to 1.5 r) would** increases flow **to $(1.5)^4$ = 5 times**Q

117. A i.e. Parallel to the long axis of blood vessel; C i.e. Increases with increase in axial velocity of fluid; D i.e. Poiseuille-Hagen equation correlate flow with viscosity; E i.e. Depend upon viscosity *[Ref: Ganong 24/e p. 573-75]*

☆

- Flowing blood creates a **shear stress (γ)** on the endothelium ***that is parallel to the long axis of vessel***Q. γ is **proportional to viscosity (η) times the shear rate**Q (dy/dr, ie the rate at which the axial velocity increases from the vessel wall toward the lumen). $\gamma = \eta\,(dy/dr)$.
- Changes in shear stress, cyclic strain & stretch *activate endothelial genes* such as endothelin 1, growth factors (PDGF α/β, TGF β) and integrins etc.
- **Poiseuille- Hagen formula correlates flow (F) with viscosity (η)**Q, pressure difference b/w two ends of tube ($P_A - P_B$), radius (r) & length (l) of tube. $F = (P_A - P_B) \times (\pi/8) \times (1/\eta) \times (r^4/L)$.

118. D i.e. Effective velocity in small vessels is less *[Ref: Ganong 23/e p 539-42; Berne & Levy 6/e p 331-34; Gabriel p 134-35]*

119. D i.e. Increase in diameter of blood vessels

- Probability of **turbulence** increases with **Reynolds number** > 3000, increase in **velocity** (above critical level), **density** of blood and **diameter** of vessel or with **decrease in viscosity**.
- Average **velocity of flow is inversely proportional to the total cross sectional area** of the vessel. Therefore the **average velocity** of flow is high in aorta **declines steadily in smaller vessels** and is lowest in capillaries. So the cause of laminar flow in small vessels mainly is **large area of cross section and less effective velocity**[Q].

120. A i.e. Local hormones *[Ref: Ganong 22/e P- 577, 603, Guyton 10/e P/162]*

Precapillary sphincter relaxation is mediated by **local hormones**[Q], circulating substances, end product of metabolisms & H_2 ions as there is **no neural innervations.**

121. A i.e. 250 ml/min **122. D i.e. 800** **123. A i.e. 55ml/100 gm/min**

124. A i.e. Liver > Kidney > Brain > Heart

- **Overall total blood flow** in various organs is **liver (1500 ml/min) > kidney > skeletal muscle (840)**[Q] **> brain > skin** (460ml/min) **> heart/ myocardium/coronary (250ml/min)**[Q].
- **Coronary flow is maximum during diastole**[Q]**. Adenosine increases it by coronary vasodilatation esp. during ischemia.**
- **Brain** blood supply is **750 ml/min or 54 ml/100gm/min**[Q].

Overall Blood Flow and Oxygen Consumption by Various Organs

Over all (ml/min)	
Blood Flow	**O_2 Consumption**
Liver > kidney > skeletal ms > Brain > skin > Heart [Q]	Liver > skeletal ms> Brain > Heart

Per unit mass (ml / 100 gm/min)	
Blood flow	**O_2 consumption**
Kidney >Heart > liver > Brain	***Heart***[Q] > Kidney > Brain

Resistance	
Absolute	Per/kg
Heart : Max	Skeletal ms : Max
Liver : Min	Kidney : Min

A-V O_2 difference (ml/L)
Heart : Max[Q]
Kidney : Min

Effects of Exercise on Cardiac Output

Cardiac output	Quiet standing	Exercise	Effect
Cardiac output ml/min	5900	24,000	↑↑[Q]
Blood flow to:			
Active skeletal muscle	650	20,850	↑↑
Heart	250	1000	↑↑[Q]
Brain	750	750	Unchanged
Skin	500	500	Unchanged
Inactive skeletal muscle	650	300	↓
Kidney, Liver, GIT ect.	3100	600	↓↓[Q]

Resting blood flow and O_2 consumption of various organs in a 63-kg adult man with a mean arterial blood pressure of 90 mm Hg and an O_2 consumption of 250 mL/min

Region	Mass (kg)	Blood Flow		Ateriovenous Oxygen Difference	Oxygen Consumption		Resistance (R units)*		Percentage of Total	
		mL/min	mL/100 g/min	mL/L	mL/min	mL./100 g/min	Absolute	per kg	Cardiac Output	Oxygen Consumption
Liver	2.6	**1500**	57.7	34	51	2.0	3.6	9.4	27.8	20.4
Kidneys	0.3	1260	420.0	14	18	6.0	4.3	1.3	23.3	7.2
Brain	1.4	750	**54.0**[Q]	62	46	3.3	7.2	10.1	13.9	18.4
Skin	3.6	462	12.8	25	12	0.3	11.7	42.1	8.6	4.8
Skeletal muscle	31.0	**840**[Q]	2.7	60	50	0.2	6.4	198.4	15.6	20.0
Heart muscle	0.3	**250**	84.0	114	29	9.7	21.4	6.4	4.7	11.6
Rest of body	23.8	336	1.4	129	44	0.2	16.1	383.2	6.2	17.6
Whole body	63.0	5400	8.6	46	250	0.4	1.0	63.0	100.0	100.0

125. A i.e. Skin

126. C i.e. Opening of Ca^{2+} channels

[Ref: Guyton 10/e P-293]

The capacity of tissues to regulate their own blood flow is referred to as autoregulation. This capacity is well ***developed in kidney,***Q ***also seen in mesentry, skeletal muscle***Q***, brain***Q***, liver***Q***, & myocardium. But no autoregulation is seen in skin***Q.

Autoregulation of GFR & Renal Blood Flow

Myogenic autoregulation

Ability of individual bloods vessels to resist stretching during increased arterial pressure.

Stretching of vascular wall
(when arterial pressure ↑ es)
↓
↑Movement of Ca^{2+} from ECF into cellQ
↓
Contraction of smooth muscle
↓
- Prevent overdistension of vessel
- ↑es vascular resistance

↓
Prevent ↑ in renal blood flow & GFR

Tubulo glomerular feed back

This feed back mechanism links changes in *sodium chloride conc at the macula densa* with the control of renal arteriolar resistance. This ensures a constant delivery of NaCl to the distal tubule.

127. A i.e. PGI_2 & B i.e. PGE_2

PGE_2 and PGI_2 cause renal vasodilation, increasing renal blood flow and release reninQ.

128. B i.e. Autoregulatory *[Ref: Sembulingum 3/e P- 516-17;Ganong 22/e P-620- 21]*

129. A i.e. Coronary blood flow is directly related to perfusion pressure & inversely related to resistance

Factors regulating Coronary Blood Flow

Auto regulation (Chemical Regulation)

- **Need for O_2** (i.e. hypoxia) is the most important factor maintaining blood flow (by causing vasodilation)
- **Metabolites** eg *adenosine, K^+, H^+, CO_2* causes vasodilation & increase blood flow

Neural Regulation

- **Nervous factors**: *sympathetic stimulation increases* and parasympathetic stimulation decreases coronary blood flow.
- **Coronary perfusion pressure** is the balance between mean arterial pressure & resistance offered to blood flow in heart. The ***mean arterial pressure particularly in aorta plays an important role in maintaining circulation where as resistence decrease it***Q.

130. B i.e. Hypoxia causes Vasoconstriction, C i.e. Blood volume in lungs is 450 ml; E i.e. It has low resistance

131. D i.e. Distended pulmonary veins in the lower lobes

132. B i.e. Pulmonary vasoconstriction in hypoxia

133. A i.e. Zone 1

134. D i.e. Most blood is in pulmonary capillaries

135. A i.e. Increase in the number of open capillaries

136. B i.e. Resistance low, Capillary pressure low

[Ref: Berne & Levy 6/e p 421-23; Guyton 11/e 486-87; Lange: Pulmonary physiology 6/e p 95-97; John, West 8/e p 36-41; Ganong 23/e 602-04]

- **Lung contains 450 ml (9% of total) blood volume of** which only **70 ml is in pulmonary capillaries** and rest is equally divided b/w arteries and veins.
- Pulmonary circulation is low pressure **low resistance system. Pulmonary vascular resistance is only one tenth**Q. **Pulmonary microcirculation** is characterized by ***remarkably low vascular resistance and low pressure and is very pulsatile***Q. **Hypoxia causes vasoconstriction in pulmonary small arteries & arterioles**Q.
- **Perfusion & ventilation both decrease from base to apex of lung**Q. **Both V & P are more in lower lobes but V/P ratio is highest in apex**Q. V/P ratio is **0.8** for whole lung at rest.
- **Zone 1 of no blood flow is physiological (alveolar) dead space**Q.
- **During heavy exercise** the cardiac output (CO) increases upto three folds while **pulmonary arterial pressure rises very little because** pulmonary circulation can accommodate significant amount of blood by phenomenon of **recruitment** (i.e. increasing the number of open capillaries conducting blood) and **distension** (i.e. increase in caliber of already open vessel).

137. B i.e. Contribute to gaseous exchange *[Ref: Berne & Levy 6/e p 422-23; Guyton 11/e p. 483; Phodes & Bell Medical physiology 3/e p-371; Miller : Lung function 6/e p 28]*

Bronchial circulation *does not take part in gaseous exhange*Q. Gaseous exchange takes place in pulmonary circulation.

138. B i.e. Umbilical Vein

- **Umblical vein and pulmonary veins carry oxygenated blood**Q. Whereas **umbilical and pulmonary arteries carry deoxygenated blood**Q.

- Deoxygenated blood (with 62% O_2 saturation) leave via **umbilical arteries** to be oxygenated at placenta whereas, **umbilical veins** carry oxygenated blood from the placenta with HbO_2 saturation of ~ 80% (as compared to 98% saturation in adults arterial circulation).
- **Right ventricle** pump deoxygenated blood through **pulmonary artery** into pulmonary capillaries where it is oxygenated. And then oxygenated blood is carried through **pulmonary** veins to left atrium.

139. A i.e. Portal vein *[Ref: BDC- 4/e vol II p 253]*

Blood supply of liver through: ***Portal vein is 80%***[Q] and Hepatic artery is 20%

140. C i.e. Sinusoids *[Ref: Davidson 17/e P 498]*

Wedged Hepatic Venous Pressure

It is the pressure recorded by a catheter wedged in a hepatic vein. It reflects the ***contribution of hepatic sinusoids to portal venous pressure.***[Q] It is elevated in sinusoidal & presinusoidal portal hypertension,

Portal venous pressure = Wedged hepatic venous pressure – free hepatic venous pressure.

141. A i.e. Tight endothelial function

142. B i.e. Foot process of astrocytes

Blood brain barrier (BBB) is formed by **tight junction of endothelial cells and foot process of astrocytes**[Q], limiting filtration of protein across capillaries.

143. A i.e. Correlates with heart rate

144. B i.e. Has constant relation to external cardiac work

145. E i.e. Directly proportional to mean arterial pressure

[Ref: Guyton 11/e 235-37; 249-53; Fawzy G. Cardiac anesthesia : Principles and clinical practice p. 25; Cardiovascular physiology – Heller (lange) 5/ed pg-62-64; Internal medicine 5/ed pg- 192-193; Textbok of physiology Gabriel (oxford) p-113; Ganong 23rd/e p. 519]

- **Myocardial O_2 demand / consumption** is primarily determined by **heart rate, contractility of myocardium (or ventricles) (i.e. inotropy), intramyocardial wall tension** (which is directly proportional to **after load** or intra cavitatory pressure and **preload** or ventricular radius and inversely proportional to **myocardial muscle mass or wall thickness)** and **ventricular work per beat** (i.e. **stroke volume X mean arterial pressure**). For left ventricle mean arterial pressure of aorta and for right ventricle MAP in pulmonary artery is used.
- ***Myocardial O_2 demand is not negligible at rest***[Q]. It has a **constant relation (not directly proportional) to external cardiac work (during ejection phase of cardiac cycle).** Myocardial O_2 demand is ***directly proportional to heart rate but has no relation to duration of systole***[Q]

146. A, B, C, D > E i.e. Preload, Afterload, Intramyocardial tension, Myocardial muscle mass > Blood Hb concentration

- Anemia, anxiety, arterio-venous fistula (AVF), beriberi, hyperthyroidism, paget's disease, pregnancy, and pulmonary disease commonly cause **high cardiac output** due to **reduced total peripheral resistane.**
- Anemia decreases total peripheral resistance by reducing viscosity of blood (d/t decreased RBC concentation) and causing local vasodilation (d/t diminished delivery of O_2 to tissue).
- **Long term increased work load** (but not so much excess that damages the heart) causes the **heart muscle to increase in mass and contractile strength** in the same way that heavy exercise causes skeletal muscle to hypertrophy.

147. D i.e Coronary circulation *[Ref: Ganong 22/e P-634]*

During exercise blood is shunted from regions that do not require immediate support to areas with increased demands. (e.g. skeletal muscles, heart)[Q].

148. A i.e. Regular 3 minute exercise

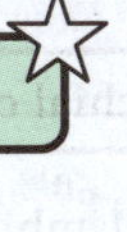

Regular 3 minute exercise have been well documented to bring about an increase in the aerobic capacity

149. C i.e. Epinephrine from medulla *[Ref: Harrison 16/e P- 1377; Schwartz 8/e P-324; Ganong 22/e P- 667]*

In cardiac transplantation, the recipient heart remains denervated, so cardiac function differs from that of the innervated heart during both rest & exercise

150. A i.e. Venoconstriction with decreased blood flow *[Ref: Ganong 22/e P-634]*

During vigrous exercise, constriction of vessels in splanchnic organ, and decreased blood ' storage' in liver & other portion of splanchnic bed occursQ, which may increase the volume of actively circulating blood, perfusion the muscles by as much as 30%. Contraction of the capacitance vessels in the viscera can pump a litre of blood into the arterial circulation, in less than a minute.

151. B i.e. Brain *[Ref Ganong 22/e P-599]*

The direct vasodilator action of CO_2 is most pronounced, in the skin and brainQ

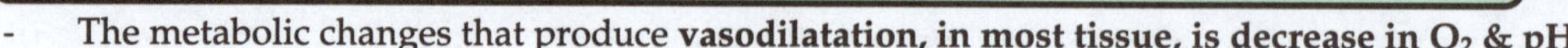

- The metabolic changes that produce **vasodilatation, in most tissue, is decrease in O_2 & pH**
- ↑ CO_2 is associated with ***cutaneous & cerebral vosodilatation***Q, but vasoconstriction elsewhere & usually a slow rise in BP.

152. D i.e. There is fall in systemic capillary hydrostatic pressure

Edema normally occurs due to increased hydrostatic pressure that pushes fluid out or due to reduced oncotic pressure that fails to pull the fluid. **Acute heart failure** is usually predominantly systolic and sudden reduction in cardiac output often result in systemic hypotension without peripheral edema. Acute heart failure is associated with a fall in hydrostatic pressure and therefore explains lack of peripheral edema.

153. D i.e. Aortic stenosis *[Ref: Ganong 24/e p. 542; Guyton 9/e P114, Braunwal 6/e P 479, 480,1675]*
154. B i.e. b

- In pressure volume curve, **during diastole in period of ventricular filling** (from d→a) **pressure increases. Pressure rises sharply to reach diastolic BP during isometric contraction** (form a→b)Q and (from b→c) during **period of ejection**. At C, the aortic valves close and pressure falls during **isovolunetric relaxation** (from c→d).
- In **AS,** pressure-volume (P-V) curve is shifted to the **left,** whereas in **MR and AR,** PV curve shifts to **right.**

Pressure Volume Curve (P-V Curve)

P-V curve denotes the pumping mechanics of the left ventricle (since left ventricle is the main chamber, all studies are referred to the left ventricle). **P-V Curve is shifted to left** (i.e. more pressure would be created for the same volume). When contractility of the chamber increases

- Increased sympathetic activity
- Concentric hypertrophy of the chamber
- Decreased compliance of the chamber

In aortic stenosis – there is ***pressure overload***Q, leading to ***concentric hypertrophy*** of the muscle causing *increased contractility* and *decreased compliance* of the left ventricle. The ***P-V curve shifts to left.***Q

In MR & AR there is *volume overload* leading to dilated left ventricle. Decreased contractility & increased compliance caused ***right shift of curve.***Q
In MS – there is *pressure overload* but only *in left atrium.*

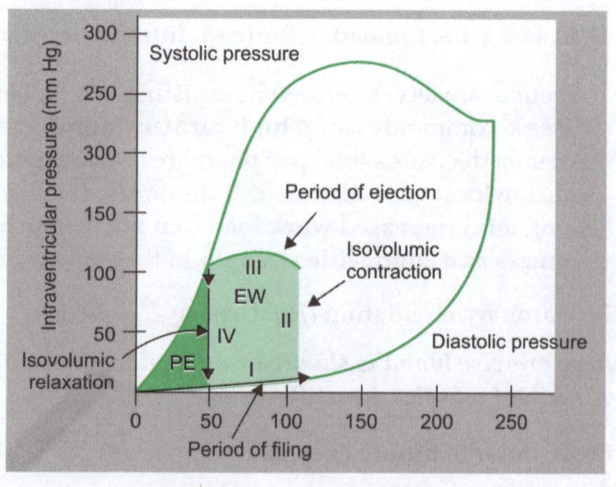

Left ventricular volume (ml)

155. D i.e. 60%

EDV=End-Diastolic volume (point a)=130 ml
ESV= End-Systolic volume (point d)= 50 ml
SV = Stroke volume= EDV=ESV= 130-50=80 ml

So, **Ejection Fraction** $= \frac{SV}{EDV} = \frac{80}{130} = 0.6 = 60\%$

Circulating Body Fluid

156. C i.e. Bone marrow

Bone Marrow

- It is one of the **largest and most active organ** approaching weight & size of liver. *Active* cellular marrow is called **red marrow,** inactive fatty marrow is K/a **yellow marrow**
- **Bone marrow is source of all blood cells in adults**[Q]. However, liver and yolk sac produce blood cells in fetal & neonatal life

Precursor/Lineage	Form
Erythroid	RBC
Megakaryocyte	Platelett
Myeloid	Neutrophil, Monocyte, Eosinophil, Basophil
Lymphoid	Lymphocytes[Q] (B & T cells)[Q]

★ **Both B & T lymphocyte origin in bone marrow in adults** (yolk sac & liver in fetus). But they **mature in Bone marrow (B=B cells)** and **Thymus (T=Thymus)** respectively

- Normally **75% marrow cells belong to white blood producing myeloid series** & only 25% are maturing RBCs. Even though in circulation RBCs are 500 times more than WBCs d/t the fact that average life span of WBCs is short and RBC is long.
- Cellularity & RBC production after 15 years onward is *Vertebrae > sternum > rib > femur shaft > tibia shaft*

157. B i.e. Lymph node **158. A i.e. Yolk sac** **159. A i.e. Flat bones**

[Ref: Guyton 11/e p. 420; Ganong 22/e p. 515-16; Chaudhary 5/e p-20-21]

The marrow of the long bones *except for the proximal humerus and tibia* (Guyton) / *upper humerus & femur* (Ganong) becomes inactive (fatty) and produces no more red blood cells after about age **20 years.** ***Beyond this age most RBC are produced in marrow of membranous flat bones such as vertebrae, sternum, ribs & ilia***[Q].

Erythropoesis

It starts in 3rd *week* of intra uterine life. Upto middle trimester of gestation blood is formed out of medullary cavity ***(extramedullary erythropoesis).***

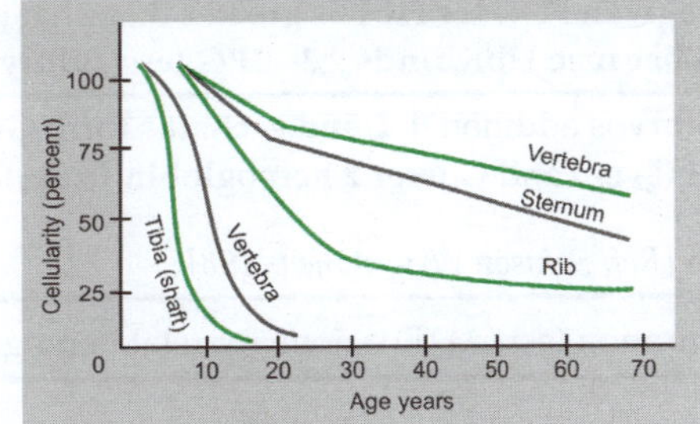

Before birth

Age	Site
3weeks – 3 months (Intra vascular phase)	***Mesoderm of yolk sac***[Q] within the *blood vessel.*
3-5 months (Hepatic phase)	***Liver (main), spleen & lymph nodes***[Q] (±)
5-9 months (Myeloid phase)	***Red bone marrow***[Q] ★ All marrow of **long & flat bones** is red at this stage

After birth

Age	Site
Birth –5 years (myeloid phase)	***Red bone marrow***[Q] ★ All marrow of long & flat bone is red at this stage.
5-20 years	***Red bone marrow***[Q] of all flat & long bones ★ There is gradual decrease of red marrow in long bones and so gradually increasing production from flat bones
>20 years	- Red marrow of **flat membranous bones** such as ***vertebrae, sternum, ribs & iliam***[Q]. - Very little production in upper humerus, tibia & femur

160. C i.e. Spleen *[Ref: Lippincott's 3/e P-280, Chaudhuri 5/e P-33]*

Breakdown of heme to bilirubin occurs in macrophages of the reticuloendothelial system ***mainly in the spleen***[Q] also in the liver and bone marrow.

161. B i.e. Inhibit heme oxygenase *[Ref: Care of newborn by meharban sing /189, Ghai 5/e P151]*

Tin & Zn porphyrins and mesoporphyrins ***inhibits the activity of heme oxygenase*** Q and *decrease formation of bilirubin*

Best method for Estimation of Hb come in blood is – ***Cyanmethhemoglobin method***Q

162. B i.e. Hemopexin

Heme Binding Proteins - haptoglobin (1st) and hemopexin (2nd line of defense) inhibit heme loss from plasma by binding heme (so preventing free heme in plasma).

163. A i.e. It is stored in ferritin *[Ref Ganong 22/e P- 477]*

Iron

Fe^{2+}	Fe^{3+} ferric	Transferrin	Ferritin
- ***Absorbed in this form in duodenum*** - ***Excreted in stool***Q	- Present in this form in diet - *Stored in this form*	***Iron transport protein in plasma***Q	***Principle storage form in tissue***Q

★ Iron is deposited in all cells of body specially in reticuloendothelial cells & liver hepatocytes.

164. C i.e. $\alpha 2\delta 2$

165. B i.e. It is made up of 2 alpha and 2 gamma subunit

166. B i.e. HbF

167. C i.e. Zeta and epsilon chains *[Ref: Ganong 24/e p. 559; Bijlani 3/e Pg 271 , Lehninger's 4/e p 173]*

- ***Embryonic hemoglobin contains epsilon & alpha ($\varepsilon_2\alpha_2$); or epsilon & zeta ($\varepsilon_2\zeta_2$); or zeta & gamma ($\zeta_2\gamma_2$) chains***Q.
- **Fetal hemoglobin (HbF)** differs from adult hemoglobin (HbA) in that **it has gamma (γ) chains in place of beta (β) chains. So HBF is $\alpha_2\gamma_2$, whereas HbA is $\alpha_2\beta_2$ tetramer**Q.
- 2,3 BPG greatly reduces the affinity of Hb to O_2. SO the **O_2 content** (at a given PO_2) **for HbF is greater** than that of adult hemoglobin **because HbF binds 2,3- BPG less avidly**Q.

Hemoglobin type	Tetramer (globin) chain
Adult Hb A	$\alpha_2\beta_2$ = most common Q
Adult Hb A2	$\alpha_2\delta_2$ = 2nd mc Q
Fetal Hb F	$\alpha_2\gamma_2$
Embryonic Hb (EHb)	
EHb Gower 1	$\zeta_2\varepsilon_2$
EHb Gower 2	$\alpha_2\varepsilon_2$
EHb Portland	$\zeta_2\gamma_2$

- In young embryos additional **ζ and ε chains** form **Gower 1 hemoglobin ($\zeta_2\varepsilon_2$)** and **Gower 2 hemoglobin ($\alpha_2\varepsilon_2$).**

168. B i.e. Fetal Hb *[Ref: Samson Wright 3/e p-198]*

Alkali denaturation test (ADT) – done for fetal hemoglobin. ***HbF is alkali denaturation resistant***Q.

169. A i.e. 6000 per cu mm *[Ref: Paul 2/ep 57-58]*

Neubauer (Hemocytometer) Square Chamber

This counting grid carved in glass is **3mm x 3mm** is size with **9 subdivision squares 1mm x 1mm**. For counting of

TLC (WBC-Number)

Four corner squares are usedQ.
Volume of 4 corner squares is 0.4 cu.mm **(=4 x.01 cu mm)**

$$\text{Number of WBCs} = \frac{\textbf{Cell count in 4 corner squares} \times \textbf{Dilution Factor}}{\textbf{0.4}}$$

$$\mathbf{WBCs = \frac{25+35+40+20}{0.4} \times 20 = 6000\,cells\,/\,dL^{Q}}$$

RBC & Platelets

Big central square is used which is split in 25 square of 0.2 mm. Each of these 25 squares are subdivided into 16 small squares. (So=25 x 16=400 total)

170. A i.e. C (Eosinophils) *[Ref: Guyton 11/ep 436, Ganong 24/ep 558]*

Parasitic infestations (=worm infections) causes eosinophilia (i.e. increased count of eosinophils)Q.

Identification of RBC & WBCs In Lab

RBCs (Erythrocytes)

Most numerous (4.8-5.5 million/mL), **biconcave disks (doughnut with a hole)** with **no nucleus** and small (8 μm dia) size.

WBCs (Leukocytes)

Much less in number **(5-10 thousand/mL)** with **~700:1 RBC: WBC ratio.** On the basis of **cytoplasmic appearance** it can be divided into 2 groups

Granular Leukocytes

Feature	Neutrophil	Eosino (Acido) phil	Basophil
Size	10-12 nm	10-12 μm	8-10 μm
Count	**Most (70%)**	2-4%	<1%
Cytoplasm (Granules)	**Lightly stained with very fine pale lilac, granules**	**Red-Orange large, uniform granules** that do not block nucleus	**Large blue-black round granules that block bilobed nucleus**[Q]
Nucleus	**Multiple (2-5) finely connected lobes** they are rarely uniform in size	**Mostly 2 (but may be 3) connected & more uniform, rounded nuclear lobes**[Q]	

Agranular Leukocytes

With **relatively clear cytoplasm**, this group includes -

- **Lymphocytes** 20-25 % of the WBCs, stains dark and is round or **slightly indented** with the **cytoplasm appearing as a rim around the nucleus.** The round, uniform nucleus and **small amount of cytoplasm surrounding it are the best identifying characteristics.**
- **Monocytes** comprise 3-8% of the WBCs, and **largest 12-20 μm** in diameter. The nucleus is indented or kidney shaped, not rounded, and **surrounded by foamy cytoplasm. Their size is the most easily identifiable characteristic.**

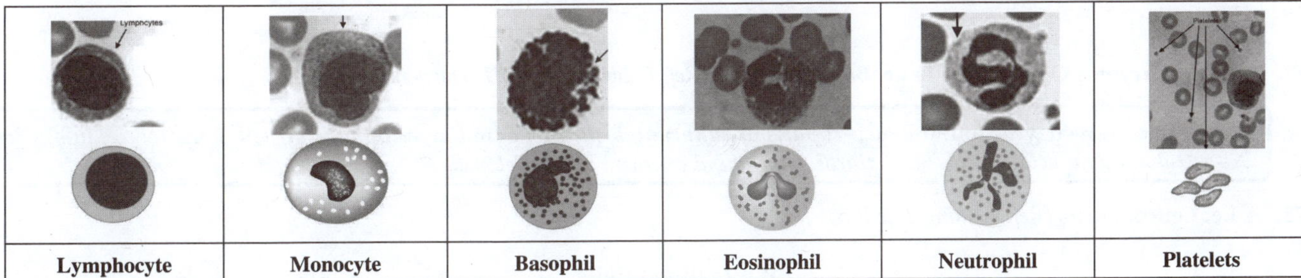

171. C i.e. Multiple myeloma *[Ref Ganong 22/e P- 585]*

> **In multiple myeloma,** M protein increase in the blood, this may cause cryoglobulinemia which leas to increase in viscosity of blood

172. A i.e. Low molecular weight and high blood concentration *[Ref: Guyton 10/e P46, 189]*

Osmotic pressure is determined by the number of particles in solution and not by the mass of the particle, that means 1 gm of a heavy molecular weight protein will contain a lesser no. of particles than 1 gm of a light molecular weight protein, & consequently will have a lesser osmotic pressure.

Plasma protein	MW	Concentration	Contribution to plasma osmolality
Albumin	69,000	3.5-5 gm%	80%
Globulin	1,40,000	2.0 gm%	20%
Fibrinogen	4,00,000	0.3 gm%	0%

Of the there major types of plasma protein, albumin with minimum molecular weight contributes. max to plasma oncotic pressure.

173. B i.e. Contractile protein *[Ref: Guyton 10/e P 419]*

> **Thrombosthenin** – is a ***contractile protein found within platelets.***[Q] It helps the platelets to contract during clot formation. Other contractile proteins found within platelets are- (i) Actin, (ii) Myosin

174. A i.e. Bone marrow; C i.e Thymus

Lymphoid Organs

Primary / Central	Secondary/ Peripheral
- Bone marrow[Q] - Thymus[Q]	- Bone marrow, Spleen, Lymph node - Payers patches, Waldeyer's ring (tonsils & adenoid)

★ Bone marrow serve as both central & peripheral lymphoid organ.

175. D i.e It takes part in intrinsic enzymatic reaction *[Ref: Ganong 22/e P- 521-525]*

Cytokines

- They are ***polypeptide***[Q] in nature.
- Induced their effect in three ways: ***Autocrine, paracrine & endocrine effects.***[Q]
- Mediates natural immunity
- Affects ***leucocytic movement***[Q]
- Requlate lymphocytic growth activation & differentiation.
- Activate inflammatory cells & stimulate hematopoesis.

176. A i.e. T cells

Lymphocyte

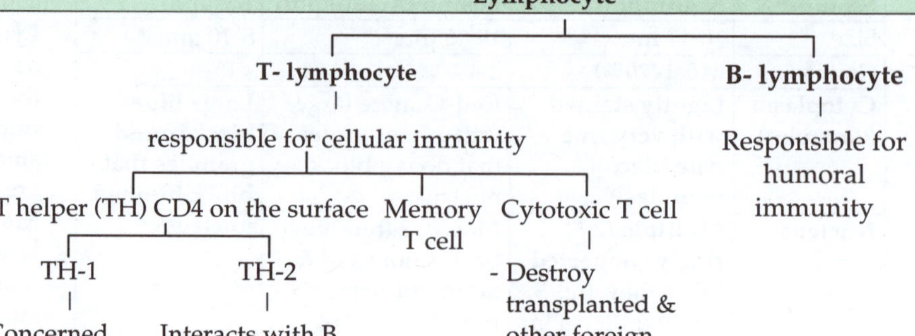

177. A i.e. Eukaryotes C i.e. Plants D i.e. Bacteriophage *[Ref: Robbins 7/e P- 61; Harper 26/e P- 621]*

Lysozyme is an enzyme found in ***neutrophils of eukaryotes, plants; & in bacteriophage virus***[Q]. It *hydrolyzes link between N- acetyl muramic acid & N acetyl D glucosamine found* in certain *bacterial walls*.

178. A i.e. Leucocytosis *[Ref: Ganong 22/e P-516]*

White Blood Cells

Granulocytes (Polymorphonuclear Leukocyte, PMNs)	Non- granular lecocytes
- Neutrophils (60-70%) - Eosinophils (1-4%) Mn: **"BEN"** - Basophils (0.2 – 1%)	- Lymphocytes (25-30%) - Monocytes (2-8%)

★ Tissue **macrophage** are derived from monocytes; and **mast cells** are related to basophils.

G-CSF: Granulocyte colony stimulating factor
GM-CSF: Granulocyte- Monocyte colony stimulating factor.

Thus G –CSF or GM-CSF will stimulate the synthesis of either granulocytes or monocytes hence leucocytosis is seen

179. B i.e. IL6; C i.e. IL 1; D i.e. TNFα *[Ref: Ganong's 24/e p. 73; Jawetz 26/e p. 130]*

Macrophage release **tumor necrosis factor (TNF)α, interleukin (IL)1/6/8/10/12/23, GMCSF** (granulocyte-macrophage colony stimulating factor), **GCSF**, transforming growth factor β **(TGF β)**, **VEGFA** and chemokines like IL8 (CXCL 8), rantes (CCL5), CXCL 9/10/11.

180. B i.e. Myeloperoxidase; C i.e. Lysozyme; E i.e. Cathepsin G. *[Ref: Chandrasoma Taylor 3/e P-409]*

Neutrophils secrete **myeloperoxidase, lysozyme** and **cathepsin G**[Q].

181. A i.e. It is a large glanular lymphocyte; B i.e. Releases granzymes and perforins; E i.e. Can kill virus infected and cancer cells *[Ref: Best & Taylor 13/e p. 375-76, 1226; Jawetz 26/e p. 125-26]*

Natural Killer (NK) cells are **large granular lymphocyte**[Q] which **kill virus infected cells and cancer cells mainly by cell** mediated immunity **using perforin and granzyme**[Q]. They **do not depend on thymus or antibody for killing**[Q] (although play role in ADCC).

182. B i.e. Kalazar; C i.e. TB; D i.e. Brucellosis *[Ref: Harrison 17/e p. 355; Harsh mohan 5/e p. 411]*

Absolute monocyte count > *800/μl* is called **monocytosis**, and it is associated with

- ***Tuberculosis (TB), Brucellosis, kalazar (visceral leishmaniasis)***[Q], subacute bacterial endocarditis, Rockey mountain spotted fever, & Malaria
- Malignancies , leukemia, myeloprotiferative syndromes, hemolytic anemias, chronic idiopathic neutropenias , & granulomatous diseases such as sarcoidosis, regional enteritis (IBD) and collagen vascular diseases.

183. B i.e. Neutrophil; C i.e. Macrophage; D i.e. Basophils; E i.e. B- Cells *[Ref: Robbins 7/e 202, 522; Harrison 15/e P- 1815]*

Sources of **Tumor Necrosis Factor (TNF)**

TNF - α

- ***Monocytes /macrophage***[Q]
- ***Basophils***[Q], Eosinophils
- Mast cell
- Natural killer (NK) cells
- Keratinocytes, Fibroblast
- Thymic epithelial cells
- ***T and β- cells***[Q]

TNF - β

- T cells
- B - cells

184. A i.e. 6 Hours *[Ref: Ganong 22/e P-516]*

The average half life of neutrophils in the circulation *is **6 Hours.***[Q]

To maintain normal circulating blood level, production of 100 billion neutrophils /day is necessary.

Half life of transfused platelet is 4 days[Q]

185. B i.e. Carries protein; D i.e. Fat absorption; E i.e. preventive role in infection. *[Ref: Bijlani 2/e P 174- 75]*

Lymphatics

k/as second circulatory system.

Feature

- Network of blind ended thin endothelial tubes.
- Endothelial lining is not fenestrated
- Unidirectional flow (d/t valves)
- All lympatics eventually open into venous system
- Intercellular junction are permeable to large molecules.
- Basement membrane is discontinuous.

Function

- ***Collects proteins, lipids & other large molecules***[Q] which leaks out of capillaries into interstitial space & returning these to circulation. This
  - Help to conserve these substance
  - Restore blood volume & composition
  - ***Prevent rising of osmotic pressure in interstitial spaces***[Q]
- ***Absorption of lipid in small intestine.***[Q]
- Carry large undesirable particulate matter and bacteria to the nearest lymph node where they can be handled by macrophage or lymphocytes (essential role in *defence mechanism of body)*[Q]

186. C i.e. VIII **187. D i.e. XII** *[Ref: Guyton 11/e p. 464; Ganong 22/e P--544]*

- **Vit K dependent factors:** ***factor II (prothrombin), VII, IX, X protein C and S***[Q]
- **Vit K is a necessary cofactor for the enzyme that catalyzes carboxylation of glutamic residue in these proteins, necessary for their action.**
- ***PT is first to be prolonged in Vit K deficiency.***[Q] (factor VII has short t1/2)

188. A i.e. Hemophilia *[Ref: Ganong 22/e P—544; Harrison 16/e P-680 ,681]*

Hemophilia A is a disorder of coagulation that occurs due to deficiency or reduced activity of factor VIII[Q].

189. B i.e. PT is increased *[Ref Ganong Physiology 23rd/e p. 531-35; 22/e P- 540-45; Harrison 16/e P-680,681;Chaudhuri 5/e P-58]*

Hemophilia A occurs d/t deficiency of factor VIII. Factor ***VIII is involved in intrinsic pathway which is measured by PTT.*** Q

190. D i.e. Factor VII *[Ref: Ganong 23rd/e p. 531- 35; Robbins 7/ed pg-128; clinical hematology 4/ed pg-355]*

Factor 7 is involved in extrinsic pathway and factors 8, 9, 11 and 12 are involved in extrinsic pathway of coagulation Q.

191. B i.e. Factor VII *[Ref: Ganong 22/e p. 539- 40, 542- 53; Guyton 11/e p. 293, 458- 65; Chandrasoma Taylor 3/e p- 426]*

Serum has essentially the same composition as plasma except that

- ***its clotting factor II,V, VIII and fibrinogen (I) have been removed*** Q
- it has a ***higher serotonin*** Q content b/o breakdown of platelets during clotting.

Plasma

It is the extracellular *fluid portion of blood* that contains immense number of ions, inorganic & organic molecules. It is rich in clotting factors, and can clot

Plasma = Whole blood – Cellular component

★ Since ***test tube (invitro) clotting activates only intrinsic pathway, the factor VII (7) that is exclusve to extrinsic system is not consumed*** Q.

Serum

It is the *fluid that remains after clot retraction*, i.e., if the whole blood is allowed to clot in a tube and clot is removed, the remaining fluid is serum. Serum *cannot clot*.

Serum = Whole blood – Clot
Serum = Plasma – Clotting factors 1, 2, 5 & 8

192. B i.e. 8-12

Half life of clotting factors (in hours) in increasing order is Factors III (6hrs), **Factor VIII (8-12 hrs)** Q, Factor V & IX (24 hrs), WVF (30 hrs), Factor X (45-50 hrs), Factor II (60 hrs), Factor XI (50-84 hrs), **Factor I (100-150 hrs) and Factor XII (150 hrs), (Mn: Factor 8 has half life of 8-12 hours)** Q.

193. A i.e. Factor XIII *[Ref: Ganong 24/e p. 577]*

Factor XIII (B) helps in bridging the fibrin in a clot and stabilizes the clot by covalently cross linking fibrin Q. It requires Ca^{++}.

194. C i.e. Thrombin

195. A i.e. Factor XIII *[Ref: Ganong 23rd/e p. 531- 35; 22/e p. 543; Harrison 17/e p. 364; Guyton 11/e p. 459- 50]*

- **Factor XIII (13)** also known as **fibrin stabilizing factor**, when gets activated (by *thrombin*) cause ***formation of covalent cross linkages and provide three dimensional strength to fibrin meshwork (stbilization)*** Q
- Factor XIII (a) converts a loose mesh of *interlacing fibrin strands to a tightly* dense aggregate by formation of multiple **covalent bonds** between fibrin monomers and cross linkages between fibrin fibers. This also requires *calcium*.

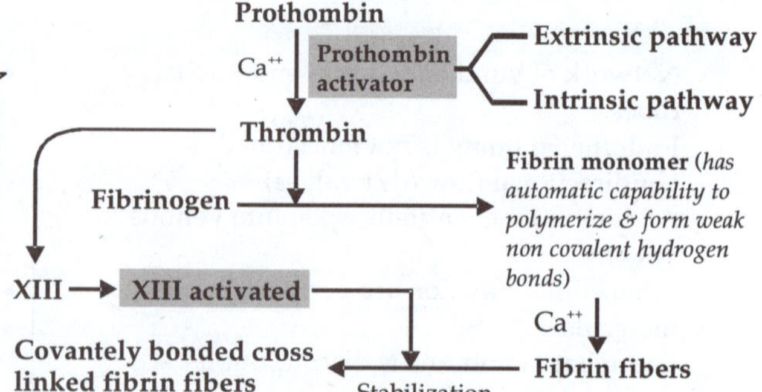

196. A i.e. Antithrombin III

197. C i.e. Cerebral circulation

198. D i.e. Vascular endothelium is smooth & coated with glycocalyx *[Ref: Ganong 24/e p. 566-69; Guyton 12/e p. 456]*

- Blood clotting is prevented by endothelium d/t their *smoothness and its glycocalyx- thrombomodulin layer* Q. Thrombomodulin, ***a thrombin binding protein, is expressed by all endothelial cells except those in the cerebral microcirculation*** Q.
- Vascular endothelium is ***smooth and is coated with a layer of glycocalyx (mucopolysaccharide)*** Q which prevents activation of intrinsic system and repels clotting factor & platelets, thereby *preventing clotting of blood with in vessels.*
- ***Antithrombin (AT) III is the most important anticoagulant in blood which prevents clotting of blood in normal vascular system*** Q. **Heparin** is powerful anticoagulant but its concentration in blood is low, so by itself it has **little or no anticoagulant property in normal vascular system**. However, heparins binding with ATIII increases effectiveness of AT III upto 1000 times. **Fibrin** (not fibrinogen) also has **antithrombin action during clot formation**.

199. D i.e. Alpha-2 macroglobulin >> B i.e. Heparin cofactor II *[Ref: Harper 27/e p. 611; Devlin 5/e p. 1041]*

- There are **4 naturally occurring thrombin inhibitors** in normal plasma
  - **Antithrombin III**Q is most important & contributes ~75% of antithrombin activity. It also inhibits factors IXa, Xa, XIa, XIIa and VIIa complexed with tissue factors.
  - **α_2-macroglobulin**Q contributes most of remainder antithrombin activity.
  - **Heparin cofactor II** and **α_1 antitrypsin** are minor inhibitors under physiological conditions
- **Heparin** (acid proteoglycan) binds to **cationic site of antithrombin III and greately potentiates its activity**Q. So, strongly cationic polypeptide such as **protamine** strongly bind to heparin & inhibit its anticoagulant effect.
- Contrary to heparin (which acts through antithrombin III), direct thrombin inhibitors such as **bivaluridin, lepirudin,** and **argatroban** directly inhibits the active site of thrombin. So they have no effect on factors 9, 10, 11, 12 and 7.
- **Thrombin** catalyzes *conversion of fibrinogen to fibrin,* and is also involved in a regulatory mechanism of coagulation in this way. Thrombin forms a complex with *thrombomodulin,* a glycoprotein on endothelial surface which *activates protein C (APC)* → activated protein C combines with protein S *and degrade factor Va and VIIIa* limiting their action in coagulation. So deficiency of either protein C or protein S can cause venous thrombosis.
- **Factor V leiden**, has a *glutamine residue in place of arginine at position 506,* which makes it *resistant to inactivation by APC.* So this condition has *increased risk of venous thrombosis.*

200. D i.e. Vasoconstriction and platelet aggregartion

201. A i.e. Platelet adhesion to exposed endothelium B i.e. Clot retraction C i.e. Activation of prothrombinase complex D i.e. Vasoconstriction *[Ref: Harper's Biochemistry 26/e P- 601; Ganong 22/e P- 542; Guyton 10/e P- 418 – 23]*

Thromboxane (TX) A_2 causes vasoconstriction & platelet aggregationQ. Whereas prostacycline (PGI_2) has reverse action ie vasodilatation & inhibition of platelet aggregation.

Role of Platelets in Hemostasis

- ***Vasoconstriction***Q d/t **release of *TXA_2* and *serotonin***
- **Adherence**: The glycoprotein of cell membrane platelet cause adherence to exposed endothelium (but repulses to normal endothelium)
- **Platelet plug formation or aggregation** closing small vascular holes **due to thromboxane A2 (TxA_2)**Q.

↓

- **Conversion of prothrombin to thrombin:** ***Activation of prothrombinase complex***Q (consisting of platelet anionic phospholipids Ca^{++}, factor Va, factor Xa and prothrombin) on the surface of activated platelet l/t conversion of prothrombin into thrombin
- **Stabilization of fibrin:** Fibrin stabilization factor released from platelet cause stablization of fibrin (Polymerization of fibrin)
- Thrombin causes conversion of fibrinogen to fibrin

↓

- **Fibrinous organization of blood clot** d/t growth factors secreted by platelet
- **Clot retraction & contraction** d/t contractile proteins actin, myosin and thrombosthenin

202. D i.e. ABO [H] antibodies are invariably present in plasma when person RBC lacks the corresponding antigen.

203. A, B, C i.e. Found on RBC membrane; Glycprotein in nature; Highly immunogenic

204. D i.e. AO *[Ref: Best & Taylor 13/e p 379; Guyton 12/e p. 445-46; Ganong 24/e p. 560-61; Ananthanarayanan 8/e p. 185-86; Lippincott 4/e p. 165]*

- **Highly immunogenic ABO blood group antigen** is due to **complex oligosaccharide (glycoprotein) found on RBC membrane.** It is inherited as **medelian autosomal dominants**Q.
- **ABO blood group** system remains the most important blood group system in clinical practice because **ABO [H] antibodies are invariably present in plasma when person's RBC's lack the corresponding antigen.** And because of these preformed antibodies the reaction is immediate.
- Genotype of a person with **A blood group** may either be **AA (homozygous)** or **AO (heterozygous)**. The genotype in **B blood group** may be **BB (Hamozygous)** or **BO (heterozygous);** in **AB** blood group **AB** and in blood group **O** the genotype is **OO.**

205. **D i.e. Nerve growth factor** *[Ref: Trocia M et al. Nerve growth factor inhibits apoptosis in memory B cells J Biochem 2001; 19;276(42):39027-36]*

- **Nerve growth factor inhibits apoptosis in memory B cells**Q via inactivation of p^{38} MAPK, prevention of antiapoptotic factor Bcl-2 phosphorylation (i.e. maintaining its integrity) & cytochrome c release

- Although other growth factors like FGF, PDGF and IGF can also prolong the survival, it is the *nerve growth factor that is most important in immortalization of memory cells.*

Growth factor → activate P13 kinase → activate Akt → inactivates procaspase 9 & inhibit Fast synthesis

206. **C i.e. Oestrogen** *[Ref: A.K. Jain clinical hematology 2/e P 150, water & Emile P664]*

Erythropoiesis is promoted by **ACTH, Prolactin, TSH (thyroxine stimulating hormone) but not oestrogen**Q.

207. **B i.e. Hints at serious heart ailment**

Ventricular extrasystole (premature beat) in the **absence of ischemic heart disease is usually benign**Q.

208. **B i.e. Brilliant Cryesyl blue** *[Ref: Samson Wright 13/e P 33,34]*

Reticulocytes- They young red cells are so called because on vital staining with cresyl blue a network of reticulum is apparent in the cytoplasm as clumps of small dots or as a faint thread connecting two small nodes. **Staining solution include:** ***Brilliant Cresyl blue***Q (Supravital staining), Sodium citrate, NaCl, Distilled H_2O

★ Myeloid: Erythroid ratio in Red bone marrow is ***3 : 1*** Q

209. **E i.e. None** *[Ref: Ganong 22/e P- 539]*

Plasma – is fluid portion of blood, containing an immense number of ions, inorganic molecules & organic molecules that are in transit to various part of the body.
Serum - If whole blood is allowed to clot and the clot is removed, the remaining fluid is serum.

- It has same composition as plasma except *its fibrinogen, factor 2,5,& 8 have been removed*
- It has high serotonin content d/t breakdown of platelets during clotting.

210. **D i.e. Used to increase oxygen delivery to tissue** 211. **B i.e. Plasma expander**
212. **C i.e. Plasma expander** *[Ref: KDT 5/e P-582-584; Trauma Management by Asensio P-70-82]*

Plasma expanders are high molecular weight substances which exert colloidal osmotic pressure and when infused intravenously retain fluid in the vascular compartment. **Substances employed as Plasma expanders include:** Human albumin, ***Dextran***Q, ***Hydroxyethyl starch (Hetastarch)***Q, Degraded gelatin polymer, Polyvinyl pyrrolidane.

213. **C i.e. Bicarbonate** *[Ref: O.P Ghai 4/e P 182]*

Composition of Ringers lactate: ***Calcium chloride***Q, ***Potassium chloride***Q, ***Sodium chloride***Q, ***Sodium lactate***Q.

Chapter -5 DIGESTIVE SYSTEM

QUESTIONS

Saliva, Oesophagus and Stomach

1. **Lysozyme is present in-** *(NBE P 13)*
   A. Saliva
   B. Human milk
   C. Tears
   D. Mucus
2. **Maximum potassium ions secretion is seen in:**
   A. Saliva *(AIIMS 09)*
   B. Gastric secretions
   C. Jejunal secretions
   D. Colonic secretions
3. **Highest concentration of potassium is in?**
   A. Bile *(AIIMS 09)*
   B. Pancreatic juice
   C. Terminal ileal secretions
   D. Rectal fluid
4. **Salivary amylase is inactivated by-** *(NBE P 13)*
   A. Enteropeptidase
   B. Low pH of stomach
   C. High pH of intestine
   D. None
5. **A man cannot digest carbohydrate. The enzyme deficient is-** *(NBE P 13)*
   A. Lipase
   B. Amylase
   C. Pepsin
   D. Trypsin
6. **Which of the following is not true about the salivary gland output in SjÖgren's syndrome?** *(AIIMS 16)*
   A. Increase in sodium concentration
   B. Increase in phosphate concentration
   C. Decreased output of salivary glands<0.5ml/min
   D. Increase in IgA concentration
7. **Effect of aceytylcholine on LES-** *(NBE P 13)*
   A. Contraction
   B. Relaxation
   C. No effect
   D. Contraction followed by relaxation
8. **Lower esophageal sphincter:** *(AIIMS 04)*
   A. Has no tonic activity
   B. Has a tone which is provided by the sympathetic system
   C. Relaxes on increasing abdominal pressure
   D. Relaxes ahead of the peristaltic wave
9. **Rennin is present in-** *(NBE P 13)*
   A. Gastric juice
   B. Liver
   C. Kidney
   D. Lung
10. **Normal gastric juice contains *all except:***
    A. Na^+ *(AI 05, AIIMS 06)*
    B. K^+
    C. Ca^{++}
    D. Mg^{++}
11. **Pepsinogen is secreted by-** *(NBE P 13)*
    A. Parietal cells
    B. Mucus cells
    C. Chief cells.
    D. Oxyntic cells
12. **Intrinsic Factor of Castle is secreted by which of the following cells in gastric glands:** *(NBE P 15, 13; AI 09)*
    A. Chief cells *(DNB 15, 14)*
    B. Parietal (Oxyntic) cells
    C. Enterochromaffin cells
    D. B cells
13. **Goblet cells secrete-** *(NBE P 13)*
    A. HCI
    B. Pepsin
    C. Mucus
    D. Serolonin
14. **Which of the following enzymes is stable at acidic low pH:** *(AI 07)*
    A. Pepsin/pepsinogen
    B. Trypsin
    C. Chymotrypsin
    D. Carboxypeptidase
15. **Chymotrypsinogen in activated into chymotrypsin by**
    A. Trypsin *(AIIMS 01)*
    B. Pepsin
    C. Fatty acids
    D. Bile salts
16. **Trypsinogen is converted to trypsin by-** *(NBE P 13)*
    A. Pepsin
    B. Enterokinase
    C. HCL
    D. None
17. **Pancreatic secretion contain -** *(NBE P 14; PGI 04)*
    A. Trypsin & Lipase
    B. Enteropeptidase
    C. Pepsin
    D. Renin
18. **All of the following are secreted proenzyme form except:** *(NBE P 14,13; Delhi 06)*
    A. Trypsin
    B. Chymotrypsin
    C. Pepsin
    D. Ribonuclease/Amylase
19. **Following are gastrointestinal hormones except :**
    A. CCK- PZ *(DNB 14,13)*
    B. GIP
    C. Motilin
    D. Chymotrypsin

20. Chymotrypsinogen is a *(AIIMS 11, 06)*
A. Zymogen
B. Carboxypeptidase
C. Transaminase
D. Elastase

21. All of the following are trypsin inhibitors, Except: *(AI 08)*
A. Alpha – 1 antitrypsin
B. Alpha – 1 – antiproteinase
C. Enterokinase
D. Egg – white

22. Cephalic phase of gastric secretion- *(NBE P 13)*
A. On food entering stomach
B. On food entering intestine
C. On seeing food
D. On stress

23. Cephalic phase of gastric secretion- *(NBE P 13)*
A. 20%
B. 70%
C. 10%
D. 100%

24. Cephalic phase of gastric secretion is mediated by *(AI 02)*
A. Neurohormones
B. Parasympathetic
C. Sympathetic
D. Gastrin

25. The gastric phase of gastric HCl secretion is brought about by *(NBE P 15,13; AIIMS 03, 14, 15)*
A. Neural factors
B. Gastrin Hormonal factors
C. Gastric distension
D. Presence of proteins in the stomach

26. Which of these statements are correct regarding acid secretion in stomach: *(PGI 06, 02)*
A. Gastrin increases acid secretion
B. Secretin decreases acid secretion
C. H_2 blockers decrease acid secretion
D. Total acid secretion reflexes functional parietal cell mass
E. Somatostatin increases acid secretion

27. Gastric secretion is increased by all except- *(NBE P 13)*
A. Histamine
B. Acetylcholine
C. Gastrin
D. HCL

28. HCL secretion is stimulated by: *(NBE P 14; PGI 08)*
A. Secretin
B. Somatostatin
C. Histamine & Gastrin
D. VIP

29. Gastric secretions stimulated by all of the following except: *(NBE P 13, 14, 15; AIIMS 14, 15)*
A. Secretin
B. Gastric (antral) distension
C. Gastrin
D. Vagal stimulus

30. Gastrin is produced by: *(NBE P 15,14,13)*
A. Pancreas
B. Gastric antral cells
C. Pituitary
D. All

31. Gastric secretion is : *(NBE P 13; UP 02, UPSC 09)*
A. Inhibited by curare
B. Stimulated by nor adrenaline
C. Increased by stomach antral distention
D. Stimulated by an increase in tonic activity

32. Which of the following is TRUE regarding gastric emptying: *(NEET 14, AIIMS 08)*
A. Decreased by CCK.
B. Decreased by gastrin
C. Increased by secretin
D. Decreased by insulin.

33. Stimulation for gastric emptying : *(DNB 01)*
A. Secretin
B. CCK
C. Gastrin
D. Distension

34. Gastric emptying sequence into duodenum- *(NBE P 13)*
A. Fat>protein>carbohydrate
B. Fat<carbohydrate<protein
C. Protein<fat<carbohydrate
D. Protein>fat>carbohydrate

35. Physiological gastrectomy is: *(PGI 2K)*
A. Ligate all major arteries
B. Antrectomy
C. Upper 1/3 of stoma resected
D. Ligation of 4-out of five arteries

36. Figure below represents the pH of the digestive juices aspirated from the alimentary tract as a function of position along the alimentary tract during digestion of a meal: *(AI 03)*

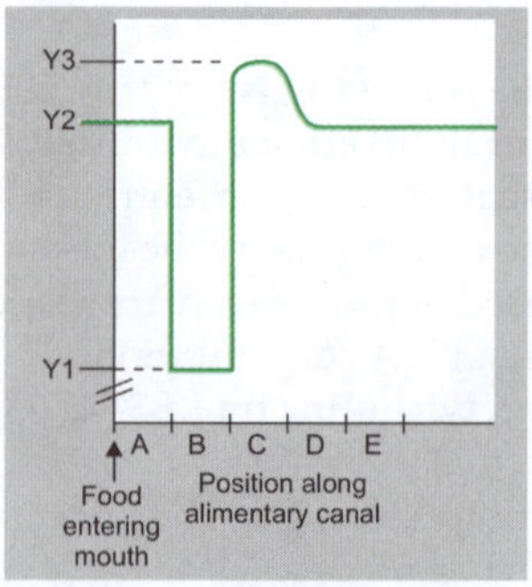

A. A typical value for Y2 is 9.0
B. A typical value for Y3 is 10.0
C. The segment C represents the pylorus
D. The digestive enzymes active in segment A are inactivated in segment B.

Pancreatic Secretions

37. Pancreatic lipase hydrolyses ester linkage of triacid glycerides at position- *(NBE P 13)*
A. 1&2
B. 1&3
C. 2&3
D. Only 3

38. Amount of water lost in stools- *(NBE P 13)*
A. 50ml ☐
B. 200ml ☐
C. 300ml ☐
D. 350ml ☐

39. Daily pancreatic secretion- *(NBE P 13)*
A. 1.5L ☐
B. 2.5 L ☐
C. 5.0 L ☐
D. 10 L ☐

40. True about secretin is: *(PGI 02)*
A. Increased gallbladder contraction and HCO_3 rich pancreatic fluid ☐
B. Increased gastrin secretion ☐
C. Gastric hypermotility ☐
D. Increase enzyme rich pancreatic fluid ☐

41. All are true about secretion except: *(PGI 08, 15)*
A. Inhibits gastric emptying *(NBE P 14, 13)* ☐
B. Increases bicarbonate rich pancreatic secretion ☐
C. Potentiates action of CCK ☐
D. ↑ ses bile salt & bile acids ☐
E. Increases bile secretion ☐

42. The duodenum secretes a hormone which has following effects except: *(DNB 14,11, AI 09)*
A. Causes copious pancreatic juice rich in bicarbonate and poor in enzymes ☐
B. Increases gastric motility ☐
C. Causes gall bladder to contract and sphincter of oddi to relax ☐
D. Leads to meagre flow of pancreatic juice rich in enzymes ☐

43. Actions of cholecystokinin include all of the following except: *(AIIMS 14)*
A. Contraction of gall bladder ☐
B. Secretion of pancreatic juice rich in enzymes ☐
C. Increases the secretion of enterokinase and augments the action of gastrin ☐
D. Stimulated gastric emptying ☐

44. Which of the following statements, regarding 'secretin' is least correct? *(AI 08)*
A. Increases bicarbonate rich secretion ☐
B. Inhibit gastric acid secretion ☐
C. Increases gastric acid secretion ☐
D. Causes contraction of pyloric sphincter ☐

45. Most potent stimulus for secretin is - *(NBE P 13)*
A. Dilatation of intestine ☐
B. Acid chime/Acid ☐
C. Protein ☐
D. Fat ☐

46. Pancreatic juice rich in water and electrolytes poor in enzymes is secreted in response to : *(NBE P 14)*
A. Pancreatozymin ☐
B. Cholecystokinin ☐
C. Secretin ☐
D. Proteins ☐

47. Secretin does not cause : *(UP 08, AI 10)*
A. Bicarbonate secretin ☐
B. Auguments the action of CCK ☐
C. Contraction of pyloic sphincter ☐
D. Gastric secretion increase ☐

48. I cells secrete- *(NBE P 13)*
A. Secretin ☐
B. Gastrin ☐
C. CCK ☐
D. Motilin ☐

49. Best stimuli for CCK secretion is: *(NBE P 13)*
A. Acid ☐
B. Protein ☐
C. Bile ☐
D. Fat ☐

50. Fat in the duodenum lumen : *(AI 09)*
A. Stimulates gall bladder contraction ☐
B. Inhibits gall bladder contraction ☐
C. Inhibits CCK secretion ☐
D. Releases Secretin ☐

51. CCK-PZ causes all of the following except :
A. Gall bladder contraction *(AI 10)* ☐
B. Pancreatic enzyme secretion ☐
C. Increased gastrin secretion ☐
D. Decreased lower esophageal sphinictor ☐

52. Gallbladder contraction is stimulated by OR The most important hormone that increases gallbladder contraction after a fatty meal is: *(NBE P 15; AIIMS 14)*
A. Gastrin ☐
B. Secretin ☐
C. Vagus ☐
D. Cholycystokinin ☐

Gall Bladder & Bile

53. Which is/are not present in bile: *(PGI 12)*
A. Bile salt ☐
B. Bile pigment ☐
C. Cholesterol ☐
D. Phospholipids ☐
E. Cholecystokinin ☐

54. Secretion of bile into bile canaliculus is by-
A. Osmotic gradient *(NBE P 13)* ☐
B. Facilitated diffusion ☐
C. Active transport across the membrane ☐
D. Simple diffusion ☐

55. Most important stimulant for bile secretion is:
A. Cholecystokinin *(AIIMS 05, Jipmer 09)* ☐
B. Secretin ☐
C. Bile acid ☐
D. Bile salt ☐

56. Bilirubin is secreted by: *(AIIMS 08, DNB 13)*
A. Bile Salts ☐
B. Bile pigments ☐
C. Secretin ☐
D. CCK. ☐

57. Maximum contraction of gall bladder is seen with:
A. CCK *(PGI 2K)* ☐
B. Secretin ☐
C. Gastrin ☐
D. Enterogastrone ☐

58. Bilirubin is derived from: *(PGI 02)*
A. Myoglobin
B. Hemoglobin
C. Muscle
D. Cholesterol
E. Amino acids

59. In blood bilirubin is with- *(NBE P 13)*
A. Protein
B. Steroid
C. Vitamin
D. Carbohydrates

60. Role of bile salts- *(NBE P 13)*
A. Vit B12 absorption
B. Formationof lipid bilayer
C. Emulsification of lipids
D. Fatry acid degradation

61. Bile acid has a detergent action due to:
A. Formation of soap *(AIIMS 07)*
B. Formation of zwitter ion
C. Amphipathic nature of bile acids
D. Formation of medium chain triglycerides.

Liver

62. Fat is maximum snythesised in- *(NBE P 13)*
A. Liver
B. Adipose tissue
C. Intestine
D. Muscle

63. Function of hepatic stellate cells is/are:
A. Formation of sinusoids *(PGI 01)*
B. Vit-A storage
C. Increases blood perfusion
D. Phagocytosis

64. Liver synthesizes all, except: *(AIIMS 07)*
A. C3 complement component
B. Hap Toglobin
C. Fibrinogen
D. Immunoglobulin

65. Conjugated hyperbilirubinemia in infancy is seen in:
A. Gilbert syndrome *(PGI 06)*
B. Criggler- najjar syndrome
C. Dubin- johnson syndrome
D. Rotor syndrome
E. Neonatal hepatitis

66. Abnormal synthesis function of liver:
A. ↑ PT *(PGI 06)*
B. Hyperbilirubinemia
C. Acute phase reactant
D. Kupffer cells

Motality

67. Gastro-colic reflex is related to: *(AIIMS 03, Orissa 08)*
A. Mass peristalsis
B. Segmental movement
C. Pendular movement
D. Colonic cases

68. All of the following statements are true for 'Intestinal Motility' except: *(NBE P 15,14; AI 07)*
A. Does not depend on Gastric motility
B. Increased by Distension
C. Increased by Acetylcholine
D. Increased by cholecystokinin

69. Intestinal motility is increased by- *(NBE P 13)*
A. Secretin
B. Gastrin
C. CCK
D. None

70. After a meal rich in carbohydrate, insulin secretion is stimulated by: *(Jipmer 03, WB 05)*
A. CCK
B. Serotonin
C. VIP
D. GLP-1 (7-36) amide

71. Major regulator of interdigestive myoelectric complexes *(NBE P 14, 15; TN04, SGPGI 03, UP 05)*
A. VIP
B. GIP
C. Motilin
D. Neurotensin
E. GRP

72. Motilin secretion decreased in- *(NBE P 13)*
A. Thirsty
B. Starving
C. Ingested meal
D. Interdigestive state

73. Myentric plexus is present in- *(NBE P 13)*
A. Muscularis externa
B. Submucosa
C. Mucosa
D. Serosa

74. Small intestinal peristalsis is controlled by :
A. Myentric plexus *(NEET 13, Kerala 04)*
B. Meissners plexus
C. Vagus nerve
D. Para sympathetic system

75. Pacemaker of the G.I.T. is located in: *(PGI 08, 15)*
A. Cardiac end of stomach
B. Long muscle of small intestine
C. Pyloric end of stomach
D. Central control of CBD origin
E. Fundus of stomach

76. Chyme is propelled forward in small intestine by
A. Segmentation *(PGI 08, 14)*
B. Haustrations
C. Migratory motor complexes (MMC)
D. Peristalsis

77. Major initiating response for peristalsis is- *(NBE P 13)*
A. Hormonal
B. Local stretching of gut
C. Neural
D. None

78. What is responsible for clearing & flushing food from the intestinal lumen in the interdigestive period-

A. Gastrin (NBE P 13) ☐
B. Migration motor complexes ☐
C. Secretin ☐
D. CCK ☐

79. Migratory motor complexes in the gut reappear after intervals of: *(AIIMS 16)*
A. 90 mins ☐
B. 120 mins ☐
C. 60 mins ☐
D. 150 mins ☐

80. Enterogastric reflex is caused by all, except:
A. Duodenum distension *(PGI 08, AIIMS 04)* ☐
B. Alkaline pH in duodenum & hormones ☐
C. Increased osmolality of chime ☐
D. Products of protein digestion & H^+ ions bathing duodenal mucosa ☐

81. Factors responsible for causing diarrhoea after vagotomy are A/E: *(NEET 13, PGI 08)*
A. Rapid gastric emptying ☐
B. Hypoacidity in duodenum ☐
C. Irregular peristalsis ☐
D. None ☐

82. All of the following are true about basal electrical rhythm of intestines except: *(AIIMS 15)*

A. Tone of contraction is related to amplitude of the stimulus ☐
B. Tone of contraction is related to frequency of stimulation ☐
C. Frequency of contraction is 6 per minute ☐
D. Threshold of contraction is –50 mV ☐

83. Slow waves/BER maximum in- *(NBE P 13)*
A. Stomach ☐
B. Ileums ☐
C. Colon ☐
D. Rectum ☐

84. Maximum postprandial motility is seen in:
A. Ascending colon *(AIIMS 11, 08)* ☐
B. Transverse colon ☐
C. Descending colon ☐
D. Sigmoid colon ☐

85. While doing sigmoidoscopy, if the rectum is inflated with gas increased peristalsis is seen in: *(AIIMS 01)*
A. Whole colon ☐
B. Proximal colon ☐
C. Distal colon ☐
D. Whole intestine ☐

Small & Large Intestine

86. Best absorbable monosaccharide- *(NBE P 13)*
A. Glucose ☐
B. Mannose ☐
C. Fructose ☐
D. Lactose ☐

87. The amount of water absorbed in the intestine in a day is: *(NBE P 13, AIIMS 05)*
A. 5 lit. ☐
B. 1 lit. ☐
C. 10 lit. ☐
D. 8 lit. ☐

88. Maximum water & electrolyte reabsorption in the Gastrointestinal tract occurs in OR Resection of which intestional segment causes marked electrolyte imbalance: *(NBE P 15,13; AI 11, 10)*
A. Stomach ☐
B. Jejunum ☐
C. Ileum ☐
D. Colon ☐

89. Maximum absorption of bile occurs at - *(Bihar 03)*
A. Jejunum ☐
B. Duodenum ☐
C. Ileum ☐
D. Colon ☐

90. Which of the following is absorbed in the colon -
A. Iron *(AMU 04, Jhar 06, MP 05)* ☐
B. Proteins ☐
C. Bile salts ☐
D. Electrolytes ☐

91. Which of the following secretions has a very high pH?
A. Gastric juice *(AI 06)* ☐
B. Pancreatic juice ☐
C. Bile in gall bladder ☐
D. Saliva ☐

92. The final sugars in intestinal chyme are: *(Delhi 06)*
A. Glucose & fructose ☐
B. Ribose & mannose ☐
C. Ribose & xylulose ☐
D. Xylulose & fructose ☐

93. The only Sugar normaly absorbed in the intestine against a concentration gradient is OR Which is maximally absorbed from GIT:
A. Xylose *(NBE P 15,13, Jipmer 04)* ☐
B. Mannose ☐
C. Glucose (Flexose) ☐
D. Ribose (Pantose) ☐

94. All of these are required for digestion of dietary fat:
A. Bile pigments *(PGI 02)* ☐
B. Gastric lipase ☐
C. Colipase ☐
D. Bile salts ☐
E. Pancreatic lipase ☐

95. True about fat absorption *(PGI 2K)*
A. Fat in stool > 6 gm/day indicate malabsorption ☐
B. C-glycine test is most sensitive test ☐
C. Major fat absorption occurs in proximal intestine (jejunum & duodenum) ☐
D. Steatorrhea means stool fat > 10 gm/day ☐

96. Short chain fatty acid produced by bacteria are maximally absorbed in : *(NEET 15,13, Jipmer 02)*
A. Duodenum
B. Colon
C. Ileum
D. Jejunum

97. What is Intrinsic Factor related to- *(NBE P 13)*
A. Cobalmin absorption
B. Vitamin D
C. Folate absorbtion
D. Vitamin C

98. Gastric secretions are essential for absorption of-
A. Cobalamin *(NBE P 13)*
B. Fat
C. Thiamine
D. Folic acid

99. Vitamin B_{12} is absorbed in: *(NBE P 15,13; PGI 15,12,07)*
A. Duodenum
B. Jejunum
C. Ileum
D. Stomach

100. Glossitis and cheilitis seen with which Vit. deficiency:
A. Vit. B2 *(PGI 06)*
B. Vit. B12
C. Vit. K
D. Vit D
E. Vit. E

101. Iron absorption is increased by: *(AIIMS 04)*
A. Fibre diet
B. Vitamin C
C. Phosphate
D. Phytic acid

102. Iron is actively absorbed in:
A. Stomach *(NBE P 14,13; AIIMS 07, 13, 15)*
B. Duodenum and proximal jejunum
C. Large intestine
D. Ileum

103. Function of peritoneum are A/E: *(PGI 01)*
A. Lubrication
B. Hormone release
C. Pain sensitive
D. Enzymatic digestion
E. Phagocytosis

104. Which of these is the best test for assessment of intestinal malabsorption? *(AIIMS 16)*
A. D-xylose absorption test
B. Fecal fat estimation
C. Serum amylase levels
D. NBT-PABA test

Colonic Microflora

105. Which vitamins are synthesised by intestinal bacteria-
A. Vit K and D *(NBE P 13)*
B. Vit K and B
C. Vit A and D
D. Vit K and C

106. Which of the following cannot be synthesized in the body: *(PGI 12)*
A. Vit K
B. Vit C
C. Thiamine
D. Riboflavin
E. Cyanocobalamin

107. Which vitamin is synthesized in vivo in the body by humans? *(AIIMS 16)*
A. Folic acid
B. Niacin
C. Pantothenic acid
D. Cyanocobalamin

108. Which of the following is not the primary function of gut flora? *(AIIMS 11)*
A. Synthesis of short chain fatty acids
B. Decreased proliferation of epithelial cells
C. Production of vit. K
D. Fermentation of mucin

109. Most potent anti oxidant- *(NBE P 13)*
A. Vit A
B. Vit K
C. Vit E
D. Vit C

Diet

110. Which of these is the correct representation of the normal oral glucose tolerance test? *(AIIMS 16)*

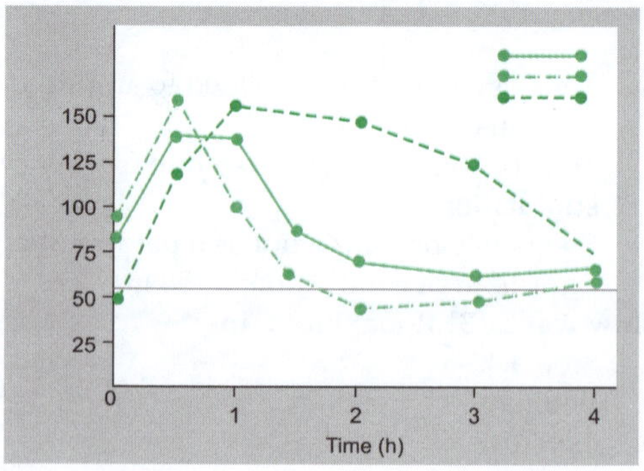

A. B
B. C
C. A
D. None of these

111. Which of the following statements about Recommended Dietary Allowances (RDA) is true
A. RDA is statistically defined as two standard deviations (SD) above Estimated Average Requirement (EAR) *(AI 09)*
B. RDA is defined as being equal to the Estimated Average Requirement (EAR)
C. RDA is defined as being equal to Adequate Intake (AI)
D. RDA is defined as the recommended minimum requirement

112. True about dietary fiber: *(PGI 07)*
- A. Soluble fiber ↑ metabolism of sugar in GIT.
- B. ↑ bulk of stool.
- C. Only soluble fibers are included in diet.
- D. ↑ GI transit time.
- E. Not prevention against colonic cancer.

113. Longest transit time in GIT is seen in: *(PGI 04,08)*
- A. Stomach
- B. Jejunum
- C. Colon
- D. Ileum

114. True about High roughage in diet is : *(AI 02)*
- A. Decreases stool transit time
- B. Increase stool transit time
- C. Normalise stool transit
- D. No effect on stool transit time

115. Which of the following plant components is not fermented (degraded) by gastrointestinal microorganisms *(AIIMS 11, AI 09)*
- A. Lignin
- B. Cellulose
- C. Hemicellulose
- D. Pectin

116. TRUE regarding action of alpha amylase *(AIIMS 04)*
- A. Breaks glucose from carbohydrate end
- B. Cleaves only at α 1-4
- C. Cleaves only at α 1-6
- D. b & c

117. Following constitute dietary fibres except:
- A. Pectin *(NBE P 15,13; AI 03)*
- B. Cellulose
- C. Hemicellulose
- D. Riboflavin / Lactulose

118. Dietary fibre contains: *(AI 04)*
- A. Collagen
- B. Pectin
- C. Proteoglycans
- D. Starch

119. Colonic bacteria, on digestion of dietary fibres would give- *(AIIMS 01)*
- A. Free radicals
- B. Glycerol
- C. Butyrate
- D. Sucrose

120. In the following food items, which one has the highest 'Glycemic Index'? *(AIIMS 03)*
- A. Corn-flakes
- B. Brown rice
- C. Ice-cream.
- D. Whole wheat bread

121. Function of Metabolism includes all except
- A. Extraction of nutrients from food *(AI 04)*
- B. Breakdown of substrate
- C. Equilibrium of biochemical with intracellular components
- D. Using building blocks for synthesis

122. Largest reserve of energy in body stored as:
- A. Liver glycogen *(PGI 07)*
- B. Muscle glycogen
- C. Adipose tissue
- D. Blood glucose
- E. Muscle protein

123. Main source of energy derived from: *(PGI 08)*
- A. Fat
- B. Glycogen
- C. Lactate
- D. Acetone

124. Which dissacharies are not broken down in git-
- A. Lactulose *(NBE P 15)*
- B. Maltose
- C. Sucrose
- D. Latose

125. During starvation, graph of three substances are plotted as below. The scale for A and B is on the left and the scale for C is on the right. Which of the substances are represented by the curve B?

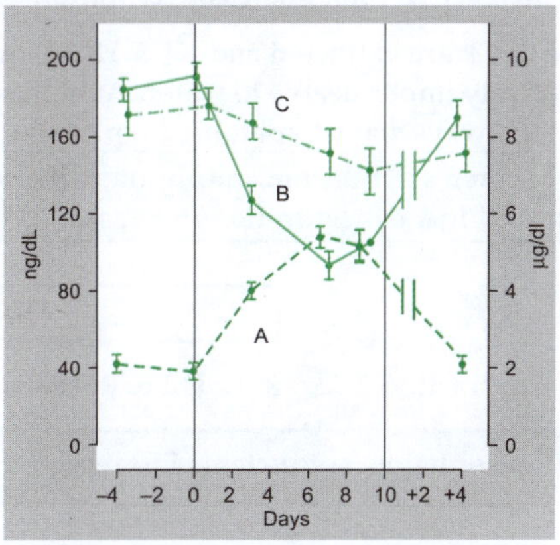

- A. RT_3
- B. T_3
- C. T_4
- D. DIT

ANSWERS & EXPLANATIONS:

Saliva

1. **A i.e. Saliva** *[Ref: Guyton 12/ep 776]*

Saliva contains thiocyanate ions and lysozyme (proteolytic) enzyme both of which destroy bacteria.

2. **A i.e. Saliva** 3. **D i.e. Rectal fluid**

[Ref: Ganong 23rd/e p. 440-42; Guyton 11th/e p. 794; Swartz 8th/ed pg- 46; Irwin- Ripe's intensive care medicine 6/e pg- 915; Berne & levy physiology 5/ed pg- 817]

- **Maximum concentration of K^+ ion** (i.e. 75 Meq/L or 80-95 mmol/l) is see ***in colonic secretions (or stool)***Q but this accounts for only a small amount of potassium because of only 100-200 ml quantity of large intestinal secretion per day.
- Whereas **saliva** has **2nd highest concentration of K^+ ions** (i.e. 25-30 meq/L at low flow rates and 15- 20 meq/L at high flow rates) but this accounts for ***overall maximum potassium ion secretion***Q because of its high (1 to 1.5 L/day) turn over.

4. **B i.e. Low pH of stomach**

Salivary amylase (Tylin) is inactivated by low pH (<4.5) of stomachQ

5. **B i.e. Amylase** *[Ref: Ganong 23/ep 453]*

Digestion of dietary carbohydrate involves salivary & pancreatic amylaseQ

6. **B i.e. Increase in phosphate concentration** *[Ref: Harrison 18/e ch 324: Ganong 24/e p 456-57]*

- **Na^+ & Cl^- are extracted** and **K^+ & HCO_3^- are added as saliva passes through duct.** Saliva is **hypotonic** because duct is relatively impermeable to water. At high secretion rates, there is less time for NaCl extraction, so tonicity of saliva rises but it **always stays hypotonic** (to plasma).
- **In Sjogren's syndrome, output of salivary gland decreases** (<0.5 ml/min), **PO_4^{-3} concentration remains same**Q, and **Na^+ and IgA concentration increases** (d/t decrease serous component of saliva).

Oesophagus and Stomach

7. **A i.e. Contraction** 8. **D i.e. Relaxes ahead of the peristaltic wave.** *[Ref: Ganong 22/e P- 490; Guyton. 10/e P-730]*

Lower oesophagus sphincter (LES) relaxes ahead of **peristaltic wave**Q allowing easy propulsion of food.

Lower Esophageal Sphincter (LES)

- The lower 3-4 cm of the esophagus is thickened to form LES. The *smooth circular muscle* fibres of gastroes ophageal function thicken to form LES.
- It is *not a true* anatomic sphincter.
- This remains ***tonically active***Q so that intraluminal pressure at lower end of esophagus is 30 mm Hg. (upper & middle portion remain relaxed). This tonic activity *prevents reflux* of gastric content into esophagus
- The tone of LES is under ***Parasympathetic***Q neural control.
  - **Vagal excitatory fibres (VEF): causes release of *acetylchoine* & esophageal sphincter contract**Q.
  - **Vagal inhibitory fibres (VIF):** causes release of *NO* and *VIP* results in *relaxation* of LES.
- The tone of LES is also influenced by some G.I hormones & other endocrinal mechanism.
- When peristaltic swallowing wave passes down the esophagus. There is ***receptive relaxation of LES ahead of the peristaltic wave***Q, which allow easy propulsion of food into the stomach.

Mechanism which Prevent GE Reflux

- ***Tonic activity of LES***Q.
- Valve like mechanism of short ***portion of esophagus that extend into the diaphragm***Q, when the gastric pressure increases this prevents reflux.
- Fibres of the ***crural portion of diaphragm***Q (skeletal muscle) surround esophagus at its lower end. They exert a pinch cock like action, preventing reflux.

9. A i.e. Gastric juice

10. C i.e. Ca^{++} *[Ref: Ganong 24rd/e p. 459-60]*

Normal gastric juice contains Mg^{2+}, Na^+, K^+, H^+ but no Ca^{++}Q. Rennin (double 'n' not Renin) = **Chymosin is proteolytic enzyme** secreted by **chief cells of stomach**. It is found in gastric juice and it **coagulates/curdle mild in very young animals.**

11. C i.e. Chief cells.

12. B i.e. Parietal (Oxyntic) Cells *[Ref: Ganong 23rd/e p. 431- 434; Gabriel p. 260-61; Guyton 11th/e p. 796; Surgical pathology of gastrointestinal tract 2/ed pg- 668, Grays 40th/e p. 1122]*

Intrinsic factor of Castle is secreted by ***parietal (oxyntic) cells*Q** and is essential for ***absorption of vitamin B_{12}*Q**; in its absence, ***Addison's pernicious (megaloblastic) anemia*Q** results.

Cells of Stomach and Secretion

The cells of the gastric glands secrete ***about 2500 ml of gastric juice daily*Q**. **Contents of Normal Gastric Juice**

- ***Cations*Q: Mg^{2+}, Na^+, K^+, H^+** (PH approx 1)
  [Mn: **M**ujhe **Na** **K**a**H**o]
- Anions: Cl^-, HPO_4^{2-}, SO_4^{2-}
- **Pepsins** - **Intrinsic** - **Mucus** - **Lipase**
  [Mn: **Pepsi in** my **lips.**]

***Parietal (Oxyntic cells)*Q**	- Present in the *body & fundus* of stomach - ***Secrete HCl and intrinsic factor*Q**
Chief (Zymogen/ Peptic) cells	- Present in the *body & fundus* - Secrete ***pepsinogen*Q**
Enterochromaffin Like cell (ECL)	- Histamine secretion - Histamine is also a trigger of parietal cell secretion via binding to H_2 histamine receptor.

★ Parietal & chief cell can also be stimulated by acetyl choline released from enteric nerve endings in fundus

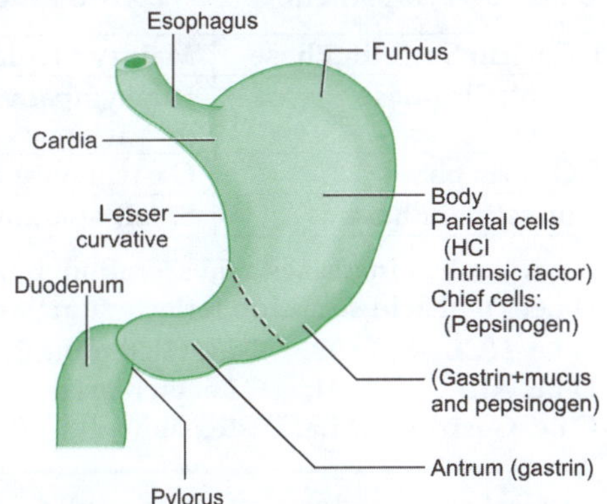

Mucus is secreted in all parts of the stomach.

13. C i.e. Mucus

14. A i.e. Pepsin *[Ref: Ganong 22/e p.471, 468]*

- Pepsin is formed from pepsinogen in stomach by HCl activation. ***Optimal pH for pepsin is 1.6 – 3.2 (acidic) at which it is stable*Q**. But its action is terminated when acidic gastric content is mixed with alkaline pancreatic juice in duodenum
- **Pancreatic enzymes** – trypsin, chymotrypsin & carboxy peptidase are ***stable in alkaline pH*Q**.

Cells with in Principal Gastric Glands in Body & Fundus

Gastric glands are simple branched tubular glands which usually open in group of 4 into a short common channel (or **gastric pit**), through which they discharge their secretions into the lumen. Each gland has 3 zones containing 4 main cell types (& secrete)

Outer zone (Luminal surface i.e. Isthmus & gastric pit)

Mucus Neck cells	***Mucus*Q** ***HCO_3^-*Q**

Globlet cells (Intestine)	**Mucus**
Brunner's Gland (Duodenum)	Mucus
Panneth Cell in crypts of Lieberkuhn (small intestine)	**Guanylin**

Middle zone (Neck & Isthmus)

Parietal or Oxyntic cell	**HClQ** **Intrinsic factor of CastleQ**

Structure of a gastric gland from the fundus and body of the stomach

Basal zone

Chief/Peptic / Zymogen cells	**PepsinogenQ**

Neuro (Entero) Endocrine cells

D cells	***Somatostatin*Q**
Enterochromaff in cells (ECC)	***Serotonin*Q**
Enterochromaff in Like cells (ELC)	***Histamine*Q**
Gastrin (G) cells.	***Gastrin*Q**

15. A i.e. Trypsin **16. B i.e. Enterokinase** **17. A i.e. Trypsin & Lipase**
18. D i.e. Ribonuclease /Amylase **19. D i.e. Chymotrypsin** **20. A i.e. Zymogen**
[Ref: Lippincott 4/e p. 64, 443, 248-49; Harper 29/e p 89, 519, 651-53; Ganong 22/e p. 468 – 69]

- **Chymotrypsinogen or prochymotrypsin is a proprotein / proenzyme / or zymogen. Chymotrypsinogen is activated to chmotrypsin by trypsin**Q. Chymotrypsin is enzyme not hormone.
- **Trypsinogen & pepsinogen** proenzymes are activated by **entero kinase and HCL** (respectively) to **trypsin & pepsin**.
- **Trypsin & lipase are pancreatic enzymes**Q

21. C i.e. Enterokinase *[Ref: Ganong 22/e p. 468; Harper 26/e p. 597; Chatterjee 7/e p. 435]*

Enterokinase (enteropeptidase), a glycoprotein enzyme of intestinal juice activates trypsinQ at pH 5.5.

22. C i.e. On seeing food **23. A i.e. 20%**
24. B i.e. Parasympathetic **25. B i.e. Gastrin Hormonal** *[Ref: Guyton 11/e p. 798 – 99; Ganong 22/e p. 494- 95]*

Gastrin Secretin Phase	Mainly Mediated by	**Accounts** For % of Total Secretion
Cephalic phase	**Parasympathetic (vagal) inputs originating from dorsal vagal complex in brain**Q **(on seeing food)**Q.	20%
Gastric phase	**Gastrin hormone mechenism**Q.	70%
Intestinal Phase	**Small amount of gastrin released by duodenum**	<10%

26. A i.e. Gastrin increases acid secretion; B i.e. Secretin decreases acid secretion; C i.e. H_2 blocker decreases acid secretion D i.e. Total acid secretion reflects functional parietal cell mass
27. D i.e. HCL **28. C i.e. Histamine & Gastrin** **29. A i.e. Secretin**
30. D i.e. All **31. C i.e. Increased by stomach (antral) distension** **32. A i.e. Decreased by CCK**
33. C i.e. Gastrin < D i.e. Distension *[Ref: Ganong 24/e P- 502-503; 469-72; Guyton 12/SAE p.447, 409-10]*

- **Gastrin** is produced by **gastric antral cells (G cells)** mainly but can also be produced by ***gastrinomas of pancreas & pituitary glands***Q. **Gastrin** (& so gastric) secretions are ***increased by gastric (antral) distension, vagal stimulus***Q and ***decreased by secretin and somatostatin***Q. ***Gastrin mainly stimulates gastric acid (HCL) and pepsin secretion***Q.
- **HCL secretion** reflects **parietal cell mass**. It is stimulated by **gastrin, acetylcholine (M3 receptor)** & **histamine (via H_2 receptors) and inhibited by low pH (acid) & H_2 blockers**Q.
- ***Gastric emptying is promoted by gastric food volume distending the stomach wall (main) and gastrin***Q. It is inhibited by **CCK (main), secretin and GIP**Q.

34. A i.e. Fat > Protein > Carbohydrate *[Ref: Ganong 241/ep 502]*

Gastric emptying is **fastest** for food rich in **carbohydrate** (few hours). **Protein rich food leaves more slowly and gastric emptying is slowest for fat rich food**Q.

Hyperosmolality of food entering duodenum **decrease gastric emptying.**

35. A i.e. Ligate all major arteries *[Ref: Ganong 22/e P- 488, 491]*
36. D i.e. The digestive enzymes active in segment A are inactivated in segment B.

Segment A	represents **mouth & esophagus**	*Salivary pH is 7*Q
Segment B	represents **stomach** (since it shows a sharp dip in pH)	Gastric pH is *1.2-1.3*Q.
Segment C	represents **duodenum** where the alkaline pancreatic/bile secretion occur, which raises pH above that of saliva	Duodenal *pH is approx 8*Q

Enzymes work efficiently only within narrow pH range. Therefore enzymes that work at pH of 7 (segment A) will be inactivated at pH of 1.5 (segment B).

Pancreatic Secretions

37. B i.e. 1&3 *[Ref: Ganong 23/ep 457]*

Fat digestion begins in duodenum by pancreatic enzymes lipase & colipase. Pancreatic lipase hydrolyses 1 and 3 ester linkage (bonds) of triglycerides (triglycerols)Q with relative ease (but bond 2 at a very low rate) producing FFAs (free fatty acids) and 2 mono acylglycerol.

Colipase is activated by trypsin and colipase activates lipase.

38. **B i.e. 200ml**

Daily secretion of Intestinal Juices		
	Daily volume (L)	pH
Saliva	1-1.5 L	6.0-7.0
Gastric secretion	1.5 – 2.5 L	1.0-3.5
Pancreatic secretion	**1 – 1.5 L**	8.0-8.3
Bile	1-0.5	7.8
Small intestine secretion	1.8 L } - 1	7.5-8.0
Brunner's gland secretion	0.2 L } - 1	8.0-8.9
Large intestinal secretion	0.2 L } - 1	7.5-8.0
Total	6.7 - 7	

39. **A i.e. 1.5L**

Daily water turnover (ml) in GIT		
Ingested		**2000**
Endogenous secretions		7000
Salivary glands	1500	
Stomach	2500	
Bile	500	
Pancreas	**1500**	
Intestine	1000	
	7000	
Total Input		9000
Reabsorbed		8800
Jejunum	5500	
Ileum	2000	
Colon	1300	
	8800	
Balance in stool		**200**

Total input of water is 9 lit and 8.8 of this fluid is reabsorbed.

40. **A i.e. Increased gallbladder contraction and HCO_3 rich pancreatic fluid**
41. **D i.e. ↑ses bile salt & bile acids**
42. **B i.e. Increases gastric motility**
43. **C i.e. Increases the secretion of enterokinase and augments the action of gastrin**

Secretin hormone stimulates copious secretion of a **very alkaline pancreatic juce that is rich in water & HCO_3^- and poor in enzymes and Cl^-** Q. It also **stimulates bile secretion (choleretics)**Q but has no role in synthesis of bile salt and bile acids. **It augments action of CCKPZ but inhibits gastrin secretion and gastric emptying & motality**Q.

44. **C i.e. Increase gastric acid secretion**
45. **B i.e. Acid chyme**
46. **C i.e. Secretin**
47. **D i.e. Gastric secretion increases**
48. **C** i.e. CCK
49. **B i.e. Protein**
50. **A i.e. Stimulates gall bladder contraction**
51. **C i.e. Increased gastrin secretion**
52. **D i.e. Cholecystokinin**

[Ref: Guyton 12/SAE p. 417; Ganong 24/e P- 468-71]

Presence of protein and fat in duodenum promotes the secretion of cholecyctokinin- pancreozymin (CCK-PZ) from the I cells of jejunum (upper small intestine)Q. CCK-PZ is not found in bile but it produces contraction of gall bladderQ.

Cholecystokinin Pancreaticozymin (CCPZ)

- Released by mucosa **of jejunum**Q **(from I cells)**Q
- **Stimuli for secretion**
  - Presence of **peptides & aminocids in small intestine**Q (main).
  - **Fatty acids, having more than 10 carbon atoms**Q, in the duodenum
- **Action**
  - Secretion of pancreatic juice **rich in enzyme**Q.
  - **Contraction of gall bladder & release of bile**Q.
  - **Inhibits gastric emptying**Q (augments contraction of pyloric sphincter)
  - Enhances **small intestinal & colonic motility**Q.
  - Augments action **of secretin**Q **in producing alkaline pancreatic juice**
  - Increases secretion of **glucagon**Q & Insulin.

Secretin

- Released from S cells of **duodenal mucosa**Q. It is structurally similar to glucagons, GIP, VIP and GLI
- **Stimuli for secretion**
  - **Acidity of chyme**Q (main)
  - **Products of protein digestion**Q.
- **Action**
  - Stimulates **bicarbonate rich**Q pancreatic secretion
  - Responsible for **adding water & alkaline component to pancreatic juice**Q.
  - **Inhibits gastric acid secretion & gastric emptying**Q **by causing contraction of pyloric sphincter**Q
  - **Augments action of CCK-PZ**Q in producing pancreatic secretion in of digestive enzyme.
  - **Stimulates bile secretion (choleretics)**Q

Gall Bladder & Bile

53. E i.e. Cholecystokinin *[Ref: Berne 6/e p. 545-48; Ganong 24/e p. 464-65]*

Bile is a micellar solution in which major solutes are **bile acids, phosphatidylcholine and cholesterol in 10 : 3 : 1 ratio.** Bile acids may be **primary** (ie synthesized by hepatocytes) **eg chenodeoxy cholic acid & cholic acid**; or secondary bile acids (ie formed by bacterial action in colon) eg lithocholic acid & ursodeoxycholic acid (formed from chenodeoxy CA) and deoxy cholic acid (formed from cholic acid). Bile also contains glucronides **of bile pigments bilirubin and biliverdin** (responsible for golden yellow color) as well as **alkaline electrolyte solution** resembling pancreatic juice.

54. C i.e. Active transport across the membrane **55. D i.e. Bile salt** **56. A i.e. Bile salts** **57. A i.e. CCK**

- **Secretion of bile into bile canaliculus is by active transport across the membrane**Q. Bile substances that are **actively secreted** into bile **across canalicular membrane are bile acids (primary force),** conjugated bilirubin, cholesterol & xenobiotics.
- Substances that increase the secretion of bile are called as **cholerectics**Q. **Bile salts** are amongst the **most important physiological cholerection**Q. Most potent stimulus for causing **gall bladder contraction is CCK-PZ**Q.

Cholagogues

Substances that cause **contraction of gall bladder**Q
- **Cholecytokinin**Q.
- **Fatty acids**Q } by ↑ing CCK-Pz
- Amino acids } by ↑ing CCK-Pz

Choleretics

Substances that **increase secretion of bile**Q
- **Secretin**Q
- **Vagal stimulation**Q
- **Bile salts**Q **(Most potent stimulus)**Q.

58. A i.e. Myoglobin; B i.e. Hemoglobin. *[Ref: Harper's 26/e P- 278]* **59. A i.e. Protein**

The **daily bilirubin** formation in human is approx. 250- 350mg, deriving mainly ***(70-80%) from hemoglobin***Q but also from ineffective erythropoiesis and from various other *heme proteins such as* ***cytochrome P450*** and ***myoglobin***Q.

1 gm of Hemoglobin yields ***35mg of bilirubin***Q.

Heme (in RBC Hb, Myoglobin, Cytochrome P450) is broken by Heme oxygenase into

↓

Biliverdin (By Biliverdin-Reduce into)

↓

Bilirubin (Unconjugated): In blood it is transported in bound from with albumin (i.e. Bilirubin-Albumin Complex) to liver where there is carrier mediated uptake.

↓

Conjugated with Glucuronic acid (to form **Conjugated-Bilirubin) by UDP-GT1AI and excreted into bile**. In intestine, it is deconjugated by bacterial **β-glucuronidase** into **Urobilinogen (80%** of which **is excreted in feces, 20%** reabsorbed to **enter enteroheaptic circulation** and small amount excreted in urine)

60. C i.e. Emulsification of lipids **61. C i.e. Amphipathic nature of bile acids** *[Ref: MTx]*

Bile acids (bile salts) have **detergent (emulsification) action** on the lipids due to their **amphipathic nature**Q. They make ingested lipids soluble & smaller by **forming micelles**, so that they can be transported to enterocytes for **digestion.**

Liver

62. A i.e. Liver *[Ref: Guyton 12/ep 822]*

In Lipid metabolism, liver causes-
1. **Synthesis of TGs** (mainly from carbohydrates >>> proteins)
2. Synthesis of other lipids (mainly **cholesterol & phospholipids)** from fatty acids (FA)
3. **Degrading FAs** into compounds that can be used energy

Synthesis of fat	Liver (maximum)Q >>> Adipose tissue
Storage of fat	Adipose tissue (maximum)>>> liver

63. **B i.e. Vit – A storage** *[Ref: Robbins 7/e P-878]*

Hepatic Cells

Hepatic Stellate cell (also called ***Ito cells***)

- Are of mesenchymal origin, found in *space of Disse.*
- Play a role in the ***storage and metabolism of Vit A***[Q].
- They *transform into collagen producing myofibroblast* when there is inflammation and fibrosis of liver.

Kupffer Cells

They have ***phagocytic function***[Q].

64. **D i.e. Immunoglobulin** *[Ref: Ganong 22/e p. 541; Guyton 11/e p. 854-57; Harper 27/e p. 585- 91]*

Alpha (α) and beta (β) globulins are produced by hepatocytes (liver), where as immunoglobins or gamma globins are produced by B- lymphocyte (plasma cell)[Q].

65. **C i.e. Dubin Johnson syndrome; D i.e. Rotor syndrome; E i.e Neonatal hepatitis** *[Ref: Harrison 16/e p. 1820 – 21; ODG 5/e p. 174]*

Disorders of Bilirubin Metabolism l/t

Unconjugaed hyperbilirubinemia

- Hemolysis
- ***Physiological neonatal jaundice***[Q]
- Breast milk jaundice
- Drug eg pregnanediol, novobiocin, chloramphenicol, gentamycin (inhibital UGT 1A)
- Transient familial neonatal hyper bilirubinemia (Lucey – Driscoll syndrome)
- ***Crigler – Najjar syndrome type I, & II***[Q]
- ***Gilbert's syndrome***[Q].

Mixed or Predominantly Conjugated hyper bilirubinemia

- ***Dubin Johnson syndrome***[Q]
- Rotor syndrome
- Benign recurrent intra hepatic cholestasis (BRIC)
- Progressive familial intrahepatic cholestasis (FIC)
- Biliary atresia
- ***Neonatal hepatitis***[Q], sepsis

66. **A i.e. ↑ PT B i.e., Hyperbilirubinemia; C i.e. Acute phase reactant** *[Ref: Ganong 22/e p. 500- 01; Guyton & Hall 11/e p. 861 – 64; Harrison 16/e p. 1810- 13]*

Liver abnormalities are diagnosed by **assessing prothrombin time (PT↑), direct & total serum bilirubin (hyperbilirubinemia), albumin, & levels of acute phase reactants (serum alanine & aspartate amino transferase=ALT & AST)**[Q]

Motility

67. **A i.e. Mass persistalsis** 68. **A i.e. Does not depend on gastric motality** 69. **C i.e. CCK**
[Ref: Berne 6/e p. 533; Guyton 11/e p. 776, 784-90, 822; Ganong 24/e p. 498-505]

- After a meal, **gastrocolic reflex** (i.e. **increased colonic motality) develops** in form of a contraction ring appearing & moving (like small intestinal peristalsis waves) aborally in colon for large distance resulting in movement of feaces from splenic flexure to rectum in single attempt (k/a **mass peristalsis).**
- **Intestinal motality depends on gastric motality**[Q]. It is increased by **distension, ACh, CCK, gastrin, motilin, substance P & serotonin**[Q].

70. **D i.e. GLP-1 (7-36) amide** 71. **C i.e. Motilin** *[Ref: Ganong 22/e p. 486 – 87; Guyton 11/e p. 776]*

- ***Glucagon derivative GLP- 1 (7-36) amide (most potent) > gastric inhibitory peptide (GIP) also known as glucose – dependent insulinotropic polypeptide >> gastrin, CCK, secretin and glucagon stimulates insulin secretion***[Q]. But only GLP-1 (7-36) amide & GIP stimulate insulin secretion when adminstered in dose that produce blood levels comparable to those produced by oral glucose.
- **Motolin** is secreted by *entero chromaffin cells & M_0 cells in stomach, small intestine and colon* during fasting. It is *released cyclically* (so ↑ed levels) at intervals of *90- 100 minutes in a fasted person* which stimulates *waves of gastrointestinal motality* called **myoelectric interdigestive cmplexes** (MIC). *Erythromycin* binds to motolin receptors so its derivatives may be of value in treating decreased intestinal motality.

- **Neurotensin** is produced by neurons & cells of ileum. Its release is stimulated by fatty acid and it increases ileal blood flow and inhibits gastro intestinal motality.

- **GIP** is produced by ***K cells in mucosa of duodenum & jejunum. Its secretion is stimulated by glucose & fat***Q in duodenum. It is named so because in large doses it inhibits gastric secretion & motality. However in small dose (that are seen after meal) it does not have significant gastric inhibitory activity.

72. **C i.e. Ingested meal** *[Ref: Ganong 24/ep 472, 498]*

Motolin, a 22 amino acid polypeptide hormone, is secreted by **Entero chromaffin cells and Mo cells in stomach, small intestine & colon**. It acts on G protein receptors on enteric neurons in duodenum & colon and **produce smooth muscle contraction in stomach and intestine in period between meals**Q. **Erythromycin** binds to motolin receptors so in future may derive compounds to treat decreased gastric motility.

- During fasting between periods of digestion, motor activity of gi smooth muscles migrate at rate of 5 cm/min from stomach to distal ileum **(MMC)** to clear luminal contents for next meal.
- **Motilin (blood level) increase at** interval **of ~100min in interdigestive state** (during contractile phase of MMC). It **initiate & migrating motor complex**Q.

Ingestion of food (meal) suppress/decrease motolin releaseQ, so **MMC** is abolished (& peristalsis returns) until digestion & absorption are complete.

73. **A i.e. Muscularis externa**

74. **A i.e. Myentric plexus** *[Ref: Ganong 24/e p. 473]*

Myenteric (Auerbach's) plexus is situated **in outer (external) muscular layer in muscularis externa** between and **innervates** ***outer longitudinal & middle circular muscular*** **layers**Q and is ***primarily concerned with motor control***Q. **Submucosal (meissner's) plexus** situated between middle circular layer and mucosa is primarily concerned with ***control of intestinal secretion***Q as it innervates glandular epithelium, intestinal endocrine cells & submucosal blood vessels.

75. **C i.e. Pyloric end of stomach** *[Ref: Ganong 24/e P- 498-99; Schwartz 8/e P- 946-47]*

About option B: Pacemaker cells (interstitial cells of Cajal) are present in ***Circular muscle layer***Q.
About option A & C : As they are ***absent in*** **esophagus and proximal portion of stomach, cardiac end and fundus of stomach** can be ruled out. Peristalsis occurs from esophagus to rectumQ.

76. **D i.e. Peristalsis** 77. **B i.e. Local stretching of gut** 78. **B i.e. Migration motor complexes** 79. **A i.e. 90 mins**
[Ref: Ganong 24/e P- 497-505; Guyton 10/e 461-62; Sembulingum 3/e P- 217]

Peristalsis ***propels the small intestinal content (chyme)***Q toward the large intestine. **It is a reflex response that is initiated when gut wall** ***is stretched*** **by contents of lumen**Q**.** It occurs in all part of g.i tract from oesophagus to rectum *propelling the content forward*. It can be increased or decreased by autonomic input to gut but its occurrence is independent of extrinsic innervation. It is blocked only if the *segment is reversed before it is sutured back* (not by removed of intestine segment & resuturing in original position).

Bowel Movements

Peristalsis	**Segmentation Contraction**	**Migrating Motor Complex**
Peristalsis ***propels the small intestinal content (chyme)*** **toward the large intestine**Q**.** It is a reflex response that is initiated when gut wall *is stretched* by contents of lumen. It occurs in all part of g.i tract from oesophagus to rectum *propelling the content forward*. It can be increased or decreased by autonomic input to gut but its occurrence is independent of extrinsic innervation. It is blocked only if the *segment is reversed before it is sutured back* (not by removed of intestine segment & resuturing in original position). **Peristaltic Rush** - *Very intense* peristaltic wave, occur *when intestine is obstructed.* - Not seen in normal individual	- Ring like contraction, which occur regularly or irregularly but in rhythmic fashion. - They move the chyme to & fro and increase its exposure to mucosal surface. - Helps in ***mixing of chyme with digestive juices***Q. - Retard movements of intestinal contents to provide time for digestion & absorption. **Haustration** ***Mixing movements in colon***Q.	- *During fasting between periods of digestion*, the pattern of electrical and motor activity in G.I smooth muscle becomes modified so that cycles of motor activity migrate from the stomach to distal ileum. Each cycle is called *migrating motor complex. (MMC)* - **They may** ***clear the stomach and small intestine*** **of luminal contents in preparation for the next meal**Q**.** - They cause moderately active peristaltic waves to *sweep excess digestive secretions into colon* & prevent their accumulation in upper GIT. - **MMCs occur at intervals of 90 minutes & migrate at rate of 5 cm/min**Q**.** Gastric & pancreatic secretion and bile flow increase during each MMC. They are immediately stopped by ingestion of food (whereas peristalsis, BER & spike potential return)

80. **B i.e. Alkaline pH in duodenum & Hormone**

81. **D i.e. None** *[Ref: Bailey & Love 24/e P-1044; Schwartz 8/e P-988; Sembulingum 3/e P- 215, Guyton 11/e P. 785-86]*

- **Enterogastric reflex** leading to stoppage of gastric emptying is caused by ***duodenal distension, acidity (i.e. H^+ not alkalinity) & high osmolarity of duodenal chyme and presence of protein & fat breakdown products in duodenum***^Q^.
- **Post vagotomy diarrhea** is caused by **irregular peristalisis, rapid gastric emptying and decreased gastric acid secretic (i.e. hypoacidity in duodenum)**^Q^.

82. **A i.e. Tone of contraction is related to amplitude of the stimulus**

- **Muscle contraction in intestine** is mostly caused by **spike potential (super imposed on BER)** and only very rarely by BER itself (alone). The **tone of contraction depends on frequency of stimulus rather than amplitude**^Q^.
- In figure (given in Q) threshold for AP & contraction is -50mV. And 1 contraction per 10 seconds implies that frequency is 6 contractions per minute.

Pacemaker (Interstital) Cell of Cajal

- Are *stellate* mesenchymal cells with smooth muscle like features that send long multiple branched processes into intestinal smooth muscles
- Pacemakar cells are ***absent in esophagus and proximal portion of stomach***^Q^.
- In stomach and small intestine they are located in ***outer circular muscle layer***^Q^ near myentric plexus.
- In the colon they are at the ***submucosal border of circular muscle layer***^Q^.
- In stomach & small intestine, pacemaker frequency is in descending gradient and the pacemaker with highest frequency usually dominates (like heart)

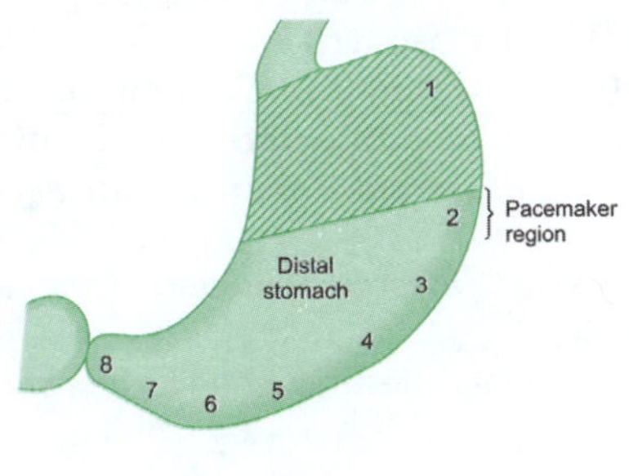

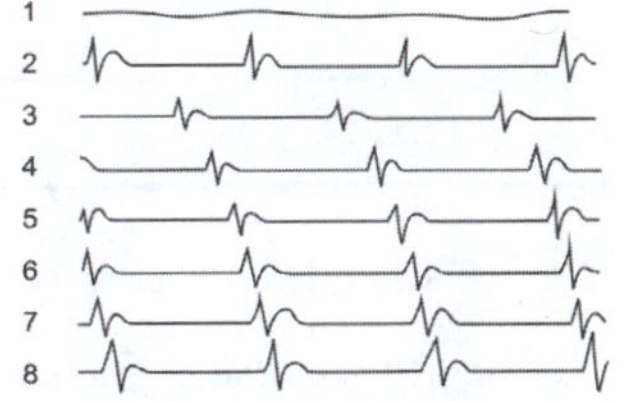

Regional myoelectric patterns in the stomach

Basic Electrical Rhythm (BER)

- **Cajal cells produce basic electrical rhythm (BER)**^Q^, which is spontaneous rhythmic fluctuation in **membrane potential between about *– 65 and –45mv***^Q^.
- **BER rarely cause muscle contraction, but *spike potential* superimposed on the most depolarizing portion of the BER waves do increase muscle tension**^Q^
- **Depolarization** of each spike is d/t ***Ca^{++} in flux***^Q^ and repolerization portion is d/t ***K^+ efflux***^Q^

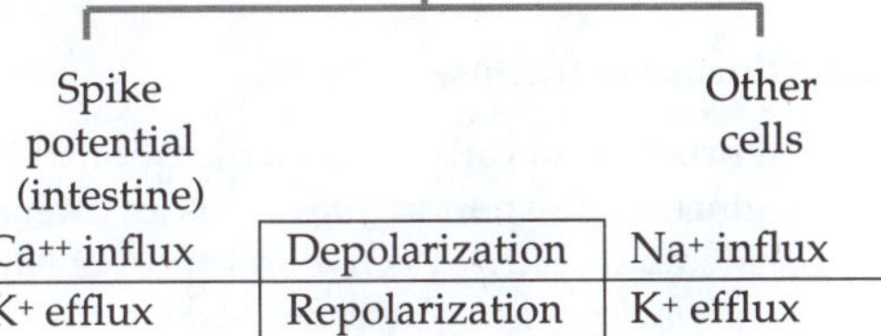

- Number of spikes & tension is **increased** by *acetyl choline* and **decreased** by *epinephrine.*
- **BER cordinates peristaltic & other motor activity such as rhythm of segmentation etc.** After vagotomy or stomach wall transection, peristalsis (in stomach) becomes irregular & chaotic.

83. **C i.e. Colon**

84. **D i.e. Sigmoid colon** *[Ref: Ganong 24/e p 505, 499; Berne & Levy 6/e p 534-36; Timothy R Koch – Colonic disease pg- 339]*

Colonic motality is minimal in fasting period. Eating stimulates colonic contractions. *Fat component* of meal is major *stimulus* to colonic contractions. ***Protein ingestion inhibits colonic contraction. Maximum postprandial increase in motality is seen in sigmod coln > descending colon > transverse colon***^Q^.

BER Rate/minute	Part
4/min	**stomach**
12/min	duodenum & proximal jejunum
8/min	distal ileum
9/min	caecum
16/min	**sigmoid colon (maximum)**^Q^

85. **C i.e. Distal colon** *[Ref: Sembulingum 3/e P-219; Guyton 10/e P 737, 710]*

When the *rectum is inflated with gas (CO_2) in* ***sigmoidoscopy***, *nerves are stimulated* and causes increased *peristalsis in* the descending colon, sigmoid ***(distal colon)***^Q^ and rectum.

Small & Large Intestine

86. A i.e. Glucose

Hexose sugars (glucose> fructose) are best absorbable (most rapidly absorbed) monosaccharide[Q]. These are mainly absorbed in **small intestine (proximal part of jejunum)**[Q].

87. D i.e. 8 lit **88. B i.e. Jejunum** **89. C i.e. Ileum** **90. D i.e. Electrolytes**

[Ref: Ganong 23/e 441, 452; Swartz 8/e p 1021-24

- **Total input of water is 9 lit and 8.8 of this fluid is reabsorbed (the nearest answer is 8 liters).**
- Out of this **9 lit** (2 lit water ingested +1.5 lit saliva + 2.5 lit gastric juice + 0.5 lit bile + 1.5 lit pancreatic juice + 1 lit small intestine secretion) **85% is absorbed in small intestine (mostly jejunum) and only 5-10% (1-1.5 lit) is absorbed in colon (large intestine)**[Q]**. Water and electrolyte (NaCl) reabsorptions** are linked.

Content	Maximum absorption
Calcium, Iron	**Duodenum**[Q]
Water, Electrolyte (Na^+, Cl-), Amino acids, **Fats** (TG,Ch),Sugar (mono & disaccharide), **water soluble vitamins (except B_{12}), Fat soluble vitamins**	**Jejumun**[Q]
Bile, Bile salts, B_{12} (vitamin)	**Ileum**

- ***Ca^{2+}, Cl^-, Fe^{2+}, SO_4^{2-}, long chain fatty acids and vitamins (except B_{12}) are mainly absorbed in upper small intestine (i.e., jejunum & duodenum)***[Q].
- ***Sodium (Na^+) is mainly absorbed is upper & lower small intestine (jejunum, ileum) and colon***[Q]. And K^+ in upper mid & lower small intestine.
- **Sugars and amino acids** are mainly absorbed in mid small intestine whereas ***bile salts, and vitamin B12 in lower small intestine (ileum)***[Q]

91. B i.e. Pancreatic juice *[Ref: Guyton 11/e P-794]*

'Pancreatic juice is essentially alkaline with a pH as high as 8.0 to 8.3.

92. A i.e. Glucose & fructose **93. C i.e. Glucose** *[Ref: Ganong 22/e p. 470]*

- Final products of carbohydrate digestion in intestinal chyme are ***glucose & fructose***[Q].
- The glucose transport in intestine is an example of **secondary active transport** i.e., the energy of glucose transport is provided indirectly by active transport of Na^+ out of cell. Because glucose & Na+ share the same *cotransporter (symport)* the *sodium dependent glucose transporter (SGLT, Na+ - glucose cotransporter*, cross cell membrane *12 times*), the high concentration of Na+ on mucosal surface of cells facillitate & low concentration inhibit hexose sugar influx into epithelial cells.

94. C i.e. Colipase; D i.e. Bile salts; E i.e. Pancreatic lipase *[Ref: Ganong 24/e P- 483-85, 465, 513; Lippincotts 2/e P 1.164]*
95. A i.e. Fat in stool > 6 gm /day indicate malabsorption; C i.e. Major fat absorption occurs in proximal intestine.
96. B i.e. Colon *[Ref: Harrison 16/e P- 1768, 238]*

The lingual & **gastric lipase** is of *little importance in fat digestion except* in pancreatic insufficiency. **Digestion of dietary fat requires pancreatic lipase, colipae & bile salts (i.e. salts of bile acids).** Whereas, **bile pigments (bilirubin & biliverdin)** are breakdown products of haemoglobin (heme), give *golden yellow* color to bile and are secreted in bile in *water soluble glucuronide conjugates.*

97. A i.e. Cobalmin absorption **98. A i.e. Cobalamin** **99. C i.e. Ileum** *[Ref: Ganong 22/e P- 477, 496]*

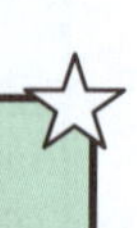

Most vitamins are absorbed in upper small intestine but ***vitamin B_{12} is absorbed in the ileum***[Q]***. Intrinsic factor is secreted by parietal or oxyntic cells of gastric mucosa***[Q] and **is estimated for vitamin B12 absorption**[Q].

100. A i.e. B_2 *[Ref: Harrison 16/e p. 404]*

Riboflavin (vit B_2) deficiency *manifests principally as* ***mucocutaneous lesions of mouth an skin such as glossitis & cheilitis***[Q].

101. B i.e. Vitamin C

102. B i.e. Duodenum and proximal jejunum
[Ref: Robbins 7/e p. 644; Ganong 22/e P- 477; KDT 5th/e P-546; Harrison 16/e p. 588; OP Ghai 6/e p. 300]

Iron is actively absorbed (via DMT 1) in proximal small intestine (duodenum & upper jejunum)Q . Its absorption is increased by ascorbic acid (vit C)Q.

103. B i.e. Hormone release *[Ref: Bailey & Love 24/e P-1133]*

Function of Peritoneum

- ***Pain perception*Q** (parietal peritoneum)
- Allow visceral movement
- ***Visceral lubrication*Q**
- Fluid and particulate absorption
- Inflammatory & Immune response ***(Phagocytosis)*Q.**
- Fibrinolytic activity
- Storage of fat.

104. A i.e. D-Xylose absorption test *[Ref: Harrison 18/e Chapter 294]*

Daily fecal fat averages 15-25gm/d with small intestinal disease & exceeds 40gm /d with pancreatic exocrine insufficiency. Evaluation of fat malabsorption:

1. Quantitative estimation of fecal fat is
- Gold standart test for diagnosis of fat MalabsorptionQ
2. Sudan III Quantitative Test is Best for ScreeningQ

Best test for diagnosis of Intestinal Malabsorption (& document integrity of intestinal mucosa) → **D-Xylose Test**

NBT-PABA, Bentiromide test and Serum Amylase tests for → **Pancreatic Malabsorption**

1. Oral glycine-1 shows **Bile acid Malabsorption**
2. **Schilling Test** is for Malabsorption of **Vitamin B12**

Colonic Microflora & Antioxidants

105. B i.e. Vit K and B

106. B i.e. Vit C; C i.e. Thiamin; D i.e. Riboflavin; E i.e. Cyanocobalamin *[Ref: Harper 29/e p. 525, 532; Chatterjea 8/e p. 173]*

Vitamins cannot be synthesized by body and must therefore be supplied in the diet. Although ***vitamin K_2 (menaquinones) & biotin are synthesized by intestinal bacteria*Q of most higher animal species.**

107. B i.e. Niacin

Humans can produce some vitamins from their precursors consumed in food eg **vitamin A (from beta carotene) and niacin (from amino acid tryptophan).**
Vitamin D is synthesized in skin from UV sunlight.

108. B i.e. Decreased proliferation of epithelial cells *[Ref: Berne & Levy 6/e p 533, 538-39; Ganong 24/e p 473,485; Jawetz 23/e p 198-99]*

Gut (colonic) microflora synthesize short chain fatty acids (SCFAs) by fermenting complex carbohydrate, resistant starches and other components of dietary fibers & mucin that escape digestion in upper git. They also **produce vitamin K and biotin**, *detoxify xenobiotics, increase & maturate immunity, preventing allergy and growth of pathogenic bacteria.* They **promote development of normal colonic epithelium and stimulate intestinal epithelial cell differentiation (ie increase not decrease proliferation of epithelial cells)**

109. C i.e. Vit E *[Ref: Guyton 12/e p 855]*

Vitamin E (tocopherol) is the most potent (important) antioxidant in the bodyQ.

GTT & Diet

110. C i.e. A

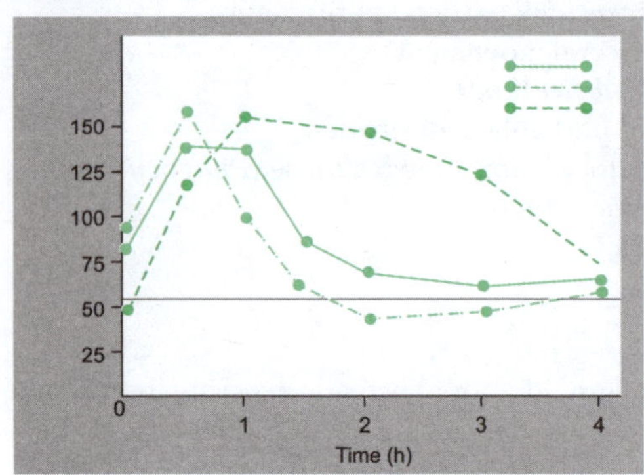

A = Normal; B = Excessively rapid carbohydrate absorption; C = Liver Disease

According to WHO

Plasma Glucose	Condition	Means
< 100 mg/dl	Fasting	**Normal**[Q]
110-125		Borderline
>125 mg/dl		**Diabetic**[Q]
<180 mg/dl	**1 Hour GTT**	Normal
< 140 mg/dl	**2 Hours GTT**	Normal
140-200		Borderline
>200 mg/dl	(Glucose Tolerance Test)	**Diabetic**[Q]

111. A i.e. RDA is statistically defined as two standard deviations (SD) above Estimated Average Requirement (EAR) *[Ref: Park's 20/ed pg- 547; Lippincott 4th/e p. 357-58]*

Recommended dietry allowance (RDA) is set at 2 SD above estimated average requirement (EAR)[Q].

112. A i.e., Soluble fibers increases metabolism of sugar in GIT B i.e., Increases bulk of stool
113. C i.e. Colon
114. A i.e. Decreases stool transit time
115. A i.e. Lignin
116. B i.e. Cleaves only at (α 1-4)
117. D i.e. Riboflavin/Lactulose
118. B i.e. Pectin

[Ref: Ganong 22/e P- 508-510; Lippincott 4/e p. 365- 68; Advanced human nutrition 1/e p. 89; Bhagvan: Medical Biochemistry 3/e p. 154; Harper's 26/e P-474]

- Dietary Fiber consists of all plant cell wall components that cannot be digested by animals' own enzymes. These include : **1) Cellulose**[Q] **2) Hemicellulose** [Q] **3) Lignin**[Q] **4) Gums**[Q] **5) Pectins**[Q] **6) Pentosans**[Q]
- **High fiber diet aids water retention during passage of food along the gut, producing larger & softer faeces; thereby also reducing the stool transit time**[Q]**. Colon has the longest transit time**[Q].
- A high fiber diet is associated with reduced incidence of : **a) diverticulosis**[Q] **b) cancer colon** [Q] **c) cardiovascular disease**[Q] **d) diabetes mellitus**[Q]

- **Lignin,** a non carbohydrate type of dietary fiber is **neither digested/hydrolyzed** (by endogenous human enzymes) **nor fermented/degraded** by gastro intestinal microorganisms.

Type of fibre		**Digestion / Hydrolysis** by enzymes in small intestine	Digestion / **Fermenttion** by colonic bacteria
Soluble "PAG"	Pectin Aliginates Gums	**Not digested**	**Fermented**
Insoluble "HCL"	Hemicellulose Cellulose	**Not digested**	**Fermented**
	Lignin	**Not digested**	**Not fermented**

- **α Amylase** is a *carbohydrate digesting* enzyme found in *saliva, pancreatic juice* and *intestinal juice. This enzyme hydrolyses α-1→4* ***glycosidic bonds.***

119. C i.e Butyrates: *[Ref. Harper 25/e P-656]*

In herbivores, such as ruminants, fiber (mainly as cellulose) is a major source of energy after it has been *digested by colonic microorganisms to* ***small chain fatty acids (acetate, propionate and butyrate)***[Q] which are absorbed into the portal vein. Colonic fermentation may also contribute to human energy requirements.

120. A i.e. Corn-flakes *[Ref. Journal of Nutritional Physiology & Biochemistry: Zeitschrift fur Natuforschung]*

Glycemic index in decreasing order (ie healthiness of food in increasing orders) is glucose (100), baked potato & corn flakes (85), white bread (70) and **brown rice** (55).

121. A i.e. Extraction of nutrients from food: *[Ref: Sembulingum 3/e P-295-97]*

Extraction of nutrients from food is not metabolism. Metabolism is oxidation of nutrients from food to produce energy.[Q]

Metabolism is a combination of two processes, namely: Anabolism: synthetic reactions that build up substances. Catabolism: reactions involving breakdown or oxidation of fuel molecules (breakdown of substrate). Both catabolism and anabolism proceed only until equilibrium is achieved. Equilibrium is a mechanism for biological control of rate at which these reactions occur.

122. C i.e. Adipose tissue *[Ref: Lippincott 4/e p. 189, 329]*

Fatty acid stored in adipose tissue in form of neutral TAG, serve as the body's major fuel storage reserve[Q].

123. B i.e. Glycogen *[Ref: Lippincott 4th/ed pg--360; Harper 28th/ed pg- 173,365-67]*

124. A i.e. Lactulose

Main source of energy in humans is carbohydrate. The primary role of dietary carbohydrate is to provide enegy[Q]**. Lactulose is not broken dowin in GIT.**

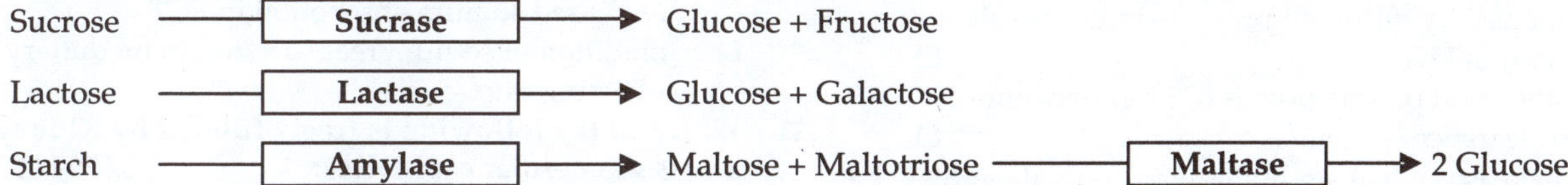

125. B i.e. T3 *[Ref: Ganong 24/e p. 345]*

With starvation, there is **marked reduction in T_3 levels with a reciprocal rise in RT_3** (in thyroid profile).

A = RT_3; B=T_3; C=T_4

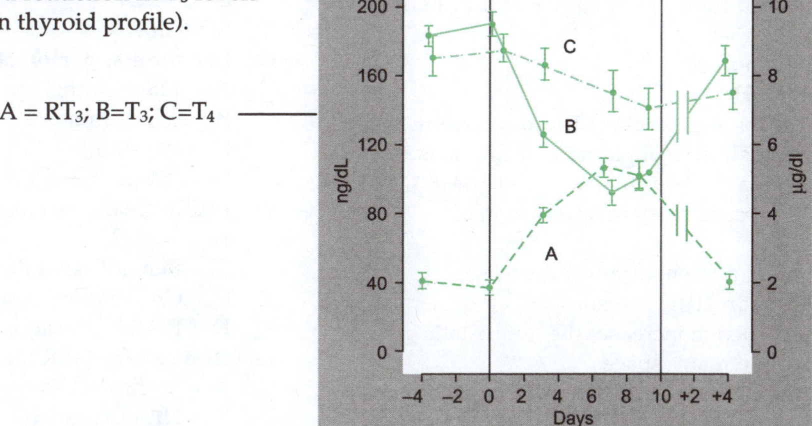

Chapter -6 EXCRETORY SYSTEM

QUESTIONS

Nephron & Glomerular Filtration

1. **All of the following structures lie in the renal medulla, Except:** *(AIIMS 08)*
   A. Juxtaglomerular apparatus ☐
   B. Loop of Henle ☐
   C. Collecting duct ☐
   D. Vasa Recta ☐
2. **Which of the following causes increase in both GFR and renal plasma flow-** *(NBE P 13)*
   A. Increased plasma colloid osmotic pressure ☐
   B. Dilatation of afferent arteriales ☐
   C. Constriction of a afferent arterioles ☐
   D. Increased tubular pressure ☐
3. **True about nephron /kidney is all except** *(PGI 15,13; NBE P 14,15)*
   A. Each kidney contains 1 million nephrons ☐
   B. DCT is 5mm long, 15% nephrons are juxtamedullary, filtration pressure in glomeruli is 10 to 15 mm HG. ☐
   C. Effective renal plasma flow is 625 ml/min and inulin clearance is same ☐
   D. GFR increases when afferent arteriotes dilate and renal blood flow increases ☐
4. **Two substances that can probably be used to determine filtrarion fraction are -** *(NBE P 14,13)*
   A. Insulin and'mannitol *(PGI 15,13,08)* ☐
   B. Urea and diodrast ☐
   C. PAH and phenol red ☐
   D. Inulin and PAH ☐
5. **All are correct about glomerular filtration, except:**
   A. Glucose concentration of glomerular filtrate is same as plasma *(AIIMS 11)* ☐
   B. Glomerular oncotic pressure is less than of filtrate ☐
   C. Constriction of afferent arteriole decreases glomerular hydrostatic pressure ☐
   D. Ureteric obstruction increases the hydrostatic pressure of Bowman's space ☐
6. **All of the following statements about Renal physiology are true, Except:** *(AI 09)*
   A. Distal tubule always receives hypoosmotic solution ☐
   B. The kidneys receive 5% of the cardiac output ☐
   C. GFR is controlled by resistance in afferent and efferent arterioles ☐
   D. The Glomerulus receives capillaries from the afferent arteriole ☐
7. **Relaxation of mesangial cells of kidney is brought about by -** *(NBE P15,14,13; AIIMS 15; Jipmer 02)*
   A. cAMP/Dopamine ☐
   B. Endothelin ☐
   C. PGF2 ☐
   D. Vasopressin & Angiotensin II ☐
8. **Following cells are responsible for acid secretion in kidney-** *(Jipmer 02)*
   A. I cells ☐
   B. P cells ☐
   C. Mesangial cell ☐
   D. Pericytes ☐
9. **Which of the following does NOT form a filtration barrier in nephrons:** *(NBE P 14; AI 08)*
   A. Podocytes ☐
   B. Mesangium ☐
   C. Endothelial cell ☐
   D. Basement membrane ☐
10. **All of these are actions of Atrial Natriuretic Peptide except:** *(AIIMS 15)*
    A. Afferent arteriole dilation ☐
    B. Mesangial constriction ☐
    C. Decreased sodium absorption in PCT ☐
    D. Inhibition of sodium reabsorption in medullary collecting duct ☐
11. **Which of the following is freely filtered by Kidney across glomerular capillaries:** *(PGI 09, 07)*
    A. Albumin (across glomerular capillaries) ☐
    B. Globulin ☐
    C. Creatinine ☐
    D. HCO_3 ☐
    E. Glucose ☐
12. **In a normal person at resting condition GFR is:**
    A. 125 ml/min *(PGI 03)* ☐
    B. 90 ml/min ☐
    C. 60 ml/min ☐
    D. 150 ml/min ☐
13. **Inulin clearance closely resembles -**
    A. G. F. R. *(NBE P 14)* ☐
    B. Renal Plasma flow ☐
    C. Creatinine clearance ☐
    D. P.A.H. clearance ☐
14. **Best test for GFR measurement is with:**
    A. Inulin *(NBE P 15,13; PGI 03, 15)* ☐
    B. Hippuric acid ☐
    C. Creatinine ☐
    D. PAH ☐
15. **In the formula for urea clearance, C = U × V/P, what does U stands for:** *(AIIMS 15)*
    A. Urinary concentration in g/24 hour ☐
    B. Urinary concentration in mg/ml ☐
    C. Urine osmolarity ☐
    D. Urine volume per minute ☐
16. **If the interstitial hydrostatic pressure is 2 mm Hg,interstitial oncotic pressure is 7 mm Hg and capillary hydrostatic pressure is 25 mm Hg. What**

should be the capillary oncotic pressure to allow a net filtration pressure of 3 mm Hg? *(AIIMS 15)*
A. 20 ☐
B. 21 ☐
C. 23 ☐
D. 27 ☐

17. What is implied, if a drug has more renal clearance than the GFR : *(AIIMS 2K)*
A. Drug is reabsorbed in the tubules ☐
B. Drug is secreted in the tubules ☐
C. Drug is excreted in bile ☐
D. Drug is neither secreted, nor resorbed. ☐

18. Which of the following statement is true?
A. Fluid coming from the descending limb of loop of Henle is hypotonic *(AIIMS 11, 08)* ☐
B. Descending limb of loop of henle is permeable to solutes ☐
C. If clearance of a substance is greater than GFR, then tubular secretion must be present ☐
D. Clearance of a substance is always more than GFR if there is tubular secretion. ☐

19. A substance is present in concentration of 2 mg% in the afferent arteriole and zero mg% in the efferent. True about the substance is: *(AIIMS 02)*
A. It is free filtered in glomerulus ☐
B. Secreted in cortical nephron ☐
C. Absorbed in PCT ☐
D. Impermeable in loop of Henk ☐

20. The renal plasma flow (RPF) of a patient was to be estimated through the measurement of Para Amino Hippuric acid (PAH) clearance The technician observed the procedures correctly but due to an error in the weighing inadvertently used thrice the recommended dose of PAH The RPF estimated is likely to be *(AI 03)*
A. False-high ☐
B. False-low ☐
C. False-high or false-low depending on the GFR ☐
D. Correct and is unaffected by the PAH overdose ☐

21. A negatively charged molecule is filtered with more difficulty compared to a positive one because-
A. Presence of negatively charged sialoproteins on the filtering membrane *(NBE P 13)* ☐
B. Negatively charged molecules are larger ☐
C. Postivelyl charged proteins on filtering membrance ☐
D. Urine is acidic ☐

22. The main cause of minimal change ds is: *(NBE P 13)*
A. Increase in pore size ☐
B. Loss of negative charge on membrane ☐
C. Loss of cells ☐
D. Decreased circulation ☐

23. Substrate which is both secreted & filtered-
A. Uric Acid *(NBE P 13)* ☐
B. Glucose ☐
C. Urea ☐
D. Na+ ☐

Proximal Convoluted Tubule

24. Transport maximum (Tm) means - *(WB 03, Jipmer 02)*
A. Maximum reabsorption & secretion ☐
B. Maximum amount of glomerular filtration /min ☐
C. Substance cleared from plasma/min ☐
D. Amount of toxic substances excreted /min ☐

25. Which of the following has no Tm value -
A. Albumin, arginine *(AIIMS 07, DNB 14)* ☐
B. Betahydroxybutyrate, glucose ☐
C. Glucose haemoglobin, phosphate ☐
D. Sulfate, Uric acid ☐
E. Urea ☐

26. Tubular maximum for kidney in practice is actually less than the calculated value because -
A. Different nephrons have different transport maximum *(AP 08, TN 07)* ☐
B. Depends on GFR ☐
C. Depends on renal blood flow ☐
D. Depends on blood Pressure ☐

27. Which of following is not absorbed in PCT:
A. Bicarbonate *(AIIMS 10)* ☐
B. Sodium ☐
C. Phosphate ☐
D. H^+ ☐

28. Bicarbonate (HCO_3^-) is maximally absorbed from:
A. PCT (Indirectly) *(AIIMS 07, 03,15,13)* ☐
B. PCT (actively) *(NBE P 15,14,13)* ☐
C. Collecting duct ☐
D. Thick ascending loop of Henle ☐

29. Active reabsorption of glucose occurs in the -
A. Distal tubule *(NBE P 15,13; AP 08)* ☐
B. Proximal tubule ☐
C. Loop of henle ☐
D. Collecting ducts ☐

30. In the presence of vasopressin the greatest fraction of filtered water is re-absorbed which part of the nephron: *(AI 03, 01)*
A. Proximal tubule ☐
B. Distal tubule ☐
C. Loop of Henle ☐
D. Collecting duct ☐

31. Which one of the following statements regarding water reabsorption in the tubules? *(AI 05)*
A. The bulk of water reabsorption occurs secondary to Na^+ reabsorption. ☐
B. Majority of facultative reabsorption occurs in proximal tubule. ☐
C. Obligatory reabsorption is ADH dependent. ☐
D. 20% of water is always reabsorbed irrespective of water balance. ☐

32. The Principal site of absorption of Sodium is:
A. Proximal convoluted tubule *(AI 10; AIIMS 14)* ☐
B. Distal convoluted tubule ☐
C. Loop of Henle (thick portion) ☐
D. Collecting duct ☐

33. The main site of bicarbonate reabsorption is:
A. Proximal convoluted tubule.
B. Distal convoluted tubule. *(AI 05)*
C. Cortical collecting duct.
D. Medullary collecting duct.

34. As fluid comes down the PCT, what is true-
A. Concentration of urea falls *(NBE P 13)*
B. Concentration of HCO_3 falls
C. Concentration of Na+ increases
D. Concentration of inulin decreases

35. Following are true about HCO_3-except: *(PGI 08)*
A. Extracellular concentration 25 m mol
B. Intracellular concentration 10 m mol
C. 7.5% solution gives 2 nmols
D. In kidney, HCO_3- is produced by carbonic anhydrase

36. The most sensitive index for renal tubular function is:
A. Specific gravity of urine *(AIIMS 09)*
B. Blood urea
C. GFR
D. Creatinine clearance

37. A/E – are absorbed in the DCT: *(AIIMS 07)*
A. Water
B. Potassium
C. Chloride
D. Sodium

38. Major portion of glomerular filtrate is absorbed in -
A. Loop of henle *(AI 04)*
B. Distal convoluted tubule
C. Collecting duct
D. Proximal segment

39. Which of the following is true about Nephron function: *(AI 09)*
A. Ascending thick limb is permeable to water
B. Descending thin limb is impermeable to water
C. Osmolality of intra-tubular content in DCT is more than surrounding interstitution
D. Osmolality of intratubular content in PCT is isotonic to surrounding interstitium

40. Which of the following occurs along with glucose transport into renal tubular cells: *(AI 08, 01)*
A. Sodium symport/Cotransport *(NBE P 15,13)*
B. Sodium anteport
C. Potassium transport
D. Amino acid transport

Loop of Henle

41. Counter current mechanism,all are true except-
A. Occurs due to opp flow in vasa recta and loop of henle *(NBE P 13)*
B. Seen in medullary nephron
C. Helps in creating osmolarity gradient
D. Urea has no role

42. Countercurrent mechanism in the kidney is responsible for- *(NBE P 13)*
A. Absorption of glucose
B. Maintenance of blood flow
C. Osmotic gradient in medulla
D. Secretion of uric acid

43. Substance involved in countercurrent mechanism for maintaining medullary gradient- *(Orissa 04)*
A. NaCl but no urea *(NBE P 15,14,13)*
B. Urea
C. NaCi, urea but not Water
D. NaCl, urea, water

44. The high sodium content of the filtrate in renal medulla is because: *(AIIMS 06)*
A. At the loop of Henle, there is counter current mechanism
B. Increased blood flow to vasarecta
C. Increased excretion of Na^+ from PCT
D. Increased absorption of Na from PCT

45. Renal medullary hyperosmolarity is due to:
A. Increased Na^+ *(PGI 15,14, 04, 03)*
B. Increased Na content
C. Increased Glucose
D. Increased urea
E. Increased Potassium

46. The prime driving force for counter current multiplier system is: *(AI 06)*
A. Medullary hyperosmolarity
B. Reabsorption of Na^+ in thick ascending limb
C. Action of ADH via aquaporin channels
D. Urea recycling

47. Countercurrent mechanism is not seen in: *(AIIMS 16)*
A. Kidney
B. Testes
C. Eye
D. Intestine

48. Which of the following is not a component of counter current multiplier mechanism? *(AIIMS 14)*
A. Vasa-recta
B. Thick ascending limb of loop of Henle
C. Thin descending limb of loop of Henle
D. Collecting duct

49. Loop of Henle handles the following ions except:
A. Na^+ *(PGI 07, 14)*
B. K^+
C. Cl^-
D. Urea

Distal Convoluted Tubule & Collecting Duct

50. Macula densa in kidney is located in relation to -
A. PCT *(NBE P 15,13; UPSC 07)*
B. DCT
C. Afferent arteriole
D. Efferent arteriole

51. The tubuloglomerular feedback is mediated by: *(AI 06)*
A. Sensing of Na^+ concentration in the macula densa
B. Sensing of Cl^+ concentration in macula densa
C. Sensing NaCl concentration in the macula densa
D. Opening up of voltage gated Na^+ channels in afferent arteriole

52. Where in the kidney does acitve reabsorption of sodium ions occur - *(AMU 01, UP 05)*
- A. Collecting duct ☐
- B. Distal tubule ☐
- C. Ascending limb of Henle ☐
- D. All of the above ☐
- E. Only B and C ☐

53. K+ secretion from loop of henle is decreased by-
- A. Furosemide *(NBE P 13)* ☐
- B. Thiazide ☐
- C. Spironolactone ☐
- D. Acetazolamide ☐

54. Alodosterone mainly acts upon- *(NBE P 13)*
- A. PCT ☐
- B. Loop of Henle ☐
- C. Glomerulus ☐
- D. Collecting duct ☐

55. Where does ADH not act- *(NBE P 13)*
- A. PCT ☐
- B. Collecting duct ☐
- C. Collecting tubules ☐
- D. DCT ☐

56. All of these are correct of renal physiology *except*:
- A. Sodium absorption occurs in DCT *(PGI 02)* ☐
- B. Potassium is both secreted and absorbed in tubules ☐
- C. Glucose is reabsorbed in DCT ☐
- D. Hb is not excreted as it is a large molecule ☐
- E. Amino acids are reabsorbed in CD ☐

57. The Principal site of acidification of urine is:
- A. Distal convoluted tubule *(AI 04)* ☐
- B. Proximal convoluted tubule ☐
- C. Loop of Henle ☐
- D. Collecting duct ☐

58. Which one of the following is not responsible for concentration of urine in the kidney - *(DNB 13)*
- A. Aldosterone ☐
- B. AngiotensinII ☐
- C. Vasopressin ☐
- D. Epinephrine ☐

59. Several hormones regulate the tubular reabsorption of water and electrolytes at different sites in the nephron. Which of the following combination is correct? *(AIIMS 03)*
- A. Angiotensin in distal tubule ☐
- B. Aldosterone in collecting ducts ☐
- C. ADH in proximal tubule ☐
- D. ANP in loop of Henle ☐

60. Functionof vasopressin- *(NBE P 13)*
- A. Absorption of water in PCT ☐
- B. Absoption of water in loop of henle ☐
- C. Absorption of water in collecting duct ☐
- D. Absorption of Na^+ in PCT ☐

61. ANP acts at which site- *(NBE P 13)*
- A. Glomerulus ☐
- B. Loop of Henle ☐
- C. PCT ☐
- D. Collection duct ☐

62. Peristalsis of ureter depends on *(AIIMS 07)*
- A. Sympathetic flow ☐
- B. Parasympathetic flow ☐
- C. Sympathetic and Parasympathetic flow ☐
- D. Pacemaker in smooth muscle of renal calyces ☐

63. Hypertonic urine is excreted due to absorption of water in: *(AIIMS 03)*
- A. Collecting ducts ☐
- B. DCT ☐
- C. Ascending part of loop of Henley ☐
- D. Descending part of loop of Henley ☐

64. Urinary concentrating ability of the kidney is increased by: *(AI 05)*
- A. ECF volume contraction. ☐
- B. Increase in RBF. ☐
- C. Reduction of medullary hyperosmolarity. ☐
- D. Increase in GFR. ☐

65. Substance that is completely reabsorbed from the kidney- *(NBE P 13)*
- A. Na^+ ☐
- B. K^+ ☐
- C. Urea ☐
- D. Glucose ☐

66. Least reabsorption out of- *(NBE P 13)*
- A. Glucose ☐
- B. Urea ☐
- C. Na^+ ☐
- D. HCO_3 ☐

Urine

67. Elimination of waste product from a normal person requires minimal amount of urine of: *(PGI 05)*
- A. 100 ml ☐
- B. 500 m ☐
- C. 200 ml ☐
- D. 2000 ml ☐

68. Normal excretion of protein in urine per day is:
- A. 100 mg *(AI 04)* ☐
- B. 150 mg ☐
- C. 400 mg ☐
- D. 600 mg ☐

69. The urge for micturition is felt when the bladder is filled with - *(DNB 05)*
- A. 100-200cc of urine ☐
- B. 200-300cc of urine ☐
- C. 500-700cc of urine ☐
- D. 700-800cc of urine ☐

70. In a normal adult the marked desire for micturition is felt - *(AIIMS 06, DNB 09)*
- A. When about 100-200 cc f urine has collected in the bladder ☐
- B. When about 300 - 400 cc of urine has collected in the bladder ☐
- C. When about 600-800 cc of urine has collected - in the bladder ☐
- D. When about 1000 cc of urine has collected in the bladder ☐

71. True statement among the following is - *(DNB 06)*
A. Bladder emptying cannot occur if volume < 100 ml.
B. Bladder muscles contains intrafusal fibres
C. Pressure increase in blader very linerly with time
D. One time of fluid, intake :results in complete excretion in 1 hour

Water and Acid Base Balance

72. Daily loss of water from skin in absence of sweating is OR Insensible water loss per day is:
A. 1 litre *(NBE P 15,13; AIIMS 04)*
B. 1.5 litres
C. 200-300 ml
D. 500-700 ml

73. Findings of Syndrome of Inappropriate Antidiuretic Hormone Secretion (SIADH) includes *(PGI 12)*
A. ↑Urine Na+
B. ↑Serum Na-
C. ↑Urine osmolality
D. ↑Serum osteolality
E. Postural hypotention

74. True about free water clearance is: *(AIIMS 07)*
A. Regulated by ADH
B. Regulated by aldosterone
C. Increased by furosemide
D. None of the above

75. In metabolic acidosis, which of the following changes are seen: *(AI 02)*
A. Increased K^+ excretion
B. Decreased K^+ excretion
C. Increased Na^+ excretion
D. Increased Na^+ reabsorption

76. All of the following statements are correct about potassium balance, except: *(AI 03)*
A. Most of potassium is intracellular
B. Three quarter of the total body potassium is found in skeletal muscle
C. Intracellular potassium is released into extra-cellular space in response to severe injury
D. Acidosis leads to movements of potassium from extracellular to intracellular fluid compartment.

77. Anion gap is mostly due to: *(AI 06)*
A. Proteins
B. Sulphates
C. Phosphates
D. Nitrates

78. Metabolic alkalosis is seen in all except - *(AI 08)*
A. Thiazide diuretics
B. Uretersigmoid_ostomy
C. Prolonged vomiting
D. Systemic antacid therapy

79. Increased anion gap is seen in: *(PGI 03)*
A. Enterocutaneous fistula
B. Illeostomy fistula
C. Lactic acidosis
D. DKA
E. Cardiac failure

80. Normal anion gap metabolic acidosis is seen in:
A. Diarrhoea *(AIIMS 02)*
B. Renal failure
C. Lactic acidosis
D. Diabetic ketoacidosis

81. In severe exercise, decrease in pH is due to-
A. Respiratory acidosis *(NBE P 13)*
B. Lactic acidosis
C. H+ retension
D. HCO_3 excretion

82. Blood buffers are: *(PGI 02)*
A. Bicarbonate
B. Plasma proteins
C. Phosphates
D. Hemoglobin
E. Oxygen

83. A newly posted junior doctor had difficulty in finding out base deficit/excess for blood in a given patient. An experienced senior resident advised a quick method to determine acid base composition of blood based on PCO_2. Which of the following is the likely method he suggested to predict acid base composition of blood? *(AI 04)*
A. Red ford normogram
B. DuBio's normogram
C. Goldman constant field equation
D. Siggard-Andersen normogram

84. If you calculate the plasma osmolality of a child with plasma Na^+ 125 mEq/*l*, glucose 108 mg/ dl, and BUN (blood urea nitrogen) 140 mg/ dl, the most appropriate answer would be:
A. 300 mOsm/kg *(AIIMS 03)*
B. 306 mOsm/kg
C. 312 mOsm/kg
D. 318 mOsm/kg

Endocrine Functions Of Kidney

85. Erythropoietin is secreted from- *(NBE P 13)*
A. Juxtraglomerular cells
B. Macula densa
C. Interstitial cells
D. Glomerulus

86. Erythropoietin secretion occurs when: *(NBE P 13)*
A. ↓ Tissue pO_2 concentration
B. ↑ Tissue pH
C. ↑ Tissue pCO_2 concentration
D. ↑ Hemoglobin

87. Erythropoietin is secreted by A/E: *(PGI 05)*
A. Hemangioblastoma
B. Hepatoma
C. Renal cell carcinoma
D. Adrenocortical tumours

88. True about function of Angiotensin II: *(PGI 10)*
A. Constriction of afferent arteriole
B. Autoregulation of GFR
C. Secreted from endothelial
D. Release aldosterone
E. Increased sodium and water reabsorption

89. Which is true about rennin: *(PGI 03)*
A. It helps to convert angiotensinogen to Angiotensin-I
B. Secreted by PCT
C. ↑ GFR causes ↑ secretion of rennin
D. ↓ plasma Na^+ & H_2O

90. True regarding rennin angiotensin system is A/E *(PGI 09)*
A. Angiotonin is octapeptide
B. ACE splits Leucine-valine bond
C. Aspartic acid is essential for rennin activity
D. PRA is better than PRC
E. Catalysis site of ACE contain Zn^{++}

91. Physiologically inactive form is *(WB 09)*
A. Angiotensin I
B. Angiotensin II
C. Angiotensin III
D. Angiotensin IV

92. True is all except *(PGI 09)*
A. Renin - liver
B. Renin- kidney
C. Renin substrate – liver
D. ACE- lung endothelium
E. Angiotensinogen – Renal

93. Angiotensin II causes all of the following, Except: *(AIIMS 11, AI 09)*
A. Stmulation of Thirst
B. Increased ADH secretion
C. Vasodilatation
D. Aldosterone secretion

94. Which causes raised angiotensin in blood- *(NBE P 13)*
A. Increased blood volume
B. Raised cardiac output
C. Decreased blood pressure
D. Increased sympathetic tone

95. A/E one results in increased secretion of Renin *(AIIMS 14,13; NBE P 14, 13)*
A. Renal ischemia, and sympathetic nerve stimulation
B. Decreased amount of Na^+ in DCT.
C. Decreased amount of Na^+ in PCT.
D. Narrowing of afferent arterioles (or low pressure)

96. Renin is secreted by : *(NBE P 15,14,13; AIIMS 07, 13)*
A. PCT
B. DCT
C. Collecting duct
D. Juxatglomerular apparatus

97. Macula densa in kidney is located in relation to - *(NBE P 15,13)*
A. PCT
B. DCT
C. Afferent arteriole
D. Efferent arteriole

98. Lacis cells are located at- *(NBE P 13)*
A. JGA
B. Proximal tubule
C. Distal tubule
D. Loop pf henle

99. True about juxta-glomerular apparatus of kidney: *(PGI 2K)*
A. Important source of angiotensiogen
B. Important source of rennin
C. Consist of macula densa
D. Consist of afferent arteriole forming lacis cell

100. Juxtaglomerular apparatus lies in relation to: *(AIIMS 07)*
A. Proximal convoluted tubule
B. Ascending loop of Henle
C. Descending loop of Henle
D. Glomerulus

101. Vasopressin acts by: *(PGI 08)*
A. Water transport across collecting duct
B. Water absorption at medullary ducts
C. Water secretion at loop of Henle
D. Water transport at PCT

102. Which one of the following is not a transport or binding protein? *(AIIMS 05)*
A. Erythropoietin
B. Ceruloplasmin
C. Lactoferrin
D. Transnsferrin

ANSWERS & EXPLANATIONS:

Nephron & Glomerular Filtration

1. **A i.e. Juxtaglomerular apparatus** *[Ref: Ganong 23rd/e p. 640-43; Gabriel C Ezeilo p. 208-10; Guyton 11th/e p. 309]*

Loop of Henle, collecting duct & vasa recta lie in renal medulla (pyramid) whereas, **JG apparatus (JG cells, lacis cells, macula densa of DCT)** lie in **renal cortex.**

2. **B i.e. Dilatation of afferent arteriales** 3. **C i.e. Effective renal plasma flow is 625 ml/min & inulin clearance is same**
4. **D i.e. Inulin & PAH** *[Ref: Ganong 24/e p. 675-80; Guyton 11/e p. 308-13]*

- Each kidney contains **1-1.3 million nephrons**Q. **PCT** is **15mm** and **DCT is 5mm long, 15% are juxtamedullary and 85% are cortical nephrons**Q.
- ***GFR increases with afferent arteriole dilation and increased renal blood flow***Q. **Normal GFR measured by inulin clearance (best) or creatinine clearance is 125ml/min** (7.5 l/hr or 180 l/day). **Net filtration pressure is 10 to 15mm Hg.**
- **Renal plasma flow** (RPF) i.e. renal blood flow or circulation can be measured by **infusing PAH (P-aminohippuric acid). Effective RPF is 625 ml/min and actual RPF is 700 ml/min**Q.
- Because **filtration fraction** is GFR/RPF (i.e. 0.16 to 0.20). It can be measured by **inulin/creatine (for GFR) and PAH (for RPF)**Q.

5. **B i.e. Glomerular oncotic pressure is less than of filtrate** 6. **B i.e. The kidneys receive 5% of the cardiac output**
[Ref: Guyton 12/e p. 314-15; 11th/e p. 314, 319; Ganong 23rd/e p. 653- 57; Gabriel p. 220, 211- 13; Disease of kidney & urinary tract 8/e pg-10]

- **Kidney** ***receives 25% of cardiac output at rest***Q **(i.e. 1.2 to 1.3 litres blood per minute).**
- **Glucose is freely filtered across glomerular capillary membrane** and therefore ***glucose concentration of glomerular filtrate is same as that of plasma***Q.
- **Glomerular (capillary) oncotic pressure (d/t plasma protein content) is higher than that of filtrate oncotic pressure in Bowman's capsule** (with almost O protein content).
- ***Constriction of afferent arteriole decreases glomerular hydrostatic pressure (& GFR)***Q, whereas afferent arteriole dilation & efferent arteriole constriction increase it.

7. **A i.e. C-Amp & Dopamine** 8. **A i.e. I cells** 9. **B i.e. Mesangium** *[Ref: Ganong 24/ 707; Robbins 7/ 957-958; MTx]*

- ***Mesangial cells do not form filteration barrier***Q. ***Relaxation of mesangial cells*** is brought about by ***C-AMP, ANP, dopamine and*** PGE_2Q.
- ***Intercalated (I) or brown cells secrete acid & transport*** HCO_3^- ***in kidney***Q.

Specialized Cells of Nephron

In Glomerulus

Stellate /Mesengial cells are *contractile*, locate between basal lamina & endothelium and regulate GFR. Agents causing their

Contraction
- Endothelins
- Angiotensin II
- Vasopressin
- Norepinephrine
- Platelet activating factor
- Platelet derived growth factor
- PGF_2
- Thromboxane A_2
- Leukotrienes C_4 & D_4
- Histamine

Relaxation
- **Dopamine**
- **ANP**
- ***C AMP***Q
- PGE_2

In Collecting Duct

Principal (P) cells
Are more numerous relatively taller cells with few organelles. They are involved in *Na^+ reabsorption & vasopressin stimulated water reabsorption*

Intercalated (I) or Brown cells
Are present in smaller number, have more microvilli, cytoplasmic vesicles, & mitochondria. They are concercerned with ***acid secretion & HCO_3^- transport***Q

★ **Type I medullary interstitial cells** contain lipid droplets & secrete prostaglandin *PGE_2*

★ **Podocytes** form epithelium of Bowman's capsule which along with capillary endothelium forms filterating membrane. These layers are separated by basal lamine.

Mesangial Cells

- Mesenchymal origin
- ***Support***Q the entire glomeular tuft.
- ***Secrete mesangial matrix***Q.
- are ***contractile***Q
- are ***phagocytic***Q
- ***Capable of proliferation***Q

Filteration Barrier

The glomeular capillary wall is the *"Filtering membrane"* of nephron. It consists of following structures:

1. Fenestrated ***endothelial cells***Q
2. Glomerular basement membraneQ (Consist of ***Type IV collagen***Q)
3. ***Visceral epithelial cells***Q (Podocytes).

10. B i.e. Mesangial constriction

ANP, BNP and CNP (on injection) **increase Na^+ excretion (i.e. cause natriuresis) by dilating afferent arterioles and relaxing mesangial cells**Q.

Natriuretic Peptide (NP)	Isolated from
Atrial NP (ANP)	**Heart (Atria), Brain**Q
Brain (B type) NP (BNP)	**Ventricle (main), Brain**
C- type NP (CNP)	Brain, Pituitary, Kidney, Vascular endothelium

11. E i.e. Glucose; C i.e. Creatinine *[Ref: Ganong 22/e p. 705-07; Guyton & Hall 11/e p. 316 –18; Sembulingam 4/e p. 290-93]*

Electrolytes such as **sodium (Na^+), water** and small orgaic compounds like **glucose, inulin** and **creatinine** are freely filtered across glomerular capillaries (i.e. filterability =1).

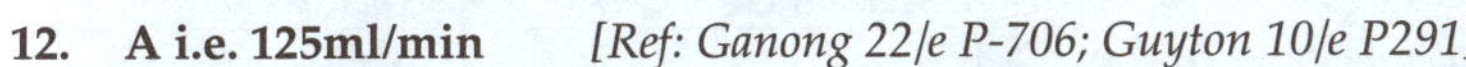

12. A i.e. 125ml/min *[Ref: Ganong 22/e P-706; Guyton 10/e P291]*

GFR in an normal person at resting condition is ***125ml/min or 7.5 L/hour or 180L/day***Q. Whereas the normal urine volume is about 1L/day. Thus 99% of filtrate is reabsorbed.

13. A i.e. GFR

14. A i.e. Inulin *[Ref: Ganong 24/e P-679]*

InulinQ is the standard substance and extensively used *to measure GFR*. **Clearance of creatinine (C_{Cr})** can also be used for GFR measurement. However, *clearance of creatinine will be slightly higher than inulin* **because of some tubular secretion**. P_{CR} (plasma creatinine) is an index of renal function.

15. B i.e. Urinary concentration in mg/ml

Renal Circulation

- Kidney receives ***1.2- 1.3 L/min blood***Q **(25% of cardiac output) at rest.**Q
- **Renal plasma flow (RPF)** equals the amount of substance excreted per unit of time divided by arteriovenous difference for the substance across the kidney (as long as hematocrit is same).

$$RPF = \frac{U_C \times V}{S_{RAC} - S_{RVC}}, \quad \textbf{Excretion ratio} = \frac{S_{RAC} - S_{RVC}}{S_{RAC}}$$

U_C = Concentration of substance in urine (mg/mL)Q, V = Urine flow (ml/min), S_{RAC} & S_{RVC} = substance renal arterial & venous concentrations respectively.

- RPF can be measured by infusing ***p-amino hippuric acid (PAH)***Q. As excretion ratio of PAH is high (0.9) and its 90% is removed from artery in a single circulation through kidney. And its renal arterial concentration is equal to plasma concentration, so RPF by PAH can also be measured by this formula, which is k/a **effective renal plasma flow (ERPF)**

$$\textbf{ERPF} = \frac{U_{PAH\ conc.} \times V}{PAH\ \ plasma\ \ concentration} = \sim 625\ mL/min^{Q}$$

$$\textbf{Actual RPF} = \frac{ERPF}{Excretion\ ratio} = \frac{630}{0.9} = 700 ml/min^{Q}$$

Glomerular Filtration

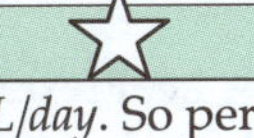

- Normal GFR is ***125ml/min***Q or *7.5L/hour or 180L/day*. So per day kidney filters fluid equal to *4 times of total body water, 15 times of ECF, & 60 times of plasma* volume.
- ***Inulin***Q **& creatinine can be used to measure GFR**
- $GFR = K_f\left[(P_{GC} - P_T) - (\pi_{GC} - \pi_T)\right]$

Kf = glomerular ultrafiltration cofficient (it is product of permeability & effective filtration area)

P_{GC} & P_T = Hyprostatic pressure (P) in glomerular capillary (gc) & tubule (t) respectively

π_{GC} & π_T = Osmotic pressure (π) of plasma in glomerular capillary (GC) & tubule (T) respectively.

- Net filtration pressure (P_{UF}) is ***15 mm Hg***Q

$$P_{UF} = P_{GC} - P_T - \pi_{GC}$$

	Afferent end (mmHg)	Efferent end (mmHg)
P_{GC}	45	45
PT	10	10
π_{GC}	20	35
P_{UF}	*15*Q	0

★ PT = Pressure in Bowman's capsule

- **Filtration fraction is ratio** of GFR/RPF, and is normally *0.16- 0.20*

16. **A i.e. 20** *[Ref: Ganong 24/e p. 680]*

Net Filtration Pressure (P_{UF}) =	**Hydrostatic Pressure in Glomerular Capillary (P_{GC}) – Hydrostatic Pressure in tubule interstitium (P_T) - Glomerular Capillary Oncotic or Osmotic Pressure (Π_{GC})**

or **$PUF = P_{GC} - P_T - \Pi_{GC}$** ; $3 = 25 - 2 - \Pi_{GC}$
; $3 = 23 - \Pi_{GC}$

So $\Pi_{GC} = 20$

17. **B i.e. Drug is secreted in the tubules** *[Ref: Gabriel C Ezeilo p. 212-15; Guyton 11th/355-56; Ganong 23rd/645-47; KDT 5/e P 27]*
18. **C i.e. If clearance of a substance is greater than GFR, then tubular secretion must be present**

If a drug is *more in renal clearance* than the amount filtered by glomerulus it *has to be secreted in renal tubules*
Tubular secretion – This is the *active transfer of organic acids and bases* in the proximal tubules.
If renal clearance of drug is greater than 120 ml/min (GFR), additional tubular secretion can be assumed to be occurring.

If renal clearance is *more than GFR*	**Tubular secretion**[Q]
If renal clearance is *less than GFR*	**Tubular reabsorption**[Q]

19. **A i.e. It is freely filtered in glomerulus** *[Ref: Ganong 22/e P- 684]*

If the substance is O mg% in efferent arteriole, it means that all of it has freely filtered in glomerulus.

20. **B i.e. False –low**

At **low plasma PAH concentration**, the measured RPF (renal plasma flow) is accurate. Whereas, **at high (>30mg/dl) plasma PAH concentrations the estimated RPF is falsely low** because of saturated secretary mechanism & TM.

21. **A i.e. Presence of negatively charged sialoproteins on the filtering membrane**
22. **B i.e. Loss of negative charge on membrane** *[Ref: Mtx; Ganong 23/ep 646]*

The **negative charges of basement membrane & podocytes restrict and repel large negatively charged and attract positively charged molecules**[Q]. ***Negatively charged large molecules are filtered less easily than positively charged molecules of equal molecular size***[Q], and even neutral molecule are filtered much more easily than negatively charged molecules of same size. So, negatively changes. **Main cause of minimal change nephropathy (disease) is loss of negative charge on basement membrane**[Q].

23. **A i.e. Uric Acid** *[Ganong 23/ep 648-50]*

Substrate which are both filtered (secreted) & absorbed are Creatinine, Uric acid & potassium (K^+)[Q]. Mn "Sec UK or CUK".

Proximal Convoluted Tubule

24. **A i.e. Maximum reabsorption & secretion**
25. **E i.e. Urea** *[Ref: Guyton 11/e p. 330 – 32; Ganong 24/e p. 682-83]*
26. **A i.e., Different nephrons have different transport maximum**
27. **D i.e. H^+**

Transport maximum (T_m) means ***maximum reabsorption & secretion***[Q]. T_m for kidney in practice is actually less than the calculated value ***because not all nephrons have same T_m***[Q]. Passively absorbed **substances e.g.** ***urea, chloride and water do not exhibit T_m***[Q].

Actual renal threshold for glucose is less than its predicted value.

28. **A i.e. PCT (indirect)** 29. **B i.e. Proximal tubule** 30. **A i.e. Proximal tubule**
31. **A i.e. The bulk of water reabsorption occurs secondary to Na^+ reabsorption** 32. **A i.e. Proximal convoluted tubule**
33. **A i.e. Proximal convoluted tubule** 34. **B i.e. Concentration of HCO_3 falls**
[Ref: Ganong 24/e P- 685, 22/e p. 717; Guyton 12/SAE p. 480-90; Sembulingum 3/e P- 254-55]

- **Proximal convoluted tubule (early part)** reabsorbs **almost all of glucose, amino acids, protein, lactate & inorganic phosphate and most of bicarbonate/ HCO_3^- (80-90%), Na^+ (60%), H_2O, K+ and Cl^-** Q. PCT is also an important site for **secretion of organic acids and bases such as oxalate, urate, bile salts, H+ and catecholamines, along with toxins, drugs eg penicillin, salicylates and PAH. So its' a work horse of nephron** Q.
- **Absorption of HCO_3-in PCT is indirect i.e. coupled with H^+ Secretion** Q
- **Greatest fraction of filtered water (60-70%) is reabsorbed in proximal tubule irrespective of presence or absence of vasopressin** Q. **Proximal convoluted tubule** reabsorbs approximately 50-60% of water (bulk of water), which is **secondary (obligatory) to Na^+ reabsorption** Q.

35. **C i.e. 7.5% solution gives 2n mols** *[Ganong 22/e P-686, 720]*

Concentration of bicarbonate
- Intracellular : ***10 mmol/L*** Q
- Extracellular : ***27 mmol/L*** Q

- **In kidney** bicarbonate is produced by ***carbonic anhydrase*** Q.

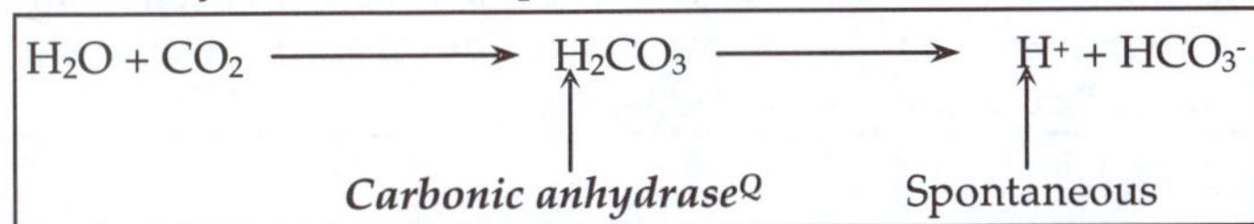

36. **A i.e. Specific gravity of urine**

The *main function of renal tubules is concentration of urine* and this can be measured by *specific gravity of urine.*

37. **B i.e. Potassium** *[Ref: Ganong 22/e P- 724]*

Potassium once filtered in the tubular fluid is reabsorbed only *in the proximal tubules*. Nowhere else it is reabsorbed so it is not reabsorbed in the DCT, rather ***it is secreted into the tubular fluid in DCT*** Q.

Water reabsorption in DCT: ***Early part*** **of distal tubule is** ***impermeable*** **to water.** ***Late DCT*** **becomes** ***permeable*** **under the** ***influence of ADH.***

38. **D i.e. Proximal segment** 39. **D i.e. Osmolality of intratubular content in PCT is isotonic to surrounding interstitium**
[Ref: Ganong 24/e P-681-91]

Major portion of glomerular filtrate is absorbed in proximal segment (mainly PCT) Q. ***Osmolality of intratubular content in PCT is isotonic to surrounding interstitium*** Q.

40. **A i.e. Sodium symport** *[Ref: Ganong 22/e P-470, 710]*

Glucose and Na^+ *share the same* ***Co-transporter (or symport) – the sodium dependent glucose transporter: (SGLT – sodium glucose co- transporter)*** Q.

Counter-Current Mechanism, Loop of Henle, DCT, CD

41. **D i.e. Urea has no role** 42. **C i.e. Osmotic gradient in medulla** 43. **D i.e. NaCl, Urea, Water**
44. **A i.e. At the loop of Henle there is counter current mechanism**
45. **A i.e. Increased Na^+ ; D i.e. Increased urea; E i.e. Increased K^+**
46. **B i.e. Reabsorption of Na+ in thick ascending limb** *[Ref: Ganong 24/e p. 687-89; Guyton 12/SAE p. 482-87; MTx]*

- **Counter current mechanism** is seen in **medullary nephrons[Q], are occurs due to opposite flow in loop of Henle & vasa-recta[Q]. Counter current multiplier at Loop of Henle generate and counter current exchanger at vasa-recta of medullary capillaries maintain medullary osmotic pressure gradient[Q]**
- **Renal medullary hyperosmolarity** is maintained by counter current mechanism l/t **↑Na^+, Cl^-, Urea & K^+ conc[Q]**. The **Counter current multiplier mechanism at the loop of Henle** is responsible for development of hyper osmolarity of medullary interstitial fluid and medullary gradient. **Hyperosmolarity is due to high Na^+ conc. of the filtrate in renal medulla[Q].**
- **'The operation of each loop of Henle as a counter current multiplier depends on the active transport of Na+ and Cl- out of its thick ascending limb,** high permeability of its thin descending limb to water and the inflow of tubular fluid from the proximal tubule with outflow into the distal tubule'. **The prime driving force for counter current multiplier is reabsorption of Na+ in thick ascending limb. The prime objective for counter current multiplier system is to produce Medullary hyperosmolarity.**

47. C i.e. Eye *[Ref: Ganong 24/ep 419, 687]*

Counter current mechanism (CCM) is a system in which *inflow and outflow run parallel & opposite (i.e. counter to) each other in close proximity to create a concentration gradient*. It is seen in many mammalian organs e.g. **kidney, testis** (b/w spermatic arteries & pampiniform plexus) and **gut** (hair pin arrangement of arteries & vein in **intestinal villi** where O_2 directly diffuses from arterioles to veins).

48. A i.e. Vasa-recta

Loop of Henle (& collecting duct)	Involved in **Counter Current Multiplier Mechanism**
Vasa recta	Involved in **Counter Current Exchanger Mechanism.**

Maintenance of Osmolarity

Medullary Gradient

- The osmolarity of cortical interstitium is same as that of plasma (300 mosm/L). However osmolality of medullary interstitium is very high (1200 mosm/L)
- Gradual increase in the osmolarity (from 300 to 1200 mosm/L) of medullary interstitium is called medullary gradient
- Counter – current mechanism is responsible for maintenance of medullary gradient i.e. **hypeosmotic renal medullary interstitium.**

***Factors responsible for Medullary Interstitium Hyperosmolarity**

1. Active transport of *Na^+ & co-transport of Cl^-, K^+*[Q] & other ions out of thick ascending limb of loop of Henle into medullary interstitium.
2. ***Passive diffusion of urea***[Q] from inner medullary collecting ducts into the medullary interstitium.
3. ***Diffusion of only small amount of water from medullary tubules***[Q] into medullary interstitium *(far less than resorption of solutes into medullary interstitium)*
4. **Active transport of ions from collecting duct** into **medullary interstitium**.

Counter Current Mechanism

Counter current flow is flow in which the inflow runs parallel to, counter to, & in close proximity to the outflow for some distance.

Counter Current Multiplier

- Is formed by ***the loop of Henle***[Q]. Loop of Henle multiplies the Na^+ concentration within medulla, by retaining the new Na^+ coming from glomerular filtrate.
- ***Gradient of increasing osmolality*** along the medullary pyramid is ***produced***[Q] by operation of the ***loops of Henle***[Q] as counter current multipliers. It acts by

Active transport of Na+ and Cl- out of its thick ascending loop	**High permeability of the thin descending limb to water**	**Additional inflow of tubular fluid into the proximal tubule.**
This initiates the increased osmolarity of the renal medulla	This allows osmosis of water out of the descending limb thus achieving hyperosmotic fluid in the descending limb	This causes the hyperosmotic fluid initially formed in the descending limb to flow into ascending limb. Once this fluid is in ascending limb, further active transport enhances the medullary osmolarity.

These steps are repeated over and over, with the net effect of adding more and more solute to medulla and creating a hyperosmotic renal medulla.

Counter Current Exchanger

- Formed by the ***vasa recta***[Q]. Vasa recta retains the Na^+ and urea in the medullary interstitium & removes water from it. Since Na^+ & urea are exchanged for water between ascending & descending limb of vasa recta it is called exchanger.
- ***Gradient is maintained***[Q] by the operation of ***vasa recta***[Q] as counter current exchanger.
  - The *solutes diffuse out* of the vessels conducting blood towards the cortex and *into the* vessels *descending* into the pyramid
  - *Water diffuses out* of the descending vessels & *into ascending* vessels
  - Therefore, the solute (Na^+, Cl^-, K^+, Urea) tends to recirculate in medulla and water tends to bypass it, so that hypertonicity is maintained
  - It is a *passive process* and could not maintain gradient if the process of counter current exchanger were to cease.

Loop of Henle as a counter current multiplier producing a gradient of hyperosmolarity in the medullary interstitium (MI).

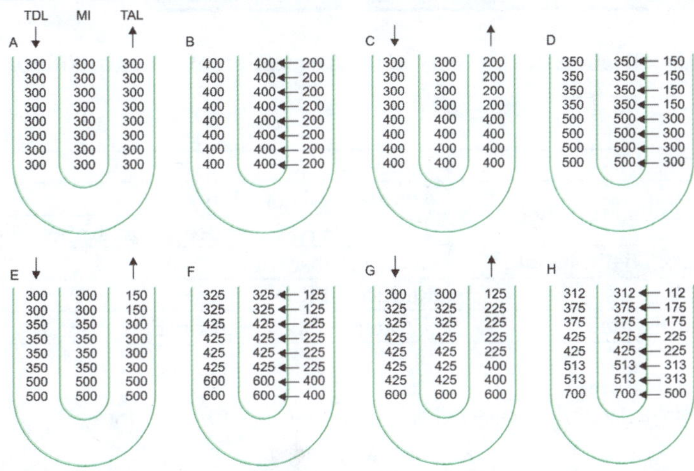

TDL, thin descending limb; TAL, thick ascending limb. The process of generation of the gradient is illustrated as occurring in hypothetical steps, starting at A, where osmolality in both limbs and the intestitium is 300 msom/kg of water. The pumps in the thick ascending limb move Na+ and Cl- into the interstitium, increasing its osmolality to 400 Mosm/kg, and this equilibrates with the fluid in the thin descending limb. However, isotonic fluid continues to flow into the thin descending limb and hypotonic fluid out of the thick ascending limb. Continued operation of the pumps makes the fluid leaving the thick ascending limb even more hypotonic, while hypertonicity accumulates at the apex of the loop.

Vasa recta as counter current exchangers in the kidney.

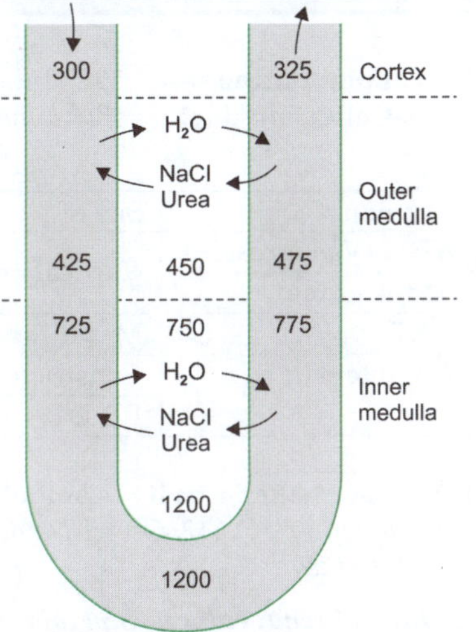

NaCl and urea diffuse out of the ascending limb of the vessel and into the descending limb, whereas water diffuses out of the descending and into the ascending limb of the vascular loop.

49. D i.e. Urea *[Ref: Ganong 22/e P- 714; Sembulingum 3/e P- 258]*

> In the ***thick ascending limb***, a carrier co-transports ***one Na^+, one K^+ and $2Cl^-$***Q from the tubular lumen into the tubular cells.

50. B i.e. DCT **51. C i.e. Sensing NaCl concentration in the macula densa** *[Ref:Guyton 11th/323, 324; Ganong 22/e p 700-13]*

> **'To perform the function of auto regulation, the kidneys have a feed back mechanism (tubuloglomerular feed back) that links changes in sodium chloride concentration at the macula densa (tubular component) with the control of renal arteriolar resistance (glomerular component). Macula densa is located in DCT**Q.

52. D i.e. All **53. C i.e. Spironolactone** **54. D i.e. Collecting duct**
55. A i.e. PCT **56. C i.e. Glucose is reabsorbed in DCT; D i.e. Hb is not excreted ..; E i.e.Amino acids are reabsorbed...**
[Ref: Ganong 22/e P- 709, 711;Chaudhuri 5/e P- 406, 412; Shinde & Chatterjea 6/e P-658]

> - **Na^+ reabsorption occurs in all parts of nephron except descending limb of LH**Q. **K^+ reabsorption takes place in PCT (maximum) and thick ascending limb of LH**Q. K^+ is secreted in thin descending limb of LH & DT.
> - **Glucose, amino acids, bicarbonates and Na^+ are reabsorbed maximally in early PCT**Q.

- **Potassium sparing (retaining) natriuretics** are diuretics which prevent **loss of K^+** (unlike other diuretics) **by inhibiting aldosterone (so Na^+-K^+ Exchange) in collecting duct (e.g. spironolactone)**Q or by inhibiting ENaCs (e.g. **amiloride**).
- **Hemoglobinuria –** *excretion of free Hb* following increased plasma level of free Hb (Hemoglobinemia). There is *renal threshold for Hb*. When this threshold is exceeded, hemoglobinuria results. If the kidneys are normal, *the threshold is about 155mg% of blood plasma*. But it may be lowered when kidneys are damaged. Hb excretion is ***not related to its molecular structure***Q.

57. **D i.e. Collecting duct** *[Ref: Ganong 22/e P- 720; Chaudhuri 5/e P- 411]*

Acidification of tubular fluid occurs in distal nephron, particularly the collecting duct, (CD).

58. **D i.e. Epinephrine**
59. **B i.e. Aldosterone in collecting duct**
60. **C i.e. Absorption of water in collecting duct**
61. **D i.e. Collection duct** *[Ref: Guyton 10/e P 290, 304, 305, 335]*

Hormone	Site of Action in kidney	Effect
ADH (Vasopressin)	**Cortical collecting duct & Distal tubule**Q	↑ Water reabsorption
Aldosterone		↑ Water & NaCl reabsorption, K^+ Secretion
ANP	**Medullary collecting duct & Distal tubule**Q	↓NaCl reabsorption
Angiotensin II	Constricts Afferent Arterioles	Reduce GFR
	PT, DT, CD & Thick ascending limb	↑Water & NaCl reabsorption

62. **D i.e. Pacemaker activity in smooth muscles of renalcalyces**
[Ref: Guyton 11/e p. 312; Georgl Tanner: Medical Physiology 2/e p. 423, www.pubmedcentral.nih.gov/articlerender.fegi?arcidz1168135]

- ***Walls of renal calyces & pelvis contain specialized smooth muscle with inherent pacemaker activity***Q. Urine flowing from collecting duct into renal calyces stretches it and increases their inherent pacemaker activity which inturn ***initiates peristaltic contractions***Q that spread to renal pelvis & then downwards along the length of ureter.
- Walls of ureter contain smooth muscle and are innervated by both parasympathetic and sympathetic nerves as well as by intramural plexus of neurons. As with other smooth muscles, ***peristaltic contractions in ureter are enhanced by parasympathetic stimulation & inhibited by sympathetic stimulation***Q

63. **A i.e. Collecting duct***[Ref: Ganong 22/e P-716]*

Osmolality of urine depends on the action of vasopressin on the collecting ductsQ**.**

64. **A i.e. ECF Volume Contraction** *[Ref: Guyton 10/e P 315]*

- The kidney has the ability to form urine that is more concentrated than the plasma. **When there is contraction of ECF volume, the urinary concentrating ability of kidney increases and it forms a concentrated urine with a smaller volume, thereby maintaining homeostasis**Q**.**
- Reduction in medullary hyperosmolarity leads to loss of oncotic pressure gradient which is essential to produce concentrated urine
- Increase in RBF and ↑ GFR indicate an adequately filed vascular system and hence likely to decrease ADH secretion. therefore decreases kidney's concentrating ability.

Prerequisite for excreting a concentrated urine

1. **High level of ADH:** ADH increases permeability of distal tubules & CT to water thus allowing these segments to absorb water.
2. **High osmolarity of renal medullary interstitial fluid:** Provides the osmotic gradient necessary for water reabsorption to occur

Mechanism

ECF volume contraction / water deficit
↑ Plasma osmolality
↑ Secretion of ADH from post pituitary
↑ Permeability of late distal tubule & CD
↑ Reabsorption of water from tubular lumen
↓
Passage of concentrated urine

65. **D i.e. Glucose**
66. **B i.e. Urea** *[Ref: Ganong 24/ep 688]*

In kidney, glucose & bicarbonate (HCO_3-) are completely (100%) reabsorbedQ > **Water & Na^+** (99.4%)> **K^+** (99.3%)> **CI-** (99.2%)> Uric acid (98%)>>> **urea (58%)**Q.

Urine

67. **B i.e. 500ml** *[Ref: Chaudhuri 5/e P- 420; Harrison 16/e P- 259; Ganong 22/e p. 707, 726-727]*
68. **A i.e. 100 mg**
69. **A i.e., 100 – 200 ml of urine**
70. **B i.e. When about 300-400 ml of urine is collected in bladder**
71. **A i.e., Bladder emptying cannot occur if volume is <100 ml**

- The minimum volume necessary to remove all waste products, with a normal diet, is **500ml /day**[Q] and is called obligatory volume. **Oliguria**[Q] is urinary output less than **500ml**[Q] in 24 hrs.
- The amount of protein in urine is normally **less than 100mg/ day**[Q]. Most of this is not filtered and comes from shed tubular cells.
- **First urge to void** is felt at a bladder volume of ~ **150 ml**[Q], and a marked sense of fullness at about **400 ml**[Q]. In adult the volume of urine that normally initiates a reflex contraction is about **300- 400 ml**[Q].

Water and Acid Base Balance

72. **C i.e. 200 – 300 ml** *[Ref: Guyton 12/e p. 355]*

Same amount of solute can be excreted **per 24 hour in urine volume of 500 ml** (with concentration of **1400 mOsm/kg**) **or in 23.3 lit volume (with concentration of 30 mOsm/kg)**[Q].

Daily intake and output of water (ml/day)

Intake

Intake	Normal	Prolonged Heavy Exercise
Fluid ingested From metabolism	2100 200	- 200
Total intake	2300	-

Output

Output	Normal	Prolonged Heavy Exercise
Insensible – skin	**350**[Q]	**350**[Q]
Insensible – Lungs	350	650
Sweat	**100**[Q]	5000
Feces	100	100
Urine	1400	500
Total output	2300	6600

73. **A, C i.e. ↑Urine Na^+, ↑Urine osmolality** *[Ref: Harrison's 18th/2908-10; Berne & Levy 6/e p 598; Best & Taylor 13/e p 850-53; Williams Endocrinology 12/e p 1698; Guyton 11/e p. 357- 60]*
74. **A i.e. Regulated by ADH**

- **Concentration and dilution of urine i.e. free water and osmolar clearances are regulated by antidiuretic hormone (ADH) or vasopressin**[Q].
- **SIADH** is characterized by relatively **excessive ADH levels, euvolemia, hypoosmolality (decreased osmolality)** of **serum, hyponatremia (↓serum Na^+), inappropriately high urine osmolality and elevated urinary Na^+ excretion**[Q].

75. **B i.e. Decreased Potassium excretion** *[Ref: Ganong 22/e P- 8, 720; Harrison 16/e P- 258]*
76. **D i.e. Acidosis leads to movement of potassium from extracellular to intracellular fluid compartment.**

98% potassium (K^+) is intracellular & about 3/4 th of total body K^+ lies in skeletal muscles[Q]**. Severe injury and metabolic acidosis cause hyperkalemia ie l/t movement of K^+ from intra to extracellular space** [Q]**.**

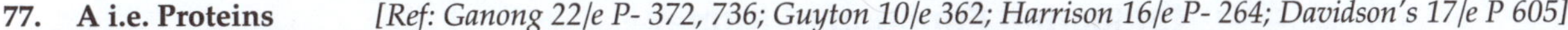

77. **A i.e. Proteins** *[Ref: Ganong 22/e P- 372, 736; Guyton 10/e 362; Harrison 16/e P- 264; Davidson's 17/e P 605]*
78. **B i.e. Uretersigmoidostomy**
79. **C i.e. Lactic acidosis; D i.e. DKA, E i.e. cardiac failure**
80. **A i.e. Diarrhoea**
81. **B i.e. Lactic acidosis**
82. **A i.e. Bicarbone; B i.e. Plasma Proteins; D i.e. Hemoglobin**

- **Anion gap is mostly due to proteins**[Q]**. Normal anion gap metabolic acidosis** is seen in **diarrhea, uretero sigmoidostomy and renal tubular acidosis**[Q]. High anion gap metabolic acidosis is seen in **lactic acidosis (d/t cardiac failures shock, acute respiratory failure) and diabetic ketoacidosis**[Q]**.**
- **Buffers in blood** include **bicarbonates, plasma proteins and hemoglobin**[Q]**.**

Anion Gap (AG)

- The concentration of anions and cations in plasma must be equal to maintain electrical neutrality. However, only certain cations (Na^+) and anions (Cl^-, HCO_3^-) are routinely measured in clinical laboratory. Anion gap (AG) represents the unmeasured anions in the plasma (difference between 'unmeasured cations & unmeasured anions'). It is *calculated*[Q] as follows:
  $AG = [Na^+] - [HCO_3^- + Cl^-]$
- The most important unmeasured cations: Ca^{2+}, Mg^{2+}, K^+. **The most important unmeasured anions: Proteins** (Albumin), sulphate, phosphates. **Proteins are present in our body in much more quantities** as compared to other unmeasured anions.
- Represents ***unmeasured anions in plasma***[Q]. AG is mostly due to ***proteins***[Q]. Normal AG is ***10 –12 mmol /L***[Q]***. Decrease in serum albumin by 1g/dl decreases AG by 2.5meq/L***[Q].

Metabolic Acidosis (MA)

High – Anion Gap MA	Non – Anion Gap MA
1) **Lactic acidosis**[Q] - Shock - **Cardiac failure**[Q] - Acute Respiratory failure - Metformin therapy 2) **Ketoacidosis**[Q] - **Diabetic**[Q] - **Alcoholic**[Q] - **Starvation**[Q] 3) Ingested toxins - **Ethylene glycol (antifreeze)**[Q] - **Methanol**[Q] - **Salicylates**[Q] 4) **Renal failure**[Q] (acute & chronic)	1) **Gastrointestinal bicarbonate loss** - **Diarrhoea**[Q] - **External pancreatic drainage**[Q] - **Ureterosigmoidostomy**[Q] - Drugs : Mg SO_4 $CaCl_2$ Cholestyramine 2) **Renal tubular acidosis**[Q] 3) **Ingestion of Ammonium chloride**[Q] 4) Carbonic anhydrase inhibitor

83. **D i.e. Siggard – Anderson normogram** *[Ref: Ganong 24/e P- 717-18]*

Siggard Anderson Curve Nomogram is used to determine **acid- base composition of blood (pH,** plotted on horizontal axis) **on the basis of P_{CO_2}**[Q] (plotted on vertical axis).

84. **B i.e. 306 mOsm/kg** *[Ref: Ganong 22/e P- 6]*

Osmolality (mOsm/kg) = 2[Na+ in mEq/l] + 0.055 [Glucose in mg/dl]+ 0.36 [BUN in mg/dl]

$$\textbf{Osmolality} = 2 \times [Na^+] + \frac{[Glucose]}{18} + \frac{[BUN]}{2.8}$$

Putting the values (of question) in equation

$$\text{Osmolality} = 2 \times 125 + \frac{108}{18} + \frac{140}{2.8} = 306 \text{ mOsm/kg}$$

Endocrine Function of Kidney

85. **C i.e. Interstitial cells**

86. **A i.e. ↓ Tissue PO_2**

87. **Di.e. Adrenocortical tumour concentration** *[Ref: Ganong 24/e P- 709; Harrison 16/e P- 627]*

The only physiological stimulus for erythropoietin secretion is **hypoxia or decreased partial pressure of oxygen**[Q]. Tumors producing erythropoietin include **RCC_A, hepatoma and cerebellar hemangioblastoma**[Q].

Erythropoietin

Structure & Sources

- It is a ***glycoprotein***Q (165aa + 4 Oligosacchride chains)
- Most important source in *adult* ***is Kidney***Q. Most important source in *fetal/ neonatal* life ***is Liver***Q.
- Erythropoietin increases the number of erythropoietin – sensitive committed stem cells in bone marrow that are converted to RBC. In the absence of erythropoietin, Erythroid ***stem cells show apoptosis***Q
- Erythropoietin is **mostly inactivated in liver**Q after circulation $t^1/_2$ of **5 hours**. However, RBC count increases after 2-3 days, as it is a slow process.

Stimuli for Secretion

- **Hypoxia**Q
- Cobalt salts / Androgen
- Alkalosis of **high altitude**Q
- Catecholamines
- Adenosine

Erythropoietin Production

Tumors producing erythropoietin	Normal source
- **Renal cell carcinoma**Q (3% of cases) - **Hepatoma**Q (10%) - **Cerebellar haemangioblastoma**Q (15%)	- **85% by interstitial cells in peritubular capillary bed of kidney**Q - **15% by perivenous hepatycytes of liver**Q

- Erythropoietin can also be extracted from **salivary gland & spleen** (but do not contain mRNA so do not produce it)
- It is also produced in **brain, uterus & oviduct**. But in cases of renal failure, all other tissues cannot compensate and anemia develops.

88. A, B, C, D, E i.e. Constriction of afferent arteriole, Autoregulation of GFR, Secreted from endothelial, Release aldosterone, Increased sodium and water reabsorption 89. A i.e. It helps to convert angiotensinogen to angiotensin I

90. B & D i.e. ACE splits Leucine- valine bond & PRA is better than PRC

91. A i.e. Angiotensin I 92. A & E i.e. Renin – liver & Angiotensinogen – Renal

[Ref: Ganong 23/e p. 670; Guyton 11/e 201-2, 223-24, 907; Robbins 7/e p 527; Harrison 16/e P-627]

- **Renin** an acid protease which **converts angiotensinogen to angiotensin I**Q, is secreted from **distal convoluted tubules of kidney**Q. **Increased GFR reduces rennin secretion**Q.
- **Angiotensin II** is formed from physiologically inactive angiotensin I by **ACE** (angiotensin converting enzyme) present in **endothelium of lung capillaries**Q. **It increases aldosterone secretion**Q from zona glomerulosa **resulting in increased sodium & water reabsorption**Q. It is a potent vaso (especially) **arteriolar constrictor**Q resulting in rise in BP & total peripheral resistance. In kidney angiotensin II causes renal **vaso** (afferent **arteriolar) constriction**Q, **contraction of mesanglial cells with resultant decrease in GFR**Q. **It is dipsogenic (i.e. increases thirst), increases secretion of vasopressin (ADH) and ACTH and decreases rennin secretion.**

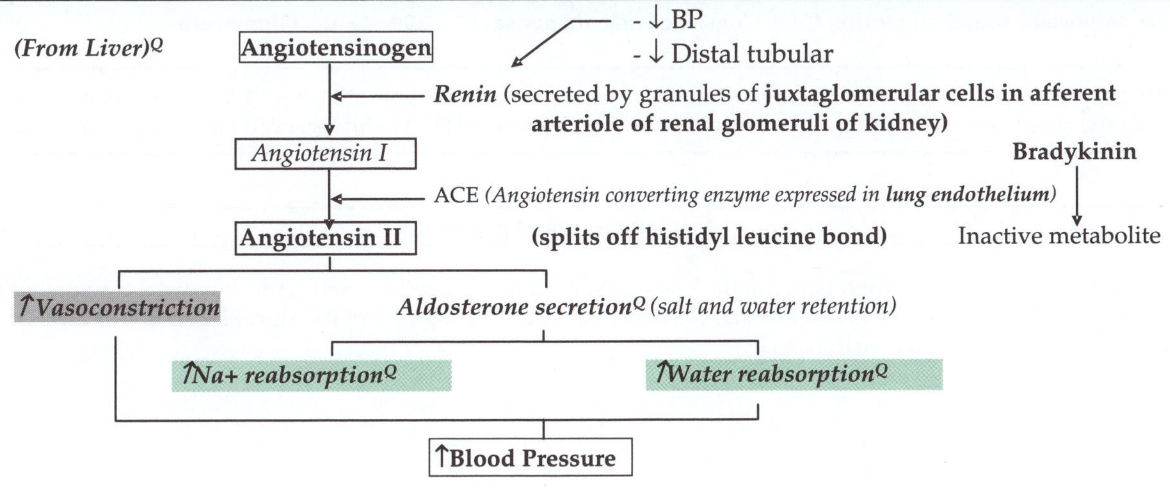

<u>**Renin – Angiotensin System**</u>

93. C i.e. Vasodilatation *[Ref: Ganong 23rd/e p. 669- 73; Board Review series, physiology 4/ed pg- 92- 93]*

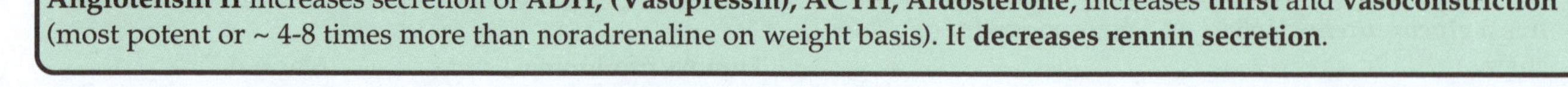

Angiotensin II increases secretion of **ADH, (Vasopressin), ACTH, Aldosterone**, increases **thirst** and **vasoconstriction** (most potent or ~ 4-8 times more than noradrenaline on weight basis). It **decreases rennin secretion.**

94. D i.e. Increased sympathetic tone > C i.e. Decreased blood pressure **95. C i.e. Decreased amount of Na^+ in PCT**

96. D i.e. Juxta glomerular apparatus *[Ref: Ganong 24/e P-706]*

***Renin is secreted by JG cells of Juxta glomerular (JG) apparatus*[Q]. Renin secretion is increased by renal ischemia, narrowing (or low pressure) in afferent arterioles & increased sympathetic activity whereas its decreased by increased Na^+ & Cl^- reabsorption across macula densa[Q].**

Factors Affecting Renin Secretion

Renin secretion depends upon the rate of transport of Na^+ and Cl^- across the *macula densa. Macula densa is a part of DCT*. Decreased delivery of Na^+ & Cl^- to distal tubule is associated with increased rennin secretion (inversely proportional).

Stimulatory

- ↑ed **sympathetic activity** via renal nerves
- ↑ed circulating **catecholamines**
- ***Prostaglandins*[Q]**
- Other conditions increasing secretions
  - **↓ Central venous pressure (↓CVP)**
    - Na^+ depletion in DCT, diuretics
    - Hemorrhage, upright posture, dehydration , **hypotension**[Q], CHF, cirrhosis
  - **↓ Renal arteriolar pressure**
    - Constriction of renal artery and aorta
  - **↑ Activity of renal nerves**
    - Psychological stimuli

Inhibitory

- ↑ed **afferent arteriolar pressure**
- ↑ed **Na^+ & Cl^- reabsorption at macula densa**
- ***Angiotensin II*[Q]**
- ***Vasopressin*[Q]**
- Prostaglandin inhibitors such as indomethacin &- B- blockers eg propranolol
- **Pepstatin** peptide & **Enalkiren** prevent rennin from generating angiotensin I.

97. B i.e. DCT **98. A i.e. JGA** *[Ref: Ganong 23rd/e p. 674; Guyton & Hall 11/e p.324-25, 10/e p.293]*

99. B i.e. Important source of rennin; C i.e. Consist of macula densa **100. D i.e. Glomerulus**

Juxta means next to or near. And so is the situation of juxta glomerular apparatus, which *lies at hilum of glomerulus*[Q]. **JG apparatus consists of JG cells, macula densa (located in relation to DCT) and lacis cells.** It is important *source of renin*[Q].

Juxtaglomerular Apparatus

Its a microscopic structure found between the vascular pole of renal corpuscle and returning distal convoluted tubule of same nephron. It *regulates renal blood flow and glomerular filtration rate* because of its critical location – ***at hilium of glomerulus*[Q]**. JG apparatus consists of

Juxta glomerular (JG) cells

- Are epitheliod cells located in the *media of afferent arterioles as they enter glomeruti*[Q].
- Also known as **granular cells**. They *secrete renin*[Q].
- **Intra renal baroreceptor mechanism** decrease renin secretion when arteriolar pressure at JG cells increase and vice versa
- Low pressure on JG cells stimulate renin secretion, which inturn increase BP and maintain GFR via *renin angiotensin system*

Macula densa

- It is ***modified region of distal convoluted tubular (DCT) epithelium at the point where afferent arteriole enters glomerulus and efferent arteriole leaves it***[Q]. This location marks the start of DCT
- ***Macula densa senses sodium chloride concentration***[Q]. Renin secretion is inversely proportional to the amount of Na^+ & Cl^- entering DCT from loop of henle, where Macula cells are located. These electrolytes enter macula cells via Na^+ - K^+ - $2Cl^-$ cotransporter. Possibly NO mediates signal b/w macula densa & JG cells for renin secretion.

Lacis cells

- Also k/a **extraglomerular mesengial cells**
- They are ***agranular cells,*** strategically located between macula densa and JG cells ***at junction between afferent and efferent arterioles***[Q]. And so it may mediate signals b/w them
- They also contain renin
- Contain ***actin & myosin,*** allowing them to contract & modulate action of JG apparatus when ***stimulated by renal sympathetic nerves***

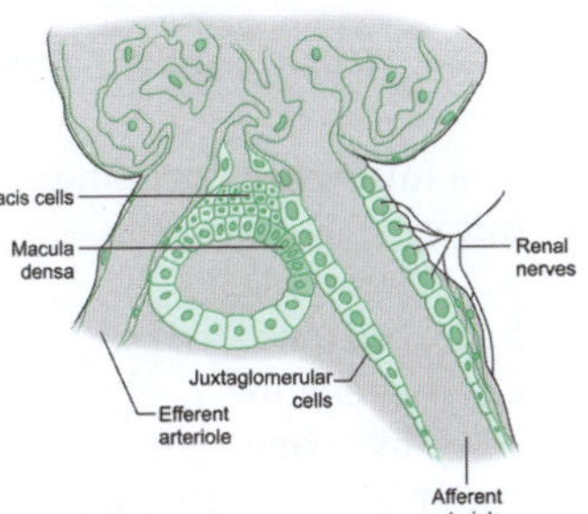

101. A i.e. Water transport across collecting duct *[Ref: Ganong 22/e P- 716 244; Guyton 10/e P 302]*

Vasopressin acts ***by increasing permeability of collecting ducts***[Q]. to water. The key to the action of vasopressin on collecting duct is ***aquaporin –2***. The overall effect is *retention of water* in excess of solute which results in *decrease effective osmotic pressure.*

102. A i.e. Erythropoietin *[Ref: Ganong 22/e P-188; Harper 26/e P-609, 620]*

Erythropoietin is a plasma protein that act as a *hormone*. Its a ***major regulator of human erythropoiesis***[Q].

Ceruloplasmin ***transport copper***[Q]. Transferrin transports ***iron***[Q]. Lactoferrin ***binds iron***[Q].

Chapter -7 ENDOCRINE SYSTEM

QUESTIONS

Receptors & Second Messengers

1. **The following hormone does not have any intracellular receptor:** *(AI 01)*
   A. Vitamin D3 ☐
   B. Cortisone ☐
   C. Adrenaline ☐
   D. Thyroxine ☐
2. **Among the following all are hydrophilic hormones that act on cytosolic receptors except one which is a lipophilic hormone that acts on nuclear receptor:**
   A. Thyroxine *(AIIMS 11,14,13)* ☐
   B. Epinephrine/Adrenaline ☐
   C. GH ☐
   D. ACTH ☐
3. **Intracellular receptors are found in A/E:** *(PGI 06,15)*
   A. Insulin & Glucagon ☐
   B. Corticosteriods ☐
   C. Androgen ☐
   D. Thyroxine ☐
4. **Which hormone acts on cytoplasmic membrane receptor-** *(NBE P 13)*
   A. TSH ☐
   B. Thyroxine ☐
   C. Androgen ☐
   D. Cortisol ☐
5. **cGMP is second messenger for which hormone(s):**
   A. Somatostatin *(AIIMS 14, 13; PGI 09, 15)* ☐
   B. Atrial natriuretic factor (ANF) & NO ☐
   C. Angiotensin II ☐
   D. Antidiuretic hormone (ADH), Insulin, GH ☐
6. **cAMP action mediates all except-** *(NBE P 13)*
   A. Glucagon ☐
   B. Follicle stimulating hormone ☐
   C. Leutinizing hormone ☐
   D. Estrogen ☐
7. **Steroid receptor super family is present in:**
   A. Vitamin D_3 *(PGI 12,06)* ☐
   B. Insulin ☐
   C. Glucagon ☐
   D. Thyroid ☐
8. **All are second messengers except;**
   A. Guanylyl cyclase *(AIIMS 12; PGI 13)* ☐
   B. c AMP/CGMP ☐
   C. IP3 ☐
   D. DAG ☐
9. **Regarding nitric oxide false is** *(AIIMS 07)*
   A. Derived from endothelium ☐
   B. Acts by increasing c-AMP levels ☐
   C. Vasodilator ☐
   D. Derived from arginine ☐
10. **True about intracellular receptors:** *(PGI 05)*
    A. Mainly on nuclear surface ☐
    B. Steroids act on them ☐
    C. Estrogen does not act on it ☐
    D. GH act on it ☐
11. **Hormone synthesized as peptide precursor is/are:**
    A. Insulin *(PGI 09)* ☐
    B. PTH ☐
    C. Renin ☐
    D. Thyroid hormone ☐
    E. Angiotensin II ☐
12. **All the following mediate their action using cAMP as second messenger except:** *(AIIMS 09)*
    A. Corticotropin ☐
    B. Dopamine ☐
    C. Glucagon ☐
    D. Vasopressin ☐
13. **Which of the following is a membrane bound enzyme that catalyzes the formation of cyclic AMP from ATP?**
    A. Tyrosine Kinase *(NBE P 15, 13; AI 10)* ☐
    B. Polymerase ☐
    C. ATP synthase ☐
    D. Adenylate cyclase ☐
14. **Following modification occurs in Gs subunit which leads to watery diarrhea in cholera** *(AIIMS 11)*
    A. ADP ribosylation ☐
    B. ATP-ADP transfer ☐
    C. Phosphorylation ☐
    D. Dephosphorylation ☐
15. **Cholera toxin:** *(AIIMS 06)*
    A. Increases the levels of intracellular cyclic GMP ☐
    B. Acts through the receptor for opiates ☐
    C. Causes continued activation of adenylate cyclase ☐
    D. Inhibits the enzyme phosphodiesterase ☐
16. **CAMP acts through:** *(PGI 06)*
    A. Activation of protein kinase ☐
    B. Activation of adenylate cyclase ☐
    C. ↑ Ca^{2+} release. ☐
    D. PIP3 pathway ☐
17. **Which one of the following acts as second messenger?**
    A. Mg^{++} *(AIIMS 06)* ☐
    B. Cl^- ☐
    C. Ca^{++} ☐
    D. PO_4^{3-} ☐
18. **Which set of hormones have nuclear receptor:**
    A. Estrogen, Thyroxin & Glucagon *(PGI 08)* ☐
    B. Estrogen, Thyroxin & TSH ☐
    C. Estrogen, TSH & Gonadotropin releasing hormone (GnRH) ☐
    D. Retinoic acid, Thyroxin & Luteinizing hormone (LH) ☐
    E. Testosterone, cortisol & Estogen ☐

19. All of the following bind to the steroid receptors except: *(AIIMS 08)*
A. Steroids ☐
B. Transcriptional mediators ☐
C. Transcriptional receptors ☐
D. Steroid response elements ☐

20. C terminal end of androgen receptor is concerned with: *(AI 07)*
A. Ligand binding ☐
B. Increasing biological half life ☐
C. Increasing the affinity of receptor to DNA ☐
D. Increasing the level of transcription ☐

21. Aldosterone receptors are present in all except:
A. Liver *(AIIMS 07)* ☐
B. Colon ☐
C. Hippocampus ☐
D. Distal nephron ☐

22. True about membrane receptors: *(PGI 2K)*
A. Barrier function ☐
B. For specific action ☐
C. Molecular transport ☐
D. None ☐

23. Receptors on cell membrane that activate ion channel after binding with agonists are
A. Nicotonic Cholinergic *(PGI 03)* ☐
B. Muscarinic Cholinergic ☐
C. Optoid μ receptors ☐
D. $GABA_A$ ☐
E. $GABA_B$ ☐

24. Action of α - subunit of G protein is: *(AIIMS 08)*
A. Breakdown of GTP to GDP ☐
B. Conversion of GDP to GTP ☐
C. Internalization of receptors ☐
D. Binding of agonist ☐

25. Following are true about G protein except: *(PGI 08)*
A. G channels ☐
B. Phosphorylase formation ☐
C. Made up of 4 units ☐
D. Related to ras oncogene ☐

26. True about G-protein receptor complex:
A. It interacts transmembrane domain.
B. GTP to GDP *(PGI 08)* ☐
C. Adenyl cyclase activation leads to increased cAMP ☐
D. GPCR has no phospharylation property ☐
E. Helical structure ☐

27. True statement about the G-protein coupled receptor is:
A. It binds to ligands at the cell surface *(AIIMS 08)* ☐
B. Association of all the three subunits (alpha, beta and gamma) is essential for its action ☐
C. G-protein acts as inhibitory and excitatory as alpha subunit exists in two forms ☐
D. GTP binds to G protein in resting state ☐

28. If there is a Gs alfa subunit gain-of-function mutation, this results in: *(AI 11)*
A. Decreased cAMP ☐
B. Decreased IP3 ☐
C. Increased GTPase activity ☐
D. Increased cAMP ☐

29. Adrenaline, noradrenaline and dopamine act through *(AIIMS 11, 06)*
A. Single pass receptors ☐
B. Four pass receptors ☐
C. Seven pass receptor ☐
D. Ligand gated channel ☐

30. True about Second messenger: *(PGI 11)*
A. Bind first messenger ☐
B. Integral protein ☐
C. Hormone secreted by stimulation of other hormones ☐
D. Substance that increase or decrease function ☐
E. Intracellular receptor ☐

31. Various cells respond differentially to a second messenger (such as increased cAMP) because they have different.
A. Receptors *(AIIMS 03)* ☐
B. Enzymatic composition ☐
C. Nuclei ☐
D. Membrane lipid ☐

32. ANF is mediated by (ANF: Atrial natriuretic factor):
A. Inositol phosphate *(AIIMS 07)* ☐
B. DAG ☐
C. CyAMP ☐
D. CyGMP ☐

33. Which of the following act through tyrosine kinase receptor: *(PGI 01)*
A. Insulin ☐
B. Glucagons ☐
C. GH ☐
D. FSH ☐

34. cAMP action mediates all except: *(PGI 2K)*
A. Glucagon ☐
B. FSH ☐
C. LH ☐
D. Estrogen ☐

35. CyAMP acts as a second messenger of:
A. FSH *(AIIMS 05)* ☐
B. Thyroxine ☐
C. Growth hormone ☐
D. Insulin ☐

36. Cyclic GMP is the second messenger of:
A. Growth Hormone *(AIIMS 04)* ☐
B. Follicle Stimulating Hormone (FSH) ☐
C. Insulin ☐
D. Thyroxin ☐

37. Which one of the following molecules is used for cell signaling? *(AI 05)*
A. CO_2. ☐
B. O_2. ☐
C. NO. ☐
D. N_2. ☐

38. All are second messengers except: *(AIIMS 08)*
A. Guanylyl cyclase ☐

B. cAMP ☐
C. IP3 ☐
D. DAG ☐

39. Which of the following function as second messengers: *(PGI 05)*
A. CAMP ☐
B. DAG ☐
C. IP3 ☐
D. Ca^{2+} ☐
E. Mg^{2+} ☐

40. Second messengers is/are: *(PGI 12)*
A. Mg^{+2} ☐
B. PO_4^{3-} ☐
C. cAMP ☐
D. Ca^{2+} ☐
E. Cl^- ion ☐

Calcium Metabolism & Parathyroid Gland

41. A small Ca^{+2} binding protein that modifies the activity of many enzymes and other proteins in response to changes of Ca^{2+} concentration, is known as: *(AI 04)*
A. Cycline ☐
B. Calmodulin ☐
C. Collagen ☐
D. Kinesin ☐

42. Parathyroid hormone is responsible for all actions except: *(PGI 07)*
A. Absorption of phosphorous increase ☐
B. Vit D absorption increases ☐
C. Mobilizes calcium from bone ☐
D. Increase intestinal absorption of calcium ☐

43. Calcium absorption is from: *(PGI 09)*
A. Proximal small intestine ☐
B. Distal ileum ☐
C. Middle small intestine ☐
D. Ascending colon ☐

44. Calcium absorptionis increased by- *(NBE P 13)*
A. Proteins ☐
B. Bile ☐
C. Acid ☐
D. Phosphates ☐

45. True of the following: *(PGI 01)*
A. Calcium reabsorbed in DCT ☐
B. 90% calcium excreted by glomerulus ☐
C. Parathormone (PTH) promotes absorption of Ca^{++} from intestine ☐
D. PTH promote action of calcitonin ☐

46. Which of the following is considered the active form of calcium: *(AI 08)*
A. Ionised Calcium ☐
B. Albumin bound Calcium ☐
C. Phosphate bound Calcium ☐
D. Protein bound Calcium ☐

47. Calcium absorption from gut is increased by all except: *(AIIMS 16)*
A. Phytates ☐
B. Vitamin D ☐
C. Alkaline pH in gut ☐
D. Protein in diet ☐

48. True statement about calcium : *(PGI 04; 15,13)*
A. Absorbed in upper small intestine ☐
B. Absorbed in lower small intestine ☐
C. Absorption increased by alkaline pH ☐
D. Absorption increased by acidic pH ☐

49. Calcium sensing receptors is/are present at: *(PGI 13,14)*
A. PCT ☐
B. DCT ☐
C. Loop of Henle ☐
D. Apical brush-border membrane of the intestinal enterocyte ☐
E. Epithelium of intestine ☐

50. Which of the following would you expect to find in a patient whose diet has been low in calcium for 8 weeks?
A. Increased phosphate levels *(AIIMS 07)* ☐
B. Raised calcitonin levels ☐
C. Increased parathormone secretion ☐
D. Activation of 24-25 dihydrocholecalciferol ☐

51. True about Parathyroid hormone: *(PGI 12)*
A. It is steroidal in nature ☐
B. Stimulate 1, 25 D3 formation ☐
C. Inhibits Ca^{2+} absorption from the intestines ☐
D. Increases the resorption of bone ☐

52. Secondary hyperparathyroidism due to Vit D deficiency shows: *(AI 01)*
A. Hypocalcemia ☐
B. Hypercalcemia ☐
C. Hypophosphatemia ☐
D. Hyperphosphatemia ☐

53. Which hormone regulate (s) serum calcium level:
A. PTH *(PGI 13)* ☐
B. Calcitonin ☐
C. Adrenaline ☐
D. 1, 25-Dihydroxy-cholecalciferol ☐
E. Procalcitonin ☐

54. Which of these can cause hypocalcemia:
A. Thyroxine *(AIIMS 02)* ☐
B. Calcitonin ☐
C. Parathyroid hormone ☐
D. Choloecalciferol ☐

55. Hypocalcemia due to calcitonin is by: *(PGI 09)*
A. Increased excretion in kidney ☐
B. Decreased bone resorption ☐
C. Decreased intestinal absorption ☐
D. Decreased renal reabsorption ☐

56. Osteoclasts are inhibited by action on specific receptor:
A. Parathyroid hormone. *(AIIMS 03, AI 05)* ☐
B. Calcitonin. ☐
C. 1,25-dihydroxycholecalciferol. ☐
D. Tumor necrosis factor. ☐

57. Sudden decrease in serum calcium is associated with: (AI 02)
A. Increased thyroxine and PTH secretion
B. Increased phosphate
C. Increased excitability of muscle and nerve
D. Cardiac conduction abnormalities

58. In tetany hyperexcitability is due to (PGI 04)
A. Low Ca^{++} causes ↑ permeability to Na+
B. Prevent K^+ release
C. Prevent Na^+ & K^+ release
D. ↓Ca^{++} produce generation of AP

59. Hypocalcemia is characterized by all except:
A. Numbness and tingling of circumoral region
B. Hyperactive tendon reflexes and positive Chvostek's sign. (AIIMS 03)
C. Shortening of Q-T interval in ECG.
D. Carpopedal spasm

60. Which of the following organ is not involved in calcium metabolism: (PGI 01, 10)
A. Lung
B. Liver
C. Spleen
D. Skin
E. Kidney

61. Which of the following organs is not involved in calcium homeostasis? (AI 06)
A. Kidneys
B. Skin
C. Intestines
D. Lungs

62. All are true about Vitamin D except: (AIIMS 08)
A. 25-hydroxylation occurs in the liver(NBE P 15,13)
B. 1-α hydroxylation occurs in the kidneys
C. In the absence of sunlight, the minimum daily requirement is 400-600 IU
D. William's syndrome consists of mental retardation, obesity and precocious puberty

63. Increased calcium levels lead to- (NBE P 13)
A. Increased 1,25 dihydroxycholecalciferol
B. Increased 24,25 dihydroxycholecalciferol
C. Decreased calcitonin
D. Increased parathormone

64. Active form of vitamin D is: (AIIMS 07)
A. Cholecalciferol
B. 24, 25 (OH)2 vit-D
C. 1,25(OH)2 vit-D
D. 25-OH vit – D

65. Function of Phospholamban is : (AIIMS 2K)
A. Regulates Na K Pump
B. Transports calcium out of the mitrochondria
C. Binds actin with myosin
D. Collects calcium into the sarcoplasmic reticulum

66. Hypercalcemia associated with malignancy is most often mediated by: (AI 05)
A. Parathyroid hormone (PTH).
B. Parathyroid hormone related protein (PTHrP)
C. Interleukin – 6 (IL-6).
D. Calcitonin.

67. Which of the following hormones is an example of a peptide hormone? (AIIMS 05)
A. Parathormone
B. Adrenaline
C. Cortisol
D. Thyroxine

68. Regarding transport of Ca++ across a membrane following are true: (PGI 03)
A. Ca^{++} calmodulin binding
B. It is a passive mechanism
C. Required hydrolysis of A.T.P.
D. It is a symport
E. It is an active process

69. Which one one of the following acts to increase the release of Ca^{2+} from endoplasmic reticulum:
A. Inositol triphosphate (AIIMS 04, AI 05)
B. ↓Parathyroid hormone
C. 1, 25-dihydroxy cholecalciferol
D. Diacyglycerol

Carbohydrate Metabolism & Pancreatic Hormone

70. ALL are true regarding pancreas except (AI 12, AIIMS 07,15,14,13; PGI 11, 10, 08)
A. Delta (D) cells secrete somatostatin
B. Insulin & amylin are secreted by beta (B) cells whereas glucagon is secreted by alpha (A) cells.
C. Pancreatic polypeptide hormone is secreted by F (PP) cells.
D. PP is secreted by D1 cells.

71. The mechanism that protects normal pancreas from autodigestion is : (AIIMS 03)
A. Secretion of biocarbonate.
B. Protease inhibitors present in plasma.
C. Proteolytic enzymes secreted in inactive form
D. The resistance of pancreatic cells.

72. All of the following enzymes are active within a cell except
A. Trypsin (AIIMS 05)
B. Fumerase
C. Hexokinase
D. Alcohol dehydrogenase

73. All are true about exocrine functions of pancreas EXCEPT: (AIIMS 07)
A. Osmolality is ½ of the osmolality of blood
B. Secretes 1½ litre of the alkaline fluid daily
C. Secretin enhances bicarbonate secretion
D. Secretion is rich in enzymes.

74. After 5 days of fasting a man undergoes oral GTT, true is all except : (AI 01)
A. GH levels are increased
B. Increased glucose tolerance
C. Decreased insulin levels
D. Glucagon levels are increased

75. A/E the following changes are seen on the 5th day of fasting:
A. Increase in FFA levels. (AIIMS 04)

B. Decreased glucose tolerance ☐
C. Decreased growth hormone ☐
D. Decreased level of Insulin ☐

76. Noble prize for sequencing insulin aminoacid sequence & molecular structure was given to:
A. Banting & Macleod *(AIIMS 11)* ☐
B. Sanger ☐
C. Charles Best ☐
D. Paul Berg ☐

77. Human insulin differs from beef insulin by how many number of amino acid residues: *(AI 05)*
A. 1 ☐
B. 2 ☐
C. 3 ☐
D. 4 ☐

78. Half life of insulin is- *(NBE P 13)*
A. 1-2min ☐
B. 4-6min ☐
C. 10-12min ☐
D. 12-16min ☐

79. Insulin is secreted along with the following molecule in a 1: 1 ratio: *(PGI 06)*
A. Pancreatic polypeptide ☐
B. Glucagon ☐
C. GLP-1 ☐
D. Somatostatin ☐
E. C- peptide ☐

80. Glucose mediated insulin release is mediated through: *(AI 02)*
A. ATP dependent K^+ channels ☐
B. cAMP ☐
C. Carrier modulators ☐
D. Receptor phosphorylation ☐

81. Insulin secretion is inhibited by: *(AI 10)*
A. Secretion ☐
B. Epinephrine ☐
C. Growth hormone ☐
D. Gastrin ☐

82. Insulin secretion is/are increased by all except:
A. Gastrin *(PGI 10)* ☐
B. Secretin ☐
C. VIP ☐
D. GIP ☐
E. CCK ☐

83. Insulin secretion is decreased by: *(PGI 03)*
A. Glucagon ☐
B. Glucose ☐
C. Adrenaline ☐
D. Vagal stimulation ☐

84. Rapid infusion of insulin causes *(AIIMS 10)*
A. Hyperkalemia ☐
B. Hypokalemia ☐
C. Hypernatremia ☐
D. Hyponatremia ☐

85. All of these cause hyperglycemia except:
A. GH *(PGI 02)* ☐
B. Cortisol ☐
C. Catecholamines ☐
D. Insulin ☐
E. Glucagons ☐

86. True about Insulin action is: *(PGI 2K)*
A. Causes neoglucogenesis . ☐
B. Not useful for growth & development ☐
C. Required for transport of glucose, aminoacid, K+ & Na^+ ☐
D. Catabolic hormone ☐

87. In fetus the insulin secretion begins by:
A. 3rd month *(AIIMS 05)* ☐
B. 5th month ☐
C. 7th month ☐
D. 9th month ☐

88. Increased ratio of insulin to glucagon causes:
A. Decreased levels of cyclic AMP *(AI 06)* ☐
B. Decreased levels of lipoprotein lipase ☐
C. Decreased amino acid synthesis ☐
D. Enhanced lipolysis in adipose tissue ☐

89. Insulin promotes lipogenesis by all of the following ways except: *(AIIMS 08)*
A. Decreasing intracellular cAMP ☐
B. Increasing the transport of glucose into the cell ☐
C. Inhibits pyruvate dehydrogenase ☐
D. Increases activity of acetyl-CoA carboxylase ☐

90. Insulin secretion seen in *(PGI 04)*
A. Glucose ☐
B. Vagal stimulation ☐
C. Acetylcholine ☐
D. Adrenaline ☐
E. Calmodulin ☐

91. Diet devoid of carbohydrates causes: *(PGI 04)*
A. Ketosis ☐
B. DM ☐
C. No effect ☐
D. Obesity ☐

92. A patient presents with hepatomegaly and hypoglycemia not responding to epinephrine. Most probable diagnosis is
A. Gaucher's disease *(AIIMS 10, PGI 10)* ☐
B. Von Gierke's disease ☐
C. Anderson's disease ☐
D. Pompes disease ☐

93. All are actions of insulin except OR insulin increases all except one which is decreased.:
A. Gluconeogenesis *(AI 2K, NBE P 15,13)* ☐
B. Glycolysis ☐
C. Glycogenesis ☐
D. Lipogenesis ☐

94. The hormone using an enzyme receptor for its action:
A. Insulin *(AI 2K)* ☐
B. Steroid ☐
C. Oestrogen ☐
D. Thyroxine ☐

95. Not done by insulin: *(AIIMS 10, 09)*
A. Glycogen synthesis ☐
B. Glycolysis ☐
C. Lipogenesis ☐
D. Ketogenesis ☐

96. **What is role of insulin in lipid metabolism:**
A. Active lipoprotein lipase *(PGI 08)* ☐
B. Increase lipolysis ☐
C. Activate hormone sensitive lipase ☐
D. Activate Acetyl CoA carboxylase ☐
E. Decrease free fatty acid level ☐

97. **Insulin increases the activities of all of the following enzymes, EXCEPT**: *(Jipmer 04, AI 05)*
A. Glucokinase ☐
B. Pyruvate carboxylase ☐
C. Glycogen synthase ☐
D. Acetyl-CoA carboxylase ☐

98. **GLUT2 is present mainly in-** *(NBE P 15,13)*
A. Beta cells of pancreas ☐
B. Placenta ☐
C. Skeletal muscle ☐
D. Cardiac muscle ☐

99. **Which of the following glucose transporter is/are used by brain:** *(AIIMS 15, 13PGI 12)*
A. GLUT1 & 3 ☐
B. GLUT 2 ☐
C. GLUT 4 ☐
D. GLUT 5 ☐

100. **Glucose transporter in myocyte?** *(AIIMS 14,12)*
A. GLUT 1 *(NBE P 15, 13)* ☐
B. GLUT 2 ☐
C. GLUT 3 ☐
D. GLUT 4 ☐

101. **Insulin mediated glucose uptake occurs through**
A. GLUT- 1 *(NBE P 15, 13; AIIMS 09)* ☐
B. GLUT -2 ☐
C. GLUT- 3 ☐
D. GLUT -4 ☐

102. **Insulin mediated glucose uptake is/are used in:**
A. Adipose tissue & Skeletal muscle *(PGI 12,15)* ☐
B. Kidney *(NBE P 15, 13)* ☐
C. Brain ☐
D. Intestine ☐

103. **Insulin does not facilitate glucose uptake in the following except** : *(AIIMS 14,08; NBE P 15, 13)*
A. Liver ☐
B. Heart ☐
C. RBC ☐
D. Kidney ☐

104. **Insulin acts on glucose metabolism by**: *(PGI 2K)*
A. ↑ permeability of glucose across cell membrane ☐
B. ↑ permeability across cell membrane against glucose gradient ☐
C. ↑ permeability of renal cells ☐
D. ↑ glucose transport to brain ☐

105. **Na dependent glucose transport is /are inhibited by:**
A. Oubain *(PGI 08)* ☐
B. Na azide ☐
C. Phlorhizine ☐
D. Phloretin ☐

106. **Sodium channels are specifically blocked by -**
A. Nifedipine *(AIIMS 05)* ☐
B. Tetradotoxin ☐
C. Tetra Ethyl lead ☐
D. Choline ☐

107. **Tetrodotoxin blocks** *(UP 2K)*
A. γNa^+ during action potential ☐
B. γK^+ during action potential ☐
C. γNa^+ during resting state ☐
D. γK^+ during resting state ☐

108. **To synthesize insulin on a large scale basis, the most suitable starting material obtained fro the beta cells of the pancreas is**: *(AIIMS 03, UP 04)*
A. Genomic DNA ☐
B. Total cellular RNA ☐
C. CDNA of insulin ☐
D. MRNA of insulin ☐

109. **Insulin resistance is seen in patients with liver disease due to:** *(AIIMS 13)*
A. Damaged hepatocytes ☐
B. Hepatic steatosis ☐
C. Impaired insulin release ☐
D. Low C peptide level ☐

110. **Ist response to hypoglycemia-** *(NBE P 13)*
A. Decreased insulin ☐
B. Increased glucagon ☐
C. Increased cortisol ☐
D. Increased nor epinephrine ☐

111. **In surgical stress all hormone is increased except:**
A. Adrenaline *(PGI 11)* ☐
B. ACTH ☐
C. Epinephrine ☐
D. Cortisol ☐
E. Insulin ☐

112. **Stress-induced hyperglycemia is due to**:
A. Glucocorticoids *(PGI 02)* ☐
B. GH ☐
C. Thyroxine ☐
D. Epinephrine ☐
E. Insulin ☐

113. **Which of the following hormones are increased due to stress during surgery, especially in DM**:
A. Epinephrine *(PGI 2K)* ☐
B. GH ☐
C. Glucocorticoids ☐
D. Thyroxine ☐

114. **Endogenous triglycerides are maximum in**:
A. VLDL *(DNB 06, AI 04)* ☐
B. Chylomicron ☐
C. LDL ☐
D. HDL ☐

Pineal Gland & Pituitary Gland

115. **Melatonin is secreted by**: *(AI 02)*
A. Hypothalamus ☐
B. Adrenal cortex ☐
C. Pineal gland ☐
D. Melanocytes ☐

116. Exposure to darkness leads to increased melatonin secretion. It is brought about by: *(AIIMS 03)*
- A. Decreasing the activity of suprachiasmatic nuclei ☐
- B. Increasing the serotonin N-acetyl transferase ☐
- C. Decreasing the hydroxy-indole-o-methyl transferase, activity ☐
- D. Blocking the release of norepinephrine from sympathetic nerve terminals ☐

117. Acidophils secrete- *(NBE P 13)*
- A. GH ☐
- B. TSH ☐
- C. ACTH ☐
- D. FSH ☐

118. Hypothalamus controls the hormone secretion of-
- A. Anterior hypophysis *(NBE P 13)* ☐
- B. Posterior hypophysis ☐
- C. Kidney ☐
- D. Pineal gland ☐

119. Hypothalamus increase release of all hormones from the pituitary except- *(NBE P 13)*
- A. TSH ☐
- B. FSH ☐
- C. CRH ☐
- D. Prolactin ☐

120. Basophilic cells of pituitary secretes A/E: *(PGI 02,15)*
- A. Prolactin & GH *(NBE P 15, 14)* ☐
- B. TSH ☐
- C. ACTH ☐
- D. LH ☐

121. Hormone secreted by anterior pituitary/ adenohypophysis are A/E: *(NBE P 15, 13, 14)*
- A. Oxytocin - Vasopressin *(AIIMS 15,13; PGI 03, 14)* ☐
- B. TSH, LH, FSH ☐
- C. Gonadotropns ☐
- D. ACTH ☐

122. Posterior pituitary secretes: *(NBE P 14; PGI 13)*
- A. Oxytocin & ADH ☐
- B. Prolactin ☐
- C. MSH ☐
- D. FSH ☐

123. Herring body is seen in- *(NBE P 13)*
- A. Pars intermedia ☐
- B. Pineal gland ☐
- C. Pars nervosa ☐
- D. Adenohypophysis ☐

124. ACTH level is highest during: *(PGI 13, 09)*
- A. Early morning ☐
- B. Evening ☐
- C. Afternoon ☐
- D. Night ☐

125. ACTH is increased in all except- *(NBE P 13)*
- A. Exercise ☐
- B. Emotions ☐
- C. Evening ☐
- D. Tumors ☐

126. Acromegaly is due to excess of: *(PGI 14)*
- A. Somatomedin ☐
- B. Growth hormone ☐
- C. Somatostatin ☐
- D. Insulin ☐

127. Somatomedin mediates: *(AIIMS 10, 09)*
- A. Deposition of chondroitin sulfate ☐
- B. Lipolysis ☐
- C. Gluconeogenesis ☐
- D. Decreased rate of glucose uptake by cells ☐

128. Growth hormone level decreased in- *(NBE P 13)*
- A. Hypoglycemia ☐
- B. Fasting ☐
- C. Sleep ☐
- D. Exercise ☐

129. Secretion of Prolactin is affected by: *(NBE P 15, AI 04)*
- A. GnRH analogue ☐
- B. Dopamine ☐
- C. Serotonin ☐
- D. FSH ☐

Posterior Pituitary Hormone

130. Pituicytes are seen in- *(NBE P 13)*
- A. Anterior lobe ☐
- B. Posterior lobe ☐
- C. Intermediate lobe ☐
- D. All ☐

131. True about milk secretion is A/E: *(NBE P 15,13; PGI 10)*
- A. Neuroendocrine part of post pituitary is involved ☐
- B. Secretion by contraction of lactiferous sinus ☐
- C. Oxytocin hormone cause ejection of milk ☐
- D. Prolactin cause contraction of Myoepithelial cells and not affected by emotion ☐

132. Which is wrongly matched pair about vasopressin receptor: *(AIIMS 10)*
- A. V1-Vascular smooth muscles ☐
- B. V2-collecting ducts ☐
- C. V3-anterior pituitary ☐
- D. V4-CNS ☐

133. When NaCl is injected in the internal carotid artery, it causes release of ADH by acting on: *(AIIMS 01)*
- A. Paramedian nucleus ☐
- B. Anterior pitutary ☐
- C. Paraoptic nucleus ☐
- D. Supraoptic nucleus ☐

134. Greatest stimulator for ADH secretion:
- A. Hyperosmolarity *(PGI 06)* ☐
- B. Hyponatremia ☐
- C. Hypotension ☐
- D. Hypovolemia ☐

135. All of the following are true for ADH except:
- A. Post-operative increase in secretion ☐
- B. Neurosecretion *(AIIMS 12)* ☐
- C. Increased secretion when plasma osmolality is low ☐
- D. Act on disal tubule and icrease permeability ☐

136. In which of the following form the Anti diuretic hormone (ADH) is circulated in plasma: *(AI 04)*
- A. Bound to neurophysin-I
- B. Bound to neurophysin-II
- C. Bound to plasma albumin
- D. Free form

137. A/E are caused by accidental transection of pituitary stalk: *(AIIMS 02)*
- A. Diabetes mellitus
- B. Polyuria
- C. Galactorrhea
- D. Diabetes insipidus

138. Which of the following is most important in sodium and water retention- *(NBE P 13)*
- A. Rennin angiotensin system
- B. ANP
- C. BNP
- D. Vasopressin

Thyroid Gland

139. In Thyroid follicle for how long Thyroxine is stored- *(NBE P 13)*
- A. 2-3 weeks
- B. 2-3 days
- C. 2-3 months
- D. 2-3 years

140. Thyroid hormones in blood is transported by: *(PGI 01)*
- A. Albumin
- B. Globulin
- C. Prealbumin
- D. Transferrin
- E. Ceruloplasmin

141. Regarding thyroid hormone all are true except: *(AI 2K)*
- A. T_3 is more avidly bound to nuclear receptors than T_4
- B. T_4 has the maximum plasma concentration
- C. T_3 is more active than T_4
- D. T_4 has shorter half life than T_3

142. Wolf chaifoff effect is due to- *(NBE P 13)*
- A. Suppression of TSH secretion
- B. Decreased iodination of MIT
- C. Decreased T_3 to T_4 conversion
- D. Iodine intake

143. Sodium iodine symporter is not present in: *(AIIMS 15)*
- A. Pituitary gland
- B. Placenta
- C. Parotid
- D. Thyroid

144. Iodine uptake is seen in following organs: *(PGI 03; NBE P 15,14)*
- A. Ovary
- B. Thyroid
- C. Parathyroid
- D. Salivary gland
- E. Mammary gland

145. Thyroxine injected to rat produces A/E: *(PGI 2K)*
- A. ↓↓ lipolysis
- B. ↑↑ O2 consumption
- C. ↓ BMR
- D. ↑ myocardial contractility

146. TRH stimulation testing is useful in diagnosis of disorders of following hormones : *(AI 02)*
- A. Insulin
- B. ACTH
- C. Growth hormone
- D. PTH

Kidney & Adrenal Gland

147. Which of the following hormone is not secreted by the kidney: *(AI 07; PGI 09,07,06)*
- A. Renin
- B. Angiotensin I/ Vasopressin / Angiotensinogen/ 25-hydroxy vit D (cholecalciferol)/ Granulocyte – Monocyte – CCF
- C. Erythropoietin
- D. 1, 25 DHCC

148. All of the following statements about adrenals are true except: *(AI 07)*
- A. Chromoffin granules are seen in pheochromocytoma
- B. Adrenal medulla normally secretes epinephrine & in excess of norepinephrine
- C. Tumours of adrenal medulla secrete epinephrine in excess of norepinephrine
- D. Adrenal medulla is not essential for life

149. Hormones secreted by adrenal medulla are: *(PGI 02, 13)*
- A. Glucagons
- B. Cortisol
- C. Norepinephrine
- D. Insulin
- E. Aldosterone

150. Destruction of zone glomerulosa will deplete- *(NBE P 13)*
- A. Aldosterone
- B. Cortisol
- C. Testosterone
- D. Catecholamines

151. Major adrenal androgen is- *(NBE P 13)*
- A. Testosterone
- B. 11-hydroxy derivative of androstenedione
- C. 17-ketosteroid dehydroepiandrosterone
- D. Cortisol

152. In the following sections of the adrenal gland, what hormone is secreted by the region marked as "A"?

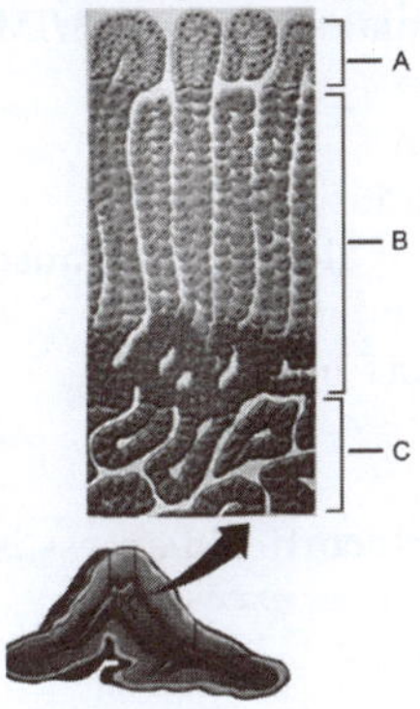

A. Aldosterone (AIIMS 16)
B. Cortisol
C. Testosterone
D. Epinephrine

153. Mineralocorticoid receptors are present in all of the following sites, Except: (AI 11, AIIMS 08)
A. Hippocampus (NBE P 15,14, 13)
B. Kidney
C. Colon
D. Liver

154. What is effect of cortisol on metabolism: (PGI 08)
A. ↑ Neoglucogenesis
B. ↑ Lipogenesis
C. ↑ Proteolysis
D. ↑ Protein anabolism in liver
E. ↑ Glycolysis

155. Effect of steroids on calcium- (NBE P 13)
A. Increased plasma level
B. Increased absorption from gut
C. Increased excretion from kidney
D. None

156. Anti-Inflammatory action of steroids due to-
A. Inhibiton of phospholipas A2 (NBE P 13)
B. Inhibhition of cyclooxegenase
C. Increased activity of lipolipase
D. Inhbhition of lipo oxegenase

157. Diurnal variation in Eosinophil count is related to:
A. Cortisol (AI 12)
B. Thyroxine
C. Growth hormone
D. Testesterone

158. In Cushing syndrome, which of the following are seen: (AI 09)
A. ↑Aldosterone
B. ↓ Aldosterobe
C. ↑ Epinephrine
D. ↓ Epinephrine
E. Edema

159. Aldosterone synthesis is inhibited by: (PGI 03)
A. Renin
B. Endothelin
C. Dopamine
D. Endorphin
E. Hypernatremia

160. Hyperaldosteronism is associated with all except
A. Hypermatrenia (AIIMS 10, NBE P 13)
B. Hypokalemia
C. Hypertension
D. Metabolic acidosis

161. Excess secretion of aldosterone causes all except
A. Increased ECF (AIIMS 08)
B. Very High Na+ in plasma
C. Increased BP
D. Natriuresis

162. Apparent mineralocorticoid excess is d/t
A. Sgk gene (WB 09, TN 08)
B. CYP $11B_2$
C. $CYP11A_1$
D. 11-β hydroxysteroid dehydrogenase

163. Least mineralocorticoid activity is seen in
A. Aldosterone (AIIMS 09)
B. Deoxycortisone
C. Dexamethasone
D. 9 α Flurotisol

164. Epinephrine action in liver: (PGI 08)
A. Glycogenoloysis
B. Gluconeogenesis
C. Glycolysis
D. Lipolysis

Reproductive Hormones

165. Beta HCG is secreted by- (NBE P 13)
A. Ovary
B. Pituitary
C. Corpus luteum
D. Placenta

166. What is thelarche? (NBE P 13)
A. Pubertal breast enlargement in girls
B. Breast enlargement in pregnancy
C. Hormone induced breast enlargement in boys
D. Post hormonal therapy breast enlargement in postmenopausal females

167. Which of the following sugar is/are found in amniotic fluid:
A. Mannose (PGI 13)
B. Sucrose
C. Glucose
D. Fructose
E. Galactose

168. Which of the following is 21-Carbon or C-21/17-OH steroid: (PGI 14, 15; NBE P 15,13; AIIMS 14)
A. Testosterone
B. Estrogen
C. Androgen
D. Progesterone & Corticosteroid

169. A middle aged woman on oral contraceptives for many years, developed neurological symptoms such as depression, irritability, nervousness and mental confusion. Her hemoglobin level was 8g/dl. Biochemical investigations revealed that she was excreting highly elevated concentrations of xanthurenic acid in urine. She also showed high levels of triglycerides and cholesterol in serum. All of the above findings are most probably related to vitamin B6 deficiency caused by prolonged oral contraceptive use except : (AI 04)
A. Increased urinary xanthurenic acid excretion
B. Neurological symptoms by decreased synthesis of biogenic amines
C. Decreased hemoglobin level
D. Increased triglyceride and cholesterol level

170. Before the onset of puberty, the GnRH neurons are under the inhibitory control of : (AI 04)

A. Glycine ☐
B. Glutamate ☐
C. Gamma amino butyric acid (GABA) ☐
D. Beta-endorphin ☐

171. Which of the following is not seen in humans:
A. Estrous cycle *(AI 10)* ☐
B. Menstrual cycle ☐
C. Endometrial cycle ☐
D. Ovarian cycle ☐

172. Ovulation is associated with sudden preovulatory (surge) rise in: *(NBE P 15,14,13; AIIMS 04, 08, 15)*
A. Prolactin/ GnRH/FSH ☐
B. Testosterone ☐
C. LH ☐
D. Oxytocin ☐

173. Ovulation in a women with 28 day cycle occurs at-
A. 14 days prior to menstruation *(NBE P 13)* ☐
B. Just before LH surge ☐
C. Just after corpus leuteal maturation ☐
D. Due to progesterone rise ☐

174. Positive feedback action of estrogen for inducing luteininzing hormone surge is associated with which of the following steroid hormone ratios in peripheral circulation: *(AI 12,03)*
A. High estrogen : low progesterone ☐
B. Low esterogen : high progesterone ☐
C. Low esterogen : low progesterone ☐
D. High esterogen : high progesterone ☐

175. Corpus luteum is maintained in pregnancy by : *(AI 07)*
A. Progesterone *(NBE P 15,14,13)* ☐
B. LH ☐
C. FSH ☐
D. Estrogen ☐

176. Sertoli cells in the testis have receptors for:
A. FSH *(AIIMS 07)* ☐
B. LH ☐
C. Inhibin ☐
D. GnRH ☐

177. Follicular stimulating hormone receptors are present on: *(AIIMS 06)*
A. Theca cells ☐
B. Granulose cells ☐
C. Leydig cells ☐
D. Basement membrane of ovarian follicle ☐

178. Ovarian reserve is best indicated by *(AIIMS 10)*
A. LH ☐
B. FSH ☐
C. LH/FSH ratio ☐
D. Estrogen ☐

179. Luteal phase dominant hormone- *(NBE P 13)*
A. Estrogen ☐
B. Progesterone ☐
C. Prolactin ☐
D. Oxytocin ☐

180. The laboratory report shows values of gonadotropin and ovarian hormones of the blood sample taken, on day 20 of the menstrual cycle of a young woman. Whether her cycle was ovulatory or not may be validly assessed by the reported serum level of :
A. FSH *(AIIMS 02)* ☐
B. LH ☐
C. Oestradiol ☐
D. Progesterone ☐

181. Estrogen is secreted during pregnancy, mostly by-
A. Maternal ovary *(NBE P 13)* ☐
B. Fetal ovary ☐
C. Pituitary ☐
D. Hypothalanmus ☐

182. Most common end product of progesterone metabolism found in urine is: *(AIIMS 13)*
A. Pregnanetriol ☐
B. Pregnenolone ☐
C. Pregnanediol ☐
D. 17 hydroxypregnenolone ☐

183. There is a mid-cycle shift in the basal body temperature (BBT) after ovulation in women. This is caused by :
A. FSH-peak *(AIIMS 03)* ☐
B. LH-peak ☐
C. Oestradiol ☐
D. Progesterone ☐

184. In post ovulatory phase thickness of endometrium is because of- *(NBE P 13)*
A. Progesterone ☐
B. Oestrogen ☐
C. FSH ☐
D. LH ☐

185. The gene coding for androgen receptors is located on
A. Short arm of X- chromosome *(AI 09)* ☐
B. Short arm of Y- chromosome ☐
C. Long arm of X- chromosome ☐
D. Long arm of Y- chromosome ☐

186. The enzyme associated with the conversion of androgen to oestrogen in the growing ovarian follicle is
A. Desmolase *(AI 04)* ☐
B. Isomerase ☐
C. Aromatase ☐
D. Hydroxylase ☐

187. Estrogen action on carbohydrate metabolism:
A. Increases uptake of glucose through increase in insulin sensitivity *(AIIMS 09)* ☐
B. Glycolysis increases ☐
C. Increasing central adipose deposition ☐
D. Worsening of NIDDM ☐

188. Cause of vasodilation in spider nevi
A. Testosterone *(AIIMS 10)* ☐
B. Estrogen ☐
C. FSH ☐
D. Hepatotoxin ☐

189. FSH acts on which of the following:
A. Granulosa cell *(AIIMS 02)* ☐
B. Theca interna ☐
C. Endometrium ☐
D. Myometrium ☐

190. Sertoli cells play a key role in which of the following process: *(AI 09)*
- A. Spermiogenesis
- B. Testosterone secretion
- C. Secretion of seminal fluid
- D. Production of germ cells.

191. Sertoli cells secrete: *(AI 04; NBE P 15)*
- A. Testosterone
- B. Estrogen
- C. Androstenedione
- D. Inhibin

192. Sertoli cells have receptors for: *(NBE P 15; AI 04)*
- A. Inhibin
- B. Luteinizing hormone
- C. Follicle stimulating hormone
- D. Melatonin

193. Sertoli cell feedback mechanism involves- *(NBE P 13)*
- A. Decreased LH
- B. Decreased FSH
- C. Decreased TRH
- D. Decreased CRH

194. Blood testis barrier is located between: *(AIIMS 13)*
- A. Sertoli and sartoli cells
- B. Leydig and myoid cells
- C. Sertoli germ cells
- D. Sertoli spematid

195. Testosterone production is mainly contributed by:
- A. Leydig cells *(NBE P 15,13; AI 06)*
- B. Sertolie cells
- C. Seminiferous tubules
- D. Epididymis

196. Which of the following statements can be regarded as primary action of Inhibin? *(NBE P 14; AI 05)*
- A. It inhibits secretion of prolactin.
- B. It stimulates synthesis of estradiol.
- C. It stimulates secretion of TSH.
- D. It inhibits secretion of FSH.

197. Ovary produces all except- *(NBE P 13)*
- A. Gonadotropin
- B. Progesterone
- C. Estrogen
- D. Inhibin B

198. Males and females show difference in the age of onset of puberty. The difference in the age of onset of puberty amongst males may be explained by:
- A. Increased Activin – A levels *(AI 07)*
- B. Decreased Follistatin levels
- C. Increased Inhibin levels
- D. Easily releasable FSH pool

199. Semen is released by- *(NBE P 15,13)*
- A. Epididymis *(AIIMS 14,12)*
- B. Testes
- C. Vas deferens
- D. Prolactin

200. Sperms become motile in: *(NBE P 15,13; AIIMS 12)*
- A. Prostate *(AI 06)*
- B. Seminal vesicles
- C. Epididymis
- D. Vas deferens

201. Capacitance of sperms takes place in: *(NBE P 15, 13)*
- A. Seminiferous tubules *(AIIMS 10, 09)*
- B. Epididymis
- C. Vas deference
- D. Uterus

202. Spermatogenesis is maintained by all hormone(s) except: *(NBE P 14, 13)*
- A. Testosterone *(PGI 08)*
- B. FSH
- C. LH
- D. Prolactin & Gonadotropin Releasing Hormone (GnRH)

203. Dihydrotestosterone acts on- *(NBE P 13)*
- A. Pituitary
- B. Exterrnal genitalia
- C. Internal genitalia
- D. Tests

204. Negative feedback in spermatogenesis by- *(NBE P 13)*
- A. ABP
- B. Inhibin
- C. Progesterone
- D. None

205. Prolonged administration of testosterone in a man causes: *(AIIMS 10)*
- A. Azoospermia
- B. Increased GnRH
- C. Increased sperm mobility
- D. Increased spermiogenesis

206. Which of the following hormones is mainly responsible for skeletal maturation: *(AIIMS 02)*
- A. Testosterone
- B. Estrogen
- C. Growth hormone
- D. Testosterone/estrogen ratio

207. Change in sex hormone binding globulin will most affect levels of which of these hormones? *(AIIMS 16)*
- A. Testosterone
- B. Estrogen
- C. Progesterone
- D. DHEA

208. In contraction stress test, positive interpretation is:
- A. Early deceleration *(AIIMS 2K)*
- B. Early acceleration
- C. Persistent late deceleration
- D. Variable deceleration

209. Change in sex hormone binding globulin will most affect levels of which of these hormones? *(AIIMS 16)*
- A. Testosterone
- B. Estrogen
- C. Progesterone
- D. DHEA

210. Antibodies against sperms may develop after:
- A. Trauma *(NBE P 14, 13)*
- B. Infection
- C. Vasectomy
- D. Orchidectomy

211. The commonest cause of primary amenorrhea with ambiguous genitalia in a female with 46XX chromosome: *(AIIMS 2K)*
A. 21 hydroxylase def. ☐
B. 17 hydroxylase def. ☐
C. 11 hydroxylase def. ☐
D. Desmolase hydrolase def. ☐

212. Velocity of human sperm- *(NBE P 13)*
A. 1-3 mm/min ☐
B. 4-6mm/min ☐
C. 6-9 mm/min ☐
D. 10-13 mm/min ☐

213. PGs in semen are secreted by- *(NBE P 13)*
A. Prostate ☐
B. Seminal vesicle ☐
C. Sperms ☐
D. Testes ☐

214. Not found in seminal fluid: *(PGI 13)*
A. Fructose ☐
B. Prostaglandins ☐
C. Spermine ☐
D. Citric acid ☐
E. Inositol ☐

215. Which of the following organs secretes zinc in large amount in man? *(AIIMS 06)*
A. Seminal vesicle ☐
B. Prostate ☐
C. Epididymis ☐
D. Vas ☐

216. Immune rejection in fetus is prevented by- *(NBE P 13)*
A. HCG ☐
B. HPL ☐
C. Oestrogen ☐
D. Progesterone ☐

217. True about placental hormone is A/E *(AI 10)*
A. hCS is diabetogenic ☐
B. hCG rise l/t nausea ☐
C. Progesterone production require fetal steroidogenic tissue ☐
D. Luteal – placental shift at 8-10 weeks ☐

218. Intrauterine growth of fetus is affected by: *(PGI 10)*
A. Growth hormone ☐
B. Insulin ☐
C. Thyroxine ☐
D. Glucocorticoids ☐
E. Parathormone ☐

Stress

219. Which of the following increases during surgical stress- *(NBE P 13)*
A. Cortisol ☐
B. Glucagon ☐
C. Insulin ☐
D. Gastrin ☐

220. Stress induced hyperglycemia is mediated through which hormone: *(PGI 05)*
A. Insulin ☐
B. Glucagon ☐
C. Thyroxine ☐
D. Epinephrine ☐
E. Cortisol ☐

221. During stress increased stimulation of cortisol release cause: *(PGI 04)*
A. Neoglucogenesis ☐
B. Glycolysis ☐
C. Protein breakdown ☐
D. Glucose utilization ☐
E. Lipolysis ☐

222. In stress which hormone is increased *(PGI 04)*
A. Insulin ☐
B. Vasopressin ☐
C. Adrenaline ☐

Nitric Oxide

223. Mechanism of action of Nitric oxide is through: *(AI 2K)*
A. cGMP ☐
B. cAMP ☐
C. Ca^{++} ☐
D. Tyrosine ☐

224. NO is synthesized by: *(AIIMS 09)*
A. Uracil ☐
B. Aspartate ☐
C. Guanosine ☐
D. Arginine ☐

225. Nitric Oxide Synthase : *(AI 02)*
A. Is inhibited by Ca^{++} ☐
B. Catalyzes a dioxygenase reaction ☐
C. Accepts electrons from NADH ☐
D. Requires NADPH, FAD, FMN & Heme iron ☐

226. True statement regarding Nitric oxide is: *(AI 09)*
A. NO is synthesized from arginine ☐
B. NO is spontaneous produced from NO_2 ☐
C. NO causes vasoconstriction ☐
D. NO is released from mitochondria ☐

227. True about nitric oxide: *(PGI 01)*
A. Free radical ☐
B. Vasodilator ☐
C. Oxidizing agent ☐
D. Catalyst ☐
E. Platelet aggregator ☐

228. The primary action of Nitric oxide (NO) in the gastrointestinal tract is: *(AI 10)*
A. Vasodilatation ☐
B. Vasoconstriction ☐
C. Gastrointestinal smooth muscle relaxation ☐
D. Gastrointestinal slow smooth muscle contraction ☐

ANSWERS & EXPLANATIONS:

Receptors and Second Messengers

1. C i.e. Adrenalin 2. A i.e. Thyroxine 3. A i.e. Insulin & Glucagon 4. A i.e. TSH

Group II (Hydrophilic) Hormones that bind to Cell surface/ Cell Membrane Receptors

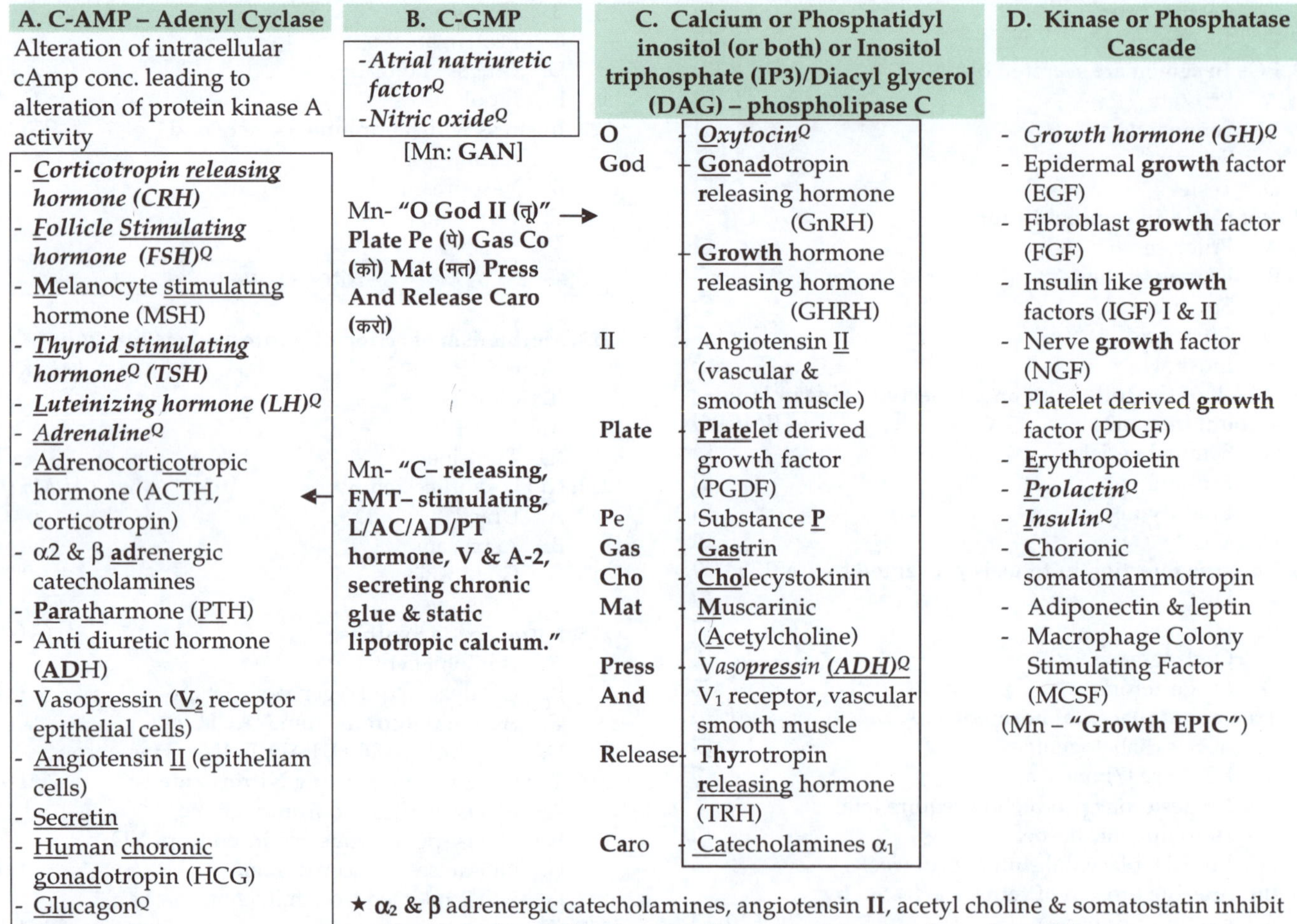

Second Messenger is

A. C-AMP – Adenyl Cyclase

Alteration of intracellular cAmp conc. leading to alteration of protein kinase A activity

- ***Corticotropin releasing hormone (CRH)***
- ***Follicle Stimulating hormone (FSH)***Q
- **M**elanocyte stimulating hormone (MSH)
- ***Thyroid stimulating hormone***Q ***(TSH)***
- ***Luteinizing hormone (LH)***Q
- ***Adrenaline***Q
- Adrenocorticotropic hormone (ACTH, corticotropin)
- α2 & β adrenergic catecholamines
- **Para**tharmone (PTH)
- Anti diuretic hormone (ADH)
- Vasopressin (V2 receptor epithelial cells)
- Angiotensin II (epitheliam cells)
- Secretin
- Human choronic gonadotropin (HCG)
- GlucagonQ
- **Soma**tostatin
- Lipotropin
- Calcitonin

Mn- **"C– releasing, FMT– stimulating, L/AC/AD/PT hormone, V & A-2, secreting chronic glue & static lipotropic calcium."**

B. C-GMP

- *Atrial natriuretic factor*Q
- *Nitric oxide*Q

[Mn: **GAN**]

Mn- **"O God II (तु)" Plate Pe (पे) Gas Co (को) Mat (मत) Press And Release Caro (करो)**

C. Calcium or Phosphatidyl inositol (or both) or Inositol triphosphate (IP3)/Diacyl glycerol (DAG) – phospholipase C

O	- *Oxytocin*Q
God	- **Gonad**otropin releasing hormone (GnRH)
	- **Growth** hormone releasing hormone (GHRH)
II	- Angiotensin II (vascular & smooth muscle)
Plate	- **Plate**let derived growth factor (PGDF)
Pe	- Substance **P**
Gas	- **Gas**trin
Cho	- **Cho**lecystokinin
Mat	- **M**uscarinic (Acetylcholine)
Press	- V*asopressin (ADH)*Q
And	V1 receptor, vascular smooth muscle
Release	- Thyrotropin releasing hormone (TRH)
Caro	- Catecholamines α1

D. Kinase or Phosphatase Cascade

- *Growth hormone (GH)*Q
- Epidermal **growth** factor (EGF)
- Fibroblast **growth** factor (FGF)
- Insulin like **growth** factors (IGF) I & II
- Nerve **growth** factor (NGF)
- Platelet derived **growth** factor (PDGF)
- **E**rythropoietin
- ***Prolactin***Q
- ***Insulin***Q
- **C**horionic somatomammotropin
- Adiponectin & leptin
- Macrophage Colony Stimulating Factor (MCSF)

(Mn – **"Growth EPIC"**)

★ **α2 & β** adrenergic catecholamines, angiotensin **II**, acetyl choline & somatostatin inhibit adenyl acyclase (H1) whereas others stimulate adenyl acyclase (H5).

Group I (Lipophilic) Hormones that bind to Intracellular Receptors

Ligand – receptor complex directly provides the signal to specific genes whose rate of transcription is there by affected.

At Cytoplasmic Receptors

- *Glucocorticoids & mineralocorticoids*Q
- *Androgens (testosterone), estrogen & progestins*Q
- *Retinoic acid (retinoids)* Q
- Vit D_3 (1, 25-$(OH)_2$ D_3) Q

At Nuclear Receptors

Includes *Thyroid* (T_3 & T_4) *hormones*Q

5. **B i.e. Atrial natriuretic factor & Nitric Oxide (NO)** 6. **D i.e. Estrogen** 7. **A i.e. Vitamin D_3 ; D i.e. Thyroid**
8. **A i.e. Guanylyl cyclase** 9. **B i.e. Acts by increasing C- AMP** 10. **A i.e. Mainly on nuclear surface; B i.e. Steroid act**
[Ref: Harper 28/e 428, 445-48; Gabriel p 281; Guyton 11/e 910-15; Ganong 23/e p. 50-54; anesthesia volume for detail]

- **Cyclic AMP, C-GMP, IP_3/DAG** are ***secondary messengers. C-GMP acts on nitric oxide (NO) and ANF (atrial natriuretic factor)***Q as second messenger.
- **Intra cellular receptors (steroid receptor super family)** is present in **thyroxine (nuclear receptor)** and **gluco/mineralo-corticoids, androgen estrogen, progestin, retinoic acid and vitamin D_3 (all cytoplasmic receptors).**
- **3 classes of second messengers** include **(1) cyclic nucleotides (i.e. cAMP & cGMP)**; (2) **IP_3** (inositol triphosphate) & **DAG** (diacylglycerol) and (3) **calcium ion (Ca^{2+})**. ***Adenyl and guanyl cyclases are not second messengers***Q, they catalyze formation of cAMP & cGMP respectively.

11. **A, B, C, E i.e. Insulin, PTH, Renin, Angiotensin II** *[Ref: Berne & Levy 6/e p-656-58; Guyton 11/e 907-224; Gabriel p 280-81]*

- **Sterod hormones** are synthesized from ***cholesterol***Q and example includes **adrenocortical hormones** (i.e. ***cortisol & aldosterone***Q), **sex hormones** (i.e. ***testosterone, estrogen & progesterone)***Q and **vitamin D3 = 1, 25- (OH)2 cholecalciferol** (a secosteroid because one of the rings of steroid nucleus , the B ring, is open)
- **Amine hormones** are derived from aminoacid **tyrosine** and examples include ***catecholamines (adrenaline /epinephrine and noradrenaline/nor epinephrine)***Q from adrenal medulla, **thyroid hormones** (triiodothyronine = ***T3, tetraiodothyronine = T4 = thyroxine)***Q and prolactin inhibiting factor /PIF (dopamine) from hypothalamus.
- All remaining hormones are either **low molecular weight proteins (i.e. poly peptides)** or **glycoproteins**. They are ***synthesized initially as larger peptide precursor***Q (eg prepro-insulin) and then cleaved off until the final smaller active molecule is produced. Some are also coupled with carbohydrates to form glycoproteins.

12. **D i.e. Vasopressin** *[Ref: Ganong 23rd/e p. 139-40, 342, 337, 279-80; KDT 6/ed pg-25; Katzung 10/ed pg-25]*

- **Dopamine** has *5 receptors*, al of which use C-AMP as second messenger. Receptors **D_1 & D_5** ***act by increasing C AMP whereas D2, D3, & D4 by decreasing it***Q.
- **Vasopressin (ADH)** has 2 receptors of which **vasopressin receptor 1 (V_1)** ***in vascular smooth muscles act via IP3/DAG mechanism***Q whereas **antidiuretic receptor 2 (V_2)** in tubular epithelial cells (important for water reabsorption) acts through ***C AMP-adenyl cyclase system***Q

Second Messenger

c AMP	**IP_3 / DAG**
- 5 HT 1 - ***Dopamine D_1, D_2, D_3, D_4, D_5***Q - Histamine H_2 - Muscarinic M_2 - GABA B - α_2 and β adrenergic - **V_2 (ADH) receptor**Q - Angiotensin II (epithelial cells)	- 5HT 2 - Histamine H_1 - Adrenergic $\alpha 1$ - Muscarinic M_1, M_3 - ***V_1 (Vasopressin) receptor***Q - Angiotensin II (Vascular & smooth muscle) - Thrombinane - Lithium

13. **D i.e. Adenylate cyclase** *[Ref: Ganong 22/e P-44-46]*

- Adenylate cyclase is an enzyme that occurs on the surface of cell membranesQ
- It belongs to the family of cell membrane receptors that are linked to the effecter through one or more GTP activated G-proteins (G-protein coupled receptor) Q
- **Cycle AMP is an important second messenger that is formed from ATP by the action of enzyme adenelyl cyclase.**Q
- Cyclic AMP acts by activating a cyclic nucleotide – dependent protein kinase (protein kinase-A) which catalyzes the phosphorylation.

14. **A i.e. ADP ribosylation** 15. **C i.e. Causes continued activation of adenylate cyclase**
16. **A i.e., Activation of protein kinase** *[Ref: Harper 29/e p 732-33; Ganong 22/e P- 43; Harrison 16/e P- 755]*

Cholera toxin (A1 subunit) catalyzes ***ADP ribosylation of Gsα subunit and causes persistent activation of adenyl cyclase***Q. This results in **elevation of cAMP**, which ***activates protein kinase A***Q and causes **phosphorylation of CFTR and Na^+ - H^+ exchanger**. This inturn leads to **inhibition of Na^+ absorption and enhancement of Cl^- secretion**. Thus massive amounts of NaCl accumulate inside intestine lumen contributing to **liquid stools (watery diarrhoea) characteristic of cholera**.

17. **C i.e. Ca++** *[Ref: Harpers illustrated Biochemistry 28/e p. 428; 27/e P-471,445; 26/e P-463,437;Ganong 22/e P-42- 45]*

Ligand binding to receptor activates **phospholipase**- C (PLC) on the inner surface of membrane via G_q. The B_1 & B_2 forms of PLC are activated by G protein and catalyze hydrolysis of **PIP_2** (phosphatidyl inositol 4, 5 diphosphate) to form **IP_3** (Inositol 1, 4, 5 – triphosphate) and **DAG** (Diacyl glycerol)
The ***IP_3 diffuses into sacroplasmic reticulum & releases calcium into the cytoplasm*Q*. DAG is also a 2nd messenger and it activates protein kinase - C***

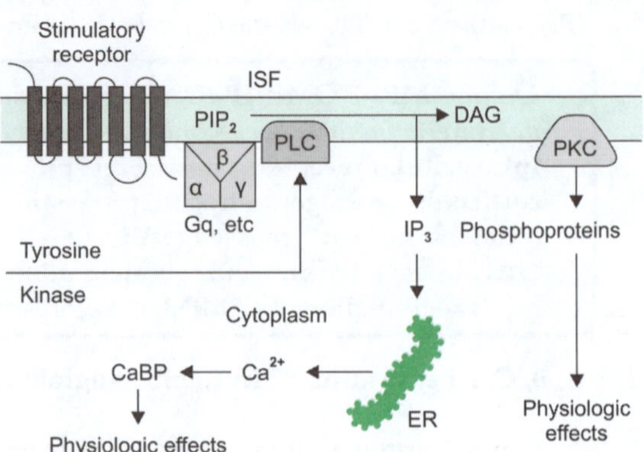

- Tyrosine kinase linked receptors can convert $PIP_2 \rightarrow IP_3$ & DAG by activating *PLCY₁*
- IP_3 receptor resemble *ryanodine receptor* (a Ca++ channel in sarcoplasmic reticulum of skeletal muscle) except that IP3 receptor is half as large.

18. **E i.e. Testosterone, cortisol & Estogen** (nearest answer) *[Ref: Harper 28/ed p. 457; Lehninger 5/e p. 422-456]*

Glucagon, TSH, GnRH &LH all bind to cell surface receptors. So **nuclear receptors (here it means intracellular steroidal receptors i.e. both nuclear & cytoplasmic receptors)** are used by testosterone, cortisol and estrogen (answer of exclusion).

19. **B i.e. Transcriptional mediators** *[Ref: Harper 27/e p-464- 66, 476- 80, Molecular cell biology December 19(12); 8383-8392; L costanzo physiology 3/e p-363]*

Steroid receptors bind to hormones, ***hormone response elements (HRE), and transcription coregulator proteins such as co-repressors (NCoR, SMRT), co- activators (CBP, P-300) and mediator related protein*Q.**

20. **A i.e. Ligand binding**

Androgen receptor belongs to *nuclear receptor super family*. At **carboxy (C) terminal** of nuclear receptor, a ***multifunctional ligand binding domain (LBD=E domain) is located***Q.

21. **A i.e. Liver** *[Ref: Harper 27/e p-476-78, 467; http://en.wikipedia.org/wiki/mineralocorticoid-receptor;http://www.lib.bioinfo.pl/meid:35592]*

- **Aldosterone** (or **mineralocorticoid**) **receptor** (MR, MLR, MCR) is expressed in ***central nervous system (hippocampus), heart, kidney, colon, brown adipose tissue and sweat glands but not not in liver***Q.

- It is a *steroid hormone receptor* that belongs to *nuclear receptor subfamily 3, group C, member 2 (NR3C2)*. It is activated by *mineralocorticoids eg. aldosterone & deoxycorticosterone*, as well as by *glucocorticoids* (such as cortisol & cortisone) and some *progestins*.
- Its activation in epithelial cells leads to expression of proteins regulating ionic and water transport (mainly epithelial sodium channels. ENaC, Na^+ - K^+ pump, serum & glucocorticoid induced kinase or SGK1) resulting in absorption of Na^+ causing increased ECF volume & BP, and an excretion of K^+ to maintain a normal salt concentration in body.

22. **B i.e. For specific action; C i.e. Molecular transport** 23. **A i.e. Nicotinic cholinergic receptor (D) $GABA_A$ receptor**
[Ref: Goodman & Gilman 10/e P34, 35; KDT 5/e p. 42; Harper's 27/e P-445; 26/e P-435-436]

- **Cell membrane receptors** bind to specific **molecule and transport** it via endo/exo-cytosis giving **specificity to process.**
- **Cell surface receptors with intrinsic ion channel** include ***nicotinic cholinergic, glutamate, glycine, $GABA_A$ and $5HT_3$ receptors*Q.**

24. **A i.e. Breakdown of GTP to GDP** 25. **C i.e. Made up of 4 units**
[Ref: Ganong 22/e P- 41-44, Guyton 11/e p. 911; KDT 6/e p. 45-48]

G protein is made up of ***3 subunits - α, β, and γ*Q.** And the intrinsic **GTPase activity of α subunit** *converts GTP to GDP*Q.

26. A i.e. It interacts transmembrane; B i.e. GTP to GDP; C i.e. Adenyl cyclase activation ..; E i.e. Helical structure
27. A i.e. It binds to ligands at the cell surface

G protein coupled receptor (GPCR) ***binds to the ligand at the cell surface***Q. It is a **seven transmembrane domain (7TM)** or **haptohelical** or **serpentine receptor. Separation of α subunit from β, γ subunits brings about biological effect**Q. βγ subunits acts on *adenyl acylase (↑ing cAMP, stimulating PKA and phosphorylating receptor)*Q. On ligand removal, the intrinsic **GTPase activity of α subunit** inactivates itself by ***converting its bound GTP into GDP***Q.

28. D i.e. Increased cAMP *[Ref: Harper 28/e 448]*

Gs-α subunit gain would cause **increased adenyl cyclase level** – ultimately resulting in ***increased c-AMP level***Q, (because adenyl cyclase converts ATP to c-AMP).

29. C i.e. Seven pass – receptor *[Ref: Guyton 11/e p. 910- 13; Ganong 24/e p. 58-59]*

Catecholamines (epinephrine, norepinephrine and dopamine) act through G **protein coupled receptors (GPCRs)**, which span the cell membrane 7 times; hence also referred to as **seven pass (seven helix) or serpentine receptors.**

30. D i.e. Substance that increase or decrease function
31. B i.e. Enzymatic composition
32. D i.e. CyGMP
33. A i.e. Insulin
34. D i.e. Estrogen
35. A i.e. FSH
36. C i.e. Insulin
37. C i.e. NO
38. A i.e. Guanylyl cyclase
39. A i.e. CAMP B i.e. DAG C i.e. IP_3 D i.e. Ca^{++}
40. C, D i.e. cAMP, Ca^{++}
[Ref: Berne & Levy 6/e p 34-42; Best & Taylor 13/e p 821-25; Ganong 24/e p 54-63; Lehninger 4/e p434; Harper 27/e p 445-52, 428; Lippincott 4/e p 422-43; Guyton 12/e p 888-91; KDT 6/e p 231-32]

- **Second messengers** (concept proposed by E.W. **Sutherland**) are **intracellular signaling molecules** mediating intracellular hormone / ligand (1st messenger) function.
- Second messengers respond differentially to a hormone or drug because of receptors but ***cells respond to second messengers differentially because of different enzymatic composition***Q.
- ***A surprising finding in mid 1980s was the role of nitric oxide (NO) as an important biological messenger***Q.
- NO is a short lived messenger that act by ***stimulating a guanyl cyclase raising cGMP and stimulating protein kinase G***Q.
- ***C- AMP, C- GMP, IP_3, DAG, Ca^{++} and protein kinase***Q function as **second messengers.**

Calcium Metabolism and Parathyroid Gland

41. B i.e. Calmodulin *[Ref: Harper's 27/e P- 471, 579; Ganong 24/e p. 57-58]*

Calmodulin is a small Ca^{++} binding protein that modifies activity of many enzymes/ proteins in response to changes of Ca^{++} concentration.

42. A i.e. Absorption of phosphorus increase
43. A i.e. Proximal small intestine
44. A i.e. Proteins
45. C i.e. Parathormone (PTH) promotes absorption of Ca^{2+} from intestine

Parathyroid hormone increases phosphate excretion in urine due to ***decrease in reabsorption of phosphate in the proximal tubules***Q. **PTH** *promotes absorption* of ***calcium from intestine***Q ***(mainly proximal small intestine)***Q via activation of vitamin D (1,25, dihydroxy cholecalciferol).

Parathyroid Hormone (PTH)

Bone	Kidney	Intestine
- PTH acts directly on bone to increase bone *resorption*Q, - On a longer times cale, PTH stimulates osteoclast & osteoblast, with the *effect on osteoclast predominating* so more Ca^{2+} is mobilized from bone.	- **↓PO_4^{3-} reabsorption**Q. - ↑Ca^{2+} reabsorption **in distal tubule**Q	↑Ca^{2+} absorption **(via activation of Vit D)**Q, mainly from **proximal small intestine.**Q

46. A i.e. Ionised calcium **47. C i.e Alkaline pH in gut**
48. A i.e. Absorbed in upper small intestine; D i.e. Absorption increased by acidic pH **49. A,B,C i.e. PCT, DCT, LH**
[Ref: Ganong 24/e p. 56-58, 377-78;Berne 6/e p. 700-2, 628-32; Harper 26/e p. 444; Chatterjee 7/e p. 875; Harrison 17/e p. 286]

- ***Free ionized calcium is physiologically active form of calcium***Q, that is a vital second messenger and is necessary for blood coagulation, muscle contraction and nerve function.
- ***Calcium is absorbed in upper small intestine (duodenum & proximal jejunum) and the absorption is increased by acidic pH***Q.
- **Calcium sensing receptors** (CaSRs) are present in **PTH secreting cells of parathyroid glands, calcitonin secreting parafollicular cells in thyroid gland** and **calcitriol (Vit D) producing cells of proximal tubules** (i.e. in the cells producing **hormone involved in regulation of serum calcium).** Ca SRs are also present in ***thick ascending limb of loop of Henle and distal tubule (DCT)***Q to directly regulate Ca^{++} homeostasis. **Small intestine cells lack CaSRs**Q.
- The active transcellular Ca^{++} absorption is facilitated in enterocytes and nephrons by **epithetial Ca^{++} channels TRPV 5 and 6** (on apical epithelium), **calbindin D9k** (in cytoplasm) and **plasma membrane Ca ATPase (PMCA;** in basolateral membrane). **The sodium/calcium exchanger (NCX)** also transport calcium out of enterocytes.

Absorption of Calcium is

Decreased by	Increased by
- ***Achlorhydria***Q	- **Protein**Q (also **increase Mg** absorption)
- Taking drugs that inhibit gastric acid secretion	- **Hypocalcemia**
- Pancreatic & biliary non sufficiency where ingested calcium remains bound to unabsorbed fatty acid etc.	- **Acidic pH in stomach**
- ***Phosphates & oxalates***Q	- **Lactose**Q
- **Alkalis (Alkaline pH)**Q	- **PTH & Vit D**Q
- **Hyper calcemia (↑Ca^{++})**	
- **High Mg^{++}, PO_4^{-3},**	
- **Phytic acid,** Caffeine, Dietary fibers	

50. C i.e. Increased Parathormone secretion **51. B, D i.e. Stimulate 1, 25 D3 formation, Increases the resorption of bone**
[Ref: Best & Taylor 13/e p -886-888; Ganong 24/e p 381-84; Guyton 12/e p 962-66]

- Synthesis & secretion of parathyroid hormone (PTH) are regulated primarily by **serum ionized calcium concentration** sensed by ***calcium sensing receptor (CaSR) located on chief cell of parathyroid gland.*** When ionized **serum Ca^{++} levels decrease below 1.3mM** (eg d/t prolonged low calcium diet), **PTH synthesis and secretion increases** (to restore Ca^{++} levels). Whereas when extracellular serum Ca^{++} increases above 1.3 mM, PTH decreases & serum calcium diminishes.
- **Parathyroid hormone (PTH)** is a **84 aminoacids linear polypeptide hormone.** PTH **stimulates 1, 25, dihydroxycholecalciferol [1, 25 $(OH)_2$ D_3] formation, promotes absorption of calcium mainly from proximal small intestis and increases bone resorption**. PTH also **increases reabsorption of calcium in distal tubules** (via **TRPV6** = Transient Receptor Potential Vanilloid type 6 channels) and **decreases reabsorption of phosphate in proximal tubules** (via Na-Pi IIa). ***In nutshell it increases serum calcium & decreases serum phosphate***Q.

52. C i.e. Hypophosphatemia *[Ref: Ganong 22/e P-392, 391]*

PTH ***increases phosphate excretion in urine causing hypophosphatemia***Q. **This phosphaturic action is due to decreased reapsorption of phosphate in distal tubules.**

Secondary Hyperparathyroidism d/t –Vit D deficiency

- This results from decreased serum Ca^{2+}.
- The released parathyroid hormone *directs its activity to increase serum* Ca^{2+} at the cost of of *loss of phosphate* from the body – ***hypophosphatemia***Q.
- PTH mobilizes both Ca^{2+} & phosphate from the bone to increased level of both in blood initially, while it reabsorbs the filtered Ca^{2+} from renal tubules, it fails to reabsorb phosphate which is lost in urine.

53. A i.e. PTH; B i.e. Calcitonin; D i.e. 1, 25 DHC *[Ref: Ganong 24/e p377-87]*

Serum calcium level is regulated by **parathormone (PTH), vitamin D (i.e. 1, 25 dihydroxy chole calciferol) and calcitonin. Vit D and PTH increase whereas calcitonin decreases serum Ca^{++} level.**

54. B i.e. Calcitonin **55. B i.e. Decreased bone resorption** **56. B i.e. Calcitonin** *[Ref: Ganong 22/e p. 393-394; KDT 5/e P-301]*

Calcitonin, a hormone secreted by **parafollicular cells or C cell**Q of thyroid gland, **lowers the serum calcium level**Q. **Calcitonin exerts its Ca^{2+} lowering effect (hypocalcemia) by inhibiting bone resorption.** This action is **direct and calcitonin inhibits the activity of osteoclast**Q. It also increases Ca^{2+} excretion in urine.

Effect of Hormone on Calcium & Phosphate Level

Hormone	Serum Calcium	Serum phosphate	Bone cells on which their receptors are present
Vit D	IncreasesQ	IncreaseQ	Osteoblast
PTH	IncreasesQ	DecreaseQ	Osteoblast
Calcitonin	DecreasesQ	DecreaseQ	**Osteoclast**Q

57. C i.e. Increased excitability of muscle and nerve.
58. A i.e. Low Ca^{++} Causes↑ Na^{+} permeability *[Ref: Ganong 22/e P- 59; Gyuton 10/e P 315]*

- A ***decrease in extra cellular Ca^{++} Concentration increases the excitability of nerve and muscle cells by decreasing the amount of depolarization necessary to initiate the change in Na^{+} & K^{+} conductance that produce the action potential***Q. In fact Ca^{++} needs to fall only 50% below the normal before spontaneous discharge occur from peripheral nerves, often causing tetany. Conversely, an ***increase in ECF Ca^{++} stabilizes the membrane by decreasing excitability***Q.
- The voltage gated calcium channels are slightly permeable to Na^{+} as well as Ca^{++}; when they are activated both Na^{+} and Ca^{++} flow to interior of the fiber. *When there is deficit of Ca^{2+} in ECF, Na^{+} channels become activated (opened) by very little change of membrane potential* (from its very negative resting level to a less negative level). Therefore nerve fibers become highly excitable. Sometime discharging repetitively without provocation rather than remaining in resting stage.
- **Decreasing the external Na^{+} concentration** ***decreases the size of action potential***Q but has little effect on RMP. **Increasing the external K^{+}** concentration ***decreases the RMP***Q.

59. C i.e. Shortening of QT interval in ECG. *[Ref: Harrison 16/e P-2263; Schwartz 7/e P-69; Ganong 22/e P-382]*

QT interval (ventricular depolarization + repolarization) on ECG ***is prolonged in hypocalcemia***Q.(as Ca^{2+} is necessary for contraction) and is ***shortened in hypercalcemia***Q.

60. C i.e. Spleen **61. D i.e. Lungs**
62. D i.e. Williams syndrome consists of mental retardation, obesity & precocious
63. B i.e. Increased 24,25 dihydroxycholecalciferol **64. C i.e. 1, 25 $(OH)_2$ vitamin D**
[Ref: Harrison 17/e p. 2138; 16/e p- 385, 1382, 2258, 2246; Harper 27/e p- 453, 492 , Shils – Modern nutrition in health & disease 9/e p-287, Ganong 22/e p. 387- 89; Braunwald's 8/e p-1085; Chatterjee Shinde 6/e p. 151; Guyton 11/e p. 983-85]

- **Spleen (>> Lung) are not involved in calcium metabolism (homeostasis)**Q**. But skin, kidney, liver and intestines** are involved in calcium metabolism.
- In **liver vit D_3 (cholecalciferol)** is hydroxylated to form **25, hydroxy cholecalciferol (calcidiol)**Q, which is released in circulation bound to a globulin, the **main storage form of vitamin D. In kidney** calcidiol undergoes either **1 hydroxylation to form active metabolite 1, 25 dihydroxy cholecalciferol (calcitriol)**Q or 24 hydroxylation to yield an inactive (probably) metabolite **24, 25 dihydroxy cholecalciferol (24- hydroxy calcidiol). When calcium level is high, minor pathway becomes main i.e. little calcitriol is produced and kidney mainly produce relatively inactive 24, 25 dihydroxy cholicalciferol**Q**.**

- **William's syndrome** is **autosomal dominant idiopathic hyper calcemia of infancy**Q. It is characterized by **multiple congenital developmental defects such as supravalvular aortic and peripheral pulmonic stenosis, mental retardation, an elfin facies, loquacious personality and hoarse voice, in association with hyper calcemia**Q d/t abnormal sensitivity to vitamin D. It is probably d/t mutations involving elastin locus on chromosome 7 (7q 11.23). Other clinical features are feeding difficulties, failure to thrive, gastrointestinal problems such as vomiting, constipation, & colic along with auditory hyperacusis, inguinal hernia, outgoing & engaging personality, strabismus, dental development abnormalities (eg. Microdontia enamel hypoplasia & malocclusion) and narrowing of peripheral systemic and pulmonary arteries.

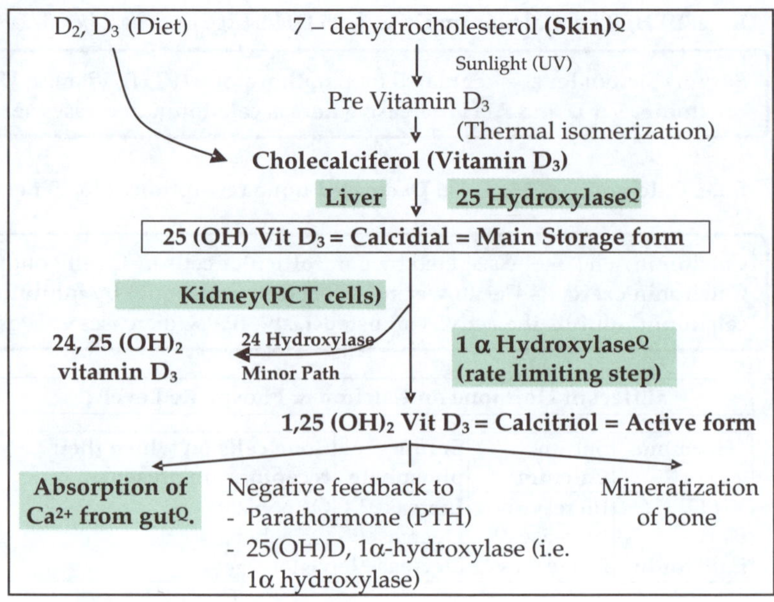

65. **D i.e. Collects calcium into the sarcoplasmic reticulum.** *[Ref: Pretest physiology 9/e Q NO – 15]*

Phospholamban is a protein contained within the sarcoplasmic reticulum that **inhibits the activity of sarcoplasmic calcium pump**Q. **Inactivation of phospholamban results in an increase in calcium sequestration by sarcoplasmic reticulum.**Q

- In cardiac muscle, the rapid sequestration of Ca^{2+} shortens the duration of contraction.
- In smooth muscle, sequestration causes the muscle to relax.
- Phospholamban has little effect on skeletal muscle contraction.

66. **B i.e. Parathyroid hormone related protein (PTHrP)** *[Ref: Harrison 16/e P-566]*

Hypercalcemia related to malignancy is also k/a **Humoral hypercalcemia of malignancy (HHM)** is most often associated with **over production of PTHrP (Parathyroid hormone related protein)**Q.

67. **A i.e. Parathormone** *[Ref: Harper 26/e P-438; Shinde 6/e P 490]*

Hormones can be classified chemically into three major groups

Steroid	Amino acid derivatives	Peptide /Protein
- Glucocorticoids	Derived from *tyrosine*	- ***Parathormone***Q
- Mineralocorticoids	- Catecholamines	- Calcitonin
- Estrogen	- Thyroid hormone	- Insulin
- Progesteron		- Glucagon
- Androgen		- Pituitary hormones

68. **C i.e. Required hydrolysis of ATP, E i.e. It is an active process**
69. **A i.e. Inositol triphosphate** *[Ref: Ganong 24/e P-56-58; Sembulingum 3/e P- 19; NMS Biochemistry 4/e P 263]*

- **Calcium can enter cell from ECF passively** down its electrochemical gradient. But the movement of calcium **outside of cytosol (ie across the plasma membrane or the membrane of internal store** ie ER & mitochondria) is against electrochemical gradient so is an **active process requiring hydrolysis of ATP**Q.
- ***Inositol triphosphate (IP_3) diffuses to the endoplasmic reticulum, where it triggers the release of calcium into cytoplasm***Q. **IP_3** is the major second messenger that causes release of Ca^{++} from ER through the IP_3 receptor activation (a ligand gated channel). So **one second messenger (IP_3) causes release of another second messenger (Ca^{++})**Q.

Carbohydrate Metabolism & Pancreatic Hormone

70. D i.e. PP is secreted by D1 cells **71. C i.e. Proteolytic enzymes secreted in inactive form** **72. A i.e. Trypsin**
73. A i.e. Osmolality is ½ of the osmolality of blood *[Ref: Ganong 23/e 328-30, 316; Berne & Levy 6/e p 675-76; Guyton 12/e p. 939; Robbin's 7/e 940-41]*

- **Pancreas** is composed of 2 types of tissue (1) **exocrine acini** constituting 80% of gland, which secrete *digestive enzymes* e.g. **trypsin** and **chymotrypsin** into the duodenum, and (2) **endocrine islets of Langerhans**, which secrete *hormones* directly into blood (and constitute 2-3% of gland). Remainder volume is constituted by ducts & blood vessels.
- **Pancrease (exocrine part) secretes enzymatically inert proenzymes (eg trypsinogen) to prevent self digestion[Q].**
- Pacreatic exocrine secretion is **isotonic with blood plasma[Q].** It is ***alkaline with 1.5 lit/day secretion rich in enzymes[Q]***. Secretin enhances its bicarbonate component.

Islets cell type		Secretion
A cells	Alpha (α)	Glucagon[Q]
B cells	Beta (β)	Insulin[Q] & amylin
D cells	Delta (δ)	Somatostatin[Q]
F cells	PP cells	Pancreatic polypeptide[Q]
D1 cells		VIP

74. B i.e. Increased glucose toterance **75. C i.e. Decreased growth hormone** *[Ref: Shinde Chatterjee P-465]*

On 5th day of fasting, blood glucose level will be low and all the physiological changes will work in the direction of increasing the blood glucose level. So **glucagon and growth hormone (GH) are increased[Q].** Whereas, **insulin and glucose tolerance is decreased[Q]. FFA levels are also increased[Q].**

76. B i.e. Sanger **77. A i.e. 1** **78. B i.e. 4-6min** **79. E i.e. C – Peptide**
80. A i.e. ATP dependent K^+ channels **81. B i.e. Epinephrine** **82. C i.e. VIP**
83. C i.e. Adrenalin **84. B i.e. Hypokalemia** **85. D i.e. Insulin**
86. C i.e. Required for transport of glucose, aminoacid, K^+ & Na^+ **87. A i.e. 3rd month**
88. A i.e. Decreased levels of cyclic AMP **89. C i.e. Inhibits Pyruvate dehydrogenase**
90. A i.e. Glucose B i.e. Vagal Stimulation C i.e. Acetyl choline *[Ref: Lehninger 5/e p 903-904,93-44; 292; Ganong 23/e 319-28; Guyton 11/e 366, 968-69; Greenspn Endocrinology 8/e p 115; Gabriel p 312]*

- Nobel prize for **sequencing insulin aminoacid sequence & molecular structure** was given to **Sanger[Q].**
- Insulin is secreted along with **C-peptide in a 1:1 ratio[Q]. Pork insulin differs from human insulin by only 1 aminoacid residue[Q]. Half life of human insulin is 5 minutes[Q].**
- **Glucose mediated insulin release** is mediated through **ATP dependent K^+ channels[Q].**
- **Insulin secretion** is **inhibited by epinephrine (adrenaline)[Q]** and **increased by gastrin, secretin, GIP, CCK[Q], glucose, vagal stimulation and acetyl choline[Q].**
- **Insulin** promotes the **transport of K^+ (potassium) and phosphate (PO4) into cells leading to hypokalemia and hypophosphatemia[Q]**, (i.e. ↓ K^+ & ↓PO^{3-}_4).
- Insulin secretion begins in fetus by **3rd month[Q].** Insulin is required for **transport of glucose, Na^+, K^+ and aminoacids[Q].** Increased insulin to glucagon ratio causes **decreased level of cyclic AMP[Q]. Insulin promotes lipogenesis by activating pyruvate dehydrogenase in adipose tissue[Q] (but not in liver).**

91. A i.e. Ketosis *[Ref: Ganong 22/e P-289-300; Harper 26/e P-189]*

Three conditions lead to deficient intracellular glucose supplies & hence to **ketoacidosis: Starvation, DM (Diabetes Mellitus) and high fat low carbohydrate diet[Q].**

Low Carbohydrate Diet

- Cause defective intracellular glucose supply, and most of the calories are supplied by fat.
- When there is high rate of fatty acid oxidation the *ketone bodies are* formed in hepatic mitochondria to provide calories (ATP) & they accumulate in blood ***(ketosis)***[Q]. Ketone bodies are important fuel in extrahepatic tissue. Small amount of glucose abolishes the ketosis & for this reson *carbohydrate* is said to be ***antiketogenic***[Q].

92. B i.e. Von Gierke's disease **93. A i.e. Gluconeogenesis** **94. A i.e. Insulin** **95. D i.e. Ketogenesis**
96. A, D, & E i.e. Active lipoprotein lipase, Activate Acetyl CoA carboxylase, & Decrease free fatty acid level
97. B i.e. Pyruvate carboxylase *[Ref: Harper's 28/e p. 221-23, 170-71, 416, 150; Lippincott's 5/e p. 347; Chatterjea 7/e p. 549; Ganong 23/e p. 318-19; Satyanarayan 3/e p 671-72; Harrison's 17th/e p. 221-23]*

- **Insulin** acts through **activation of receptor tyrosine kinase activity**[Q] **(an enzyme receptor). Insulin prevents ketogenesis and diabetes mellitus (i.e. lack of insulin) promotes ketogenesis**[Q].
- **Insulin increases lipogenesis (i.e. FA, TG & glycerol P synthesis) and decrease lipolysis and so free fatty acid level**[Q]
- **Insulin activate acetyl CoA carboxylase (rate limiting enzyme of FA synthesis), activate lipoprotein lipase (so increasing TG synthesis) but inhibits hormone sensitive lipase.**[Q]
- **Insulin decreases gluconeogenesis by inactivating pyruvate carboxylase**[Q] **etc and increases glycolysis by inducing phosphofructokinase and pyruvate kinase enzymes**[Q].
- Patient with **hepatomegaly & hypoglycemia not responding to epinephrine** most probably has **von Gierke's disease.**

98. A i.e. Beta cells of pancreas **99. A i.e. GLUT1 & 3** **100. D i.e. GLUT 4**
101. D i.e. GLUT-4 **102. A i.e. Adipose tissue & Skeletal muscle** **103. B i.e. Heart**
104. B i.e. ↑ permeability across cell membrane against glucose gradient
[Ref: Harper's 28/e P- 171; 26/e P-160, Lippincott's 3/e P-95, 310, Ganong 24/e P 434]

- Insulin increases glucose uptake by increasing the number of glucose transporter in cell membrane. **Direct insulin stimulated glucose uptake** is **mediated by Glut 4** and is seen only in: 1) Muscle: **Skeletal muscle**[Q] and **cardiac muscle**[Q] 2) **Adipose tissue**[Q]**. Insulin acts on glucose metabolism by increasing permeability of glucose across cell membrane**[Q]**.**
- **GLUT 3** is used by **brain** (placenta & kidney) and **GLUT 1** is used by **blood brain barrier (BBB, brain,** placenta, kidney, colon & RBC).

Glucose Transporters In Mammals

Facilitated Bidirection Diffusion	Function	Major Sites of Expression	Km
GLUT 1	Basal glucose uptake	- Placenta, **blood – brain barrier,** ***brain***[Q]**,** *RBC, kidney, colon & other organs*	1-2
GLUT 2	B cell glucose sensor; transport out of intestinal & renal epithelial cells.	- **B cells of islets**[Q], Liver, **Small intestine, Kidney**	12-20
GLUT 3	Basal glucose uptake	- Brain, placenta, kidney	<1
GLUT 4	***Insulin stimulated glucose uptake***[Q]	- ***Skeletal & cardiac muscle***[Q] ***Adipose tissue***[Q]	5
GLUT 5	**Fructose transport**	- Jejunum, Sperm	1-2
GLUT 6	None	- ***Brain***[Q], spleen, kidney	-
GLUT 7	***Glucose 6-PO_4 transporter in endoplasmic reticulum***	- Liver	-
Secondary Active Transport Na+ glucose cotransport (unidirectional -transporter)			
SGLT-1	*Active uptake of glucose against concentration gradient*	Small intestine, renal tubule	0.1 - 1.0
SGLT-2		Renal tubule	1.6

105. C i.e. Phlorhizine **106. B i.e. Tetradotoxin** **107. A i.e. γ Na+ during action potential**
[Ref: Ezeilo p. 13, 28, 271, 293, 296; Shinde & Chatterjea 7/ed pg-134, 571; Ganong 23rd/e p. 453-54, 676]

Phlorizin inhibits Na dependent glucose transport[Q]. Whereas phloretin inhibits Na^+ independent GT (GLUT2). **Tetrodotoxin** blocks **sodium channels during action potential**[Q].

108. D i.e. mRNA of insulin *[Ref: Lehninger 4/e P 318-19]*

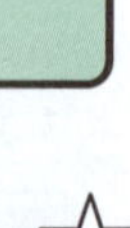

Insulin is synthesized on a large scale basis from complementary DNA's (cDNA), using recombinant technology. But cDNA is not the starting material. ***cDNA are derived from mRNA***[Q].
Thus mRNA is starting material for insulin synthesis on a large scale basis.

- Construction of cDNA from mRNA
- This duplex DNA is inserted into an appropriate cloning vector which produces large number cDNA clones. This method of producing DNA clones from RNA is *Recombinant DNA technology*.

mRNA (from specific cells of an organism)
↓ Reverse transcriptase
Complementary DNA strand
↓
mRNA – DNA hybrid
↓
mRNA is degraded by alkali
↓ DNA polymerase I
Double stranded DNA (cDNA)

109. B i.e. Hepatic steatosis *[Ref: Berne 6/e p. 672, 686, 791]*

Insulin resistance in patients with liver involvement (eg d/t obesity) is because of **lipotoxicity leading to hepatic steatosis or fatty liver** and **nonalcoholic steatotic hepatitis (NASH).**

110. A i.e. Decreased insulin *[Ref: Harrison 17/e p. 2305]*

Decreased insulin is the first (1st) response to hypoglycemia[Q] followed successively by **increase in glucagon, epinephrine, cortical & GH.**

111. E i.e. Insulin: **112. A i.e. Glucocorticoids; B i.e. GH; D i.e. Epinephrine**
113. A i.e. Epinephrine; B i.e. GH; C i.e. Glucocorticoid.
[Ref: CSDT 11/e p 103-105; Best & Taylor's 13/e p 831, 840, 874; Lippincott's 2/e P-30; Lee's 386, Sampson &Wright 3/e P 519-520]

Glucagon, catecholamines (epinephrine & norepinephrine), cortisol, ACTH, GH (growth hormone) are increased in stress (infection, surgery, hypoglycemia) whereas, insulin is suppressed (decreased)[Q]**.**

114. A i.e. VLDL *[Ref: Ganong 22/e P-302]*

- **Maximum triglycerides** are in **chylomicrons**[Q]
- **Exogenous (Dietary) triglycenrides** are maximum in **chylomicrons**[Q]
- **Endogenous triglycerides** are maximum **in VLDL**[Q]

Pineal Gland & Pituitary Gland

115. C i.e. Pineal gland *[Ref: Ganong 22/e P-462]*

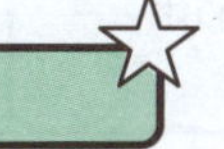

Melatonin is synthesized & secreted by pineal gland[Q]**.**

116. B i.e. Increasing the serotonin N- acetyl transferase *[Ref: Ganong 22/e P-463-64]*

Increased in N-acetyl transferase of hydroxy indole-o-methyl (HOM) transferase activity in darkness l/t increased melatonin secretion[Q]

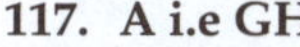

117. A i.e GH **118. A i.e. Anterior hypophysis > B ie. Posterior hypophysis** **119. D i.e. Prolactin**
120. Ai.e. Prolactin & GH **121. A i.e. Oxytocin - Vasopressin** **122. A i.e. Oxytocin & ADH**
123. C i.e. Pars nervosa *[Ref: Ganong 22/e P- 396, BDC 4/e Volume 3 P 99; Guyton 12/ep 898]*

Most anterior pituitary hormone secretion is increased by hypothalamus. But **prolactin is under its inhibitory control (prolactin inhibitory hormone=PIH).** Growth hormone has both GHRH & GH IH (i.e. releasing & inhibitory control). RH = Releasing Hormone & IH = Inhibitory Hormone.

Pituitary gland

Adenohypophysis (Anterior Pituitary)

- Develops as an *upward growth* called *Ratheke's pouch* from ectodermal roof of the stomodeum.

Hormones secreted	**Hypothalmic control**
TSH[Q]	**TRH**
ACTH[Q]	**CRH**
FSH[Q]	**GnRH**
LH[Q]	
Prolactin[Q]	PIH
Growth hormone	GRRH, GHIH

Neurohypophysis / Pars Nervosa (Posterior Pituitary)

- Develops as a downward growth from the *floor of diencephalons* & connected to hypothalamus by neural pathways.
- Oxytocin & ADH is synthesized in supra- optic and ***paraventricular nuclei of of hypothalamus***[Q] in ribosomes of cell bodies. After removing leader sequences in ER, **Secretary granules (Herring bodies)** are packed in golgi apparatus and transported **by axoplasmic flow to pars nervosa**[Q]. **Herring bodies** store ie hormones secreted by post. Pituitary

  - ***Oxytosin***[Q]
  - **Arginine vasopressin *(ADH)***[Q].

Hormone secreting cells of Anterior Pituitary

Acidophillic Cells		***Basophillic Cell***[Q]	
Cell type	Hormone	Cell type	Hormone
Somatotrope	**Growth hormone**	Corticotrope	**ACTH**
		Thyrotrope	**TSH**
Lactotrope	**Prolactin**	Gonadotrope	**FSH, LH**

★ **Melanocyte stimulating hormone (MSH)** is secreted by ***intermediate pituitary gland***[Q]. However, intermediate lobe is rudimentary in humans & it appears that MSH is not secreted in adults.

124. A i.e. Early morning *[Ref: Ganong 22/e P-373]* **125. C i.e. Evening**

- **ACTH level** is ***highest during early morning***[Q]. About 75% of daily output occurs *between 4 AM and 10 AM*. Secretion is *least in the evening*. The biological clock responsible for diurnal variation of ACTH is located in ***suprachiasmatic nuclei of hypothalamus***[Q].

- **ACTH secretion is increased** in **stress** (1. mental or emotional stress, endogenous depression, 2. physical stress or illness, exercise), alcohol abuse, obesity and ACTH producing tumors.

126. B i.e. Growth hormone *[Ref: Ganong 22/e P-409, 402]*

Tumors of somatortopes of the anterior pituitary secrete large amount of growth hormone, leading in **children to gigantism** and in **adults to acromegaly**.
Hypersecretion of GH is accompamied by hypersecretion of prolactin in 20 – 40% of patient with acromegaly.

Somatomedian: are polypeptide growth factors secreted by liver & other tissues. The effect of growth hormone on growth, cartilage and protein metabolism depend on interaction between GH & somatomedian.

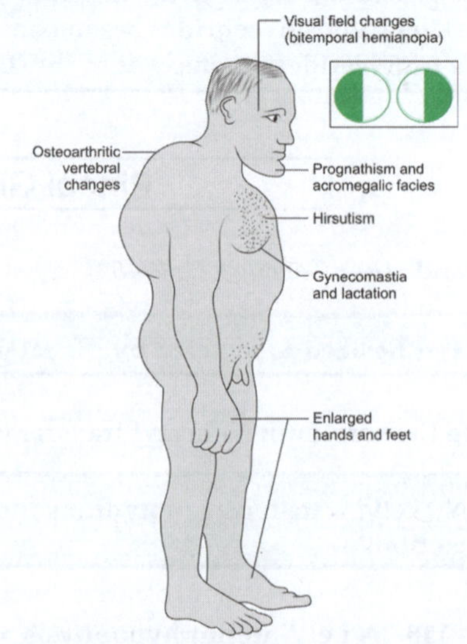

127. A i.e. Deposition of chondroitin sulfate *[Ref: Ezeilo p. 288, 310; Guyton 11th/e p. 923-24; Ole Holger petergson 5/ep – 247; Hans Hess: vol 17/pg- 223 (both on books, google.com) Ganong 23rd/e p. 382-84; 318, 321]*

Growth hormone exerts much of its effects (especially on growth, cartilage & protein metabolism) through intermediate polypeptide growth factors also k/a somatomedin or insulin like growth factor secreted by liver & other tissues. The first of somatomedin isolated was called sulfation factor because it **stimulated incorporation of sulfate into cartilage (i.e. deposition of chondroitin sulfate)**[Q] and collagen formation.

128. C i.e. Sleep *[Ref: Ganong 24/ep 330]*

Stimuli Affecting Growth Hormone (GH) Secretion

Decreasing GH	Increased GH Secretion
REM SleepQ, Glucose, Cortisol, Free fatty acids, GH, IGF-1, Medroxy progesterone	- **Going to sleep, Hypoglycemia, Fasting, Exercise**Q**, Stress** - 2-deoxyglucose, Protein meal, Arginine infusion, ↑ blood level of amino acids, Lysine vasopressin, **Pyrogen**, Glucagon - L Dopa & α adrenergic agonists, Apo morphine (dopamine receptor agonist), Estrogen & Androgen

129. B i.e. Dopamine *[Ref: Ganong 22/e P- 423]*

Dopamine acts as **hypothalamic prolactin inhibiting hormone**Q and decreases prolactin secretion.

L – DOPAQ	Decreases prolactin release by formation of dopamine
BromocriptineQ (& Dopamine agonists)	Inhibits prolactin releas by stimulating dopamine receptors.
ChlorpromazineQ (& Dopamine antagonist)	Enhances prolactin release by blocking dopamine receptors

Factors enhancing prolactin secretion: [Mnemonic: **Nu PETS SHOP]**		
Nu – Nursing	S – **Stress**Q	S – Sexual intercourse
P – **Pregnancy**Q	S – **Strenuous excercise**Q	H – Hypoglycemia
E – **Estrogen**Q	S – **Breast stimulation**Q in non- lactating women	H – **Hypothyroidism**Q
T – **TRH**Q		O – **Opiates**Q
S – **Somatiostatin**Q	S – **Sleep**Q	P – **Phenothiazine**Q

Posterior Pituitary Hormone

130. B i.e. Posterior lobe

Pituicytes are glial cells of posterior pituitary which assist in storage & release of ADH & oxytocin hormone.

131. D i.e. Prolactin cause contraction of Myoepithelial cells and not affected by emotion

Milk secretion (ejection or let down) a **neuroendocrinal reflex**Q is caused by **oxytocin secreted from posterior pituitary**Q. Oxytocin, **whose secretion is affected by emotions**Q & genital stimulation, cause **contraction of myoepithelial cells**Q that lie outside the alveoli and hence l/t milk ejection.

132. D i.e. V4-CNS *[Ref: Ganong 23/e 279, 665-66; Guyton 11/e 358-62, 928-29; 734, 1040-41; Katzung 10/e p 614-15]*
133. D i.e. Supraoptic nucleus **134. A i.e. Hyperosmolarity** **135. C i.e. Increased secretion when plasma osmolality is low**
136. D i.e. Free form **137. A i.e. Diabetes mellitus**

- **ADH** is formed primarily in **supraoptic nuclei**Q, whereas **oxytocin** is formed mainly in **paraventricular nuclei**Q of hypothalamus. Both hormones are secreted in **free form** or loosely bound to **neurophysin (II & I** respectively but then immediately gets detached) to **circulate in blood as free hormone forms**Q.
- **Hyperosmolarity is the greatest stimulator for ADH secretion**Q. So **injection of hyperosmolar (concentrated) electrolyte solution in artery supplying hypothalamus (supraoptic nucleus mainly) cause release of ADH**Q.
- **Neurosecretion of posterior pituitary hormone ADH (antidiuretic hormone or vaspression)** mainly from **supraoptic nuclei of hypothalamus is increased with increased plasma osmolality (hyperosmolality)** and is decreased with decreased plasma osmolality. **Surgery, exercise, stress, pain also increaseADH secretion**Q**. ADH increases the permeability of distal tubule & collecting ducts to water**Q **therefore retaining water in excess of solute.**
- **Vasopressin (ADH)** has 3 receptor – **V_{1A} receptor** in **vascular smooth muscles**Q, (causing vasoconstriction), liver (glycogenolysis) and area postrema of brain (decreasing cardiac output); **V_{1B} or V_3 receptor in anterior pituitary**Q (increasing ACTH secretion); and V_2 receptor in **principal cells of collecting ducts**Q (augmenting movement of water through water channel **aquaporin-2)**.
- **Diabetes mellitus** results from **complete or absolute lack of insulin d/t reduction in β -cell mass of pacrease**Q. It has nothing to do with pituitary.

Hypothalamus mediated response	Part of hypothalamus responsible	
Response to heat[Q]	Anterior hypothalamus	Preoptic
Response to cold[Q]	**Posterior hypothalamus (Shivering center)**	area
Circadian rhythm[Q]	**Suprachiasmatic nucleus**[Q]	
GnRH is secreted[Q]	Arcuate nucleus	
Oxytocin released[Q]	Paraventricular nucleus	
ADH released[Q] mainly	**Supraoptic nucleus**[Q]	
Satiety centre[Q]	Ventromedial hypothalamus	
Food intake is governed[Q]	Ventromedial hypothalamus	
Feeding (hunger) and thirst centre[Q]	Lateral hypothalamus	

Magnocellular neurons of Supraoptic nuclei & Paraventricular nuclei of hypothalamus form precursor molecule i.e.

- **Signal peptide + AVP + Neurophysin II + Glycopeptide (copeptin)**
- **Signal peptide + Oxytocin + Neurophysin I**

Signal /leader sequence removed in **ER**, packaged into secretory granule (**Herring bodies**) in GA and transported through axon by axoplasmic flow to reach nerve endings in posterior pituitary in several days.

Cleaved during transport and so storage granules contain free ADH/oxytocin, corresponding neurophysin & glycol peptide (in vasopressin neurons) which are released in circulation.

138. D i.e. Vasopressin

Thirst -ADH (Vasopressin) Mechanism

It is the **major (most important) regulator of body Na^+ and water balance**[Q], maintaining **near perfect Na^+ balance** in body (even in absence of aldosterone)

Aldosterone (Renin-Angiotensin System)

- It is a **weak regulator of Na^+-water b/o mineralo-corticoid escape** i.e.
  1. ↓ Na^+ with normal ECF volume is weak stimulator of aldosterone
  2. Aldosterone ↑ tubular reabsorption of both Na^+ & water and so expansion of ECF volume produces natriuresis
- **Aldosterone is key regulator of external K^+ balance**[Q] (absence of which may r/i fatal hyperkalemia

Thyroid Gland

139. C i.e. 2-3 months

140. A i.e. Albumin; B i.e. Globuin; C i.e. Prealbumin *[Ref: Ganong 23/e P- 305.; Guyton 10/e P 833]*

In thyroid follicles, thyroid hormones (thyroxin, T_3) are stored for 2-3 months[Q] (i.e. in amounts sufficient to supply normal requirements for 2-3 months).

- Thyroid hormones in blood is transported combined with plasma proteins. Normally 99.9% of T_4 (&T_3) in plasma is protein bound. Plasma protein which bind T_4 & T_3 are: 1) ***Albumin***[Q] 2) Thyroxine binding ***prealbumin***[Q] (TBPA) (new called transthyretin) 3)Thyroxine binding ***globulin***[Q] (TBG): affinity to bind T_4 is maximum.
- ***Transferrin***[Q] [apotrans ferrin (β -globulin) + Fe]: ***transport iron to plasma***[Q]. ***Ceruloplasmin***[Q] [Copper binding protein] transport Cu to plasma.

Protein	Plasma Concentration (mg/dl)	Amount of Circulating Hormone bound (%)	
		T_4	T_3
TBG[Q]	2	*67*[Q]	46
Transthyretin[Q] (TBPA)	15	20	1
Albumin[Q]	3500	13	53

141. D i.e. T4 has shorter half life than T3 *[Ref: Ganong 22/e P-319; KDT 5th/e P-228]*

Plasma ***T1/2 of T_4 is more (6-7 days)***[Q] than T_3 (1-2days).

142. D i.e. Iodine intake *[Ref: Ganong 24/ep 309]*

Iodine is **fastest acting thyroid inhibitor**[Q]. So **excessive iodine intake** inhibits its own transport in thyroid cells, alter redox potential of cells, **interfering iodination and thus reducing T_3/T_4 synthesis (Wolff-Chaikoff effect)** .
All aspects of thyroid hormone synthesis are affected but **most important effect is thyroid constipation (i.e. inhibition of thyroid hormone release)**[Q].

143. A i.e. Pituitary **144. B i.e. Thyroid; D i.e. Salivary gland; E i.e. Mammary Gland.** *[Ref:Ganong 24/e P- 341]*

Iodine uptake i.e. **sodium-iodine symporter (Na-I symporter)** is seen in **thyroid gland, salivary gland, mammary gland**[Q], **gastric mucosa, placenta, ciliary body of eye & choroids plexus.**

145. A i.e. ↓↓ Lipolysis, C↓BMR *[Ref: Ganong 22/e P-324; Chaudhuri 5/e P- 262-263]*

Thyroxine increases BMR, Lipolysis, O_2 consumption and myocardial contractility[Q].

146. C i.e. Growth hormone *[Ref: Harrison 16/e P-2090, 2096]*

About 60% of patients with GH – secreting tumours may exhibit ***paradoxical GH response to TRH stimulation.***
TRH induced GH stimulation may occur ***in acromegaly**[Q]**, renal failure & depression.***

Kidney & Adrenal Gland

147. B i.e. Angiotensin I *[Ref: Berne & Levy 6/e p 699, 655; Ganong 23/e 670; Guyton 11/e p 907; Gabriel p-145, 227]*

- **Kidney** produces **rennin (& so angiotensin I), erythropoietin and 1, 25-dihydroxy vitamin D3 (Cholecalciferol)**[Q], Mn "**RED3**". Erythropoietin (peptide) increases erythrocyte production; rennin (peptide) converts angiotensinogen to angiotensin I and 1,25 $(OH)_2$ vitamin D (steroid) causes bone mineralization by increasing intestinal Ca^{++} absorption.
- **Liver** produces **25-hydroxy vitamin D (calcifediol), vitamin D binding protein (DBP), angiotensinogen**[Q], insulin like growth factor type I (IGF-1) & testosterone.
- **ACE (angiotensin converting enzyme)** and so **angiotensin II** is produced in **endothelium** of mainly **lungs** (but conversion also occurs in many other parts).

Angiotensinogen (Liver)
↓ **Renin (Kidney)**
Angiotensin I
↓ **ACE (Lung-endothelium)**
Angiotensin II (Lung- endothelium)

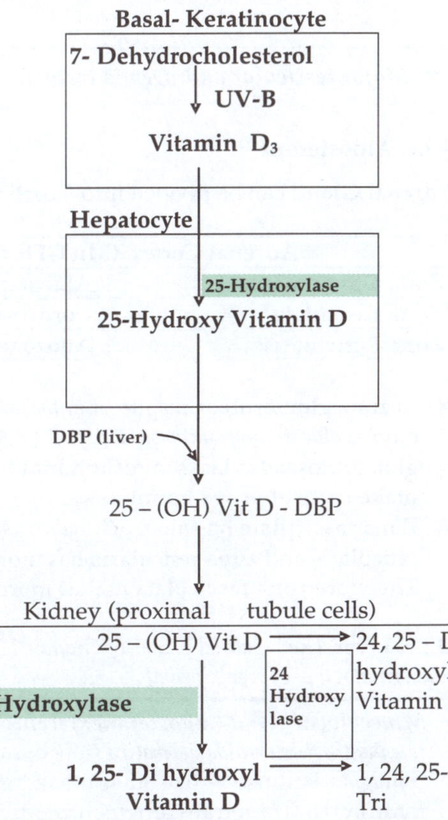

- **Heart** produces **atrial natriuretic peptide (ANP); adipose tissue** produce leptin & adiponectin; **Stomach** produce gastrin, somatostatin & ghrelin; **intestines** produce **secretion**, cholecystokinin (CCK), glucagons like peptide (GLP) 1, and 2, motilin and glucose dependent insulinotropic peptide (GIP; gastric inhibitory peptide); **adipose tissue & mammary glands** produce estradiol 17 β-; **liver & sebaceous gland** produce testosterone and **genital skin and prostate** produce 5-Dihydrotestosterone (DHT).
- Granulocyte & granulocyte – macrophage colony stimulating factors (**GCSF & GM – CSF respectively**) are hemopoietic growth factors (like erythropoietin). G – CSF is relatively specific and induces mainly granulocytes. GM – CSF induces granulocytes, macrophages, and eosinophils.

148. B i.e. Adrenal medulla normally secretes epinephrine & in excess of..

149. C i.e. Norepinephrine

150. A i.e. Aldosterone *[Ref: Harrison 16/e P-2148; Ganong 22/e P-356]*

151. C i.e. 17-ketosteroid dehydroepiandrosterone

Adrenal medullary hormones (adrenaline, norepinephrine, dopamine) are not essential for lifeQ, but they help to prepare the individual to deal with emergencies. **Adrenal cortex is essential for life**Q. **The mineratocorticoids & Glucocorticoids are essential for life**Q. **In health, 80% of output from adrenal medulla is epinephrine & only 20% is noradrenalin**Q.

Pheochromocytoma are catecholamine secreting ***tumour of chromaffin cells***Q derived from adrenal medulla or extradrenal sources (chromaffin cells in or about sympathetic ganglia)

Adrenal	Extra adrenal
Most of them secrete *nor epinephrine* in greater amount ***[Na: Adr= 20:1]***Q.	Most of them *exclusively* secrete ***Nor epinephrine***Q.

Hormones of Adrenal Gland

Adrenal Cortex

Zona glomerulosa	Zona faciculate	Zona reticularis
- **Mineralocorticoids**Q - **Aldosterone**Q - Deoxycorticosterone	- **Glucocorticoids**Q - **Cortisol**Q - Corticosterone	**Androgens eg.** - **17 Ketosteroid- DHEA (Dehydro Epi Androsterone)**Q **is major adrenal androgen** - Androstenedione.

★ ***Major testicular androgen is testosterone***Q

Adrenal Medulla

- ***Norepinephrine***Q
- Epinephrine
- Dopamine

★ Adrenals may also secrete *small amount of estrogen,* although most of the estrogen that are not formed in the ovaries are produced in the cirulation from adrenal androstenedione.

152. A i.e. Aldosterone

Adrenal Gland can be divided into 3 **cortical zones & medulla**

Adrenal Cortex (Mn GFR from out to in)	
Zona Glomerulosa	**Aldosterone**Q
Zona Fasiculata	**Corticosteroids mainly**
Zona Reticularis	**Androgen (sex steroids) mainly**

Adrenal Medulla

Epinephrine & NorepienphrineQ

★ In **zone glomerulosa** inspite of *mitochondrial 11β hydroxylase (P 450 C 11 or (YP 11* ***B1****)*, a closely related mitochondrial enyme *aldosterone synthase (P 450 C 11 AS or CYP 11 B2)*, is found (gene of both enzymes found and *chromosome 8)*. Zona glomerulosa also lacks mitochondrial *17α hydroxylase (P450 C****17*** *or cYP-****17****)* that is why **it makes aldosterone but fails to make cortisol or sex hormone**Q.

★ **Zona fasciculate** has more *3β- hydroxysteroid dehydrogenase (smooth endoplasmic reticulum enzyme activity)* than zona reticularis and **zona reticularis** has more of cofactors required for expression of *17, 20 lyase activity of 17α hydroxylase*. Therefore **zona fasciculata makes more cortisol & corticosterone, & zone reticularis makes more androgen**Q.

153. D i.e. Liver *[Ref: Gabriel p. 305-6; Guyton 11th/e p. 947-50; Ganong 23rd/e p. 342-48, 355-59; Stuart: molecular & cellular pediatric endocrinology p-219; wikipedia]*

- ***Mineralocorticoid (aldosterone) receptors are not found in liver***Q. Much of Aldosterone is *metabolized in liver to tetrahydroglucuronide derivative* (inactive) and some is changed in *liver & kidney* to *18- glucuronide* also k/a *acid labile conjugate'* because unlike other breakdown products of steroids, it is converted back to free aldosterone at pH 1 by hydrolysis. 40% tetrahydroglucuronide, 5% acid labile conjugate & < 1% free aldosterone appear in urine.
- **Mineral corticoid receptors** are present in ***collecting tubules (principal cells), distal tubules & collecting ducts of kidney, sweat glands, salivary glands, and intestinal epithelium especially in colon***Q causing conservation (reabsorption) of Na^+ & water and secretion (excretion) of K^+ & HCO_3^-. These receptors are also found in ***brain (hippocampus), myocardium, muscle, vessels (peripheral vasculature) and brown adipose tissue***Q.

154. A , C, & D i.e. ↑ Neoglucogenesis, ↑ Proteolysis, & ↑ Protein anabolism in liver *[Ref: Gabriel p. 302-4; Chatterjea & Shinde 7th/e p. 556-57; Harper 28th/e p. 116, 171, 221-22, 430-31, 442- 43; Katzung 10/e p640; KDT 6th/ed pg-277]*

Glucocorticoid is anti-insulin hormone that is catabolic to peripheral tissues and anabolic to liver. So in **liver** it increases **glycogen and protein synthesis and gluconeogenesis**[Q] whereas, in peripheral tissue it causes hyper glycemia (d/t **decreased glucose uptake and decreased glycolysis)**[Q], **increased free fatty acids & aminoacids** in plasma (d/t **increased lipolysis and proteolysis respectively)**[Q]

155. C i.e. Increased excretion from kidney *[Ref: MTx: Glucocorticoids]*

Glucocorticoids (steroid) facilitate or increase free water clearance (i.e. rapid excretion of water load) and uric acid excretion. It also inhibits intestinal absorption and enhance renal excretion of Ca^{++}[Q] (esp. on large dose). So prolonged use of steroids cause **osteoporosis**[Q] **(decreased bone matrix)**[Q].

156. A i.e. Inhibiton of phospholipase A2

Anti-inflammatory action of Steroids is d/t inhibition of phospholipase A-2[Q].

157. A i.e. Cortisol *[Ref: Ganong 24/e p 366-369; Williams 7/e p 869]*

Diurnal variation in eosinophilic count is reciprocally (invrsely) related to circadian levels of cortisol[Q].

158. A i.e. ↑Aldosterone; C i.e. ↑ Epinephrine; E i.e. Edema *[Ref: Ganong 23rd/e p. 349-51; Harrison 17/e p. 2252-55; 356, 359; ACTH stimulation of adrenal epinephrine & norepinephrine vol 23, Nov 2008; Textbook of Physiology Gabriel C Ezeilo p. 307-8]*

- In **cushing syndrome** there may be **increase in ACTH (in ACTH dependent type), aldosterone (for 1-2 days), deoxycorticosterone, angiotensin secretion and even epinephrine & norepinephrine leading to hypertension and edema**[Q].

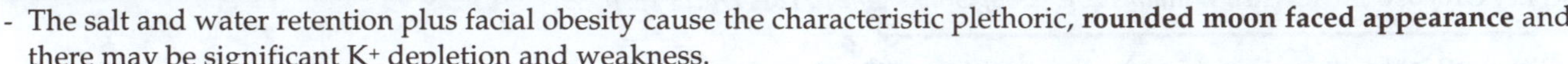

- The salt and water retention plus facial obesity cause the characteristic plethoric, **rounded moon faced appearance** and there may be significant K^+ depletion and weakness.
- Osteoporosis, precipitation of diabetes, prominent reddish purple striae on thin skin, poor wound healing, thin extremities, pedulous abdomen, buffalo hump, moon face and red cheeks are other features of cushing syndrome.
- 3 primary regulatory factors involve in **aldosterone secretion** are ***ACTH, renin (via angiotensin II) and rise in plasma K+ concentration***[Q] *(Ganong - 356).*

159. E i.e. Hypernatremia *[Ref: Ganong 23/e P-357-58; Chaudhuri 5/e P-281; Guyton 11/e P-948-952]*

Increase in plasma Na^+ inhibits aldosterone secretion & acute decline in plasma Na^+ stimulates its secretion.[Q]

160. D i.e. Metabolic acidosis

161. B i.e. Very High Na^+ in plasma *[Ref: Guyton 11th/e p. 948; Ganong 23rd/e p. 356-59; Gabriel p-305-07]*

- **Hyperaldosteronism (excess mineralocorticosteroid)** leads to ***potassium (K^+) depletion / hypokalemia and sodium (Na^+) retention, usually without edema but with weakness tetany, polyuria, hypertension and hypokalemic mild metabolic alkalosis***[Q].
- Hyperaldosteronism ***does not cause metabolic acidoss***[Q]. And plasma ***Na^+ level is elevated only slightly if at all***[Q] because water is retained with osmolically active Na^+ ions.

162. D i.e. 11 β hydroxysteroid dehydrogenase *Ref: Ganong 23rd/e p. 355*

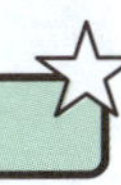

Apparent mineralocorticoid excess is d/t ***inhibition or absence of 11β hydroxysteroid dehydrogenase type 2***[Q]

163. C i.e. Dexamethasone.

Glucocorticoid (GC) & Mineralacorticoid (MC) Activity of Steroids

Adrenal Steroids	GC	MC
Cortisol	1	1
Corticosterone	0.3	15
Aldosterone	0.3	**3000**
Deoxycorticosterone	0.2	**100**
Dehydroepiandrosterone	-	-

Synthetic Steroids	GC	MC
Cortisone	0.7	0.8
Prednisolone	4	0.8
Methyl Prednisone	5	-
Dexamethasone	25 -30	-
9 α- Fluorocortisol	10	125

164. A i.e. Glycogenolysis *[Ref: Ganong 22/e P- 360; KDT 5th/e P-110]*

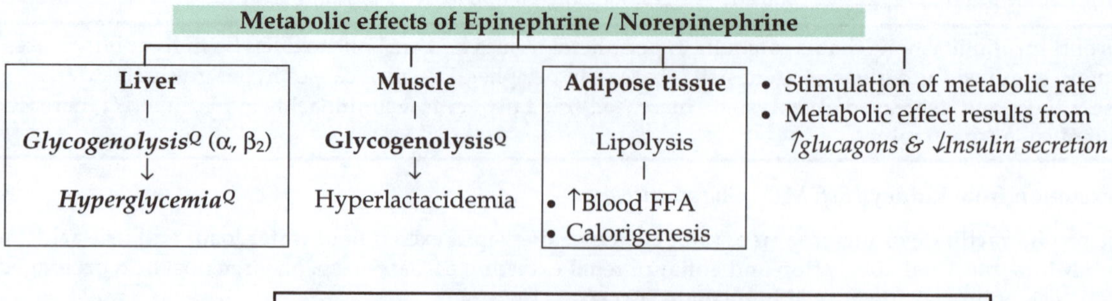

Reproductive Hormones

165. D i.e. Placenta *[Ref: Ganong 23/e p. 425]*

β-HCG (human chorionic gonadotropin) is secreted by syncytiotrophoblast of placenta^Q.

166. A i.e. Pubertal breast enlargement in girls

- **In girls, at puberty, thelarche (breast development/enlargement) is the first event^Q,** followed by **pubarche** (development of pubic & axillary hair) and then by **menarche** (first menstrual period). Estrogen is growth hormone of breast responsible for thelarche.
- **Adrenarche** ie increased secretion of adrenal androgens also occurs in humans at puberty.

167. C i.e. Glucose *[Ref: Williams 23/e p. 88; Gray's 40/e p. 181; Dutta 7/e p. 39]*

Glucose^Q is the **sugar found in amniotic fluid.**

168. D i.e. Progesterone; & Corticosteroid
[Ref: Harper's 27/e P- 446-50]

C- 21 steroids	- *Corticosteroids (gluco & mineralocorticoids)^Q* - *Progesterone^Q*	**17-Hydroxy steroids** i.e. OH gp at 17
C- 19 steroids	- **Testosterone** - **Androgen**	**17-keto steroids** i.e. Keto gp at 17
C- 18 steroid:	**Estrogen**	

169. D i.e. Increased triglyceride & cholesterol level in serum
[Ref: Lippincott's 3/e P- 376, Chatterjea 6/e P- 451, Dutta 5/e 585]

Increased triglyceride and cholesterol levels are best attributed to the metabolic effects of steroidal contraceptives^Q rather than as consequence of decreased vitamin B 6 level. Effects of OCP on lipid metabolism
- Plasma lipid and lipoproteins are increased
- Total cholesterol & triglyceride are increased.
- Use of OCP is also associated with deficiency of pyridoxine(Vit. B6).

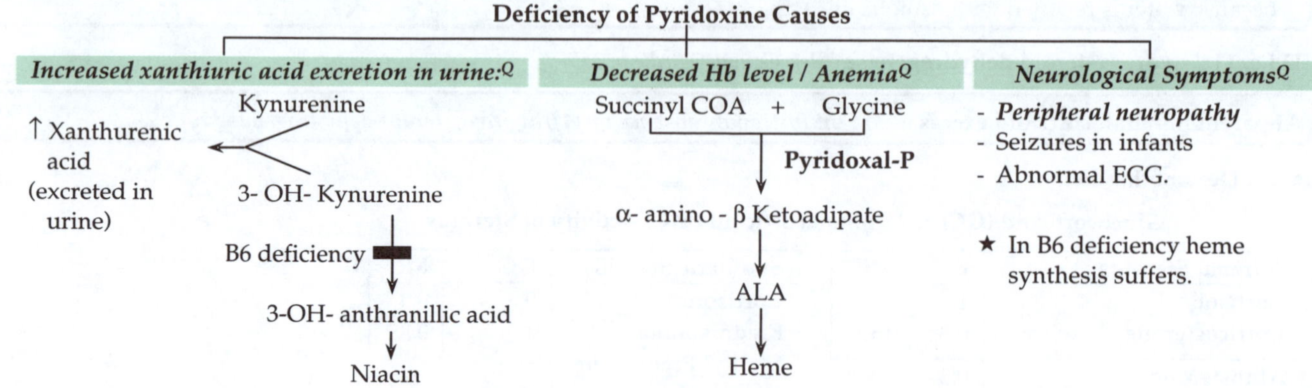

170. C i.e. Gamma amino butyric acid. *[Ref: Ganong 22/e P-419]*

> Gn RH neurosecretion has been shown to be under the control of many neurotransmitter & neuropeptides:
> - **GABA** – exerts an **inhibitory action on GnRH secretion before onset of puberty**[Q].
> - **Glutamate** – has an **excitatory effect**[Q] & whose levels increase **at the onset of puberty**[Q].

Gama amino butyric acid (GABA)[Q] appears to be an inhibitory neurotransmitter responsible for restricting LHRH release before onset of puberty in female rhesus monkey.

171. A i.e. Estrous cycle *[Ref: Levy & Berne 6/e p 776-77; Novak's 14/e p 172; William's obstetrics 23/e p 36; Ganong 23/e p. 412-17]*

> - **Humans** undergo **menstrual** cycle, **ovarian** cycle, **uterine (endometrial)** cycle, uterine **cervx** cycle, **vaginal** cycle, **anovulatory cycles** and cyclic changes in breast, **but not an estrous cycle**[Q].
> - **Mammals other than primates** donot menstruate and their sexual cycle is called an **estrous (heat) cycle**[Q]. It is named for the conspicuous period of heat (estrus) at the time of ovulation, normally the only time during which sexual interest of female is aroused.

Feature	Menstrual cycle	Estrous Cycle
Occurs in	**Menstruating** mammals in cluding humans & higher prmates	**Non menstruating** mammals other than primates
Fate of endometrium, if conception does not occur	**Shed** as menstruation	**Reabsorbed**
Females are sexually aroused & receptive	At any time of cycle unrelated to time of ovulation	Only around the **time of ovulation** (i.e. **estrous phase or heat of cycle**)

172. C i.e. LH **173. A i.e. 14 days prior to mensturation** **174. A i.e. High estrogen, low progesterone**

175. B i.e. LH *[Ref: Ganong 22/e P-434-445;Chaudhuri 5/e P-318; Shaws 12/e P-37]*

> **A surge in LH secretion triggers ovulation**[Q], and ovulation normally occurs about **9 hours after the peak of LH surge at midcycle (i.e. 14 days prior to start of next menstruation)**[Q]. **L H surge causes ovulation**[Q]. For ovulation to occur the hormone picture should be **high estrogen & low progesteron**[Q].

Action of LH **are**
- Stimulates **ovulation**[Q].
- **Formation & maintenance of corpus luteum**[Q]
- **Formation of progesterone in the corpus leutieum from the lutein cells**[Q].

176. A i.e. FSH **177. B i.e. Granulosa Cell** *[Ref: Ganong Physiology 22/e P- 446, 432; Chaudhuri Physiology 5/e P- 318]*

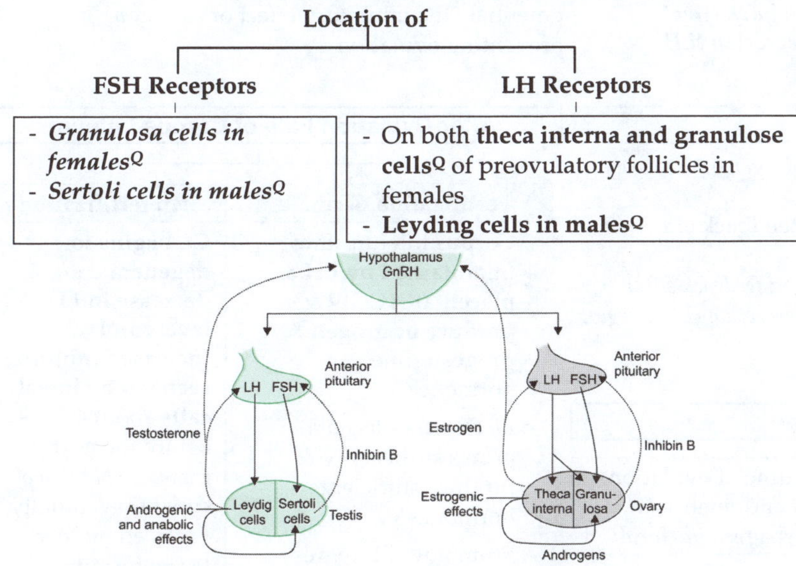

- - - Broken line = inhibitory pathway; ----- solid line = stimulatory pathway

Sertoli cells have **receptors for FSH & testosterone**[Q]

FSH stimulates the first half of spermatogenesis	**Testosterone** causes last half of Spermatogenesis

★ **FSH** is responsible for early growth of ovarian follicle in female; where as **LH** is responsible for final maturation of ovarian follicle & estrogen secretion from them. It is also responsible for ovulation, initial formation of corpus luteum and secretion of progesterone.

178. B i.e. FSH *[Ref: Harrison 17/e p 2331; Berne & Levy 6/e p 776-77; William Gynaecology (2008) 1/e p 434; Daftari Reproductive endocrinology p-250]*

Ovarian reserve can be best assessed by measuring ***FSH levels on 3rd day of menstrual cycle,*** **clomiphene citrate challenge / provocative test** (measures **FSH levels on cycle day 10** after antiestrogen clomiphene citrate 100 mg administration from day 5 to 9). **Serum inhibin B level** and **ultrasonic scanning to count** the number of **antral follicles** in ovary are other methods.

179. B i.e. Progesterone

180. D i.e. Progesterone *[Ref: Shaw's 12/e P-167]*

Whether the cycle is ovulatory or anovulatory can be studied by ***plasma level of progesterone and LH***Q.

Plasma Progesterone

- Progesterone is secreted by ***Corpus luteum***Q (which is formed after ovulation), placenta and in small amount by follicle.
- **Its concentration rises after ovulation & peaks at mid *luteal phase (around day 20)* and then declines as luteum degenerates**Q.

Plasma LH

- LH is secreted by anterior pituitary gland
- LH surge causes ovulation and formation of corpus luteum.
- Its peak *(LH surge)* is reached about ***24-36 hrs before ovulation***Q.
- After ovulation its level start falling because of negative feedback of progesterone.

181. A i.e. Maternal ovary

Estrogen is primarily secreted by **granulosa cells of ovarian (griffin) follicles (before ovulation), corpus luteum (after fertilization in early pregnancy)**Q and by **placenta (in late pregnancy (after 8 weeks).**

Hormonal Picture at the time of Ovulation / LH Surge

For ovulation to occur ***Estrogen should be high & Progesteron should be low***Q.

Estrogen

- At the time of ovulation, ova in the Graffian follicle needs to be well developed, which is accomplished by ' ***high estrogen***Q
- LH secretion is held in check by negative feedback effect of rising plasma estrogen.
- ***At 36-48 hours before ovulation estrogen feed back effect becomes positive & initiates a burst of LH secretion (LH surge)***Q

Progesteron

- Progesteron is secreted by the *corpus luteum,* which is the remnant of graffian follicles *after the ova has been released.* Thus ***progesterone would rise only after ovulation***Q.
- Large doses of progesterone *inhibit LH secretion* & potentiate the inhibitory effect of estrogen, preventing ovulation

LH Surge

- Just prior to ovulation there is an *increase in estrogen* and to *some degree progesterone* level.
- LH secretion is held in check by the negative feedback effect of rising plasma estrogen.
- But at *36 – 48 hours before* ovulation the estrogen *feedback effect becomes positive* & this initiates the *burst of LH secretion (LH Surge),* FSH secretion also peaks.
- This ***LH surge induces ovulation***Q.

Other indicators of Ovulation

- Increase in ***basal body temperature***Q at the time of ovulation
- Presence of ***secretory pattern***Q on biopsy of endometrium.
- Presence of ***thick cervical mucus***Q that forms a ***fern pattern***Q

After Ovulation Fate of Corpus Luteum

Fertilization occurs

- **Corpus** luteum stays **(maintained by LH & placental HCG)**Q & **produce oestrogen & progesterone** hormones.
- *By 8th week* placenta grows sufficiienty & produce sufficient hormones.
- From now CL regress.

No fertilization

CL begins to degenerate d/t decrease in LH levels and increased inhibin secreted by luteal calls about 4 days before the next menses *(24th day of cycle)* & eventually replaced by scar tissue forming *corpus albicans*

182. C i.e. Pregnanediol *[Ref: Ganong 24/e p. 409; KDT 6/e p. 308]*

Progesterone (21C steroid) is formed from cholesterol (→ pregnenolone) has short half life and is converted in liver to **pregnanediol (most common end product)** which is conjugated to glucronic acid and excreted in urine as sodium pregnanediol-20-glucuronide.

183. D i.e. Progesterone *[Ref: Ganong 23/e P-410-14]*

184. A i.e. Progesterone

- **Progesterone** is *thermogenic* & responsible for the ***rise in basal body temperature***Q at the time of ovulation
- Increase in basal body temperature at the time ovulation in reliable indicator of time of ovulation. The rise starts 1-2 days after ovulation. Other indicators of ovulation - ***Secretory pattern***Q on biopsy of endometrium, *Thick cervical mucus* that forms a fern pattern

Preovulatory proliferative changes in endometrium	**are d/t estrogen**
Postovulatory secretary changes in endometrium	**are d/t-progesterone (mainly)**

185. C i.e. Long arm of X-Chromosome *[Ref: Harrison 16/e P-2128]*

The androgen receptor is a typical member of the steroid/ thyroid family and is encoded by a gene on the ***long arm of X-chromosome***Q.

186. C i.e. Aromatase

187. B i.e. Glycolysis increases

[Ref: Gabriel C Ezeilo p. 366-73; Ganong 23rd/e p. 348, 371, 392, 427, 416; Diabetes & Pregnancy 2/e p. 459]

Aromatase is the enzyme that catalyzes the conversion of ***testosterone to estradiol***Q and *androstenedione to estrone.* ***Estrogen increases glycolysis***Q.

188. B i.e. Estrogen *[Ref: Harrison 17/e p 1920; Robbin's 7/e p- 882; Neena Khanna 3/e p 330]*

In **chronic liver disease** (especially **cirrhosis)** and **pregnancy**, ***impaired estrogen metabolism and consequent hyper estroenemia***Q leads to **spider angiomata /nevi** (superficial, tortous arterioles, that unlike simple telangiectases, typically fill from the center outwards and occur invariably on upper half of body) and **palmar erythema** (mottled redness of thenar & hypothenar eminences).

189. A i.e. Granulosa cells *[Ref: Ganong 22/e P-446, 432; Chaudhuri Concise Physiology 5/e P-318]*

- **FSH** acts on the ***granulose cells in female and sertoli cells in males***Q
- **LH** acts on ***both theca interna & granulose cells***Q of pre ovulatory ovarian follicles in females and ***on leydig cells in males***Q.

190. A i.e. Spermiogenesis **191. D i.e. Inhibin** **192. C i.e. FSH** **193. B i.e. Decreased FSH**

Ganong 23rd/e p. 402-3; Grays 40th/e p. 1265-67, 1317-20; Smith urology 17thed pg-686-87; Basic Histology – test & Atlas 11/ed pg-427; Gabriel p. 354-56; Chaudhari 6/ed pg-324; Endocrine physiology 11/ed pg-478

- **Sertoli cells** have **receptors for FSH & testosterone**Q**; secrete inhibin, Mullerian inhibiting (regression) factor, & androgen binding protein**Q. They are involved in **orchestration and coordination of all key events in spermatogenesis & spermiogenesis**Q.
- Spermatids donot divide but gradually mature into spermatozoa by a series of nuclear & cytoplasmic changes k/a **spermiogenesis**. All of these maturational changes **take place while spermatids remain closely associated with sertoli cells**Q. Spermiogenesis involves – golgi, cap, acrosomal and final phase. In the final phase of maturation, excess cytoplasm is detached as a residual body that is **phagocytized & degraded by sertoli cells**Q

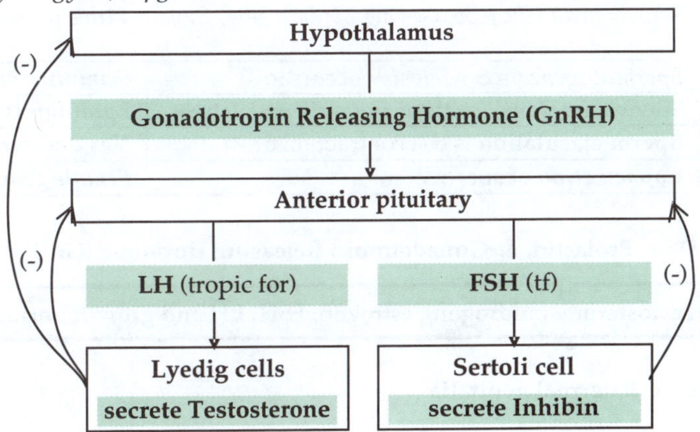

194. A i.e. Sartioli & Sertoli cells *[Ref: MTx]*

Occluding **tight junctions between sertoli cells forms the BTB (Blood Testis Barrier)[Q].**

195. A i.e. Leydig cells

196. D i.e. It inhibits secretion of FSH *[Ref Ganong 22/e P-432; Chaudhuri 5/e P- 311]*

- **'Between the tubules in the testes are nests of cells containing lipid granules, the 'Interstitial cells of Leydig' which secretes testesterone into the blood stream'**
- **Inhibin** is a polypeptide hormone and **inhibits FSH secretion[Q]** of anterior pituitary by direct action.

Testes

- Seminiferous tubules
  - Primitive germ cells
    - Mature into primary spermatocytes
  - **Sertoli cells**
    - **Secrete :**
      - **Androgen binding protein[Q]**
      - **Inhibin[Q]**
      - **MIS[Q] (contain aromatase cypia)**
    - Contribute to blood testes barrier (The spermatids mature into spermatozoa in sertoli cells)
- **Interstitial cells of Leydig**
  - **Secrete testesterone[Q]**

★ Mature spermatozoa are released from sertoli cells[Q]

★ Mature spermatozoa acquire motility during passage in the epidydimis[Q].

Inhibin	- Secreted **by sertoli cells in males & granulose cells in females[Q].** - **Inhibits FSH secretion[Q]**
Activin	- Secreted by sertoli cells in males and granulose cells in females - Stimulates FSH secretion
Relaxin	- Secreted in females by **corpus luteum in ovary and from placenta[Q].** - **Relaxes the symphysis & sacroiliac joints during pregnancy and helps in cervical ripening[Q].** - **Structurally similar to insulin & IGF[Q].**

197. A i.e. Gonadotropin *[Ref: Ganong 23/ep 632]*

Hormones produced by Ovary

- **Estrogen, Activin & Relaxin by Granulose cells[Q]**
- **Inhibin by Granulose cells & Corpus luteum**
- **Progesterone by Theca cells[Q]**

198. C i.e. Increased inhibin levels *[Ref: Sex differences in FSH regulatory peptides in pubertal age boys & girls; Journal of human reproduction vol. 19, No. 7, 1668- 1676, 1107, July 2004; Guyton 11/e p.1006-7]*

Delayed onset of puberty in boys in due to increased production of inhibin[Q], which results in greater negative feedback on FSH as compared to girls.

199. C i.e. Vas deferens

200. C i.e. Epidydmis

201. D i.e. Uterus

[Ref:Langman 10/e p.35; Ganong 23rd/e p. 404; Guyton 11th/e p. 1000]

Spermatogenesis & Meiosis[Q] occurs in	***Seminiferous tubules[Q]***
Sperms are *stored, matured* and ***gain motility in***	***Epididymis[Q].***
Sperm ejaculation is d/t contraction of	**Vas deferens[Q]**
Capacitation of sperm occur in	***Female genital tract[Q].***

Semen release (i.e. spermatozoa ejaculation) involves contraction of smooth muscles **of vas deferens[Q]** (mediated by ligand gated cation channels responding to ATP=P_2X receptors)

202. D i.e. Prolactin & Gonadotropin Releasing Hormone (GnRH) *[Ref: Guyton 11th/e p. 999; Ganong 23rd/e p. 404]*

Testosterone (androgen), estrogen, FSH, LH and growth hormones play essential roles in spermatogenesis[Q].

203. B i.e. Externral genitalia

Male Sex Hormone (Androgens)

Potent agent produced by Leydig cells of testis=Testosterone (responsible for growth of **internal genitalia** i.e. epididymis, vas deferens, seminal vesicle, **spermatogenesis, erythropoeisis & LH inhibition**

Week agents produced in small amounts by **adrenal cortex**

- **Dehydroepiandrosterone**
- **Androstenedione**

↓

Converted **by 5 α reductase to most potent Di hydro-testosterone (responsible for external genital growth** i.e. penis, scrotum, hair loss, pubertal **sexual maturity** & male behavior, and **prostate growth** in elderly).

Bone skeletal growth, muscle mass & epiphyseal fusion is caused by both. Androsterone is testosterone metabolite with $^1/_{10}$ activity.

204. B i.e. Inhibin **205. A i.e. Azoospermia** *[Ref: Berne & Levy 6/e p 766-67]*

- **Testosterone & inhibin** are involved in **negative feedback in spermatogenesis**[Q]. Because **testosterone inhibits LH secretion and inhibits FSH secretion** and both are essential for spermatogenesis.
- **Prolonged administration of testosterone** in **males** causes *azoospermia*[Q]/ **or oligospermia**[Q].

206. B i.e. Estrogen *[Ref: Nelson 16/e P-1688; Ganong 22/e P-406]*

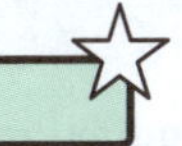

Skeletal maturation, epiphyseal fusion & cessation of growth[Q] is caused by **estrogen.**

Growth spurt at puberty occurs because of androgen & estrogens, but estrogen ultimately *terminate growth* by *causing the epiphyses to fuse* to the long bones (epiphysial closure). Once the epiphyses have closed, linear growth ceases. Patient with sexual precocity are apt to be dwarfed. On the other hand men who were castrated before puberty tend to be tall because their estrogen production is decreased & their epiphysis remain open.

These observation suggest that *estrogen*, rather than androgen, are responsible for ***bone maturation that ultimately leads to epiphyseal fusion and cessation of growth***[Q].

207. A i.e. Testosterone *[Ref: Ganong 24/ep 424]*

- **Gonadal Steroid Binding Globulin (GBG) or sex hormone binding globulin** is a glycoprotein which binds to sex hormones (in decreasing order affinity).

Dihydro testosterone (DHT) > Testosterone (65% bound)>>> Estradiol/Estrone (38%) >> Androstenedione (8%)>> Progesterone & Cortical (0%)

- **Corticosteroid Binding Globulin (CBG)** has affinity in decreasing order as following **Cortisol** (90%) >>> > **Progesterone** (18%) >>> DHT, T and Androstenedione (0%).
- **Albumin** binding in decreasing order is; Androstenedione (90%)> Progesterone (80%) > Estradiol (60%) > Testosterone (33%) > Cortical (6%).

208. C i.e. Persistent late deceleration *[Ref: Dutta 6/e P501]*

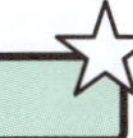

In **contraction stress (oxytocin challenge) test,** positive result means ***persistent late detection of FHR***[Q].

209. A i.e. Testosterone **210. C i.e. Vasectomy** *[Ref: Ganong 22/e P- 428]*

50% of men who have been ***vasectomized develop antibodies against spermatozoa***[Q]. This holds significance, as because of these antibodies reversal of vasectomy may not restore fertility, even when the reversal is successful.

211. A i.e. 21- hydroxylase deficiency *[Ref: Harrison 16/e P-2128, 2145; Ganong 22/e P-365]*

- **Classic 21 – hydroxylase deficiency** is **most common cause of ambiguous genitalia in new born (virilization) and primary amenorrhea**[Q]. i.e. **Pseudohermaphroditism of female child**
- **Primary amenorrhea with Virilization**[Q] in females is in: i) 21 – hydroxylase deficiency ii) 11 – Hydroxylase deficiency

212. A i.e. 1-3 mm/min **213. B i.e. Seminal vesicle** **214. E i.e. Inositol** **215. B i.e. Prostate** *[Ref: Ganong 24/e p. 422]*

Zinc is secreted by prostate; and prostaglandins from seminal vesicle[Q]**. Semen (seminal fluid) contains fructose, prostaglandins, spermine and citric acid but no inositol**[Q]**.**

Semen

Semen contains sperm and *secretions of the seminal vesicles, prostate, cowper's gland* and probably, the *urethral glands*. An average volume ejaculation is *2.5- 3.5mL*. Each mL of semen normally contains about ***100 million***[Q] sperms. *50%* of men with counts of *20-40 million* /mL and essentially all those with counts < *20 million /mL* are sterile. Morphologically abnormal & or immotile spermatozoa also correlates with infertility. Human sperm move at a speed of ***~3mm/ min***Q through the female genital tract. Sperms reach uterine tubes *30- 60 minutes after copulation.* Composition of human semen -

- Colour : white, opalescent
- Specific gravity : 1.028
- PH : *7.35- 7.50*Q
- Sperm-count : ***~100million/mL with fewer than 20% abnormal form***Q
- Contain hyaluronidase

Seminal Vesicle Secretions (contributes 60% of total volume)

- ***Fructose***Q (1.5- 6.5mg/mL)
- Flavins
- Ergothionene
- *Ascorbic acid*
- Phosphoryl choline
- ***Prostaglandins***Q

From prostate (20% of volume)

- ***Spermine***Q
- ***Citric acid***Q
- Cholesterol
- Phospholipids
- Fibrinolysin
- Fibrinogenase
- ***Zinc***Q
- *Acid phosphatase*

Buffers

- Phosphate
- Bicarbonate

216. A i.e. HCG > D i.e. Progesterone *[Ref: Multiple papers]*

Immune rejection of fetus is prevented by hCG >> Progesterone by inhibiting maternal immune responses to fetal antigensQ.

217. C i.e. Progesterone production require feta steroidogenic tissue

218. B, C, D i.e. Insulin, Thyroxine, Glucocorticoids, *[Ref: Berne & Levy 6/e p 787-91; Ghai 7/e p 1]*

- Ironically, **fetal growth hormone does not appear to regulate growth**Q, and anencephalic infants and GH-deficient children typically have normal birth weight.
- **Fetal thyroxine, insulin and glucocorticoids**Q play important role in intrauterine growth of fetus.

Stress

219. A i.e. Corticol > B i.e. Glucagon
[Ref: Ganong 22/e P-370; 374, 145, 39, 349; Morgan 3/e P- 320]

220. B i.e. Glucagon; D i.e. Epinephrine; E i.e. Cortisol

Stress induced Hyperglycemia is mediated through increased **epinephrine, cortisol and glucagon**Q causing gluconeogenesis

221. A i.e. Neoglucogenesis E i.e. Lipolysis C i.e. Protein breakdown *[Ref: Ganong 22/e P-352, 370; KDT 5/e P- 256]*

222. B i.e. Vasopressin; C i.e. Adrenaline *[Ref: Ganong 22/e P- 245]*

Vasopressin Secretion

Increased

- ↑ Effective osmotic pressure of plasma
- ↓ ECF volume
- Pain , emotion, ***stress***Q, exercise, standing
- Angiotensin II, clofibrate, carbamazapine

Decreased

- ↓ Effective osmotic pressure of plasma
- ↑ ECF volume
- Alcohol

Nitric Oxide

223. A i.e. cGMP

224. D i.e. Arginine

225. D i.e. Requires NADPH, FAD, FMN & Heme iron

226. A i.e. NO is synthesized from arginine

227. A i.e. Free radical; B i.e. Vasodilator; C i.e. Oxidizing agent; D i.e. Catalyst

228. C i.e. Gastrointestinal smooth muscle relaxation *[Ref: Berne & Levy 6/e P 100, 281; Gabriel p 145-46, 163, 248, 280; Harper 28/e 559-60, 55, 591; Guyton 11/e 564, 199-200, 332; Ganong 23/e p. 563-64, 112; Lippincott 5/e p 150-51]*

- **Nitric oxide (NO)** is synthesized from arginine (O_2, NADPH) by NO synthase (requiring FMN, FAD, heme & BH_4) in nerves and vascular endothelial cells (hence called EDRF). It **relaxes smooth muscles by increasing cyclic GMP**Q.
- **Nitric oxide (NO)** and **atrial natriuretic factor (ANF)** are hormones that **act through c-GMP**Q.
- NO (along with **VIP** and **PACAP**) are **inhibitory neurotransmitter** in enteric (gastrointestinal) neurons that **primarily mediate gastrointestinal smooth muscle relaxation via c-GMP pathway**Q.

Chapter :8 GENERAL PHYSIOLOGY

QUESTIONS

BMR

1. **Basal Metabolic Rate depends most closely on:**
   A. Lean body mass (NBE P 15,14; AI 10) ☐
   B. Body mass index ☐
   C. Obesity ☐
   D. Body surface area ☐
2. **Basal metabolic rate closely associated with?**
   A. Lean body mass (NBE P 14,13; AI 11) ☐
   B. Body surface area ☐
   C. Body mass index ☐
   D. Body height ☐
3. **Decreased Basal Metabolic Rate is seen in:**
   A. Obesity (AI 10) ☐
   B. Hyperthyroidism ☐
   C. Feeding ☐
   D. Exercise ☐
4. **BMR depends on:** (AI 05)
   A. Body weight ☐
   B. Surface area ☐
   C. Amount of adipose tissue ☐
   D. Amount of lean body mass ☐
5. **Which of the following statements is true regarding basal metabolic rate:** (PGI 01)
   A. Increased in starvation ☐
   B. It is not influenced by hormonal changes ☐
   C. It is not affected by dietary changes ☐
   D. Decreased by 50% in starvation ☐
   E. It is not affected by energy expenditure ☐
6. **Energy expenditure in Resting state depends on**
   A. Lean Body Mass (AIIMS 11, AI 09) ☐
   B. Adipose tissue ☐
   C. Resting Heart Rate ☐
   D. Exercise ☐

Aging

7. **Which of the following does not changes in the old age:**
   A. GFR, FEV_1 (AIIMS 07) ☐
   B. Glucose tolerance ☐
   C. Haematocrit ☐
   D. Blood pressure ☐

Exercise

8. **In moderate excercise the respiratory rate is increased due to response of :** (NBE P 15, 13)
   A. Propioception receptor in the joints ☐
   B. ↑PCO_2 in arterial blood ☐
   C. ↑PO_2 in arterial blood ☐
   D. J-receptor stimulation ☐
9. **Aerobic capacity is increased by:** (AIIMS 04)
   A. Prolonged exercise routine ☐
   B. Strenuous exercise ☐
   C. Regular 3 minutes exercise ☐
   D. Spurt of exercise ☐
10. **Exercise causes which of the following?**
    A. Increased blood flow to the muscles after half minute (AIIMS 07) ☐
    B. Increase in cerebral blood flow due to increase in systolic blood pressure ☐
    C. Increase in body temperature ☐
    D. Decreased O_2 consumption ☐
11. **Which of the following is TRUE regarding physiological changes in the brain during moderate exercise?**
    A. Blood flow is decreased (AI 08) ☐
    B. Blood flow is increased ☐
    C. Blood flow remains unaltered ☐
    D. Blood flow initially increases & then decreases ☐
12. **Autoregulation means** (UP 2K)
    A. Maintains the blood flow ☐
    B. Vary with change in pressure ☐
    C. Regulated by local metabolites ☐
    D. Well developed in the skin ☐
13. **In isometric exercise all are increased except:**
    A. Heart rate (AIIMS 07) ☐
    B. Cardiac output ☐
    C. Mean arterial pressure ☐
    D. Systemic vascular resistance ☐
14. **Strengthening muscle exercise-** (NBE P 13)
    A. Isotonic ☐
    B. Isometric ☐
    C. Aerobic ☐
    D. None ☐
15. **The main cause of increased blood flow to exercising muscles is :** (AIIMS 10, AI 09)
    A. Raised blood pressure ☐
    B. Vasodilatation due to local metabolites ☐
    C. Increased sympathetic discharge to peripheral vessels ☐
    D. Increased heart rate ☐
16. **All are true regarding blood supply increase in muscles during exercise, except:** (AIIMS 12)
    A. Decreased beta adrenergic stimulation ☐
    B. Local metabolites ☐
    C. Increased arterial pressure ☐
    D. Cholinergic stimulation ☐
17. **A/E are the features of exercise:** (AIIMS 09)
    A. Left shift of $Hb-O_2$ dissociation curve ☐
    B. Increase blood supply to muscle ☐
    C. Increase stroke volume ☐
    D. Increase O_2 extraction ☐

18. Physiological changes during severe exercise are:
- A. Hyperventilation in the beginning
- B. Hyperkalemia *(PGI 03)*
- C. ↓ed Pa O_2.
- D. ↓ed Pa CO_2
- E. ↓ed H_2CO_3

19. In exercising muscle; true about metabolism is: *(NBE P 13,15; AIIMS 16,14; PGI 08)*
- A. Same in aerobic and anaerobic
- B. Fatty acids used mainly
- C. Glycogen & (phospho) creatine kinase used anerobically
- D. All of the above

20. Exercise is also prescribed as an adjuvant treatment of depression. Most probably it acts by:
- A. Increasing pulse pressure *(AIIMS 05)*
- B. Improving hemodynamics
- C. Raising endorphin levels
- D. Inducing good sleep

Homeostasis

21. Living body control system correct deformity/disturbance: *(PGI 09)*
- A. Immediately
- B. Completely
- C. Incompletely
- D. With gain

22. Which of the following is not mediated through negative feed back mechanism:
- A. BP *(NBE P 15,13; AIIMS 15; AI 01)*
- B. GH formation
- C. Thrombus formation
- D. ACTH release

23. About the homeostatic mechanism of the body following are true except : *(AIIMS 02)*
- A. Values revolve around the mean
- B. Value of controlled variable is compared to the reference value
- C. Value of controlled variable oscillates near a set point
- D. System is stabilized by the positive feed back mechanism

24. Positive feed back is seen in A/E :
- A. LH Surge *(AIIMS 01)*
- B. Entry of Ca into sarcoplasmic reticulum
- C. Stimulation of gastric secretion of histamine & gastrin.
- D. Thrombolytic activity in coagulation cascade

Inflammatory Mediators

25. 'C' in CRP stands for *(AIIMS 09)*
- A. Concanavalin A
- B. Cellular
- C. C polysaccharide of pneumococcus
- D. Chondroitin sulfate in series following ARP and BRP

26. Low haptoglobin in haemorrhage is masked by concurrent presence of
- A. Malnutrition
- B. Pregnancy
- C. Obstructive biliary disease
- D. Liver parenchymal disease

27. Histamine is formed by ------ of histidine.
- A. Methylatin *(AI 08)*
- B. Reduction
- C. Oxidation
- D. Carboxylation

28. Which of the following statements about Histamine is true: *(AI 08)*
- A. Is found in Mast cells
- B. Increases gastric acid secretion
- C. Related to arousal and blood pressure
- D. All of the above

29. 'Flare' in Triple response is mediated by : *(AI 02)*
- A. Axon reflex
- B. Arteriolar dilation
- C. Histamine release
- D. Local hormones

30. Lewis Triple Response is mediated by *(AI 08)*
- A. Histamine
- B. Axon reflex
- C. Injury to endothelium
- D. None of the above

31. In Lewis Triple Response, redness when skin is scratched with a pointed object is seen due to
- A. Axon Reflex causing Vasoconstriction *(AIIMS 12)*
- B. Histamine Release due to local injury to mast cells
- C. Free Nerve Endings
- D. Endothelial Damage leading to increase in permeability

32. Which of the following statement about Bradykinin is true: *(NBE P 15,14,13; AI 08)*
- A. Causes pain
- B. Causes bronchodilation
- C. Causes vasoconstriction
- D. Decreases vascular permeability

33. O_2 consumption is minimal when temp. gradient between skin and external environment is:
- A. $< 0.5^0$ *(PGI 2K)*
- B. $< 2.5^0$
- C. $< 1.5^0$
- D. $> 3.5^0$

ANSWERS & EXPLANATIONS:

BMR

1. **A i.e. Lean body mass**
2. **B i.e. Body surface area**
3. **A i.e. Obesity**
4. **B i.e. Surface area**
5. **D i.e. ↓ 50% in saturation**
6. **A i.e. Lean Body Mass**

[Ref: Ganong 23rd/e p. 461-63; Exercise physiology Thomas Poland vol 2; Guyton 11th/e p. 886-87; Marks- essential medical Biochemistry 2/e pg-15; Manual of nutritional therapeutics 5/ep 80; Harrison 17/ed pg- 464; Chaudhuri 5/e P- 343]

Resting energy expenditure or **resting metabolic rate (RMR)** and **basal metabolic rate (BMR)** depends more closely & more logically on **metabolically active fat free- lean body mass (i.e. muscle and internal organs) than body surface area**Q. However, body surface area is a reasonable determinant of lean body mass (So RMR/BMR depends on **LBM > Body mass > BSA > Body weight > BMI > Height)**.
Obesity (i.e. excess of metabolically inactive fat /adipose tissue) **and starvation decrease BMR**Q.

Aging

7. **C i.e. Hematocrit** *[Ref: Chaudhuri 5/e P- 302]*

Hematocrit does not changes with ageQ

Exercise

8. **A i.e. Propioception receptor in the joints.** *[Ref: Ganong Review of Medical Physiology 22/e P- 681]*

- **In moderate excercise** the abrupt increase in ventilation at the start of excercise is **due to psychic stimuli and afferent impulses from proprioceptors in muscles, tendons and joints**Q.
- **Arterial pH, P_{CO2} and P_{O2} remain constant**Q during moderate exercise because increase in ventilation is proportionate to increase in O_2 consumption.

9. **C i.e. Regular 3 minute excercise**
10. **C i.e. Increase in body temperature**
11. **C i.e. Blood flow remains unchanged**
12. **A i.e. Maintains the blood flow**
13. **D i.e. Systemic vascular resistance**
14. **B i.e. Isometric**

[Ref: Ganong 22/e p. 632 – 35, 681- 83; Guyton 11/e p. 1055– 66; Fox physiology 8/e p-346; http: /www. pubmedcentral.nih.gov/ pagerender. fcgi? artid = 301529 & pageindex = 2 # page]

- **Aerobic capacity** is **increased by regular 3 minute exercise**Q (not by spurts of prolonged & strenuous exercise). Exercise increases blood flow to muscles at or even before the start of exercise. It increases O_2 consumption & body temperature.
- **Cerebral blood flow is maintained due to auto regulation (between 60- 160 mm Hg) in response to moderate exercise**Q.
- **Isometric exercise** characteristically show modest increase in heart rate and cardiac output and pronounced increase in systolic and diastolic arterial pressure. The relative increases in cardiac output and mean blood pressure are such that (calculated) **systemic vascular resistance is unchanged**Q.
- **Isotonic (or DCER= Dynamic Constant External Resistance) exercise includes** all exercises which **involve joint movement** like running, rowing etc. Whereas, **isometric exercise** are static (i.e. no **joint movement is involved)** and include yoga postures, wall press/sit. So it strengthens muscles at that angle and benefits will not carry over to joint actions beyond that range.
- **Muscle strength (endurance)** is increased both by isotonic & isometric exercises. Recent studies however report, that **strengthening occurs more in isometric exercises** (because there is no help of supporting muscles & momentum) **with a benefit of less chances of muscle injury**Q. **Muscle bulk is mainly increased by isotonic exercise.**

15. **B i.e. Vasodilatation due to local metabolites** *[Ref: Guyton 12/SAE p. 99, 208; Ganong 24/e p. 666-668]*
16. **A i.e. Decreased beta adrenergic stimulation**

- The main cause of **increased blood flow to exercising muscle** is **vasodilation due to local metabolites**Q. The most important local chemical effect is reduction of O_2 in muscle tissue. **Increased arterial pressure** above normal, **β (beta) adrenergic receptor mediated vasodilation in exercising muscle** and **α (alpha) adrenergic receptor mediated vasoconstriction** in resting muscles are other factors responsible for increased blood supply in muscles during exerc
- **Increased (not decreased) β_2 adrenergic stimulation** (in humans) and **cholinergic stimulation** (in some animals like dogs, cats) are responsible for **skeletal muscle vasodilation** whereas, **α 1 adrenergi**c stimulation cause skeletal muscle **vasoconstriction.** Epinephrine excites more of β receptors (=vasodilation), whereas α vasoconstrictor receptors are excited especially by norepinephrine.

17. A i.e. Left shift of $Hb–O_2$ dissociation Curve *[Ref: Ganong 22/e P- 681]*

18. A i.e. Hyperventilation in the beginning; B i.e. Hyperkalemia D $\downarrow P_{aCO_2}$ *[Ref: Ganong 22/e P-681–82, Guyton 10/e P479-481]*

*A right shift of Hb – O_2 dissociation curve*Q is seen in exercising muscle. Right shift occurs because of *accumulation of CO_2* **(↓ pH)**Q and *increased temperature of contracting muscle*Q.
Physiological changes during severe exercise include *hyperventilation (in the beginning),* **↑ed PaO_2, ↓$PaCO_2$, ↓pH, ↓HCO_3^-** *and hyperkalemia*Q.

19. C i.e. Glycogen and creatine kinase used anerobically *[Ref: Ganong 24/e p. 106-108; Guyton 10/e 941]*

Glycogen lactic acid system and **phosphoryl creatinine stores** (or **creatine kinase)** are used during **anaerobic exercise.**

20. C i.e. Raising endorphin level *[Ref: Kaplan & Saddok's 7/e P-106, 107]*

Exercise increases release of endogenous opioids and is associated with mood enhancement.
- *β endorphin* is the *principal endogenous opioids*
- The best documented function of endogenous opiates is in *analgesia & alteration of pain perception*

Homeostasis

21. All *[Ref: Guyton 11/e 6-8; Ganong 23/e 58-60]*

- Thousands of **homeostatic control systems** operate within living body (in all cells, organs) to maintain the constancy of internal environment. These may correct disturbance (deformity) **completely** or **incompletely (with error** & gain) mostly using negative feed back. It is corrected **immediately** (adaptive control) or after a delay.
- **Gain of a control system**: Most control systems are of **negative feed** back **nature (i.e. negative to initiating stimulus**). If some factor (eg any ion, BP etc) becomes excessive or deficient, negative feed back consists of a series of changes that return the factor towards normal mean value. The degree of ***effectiveness*** of control system to maintain constant condition is determine by the **gain of negative feedback**. For example same amount of blood volume is transfused into 2 persons with and without baroreceptor pressure control system has caused an arterior pressure to increase from normal 100 mm Hg to 125 mm Hg and 175 mm Hg respectively. This means feedback control system has caused a **correction** of -50 mmHg (i.e. from 175 to 125 mmHg) but still there is an **error** of 25 mm Hg (as there remains an increase of +25 mmHg pressure even in normal functioning control system; which also means that control system is **not 100% effective** in preventing change in this case). The gain is calculated by

$$\textbf{Gain} = \frac{\text{Correction}}{\text{Error}} = \frac{-50}{+25} = -2$$

(i.e. a disturbance that increases or decrese the arterial pressure does so only 1/3rd as much as would occur if this control system were not present)

Gain of temperature control system is much greater (-33) therefore it is much more effective than baroreceptor pressure control system.

Feed Back Mechanism

22. C i.e. Thrombus formation

23. D i.e. system is stabilized by the positive feedback *[Ref: Guyton 10/e P 6, 7]*

Positive feed back system leads to vicious cycle which destabilizes the homeostatic mechanismQ**.** So it is the negative feed back system that stabilizes the body's homeostatic mechanism. **Clotting of blood (ie thrombus formation)** is **mediated through positive feed back mechanism**Q**.**

24. **C i.e. Stimulation of gastric secretion by histamine & gastrin** *[Ref: Ganong Physiology 22/e P- P470, Guyton 10/e P6]*

Most control system of the body are negative feed back system. Release of acid in stomach by the action of gastrin is negative feed back system, as ↑in acid secretion inhibits further gastrin secretion.

Inflammatory Mediators

25. **C i.e. C polysaccharide of pneumococcus**
[Ref. Harrison 17th/e p. 568-569, 638; Tillet & Francis : Serological reactions in pneumonia; J Exp Med 1930, 52: 561-585]

- **C-reactive protein (CRP),** discovered by Tillet and Francis in 1930, is so named **because it reacts with the C polysaccharide of pneumococci.**Q

- **Acute phase proteins** (or **reactants**) are proteins that increase during acute inflammatory states or secondary to certain types of tissue damages. These include - **α1- antitrypsin, α1 acid glycoprotein, CRP, haptoglobin and fibrinogen**Q**.**
- Interleukin-1 (IL-1), a polypeptide released from mononuclear phagocytic cells, is the principal – but not the sole – stimulator of synthesis of majority of acute phase reactants by hepatocytes. Cytokine IL-6 are also involved. Nuclear factor Kappa-B (NFKB) is a transcription factor that has been involved in the stimulation of synthesis of acute phase proteins.
- CRP (a type of pentraxin protein) is synthesized by liver in response to factors released by fat cells. It binds to phosphocholine expressed on surface of dead or dying cells in order to activate classic complement pathway via C1q. Its level is mainly determined by rate of production (rises within 6 hours, peak in 48 hours & t½ is constant)

26. **D i.e Liver parenchymal disease** *[Ref: Harrison 17th/e p. 570; Gabriel p.71]*

Haptoglobin (Hp) binds extracorpuscular (i.e. extracellular) hemoglobin (Hb), preventing free Hb from entering the kidney. Hp-Hb complex is removed from plasma by **haptocytes**. Levels of haptoglobin falls rapidly in situations where hemoglobin is constantly being released from RBC such as occurs in hemolytic anemia (haemorrhage). But in case of **parenchymal liver disease**, Hp-Hb complex removal is deranged so reduction in haptoglobin level is masked.

27. **D i.e. Carboxylation**
28. **D i.e. All** *[Ref: Gannong 22/e p. 107; Guyton 11/e p. 797-98, 450, 480, 202, 529, 285-86; Chaudhary 6/e p. 318; KDT 6/e p. 151-53]*

Histamine is formed by **decarboxylation of amino acid histidine**Q, and is found **in mast cell, basophils, enterochromaffin like cells of gastric mucosa and brain**Q. It has been related to **arousal, sexual behaviour**Q, regulation of secretion of some anterior pituitary hormones, blood pressure, drinking & pain threshold.

29. **A i.e. Axon reflex** 30. **A i.e. Histamine** 31. **Histamine Release due to local injury to mast cells**
[Ref: Ganong 22/e P-593, 627; Chaudhuri 6/e P-249; BOS-Skin immune system 3/e p. 401-02; Ramdass (2007) p. 141]

Flare in triple response is caused by Arteriolar dilatation which is **mediated by the axon reflex**Q.
Histamine is primarily responsible for Lewis triple response. Axonal reflex only mediates flare part of triple response.

32. **A i.e. Causes Pain** *[Ref: Guyton 11/e p. 436, 202, 529, 322, 779, 795; Robbin's 7/e p. 65, 74-75, 69]*

Bradykinin increases vascular permeability, and causes contraction of smooth muscle (utrine, intestine, broncho-constriction), dilation of blood vessels and painQ when injected into the skin. These effects are similar to those of histamine.

33. **A < 0.5°C (still searching)**

Chapter -9 CELL PHYSIOLOGY

QUESTIONS

Cell Membrane

1. **Eukaryotic plasma membrane is made up of all except:**
   A. Carbohydrates *(AIIMS 10, 09)* ☐
   B. Triglycerides ☐
   C. Lecithin ☐
   D. Cholesterol ☐
2. **Plasma membrane is mainly composed of:**
   A. Cholesterol *(NBE P 14,13; AIIMS 04)* ☐
   B. Carbohydrate ☐
   C. Phospholipid ☐
   D. Protein ☐
3. **On weight basis, the membrane contains protein and lipid in the ratio of-** *(NBE P 13)*
   A. 1:2 ☐
   B. 1:1 ☐
   C. 2:1 ☐
   D. 4:1 ☐
4. **Which of the following is seen in association with membrane raft?** *(AIIMS 12)*
   A. Glycosylphosphatidylinositol (GPI) anchored protein ☐
   B. Mannose binding protein (MBP) ☐
   C. Guanosine triphosphate associated protein ☐
   D. Spectrin associated protein ☐
5. **Function of phospholipid in cell membrance is:**
   A. Cell to cell variation *(PGI 01)* ☐
   B. Transduction of Signals ☐
   C. Transmembrane preparation of protein ☐
   D. DNA replication ☐
   E. Enzyme activation at membrane surface ☐
6. **Membrane fluidity is increased by:** *(AIIMS05)*
   A. Stearic acid ☐
   B. Palmitic acid ☐
   C. Cholesterol ☐
   D. Linoleic acid ☐
7. **Transition temperature of lipid bilayers of cell membrane is increased by-** *(AIIMS 2K)*
   A. Cholesterol ☐
   B. Saturated fatty acids ☐
   C. Hydrocarbons ☐
   D. Unsaturated fatty acids ☐
8. **Addition of PUFA in plasma membrane causes**
   A. Membrane becomes rigid *(AIIMS 09)* ☐
   B. Increase in fluidity of membrane ☐
   C. Decrease in fluidity of membrane ☐
   D. No change in fluidity of membrane ☐
9. **True about lipid bilayer of cell wall:** *(PGI 01)*
   A. Asymmetrical arrangement of cell wall component ☐
   B. Lateral diffusion of ions ☐
   C. Symmetrical arrangement of cell wall components ☐
   D. Not made up of amphipathic lipids ☐
10. **In cell membrane, following are true except:** *(PGI 05)*
    A. Lipids are regularly arranged ☐
    B. Lipids are symmetrical ☐
    C. Protein displaced laterally ☐
    D. None ☐
11. **Which of the following membrane has the highest protein content per gram tissue:** *(AIIMS 02)*
    A. Inner mitochondrial membrane ☐
    B. Outer mitochondrial membrane ☐
    C. Plasma membrane ☐
    D. Myelin sheath ☐
12. **The transmembrane region of protein is likely to have:** *(AI 04)*
    A. A stretch of hydrophilic amino acids ☐
    B. A stretch of hydrophobic amino acids ☐
    C. A disulphide loop ☐
    D. Alternating hydrophilic and hydrophobic amino acids ☐
13. **Lipids and proteins interact in membrane by**
    A. Hydrophobic interactions *(PGI 07)* ☐
    B. Both hydrophobic and covalent interactions ☐
    C. Covalent bonds ☐
    D. H bonds ☐
14. **In leucine zipper model, Leucine residue seen after every** *(PGI 07)*
    A. 3 amino acids ☐
    B. 6 amino acids ☐
    C. 9 amno acids ☐
    D. 12 amino acids ☐
    E. 7 amino acid ☐
15. **Which important component of cell wall has carbohydrate moiety:** *(PGI 01)*
    A. Phosphoglyceride ☐
    B. Triacylglycerol ☐
    C. Sphingomyelin ☐
    D. Cholesterol ☐
    E. GM_2 Gangliosides ☐
16. **Glycophorin is present in:** *(PGI 09)*
    A. Enterocyte ☐
    B. Hepatocyte ☐
    C. RBC ☐
    D. Lymphocyte ☐
17. **RBC membrane integrity is maintained by:**
    A. Spectrin *(AIIMS 02,01)* ☐
    B. Laminin ☐
    C. Collagen ☐
    D. Elastin ☐

18. Most permeable to pure phospholipid bilayer is- *(NBE P 13)*
- A. Oxygen
- B. Na
- C. Cl
- D. Water

Transport Across Cell Membrane

19. Osmolarity is defined as- *(NBE P 13)*
- A. Number of osmole per litre
- B. Number of osmole per kg
- C. Weight of solute per litre
- D. Weight of solvent oper litre

20. Osmotic pressure of 1 mol of idea solute relative to pure water is: *(PGI 09)*
- A. 6.5 atm.
- B. 22.4 atm.
- C. 4 atm.
- D. 2 atm.
- E. 1 atm.

21. Cell volume & shape is maintained by- *(NBE P 13)*
- A. Goldman effect
- B. Gibbs-Donnan effect
- C. Singer's effect
- D. None

22. Potential developed due to movement of freely diffusible ions across a semi-permeable membrane is calculated using: *(AIIMS 16)*
- A. Nernst equation
- B. Gibbs equation
- C. Goldman-Hodgkin-Katz equation
- D. Fick principle

23. Equilibrium potential for an ion is calculated using: *(AIIMS 08, 15)*
- A. Gibbs-Donnan equation
- B. Nerst equation
- C. Goldman equation
- D. Fick law

24. The extracellular potassium concentration is 100 mEq/mmol and intracellular potassium concentration is 10 mEq/mmol. What will be the equilibrium potential for potassium according to Nernst equation? *(AIIMS 15)*
- A. 0 V
- B. –60 V
- C. –90 V
- D. +30 V

25. Fick's law of diffusion explains *(AIIMS 13, 14)*
- A. Active diffusion along concentration gradient
- B. Passive diffusion along concentration gradient
- C. Both of these
- D. None of these

26. Fick's law, flux of Geomembrane increased in: *(PGI 08)*
- A. Concentration across
- B. Temperature
- C. Increased size of molecule
- D. Weight
- E. Area

27. Resting membrane potential is mainly due to: *(NBE P 15,13; PGI 03, 15,13)*
- A. Na^+
- B. K^+
- C. Cl^-
- D. Mg^{++}

28. RMP of nerve cell is equal to which ion's equilibrium potential...?- *(NBE P 13)*
- A. K^+
- B. Cl^-
- C. Na^+
- D. Ca^+

29. Resting membrane potential of neuron is- *(NBE P 13)*
- A. +70 mv
- B. -70 mv
- C. +90 mv
- D. -90

30. What is/are effect on membrane when extracellular concentration of K+ is decreased: *(PGI 09, 08)*
- A. ↓ magnitude of RMP
- B. ↑ negativity of the membrane
- C. ↑ magnitude of RMP
- D. ↓ negativity of membrane

31. For sodium - potassium pump the coupling ratio is *(Assam 04, AIIMS09)*
- A. 1 : 1
- B. 2 : 3
- C. 3 : 2
- D. 1 : 4

32. K^+ homeostasis in human is: *(PGI 05)*
- A. Most of the K^+ are intracellular
- B. Most of the K^+ are extra cellular
- C. An essential electrolyte for different organ function.
- D. Actively secreted in the distal tubule
- E. It maintains the Na^+ K^+ ATPase activity.

33. True about Na+ - K+ pump is that: *(PGI 04, 06; WB 05; NBE P 15, 13)*
- A. Involves ATPase (enzyme) activity
- B. It can move Na^+ in and out of cell
- C. Electrically neutral
- D. Pumps out one Na+ for one K+
- E. Pumps 3 Na and 2k inside the cell

34. True statement regarding mechanism of action of Na/K ATpase: *(NBE P 15,13; PGI 12)*
- A. Pumps 3 Na out & 2K+ in
- B. Pumps 3 K out & 2 Na+ in
- C. Pumps 3 Na in & 2K+ out
- D. Pumps 2 K out & 3Na+ in

35. True regarding Na+ - K+ pump *(UP- 05, AMU –06)*
- A. Hetrodimer – homogenous
- B. Hetrodimer – hetrogenous
- C. Homodimer – hetrogenous
- D. Homodimer – homogenous

36. Intracellular binding site on Na+ - K+ pump is *(JIPMER – 06, WB – 05)*
- A. Na^+
- B. ATP
- C. PO_4
- D. Ouabain

37. Binding site present on β unit of Na+ - K+ pump is
A. Na^+ *(TN-04, KA-05)* ☐
B. K^+ ☐
C. ATP ☐
D. Glycosylation ☐

38. Which of them is TRUE about Na^+-K^+ pump:
A. K^+ is pumped against the gradient. *(AIIMS 09)* ☐
B. $2K^+$ are exchanged with $5Na^+$ ☐
C. Hypercalcemia causes arrest in Na^+ K^+ pump ☐
D. Increase in intracellular Na^+ increases action potential. ☐

39. The sodium- potassium pump is an example of:
A. Active transport *(AIIMS 06)* ☐
B. Passive transport ☐
C. Facilitated diffusion ☐
D. Osmosis ☐

40. True regarding transport across a cell membrane is :
A. Cl- with glucose symport *(AIIMS 14; AI 08)* ☐
B. Na+ with glucose anteprot ☐
C. Na+ with glucose symport ☐
D. K+ with glucose symport ☐

41. Glucose is co-transported with Na^+ ions. This is a type of- *(NBE P 13)*
A. Secondary active transport ☐
B. Primary active transport ☐
C. Facilitated diffusion ☐
D. Simple diffusion ☐

42. A cell membrane is damaged by insertion of microneedle, repair shall occur by which of the following processes?
A. Lateral movement of proteins *(AIIMS 13)* ☐
B. Resealing by lipid bilayer ☐
C. Enzymatic reaction ☐
D. Hydrophobic interaction ☐

43. Which of the following increases particle diffusion across the cell membrane? *(NBE P 13)*
A. Increasing size of particle ☐
B. Decreasing lipid solubility of substance ☐
C. Increasing lipid solubility of substance ☐
D. Decreasing size of opening in cell membrane ☐

44. All of the following transport process follow 'saturation kinetics' except: *(AIIMS 05, 13)*
A. Facilitated diffusion ☐
B. Na^+ - Ca^{2+} exchanger ☐
C. Simple diffusion ☐
D. Na^+ coupled active transport ☐

45. True about facilitated diffusion are A/E:
A. Occur in direction of concentration gradient ☐
B. Does not require energy *(PGI 08)* ☐
C. Occur in direction opposite to electrical gradient ☐
D. Facilitated by charge of molecule ☐

46. All of the following are true except: *(NBE P 15,13)*
A. Facilitated diffusion requires energy ☐
B. Active transport is an energy dependent process *(AIIMS 14,13, 08)* ☐
C. Co-transport is mediated via the use of carriers ☐
D. Glucose is transported via passive diffusion ☐

47. Active transport across the cell membrane is mediated by: *(AIIMS 01)*
A. G-proteins ☐
B. Na^+- K^+ ATPase ☐
C. Carrier protein ☐
D. Channel protein ☐

48. Which of the following statements about facilitated diffusion is true *(AI 09)*
A. It is a form of active transport ☐
B. It requires a carrier protein ☐
C. Rate of transport is proportionate to the concentration gradient ☐
D. Requires creatine phosphate ☐

49. Ionophores have following action except:
A. Abolish proton gradient *(PGI 07)* ☐
B. Inhibit ADP to ATP conversion ☐
C. Hydrophilic in character ☐
D. Abolish pH gradient ☐

50. Water travelling from extracellular to intracellular is by- *(NBE P 13)*
A. Co-transport ☐
B. Diffusion ☐
C. Filtration ☐
D. Active transport ☐

51. Transport of neutral substances across the cell membrane occurs via *(AI 08)*
A. Porins ☐
B. Lonophore ☐
C. Lipopolysaccharides ☐
D. Diffusion ☐

52. The emeiocytosis or reverse pinocytosis & exocytosis requires which ion
A. Na^+ *(NBE P 15,14,13; AIIMS 15,13,03)* ☐
B. K^+ ☐
C. Ca^{++} ☐
D. Mg^{++} ☐

53. Exocytosis *(PGI 2K)*
A. Extrusion of cell bound vesicles ☐
B. Intrusion of liquid particles ☐
C. Instrusion of solid particles ☐
D. All of the above ☐

54. Clathrin is used in : *(AIIMS 01)*
A. Receptor mediated endocytosis ☐
B. Exocytosis ☐
C. Cell to cell adhesion ☐
D. Plasma membrane ☐

55. The process by which fusion of part of a cell membrane occurs is/are : *(PGI 05)*
A. Cell division ☐
B. Endocytosis ☐
C. Exocytosis ☐
D. Virus replication ☐

56. The cell junctions allowing exchange of cytoplasmic molecules between the two cells are called-
A. Gap junctions *(NBE P 13)* ☐
B. Tight junctions ☐
C. Focal junctions ☐

57. All of the following are involved in the transmission of regulatory signals through the ECF, Except: *(AI 09)*
A. Synaptic signals through neurotransmitters ☐
B. Endocrine signals through hormones ☐
C. Direct contact through gap junctions ☐
D. G protein coupled receptors ☐

58. Nernst potential for K+ is- *(NBE P 13)*
A. +90 ☐
B. -90 ☐
C. +70 ☐
D. -70 ☐

59. The ligand-receptor complex dissociates in the endosome because: *(AI 06)*
A. Of its large size ☐
B. The vesicle looses its clathrin cost ☐
C. Of the acidic pH of the vesicle ☐
D. Of the basic pH of the vesicle ☐

Body Fluids/Extra Cellular Fluid

60. Volume of ICF in body- *(NBE P 13)*
A. 0.2×body wt ☐
B. 0.4×body wt ☐
C. 0.6×body wt ☐
D. 0.8×body wt ☐

61. The following are true about body water:
A. Water constitutes 60% of the body weight ☐
B. Plasma volume constitutes 10% of the total body water *(PGI 07)* ☐
C. ECF volume can be determined by dilution methods ☐
D. 10% is intracellular water ☐

62. True statements are : *(NBE P 13; PGI 04)*
A. Totally body water constitutes about 60% of body weight ☐
B. Most intracellular water is n the Musculoskeletal system ☐
C. Extra cellular water constitutes about 40% of body weight ☐
D. Total plasma constitutes about 10% body weight ☐
E. Extra cellular fluid can be measured by dilution method ☐

63. True statements about ions composition in body:
A. Intracellular & Extra cellular ions compositions are same *(PGI 06)* ☐
B. Phosphoru and Mg^{++} are major ions intracellularly ☐
C. Na^+, Cl^- principal ions in E.C.F. ☐
D. Kidney tightly regulates Na^+, K^+, Cl^- composition ☐

64. Predominant extracellular ions are A/E: *(NBE P 15,13; PGI 14,12,06)*
A. Na^+ ☐
B. K^+ & PO_4^- ☐
C. Cl^- ☐
D. HCO_3^- ☐

65. True statement regarding extra cellular fluid to intracellular fluid is : *(AI 08)*
A. ECF is rich K+ ☐
B. ECF is more than ICF ☐
C. ECF is rich in organic anion ☐
D. High Na:K+ ratio is seen ☐

66. ICF is- *(NBE P 13)*
A. 14L ☐
B. 20% of body weight ☐
C. 28L ☐
D. 33% of body weight ☐

67. Most osmotically active intracellular cation-
A. K^+ *(NBE P 13)* ☐
B. Na^+ ☐
C. Mg^{+2} ☐
D. Protein ☐

68. Features of ECF as compared to ICF: *(PGI 13)*
A. High K^+ ☐
B. High Na^+ ☐
C. High proteins ☐
D. High Cl^- ☐
E. Nearly equal osmolarity in both fluid ☐

69. D_2O (Deuterium oxide) is used to measure volume of *(AIIMS 03)*
A. Blood ☐
B. Total body water ☐
C. Extracellular fluid ☐
D. Intracellular fluid ☐

70. Most accurate measurement of extracellular fluid volume (ECF) can be done by using :
A. Sucrose. *(NBE P 15,13; AIIMS 03)* ☐
B. Mannitol. ☐
C. Inulin. ☐
D. Aminopyrine ☐

71. Which of the following methods is not used for measurement of body fluid volumes? *(AIIMS 05)*
A. Antipyrine for total body water ☐
B. Insulin for extracellular fluid ☐
C. Evans blue for plasma volume ☐
D. ^{125}I-albumin for blood volume ☐

72. Isotope used to measure RBC volume is- *(NBE P 13)*
A. Cr51 ☐
B. H3 ☐
C. D_2O ☐
D. I^{135} ☐

73. Interstitial fluid volume can be determined by: *(AIIMS 15)*
A. Radioactive iodine and radiolabelled water ☐
B. Radioactive water and radiolabelled albumin ☐
C. Radioactive sodium and radioactive water ☐
D. Radioactive sodium and radioactive labelled albumin ☐

74. In a study to detect extracellular fluid volume, 10 gm mannitol was injected by intravenous route and after waiting for adequate time for equilibration of levels, concentration was measured as 50 mg/100 ml. In this time, 10% mannitol was excreted. What is the calculated volume of ECF? *(AIIMS 15)*

A. 10 Litres
B. 18 Litres
C. 42 Litres
D. 52 Litres

75. In a study, dye ABC is used to measure cardiac output and blood volume. The dye is replaced with a new dye XYZ which diffuses more rapidly out of the capillaries. This would affect the study by
A. Normal cardiac output, altered blood volume
B. Altered cardiac output, normal blood volume estimation *(AIIMS 02)*
C. Both altered
D. Both normal

76. Which of the following technique is used to study current flow across a single ion channel? *(AIIMS 14)*
A. Patch clamp
B. Voltage clamp
C. Iontophoresis
D. Galvanometry

77. Osmoreceptor is located at which site -
A. Anterior hypothalamus
B. Renal medulla *(AI 11, TN 04, AIIMS 13)*
C. Carotid body
D. Atrial chamber

78. Ineffective osmols is *(NBE P 14; Jipmer 02)*
A. Na^+
B. K^+
C. Urea
D. All

79. Osmotic adaptation is A/E *(JIPMER- 04, WB 05)*
A. Due to osmolytes
B. In brain cells
C. Due to urea & glucose mainly
D. Protects against large H_2O shift

80. About Sodium, true: *(PGI 07)*
A. Normal serum level is 135- 145 mEq/L
B. Daily intake is 150 mmol of NaCl
C. Major portion is extra cellular
D. Major reserve is skeletal muscle

81. The majority of body sodium is present -
A. Extra cellular fluid *(NBE P 15)*
B. Intra cellular fluid
C. Plasma
D. Bone

Extracellular Matrix

82. Which of the following is/are extracellular matrix protein: *(PGI 09)*
A. Collagen
B. Laminin
C. Fibronectin
D. Integrin
E. Elastin

83. Which of these is not a part of extracellular matrix:
A. Laminin *(AIIMS 02)*
B. Fibronectin
C. Integrins
D. Collagen

84. Basement membrane consists of all except:
A. Laminin *(AIIMS 07)*
B. Nidogenin
C. Entactin
D. Rhodopsin

85. Triple helix is seen in : *(AIIMS 05)*
A. Collagen
B. DNA
C. Elastin
D. RNA

86. Which of the following is not seen in the interphotoreceptor matrix.: *(AI 08)*
A. Metalloproteinase
B. Sialoprotein Associated with Rods and Cones (SPARC)
C. Tissue Inhibitors of Metalloproteinases (TIMP)
D. Memicane

87. Basement membrane (or collagen) degeneration is mediated by: *(NBE P 14,13; AI 07)*
A. Metalloproteinases
B. Oxidases
C. Elastases
D. Hydroxylases

88. Type of collagen forming basement membrane of kidney:
A. I *(PGI 06)*
B. II
C. III
D. IV
E. V

89. The collagen triple helix structure is not found in:
A. Cytoplasm *(AI 03)*
B. Golgi apparatus
C. Lumen of endoplasmic reticulum
D. Intracellular vescicles

90. Defect in collagen formation is seen in:
A. Scurvy *(PGI 02)*
B. Hunter's syndrome
C. Marfan's syndrome
D. Osteogenesis imperfecta

91. Hyaluronic acid – mucopolysaccharide is present in
A. Cornea *(AIIMS 10)*
B. Mast cell
C. Vitreous humor
D. Dermis

92. Which of the following is the major proteoglycan of synovial fluid- *(NBE P 15)*
A. Chondroitin sulfate
B. Dermatan sulfate
C. Heparna sulfate
D. Hyaluronic acid

93. Viscosity of synovial fluid depends upon:
A. N-acetyl galactosamine *(AIIMS 14, 02)*
B. N-acetyl glucosamine
C. Glucuronic acid
D. Hyaluronic acid

94. Danaparoid contains: *(PGI 09)*
A. Keratin sulphate ☐
B. Chitin ☐
C. Dermatan sulphate ☐
D. Heparan sulphate ☐
E. Keratin ☐

95. Uronic acid level in urine is elevated in
A. Tyrosinosis *(AIIMS 07)* ☐
B. Maple syrup urine disease ☐
C. Nieman picks disease ☐
D. Mucopolysacchridosis. ☐

96. Products accumulated in Hunter 's syndrome are
A. Keratan sulfate *(PGI 02)* ☐
B. Dermatan sulfate ☐
C. Chondroitin sulfate ☐
D. Heparan sulfate ☐
E. Hyaluronic acid ☐

97. Elasticity of the corneal layer of skin is due to the presence of *(AI 02)*
A. Histidine ☐
B. Keratin ☐
C. Lysine ☐
D. Cysteine ☐

98. Keratin of skin and nail differ because of
A. Disulphide bond *(AIIMS 2K)* ☐
B. Covalent bond ☐
C. Vander Waal bond ☐
D. Hydrogen bond ☐

Cell Organelle

99. Force generating proteins are : *(AI 01)*
A. Myosin and myoglobin ☐
B. Dynein and kinesin ☐
C. Calmodelin and G protien ☐
D. Troponin ☐
E. Lysosomes ☐

100. Axonal transport is- *(NBE P 13)*
A. Antegrade ☐
B. Retrograde ☐
C. Antegrade & Retrograde ☐
D. None ☐

101. Rapid axonal flow in the neurons is mediated by all except *(AIIMS 07)*
A. Dynein ☐
B. Kinesin ☐
C. Neurofilaments ☐
D. Microtubules ☐
E. Lysosome ☐

102. Agranular cytoplasmic reticulum is involved in the synthesis of *(AIIMS 06)*
A. Protein ☐
B. Lipid ☐
C. Vitamin ☐
D. Carbohydrate ☐

103. Glycolysis occurs in *(AIIMS 07)*
A. Cytosol ☐
B. Mitochondria ☐
C. Nucleus ☐
D. Lysosome ☐

104. All take place in mitochondria except
A. Fatty acid oxidation *(AIIMS 07)* ☐
B. EMP pathway ☐
C. Electron transport chain ☐
D. Citric acid cycle ☐

105. All of the following occur in mitochondria except:
A. Citric acid cycle (Kreb's cycle) *(AI 07)* ☐
B. Glycogenolysis ☐
C. Fatty acid oxidation ☐
D. Electron transport chain ☐

106. All of the following metabolic functions occur in the mitochondria, Except: *(NBE P 15; AIIMS 16; AI 12)*
A. Beta-oxidation of fatty acids ☐
B. Biosynthesis of fatty acids ☐
C. Protein synthesis/ DNA synthesis ☐
D. Citric acid cycle ☐

107. Agranular endoplasmic reticulum is involved in the synthesis of: *(AI 07)*
A. Protein ☐
B. Lipid ☐
C. Carbohydrate ☐
D. Vitamin D ☐

108. Protein synthesis occurs in: *(PGI 08)*
A. Smooth ER ☐
B. Golgi bodies ☐
C. Rough ER ☐
D. Lysosomes ☐

109. Which of the following pathway occurs partly in mitochondria and partly in cytosol- *(NBE P 15)*
A. Glycolysis ☐
B. Kreb's cycle ☐
C. Ketogenesis ☐
D. Urea cycle ☐

110. Intracellular sorting and packing done for:
A. ER *(PGI 07)* ☐
B. Golgi apparatus ☐
C. Ribosome ☐
D. Cytoplasm ☐
E. Nucleus ☐

111. True regarding golgi apparatus is A/E *(WB-04)*
A. Cis is receiving end *(Jipmer 09, AMU – 03)* ☐
B. Trans is secretory end ☐
C. Non polarized structure ☐
D. Situated near nucleus ☐

112. Sequence of vesicle transport is *(TN 02, Kerala 03)*
A. ER → Trans → Cis → lysosome ☐
B. ER → Cis → Trans → Cell membrane ☐
C. ER → Lysosome → Trans → Cis ☐
D. Cis → ER → Trans → Cell membrane ☐

113. True about mitochondria is A/E:
A. Site for ATP synthesis *(NBE P 14,13; PGI 13)* ☐
B. Isolation is done by hydrolysis in alkaline pH & synthesize fat ☐
C. Protein synthesis ☐
D. Double stranded circular DNA ☐

114. Which of the following liver enzymes is predominantly mitochondrial: *(AI 10)*
- A. SGOT (AST) ☐
- B. SGPT (ALT) ☐
- C. GGT ☐
- D. Nucleotidase ☐

115. Aggrecan in: *(PGI 2K)*
- A. Receptor over platelets ☐
- B. A molecule present in osteoid tissue ☐
- C. Granules in leukocytes ☐
- D. Important component of cartilage ☐

116. Markers of plasma membrane are A/E: *(NBEP 15,14,13; PGI 09,07)*
- A. Galactosyl transferase & Glucokinase ☐
- B. 5 – Nucleotidase ☐
- C. Adenyl cyclase ☐
- D. Na^+ K^+ ATpase ☐

117. Enzyme marker for Golgi apparatus:
- A. Peroxidase *(NBE P 15,14,13; PGI 03, 14, 15)* ☐
- B. Galactosidase ☐
- C. Galactosyl transferase ☐
- D. Catalase ☐

118. Marker Enzyme of Mitochondria are/is:
- A. Na_+ - K_+ ATPase *(PGI 05)* ☐
- B. Glutamic dehydrogenase ☐
- C. Lactate dehydrogenase ☐
- D. No specific enzyme ☐

119. Catabolism of H_2O_2 is carried out by *(AI 04)*
- A. Peroxisomes *(NBE P 15,13)* ☐
- B. Mitochondria ☐
- C. Endoplasmic reticulum ☐
- D. Lysosomes ☐

120. In dividing cells, spindle is formed by : *(AI 02)*
- A. Ubiquitin ☐
- B. Tubulin ☐
- C. Laminin ☐
- D. Keratin ☐

121. Not true about microtubules is /are: *(PGI 2K)*
- A. Dynamic instability ☐
- B. Polarity ☐
- C. Charged ☐
- D. GTP not required ☐
- E. Form spindle ☐

122. Cell shape and motility are provided by *(AI 05)*
- A. Microfilaments ☐
- B. Microtubules ☐
- C. Golgi apparatus ☐
- D. Mitochondria ☐

Cell Cycle

123. True about cell cycle: *(PGI 15,14,11)*
- A. Sequence is G_1SG_2M ☐
- B. M is Meiotic phase ☐
- C. DNA synthesis occur in S phase ☐
- D. DNA synthesis occur in M phase ☐
- E. Cell divide in M phase ☐

124. The correct sequence of cell cycle is:
- A. G0-G1-S-G2-M *(AIIMS 04)* ☐
- B. G0-G1-G2-S-M ☐
- C. G0-M-G2-S-G1 ☐
- D. G0-G1-S-M-G2 ☐

125. Which parts of cell cycle are fixed in duration:
- A. G1 *(PGI 02)* ☐
- B. G2 ☐
- C. S ☐
- D. M ☐

ANSWERS AND EXPLANATIONS:

Cell Membrane

1. **Ans. B i.e. Triglycerides** 2. **D i.e. Protein** 3. **B i.e. 1:1**

[Ref: Ganong 23rd/e p. 32-34; Harper 28/e p. 407-11, 124; Guyton 10/e P-10]

Triglycerides are not found in eukaryotic plasma membraneQ. Plasma membrane is **mainly composed of protein**Q. Protein equal or exceed the quantity of lipid in nearly all membranes except myelin (an electrical insulator found on nerve fibers).

Cell membrane	Component	Percentage
Protein		55%
Lipid	**Phospholipids eg. lecithin (phosphatidylcholine), phosphatidyl ethanolamine, phosphatidyl inositol, phosphatidyl serine and sphingomyelin**Q	25%
	Cholestrol	13%
	Glyco (sphingo) lipids eg. **cerebrosides** (galactosyl & glucosyl ceramide) and **ganglioside** and other lipids Oleic acid	4%
Carbohydrate	Glycoprotein & glycolipid	3%

Ratio of Protein to Lipid in Different Membranes

Inner mitochondrial membrane	**3.2 (Max.)**
Sarcoplasmic reticulum	2.0
Outer mitochondrial membrane	1.1
Myelin	0.23

★ In almost all the membranes of the body proteins are equal or exceed the quantity of lipid. The only exception is **myelin (high lipid content provide good insulation)**Q. **Whereas, the inner mitochondrial membrane has highest protein content per gram**Q.

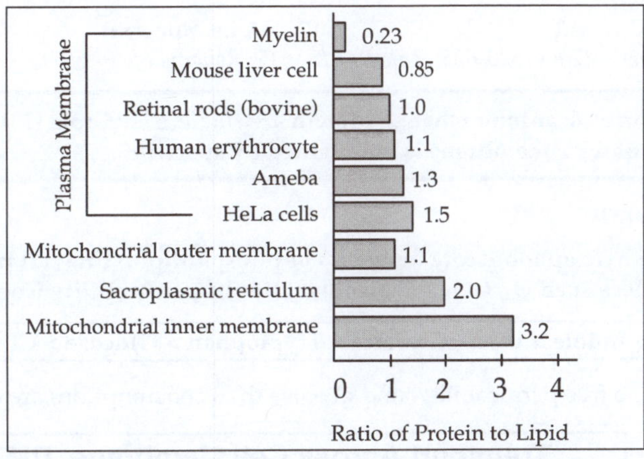

4. **A i.e. Glycosylphosphatidylinositol (GPI) anchored protein** *[Ref: Harper 29/e p. 466, 564-65; Berne 6/e p. 5-7]*

Membrane lipid rafts are cholesterol and sphingolipid (phospholipid) enriched micro-regions in the outer leaflet of plasma membrane. Lipid rafts are rich in **2 types of integral membrane protein** (1) ***GPI (glycosylphosphatidyl inositol) anchored protein***Q and (2) **proteins anchored to membrane by two covalently attached long chain saturated fatty acids** (2 palmitoyl groups or one palmitoyl and one myristoyl group).

5. **B i.e. Transduction of signals; E i.e. Enzyme activation at membrane surface**

[Ref: Harper's 27/e P-429-30; Ganong 22/e P- 9; Shinde & Chatterjee 6/e P- 13,14]

Phospholipid in cell membrane is responsible for **transduction of signals & enzyme activation at membrane surfaces**Q.

6. **D i.e. Linoleic Acid** 7. **B i.e Saturated fatty acids** 8. **B i.e. Increased fluidity of membranes**

[Ref. Harper's 27/e P-428-29; 26/e P-422, 417]

Polyunsaturated fatty acids (PUFAs) eg linoleic acid addition increases the **fluidity of membranes**Q. Whereas, **saturated FAs increase transition temperature (Tm) of lipid bilayer**Q.

9. **A i.e. Asymmetrical arrangement of cell wall component** 10. **B i.e. Lipids are symmetrical**
[Ref: Harper's 27/e P- 427; 26/e P- 416-29; Debjyoti Das: Biochemistry 8/e P-515]

In cell membrane there is asymmetrical arrangement of all cell components including lipidsQ.

11. **A i.e. Inner mitochondrial membrane** *[Ref. Harper's 27/e P-423; 26/e P-416].*

In almost all the membranes of the body proteins are equal or exceed the quantity of lipid. The only exception is **myelin (high lipid content provide good insulation)**Q. **Whereas, the inner mitochondrial membrane has heighest protein content per gram**Q.

12. **B i.e. A stretch of hydrophobic aminoacids** 13. **D i.e. Hydrogen bonds** 14. **E i.e. 7 aminoacid**
[Ref: Chatterjee 7/e p. 12-13; Harper's 27/e P-425-430; 26/e P- 450]

- **Trans membrane region of protein** is likely to have **a stretch of hydrophobic aminoacids,** while hydrophilic amino acids at ends.
- Lipids and proteins interact in membrane by **hydrogen bonds**. In leucine-zipper, leucine residue is seen after every **7 amino acid.**

15. **E i.e. Gm_2 – Gangliosides** *[Ref: Harper's 27/e P- 423-25]*

Glycolipids are widely distributed particularly in nervous tissue as brain. They **occur particularly in outer plasma membrane where they contribute to cell surface carbohydrate**Q

16. **C i.e. RBC** 17. **A i.e. Spectrin**
[Ref: Harper's 27/e P-623-625; 26/e P- 615- 617; Robbins 6/e P- 607]

Glycophorins & anion exchange protein are single & multiple (10) pass type integral proteins of RBC respectively. **Integrity of RBC membrane is maintained by spectrin**Q.

18. **A i.e. Oxygen**

- **Middle hydrophobic core (made up of phospholipid) bilayer) in cell membrane is most permeable to fat soluble substances such O_2, CO_2 and alcohol**Q. **But its permeability (coefficient) to polar substances in decreasing order is:**

H_2O > Indole > Urea =Glycerol > Tryptophan > Glucose > Cl^- > K^+ > Na^+

- **Urea** (b/o free permeability) and **glucose** (b/o consumption) are **osmotic infective.**

Transport Across Cell Membrane, RMP & Equilibrium Potential

19. **A i.e. Number of osmole per litre**

Osmolarity is numbers of **osmoles per liter** (in **1 liter**) of solution (plasma), whereas **osmolality** is numer of **osmoles per kilogram** of solvent (water). (Mn "Both Osmolar and liter end in r")Q.

20. **B i.e. 22.4** *[Ref: Garrett Biochemistry 3/ep- 37; Berne & Levy 6/e p 15-18; Ganong 23/e p. 4-6; Gabriel p 16-17; Gutyon 11/e 52, 297-98; Sabyasachi (2008) p-21-22]*

1 mol of an ideal solute dissolved in 1 kg (1000 gm) of water (i.e. 1 molal or M solution) at 1 atm pressure at 25°C yields a solution whose osmotic pressure relative to pure water is ***22.4 atm***Q.

21. **B i.e. Gibbs-Donnan effect** 22. **C i.e. Goldman-Hodgkin-Katz equation**
23. **B i.e. Nernst equation** *[Ref: Ganong 22/e p. 7, Guyton & Hall 11/e p. 58, 50, MTx]*

- **Cell is prevented from rupture (i.e. shape & volume of cell is maintained by) Donnan & Gibbs effect**Q.
- **Equilibrium potential** (i.e., membrane potential at which equilibrium b/w concentration & electrical gradient exist) for **any (one) univalent ion is calculated by Nernst equation**Q and for several different ions by **Goldmann- Hodgkin-katz equation.**

- **Cell is prevented from rupture (ie shape & volume of maintained by) Donnan & Gibbs effect**Q

24. B i.e. -60V *[Ref: Ganong 24/e p. 10; MTx]*

Nerst Equation

- Because **interior of cell is negative relative to exterior and NaCl concentration is more in ECF and K^+ concentration is more in ICF. Concentration & electrical gradients of various ions are**

Ion	CG	EG	Concentration		EP (mv)
			Out	In	
Cl^-	Inwards	Outwards	125	9	-70
K^+	Outwards	Inwards	5.5	150	-90
Na^+	Inwards	Inwards	150	15	+ 60

- **Sign of equilibrium potential is**

Positive (+) if	Negative (-) if
- **Negative (-) ion diffuse from inside to outside or** - **Positive (+) ion diffuse from outside to inside**	- (+) ion diffuse form inside to outside - (-) ion diffuse from outside to inside

(Cl^-) EMF = 61.5 log $\frac{[Cl_i^-]}{[Cl^-_0]}$
(K^+) EMF = 61.5 log $\frac{[K^+_0]}{[K^+_i]}$

For CI-ion concentration ratio is reversed (i.e. inside/outside) because valence is (-1).

Now about question

(K^+) EP $= 61.5 \log \frac{100}{10}$

$= 61.5 \times \log 10 = 61.5 \times 1$

$= 61.5 \approx 60$ mv

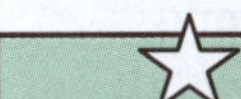

Donnan Effect

- **It is effect of a nondiffusible ion on distribution of other ions to which membrane is permeable**Q. For example a positive (+) charged non diffusible cation hinders diffusion of diffusible anion (-) & favors diffusion of diffusible cations (+).

Membrane

A	B
K^+	K^+ } Permeable
Cl^-	Cl^- }
	Protein (impermeable)

- Assuming that concentration of cations & anions are initially equal on both sides. Which means Cl^- conc. is more on side A and it diffuses down its concentration gradient from A to B, and some K^+ moves with –ve charged Cl^- because of its opposite charge. So ,

  $[K^+_B] > [K_A^+]$ and furthermore.

  $[K^+_B] + [Cl^-_B] + [Prot_B^-] > [K^+_A] + [Cl_A^-]$

  i.e., more osmotically active particles on side B than on side A.
- **Donnan & Gibbs equation** , for any pair of cations & anions of same valence, shows that in presence of a non diffusible ion, the diffusible ions distribute themselves so that at equilibrium, their concentration ratios are equal.

  $$\frac{|K_A^+|}{|K_B^+|} = \frac{|Cl_B^-|}{|Cl_A^-|} \text{ or } |K_A^+||Cl_A^-| = |K_B^+||Cl_B^-|$$

- It has 3 effects on body
- There are more osmotically active particles inside the cells because of presence of proteins (Pro-) and so **rupture of cells d/t osmosis is prevented by $Na_-^+K_-^+$ ATPase pump**Q. **(i.e. maintain cell shaped volume)**Q.
- Plasma has more protein than interstitial fluid, which affects ion movement across capillary wall.
- Because of asymmetrical distribution of ions across membrane at equilibrium, an electrical difference exists across membrane whose magnitude can be measured by Nernst equation.

Nernst Equation

- Movement of each ion across the membrane depends on its **concentration & electrical gradients**, across the membrane. For example b/o its higher concentration in ECF Cl^- ion tends to move inside the cells (**concentration gradient=CG**), where as **relative negative cell interior push Cl^- ion out of cell (electrical gradient= EG).**

Ion	CG	EG
C1	Inwards	Out wards
K^+	Outwards	Inwards
Na^+	Inwards	Inwards

- The membrane potential at which **influx & efflux of an ion are equal** (i.e., equilibrium b/w electrical & concentration gradients exist) is k/a **equilibrium potential**Q
- **Electrical gradient** that will balance a given concentration gradient (at 37°C) of univalent ion can be calculated from **Nernst equation**

$$\text{EMF (milivolts)} = \frac{RT}{FZ_I} \times \ln \frac{[C_0]}{[C_i]}$$

$$EMF = \pm 61.5 \log \frac{[C_i]}{[C_0]}$$

EMF = Electromotive force or equilibrium potential
R = Gas constant
T = Absolute temperature
F = Faraday (coulombs per mole of charge)
Z_I = Valence of ion eg Cl has –1 & Na has +1
Co = Concentration outside Ci = Concentration inside

Goldmann Equation

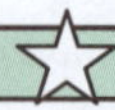

- When the membrane is permeable for several ions, the diffusion potential depends on (1) Polarity of ion (2) Permeability (P) of each ion & (3) Concentration of each ion on inside (i) & outside (0). This means the degree of importance of each ion in determining voltage is proportional to its **membrane permeability and concentration gradient.**
- **Goldman Hodgkins – Katz equation** for calculating membrane potential on the inside of membrane is EMF (mV) $= -61 \log \dfrac{CNa^{+}(i)\, P_{Na^{+}} + C_{k^{+}(i)} P_{k^{+}} + C_{Cl^{-}(0)} P_{Cl^{-}}}{C_{Na^{+}(0)} P_{Na^{+}} + C_{k^{+}(0)} P_{k^{+}} + C_{Cl^{-}(i)} P_{Cl^{-}}}$

25. B i.e. Passive diffusion along concentration gradient

26. A & E i.e. Concentration across & Area*[Ref: Ganong 23rd/e p. 5; Gabriel C Ezeilo p. 15, 141]*

According to **Fick's law of diffusion,** the net rate of diffusion is **directly proportional to available surface area across which diffusion is taking place and the concentration or chemical gradient but inversely proportional to thickness of membrane**[Q]. **Fick's law of diffusion** explains **passive diffusion along concentration gradient**[Q].

27. B i.e. K+ **28. B i.e. Cl-** **29. B i.e. -70 mv**

[Ref: Ganong 22/e P- 8, 59; Gabriel C. Ezeilo p. 27-28; Sembulingum 3/e P-142]

The potential difference between inside and outside of the cell under resting condition is known as **resting membrane potential (RMP).** ***K+ channels maintain the RMP***[Q]. **RMP of nerve cell (-70 mv) is equal to equilibrium potential of Cl-**[Q]

Tissue	RMP (-) mv
Inner Hair cell	- 150
Skeletal muscle, Ventricle[Q]	- 90[Q]
Neuron (Nerve-cells)	- 70[Q]
Thyroid	- 50
Smooth muscles, SA node	- 40 to - 30
RBC	- 10
Endocochlear Potential	+85[Q]

30. B & C i.e. ↑ negativity of the membrane & ↑ magnitude of RMP *[Ref: Gabriel C Ezeilo p. 22, 25, 27; Berne: Physiology 5/e pg-29]*

Increasing extracellular concentration of K+ ***decreases magnitude of RMP and negativity of membrane i.e. (depolarize cell)***[Q] whereas **decreasing** extracellular concentration of K+ ***increases RMP and negativity of membrane (i.e. hyperpolarize the cell)***[Q]. so relation is inverse but linear except at lower concentrations.

31. C i.e. 3 : 2 **32. A i.e. Most of the K+ are intracellular C i.e. An essential electrohyte for different organ function**

[Ref: Guyton 10/e P 338-39; Ganong 22/e P- 8, 69 35, 724; Harrison 15th/258- 62]

Most of the K+ ion are *intracellular*[Q] and it is required for *maintenance of restingmembrane potential, nerve conduction, muscle contraction* etc. For Na-K pump the coupling ration is 3:2.

33. A i.e. Involves ATPase activity **34. A i.e. Pumps 3 Na out; Pumps 2 K in** **35. B i.e. Hetrodimer hetrogenous**

36. D i.e. Ouabain **37. D i.e. Glycosylation** **38. A i.e. is K+ pumped against the gradient**

39. A i.e. Active transport *[Ref: Chaudhuri 5/e P-14; Ganong 22/e p. 33 – 35]*

- ***Na+ - K+ pump/Na+-K+ ATPase,*** is an ***electrogenic pump***[Q] that ***extrudes 3Na+ from the cell & take 2K+ into the cell.(coupling ratio is 3:2)***[Q]. It is a ***heterodimer* made up of *hetrogenous α & β units.***
- It pumps *both Na+ & K+ against their concentration gradient by* utilizing energy from the ***hydrolysis of ATP.***[Q]
- Increase in intracellular Na+, decrease the height of action potential. The pump keeps intracellular Na+ low and contributes to small amount of membrane potential.

α - Subunit (MW 1 lack)	β - Subunit (MW 55,000)

- α_1 isoform is found in membranes of most cells, α_2 in muscle, heart, adipose tissue and brain; and α_3 isoform in heart and brain
- It transports Na^+ & K^+ and spans cell membrane 10 times, with amino & carboxyl terminal both located intracellularly. It contains

Intracellular	Extracellular
- **Na+ binding site**[Q] - **Phosphorylation (Asp 376) site**[Q] - **ATP binding site**[Q]	- **K+ binding site**[Q] - Ouabain binding site[Q]

- β_1 subunit is widely distributed but absent in certain astrocytes, vestibular cells of inner ear, & glycolytic fast twitch muscles. Whereas fast twitch muscles contain only β_2 subunit
- It is a glycoprotein, has single membrane – spanning domain & **3 extracellular glycosylation site**[Q] all of which have attached carbohydrate residues.

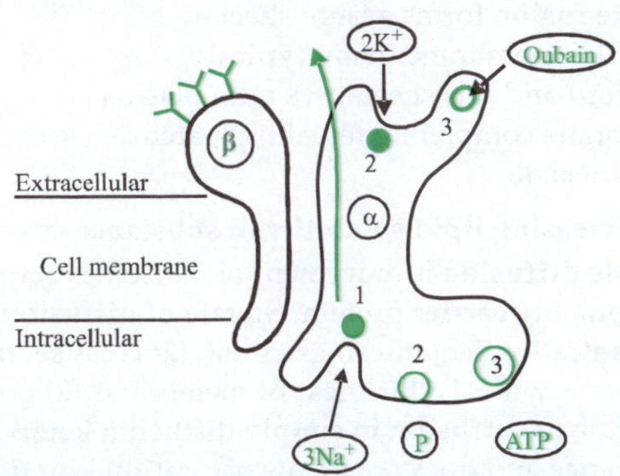

40. C i.e. Na+ with glucose symport *[Ref: Sembulingum 3/e P- 19; MTx]*

41. A i.e. Secondary active transport

Na+ is cotransported (symported) with glucose[Q].Co (Sym) transport and antiport or counter transport are secondary active transport[Q].

Transport	Osmosis	Simple Diffusion	Facilitated Diffusion	1°Active Transport	2° Active Transport
Move	**Water**[Q]	O_2, CO_2, Fat	Glucose, some aa,	Unipart of ions Na^+, K^+, H^+, Ca^{++}	- **Symport (contra sport) of glucose/aa in cell along Na+**[Q] - **Anti (counter) transport** of H^+, Ca^{++} out of cell against Na^+

Sodium Co-transport (Symport)

In this along with Na^+, another substance is carried by the carrier protein called symport. The energy is obtained from diffusion process of Na^+ due to concentration gradient across the cell membrane.

Carrier protein

It has two receptor sites on outer surface. One is for Na^+ & another site is for other substance

Substance carried by Na+ - Co – transport

- Glucose
- Amino acid
- Chloride, Iodide
- Urate

Sodium co transport of glucose

One sodium ion & one glucose molecule from ECF enter the cell.[Q]

42. B i.e. Resealing by lipid bilayer

[Ref: Berne 6/e p. 6-10; Journal of Cell Science (2002): Repairing a torn cell surface: make way lysosome to rescue]

After a cell membrane is damaged by insertion of microneedle, repair occurs by resealing of lipid bilayes through vesicle- plasma membrane fusion (in cases of small breech) or through **vesicle-vesicle fusion** (in cases of large disruption).

Repair: Lipid Bilayer Resealing

- **Calcium (Ca^{++}) entering through disruption** signals repair, initiates **depolymerization of subcortical F actin network** and triggers **accumulation of vesicles** (powered by kinesin & myosin motor proteins) at the breach site
- In small breaches, **vesicles fuse to plasma membrane (exocytotic reaction).** Whereas, in large disruptions **vesicle-vesicle fusion** forms a large sheet of vesicular membrane **(homotypical reaction)** and this sheet fuses with plasma membrane completing resealing **(patch hypothesis).**

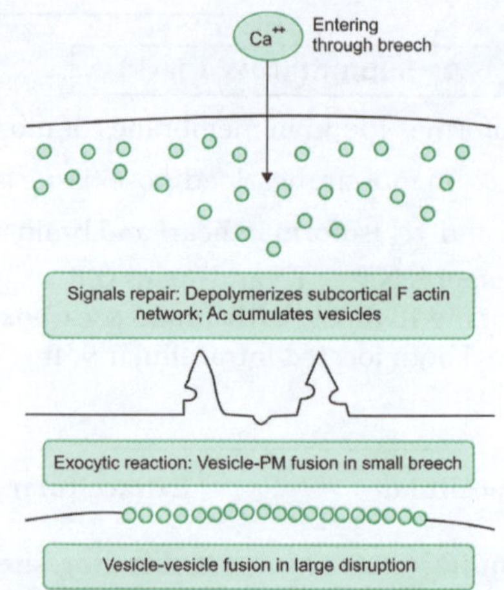

43. C i.e. Increasing lipid solubility of substance

44. C i.e. Simple diffusion *[Ref: Guyton 12/e P-45-47]*

- **Simple diffusion** is movement of molecules **across cell membrane following a concentration or chemical gradient without any carrier protein. So rate of diffusion is directly proportional to (i.e. increases with increase in) (1) concentration (chemical) gradient, (2) cross section area** of membrane & **prone size,** (3) **lipid solubility**Q. But it decreases with (1) **thickness** of membrane, (2) **polarity (charge)** of substance and (3) large particle size.
- **The rate of diffusion in simple diffusion keeps on increasing proportionately with the concentration of the diffusing substance** and does not follow **saturation kinetics.**

45. C i.e. Occur in direction opposite to electrical gradient

46. A i.e. Facilitated diffusion requires energy

47. C i.e. Carrier protein

48. B i.e. It requires a carrier protein

[Ref: Ganong 23rd/e p. 46; Guyton 11th/e p.47; Harper 28th/e p. 414- 16; Chaudhari 6/ed pg-11; Sembulingum 3/e P-17; Harper's 27/e P-430, 434; 26/e P-423]

- When carrier proteins move substances **in the direction of their chemical or electrical gradient,**Q **no energy input is required**Q and the process is called **facilitated diffusion.**
- **A carrier protein** is responsible for both the **facilitated diffusion and active transport.**Q

*Feature	Simple Diffusion	Facilitated Diffusion	Active Transport
Type	**Passive**	**Passive**	**Active**
ATP (energy) expenditure	**Not required**	**Not required**	**Required**
Concentration / Electrochemical (EC) gradient	**Along** EC gradient	**Along** EC gradient	**Against** EC gradient
Direction	Bidirectional	(Can be) Bidirectional	Unidirectional
Carrier proteins	**Not required**	**Required**	**Required**
Saturability	**Not** saturable	Saturable	Saturable
Maximum rate of transport (V_{max})	Does **Not** have V_{max}	Have V_{max}	Have V_{max}
Rate of Transport	**Proportionate** to concentration gradient over a wide range	- Proportionate only at low concentrations before carrier protein becomes saturated - After V_{max} becomes constant i.e. rate is not proportionate over a wide range	Not proportionate to concentration gradient (difference)
Competitive Inhibition (by structurally similar inhibitor)	Not inhibit	Inhibited	Inhibited
Examples	Diffusion of gasses (O_2, CO_2) in lung, movement of fat	**Glucose** uptake by muscles, some aminoacids	Na^+ / K^+ ATPase H^+ / K^+ ATPase

49. C i.e. Hydrophilic in character *[Ref: Harper's 27/e P-433-34; 26/e P-426; Shinde 6/e P-15; Thomas M. Devlin 4/e P-211, 212, 213]*

> *Ionophores are hydrophobic in nature*Q

50. B i.e. Diffusion

51. D i.e. Diffusion *[Ref: Harper 27/e p. 108-10; 439-39]*

> - **Movement of water across cell membrane occurs by osmosis (simple diffusion)**Q.
> - Transport via **simple passive diffusion** is favoured by ***small size, lipid solubility (hydrophobicity) absence of charge (neutrality), and absence of polarity (nonpolar nature)***Q.

52. C i.e. Ca^{++}

53. A i.e. Extrusion of cell bound vesicles

54. A i.e. Receptor mediated endocytosis

55. B i.e. Endocytosis C i.e. Exocytosis

[Ref: Ganong 24/e p. 47-50; 22/e p. 28; Harper 27/e p. 436-38]

> Process by which **fusion of part of cell membrane occurs are exocytosis & endocytosis.** Q **Exocytosis is extrusion of cell bound vesicles. Clathrin** is used for ***receptor mediated endocytosis***Q. **Reverse pinocytosis** requires *Ca^{++}* Q.

56. A i.e. Gap junctions

57. C i.e. Direct contact through gap junctions

[Ref: Ganong 23rd/e p. 40-38; Gabriel C Ezeilo p. 9, 37, 56, 113, 117; Lehninger 5/e pg- 374-95]

> **Gap junctions** are involved in ***transmission of regulatory protein (Signal) from cell to cell without entering ECF***Q.

58. B i.e. -90

Concentration in Nerve Cell (mmol/L of H_2O)			
Ion	Inside cell	Outside cell	**Equilibrium Potential** (mV)
Na^+	15.0	150.0	**+60**Q
K^+	150.0	5.5	**-90** Q
Cl^-	9.0	125.0	**-70** Q

Resting Membrane Potential (RMP) = -70mV Q

59. C i.e. Of the acidic pH of vesicle *[Ref: Chatterjea 7/e p. 19; Lippincott's 5/e p. 230-31]*

> **The low pH breaks the linkage between receptor –macromolecule (ligand) complex.**

Body Fluid / Extra & Intra Cellular Fluid

60. B i.e. 0.4×body wt *[Ref: Ganong 24/e P- 3-5; Guyton 12/SAE p. 47-53]*

61. A i.e. Water constitutes 60% of body weight

62. A i.e. Total body water constitutes 60% of body weight

63. B i.e. Phosphorus & Magnesium.. C i.e. Na^+ & Cl^- principal ions ECF; D i.e. Kidney tightly regulates Na^+, K^+, Cl^- …

64. B i.e. K^+ & PO_4^-

65. D i.e. High Na: K^+ ratio is seen

66. C i.e. 28L

67. A i.e. K^+

68. B i.e. High Na^+; D i.e. High Cl^- ; E i.e. Nearly equal osmolarity in both fluid

- In the average young adult male 18% of body weight is protein, 7% is mineral and 15% is fat. The remaining **60%** is **water**Q. The total blood volume is 8% of body weight.

> - **Na^+, Cl^- and HCO_3^-** are major **extra cellular** and **K^+, PO_4^{3-} & Mg^{+2}** are major intracellular ions.
> - **ECF composition** is carefully regulated by various mechanisms, but **especially by kidneys**Q

- **Osmolarity** (corrected, in mosm/L) and **osmotic pressure** (mmHg at 37° C) **are nearly equal for ECF and ICF**Q.

	ECF		**ICF**
	Plasma	**Interstitial fluid**	**Intracellular fluid**
Osmolarity	282	281	281
Osmotic pressure	5443	5423	5423

	ECF: Predominant ions	**ICF: Predominant ions**
Cation (+)	**Na^+(most abundant & osmotically active)**Q **>>>Ca^{++}**	**K^+ (most abundant & osmotically active)**Q **>>> Mg^{++}**
Anion (-)	Cl^->>> HCO_3^-	**Phosphate (PO_3^{-3})>>> Protein**
Overall	**Na^+ >Cl^- >HCO_3^->Ca^{++}**	**K^+ > PO_4^3> Mg ++> Proteins**

Total Body Water (TBW)= 60% Body Weight (BW) = 42 liters

Intracellular Fluid=28 lit

- Is 2/3rd of TBW i.e. **40% of body weight**[Q] **=0.4 × BW**[Q]
- Portion of total body fluid which remain within the cell membrane

Extracellular Fluid = 14 liters

- **Is 1/3rd of TBW i.e. 20% of body weight**[Q] **= 0.2 x BW**
- It is a general term for all the body fluids outside the cell. It consist of: interstitial fluid , plasma , lymph, cerebrospinal fluid.

In the Vascular system (Plasma)

- 25% or 1/4th of ECF = 3.5 liters
- **5% of body weight**[Q] (8% of TBW)

Outside the vascular system (Interstitial fluid)

- 75% or 3/4th of ECF = 10.5 liters
- **15% of body weight**[Q] (25% of TBW)

Composition of ECF & ICF 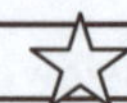

ECF (Plasma & Interstitial Fluid)

- **Contains large amounts of sodium (Na^+) & chloride (Cl^-) ions**[Q], reasonably large amounts of bicarbone (HCO_3^-) ions, but only small quantities of potassium (K^+), calcium (Ca^{++}), magnesium (Mg^{++}), phosphate (PO_4^{3-}) and organic acid ions.
- **Most abundant cation is Na+ and anion is Cl-**[Q]

ICF

- Contains **large amount of potassium (K+) and phosphate (PO_4^{3-}) ions plus moderate quantities of magnesium (Mg^{++}) and sulfate (SO_4^{--}) ions**[Q]
- Contains **only small quantities (low concentrations) of sodium & chloride**[Q].
- **Most abundant cation is K^+ and anion is PO_4^{3-} followed by protein**[Q]

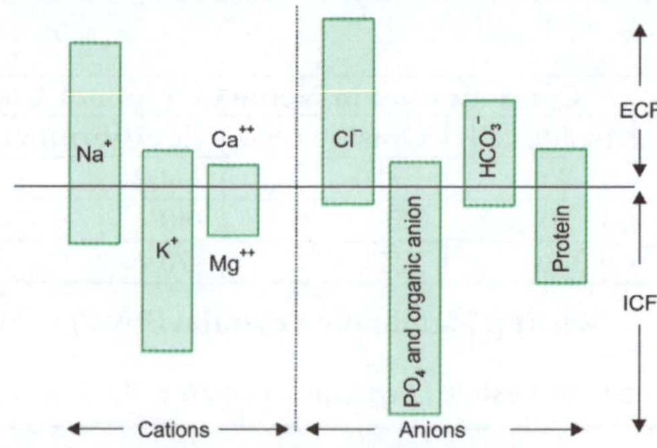

69. B i.e. Total body water **70. C i.e. Inulin** **71. D i.e. I125 – albumin for blood volume**
72. A i.e. Cr51 *[Ref: Ganong 24/e P- 2,3]*

Body Fluid/ Volume	Method of Measurement
Total body fluid (or TBW) **By Dilution Principle** **Mn : "DAT"**	- **Deuterium (^2H_2O, D_2O heavy water most commonly used)**[Q] - **Aminopyrine**[Q]**, Antipyrine** - Tritium oxide. ($3H_2O$)
Extracellular fluid volume (ECF) **Mn : "SIMaN"**	- **Inulin**[Q] **(most accurate measurement), I^{125} iothalamate** - **Mannitol**[Q]**, Na^{22}, Sucrose**[Q]**, Tiosulfate**
Plasma volume Mn : **[P E A]**	- **Evan's blue**[Q] (T-1824) = Due bound to plasma protein - **Albumin labeled with radioactive iodine**[Q] **(I^{125}), Na^{22}, Thiosulphate**
Intracellular volume (ICF) (Cannot measured directly)	Total body fluid – Extracellular fluid (= TBW - ECF)
Interstitial fluid volume (Cannot measured directly)	ECF – Plasma volume
Total Blood Volume	- **Cr_{51} labelled RBC**[Q] or $= \frac{\text{Plasma volume}}{1 - \text{Hematocrit}}$
Red Cell Volume	- Is volume occupied by all circulating red cells in the body can be determined by **TBV- PV** - Measured independently by injencting tagged RBCS and measuring the fraction of red cells that is tagged. A commonly used tag **is Cr^{51} and Fe^{59}, P^{32}**

73. D i.e. Radioactive sodium and radioactive labelled albumin

Intestinal fluid volume cannot be calculated directly. It is calculated by using **ECF volume** (which is **measured by radioactive Na**^{22}) and **plasma volume** (measured by **radioactive iodine labeled albumin)**^{Q}.

74. B i.e. 18 Litres *[Ref: Ganong 24/ep 2]*

- Out of **10 gm of injected** mannitol, 10% **(=1gm)** was **excreted**. So amount of mannitol distributed in ECF wound be 9 gm. Because at equilibrium, concentration of mannitol in ECF= 50 mg/100ml, i.e. 50 mg mannitol is distributed in 100 ml of ECF
- So 9 gm mannitol would be distributed in $\frac{100\ ml}{50\ mg}$x 9 gm = $\frac{0.1\ lit}{0.05\ gm}$x 9 gm = $\frac{10}{5}$x9 = 18 lit^{Q}

75. A i.e. Normal cardiac output, altered blood volume *[Ref: Ganong 22/e P-2; Sembulingum 3/e P- 39; Chaudhuri 5/e P- 417]*

Diffusion of Dye out of Capillaries Causes

No change in cardiac output estimation (because)	**Altered Blood volume estimation** (because)
• For the estimation of CO by dye method, the dye is injected in suitable vein & the samples are drawn from an artery. • Cardiac output is equal to the amount of indicator injected divided by its average concentration in arterial blood. After a single circulation through the heart *(so before the dye reaches the capillaries the work of estimation of CO is already complete)*	• A known quantity of substance is injected into blood vessels & allowed to mix thoroughly with the fluid. Then a sample of fluid is drawn & the concentration of substance is determined ∴ Volume of fluid in compartment = $\frac{\text{Amount of substance injected}}{\text{Concentration of substance in sample of fluid}}$ • ***For accurate estimation dye must remain within the blood vessels.***^{Q} • *If it diffuses out of capillaries* concentration of substance in sample fluid decreased & the calculated blood blood volume would be much ***higher than real volume***^{Q}

76. A i.e. Patch clamp *[Ref: Internet]*

- **Patch clamp Electrophysiological Technique** is used to **study current flow across a single or multiple ion channel**^{Q}. However, this refinement of voltage clamp (by Neher & Sakmann) made it possible to study current flow **across single ion channel for the first time.**
- It is especially useful in **excitable cells like neurons, muscle fibres, cardiomyocytes, pancreatic beta cells** and bacteria (giant spheroplasts).

77. A i.e. Anterior hypothalamus **78. C i.e. Urea** | **79. C i.e. Due to urea of glucose mainly**

80. A i.e. Normal serum level is 134- 145 m eq/lit; B i.e. Daily intake is 150 mmol of NaCl; C i.e. extracellular

81. D i.e. Bone *[Ref: Harrison 16/e p. 253 – 54; Guyton & Hall 11/e p. 293 – 96; Bailey & Love 24/e p. 56-57]*

- Typical **western diet** consumption provides approximately ***150 mmol of sodium chloride (NaCl) daily***^{Q}.
- Normal level of serum sodium is ***136 – 145 mmol/L (SI unit) or 136- 145 meq/L (conventional unit)***^{Q}.
- Na^{+} - K^{+} ATP pase pump actively transports Na^{+} out of cells. As a result, ***85- 90% of all sodium is extracellular***^{Q} and ***ECF volume is a reflection of total body*** Na^{+} ***content***^{Q}. And in the same way total body Na+ content is a reflection of ECF volume.
- ***Sodium reserve is chiefly stored in stomach wall***^{Q}, which makes it alkaline to counter balance the acidic environment. *30-40%* sodium is stored in *skeletal muscles*.
- The normal plasma osmolality is *275 – 290 milliosmoles/kg*. To maintain it, normally about *600 mosmols/day* solute must be excreted. And since maximum urine osmolality is 1200 mosmols/kg a *minimum urine out put of 500 mL/d* is required.
- **Osmoreceptor** located in ***anterolateral hypothalmus***^{Q} is stimulated by hypertonicity. **Ineffective osmols** i.e. solutes that do not contribute to shift water across cell membrane, like ***urea and glucose***^{Q} do not play a role in stimulating thirst. The average osmotic threshold for thirst is ~ *295 mosmol/kg*. **Osmotic adaptation** is a defence mechanism of brain cells ***in chronic hypo & hyper natremia against large water shifts***^{Q}. It is mediated by initialshifts of K^{+} & Na^{+} f/b synthesis, import or export of ***organic solutes (osmolytes) such as inositol, betaine & glutamine***^{Q}. In chronic hyponatremia brain cells lose & in chronic hypernatremia gain solutes.
- Sodium is the principal cation content of ECF. The total body sodium is ~ *5000 mmol*, of which 44% is in *extracellular fluid* 9% is in intracellular fluid and remaining ***47% is in bone***^{Q}.
- 98% of potassium (K^{+}) is intracellular & 2% in extracellular fluid. ***3/4 of total boy*** K^{+} ***(~ 3500 mmol) is found in skeletal mucles***^{Q}. Normal adult ingests ~ 1.0 mmol/kg of K^{+} in food. Fruit, milk & honey are rich in K^{+}.

Extracellular Matrix

82. A, B, C, E i.e. Collagen, Laminin, Fibronectin, Elastin

83. C i.e. Integrins *[Ref: Harper 28/e p. 527-35; Lippincott 5/e p. 43-51; Lehninger 5/e p. 249-54; Robbin's 7/e p. 103-106]*

- **Extracellular matrix proteins** are collagen, elastin, fibrillin, fibronectin, laminin and proteoglycans (GAGs) Mn- "Call Ela For Last Prose" Whereas cell **adhesion molecules present** in cytoplasm or cell membrane include **integrins, selectins, cadherins and immunoglobulin family CAMs**Q.
- **Integrins** are cell surface adhesion protein that provide linkage between cell outside & inside, between cell- cell and between cell & extracellular matrix.

84. D i.e. Rhodopsin *[Ref: Robbins 7/e p. 103- 06, 956, 54]*

Basement membrane is PAS (periodic acid shiff) positive amorphous structure which consist of **non fibrillar collagen (mostly type IV), laminin (most abundant glycoprotein), fibronectin, entactin (nidogen)**Q, tenascin and several other glycoproteins along with polyanionic proteoglycans (mostly heparan sulfate or perlecan).

85. A i.e. Collagen *[Ref: Chatterjea: 7/e p. 85-86]*

Due to formation of hydrogen & disulphide bonds, peptide chain assumes 3-D secondary structure by way of folding or coiling leading to formation of

α- Helix	**β- Pleated sheet**	**Triple Helix**	**Reverse turns / β- Bends**
Found in **Keratin**Q	- Silk fibers - Spider's web - Reptilian claw	- **Collgen**Q is rich, in proline & hydroxy- proline & cannot for α-helix & β pleated sheet - It forms triple helix	- Polypeptide chain of globular protein changes direction >2 times, when it folds k/a β- bends - Proline is ideally suited for 2nd residue and glycine for 3rd residue of reverse turn

86. D i.e. Memicane *[Ref: Albert & Jacobie 2/e vol 2 p.1419-21; The eye: Basic sciences in practice 2/e p. 212; Molecular biology in Medicine 3/e vol I p. 1018-38]*

Interphotoreceptor matrix has SPARC, TIMP and matrix metalloproteinases but no mimecaine (or osteoglycin).

87. A i.e. Metalloproteinases *[Ref: Robbins 7/e p. 110-11, 103, 312]*

Zinc dependent matrix metalloproteinases (MMP) degrade collagen and other extracellular matrix proteins (including that of basement membrane)Q.

88. D i.e. IV **89. A i.e. Cytoplasm** **90. A i.e. Scurvy; D i.e. Osteogenesis**

[Ref: Lipppincott 2/e P-40; Harper's 27/e P-545-49; 26/e P-535-538; Robbins 7/e p. 104]

Collagen show **triple helix**Q and is **never present free inside the cytoplasm**Q. **Scurvy, osteogenesis imperfecta**Q, Ehler – Danlos syndrome & Alport syndrome occurs d/t its deficient synthesis.

91. C i.e. Vitreous humor **92. D i.e. Hyaluronic acid** **93. D i.e. Hyaluronic acid**

[Ref. Harper's 28/e p. 535-38; Lippincott's 5/e p. 158-63; Katzung 10/e p. 547; KDT 6/e p. 600]

- **The viscosity and the plastic (thixotropic properties) of the synovial fluid is because of its hyaluronate content.**Q
- **Hyaluronic acid**, a **glycosaminoglycan** is a polymer of repeating disaccharide units (of **glucuronic acid and N-acetyl glucosamine**).

Functions of Glycosaminoglycans

Hyaluronic acid	- Viscosity of the ***synovial fluid***Q. - Tensile strength and elasticity of *cartilage and tendons* - Jelly like consistency of ***vitreous humor of eye***Q.
Chondroitin sulfate	- Tensile strength of *cartilage tendons, ligaments* and the *walls of aorta**.
Dermatan sulfate	- Pliability of skin* and heart valves*.
Keratan sulfate	- Found in **horny structures*** of body composed of dead cells - *hair, nails, claws, horn, hoofs.* - Also present in cornea*.
Heparin	- *Anticoagulant*

94. A, C, D i.e. Keratin sulphate, Dermatan sulphate, Heparan sulphate *[Ref: Gray's 40/e p 974]*

Danaproid is a **low molecular weigh (LMW) heparanoid containing chondroitin sulfate, dermatan sulfate and heparan sulfate (i.e. sulfates of chondroitin, dermatan & heparan)**Q. Other **heparinoids are ancrod, lepirudin and heparan sulfate.**

95. D i.e. Mucopolysacchridoses *[Ref. Harper's 29/e p. 599; Lippincott 2/e P-154; NMS Biochemistry 4/e P-83]*

96. B i.e Dermatan sulfate D i.e. Heparan sulfate

Uronic acid level is elevated in urine in **mucopolysaccharidosis. Dermatan & heparan sulfate** are urinary metabolites accumulated **in Hurler & Hunter's syndrome**Q.

97. B i.e. Keratin *[Ref: IADVC Textbook & Atlas of Dermatology/1st /9-10; Lehinger 2/e P 60-65, 126- 135]*

The elasticity, stability and integrity of stratum corneum of skin is due to disulfide cross linkages between the keratin moleculesQ

In the stratum corneum layer, keratohyaline granules are present. These granules form protein profilaggrin, which is degraded into filaggrin (filament aggregating protein), as granular cells transform to keratinized corneum cells. Filaggrin is a hyaline rich protein which functions as interfilamentous glue to aggregate and align the keratin filaments in keratinized cells. Keratohyaline also contain cysteine rich proteins, whose disulfide bonds contribute to the chemical inertness and strengh of the keratinized layer.

98. A i.e Disulphide bond *[Ref. Lippincott's 2/e P-18; Ref: IADVC Textbook & Atlas of Dermatology/1st /9-10; Lehinger 2/e P 60-65, 126- 135]*

The keratins are a family of closely related fibrous proteins, whose structure is nearly entirely alpha-helical.They are a major component of tissues such as hairs and skin; **their rigidity is determined by the number of disulphide bonds between the constituent polypeptide chains.**Q

Cell Organelle

99. B i.e. Dynenin and kinesin *[Ref: Comprehensive human physiology R. Gregor/86; Harper's 27/e 585; 26/e P-577; Ganong 22/e P- 14, 15]*

Microtubules guide the transport of protein & vesicular material; and **'Motors' (Denin & Kinesin) provide the force behind such movement**Q

100. C i.e. Antegrade & Retrograde

101. C i.e. Neurofilament *[Ref: The journal of cellular biology: Axonal transport of membranous & non membranous cargoes: a unified perspective: Anatomy Brown (17 march 2003)]*

- **Rapid axonal flow in neurons** is mediated by **dynein, kinesin & lysosome.** Whereas, **microfilaments >> microtubules & neurofilaments mediate slow axonal transport**Q.

- Materials destined for the axon are transported **anterogradely**, toward the axon tip, and materials destined to return are transported **retrogradely**, toward the cell body. This **bidirectional transport** process, known as **axonal transport**, is not fundamentally different from the pathways of macromolecular and membrane traffic that occur in all eukaryotic cells, but it is remarkable for its scale

102. B i.e. Lipid **103. A i.e. Cytosol** **104. B i.e. EMP pathway** **105. B i.e. Glycogenolysis**
106. B i.e. Biosynthesis of fatty acids **107. B i.e. Lipid** **108. C i.e. Rough ER** **109. D i.e. Urea cycle**

[Ref: Harper 29/e p 308-9, 155-55, 211, 207, 549-50, 122; Chattarjea 8/e p 6-9, 438; Ganong 22/e P-18; Guyton 11/e p. 21, Chaudhari 5/e p. 4; Lipponcott 4/e p. 220-225; Harper 27/e p. 100-01, 506]

- **Lipid & steroid synthesis** occurs in **smooth (agranular) cytoplasmic / endoplasmic reticulum**, whereas **protein synthesis** occurs in **rough or granular ER**.
- **Glycogenesis, glycogenolysis, glycolysis, HMP (PPP) shunt, biosynthesis of fatty acids and denovo purine synthesis occurs in cytosol (not in mitochondria)**[Q]. **Mitochondria** is primarily (**mainly**) involved in **TCA (Kreb's /citric acid) cycle, oxidative phosphorylation (ATP synthesis), electron transport (respiratory) chain, β-oxidation of fatty acids (<20 carbon)** and ketone body formation (**Keto genesis**). It is also partly involved in metabolic functions like **gluconeogenesis, urea synthesis (cycle), heme synthesis and denovo pyrimidine synthesis**[Q].
- Mitochondrial double stranded circular DNA is found in matrix and encodes mitochondrial (mt) **r-RNAs** (12 S small & 16 S large subunit), **22 t RNAs** and **13 protein subunits of respiratory chain** (out of total 67). It has high mutation rate and contains very few untranslated sequences. Although **mitochondria synthesize some proteins required for energy generating function**, the structural proteins and other proteins need to carry out cellular respiration are encoded by nuclear chromosomal DNA.

Sub cellular Sites of Metabolic Pathways

Cytosol (Main / Primary site)
- Glycolysis, Glycogenolysis & Glycogenesis[Q]
- HMP shunt (PPP pathway)[Q]
- Fatty acid synthesis[Q]
- De novo purine synthesis

Mn- Cytosolic Shunt of Pure, Fatty, & Glyco synthesis (+ lysis)[Q]

Cytosol f/b Endoplasmic Reticulum (ER) membrane
- Cholesterol synthesis[Q]

Mitochondria
- **β–oxidation of fatty acids (<20 carbons)**[Q]
- **Electron transport (respiratory) chain = ETC**[Q]
- **Tricarboxylic acid (Kreb's or citric acid) cycle = TCA**
- **Oxidative phosphorylation (ATP synthesis)**[Q]
- **Ketogenesis** (ketone body formation)

Mn BEKT- OX in Mitochondria

Peroxisome followed by mitochondria

Beta oxidation of very long chain fatty acids (≥ 20 carbons)

Microsome, Mitochondria & Peroxisome
- **Primary bile acid synthesis** (1st regulatory 7-α hydroxylase is **microsomal** enzyme; 27 hydroxylation forming chenodeoxy cholyl CoA is **mitochondrial** step).
- **Bile salts** are formed by conjugation of primary bile acids in **peroxisome.**

Mitochondria & Cytosol
- **Gluconeogenesis**[Q] (initially in mitochondria & later in cytosol)
- **Urea synthesis**[Q] (initial two steps in mitochondira & remaining in cytosol)
- **Heme (& porphyrin derivatives) synthesis** (Mitochondria → cytosol → mitochondria)
- Denovo **pyrimidine synthesis** (cytosol followed by mitochondria)

Mn- "**New Glucose, urea heme & pyrimidine**"

Microsome (≈ER)
- **Heme catabolism (degradation** ie **bilirubin production)**
- **Elongation of FA chains** (both saturated & unsaturated fatty acyl-Co As)

Nucleus
- DNA replication & transcription (mRNA synthesis)

Golgi Apparatus
- **Sorting of proteins**[Q] for their correct destination
- Synthesize & packaging of complex molecules (including glycolipids, glycoproteins & lipoproteins) such as **hyaluronic acid and chondroitin sulfate**[Q].
- Maturation of synthesized proteins, protein sorting, packaging & secretion

Endoplasmic Reticulum (ER)

Rough / Granular
- Ribosomes are attached to the cytoplasmic side of membrane
- **Function:**
  - **Protein synthesis**[Q]
  - Initial folding of polypeptide chain with formation of disulfide bond

Smooth / Agranular
- In this ribosomes are absent
- **Function**
  - **Site for steroid syntheis**[Q] in steroid secreting cells
  - Site of **detoxification** in other cells.
  - **Synthesize lipid especially phospholipids & cholesterol**[Q]
  - Provide enzymes that control glycogen breakdown when glycogen is to be used for energy.

110. B i.e. Golgi apparatus **111. C i.e. Nonpolarized structure** **112. B i.e. ER→Cis→Trans→Cell membrane**
[Ref: Chatterjea & Shinde 7/e p. 7; Ganong 22/e p. 27- 28; Guyton & Hall 11/e p. 15]

Golgi apparatus serves as a unique **sorting & packing device**Q, that receives newly synthesized proteins, all containing signal or transit peptide from endoplasmic retinaculum. It rejects proteins with no signal or transit peptide without processing and that remain as cytoplasmic protein.

113. B i.e. Isolation is done by hydrolysis in alkaline pH & synthesize fat *[Ref:Harper 28/e P-193; Chatterjea 7/e P 5-6]*

- **Mitochondria** is the 'Power house' of cell because enzymes for energy metboism and **ATP synthesis are present in mitochondria**Q. Mitochondria both **import and synthesize proteins**Q. Isolation of mitochondria is done **by ultracentrifugation**Q.**Mitochondria has double stranded circular DNA**Q.
- **Main pathway for lipogenesis (do not have fatty acid synthesis) occurs in cytosol**Q. **Fatty acid is synthesized in cytoplasm of a cell**Q.

114. A i.e. SGOT (AST) *[Ref: Vasudevan 6/e p-268-70; Lehninger 5/e p 631-33, 677-88, 873-74; Herper 28/e p 272-73, 132/35/36/43/47/87/84/85, 111-12, 488, 101, 610, 319-20, 207, 104 Clatchey: Clinical laboratory medicine 2/e p 286-88; Textbook of Hepatology 3/ep 451; Chatterjae 7/e p 625*

- **Glutamate dehydrogenase (GDH) and aparate aminotransferase (AST)/ or serum glutamate oxaloacetate transaminase (SGOT)**Q mitochondrial isoenzyme, are **liver enzymes** predominantly present in **mitochidrial matrix**.

- **AST (or SGOT)** exists in genetically distinct 2 different forms which are named a/t their location: (1) **Mitochondrial isoenzyme (80%)** is responsible for maximum AST activity of liver and ; (2) **Cytosolic or cytoplasmic isoenzyme** (20%) is responsible for most of circulating AST activity.
- AST (SGOT) is found in maximum concentration in **Heart**. ("Mn **She GOT Heart**") and then in *liver, skeletal muscle and kidney*. So elevated levels of mitochondrial AST or mitochondrial AST/Total AST ratio is indicative of necrosis of cells containing AST (and thus causing cellular leak) eg heart cell necrosis in MI or liver cell necrosis in chronic liver disease.
- SGOT (AST) and SGPT (ALT) both are found in most tissues but their relative amounts vary. ***Heart muscles are richer in SGOT whereas liver is richer in SGPT***Q.

115. D i.e. Important component of cartilage *[Ref: Harper's 27/e P-558-61; 26/e P-551]*

Aggregan is the **major proteoglycan component of cartilage**Q. It is composed of several glycosa – amino glycans (hyaluronic acid, chondroitin sulfate and keratin sulfate) and both link and core proteins.

116. A i.e. Galactosyl transferase & Glucokinase
117. C i.e. Galactosyl transferase
118. B i.e. Glutamic dehydrogenase
119. A i.e. Peroxisomes *[Ref: Harper's 28/e p. 410]*

Marker enzymes of **plasma membrane** are **adenyl cyclase, 5' nucleotidase** and **Na+ - K+ ATPase**. Mn **"ANNA"**. Whereas, marker of **golgicomplex** is **galactosyl transferase**Q and **mitochondria** is **glutamate dehydrogenase**Q.

Organelle or Fraction	Marker	Major Function
Nucleus	DNA	Site of chromosomes Site of DNA-directed RNA synthesis (transcription)
Mitochondria	**Glutamate dehydrogenase** Q	Citric acid cycle, oxidative phosphorylation
Ribosome	High content of RNA	Site of protein synthesis (translation of mRNA into protein)
Endoplasmic Reticulum	**Glucose-6-phosphatase** Q	Membrane-bound ribosomes are a major site of protein synthesis Synthesis of various lipids Oxidation of many xenobiotics (Cytochrome P_{450})

Membrane	Enzyme
Plasma	**5'-Nucleotidase**Q **Adenylyl cyclase**Q **Na+-K+ ATPase**Q
Endoplasmic reticulum	**Glucose-6-phosphatase**Q
Golgi apparatus	
Cis	GlcNAc transferase I
Medial	Golgi mannosidase II
Trans	**Galactosyl transferase**Q
TGN	Sialyl transferase
Inter mitocho-ndrial membrane	**ATP synthase**Q

Lysosome	**Acid phosphatase** Q	Site of many hydrolases (enzymes catalyzing degradative reactions)
Plasma membrane	**Na+-K+ ATPase**Q **5′-Nucleotidase**Q	Transport of molecules in and out of cells Intercellular adhesion and communication
Golgi Apparatus	**Galactosyl transferase**Q	Intracellular sorting of proteins Glycosylation reactions Sulfation reactions
Peroxisomes	**Catalase**Q Uric acid oxidase	Degradation of certain fatty acids and amino acids **Production and degradation of hydrogen peroxide**Q
Cytoskeleton	No specific enzyme markers	Microfilaments, Microtubules, Intermediate filaments
Cytosol	**Lactate dehydrogenase** Q	Enzymes of glycolysis & fatty acid synthesis

Serum Enzyme	Major Diagnostic Use
Aminotransferases - Aspartate aminotransferase (AST, or SGOT) - Alanine aminotransferase (ALT, or SGPT)	 Myocardial infection Viral hepatitis
Amylase	Acute pancreatitis
Ceruloplasmin	Hepatolenticular degeneration (Wilson's disease)
Creatine kinase	Muscle disorders and myocardial infarction
γ-Glutamyl transpeptidase	Various liver disease
Lactate dehydrogenase (isozymes)	Myocardial infarction
Lipase	Aute pancreatitis
Phosphatase, acid	Metastatic carcinoma of the prostate
Phosphatase, alkaline (isozymes)	Various bone disorders, obstructive liver disease

120. B i.e. Tubulin **121. D i.e. GTP not required** **122. B i.e. Microtubules**
[Ref: Harper's 27/e P-584-86; 26/e P-576- 78; 539- 40]

In dividing cells mitotic spindle is formed by microtubules containing α- & β tubulinsQ 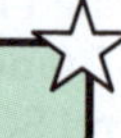

★ **Ubiquitin** is a small protein present in all eukaryotic cells, *targets many intracellular proteins for degradation.*

★ The primary components of basal lamina are three protein ***laminin, entactin and type IV collagen***Q and the *GAG heparin or heparan sulfate.* ***Laminin is a major protein component of renal glomerular and other basal laminas***Q. **Entactin** or **nidogen** is a glycoprotein containing *RGD sequence (Arg – Gly – Asp)* is the major cell attachment factor. *The negative charges of heparan sulfate* and certain sialic acid containing glycoprotein present in basal lamina repel albumin & most plasma proteins, which are negatively charged at the pH of blood. (small pore size also prevent excretion of proteins).

Cell Cycle

123. A i.e. G_1SG_2M; C i.e. DNA synthesis occurs in S phase; E i.e. Cell division in M phase

124. A i.e. GO – G I – S – G2 –M **125. B i.e. G2; C i.e. S; D i.e. M** *[Ref: Robbins 7/e P 91, 291; Gray's 40/e p. 20-23]*

Sequence of **cell cycle** is **G_0 G_1 S G_2 M**; where **'S'** is the **DNA synthesis/replication** phase and **M** is **cell division/mitosis** phase. **Time taken for S, G_2 and M phases are fixed in duration.**

NOTES

NOTES

PHYSIOLOGY

Review Notes with High Yield Text

Chapter 1. CENTRAL NERVOUS SYSTEM: REVIEW NOTES

Higher Function

Association Areas

The proportion of the various parts of the brain are similar in the brains of apes and human, **but the human brain is larger**[Q], so the **absolute size of the association area is greater**[Q].

Association areas: are part of six- layered neocortical mantle of gray matter that spreads over the lateral surfaces of cerebral hemisphere from concentric allocortical & juxta cortical rings around the hilum. **The most prominent gross feature of the human brain is immense growth of three major association areas**[Q].

i) Frontal in front of premotor area
ii) Parietal temporal occipital – b/w somatesthetic & visual cortex extending into posterior portion of temporal lobe.
iii) Temporal – from the lower portion of temporal lobe to limbic system. Speech & other intellectual function are controlled by neocortex.

★ **Brain size: Human >Chimpanzee > Monkey**[Q]. **Weight** of Human brain=1400 gm and Monkey brain = 100gm
★ The ratio b/w brain weight and body weight is more important than size of the brain as three species have brains larger than humans (the whale, elephant & porpoise)
★ The right to left differentiation is seen in chimpanzee and human. In humans left brain > Right brain

Functions & Lesions

Somatosensory area I (SI)

Primary somatosensory area (SI) is Brodmann's area 1, 2, 3 situated in **postcentral gyrus.** Ablation of SI would lead to cortical pattern of sensory loss. Lesion in this area produce contralateral impairment of:

- **Touch**[Q]
- Pressure
- Proprioception
- **Two point discrimation**[Q]
- Sterognosis
- Barognosis
- Cutaneographia

Somatosensory area II (SA II)

Lesion of somatosensory II is associated with alteration in pain sensation.

Brain Fuel

- The brain contains essentially **no fuel reserves**[Q] and must be continuously supplied with fuel from the blood. **So it is sensitive to hypoxia**[Q].
- **Brain tissue normally uses glucose**[Q] as an exclusive fuel, except during starvation
- **During starvation brain can adapt to use ketone bodies**[Q] as an energy source.

Pattern of Sensory Loss

Cortical lesion

Patients is able to recognize all sensation but localizes them poorly

- **Loss of two point discrimina-tion**[Q]
- **Asteregnosis**[Q] (loss of touch sensation)
- Sensory inattention

Thalamic lesion

Hemisensory **loss of all modalities**[Q]

Brainstem lesion

Loss of **pain & temperature** on ipsitateral face and **opposite side of body**[Q]. **(Lateral medullary syndrome)**[Q]
[Mn: TOP = Temp & Pain Opposite side]

Spinal cord lesion

Five patterns are seen depending upon whether there is:

- Complete transaction
- Hemisection
- Central cord section
- Posterior column section
- Anterior column section

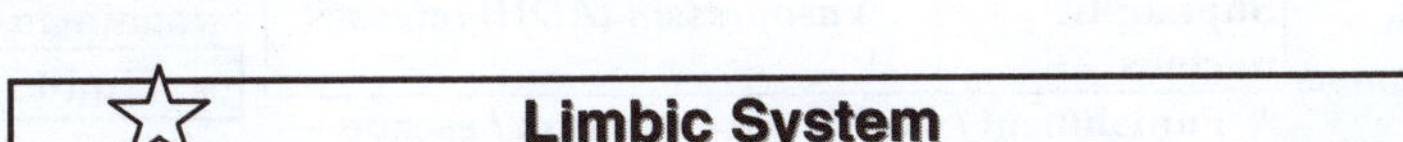

Limbic System

It is the entire neuronal circuit that *controls emotional behaviour & motivational drives* and a term that originally was used to describe bordering structures around basal region of cerebrum.

Functional Anatomy

- From physiological point of view, **hypothalmus**, located in the middle is one of the *key (central) element* of limbic system

Functions of hypothalamus

Posterior Hypothalmus

Part of hypothalmus	Vegetative & endocrinal function	Behavioural function

Functions of other parts

- **Hippocampus**

- Almost any sensory experience activates some part which inturn distribute signals to other part of limbic system. So

- **Subcortical limbic structures,** surrounding hypothalmus are Mn- " **Amy SAT Perfectly On Portions of Basal Hip**" i.e.,

  - Amygdala
  - Septum area
  - Anterior nuclei of Thalmus
  - Para Olfactory area
  - Portions of Basal ganglia
  - Hippo campus

- **Limbic cortex**, surrounds sub cortical limbic areas. It is a ring of cerebral cortex composed of Mn – **"CORPUS"**

  - Cingulate gyrus
  - Orbitofrontal cortex
  - Parahippocampal gyrus
  - Uncus
  - Subcallosal gyrus

★ Limbic system & brain stem communicate via *media forebrain bundle* & short pathways among reticular formation. The former extends from *septal & orbito frontal cortex* through middle of *hypothalmus* to brain stem *reticular formation.*

★ Most anterior & most posterior area of hypothalmus stimulates sexual drive.

★ **Fear** is produced by stimulation of *hypothalmus & amygdaloid* nuclei. Amygadala encodes memories that evoke fear.

★ **Anxiety** is related with *anterior end of temporal lobes*

★ **Violent range** occurs after removal of neocortex, & after destruction of ventromedial hypothalmic nuclei & septal nuclei (with intact cortex)

★ **Abnormal placidity** (calm) produced by b/l destruction of amygdaloid nucleus

★ Lesions of *left insula & putamen* l/t difficult **recognition of disgust** on faces or in voices

★ **Reward /satisfaction/ approach – centers** are located *along the course of medial forebrain bundle especially in lateral & ventromedial nucleus of hypothlmus*[Q] (Gyton). The most responsive area is in dopaminergic pathway ***from ventral tegmental area to nucleus accumbens***[Q]. So it includes *ventral tegmentum, medial fore brain bundle, nucleus accumbens, & frontal cortex.*

Lateral area	• **Thirst & hunger centre** - Stimulation l/t extreme hunger, voracious appetite & intense desire to search food - Damage causes lost desire for food and lethal starvation.	Stimulation increases general level of activity l/t *fighting & overt rage* $(\uparrow BP)$
Ventro medial	• **Satiety center** - Stimulation l/t satiety, decreased eating - Destruction l/t voracibus appetite • Neuroendocrinal control	Stimulation l/t *tranquility*
Mamillary body	• **Feeding reflexes** such as licking of lips & swallowing	
Dorsomedial nucleus	G I stimulation	
Perifornical nucleus	- Hunger - ↑ BP	Rage
Posterior hypothalmus	- ↑ BP - Pupillary dilation - *Shivering*[Q]	
Arcuate nucleus & Periventricular zone	- Neuroendocrinal control	Fear & punishment reaction

Anterior Hypothalmus

Paraventricular nucleus	- ***Oxytocin release***[Q] - Water conservation
Medial preoptic area	- ↓BP - ↓Heart rate - Bladder contraction
Posterior preoptic & anterior hypothlmic area	- Body temperature regulation - Panting, sweating - Thyrotropin inhibition
Supraoptic nucleus	- ***Vasopressin (ADH) release***[Q]

★ **Punishment / avoidance / aversion / escape – centre** are found in *central gray area surrounding aqueduct sylvius* (in mesencephalon), *lateral portion of posterior hypothalmus, dorsal midbrain, entorhinal cortex,* & periventricular zone of hypothalmus & thalmus.

★ **Addiction** is associated with reward centre & particularly with *nucleus accumbens*. D_3 dopamine receptor blocker reduce and agonist increase the rate of self stimulation (reward).

it acts as a channel through which incoming sensory signals can initiate behavioural reactions for different purposes.

- Becomes *hyper excitable and gives off prolonged output* signals. So in hippocampal seizures psychomotor (olfactory, visual, auditory, tactile) hallucinations cannot be suppressed as long as seizure persists.
- Provides the drive that ***causes consolidation of long term memory (i.e. translates short term memory into long term memory)***[Q]. It determines the importance of incoming sensory signal and has a *critical decision making role that the information is likely to be committed to memory*, making the mind *rehearse over & over* the new information until permanent storage takes place.
- B/L damage l/t **anterograde amnesia,** with lost ability to establish memory lasting longer then few minutes.

• Amygdala

- Corticomedial nuclei concerned with olfaction
- Basolateral nuclei is more developed in humans which is concerned with behavioural activities
- It is the ***window through which limbic system sees the place of person in the world***[Q]
- Stimulation can cause all the effects of hypothalmus puls tonic / clonic / rhythmical / circling movements, rage, escape, punishment, severe pain, fear, reward, pleasure, and even sexual activities such as erection, copulatory movements, ejaculation, ovulation, uterine activity & premature labor.
- **Kluver Bucy syndrome** d/t ***bilateral ablation of amygdala***[Q] presents with (1) loss of fear, (2) extreme curosity (3) tendency to place everything in mouth (4) forgets rapidly and (5) strong sex drive so much so that it attempts to copulate even with wrong (immature, wrong sex, different species) anmials & inanimate objects.

• Limbic cortex

- **Anterior temporal cortex** : Gustatory & olfactory behavioural association
- **Posterior orbital frontal cortex damage**: Insomnia with intense motor restlessness (unable to sit still & moving about continuously)
- **Parahippocampal gyri** : complex auditory & thought associations derived fro Wernike's area
- **Middle & posterior cingulate cortex**: sensorimotor behaviour association.

Neural Basis of Instinctive Behaviour & Emotions

Emotions

It has two aspects- sensory & expressive. **Sensory aspect** of emotions develop in the ***limbic system***[Q] where as ***expressive emotions*** develop in the ***hypothalamus***[Q] (as well as *amygdala*) Neuronal circuits exists which connects limbic system with hypothalamus eg. *Papez circuits*

Sensory

It is characterized by

I) **Cognition** is an awareness of the sensation & usually its cause (i.e. *seeing & recognizing*) eg recognizing a person who had previously insulted you.

II) **Affect** means ***development of feeling***[Q] eg. rage

III) **Conation** is the ***desire to take action***[Q] eg. desire to beat

Expressive

Expression is the motor side of emotional behaviour and has 2 sub divisions

1) **Autonomic** via sympathetic or parasympathetic system
2) **Somatic** eg act of beating

Limbic Lobe / System

- The **limbic system** or **lobe** is applied to the part of brain that consist of a rim of cortical tissue around the hilum of cerebral hemisphere and a group of associated deep structures
- It was formerly called *rhinocephalon* because of its relation to olfaction & it is phylogenetically the oldest part of cerebral cortex *(allocortex)*
- It consists of:
  1. *Cingulate gyrus*
  2. *Septal nuclei*
  3. *Hippocampal formation* - Hippocampus
     - Dentate nucleus
  4. *Amygdala*
- Cingulate gyrus & hippocampus form a 'C' which encircle upper part of brainstem
- Limbic system also contains a fibrous tract *median forebrain bundle (MFB)*
- **Papez circuit** links *limbic system to hypothalamus & thalamus* and is concerned with expressive side of emotions. It consists of:

Fornix from hippocampus → mamillary body of hypothalamus → Anterior nucleus of thalamus → Cingulate gyrus → Hippocampus again.

Sham Rage (= False Anger) Reaction

- **Sham (false) rage** is defined as an **outburst of inappropriate, uncontrolled (pathological / violent) rage** (fear & anger) on mild peripheral provocation or stimulation. It is seen in **decorticate animals (after removal of neocortex) and after destruction of venteromedial nuclei of hypothalamus** & septal nuclei, due to release of punishment centers of brain (esp in periventricular zone of hypothalamus & lateral hypothalamus) from cortical and hypothalamic inhibitory control.
- It is misnomer, as *originally* it was *thought* that the rage attacks in decorticated animals (with fore brain, diencephalic lesions) represent only a physical – motor phenomenon of anger and *lack emotional (mental) aspect*. But now its proved wrong as animals develop unpleasant feelings directed with great accuracy at the source of irritation and develop extremely persistent conditioned avoidance response.
- Sham rage (like normal rage) can also be produced by strong (in normal) or mild (in decorticated animals) ***stimulation of punishment centers of hypothalamus***[Q] and shows **features of sympathetic stimulation** like increased BP, increased heart rate, dilation of pupils and piloerection.

Punishment or Escape Centers

- **Electrical stimulation of punishment center** ie thin **zone of periventricular nuclei** (located adjacent to 3rd ventricle), adjoining **central grey area of mesencephalon and lateral hypothalamus** leads to **unpleasant (aversive) fear, anger, defence, escape , terror, punishment (even sickness & pain) reactions.**
- Most potent areas for **punishment & escape tendencies** are found in **central grey area surrounding the aqueduct of Sylvius in mesencephalon**, extending upwards into the **periventricular zone of hypothalamus & thalamus**; whereas less potent areas include **amygdale and hippocampus.**
- **Stimulation of punishment center usually inhibit the reward & pleasure centers** completely, showing that fear and punishment can take precedence over pleasure and reward

Rage & Punishment Centers

- **Rage** is an emotional behavior pattern that involves **strong stimulation of the punishment centers of hypothalamus & other limbic structures** (especially in **periventricular zone of**

Reward or Pleasure Centers

- If electrical stimulation of any area gives the animal a sense of reward, then it will stimulate the area by pressing lever again and again (sometimes even

hypothalamus and in lateral hypothalamus) and cause animal to behave in a manner that one would expect from an animal being severely punished. It causes the animal to

(1) Develop a defence posture
(2) Lift its tail
(3) Hiss, spit, growl or bite
(4) Extend its claws
(5) Develop sympathetic features like dilated pupils, wide open eyes & piloerection and
(6) Cause an immediate **savage (crudely violent) attack even on slightest provocation.**

- Normally, this rage phenomenon is held in check mainly by inhibitory signals from the **ventero medial nuclei of hypothalamus. Portions of hippocampi & anterior limbic cortex** especially in **anterior cingulate gyri and subcallosal gyri** also help to suppress the rage reaction.

thousands of time per hour) – ie **self stimulatory reward induction**. When offered the choice between eating delectable (liked) food as apposed to stimulate the reward center, the animal often chooses electrical stimulation of reward induction.

- **Major reward centers** are located **along course of the media forebrain bundle** especially in **lateral and ventro medial nuclei of hypothalamus.** Less potent reward centers which are secondary to major hypothalamic centers are found in the **septum, amygdala, certain** areas of **thalamus and basal ganglia** and extending downward into the *basal tegmentum of mesencephalon*
- Lateral nucleus, like many other areas, **with weaker stimuli giving a sense of reward and with stronger stimuli a sense of punishment.**

- ***Sexual behavior is integrated in anterior-ventral hypothalamus*[Q]**; plus **piriform cortex** (in males only) – Ganong
- **Sexual drive can be stimulated from** several areas of hypothalamus, especially the ***most anterior and most posterior portions of hypothalamus*[Q]** (Guyton)
- **Medial preoptic area (MPOA) or the most anterior portion of hypothalamus** is most important integrative nucleus involved in ***sexual behavior regulation of males in all vertebrates*[Q]**. It integrates the male sexual behavior by receiving all indirect inputs from every sensory organ and sends efferents to structures that are critical for initiation and patterning of copulation. Therefore, *stimulation of MPOA enhances sexual activity in males, whereas its damage consistently impairs male sexual behavior.*

Integrating Areas of Hypothalamus	Function
Anterior hypothalamus (response to **heat**), **Posterior** hypothalamus (response to **cold**)	**Temprature regulation** (anteriorly hot, posteriorly cold)
Suprachiasmatic nuclei	Control of **circadian body rhythm**
Punishment centers (esp periventricular zone of hypothalamus adjacent to 3rd ventricle, lateral hypothalamus & central grey area of mesencephalon) are stimulatory and **ventromedial nuclei of hypothalamus**, hippocampi, **anterior limbic cortex** (esp anterior cingulate gyri and subcallosal gyri) are inhibitory to fear (punishment)	**Defensive reactions (fear, anger, rage, punishment, fighting)= Unpleasant sensation (Aversion)**
Reward centers locatd along the course of *medial forebrain bundle*[Q] especially in **lateral and ventromedial nuclei of hypothalamus are self stimulatory**	**Calmness (Placidity, tameness & tranquility) = Pleasant sensation (Reward or satisfaction)**
	Appetitive Behavior
Lateral (superior) hypothalamus[Q]	**Thirst**
Lateral hypothalamus	**Hunger (eating) & increased activity level**
Venteromedial nucleus[Q], arcuate & paraventricular nuclei	**Satiety** (Decreased eating) & **tranquility**
Anterior ventral hypothalamus; most anterior (medial preoptic area=MPOA) & most posterior portions of hypothalamus[Q]; **piriform cortex** (in males only)	**Sexual drive**
	Neuroendocrinal control of
Preoptic area	**FSH & LH via Gn RH**
Supraoptic & paraventricular nuclei	**Vasopressin, Oxytocin**
Paraventricular nuclei	TSH (thyrotropin) via TRH ACTH & β- lipotropin (β-LPH) via CRH
Paraventricular nucleus and arcuate nucleus	GH via somatostatin & GRH
Arcuate nucleus; (hypothalamus inhibits secretion)	Prolactin via PIH & PRH
Dorsal & posterior hypothalamus	Catecholamines

Role of Hippocampus and Bilateral Lesion

- ***Hippocampus is the site where short term memory is processed and converted into long term memory***Q, by long term potentiation (LTP). Hippocampus after processing on basis of reward or punishment decides which of the short term experience is worthy to be stored long term.
- Only long term memory of **explicit (declarative) type** , which requires *symbolic rehersal in mind (verbalization or symbolic types of intelligence) is formed in hippocampus.* **Reflexive (implicit or non-declarative)** type of long term memory *is not formed in hippocampus.* So people with hippocampal lesion

Do not have difficulty in *learning physical repetitive skill* that do not require symbolic rehersing in mind such as *type writing & car driving* (i.e., implicit / non declerative/ reflexive long term memory)	Have **antegrade amnesia** i.e., long term memory prior to accident remains intact and they are ***unable to establish implicit (declarative) type of long term memory***Q

- Once the short term memory is converted to long term it is ***stored in neo cortex (not hippocampus)***Q. That's why even after removal of b/l hippocampus, patients still retain long term memories prior to removal of hippocampus.
- **Bilateral removal of hippocampal formation** severely and permanently **disrupts recent memory. Short term and long term memories** (for events that occurred prior to injury) **are unaffected**, but patient suffers **anterograde amnesia and new long term memories cannot be stored**. Therefore, patients remember events before the injury but **fail to recall new events, even with multiple exposure**, *and must be reintroduced to their therapists repeatedly*. There is **loss of declarative memory** involving *conscious recall of personal events, words and their meanings and general history*. However, these patients **retain implicit (procedural) memory**, the ability to acquire problem solving, association and motor skills and can learn some tasks. These patients if given a complex task to perform (eg mirror writing), they will not only improve during 1st training session but will also perform better on subsequent days despite their denial of having any experience with task.

Molecular Mechanism of Memory

Longterm memory

It results from *actual structural changes* instead of only chemical changes in following ways.

- ***Protein synthesis & activation of genes***Q. So aquisition of long term memory is prevented, if *within 5 minutes* the animal is anesthetized, given electric shock, subjected to hypothermia or given drug that block protein synthesis. But there is no respoonse after 4 hours.
- ***Spatial reorganization (restructuring) in synapses***Q changes their sensitivity for transmitting nervous signals by increasing vesicle release sites, number of transmitter *vesicle, number of presynaptic terminals* and changes in structure of dendritic spines that permit transmission of stronger signals. So a drug that blocks, DNA stimulation of protein replication will prevent long term memory formation.
- **Change in number of neuron & their connectivity** is often significant during first few week, months & even years of life. Even adults use this mechanism to at least some extent. So soon after birth, there is a principle of " use it or loose it "that governs final number of neurons & their synapse (i.e., the recruitment of neurons is from the already existing pool) – Guyton. But according to Ganong (270) new neurons form from stem cells through out life in 2 areas – olfactory bulb & *hippocampus*. (So it is relative answer only).

Intermediate memory

May *last for many minutes to even weeks* and will eventually be lost unless activated enough to be become long term. It results from ***temporary chemical &/or physical changes in either presynaptic terminal or post synaptic neuronal membrane*** **in two ways**

- **Habituation (negative memory)** is d/t progressive closure of Ca^{++} channels
- **Facilitation (positive memory)** is d/t *serotonin release* at facilitator synapse, which acts on its receptor on sensory terminal activating adenyl cyclase & forming c-AMP. The c-AMP activates protein kinase which phosphorylates K+ channel protein and blocks the K+ conductance out of terminal. This results in prolonged action potential & prolonged activation of Ca^{++} channel.

Short term memory

It last for *few seconds to few minutes*, but lasting only as long as person continues to think about it. It is caused by

- Continual neural activity in a *circuit of reverberating neurons*.
- ***Neurotransmitter chemicals serceted from terminal cause presynaptic facilitation or inhibition***Q. **(= changes in level of neurotransmitter at synapse).**

Working Memory

- It is a form of short term memory that keeps information available for very short periods, while person plans action according to it eg remembering a telephone number while picking up phone and dialing it.
- It involves **central executive (prefrontal cortex)** and two **rehearsal systems: a verbal system** for retaining **verbal memories** and a **visuospatial system** for retaining visual and spatial aspects of objects.

Normal Centres for Sleep

Hypothalmus

3 important group of neurons play a *critical role in regulation of sleep*

Ventro Lateral Pre optic (VL PO) area in anterior hypothalamus

- VLPO neurons contain inhibitory neurotransmitters *GABA & galanin*
- They project to & inhibit TMN and multiple distinct arousal or wakefullness centre located in brain stem, thalamus & hypothalamus suggesting that ***VLPO play a key executive role in sleep regulation***Q
- VLPO neurons are selectively activated conincident with sleep onset suggesting that it acts as a *sleep generating nucleus*
- VLPO serves as a **centre for sleep switch'** under the influence of biological (circadian) clock or SCN

Tubero-Mammilary Neurons (TMN) in posterior & lateral hypothalamus

- These *hypocretinergic & histaminergic* neurons are critical for ascending arousal system & wake fullness
- TMN are inhibited by projections from VLPO

Suprachiasmatic Nucleus (SCN)

- Located bilaterally above the optic chiasma
- These nuclei receive information about light dark cycle via special **retinohypothalmic fibers**
- SCN is responsible for **circadian rhythm** including the *sleep wake cycle & secretion of pineal hormone melatonin,* ACTH & other pituitary hormone
- SCN have 2 peaks of circadian activity.
- SCN interacts with VLPO & TMN to regulate sleep in relation to circadian rhythm.

Brainstem

- Most conspicuous stimulation are for causing almost natural sleep is the **raphe nuclei** in lower half of pons & in medulla. It is *serotonin* secreting.
- Some areas in **nucleus of tractus solitarius** can cause sleep. This is termination in medulla & pons for viscerl sensoy signals entering by vagus & glossopharyngeal nerves.

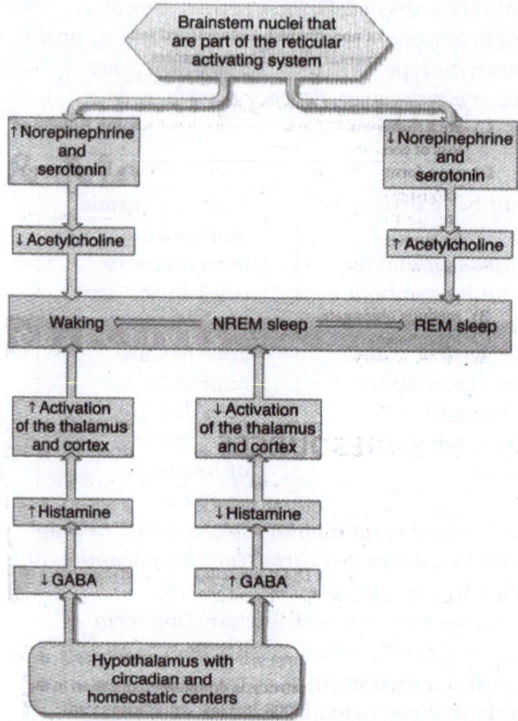

A model of how alternating activity of brain stem and hypothalamic neurons may influence the different states of consciousness.

Circadian Rhythm 

- **Suprachiasmatic nucleus (SCN) neurons of anterior hypothalamus** represent an **intrinsic (biological) circadian clock** (modulator) and demonstrate a spontaneous peak of electrical activity **at the same time every 24 to 25 hours.** The rhythm is **endogenous** and **persists even in absence of external environmental cues** (i.e. **neither stops nor becomes irregular**).
- Although circadian rhythms are **intrinsic (endogenous/inbuilt/or self sustained),** they become **entrained i.e. synchronized (adjusted) to the day-night light cycle in the environment**. The external environmental cues (factors) that can entrain (control or synchronized the timing of) circadian rhythm are called **zeit gebers (i.e. time givers). Day light** is the most important environmental cue. If not entrained, they become **progressively more out of phase** as *most circadian rhythm are longer or shorter than 24 hours.*
- Most circadian rhythms with 23-25 hours periodicity can be entrained to 24 hrs by normal environmental light dark cycle created by earth's rotation such that the periodicity of clock appears to be environmentally controlled. The entrainment

process is dependent on **suprachiasmatic nuclei (SCN)** located bilaterally above optic chiasma. Neural inputs are generated from **specialized light sensitive retinal cells** that are distinct from rods and cones and carry information about light-dark cycle via a special neural pathway-the **retinohypothalamic fibers** to SCN. Efferents from SCN entrain all circadian rhythms including sleep-wake cycle and secretion of pineal hormone melatonin.

- The **pineal gland** forms a neuroendocrine link between SCN and various circadian rhythm processes. It lies close to hypothalomns and synthesize **melatonin** (from serotonic/tryptophan) by rate limiting enzyme **N acetyl transferase**. The amount and activity of enzyme vary markedly in cyclic fashion **(inhibited by light and stimulated by darkness)** which accounts for cycling of melatonin synthesis and plasma levels. So *melatonin may transmit the information that night has arrived.*
- **Entrainment can be disrupted by isolating the subject from the environment (i.e. removing all external cues),** putting him in a **constant environment** (where there are absolutely no temporal cues) or **shifting time zones** (jet lag). Circadian rhythms in constant environment with no external cues (or in constant conditions of light or dark) becomes **free running** and **drift away slightly from** a 24 hour cycle to its **original intrinsic rhythm (free running period).** ***For sleep wake cycle it is slightly greater than 24 hours (upto 25 hours)***[Q].
- SCN have 2 peaks of circadian activity and exposure to bright light can either **delay** *(if exposed just after dark)*, **advance/accelerates** *(just before dawn)* or have **no effect** (if exposed during the usual day time) on onset of sleep period.

Cerebral Dominance or Complementary Specialization of Hemisphere 

Dominant (Categorical) Hemisphere (Mostly Left)

- It is concerned with ***categorization, symbolization and sequential analytic processes***[Q].
- It is important for

1. ***Language (written, spoken & expression) function***[Q]
2. ***Mathematical & scientific skills***[Q]
3. Reasoning
4. Right handed control (in right handed persons)
5. Hearing (right ear preference), right visual field, stereognosis (right side) and **left side olfaction.**

- **Planum temporale** an area of *superior temporal* gyrus which is located in the *floor of lateral fissure* is involved in **language related auditory processing** and correlates with **language dominance**. It is regularly larger on the left side making it dominant lobe.
- Lesions in categorical (which is in most of the times left) hemisphere leads to

1. Fluent, nonfluent and anomic **aphasia**
2. Acquired **dyslexia** (i.e. impaired ability to read and learn)
3. Patients are depressed & disturbed about their disabilities
4. **Dyscalculia** (impaired ability to perform mathematical calculations)
5. Loss of ability to thin reasonably (logically) through problems.
6. Lesion in dominant parietal cortex only l/t loss of **higher order somesthesias eg agraphesthesia** (inability to identify characters drawn on palm) and **astereognosis** (inability to identify an object only by touch)

- Understanding the spoken & printed words and expressing ideas in speech and writing (i.e. all **language functions)** depend on **dominant (categorical) hemisphere**. So damaging wernicke's area in dominant hemisphere (*mostly left*) leads to ***loss of almost all intellectual functions associated with language or verbal symbolism, such as the ability to read, the ability to perform mathematical operations (i.e. dyscalculia) and even the ability to think through logical problems***[Q].

Non-dominant (Representational) Hemisphere (Mostly Right)

- It is not less developed or non dominant; instead it is specialized in area of *visuospatial (or spatio- temporal relations*[Q]*)*
- It is important for

1. Recognition & interpretation of music **(Music awareness)**
2. Non verbal visual experiences (esp visual patterns)
3. Spatial relationships between the person & their surroundings **(Visua-spatial orientation)**
4. Significance of body language & intonations of peoples voices and probably many somatic experiences related to use of limbs & hands.
5. Identification of objects by their form and recognition of faces **(Recognition of forms, faces& body image)**
6. Three dimensional awareness **(Memory of shapes)**
7. ***Art awareness***[Q]
8. Insight & imagination
9. Left hand control (in right handed persons)
10. Hearing (left ear preference), left visual field, stereognosis (left side) and **right side olfaction**

- Lesions in representational hemisphere l/t

1. **Agnosia** (i.e. inability to recognize objects by a particular sensory modality even though the sensory modality itself is intact).
2. **Astereognosis** (i.e. inability to identify objects by feeling them)
3. Unilateral inattention & neglect
4. **Visuo- spatial defects**
5. Impaired ability to tell a story, make a joke, to get the point of a joke, & more broadly, to comprehend the meaning of differences in color and inflection of speech.

- ★ Hemisphere specialization is related to handedness (which is genetically determined). In 96% of right handed persons (which is 91% of total population), **left hemisphere is dominant** and in remaining 4% the right hemisphere is dominant.
- ★ In 70% of left handers, left hemisphere is dominant, in 15% right and in remaining 15% thre is no clear lateralization.
- ★ Left handers have above average spatial talents; a significantly disproportionately large number of musicians, artists, mathematicians are left handed. However, dyslexia is significantly more common in left handers who also have slightly but significantly shorter life span.

6. **Dysgraphia or agraphia** (i.e deficiency in the ability to write, regardless of ability to read
7. **Cortical neglect** d/t lesion in *non dominant parietal* cortex. In this, patient ignores objects and individuals on left side, draws object, that are incomplete on left and denies that his left body parts are his and fails to dress the left side of body. He denies that he has any such difficulty (**anosognosia**). He may respond to touch & pinprick on his left hand but cannot identify objects placed on left hand. The lesion is adjacent to *SI & visual association cortex*, areas important for perception of **one's body image and immediate extra personal space**

Aphasia

Is a disorder of understanding, thought and word finding

	Broca's aphasia [*Non fluent/Expressive /Motor* aphasia]	**Wernicke's aphasia** [*Fluent/Receptive/Sensory* aphasia]
Lesion site[Q]	***Inferior frontal gyrus***[Q] or Broca's area (Area 44) immediately anterior to primary motor cortex & above sylvian fissure.	In wernicke's area (supramarginal gysus) of the *parietal lobe & upper part of temporal lobe.*
Cause	d/t occlusion of superior ***branch of middle cerebral artery***[Q]	d/t occlusion of inferior division of ***middle cerebral artery***[Q].
Comprehension	***Preserved (except grammer)***[Q]	***Impaired***[Q]
Fluency	***Decreased***[Q]: Speech is *not fluent*, laboured, dysarthric & interrupted with ***many word finding pause***[Q]. It is telegraphic but informative.	Preserved or increased: Speech fluent but highly paraphasic & associated with ***neologism (Jargon aphasia)***[Q]
Naming[Q]	Impaired	Impaired
Repetition[Q]	Impaired	Impaired
Neologism[Q]	Absent	Present
Insight	Insight into condition is preserved	Not preserved

Conduction Aphasia

- A form of fluent aphasia in which patients can *speak relatively well & have good auditory comprehension but cannot put parts of words together or conjure up words*
- It was throught to be d/t lesions of ***arcuate fasciculus*** connecting Wernicke's & Brocha's areas. It now appears that it is d/t lesion in and around the **auditory cortex (areas 40, 41 and 42)**

Anomic Aphasia

- When a lesion damage ***angular gyrus*** in the categorical hemisphere without affecting Broch's & Wernicke's area, there is no difficulty with speech or undertanding of auditory information; instead there is ***trouble understanding written language or picture because visual information*** is not processed and transmitted to Wernicke's area.
- Most commonly seen in ***head trauma***[Q], ***metabolic encephalopathy*** and ***Alzheimer's disease***[Q].

Type of aphasia & site of lesion	Characteristic Naming Errors
Nonfluent (Broca's area)	"Tssair"
Fluent (Wernicke's area)	"Stool" or "choss" (neologism)
Fluent (areas 40, 41, and 42; conduction aphasia)	"Flair . . . no, swair . . . tair"
Anomic (angular gyrus)	"I know what it is . . . I have a lot of them"

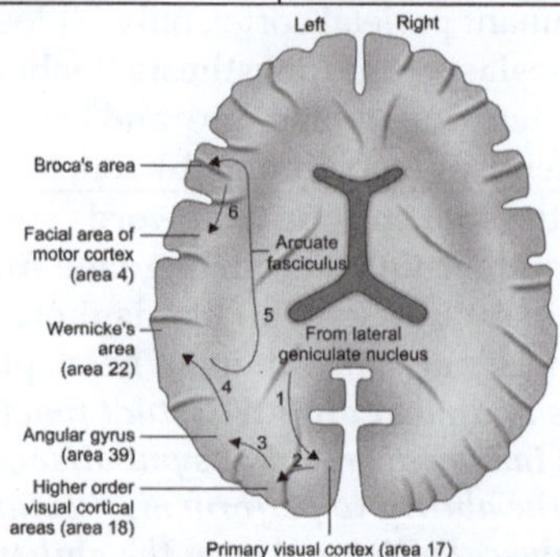

Pathway taken by impulses when a subject names a visual object projected on a horizontal section of the human brain

Vision

Stereopsis (Depth of Perception)

Binocular Components (True- stereopsis)

Binocular vision has most important role in depth perception[Q]

This is because each eye views the visual world from slightly different horizontal positions; so image of both eyes is differ from the other. Objects at different distances from the eyes project images in the two eyes that differ in their horizontal positions, giving the depth cue of **horizontal disparity** also K/a **retinal disparity / binocular disparity** or ***binasal disparity***[Q].

Monocular Components *(Pseudo)*

- Relative sizes of objects
- Degree one looks down at them
- Their shadows
- Relative movements for moving objects (*movement parallax*)
- Overlay of contours

❖ *Charles Wheatstone* discovered *stereopsis* & invented *stereoscope*.

Visual Pathway from Retina to Visual Cortex

Retinal Ganglion Cells → **Lateral Geniculate Body** → **Visual Cortex**

Retinal Ganglion Cells

These are of two kinds

M cells (Magno cells)	P cells (Parvo cells)
Large ganglion cells Project to the • Magnocellular portion of lateral Geniculate body	**Small ganglion cells** • Project to the • Parvocellular portion of lateral Geniculate body • Interlaminar portion of Lateral Geniculate body

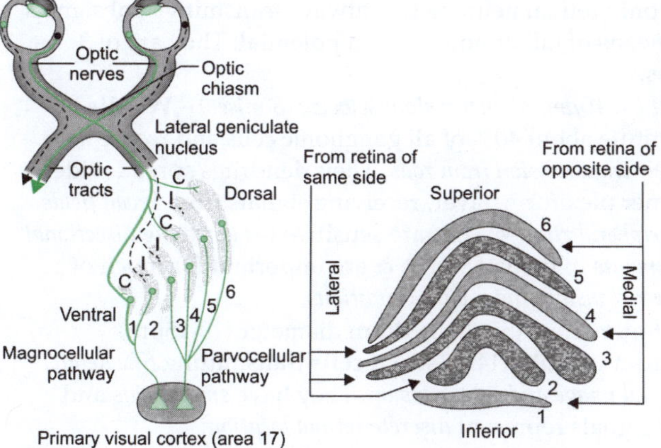

Lateral Geniculate Body

- Each Geniculate body contains six well defined layers
- Six layers divide Lateral geniculate body into three portions

Magnocellular portion (Layers 1, 2)	Parvocellular portion Layers 3, 4,5, 6)	Interlaminar portion (In between layers)
Receives projections from M cells	Receives projection from 'P' cells	Receives projection from 'P' cells
Carries signals for detection of movement depth and flicker	**Caries signals for color vision, texture shape and fine detail**	*Caries signals concerned with color vision*

- Lateral geniculate body (part of thalamus) is relay station on the visual pathway lying just posterior to the optic tract. It receives fibres from the *contralateral nasal hemiretina* and *ipsilateral temporal hemiretina*. Gray matter of this body is split into six laminae.

Visual Cortex

- Each visual cortex has 6 layers
- Visual cortex receives afferents from
  - Magnocellular pathway
  - Parvocellular pathway
  - Interlaminar portion
- These pathways mainly terminate in Layer 4 but also in layer 2 & 3

Magnocellular Parvocellular	Interlaminar pathway
Layer 4	Layer 2, 3

Blobs & Visual Pathway

- Layers 2 and 3 of the cortex contain clusters of cells about 0.2 mm in diameter, that unlike neighbouring cells contain a high concentration of the mitchcondrial enzyme 'cytochrome oxidase'.

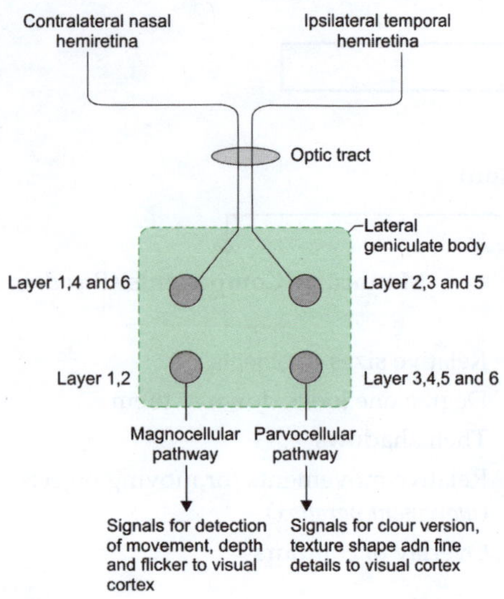

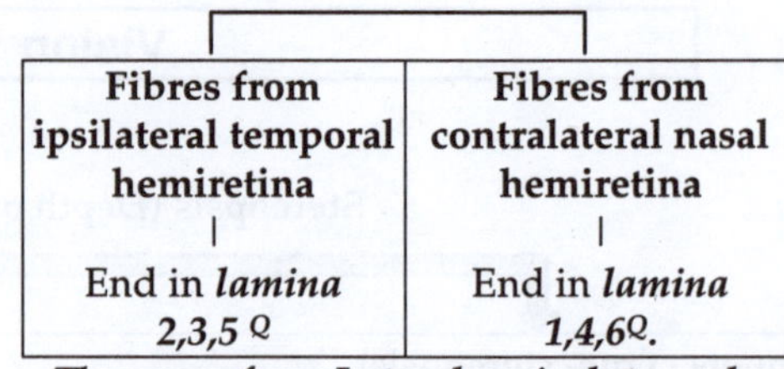

Fibres from ipsilateral temporal hemiretina	Fibres from contralateral nasal hemiretina
End in *lamina* 2,3,5 [Q]	End in *lamina* 1,4,6[Q].

- ***These clusters have been named as blobs***
- ***They are arranged in a mosaic in the visual cortex and are concerned with color vision.***

- ***The axons from Lateral geniculate nucleus that form the magnocellular pathway end in layer four (4). Many of the axons that form the parvocellular pathway also end in Layer 4. Most of the axons from Lateral geniculate nucleus thus end in Layer 4 of the visual cortex.*** *Some fibres from Lateral geniculate body terminate via the inter laminar pathway. These terminate onto layers '2' & '3' of visual cortex.*

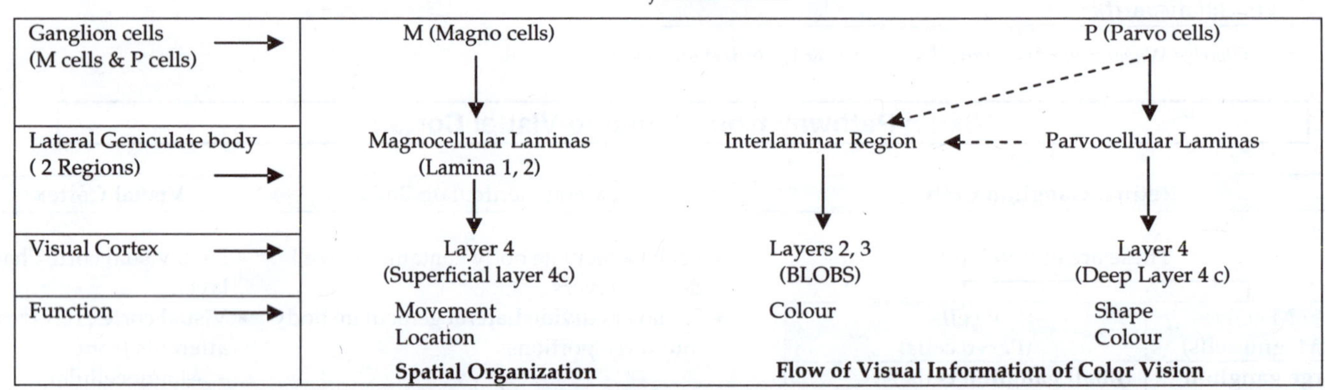

Ganglion cells (M cells & P cells) →	M (Magno cells)		P (Parvo cells)
Lateral Geniculate body (2 Regions) →	Magnocellular Laminas (Lamina 1, 2)	Interlaminar Region ← - - -	Parvocellular Laminas
Visual Cortex →	Layer 4 (Superficial layer 4c)	Layers 2, 3 (BLOBS)	Layer 4 (Deep Layer 4 c)
Function →	Movement Location	Colour	Shape Colour
	Spatial Organization	**Flow of Visual Information of Color Vision**	

Cells of Retina

Amacrine Cells

- Transmits signals *from rod bipolars to ganglionic cell* & is therefore essential component of rod pathway
- Modulates photoreceptive signals, serving to ***adjust or maintain the relative colour & luminosity inputs under changing light conditions***[Q] viz
  - at different times of day
  - directional movement detection.(**directional sensitive**)
- ***Increases visual acuity by lateral inhibition***[Q] i.e. inhibit firing of cells lateral to main neuronal pathway. However, lateral inhibition to enhance visual contract to allow high visual accuracy is primarily a function of **horizontal cells**.

Muller Cells/ Retinal Astrocyte

- Type of *glial cells help in binding* together of neural elements
- Neuroltransmitter uptake & Remove debris
- Electrical-insulation of receptor & neurons
- Store glycogen
- Do not take part in neurosensory pathway of light

★ Retinal neurons conduct their visual signals by **electrotonic graded conduction** (i.e. direct flow electric current not AP). Thus degree of hyperpolarization is directly related to intensity of illumination

Ganglion Cells

- *Multipolar cells* provide connection from bipolar neurons & amacrine cells to neurons in CNS.
- Fires continuously to some degree with or without light
- The only retinal neurons that always transmit visual signals by means of (all or none) action potential. They are of 3 types.
  - *Small (< 10μm) diameter slow velocity (8 m/sec)* – **W cells** constitute about 40% of all ganglionic cells and *receive most of their transmission from rods*. Their dendrites spread widely in inner plexiform, layer, receiving signals from *broad fields in peripheral rtina* W cells are sensitive for *detecting directional movements* in field of vision & are important for much of *crude rod vision under dark conditions.*
  - Most numerous (55%), medium diameter (10-15μm) medium velocity (14m/sec) **X cells** transmitting *fine details of visual image and colour vision*. They have *small fields* and their signals represent *discrete retinal location.*
  - Largest (35 μm) diameter, fastest velocity (50m/sec), least numerous (5%) **Y cells**. They have broad fields and respond, like many amacrine cells, to *instantaneous (rapid) change in visual image*- either rapid movement or rapid change in light intensity sending bursts of signals for only small fractions of second.

Visual Cycle

- The photosensitive pigment in the rods is called *rhodopsin* or *visual purple*. It has a peak sensitivity to light at 505nm.
- Rhodopsin consists of *11-Cis retinal* specifically bound to protein opsin.
- *Regeneration of rhodopsin* requires isomerization of all trans retinal back to 11-Cis retinal. Trans retinal after being released from rhodopsin is isomerized to 11-Cis retinal which spontaneously combines with opsin to form rhodopsin thus completing the cycle.
- Similar reactions are responsible for color vision in the cone cells

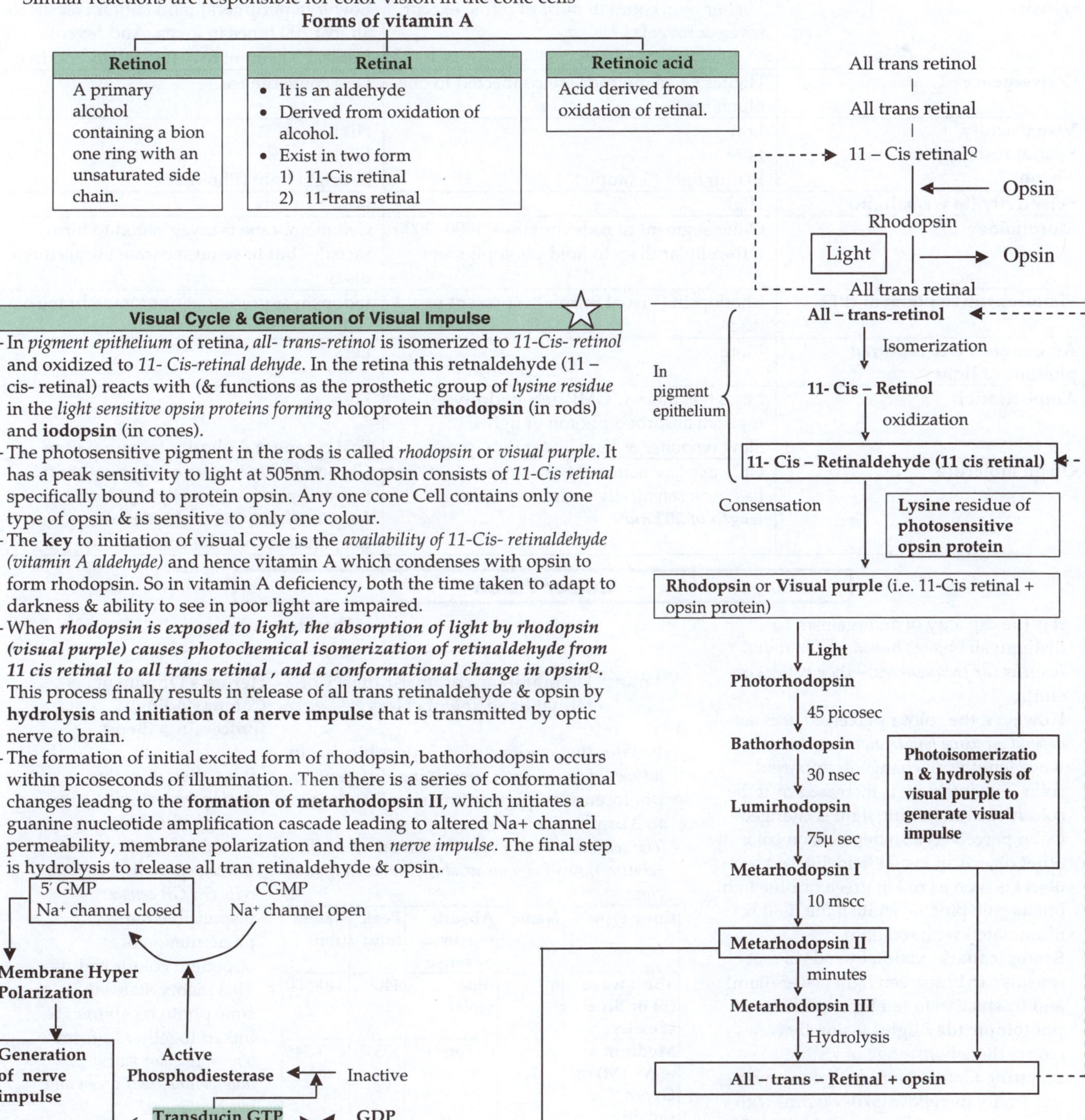

Forms of vitamin A

Retinol	Retinal	Retinoic acid
A primary alcohol containing a bion one ring with an unsaturated side chain.	• It is an aldehyde • Derived from oxidation of alcohol. • Exist in two form 1) 11-Cis retinal 2) 11-trans retinal	Acid derived from oxidation of retinal.

Visual Cycle & Generation of Visual Impulse

- In *pigment epithelium* of retina, *all- trans-retinol* is isomerized to *11-Cis- retinol* and oxidized to *11- Cis-retinal dehyde.* In the retina this retnaldehyde (11 – cis- retinal) reacts with (& functions as the prosthetic group of *lysine residue* in the *light sensitive opsin proteins forming* holoprotein **rhodopsin** (in rods) and **iodopsin** (in cones).
- The photosensitive pigment in the rods is called *rhodopsin* or *visual purple*. It has a peak sensitivity to light at 505nm. Rhodopsin consists of *11-Cis retinal* specifically bound to protein opsin. Any one cone Cell contains only one type of opsin & is sensitive to only one colour.
- The **key** to initiation of visual cycle is the *availability of 11-Cis- retinaldehyde (vitamin A aldehyde)* and hence vitamin A which condenses with opsin to form rhodopsin. So in vitamin A deficiency, both the time taken to adapt to darkness & ability to see in poor light are impaired.
- When ***rhodopsin is exposed to light, the absorption of light by rhodopsin (visual purple) causes photochemical isomerization of retinaldehyde from 11 cis retinal to all trans retinal , and a conformational change in opsin***Q. This process finally results in release of all trans retinaldehyde & opsin by **hydrolysis** and **initiation of a nerve impulse** that is transmitted by optic nerve to brain.
- The formation of initial excited form of rhodopsin, bathorhodopsin occurs within picoseconds of illumination. Then there is a series of conformational changes leadng to the **formation of metarhodopsin II**, which initiates a guanine nucleotide amplification cascade leading to altered Na+ channel permeability, membrane polarization and then *nerve impulse*. The final step is hydrolysis to release all tran retinaldehyde & opsin.

Differences between Rods & Cones 

Rods & cones differ in *number*[Q], structure, retinal distribution, photochemical molecules, ***sensitivity, wave length, acuity***[Q], color, synaptic connections & functions.

Feature	Rods	Cones
Number	90 – 100 millions	3 – 4.5 millions
Density	Higher than cones in most of retina except fovea & foveola	Lower in peripheral retina but increases to almost 200 times in fovea. And foveola (central 300μm of fovea) is totally rod free.
Convergence	Higher i.e. many rods are connected to one bipolar cells	Less convergence
Visual acuity **Spatial resolution** **Vision**	Low Low In dim light (Scotopic)	High High In bright light (Photopic)
Sensitivity (to weak light)	High	Low
Morphology	Outer segment of rods contain ~ 1000- 2000 intracellular discs to hold photopigment	Cell membrane is invaginated to form saccules but have no separate intracellular discs
Photosenstitive pigment (PP)	Rhodopsin (Visual purple) & present in disc	Iodopsin & present in outer membrane of cell
Amount of PP & captured photons of light	More	Less
Amplification	More (i.e. more C GMP gets hydrolysed for each absorbed photon of light) Slow response & long integration time	Less Fast response & short integration time
Opsin molecule	Only *one type* achromatic scotopsin that has peak sensitivity to light ***at a wave length of 505 nm***[Q]	Chromatic, *three types* of pigment that respond maximally to light at ***wave lengths of 440, 535 and 565 nm***[Q] Responsible for colour vision

Colour Vision

- It is the capacity of an organism to distinguish objects ***based on the wave lengths (or frequencies)***[Q] they reflect or emit.
- However, the colour perceived *does not depend on wave length alone*; as the same wave length can change its apparent color if its intensity is increased or if the colour of illuminating light is changed.
- Color perceived also depends on color of other objects in visual field. Eg. red object is seen as red in green or blue light but as pale pink or white if the field is illuminated with red light.
- **Scotopic (dark) vision** by rods is mot sensitive to bluegreen light (440-570nm) and insensitive to red light; whereas **phototopic (day light) vision** by cones covers the whole range of visible spectrum *(380-800 nm)* with maximum sensitivity in yellow (570-590 nm) with maximum sensitivity in yellow (570- 590 nm) region.
- This *shift of maximum sensitivity to longer*

Theories

Young- Helmholtz trichromatic theory of retinal handling of colors

- It states that colour vision is possible due to *3 types of cones*, each containing different photosensitive pigment maximally sensitive to 3 primary colors.
- *The sensation of any color is determined by the relative ratio of signals arising from each type of cone.*

Cone type	Name	Absorb maximal or sense	Peak (nm)	Range (nm)
Short wave (S) or Blue sensitive	β	Blue violet	440	440-500
Medium wave (M) or Green sensitive	γ	Green	535	450-545
Long wave (L) or Red sensitive	ρ	Yellow but also sense red	565	564-580

Hering's Opponent Colour Coding (Processing) theory

- It is called into play *during transmission through visual pathway.* Ewald hering proposed that *bipolar cells, ganglion cells & LGB cells* are responsible for phenomenon of opponent colour coding.
- This theory states that cone photo receptors are linked together to form 3 *opposing color pairs: blue/yellow, red/ green and black /white*
- Activation of one member of pair inhibits activity in other. So *no*

wave lengths, which accompanies the change from scotopic to photopic vision is k/a **purkinje shift.**

- Colours have 3 attributes: **hue, intensity & saturation (*"HIS"*)**[Q]. saturation is degree of freedom from dilution with white. **Complementary color** of any color is the color that when properly mixed with it produces white color.
- Black colour produced by absence of light is a positive sensation because *blind eye does not see black*; rather it sees nothing
- *Red* (723-647nm), *green* (575-492) and *blue* (492-450 nm) are called primary colors because mixing of these in various proportions can produce, white, any spectral & even extra spectral color purple.
- Each retina has *100 million rods, 3 million cones & only 1.6 million ganglionic cells. Thus 60 rods & 2 cones converge on each ganglionic cell & optic nerve fiber* leading from it to brain. In central retina (fovea) fewer rods & cones converge on each fiber progressively *increasing the acuity of vision. Central fovea (i.e. foveola)* has *35,000 slender cones and no rods* converging on almost exactly equal number of nerve fibers. l/t ***maximum colour vision acuity***[Q].
- *Peripheral retina has much greater sensitivity to weak light* because rods are 30-300 times more sensitive to light than cones and ~ 200 rods converge on a single optic nerve fiber in peripheral portions of retina.
- Lateral inhibition (by horizontal & amacrine cells) provide contrast detection & enhancement.
- This theory is proved by absorption spectra of retinal cones using retinal densitometry
- However, it *cannot explain* phenomenon of complementary after images, in which the extended inspection of one color will l/t the subsequent perception of its complementary color. For example if one looks at a unique red patch for about a minute & then switches the gaze to a homogenous white area they will see a greenish patch in white arch.

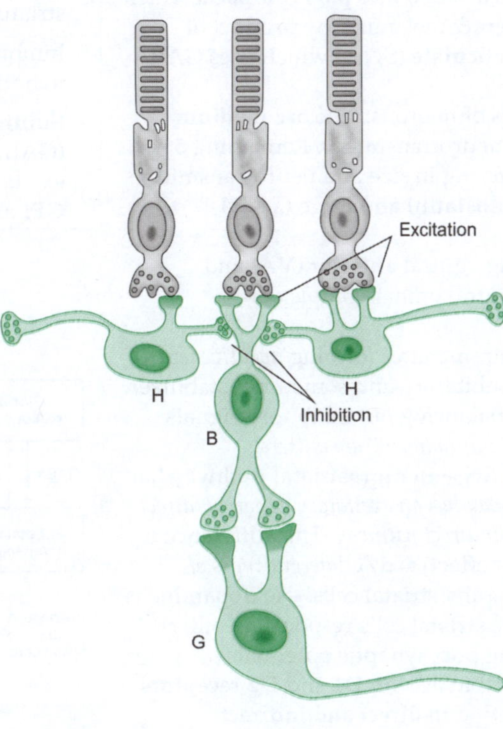

two members of a pair can be seen at the same location. That's why we don't experience bluish- yellow or reddish green where as bluish green (turquoise) and yellowish red (orange) are very commonly seen.

- This *antagonism between colors occurred in retina* as spectrally opponent processing (red Vs green and (yellow vs. blue) and spectrally nonopponent processing (black vs white).
- Mechanism: one colour cone (eg red) excites the ganglion cell by direct excitatory route through a depolarizing bipolar cell whereas, the opponent color type cone (eg green) inhibits the ganglion cell by indirect inhibitory route through a hyperpolarizing bipolar cells.
- **Retina itself begins to differentiate colors by these color contrast mechanism**[Q]**.** There fore **color analysis begins in retina** & is not entirely a function of brain.
- This theory *explains phenomenon of complimentary after images* and why a gray square on red background looks green.

Basal Ganglia or Basal Nuclei ☆

Structural Organization

- Basal ganglia is composed of 5 interactive structures on each side of brain including
  - **Caudate nucleus**, **putamen** and **globus pallidus** (= 3 large nuclear masses underlying the cortical mantle) and
  - **Subthalamic nucleus** of diencephalon and **substantia nigra** of midbrain
- The term **striatum** (or **corpus striatum**) is applied to **caudate nucleus & putamen** because of the *striated appearance* of these nuclei. The striations are produced by fiber bundles formed by the

Major Connections of Basal Ganglia

- **Afferents: 2** main inputs to basal ganglia, both of which are **excitatory (glutamate) terminate in striatum**. They originate from **layer V of** most regions of **cortex (except primary visual & auditory cortices)** with an important component originating in motor cortex (**corticostriatal pathway**) and from **intralaminar nuclei of thalamus (thalamostriatal pathway)**.
- **Efferents : 2** main **outputs** of basal ganglia, both of

anterior limb of internal capsule as it seperates the caudate nucleus and putamen

- The **putamen and globus pallidus** collectively form **lenticular nucleus.**
- **Globus pallidus** has two parts **GPi** and **GPe. Substantia nigra** (substance black d/t melanin) has 2 parts SN_{PC} and SN_{PR}

Neurotransmitters

- **Globus pallidus** has 2 parts, an **internal** and an **external segments (GPi & GPe)**; both containing inhibitory GABA ergic neuron
- **Substantia nigra (= black substance)** derives its name from its content of melanin pigment. It is divided into **pars compacta** which uses **dopamine neurotransmitter** (& melanin; a by product of dopamine synthesis) and **pars reticulate (SN_{PR})** which uses GABA as neurotransmitter.
- Striatum contains at least 4 types of neurons: **95% are medium spiny neurons using GABA** as neurotransmitter. Remaining **5%** are all **Aspiny interneurons** differing in size and neurotransmitters : **small (GABA), medium (somatostatin) and large (acetyl choline).**
- Several thalamic nuclei including **ventral anterior (VA)** and **ventral lateral (VL) nuclei** and intralaminar complex are associated with basal ganglia.
- **GABA** is *always inhibitory* neurotransmitter forming *negative feed back loops*. **Dopamine** is mostly inhibitory and sometimes stabilizer. **Glutamate** is always excitatory balancing out inhibitory signals from *GABA, dopamine & serotonin inhibitory transmitters.*
- **Dopamine neurotransmitter of SN_{PC} in nigrostriatal pathway** has an *excitatory action on direct pathway has an excitatory action on direct pathway & an inhibitory action on indirect pathway*. This difference in action of dopamine (modulatory effect) is d/t *different types of dopamine receptors* expressed by spiny striatal cells. – ie dopamine is causing its action by altering the striatal cells response to other transmitters (& not by generating post synaptic potentials). **Dopamine** is a **neuromodulator** that acts on **D1 and D2 receptors** on striatal neuron cells participating in **direct and indirect pathways** (respectively) by projecting to **GPi and GPe respectively**

Direct & Indirect Pathways

- Excitatory cortical input to striatum influences output from GPi and SN_{PR} via a direct and indirect pathway.
- The overall effect of **direct pathway** is to **enhance motor activity,** whereas **indirect pathway** reduces the activity of motor neurons in cerebral cortex.

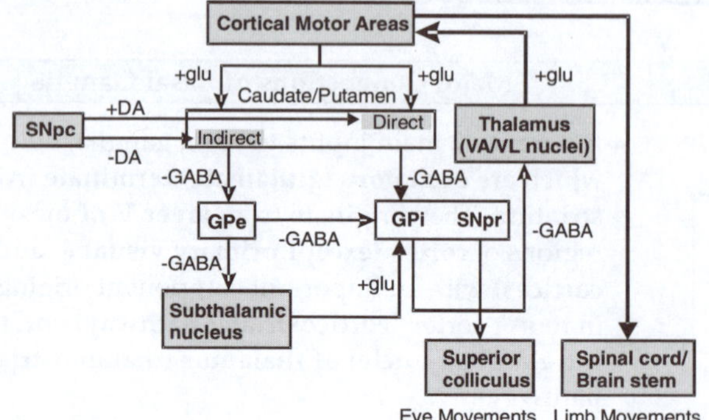

which are **inhibitory (GABA** ergic); arise from **GPi and SN_{PR} and project to thalamus.** Thalamic neuron inturn give excitatory (glutamate?) projections to *prefrontal and premotor cortex thereby, completing a ful cortical – basal ganglia-thalamic – cortical loop.*

- Connections within basal ganglia include

- **Dopaminergic** (both excitatory & inhibitory) **nigrostriatal projection** from substantia nigra pars compacta (SN_{PC}) to striatum and an inhibitory **GABA ergic reverse projection** from striatum to SN_{PR} (pars reticulata)
- Inhibitory GABA ergic projections from stritum to both GPi and GPe.
- **Subthalamic nucleus** receives an inhibitory (GABA) *input / afferent from GPe* and project **excitatory (glutamate) output / efferent to both GPi and GPe.**

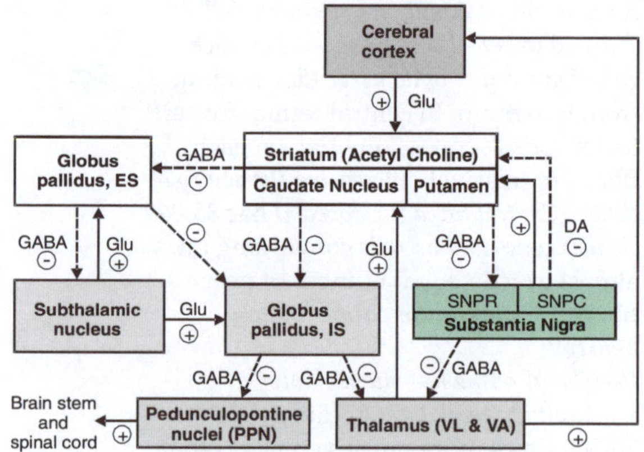

Subdivision of Striatum

- On the basis of NTs, it can be divided into **striosome** (to which limbic system projects) and **matrix** (to which cortical projections related to motor control end). Striosome synapse in SN_{PC} to influence dopaminergic nigrostriatal pathway.

- Striatal neurons disoharge before movement occurs suggesting their role in *selecting the probable movements.* **Putamen** is related to **body movement** and **caudate nucleus to eye movement.**

Control of Voluntary Movements

Corticobulbar / corticospinal system	Basal Ganglia	Cerebellum
• Tracts : - **Corticobulbar**: The nerve fibers from the motor cortex to cranial nerve nuclei. - **Corticospinal:** 80% lateral corticospinal (that cross the midline in medulla) + 20% Anterior/ ventral corticospinal tract. • **Cortical motor areas** - **Motro Cortex** *(area4)*: Where stimulation produces prompt discrete movement - **Supplementary motor area:** involve in programming motor sequences - **Premotor cortex (area 6):** Concerned with setting posture at the start of planned movement. - **Posterior parietal cortex:** *Motor responses are also produced by stimulation of somatosensory I & II* in parietal lobe • The ***corticospinal & corticobulbar system is the primary pathway for the initiation of skilled voluntary movement***Q.	• The term basal ganglia applied • to 5 structures on each side of brain: Caudate nucleus } Striatum Lenticular nucleus { Putamen, Globus pallidus } Subthalamic nucleus Substantia nigra • **Function: of basal ganglia**Q. - In **planning & programming of movements**Q. - **Convert abstract thoughts into voluntary action**Q.	Functional division • **Vestibulo cerebellum**: ***(flocculonodular lobe)***Q - ***Oldest***Q part of cerebellum - Concerned with equilibrium & learning induced changes in VOR (vestibulo occulo-reflex) • **Spinocerebellum:** Receive proprioceptive input from all body as well as copy of 'motor plan' from motor cortex, By comparing plan with performance ***it smoothes & coordinates ongoing movements***Q • **Neocerebellum**: They interact with the motor cortex in planning & programming movement.

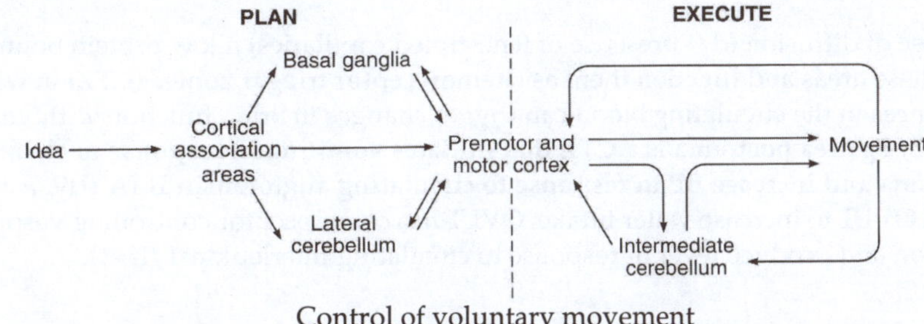

Control of voluntary movement

Blood Brain Barrier (BBB) & Blood Cerebrospinal fluid Barrier (BCSFB)

- BBB & B-CSF-B exist between the blood & brain interstitial fluid and CSF respectively to uniquely limit the exchange of substances into the brain. That is why the constituents of CSF are not the same as in ECFs (extracellular fluids) elsewhere in body.
- These barriers exist both **at the choroid plexus** [between choroid epithelium (CSF) and capillary endothelium (blood)] and at **tissue capillary membranes**. The cause of low permeability is presence of **tight junctions** b/w the adjacent endothelial cells.
- Because of the sensitivity of cortical neurons to even minor variations of ionic (K^+, Ca^{++}, Mg^{++}, H^+ etc) concentration changes, BBB is an additional defence evolved *to protect & maintain the constancy of environment of neurons in CNS*. It also *protects* brain *from endogenous & exogenous toxins* in the blood & *prevents escape of neurotransmitters in general circulation*. BBB is immature **at birth** and is breached (broken down) in areas **of injury, infection and tumors**. Tumors develop new capillary that lack light junction and contact with astrocyte – so the radioactive iodine labeled albumin penetrates tumor rapidly, making it stand out as an island of radioactivity in the surrounding normal brain. BBB is temporarily disrupted by sudden marked **increase in BP** or by IV injection of **hypertonc fluids**.
- **Blood-CSF Barrier & Blood-Brain Barriers** are ***highly permeable to water, CO_2 (carbondioxide), O_2 (oxygen)₂, and most lipid soluble (lipophilic) substances such as free forms of steroid hormones, alcohol and anesthetics***Q; slightly permeable to electrolytes like Na^+ (sodium), K^+ (potassium) and Cl^- (chloride); and almost **totally impermeable** to plasma proteins, protein bound forms of steroid hormones, protein antibodies and most non lipid soluble large organic molecules (i.e. impermeable to, in general, ***all proteins and polypeptides)***Q. It slows penetration of some smaller molecules like urea.
- *Passive diffusion* across cerebral capillaries with tight junction is *very limited* but numerous *carrier-mediated & active transport system* move substances out (more freely) as well as into the brain. Many peptide & drugs actually cross the cerebral capillaries but are transported back rapidly into blood by a **multidrug nonspecific, p-glycoprotein – ATP binding transporter** in apical membranes of endothelial cells, that transports various proteins & lipids across cell membranes. So larger (adequate) amounts of chemotherapeutic drugs, analgesics & opioid can be delivered to brain by inhibiting this transporter.

- Transporter exist for *glucose, thyroid hormone, leptin hormone (control appetite & sympathetic activity) choline, several organic acids, nucleic acid precursors and basic, neutral and acidic aminoacids* at BBB. Diffusion of glucose (the ultimate source of energy for nerve cells) across BBB would be very slow in absence of glucose transporters like **GLUT 1**. Two isoforms **GLUT 1 (55 K)** of brain capillaries/endothelium and **GLUT 1 (45 K)** of astroglia, neuron (+ GLUT-3) & microglia (+ GLUT-5) are encoded by a same gene, but they differ in the extent of glycosylation. Infants with congenital low GLUT1 develop low CSF glucose concentrations in the presence of normal plasma glucose l/t seizures and delayed development.

Circumventricular Organs

- They have **fenestrated capillaries** & because of their permeability they are said to be 'outside the blood–brain barrier'. Some of them function as **neurohemal organ** i.e. area in which polypeptides secreted by neurons enter the circulation. **Sites of brain outside the blood brain barrier** i.e. ***'Circum ventricular organ'***[Q] include:

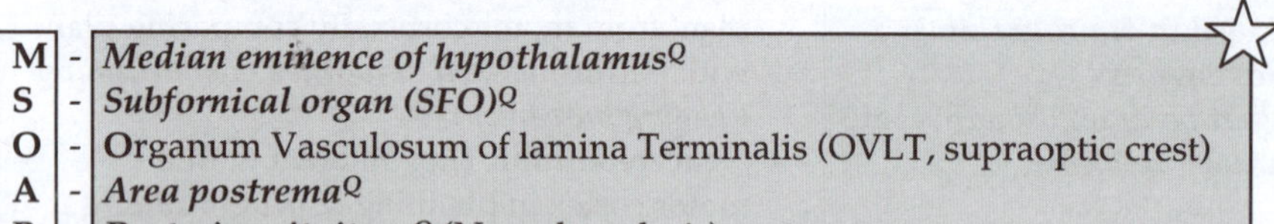

M	- ***Median eminence of hypothalamus***[Q]
S	- ***Subfornical organ (SFO)***[Q]
O	- Organum Vasculosum of lamina Terminalis (OVLT, supraoptic crest)
A	- ***Area postrema***[Q]
P	- ***Posterior pituitary***[Q] (Neurohypolysis)

[Mn: Marble **SOAP**]

- The ease of diffusion (d/t presence of fenestrated capillaries) allow protein bound dyes to stain these areas and function them as **chemoreceptor trigger zones (CTZ)** in which substances in the circulating blood can trigger changes in brain function without penetrating the BBB. **Eg area postrema is a CTZ that initiates vomiting in response to chemical changes in plasma and increase BP in response to circulating angiotensin II (A II)**[Q]. A II also acts on SFO & OVLT to increase water intake. OVLT has osmoreceptor controlling vasopressin secretion and produce fever in response to circulating interleukin-1 (IL-1).

- Althoug **pineal gland** and **anterior pituitary** have fenestrated capillaries and are outside the BBB, but both are endocrinal glands and are not part of brain
- **Subcommissural organ** closely a/w pineal gland & histologically resembling the circumventricular organs does not have fenestrated capillaries and high permeability.

Cerebellum

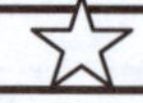

3 Layers

- It has a **3 layers** – *external molecular layer, Purkinje cell layer* (that is only one cell thick) and *internal granular layer.*

5-Types of Neuron Cells

- Cerebellar cortex contains **5 types of neurons** – ***Purkinje, granule, basket, stellate and Golgi cells***[Q].
- **Purkinje cells** are amongst *the biggest neuron* in the body have *extensive dendrites* that extends throughout *molecular layer*. ***Their axons are the only output from the cerebellar cortex and these generally pass to deep nuclei***[Q].
- ***Granule cells are excitatory***[Q]. **Granule cells** receive input from mossy fibres & innervate Purkinje cells. Their cell body lie in granular layer and **axon** on reaching molecular layer *bifurcates to form 'T'* which are called ***parallel fibres.*** (The parallel fibres synapse with many Purkinje dendrites)
- The other 3 types of neurons are *inhibitory interneurons*. The *basket cells* are located in molecular layer. They receive input from parallel fibres & each project to many Purkinje cells. Their axons form a basket around the cell body & axon hillock of each Purkinje cell they innervate.
- ***Stellate cells*** are similar to basket cells but more superficial in location.
- ***Golgi cells*** are located in granular layer & their dendrite project into the molecular layer, receive input from parallel fibres. Their cell bodies receive input via collaterals from the incoming mossy fibres & Purkinje fibres. Their axons project to the dendrites of the granule cell.

4-Deep Cerebellar nuclei

- Deep cerebellar nuclei separate external cerebellar cortex from white matter. There are **4 deep nuclei**: - **d**entate, **e**mboliform, **f**astigial & **g**lobose[Q] (Mn: 'DEFG')
- The *globose & emboliform* nuclei are sometimes lumped together as *interpositus nucleus.*

Afferents

- Its primary afferent inputs, ***the mossy & climbing fibres***[Q], send collateral to deep nuclei & pass to the cortex.
- **Two main inputs (afferents) to cerebellar cortex- *climbing fibres & mossy fibres are excitatory.***
- **Climbing fibres** come from ***inferior olivary nuclei***[Q](propioceptive input to i.o.n. comes from all over body). Each *projects to primary dendrites of a Purkinje cell*, around which it entwines like a *climbing plant.*
- **Mossy fibres** provide direct propioceptive input from all parts of the *body* plus input from the *cerebral cortex* via *pontine nucleus* to the cerebellar cortex. They end on the dendrites of

Transmitters

- **GABA** is secreted by the *stellate, basket, golgi and Purkinje cells* ($GABA_A$ receptor)
- **Glutamate** is secreted by granule cell (only neuron of CNS that has *$GABA_A$ receptor containing α-6 subunit*).

Fundamental Circuit: Summary

- **Climbing fiber** inputs exerts a *strong excitatory* effect on *single Purkinje cells*, whereas *Mossy fiber* inputs exerts a *weak excitatory* effect on *many Purkinje cells via granule cells.*
- **Granule cells** via their *parallel fibres* also excite *basket & stellate cells* which *inturn inhibit Purkinje cell* (Feed-forward inhibition)
- **Golgi cells** are excited by Mossy fiber collaterals, Purkinje cell collaterals & parallel fibres and they *inhibit* transmission from mossy fibres to granule cells
- **Purkinje cell** out put *inhibit deep cerebellar nuclei*. Nuclei also receive excitatory inputs via collaterals from mossy & climbing fibres.
- The output from deep cerebellar nuclei to brainstem & thalamus is always excitatory. Thus almost all cerebellar circuit seems to be concerned solely with modulating or timing the excitatory out.

Lesion leads to

- *Incordination*[Q] of rate, range, force and direction of movements l/t **ataxia**, asynergia, astasia, **dysmetria**, dysarthria, scaning speech, past pointing, rebound phenomenon, **dysdiadokinesia** and **nystagmus**.
- *Intentional tremors*[Q] :unlike the resting tremors of parkinsonism it is absent at rest
- Disorder of equilibrium gait & *posture*
  Hypotonia[Q]

granule cells in complex synaptic groupings called *glomeruli*. The glomeruli also contain the inhibitory endings of Golgi cell.

Efferents

- The *output* is through *purkinje cells* and *deep cerebellar nuclei*. The output of purkinje cell is inturn inhibitory to deep cerebellar nuclei. It is interesting that the ***output of deep cerebellar nuclei to the thalamus and brain stem is always excitatory***[Q]
  Thus almost all the cerebellar circuitry seems to be concerned solely with modulating or timing the excitatory output of the deep cerebellar nuclei to the brain stem & thalmus[Q]
- Most of the ***vestibulocerebellar output (i.e. from flocculo-nodular lobe) passes directly to the brainstem***[Q], but the rest of the cerebellar cortex projects to the deep nuclei which inturn project to the brainstem. Thus the deep nuclei provide the only output for the spinocerebellum & neocerebellum.
- Medial portion of spinocerebellar projects to fastigial nuclei & from there to brainstem.
- Ajdacent hemisphere portion of spinocerebellum projects to emboliform & globose nuclei and from there to the brainstem.
- Neocerebelum projects to dentate nucleus & from there to ventrolateral nucleus of thalamus.

The Orexins (Hypocretins) System

Orexins were first described in **1998** as a result of a search for an unknown regulatory peptides in *hypothalamus*. These are signal substances *used both in CNS & periphery.*

In the CNS

- All the orexinergic neurons have their origin in the lateral hypothalamus from where they project widely.
- They are believed to regulate:
- Wakefulness and paradoxical sleep,
- Appetite and food intake
- Endocrine and Autonomic processes.

In the Periphery

- Orexins and orexin receptors have been have been found in the gastro-intestinal tract and in the endocrine organs.
- The prominent peripheral effects seen so far include regulation of gastro-intestinal motility and hormone production and release, especially in the adrenal gland

Orexin (hypocretin) producing neurons occur in **hypothalamus. Orexins A and B** increase **feeding (appetite)** whereas, brains from humans with

Ghrelin

- It is a *gastrointestinal hormone* synthesized & released mainly by **oxyntic cells** of stomach (Guyton) / **P or D1 cells of fundus of stomach**. It is also produced by the *intestine & epsilon cells of pancreas* in small amounts.
- Ghrelin acts to ***stimulate hunger (appetite)***[Q]. So blood levels rise during fasting, peak just before eating and then fall rapidly after a meal (**orexigenic**). In this way, it is *counter part of hormone leptin*, produced by *adipose tissue*, which induces *satiation (i.e. is anti-orexigenic)* when present at higher levels.
- Ghrelin is also produced in **arcuate nucleus of hypothalamus** and has *marked growth hormone stimulating activity* i.e. it stimulates GH secretion from anterior pituitary gland by acting directly on receptors in pituitary.
- **G protein coupled ghrelin** receptor formerly k/a **growth hormone secretagogue (GHS) receptor** is expressed in *arcuate nucleus, lateral hypothalamus, vagal afferent cell bodies & vagal afferent endings through out gastrointestinal tract*.
- It has an important role in neurotrophy, particularly in hippocampus and is essential for cognitive adaptation to changing environment and process of learning.

★ **Growth hormone (GH)** also k/a **somatotropic hormone** or **somatotropin** exerts much of its effects through intermediate

narcolepsy have fewer orexin producing neurons in hypothalamus. The orexins most often act in an excitatory manner both via putative pre-, post- and extrasynaptic mechanisms.

The orexin system consists of

- **Orexin – A** and **Orexin B,** two closely related neuropeptides, derived from the same gene (common precursor) by alternate splicing.
- **OX-1** and **OX-2**, the two orexin receptors. At most of the projection sites both OX1 & OX2 receptors are expressed. Mutation in one of the orexin receptor genes cause **narcolepsy**.

substances called **somatomedins** secreted by **liver** (and to a much less extent, other tissues). Because many effects of somatomedins on growth are similar to those of insulin, therefore somatomedins are also called **insulin like growth factors (IGFs)**. Out of 4 somatomedins isolated, the most important is *somatomedin C* (or *IGF-1*) and pygmies of Africa & Levi-Lorain dwarf have congenital inability to synthesize significant amount of IGF-1.

★ **Cholecystokinin (CCK)** is secreted by **I cells of upper small intestine** (jejunum) and decreases feeding (antiorexigenic / aorexigenic), inhibits gastric emptying, and stimulates secretion of pancreatic juice rich in enzymes, contraction of gall bladder, secretion of glucagon & insulin and small intestine & colonic motality.

Neurotransmitter

Neuropeptide – Y (NP-Y)

- **Neuropeptide Y** (found in *brain & autonomic nervous system*), **pancreatic polypeptide** (produced by **F cells** in islets) and **polypeptide YY** (a *gastrointestinal hormone*) – are closely related as they all contain ***36 aminoacids***[Q], *end in tyrosine, are amidated at their carboxy terminals* and *all act on at least 2* of the 4 known G protein coupled receptors for these peptides : Y1, Y2, Y4 and Y5. However, neuropeptide Y is **secreted only by neurons**, whereas pancreatic polypeptide & polypeptide YY are secreted by *endocrine cells*.
- NPY is secreted by (*adrenergic, noradrenergic* & other) neurons of brain (**hypothalamus**, periaqueductal gray, medulla) and *autonomic nervous system.*
- Neurons that produce **orexigenic substances NPY** and AGRP, have their **cell bodies in arcuate nuclei and project** their axons **to paraventricular nuclei** (of hypothalamus) to antagonize melanocortin receptors (MCR-3 & MCR-4) there by inhibiting the effects of α-MSH produced by POMC neurons. **When energy stores of body are low (eg starvation)**, orexigenic neurons are activated to **release NPY**, which stimulates appetite and at the same time, firing of POMC neurons is decreased thereby *reducing the activity melanocortin pathway*, so further stimulating appetite. (Guyton -870) . When injected into hypothalamus, NPY increases food intake, and inhibitors of NPY synthesis decrease food intake. NPY m-RNA in the hypothalamus ***increases during feeding and decreases during satiety***[Q]. NPY exerts its effects through **Y-5 receptor.** Knocking out of NPY gene does not produce marked effects on feeding, pointing that other pathways are also involved, but knockout of NPY gene in leptin deficient cause them to eat less and spend more energy that have normal NPY gene Leptin, a 167 aminoaicd polypeptide, produced primarily in fat cells act on hypothalamus to decreases the activity of NPY neurons and decrease activity of POMC secreting neurons thereby causing anorexia & increased energy consumption. The anorexiant action of leptin is *antagonized by blockade of CB1 receptor* (marijuana / cannabinoids increase appetite by acting on CB1 receptor) and *inhibition of phosphatidylinositol -3-hydroxykinase* (an hypothalamic enzyme activated by leptin). Leptin also *increases activity of SOCS-3 (suppressor of cytokine signaling-3) in NPY neurons* and SOCS-3 supresses further leptin receptor signaling, suggesting a turn off mechanism.
- So NPY (& AGRP) orexigenic neurons **increase food intake and reduce energy expenditure** (which includes basal /resting metabolic rate , energy cost of metabolizing & storing food, thermic effect of exercise, and adaptive **thermogenesis**).

Neuropeptide (Slowly Acting Transmitters /Growth Factors)

- **Neuropeptides (unlike small molecule, rapidly acting transmitters)** are *not synthesized in the cytosol of presynaptic terminals.* Instead, they are produced in *neuronal cell body by ribosomes* as a part of large protein molecules, which enters ER and then golgi apparatus. In GA, the neuropeptide forming protein is *enzymatically split into smaller fragments* (some of which are either neuropeptide or its precursor) and *packaged into minute transmitter vesicles (TV)* which are released into cytoplasm. These TVs are transported by *axonal streaming of cytoplasm at a slow rate (few cm/day)* to tips of nerve fibers, where they release neurotransmitters in response to action potentials in the same manner as for small molecule, transmitter (SMT). However, these TVs *are autolyzed and not recycled & used over & over again (like SMT).*
- **Unlike SMTs**, neuropeptides are *released in much smaller quantities, are more potent* (> thousand times) and have *prolonged action.*
- Small molecule rapidly acting transmitters include acetylcholine (Class I); epinephrine, NE, dopamine, serotonin, histamine (II = amines); GABA, glycine, glutamate, aspartate (III = amino acids) ; and NO (IV).
- **Slowly acting Neuropeptides** are.
  - Hypothalamic releasing hormones (thyrotropin-RH, luteinizing hormone and somtostatin / growth hormone inhibitory factor)
  - Pituitary peptides (ACTH, LH, GH, α-MSH, α-MSH, β-endorphin, prolactin,

- Cotransmitters in autonomic neurons include, VIP (released with actyl choline) and **ATP & NPY** (with norepinephrine). The **small granulated vesicles in post ganglionic adrenergic neurons** contain ATP and norepinephrine (NE) and **large granulated vesicles** contain NPY. The **low frequency stimulation** promotes release of ATP, whereas **high frequency stimulation** causes release of NPY.
- Noradenergic postganglionic sympathetic nerves containing **NPY** are found on many blood vessels and cause **vasoconstriction** (whereas cholinergic nerves containing VIP and sensory nerves containing CGRPα & substance P cause vasoconstriction).

thyrotrophin vasopressin , oxytocin).
- Peptides acting on brain & gut (gastrin, CCK, VIP, insulin, glucagons, substance P, neurotensin, nerve growth factor, brain derived neurotropic factor, leucine & methionine-enkephalin)
- Others (angiotensin II, bradykinin, carnosine, calcitonin, sleep peptides)

★ Large precursor protein (prohormone) **propionmelanocortin (POMC)** is synthesized in *corticotropes of anterior lobe pituitary, intr mediate lobe, hypothalamus, lungs, gastrointestinal tack and placenta*. POMC processing by *prohormone convertase (PC) 1 & 2* is tissue specific and result in production of different peptides in different tissue. Anterior pituitary corticotropes expresses PC1 resulting in formation of N terminal peptide, joining peptide, **ACTH**, β-lipotropin (LPH) and a small amount of β-endorphin. In intermediate lobe &/or hypothalamus, PC-2 expression l/t production of CLIP (corticotropin like intermediate lobe peptide), γ-LPH, **melanotropins (α-, β-, and γ- MSH)** and appreciable quantities β-endorphins, but not ACTH from POMC.

Substance – P

- It is a *polypeptide* called tachykinins containing 11 aminoacid residues that is found in **intestine, *various peripheral nerves and CNS***[Q]. All 6 *mammalian tachykinin* members differ at mino terminal but have in common the carboxy terminal sequence of *Phe – X – Gly- Leumet – NH₂*, where X is Val, His, lys or phe.
- It is found in -
  - *Primary afferent neuron endings in dorsal horn of spinal cord* as mediator at the first synapse in pathways for **pain transmission**[Q].
  - *Nigrostriatal system* where its concentration is **proportional to dopamine**
  - *Hypothalmus*, where it plays a role in **neuroendocrine regulation**.
- Upon injection into the skin, it causes redness & swelling, and it is probably the ***mediator released by nerve fibers that is responsible for axon reflex***[Q]
- **In intestine it cause peristalsis**[Q]. Centrally active NK-1 receptor *antagonist has antidepressant activity* in humans

Mammalian Tachykinins

Gene	Polypeptide products	Receptors
Substance P (SP) / Neurokinn A (NKA) gene	Substance P Neurkinin A Neuropeptide K Neuropeptide α Neurokinin A (3 -10)	Substance P (NK-1) Neuropeptide K (NK-2)
NKB gene	Neurokinin B	Neurokinin B (NK-3)

★ NK 1 & 2 receptors are G protein coupled receptors. Activation of SP receptor l/t activation of phospholipase C and increased IP3–DAG.

Cutaneous pain type	Nature	Transmitted by	Neuro-transmitter	Synapse /project to
Fast (mild)	Initial, sharp, pricking & easily localizable	**Ventrolateral spinothalic tract**	*Glutamate*[Q]	Ventral posterior lateral (VPL) nucleus
Slow (severe)	Late, burning or dull & intense, diffuse & accompanied by unpleasant autonomic feelings	**Spinoreticular pathway**	*Substance P*[Q]	Centrolateral nucleus of thalmus

Neurotransmitter - & Neuromodulators

- **Excitatory amino acids**
  - ***Glutamate***[Q]
  - ***Aspartate***[Q]
- **Inhibitory amino acids**
  - ***Glycine***[Q]
  - ***GABA***[Q]

- **Pyrimidine**
  - UTP
- ***Purine***
  - Adenosine
  - ATP
- **Lipids**
  - Anandamide
- **Gases**
  - NO, CO

- **Amines**
  - Dopamine
  - NA, Adrenaline
  - Serotonin
  - Histamine
- Acetylcholine

- **Polypeptides**
  - Substance P, tachykinins
  - Vasopressin, oxytocin, CRH, GRH, TRH, GnRH, Somatostatin
  - Endothelin, Enkephain, CCK4 & 8 etc

Thirst Control

- Water intake is regulated by osmolality of plasma and decrease in ECF volume.
- Body respond to increased plasma osmolality in two ways.
  (i) By increasing ADH secretion which decrease water excretion by kidney
  (ii) By stimulating thirst centre which increase water intake.
- In both these mechanism osmoreceptors are involved.
  (iii) Supraoptic nucleus near anterior hypothalamus causes *ADH secretion.*
  (iv) *Preoptic* nucleus is centre for thirst *stimulation*[Q]
- The osmotic *threshold for thirst* is same or *slightly* (~5%) *greater than the threshold* for increased ADH secretion.
- *It is still uncertain whether the same osmoreceptors mediate both effects.*
  That means centre for ADH secretion and thirst stimulation might be same or stimulation of one can lead to both the mechanism. Thus with increase in osmolality 1st thing to occur is ADH secretion followed by thirst stimulation.
- Vasopressin secretion is regulated by **osmoreceptors**, that are situated *outside blood- brain barrier* & located in circumventricular organs primarily ***in OVLT/ supraoptic crest***[Q]

Regulation of Body Temperature

Role of Hypothalamus & Temperature Receptors

- Core body temperature can be maintained normally between 97° & 100°F in an ambient temperature of over *100°C (ie in dry air* environment between 50°-130°F) but only < 50°C in a humid atmosphere. **Environmental factors** such as *temperature, humidity (amount of moisture), wind movement and even nature of surroundings* have important role temperature regulation.
- **Hypothalamus (through temperature regulating centres) integrate all body temperature information** obtained from sensory (afferent) receptors (**primarily cold receptors**) located in the **skin** (for peripheral detection of surface temperature) and **deep tissues** (eg deep receptors found mainly in **spinal cord, abdominal viscera, in and around great veins** in thorax and upper abdomen, **extrahypothalmic portion of brain** and **hypothalamus** itself for detecting *core body temperature*).
- *Cold receptors are far more than warmth receptors in skin* (almost as many as 10 times) and deep tissues – indicating their primary concern of *preventing hypothermia (low body temperature)*. Each of the 5 inputs (from skin, spinal cord, extrahypothalmic brain, hypothalmus & other deep tissues) contributes about 20% of integrated information.
- **Anterior hypothalamic preoptic area** contains **2/3rd heat sensitive neurons** as well as 1/3rd cold sensitive neurons and therefore has the capability to serve as a **thermostatic detection and control center of body temperature**. These neurons serve as *temperature sensors for controlling body temperature*. The heat sensitive neurons increase firing rate in response to rise in body temperature (2 to 10 fold on 10° C increase), whereas cold sensitive neurons increase their firing rate when the body temperature falls.
- Bilateral **posterior hypothalamic area** (approximately at the level of mammillary bodies) **integrate the central and peripheral temperature sensory signals** (obtained *from anterior hypothalamic preoptic area and from elsewhere* in body respectively) to control the heat producing and heat conserving reactions of the body.
- For each temperature regulating response , there is **threshold core temperature** eg 37°C for sweating and vasodilation, 36.8°C for vasoconstriction, 36°C for nonshivering thermogenesis, and 35.5°C for shivering. The **reflexes activated by warmth** are controlled primarily from the **anterior hypothalamus** and reflex responses activated by **cold** are controlled from **posterior hypothalamus**, so →

Anterior Hypothalamus		**Posterior Hypothalamus**
Cutaneous vasodilation & sweating	**Stimulation (l/t)**	Shivering
Hyperthermia (upto 43°C or 109.4°F)	**Lesion (l/t)**	Hypothermia (Body temperature falls towards that of environment)

Critical Temperature Set Point For Core Temperature Control

- The critical body core temperature set point (of **37.1°C or 98.8°F**) in the hypothalamus above which rate of heat loss is greater than heat production (& sweating begins) and below which the rate of heat production is greater than that of heat loss (& shivering begins) is determined mainly by the **degree of activity of the heat temperature receptors in anterior hypothalamic pre-optic area**. All temperature control mechanisms, continually attempt to bring the body temperature back to this set point.
- Temperature signals from peripheral areas especially from **skin** & certain deep body tissues (spinal cord & abdominal viscera) also contribute slightly to body temperature regulation by **slightly altering the set point of hypothalamic temperature control centre**
- For example, hypothalamic set point for sweating increases from 36.7°C to 37.4°C when skin temperature falls from 33°C to 29°C. In other words, *sweating begins at lower hypothalamic temperature when skin temperature is higher* (than when the skin temperature is low). That's why, sweating is inhibited when skin temperature is low; otherwise the combined effect of low skin temperature & sweating could cause too much loss of body heat

Similarly cold skin drives the hypothalamic centers to the shivering threshold even when hypothalamic temperature itself is still on the hot side of normal – ie **cold skin anticipates a fall in internal body temperature and prevents this.**

Body Heat Producion
- Basal metabolic process - Foot intake - Muscular activity

★ **Epinephrine & norepinephrine** produce a **rapid but short lived** increase whereas **thyroid hormones** produce a **slowly developing but** prolonged increase in heat production
★ **Sympathetic discharge** is increased by feeding & decreases during fasting
★ **Brown fat** is source of considerable heat in infants.

Body Heat Loss at 21°C	
- Radiation	55-65%
- Conduction	10– 15%
- Vaporization of sweat	27%
- Respiration	2%
- Urination & defecation	1%

★ **Radiation** is heat transfer by infrared electromagnetic radiation between objects not in contact, whereas **conduction** is heat change between objects that are in contact. Conduction is aided by **convection** ie movement of molecules away from the area of contact

Temperature Regulating Mechanism

These reflex and semireflex thermoregulatory responses include **autonomic, endocrine, somatic and behavioral changes,** facilitating increase heat loss & decreased heat production (on exposure to heat) or decreased heat loss and increased heat production (on exposure to cold). Therefore mechanisms activated by

Heat (ie promote heat loss)
Mostly increased parasympathetic activity

Increased heat loss	Decreased heat production
- Cutaneous vasodilatation - Sweating - Increase respiration - Panting (rapid shallow breathing by mouth) in animals like dogs	-Anorexia -Apathy and inertia -Inhibition of shivering & chemical thermo-genesis

Cold (ie promote heat gain)
Mostly increased sympathetic activity

Decreased heat loss	Increased heat production
-Cutaneous vasoconstriction -Piloerection -Curling up -**Piloerection (horripilation or goose pimples)** -**Curling up in a ball (universal flexion) posture**	-Shivering -Hunger -Increased voluntary activity -Increased secretion of norepinephrine/ epinephrine -**Nonshivering thermogenesis** -**↑BMR** -Sympathetic stimulation -**Thyroxine secretion**

Physiological changes that occur during Heat Acclimatization

- Cutaneous vasodilatation causes increase in plasma volume
- ***Increased rate of sweating***[Q] (Approx. two fold)
- ***Decreased renal blood flow***[Q] (to conserve water as much is lost through sweating)
- ***Diminished loss of salt in sweat & urine***[Q] to almost none (d/t ***increased secretion of aldosterone for better conservation of body water & salt.)***[Q]

Thermoregulation in Cold
[Hypothalamus is responsible for thermoregulation[Q]]

When a person is exposed to cold, thermoregulation occurs in two phases-

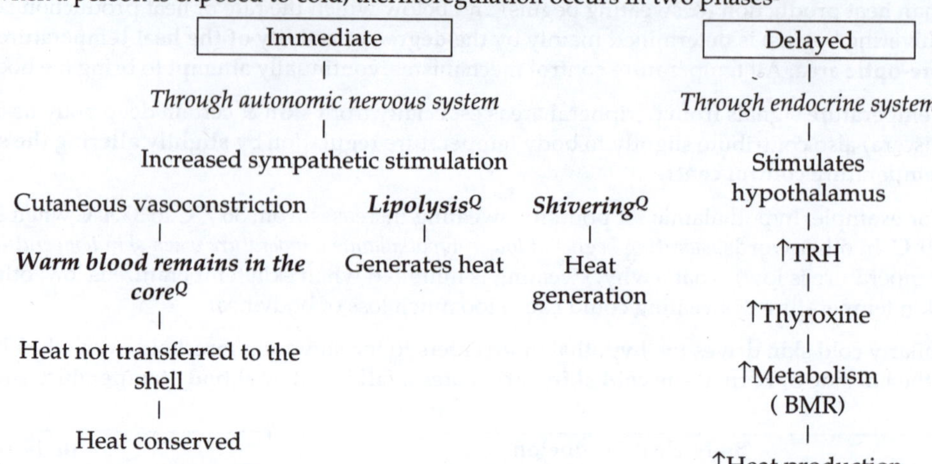

★ 'Piloerection means hairs 'standing on end'. Sympathetic stimulation causes the arrector pili muscles attached to the hair follicles to contract which brings the hairs to an upright stance. **This is not important in human beings** but in lower animals, upright protections of hairs allows them to entrap a thick layers of 'insulator air' next to the skin, so that transfer of heat to the surroundings is greatly depressed'– Guyton 11th/895

Effects of Fall of 1°C Temperature

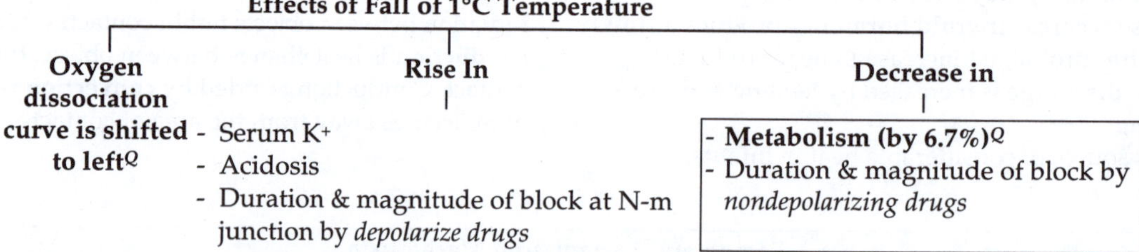

- Lesion of **Anterior hypothalamus** causes ***hyperthermia***[Q] (manifestation include cutaneous vasodilation & sweating)
- Lesion of **posterior hypothalamus** causes ***hypothermia***[Q] (manifestation include shivering)

Nerve (Axonal) Regeneration

Axonal regeneration is characterized by *development & prolongation of **growth cone (short sprouts)** from the proximal nerve stump and its extension along the rows of schwann cell column in the distal nerve stump through intact neurilemma **(ie ghost tube)**. **Axonal regeneration occurs in peripheral nervous system but not in CNS** because* of following reasons.

Feature	PNS	CNS
Rate of removal of myelin debris, cytokine release and RAG s (regeneration associated gents) expression	**Fast** an in high concentration	**Slow** and poor
Schwann cells multiply rapidly & form rows to appropriately guide sprouting proximal stump. **Dedifferentiated Schwann cells upregulate production of neurotrophins ie growth promoting factors** eg nerve growth factors (NGF), Ng CAM/L1. ***Neurilemma (endoneural tube)***[Q] is the outermost cell membrane of Schwann cell (the nucleus of which lies b/w nyelin sheath & neurilemma)	In PNS **presence of Schwann cells, Neurilemma (endoneural tube)** and **growth factors** help regeneration.	**CNS lacks Schwann cells** and single oligodendroglial cell myelinates many axons so it can't form path for growing sprouts.
Astrocytic proliferation, Formation of glial scar[Q] by astrocytes; Activation of microglia; Inflammation and invasion of immune cells provide inappropriate environment for regeneration.	Absent	**Present** [Q]
CNS myelin is axonal growth inhibitor[Q]. **Myelin associated inhibitors** include Nogo, MAG (myelin associated glycoprotein) OMgp (oligodendrocyte myelin glycoprotein) & trans membrane semaphorin 4 D	Absent	**Present** [Q]

NSAIDs inhibit **Rho A (small GTPase protein** that prevents axonal repair). Similarly, **drugs inhibiting IP_3 or PI_3** (phosphoinositide 3 kinase) pathway also promote nerve regeneration. Growth cone collapse by myelin associated inhibitors is prevented by **pertussis toxin.**

Cerebro Spinal Fluid (CSF) ☆

☆ CSF Constituents

Appearance	Clear colourless
Proteins	***20 – 40 mg/dl***Q
Sugar	***40 – 70 mg/dl***Q
Chlorides	***720 – 750 mg/dl***Q
Cell/mm^3	***Lymphocytes (0-5)***Q
DLC	60-70% lymphocytes 30-40% monocytes ***0% (None) neutrophils***Q

Substance	CSF concentration	Plasma conc	CSF/plasma ratio.
Mg^{++}	2.2	1.6	1.39
PCO_2	50.2	39.5	1.28
Creatinine	1.5	1.2	1.25
Cl^-	113	99	1.14
HCO_3^-	25.1	24.8	1.01
Osmolality	289	289	1
Na^+	147	150	0.98
Urea	12	15	0.80
Inorganic-P	3.4	4.7	0.73
Glucose	**64**	**100**	**0.64**Q
K^+	2.9	4.6	0.62
Ca^{++}	2.3	4.7	0.49
Uric Acid	1.5	5	0.3
Protein	**20**	**6000**	**0.003**
Cholesterol	0.2	175	0.001
pH	**7.33**Q	7.40	

★ All ions (Na^+, K^+, Mg^{++}, Ca^{++}, Cl^-) are in **meq/kg H_2O** except HCO_3^- ion which is in **meq/L.** All organic substances (glucose, protein, urea, creatinine, uric acid, cholesterol) &inorganic – p are in **mg/dL** whereas osmolality is in mosm /kg H_2O and PCO_2 in mmHg.

★ All +ve ions (Na^+, K^+, Ca^{++}) are more in plasma except Mg^{++} which is more in CSF

★ All –ve ions (Cl^- / HCO_3^-) are more in CSF.

Enzymes in CSF

- **Creatinine kinase (CK) BB**, **Enolase** and **Neopterin** are found in *CSF after stroke, global ischemia, hypoxia or trauma* and have been used as **markers of brain damage**.
- **Lactate dehydrogenase (LDH)** is increased in **bacterial** (than aseptic) **meningitis, intracranial & subarachnoid hemorrhage** (but not in current traumatic tap with intact RBC s) .and CNS leukemia/ lymphoma/metastatic carcinomas.
- **Adenosine deaminase** is increased in meningeal TB (d/t increased T lymphocytes containing it). **Lysozyme is** increased in both bacterial & TB meningitis.

*CSF formation*Q	50-70% is formed by ***choroids plexus***Q, remaining CSF formed around *blood vessel &* ***ventricular walls***Q
- **Volume** - **Rate of CSF formation** - Rate of CSF turnover - **Specific gravity**	- ***150ml***Q - ***550ml / day (2.3 ml/hr or 0.38 ml/min)***Q - ***Approx. 3 time /day***Q - ***1.006 – 1.007***Q
- **PH** of CSF - **CSF pressure** - Ion with maximum CSF/plasma ratio - Minimum CSF/plasma ratio - Equal CSF /plasma ratio is with.	- ***7.33***Q - ***70-180mm of water (in lumbar area)***Q ***and average is 130mm H_2O (10mm Hg)*** - ***Mg^{2+}***Q - ***Cholesterol & Protein***Q - ***Osmolality***Q

Regulation of CSF Pressure by Arachnoid Villi

- Rate of CSF formation is nearly constant, so it is seldom a factor in pressure control.
- Whereas, **arachnoid villi function like valves** that allow CSF to flow readily into blood in venous sinuses while not allowing blood to flow backward in opposite direction
- CSF flow begins when its pressure is **1.5 mmHg higher** than the pressure of blood in venous sinuses.
- The valve opens more widely, when this pressure difference is higher, which in normal conditions never allows CSF pressure to rise more than few mm Hg higher than cerebral venous sinus pressure.
- Absorption is proportional to pressure. At a pressure of **112 mm H_2O**, which is average normal CSF pressure, filteration & absorption are equal. **Below** a pressure of **68 mm H_2O, absorption stops.**

Causes of Reduced (i.e. between 3-20 mg/dl) CSF Protein

- ***Hyper thyroidism***Q
- ***Benign intracranial hypertension (pseudotumor cerebri)***Q
- ***Infants & children between 6 to 24 months of age***Q
- Acute water intoxication (increased ICP with decreased proteins)
- **CSF leaks** (such as due to trauma, ***repeated lumbar puncture***Q & pneumoencephalography) and **removal of large volumes of CSF** (eg for cytological studies).

Herniation /Coning

Refers to displacement of brain tissue away from a mass and into a compartment that it normally does not occupy.

[The cranial cavity is separated into compartments by *infolding of the dura* the true cerebral hemisphere are separated by falx and anterior & posterior fossa by the tentorium]

Uncal Herniation	Central transtentorial Herniation	Transfalcial Herniation	Foraminal Herniation
Displacement of antero medial *temporal gyrus (uncus)* into the tentorial opening l/t Sequential Compression of: - Ipsilateral *III cranial nv.* - Contralateral brainstem (later) - Whole brainstem (eventually) **Physical Sign:**	Symmetric downward movement of *upper thalamic* region through tentorial opening l/t Sequential Compression of: - Upper midbrain (first) - Pons (later) - Medulla (finally) **Physical sign:**	Displacement of *cingulate gyrus* under the falx and across the midline	Downward forcing of the *cerebellar tonsil* into the foramen magnum.

Uncal Herniation – Physical Sign

Early	*Later*	*Eventually*
- ***I/L dilated pupil***Q - Sign of supratentorial mass lesion	- ***Babinski sign***Q - I/L hemiplegia - ***Autonomic disturbance***Q	- Tetraparesis - B/L fixed dilated pupil - Erratic respiration - Death

Central transtentorial Herniation – Physical sign

Early	*Later*	*Eventually*
- Erratic respiration - Small reactive pupil - ***B/L extensor planter***Q	- Cheyne stokes respiration - Decorticate rigidity	- Fixed dilated pupil - Decerebrat eposturing

Physiological effects produced by Opiate Receptors

μ (mu)

- <u>P</u>hysical dependence
- ***<u>M</u>iosis***Q
- ***<u>C</u>onstipation***Q
- ***<u>A</u>nalgesia***Q
- <u>R</u>espiratory depression
- ***<u>E</u>uphoria***Q
- ***<u>S</u>edalion***Q
- ↑ ed secretion of GH & ***prolactin***Q

[Mnemonic: **P.M CARES**]

K (kappa)

- Miosis (lower ceiling)
- ***Diuresis***Q
- ***Analgesia***Q
- ***Dysphoria***Q
- Sedation

δ (delta)

- Analgesia
- Respiratory depression

★ Miosis is a better option as sedation is also a feature of K-receptor [Miosis is also a feature of kappa receptor but there is only slight miosis]

★ **μ receptor** is site of action of **morphine** and **endorphins**.

Thermal Receptors ☆

Cold- receptors

- Cold receptors are **inactive at 40°** but then steadily increase their firing rate as skin temperature falls to about **24°C**. As skin (subepithelial) temperature further decreases upto **10°C** the firing rate of cold receptor decreases. Below **10°C** the receptor are inactive and cold becomes an effective local anesthetic (i.e. respond to **10°C – 38°C**).
- Histologically definitive cold receptors are **nerve endings of Aδ myelinated** nerves, that branches a number of times, the tip of which protrude into the **bottom surfaces of basal epidermis.** So. it is the temperature of **subepithelial subcutaneous tissue** that determine the responses.
- Cold signals are transmitted **mainly by Aδ nerve fibres**. Some cold sensation may also travel in type C fibres as well.
- There are **4-10 times** as many cold sensitive as hot sensitive spots and the number in different areas of body varies from 15-20 cold spots/cm^2 in lips to 3-5 colds spots/cm^2 in fingers to < 1 cold spot/cm^2 in trunk.
- The receptors for moderate cold is the **cold** and **menthol sensitive receptor 1 (CMRI)**

Warmth (Heat)– receptors

- Threshold for activation is **30°C** & they increase their firing rate upto **46°C** (i.e. respond to 30-46°)
- Warmth receptor, not being identified histologically are presumed to be **free nerve endings** because heat signals are transmitted mainly by **type C nerve fibres.**

★ In addition to ending in post central gyrus, fibers from thalamus end in I/L ***insular cortex (true primary thermal receiving area)***Q

Pain receptors

- ***VR1 (vanilloid receptor 1)***Q respond to pain producing chemical capsaicin & temperature >43°C
- **VRL –1** respond to temperature > 50°C (but not to capsaicin)

Accomodation

It is a property of nerve, where a ***slowly rising (increasing) subthreshold stimulus raises (increases) the threshold of nerve to generate an action potential***[Q].

Adaptation (Desensitization)

- It is ***a progressive decrease in sensory receptor's response despite the continued presence of a stimulus***[Q].
- When a *maintained stimulus of constent strength* is appled to a receptor, the frequency of action potential in its sensory nerve declines over time. This is k/a adaptation
- It is *a characteristic of all sensory receptor* i.e., when a *continuous sensory stimulus is applied , the receptor responds at a high impulse rate at first and then at a progressively slower rate* until finally the rate of action potentials decreases to very few or often to none at all.

Electrotonic Conduction

- *Most dendrites cannot transmit action potentials,* because of few voltage gated Na^+ channels in their membranes & very high threshold for action potential. But they can *transmit signals to soma (within the same neuron) by electrotonic conduction* (EC)
- EC is *direct spread of electrical current by ion conduction* with in the fluids of dendrites but with out generation of AP.
- It is *decremental conduction,* as the dendritic membrane is thin and partially permeable to K^+ & Cl^- ions, making them leaky to electric current.
- *So the synapse that lies near soma has lesser decrement and* have far more effect in causing neuron excitation or inhibition.
- Dendrites can *summate all excitatory & inhibitory* postsynaptic potentials in the same way as soma can.

Motor Neurons

Somatic (effector organ = Skeletal ms)

UMN

Upper motor neuron (UMN) consists of *pyramidal cell & their neurons.* The pyramidal (corticospinal) system consists of the central pathway which directly *link the pyramidal cell in the 5th layer of motor cortex with the motor neurons in the brainstem & spinal cord.*

- Pyramidal system (voluntary movement)
- Extrapyramidal system (for involuntary movement: tone, posture & equilibrium)

LMN (final common pathway)

Lower motor neurons (LMN) consists of *anterior horn cells* or homologus cells in the brainstem, *their efferent nerve fibers* (which pass via the anterior spinal nerve root) *peripheral nerves* to the muscle & *the muscle fibers* innervated by these nerve fibers & their terminal branches.

Autonomic (effector organ = Cardiac & smooth muscle)

- Sympathetic
- Parasympathetic

★ Large myelinated fibers originating from **giant pyramidal (Betz) cells** (found only in primary motor cortex) are most impressive fibers in pyramidal tract. Diameter of cell is *60μm* & of fiber is *16 μm (micrometer)* with a conduction velocity of *70 m/sec.* (most rapid transmission from brain to cord). Total fibers in pyramidal tract is *1 million,* of which 3% (34,000) are from Betz cells. Remaining 97% fibers are <4*μm* diameter.

Corticospinal (Pyramidal) Tract

- It originates from *primary motor cortex* (30%), *premotor & supplementary motor area* (30%) and *somatosensory areas* posterior to central sulcus (40%)
- It passes through *posterior limb of internal capsule* (b/w caudate nucleus & putamen of basal ganglia) and then form *pyramid* of medulla.

Lateral corticospinal tract (LCT)

- **80%** of fibers of pyramidal tract ***cross in lower medulla***[Q] to opposite side & form LCT.
- Concerned with *skilled movements and ends directly on motor neurons* in humans (Ganong).
- But according to Guyton fibers finally terminate on interneurons in intermediate *regions of cord gray matter* (most) > *sensory rely neurons* in dorsal horn (few) > directly on *anterior motor neurons* that cause muscle contraction (very few)

Anterior /Ventral – corticospinal tract

- **20%** fibers do not cross to opposite side in medulla
- *Do not cross the middle until it reaches the level of muscles* it controls. At this level fiber ends on *inter neuron* that is *connected to motor neuron of both sides of body* (Ganong)
- Many (if not most) fibers *cross to opposite side of body either in neck or in upper thoracic region* (Guyton); and are concerned with control of *bilateral postural movements* (by supplementary motor cortex).

Difference

Feature	Upper Motor Neuron (UMN /pyramidal tract) lesion	Lower Motor Neuron lesion	Myopathy
Muscle atrophy (wasting)	None	*Marked*[Q]	Mild
Fascicultion	None	*Common*[Q]	None
Distribution of weakness	Pyramidal or regional	Distal or segmental	Proximal
Muscle Tone	*Increased (Spastic)*[Q]	Decreased lost (flaccid)	Normal /Decreased
Clonus	*Present*[Q]	Absent	Absent
Deep tendon reflexes (jerks)	Exaggerated /hyper *active*[Q]	Lost /Hypoactive	Nomal or hypoactive
Babinski's sign	*Present*[Q]	Absent	Absent
Plantar reflex	*Extensor*[Q]	Flexor	Flexor
Superficial abdominal reflex	Lost	Lost only when the particular neuron supplying the muscle is lost.	Normal

Pyramindal system	Extrapyramidal system
- It includes *motor cortex + the axons descending through* the pyramidal tract (PT) or cortico spinal tract. - Anterior corticospinal - Lateral corticospinal	- Denotes all those portion of the brain and brain stem, that cortribute to motor control and are not part of the direct corticospinal pyramidal system. - *Basal ganglia* - Motor nuclei of reticular formation of brain stem - Vestibular nucleus - Descending fibers which convey the impulses from these nuclei to spinal cord.
- Concerned with ***voluntary activities of body***[Q]	- Concerned with ***control of posture, tone and equilibrium***[Q]

- **Athetosis** (i.e. continuous, slow writhing movemets) and **chorea** (rapid involuntary dancing movements) occur in an involuntary, disorganized way at the start of voluntary movements. **Ballism** is involuntary flailing, intense, violent movements. **Akinesia** is difficulty in initiating movement & decreaed spontaneous unconscious movements such as swinging of arm during walking, different facial expressions related to emotional content of speech & thought and multiple gestures & fidgety actions that occur in all of us. **Bradykinesia** is slowness of movements.
- **Rigidity** differs from spasticity because in it *motor neuron discharge increases to both the agonist & antagonist muscles* and so passive motion meets with a *plastic, dead feeling continuous resistance* that has been linked to bending a lead pipe & is therefore called **lead pipe rigidity**. Sometimes a series of "catches" (i.e. resistance f/b release f/b resistance) takes place during passive motion, then it is called **cogwheel rigidity**, but the sudden loss of resistance as seen in spastic extremity (i.e. **clasp knife rigidity**) is absent in EPS lesions. **Resting tremors** d/t regular alternating 8 Hz contractions of antagonist muscles, *disappears with activity*.

Motor Neuron Disease

Is characterized by degeneration of motor neurons, either upper motor neuron or lower motor neuron or both.

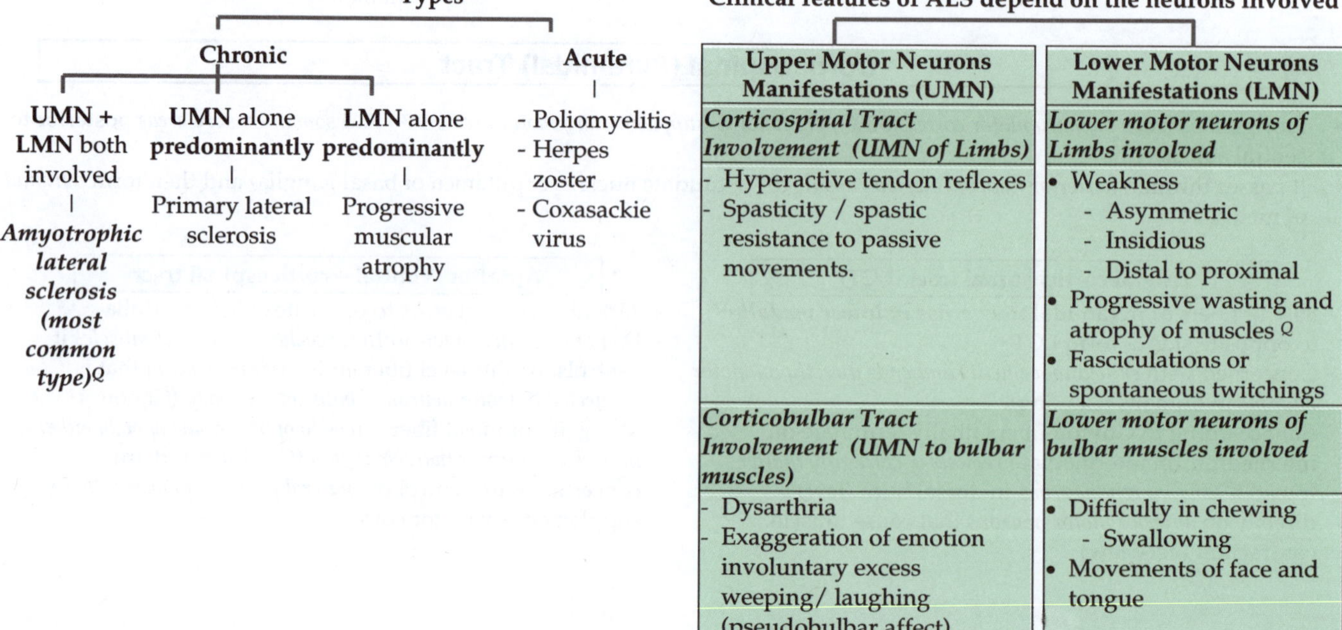

Brown – Sequard Syndrome

- It is **functional hemisection of spinal** cord usually caused by spinal cord tumors, trauma (eg pallet /bullet), degenerative disc disease and ischemia.
- Normal physiology /anatomy of tracts

- **Anterior (Ventro) lateral – spinothalamic tract** crosses the midline more or less at the level of point of entery itself and hence it **ascends contralateral** along the whole length of spinal cord to reach the brain.
- **Dorsal (posterior) column – Medial lemniscal tract (Fasciculus gracilus or fasciculus cuneatus)** ascends such that it remains **ipsilateral** along the entire length of spinal cord. Its fibers cross over to opposite side in medulla.
- **Descending Corticospinal (Pyramidal) Tract** crosses the midline to reach opposite side in medull. This means that any lesion in this tract above medulla will produce, contralateral whereas, below medulla (in spinal cord) will produce ipsilateral signs & symptoms.

- **Segmetal (LMN) signs** like radicular pain, muscle atrophy, or loss of deep tendon reflex etc are **ipsilateral unilateral**.

Clinical Presentation

- It is important to note that **lesion of descending** (from cortex to organ) **tract** like pyramidal tract **after crossing over** and **ascending tracts** (from organ to cortex like dorsal column & spinothalamic tract) **before crossing over** produce **ipsilateral** signs (and vice versa).
- This is why, in Brown- Sequard syndrome, hemisection of spinal cord (which at that level contains *already crossed ascending spinothalamic and descending pyramidal tracts and uncrossed dorsal column ascending tract)* produces.

Ipsilateral loss (on the same side of transaction)	Contralateral loss (on the opposite side of transaction)
•**Dorsal column** sensations in all dermatomes below the level of transaction i.e. - **Fine (light) touch & pressure** - **Discrete localization, two point tactile discrimination or discriminative touch** - **Proprioception, Joint position sense (static position sense & kinesthesia or dynamic proprioception /rate of movement sense)** - **Vibration** and sensation of movement against skin •Corticospinal (pyramidal) tract features below the level of transaction - **Muscle weakness, and spasticity** - **Clonus, exaggerated tendon reflex**	•**Spinothalmic sensations** are lost on contralateral side in all dermatomes begning **1 or 2 segments** (Ganong) **/2 to 6 segments** (Guyton) **below the level of transaction** i.e. - ***Pain***[Q] - ***Temperature***[Q] - Crude touch, which is poorly localized, may still persist because of partial transmission in opposite spinothalamic tract. ★ **"BS – POTS"=Brown Sequard syndrome** has **Opposite (contralateral) loss of pain & temperature** or **spinothalamic tract**.

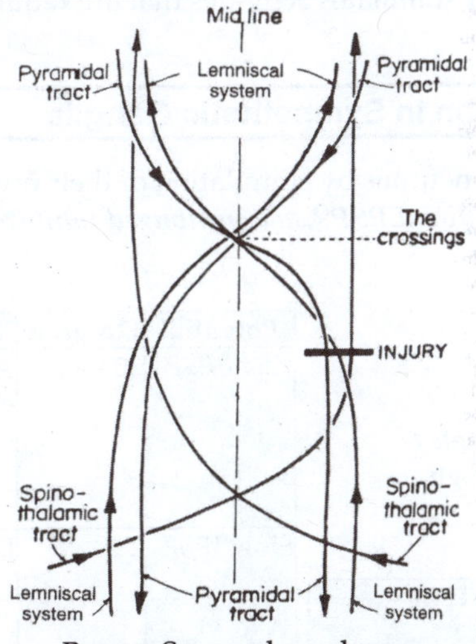

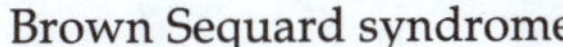
Brown Sequard syndrome

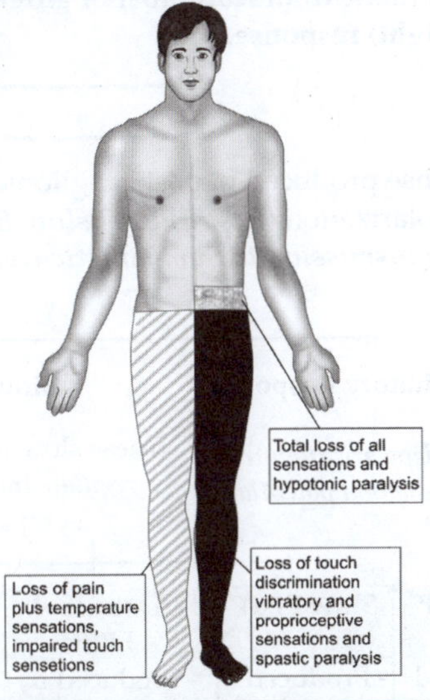

Blood Supply of Spinal Cord

- **Anterior spinal artery**: supply *anterior 2/3 of cord*
- **Posterior spinal artery**: *(a pair)*: supply *posterior 1/3* of cord [posterior column]
- **Radiacular arteries:** The largest rdicular artery arises from aorta in the lower thoracic or upper lumbar region (*artery of Adamkiewiz*) and major source of blood supply to *lower 2/3 of the spinal cord*

Clinical Features of Spinal Vascular Syndromes

Anterior spinal artery syndrome

1) Radicular / girdle pain
2) Motor signs (Flaccid quadriplegia / paraplegia below the level of lesion
3) All sensory modalities lost except vibration & position sense. [*Posterior column is spared*]
4) Impairment of bladder & bowel function

Posterior spinal artery syndrome

Loss of proprioception & vibration sense below the level of lesion[Q].

Conditioned Reflex

Conditioned reflex is a reflex response to a stimulus that previously elicited little or no response, acquired by repeatedly pairing the stimulus with another stimulus that normally does produce the response.

In Pavlov's Classical Experiment[Q] –

- Presentation of food – *Unconditioned stimulus* (US; which normally produce an **innate response**)
- Ringing of the bell – *Conditioned stimulus* (C S). After the CS & US had been paired a number of times, the CS is able to produce the response originally evoked by US. Conditioning of visceral response is called **biofeedback.**

Autonomic Nervous System (ANS)

- In **somatic nervous system** (or **somato-motor system**), the final common pathway linking the CNS to skeletal muscles is **large diameter- rapidly conducting α motor neurons (Aα)**. However, in ANS the peripheral motor portion of sympathetic & parasympathetic neurons (supplying smooth muscle, cardiac musclc & glands) are made up of two neurons; **preganglionic and postganglionic neurons.**
- The cell bodies of ***preganglionic neurons*** are located in the intermediolateral (IML) gray column of spinal cord or the homologus motor nuclei of the cranial nerves therefore ***they have a long course***[Q]. ***The cell bodies of the post ganglionic neurons are located on or near the body of viscera therefore postganglionic neurons are very short***[Q]. Each preganglionic axon diverges to an average of 8 or 9 post ganglionic neurons. ***Preganglionic: Postganglionic → 1: 8 or 9***[Q]. So the ANS output is diffuse. **Preganglionic** autonomic fibers are **myelinated B fiber**, whereas **postganglionic** fibers are **unmyelinated C** type. Conduction speed is A>B>C.
- **Parasympathetic** division is k/a **craniosacral** (involving **3, 7, 9, 10** CN & **S_2, S_3, S_4** sacral roots) or **cholinergic system** (uses ACh). It stimulates activities that conserve energy & restore body resources such as increased digestion & absorption of food and decreased heart rate. **Ciliary spheno (pterygo) palatine, submaxillary (submandibular)** and **otic ganglions** are parasympathetic ganglions of 3rd, 7th & 9th cranial nerves.
- **Sympathetic (thoracolumbar or adrenergic) system** stimulates activities that are **required during emergency (fight, fright and flight) response.**

Transmission in Sympathetic Ganglia

The response produced in post ganglionic sympathetic neurons by stimulation of their preganglionic innervations generates rapid depolarization ***(Fast EPSP)***[Q] ***slow EPSP***[Q], a ***late slow EPSP***[Q], ***and prolonged inhibitory post synaptic potential (slow IPSP)***[Q]. ***Transmission in Sympathetic Ganglia.***

Fast Excitatory Response

A *rapid depolarization* that *generate action potential*

Slow Responses

These slow responses *modulate & regulate transmission* through sympathetic ganglia

Fast EPSP	Slow EPSP	Late Slow EPSP	Slow IPSP
- Produced by ***acetyl choline via nicotinic receptor***[Q]	- Produced by ***aectyl choline***[Q] acting on a ***muscarinic receptor (M_2-cholinergic)***[Q]	- Produced by *GnRH* or a peptide closely resembling it - Very prolonged *lasting minutes* rather than milliseconds.	- Produced by ***dopamine***[Q] (via D_2 receptor) *interneurons* within ganglia. The inter- neurons that secrete dopamine are the small, intensely **fluorescent cells (SIF cells)** in the ganglia - The interneuron is excited by *M_2 muscarinic receptor*

Potential	Duration	Mediator	Receptor	Special features
Fast EPSP	30 ms	Acetyl-choline	Nicotinic cholinergic	- Rapid depolarization that generates action potential
Slow IPSP	2 s	Dopamine	D_2	- *d/t increase in K^+ conductance.* - **Dopamine** is secreted by intensely fluorescent cells (SIF cells) in ganglia
Slow EPSP	30s	Acetyl-choline	M_2 cholinergic	- d/t decrease in K^+ conductance
Late slow EPSP	4 min	Gn RH	Gn RH	Late slow EPSP has a latency of 1-5s and last for few minutes.

Some Drugs and Toxins Affecting Autonomic Activity

Site of Action	Compounds That Augment Autonomic Activity	Compounds That Depress Autonomic Activity
Sympathetic and parasympathetic ganglia	• ***Stimulate postganglionic neurons*** - Nicotine - Low concentrations of acetylcholine • ***Inhibit acetylcholinesterase*** - DFP (diisopropyl fluorophosphate) - Physostigmine (Eserine) - Neostigmine (Prostigmin) - Parathion	• ***Block conduction*** - Hexamethonium (C-6) - Mecamylamine (inversine) - Pentolinium - Trimethaphan (Arfonad) - High concentration of acetylcholine
Endings of postganglionic noradrenergic neurons	• ***Release norepinephrine*** - Tyramine - Ephedrine - Amphetamine	• ***Block norepinephrine synthesis*** - Metyrosine (Demser) • ***Interfere with norepinephrine storage*** - Reserpine - Guanethidine (Ismelin) • ***Prevent norepinephrine release*** - Bretylim (Bretylol) - Guanethidine (Ismelin) • ***Form false transmitters*** - Methyldopa (Aldomet)
Muscarinic receptors		Atropine, scopolamine
α adrenergic receptors	• ***Stimulate α1 receptors*** - Methoxamine (Vasoxyl) - Phenylephrine (Neo-Synephrine)	• ***Block α receptors*** - Phenoxybenzamine (Dibenzyline) - Phentolamine (Regitine) - Prazosin (Minipress) (block α1) - Yohimbine (blocks α2)
b adrenergic receptors	• ***Stimulate β receptors*** - Isoproterenol (Isuprel)	• ***Block β receptors*** - Propranolol (Inderal) and others (blocks β1 & β2) - Atenolol (Tnormin) and others (blocks β1) Butoxamine (blocks β2)

Galvanic Skin Response

- **Galvanic skin response (electrodermal response** = EDR, **skin conductance response** = SCR, **psychogalvanic response** = PGR) is a *measure of electrical resistance of skin* as a reflection of changes in *emotional or autonomic activity.*
- It appears as an **increase in electrical conductance** (i.e. **decrease in resistance**) of skin, measured by attaching electrodes to skin and recording changes in associated moment to moment perspiration & autonomic activity.
- **Emotional arousal** like *fear, anger, sexual feeling, startle response, orienting response, stress, anxiety & knowingly stating a falsehood (lie)* and **sympathetic activity** as by pinprick or threat of injury **produce sweating** and **increased electrical conductance** of skin l/t a similar ↑ **GSR** response. It increases to a maximum after 2 to 10 seconds after stimulation and subsides at about the same rate.
- It is used in *lie detection,behaviour therapy and hypnosis to indicate that client is experiencing emotional arousal.*
- ***GSR is decreased during relaxed states like during yoga***[Q]

Chapter 2. NERVES AND MUSCLES PHYSIOLOGY: REVIEW NOTES

Neurotransmitters

For a substance to be considered NT, it must be *present in presynaptical terminal*, is *synthesized by cell*, should be *released on depolarization* of terminal and there should be *specific receptors* for it on the post synaptic terminal (±) it can be divided into

1. Small Molecule NT	2. Large Molecule NT or Neuro-Peptides	3. Gaseous NTs
A. **Acetyl choline** B. **Aminoacids** eg **glutamate , GABA and glycine**[Q] C. **Biogenic monoamines** eg **dopamine, epinephrine** (adrenaline), **norepinephrine** (noradrenaline), **serotonin** (5 HT or 5 hydroxy tryptamine) and **histamine** D. **Purines** eg **ATP**	- **Hypothalamic hormones** & CRH, LHRH, TRH, GHRH, oxytocin, somatostatin & **vasopressin** - **Opioid peptides** eg **enkephalin,** dynorphin - **Tachykinins** eg **substance** P, neurokinin α, B, K - **VIP – glucagon family** - **Insulin**, ACTH, CCK, α-MSH, Motilin etc.	- Nitric oxide (NO) - Carbon monoxide (CO)

Excitatory aminoacid NT
- **Aspartate**
- **Glutamate**[Q] (Major ≥75%).
  Mn-"Excited AS Glue"

Inhibitory Aminoacid NT
- **GABA**[Q] (major)
- **Glycine (both excitatory & inhibitory).**
  Mn **"in habited Gay guy"**

★ Glycine is inhibitory by increasing Cl^- conductance like GABA. It is excitatory when binds to NMDA receptor and makes them more sensitive to glutamate.

Golgi Tendon – Inverse Stretch Reflex

- Golgi tendon organ is an encapsulated sensory receptor , consisting of a net like collection of knobby nerve endings among the *fasicles of a tendon*. There are ***3 –25 (usually 10-15) muscle fibers connected to each golgi tendon***[Q].
- Unlike muscle spindles, golgi tendon organs are in series with the muscle fibers, so they are ***stimulated by both passive stretch and active contraction of muscle***[Q]. It is important to note that ***spindle detects muscle length and changes in muscle length, wheres golgi tendon detects muscle tension***[Q]. So it is ***stimulated when muscle fiber is tensed by contracting or stretching muscle***[Q].
- Like primary receptor of muscle spindle, tendon **organ has both a dynamic** (intense response to sudden increase in tension) and ***static response***[Q] (steady state firing of lesser degree almost directly proportional to muscle tension).
- Impulses from tendon organ are transmitted through ***large, myelinated rapidly conducting sensory Ib nerve fibers***[Q] (~ 16 μ dia). This Ib fibers end in the spinal cord on *inhibitory interneuron*, which inturn terminate on α - motor neuron supplying the muscle from which Ib originated. They also make excitatory connections with motor neurons supplying antagonist muscles. ***Stimulation of tendon organ causes inhibition of α-motor neuron***[Q] whereas muscle spindle stimulation excites α motor neuron.
- The ***threshold of golgi tendon is low***[Q]. Since more elastic muscle fibers take up much of the stretch, the ***degree of stimulation by passive stretch is not great, and strong stretch is required to produce relaxation***[Q]. However, contraction of muscle regularly stimulate golgi tendon. It is responsible for inverse stretch reflex.

Upto an extent, the strength of reflex contraction of muscle is proportional to the magnitude of stretching. However, *when tension becomes very high there is sudden relaxation of muscle. This is k/a* ***inverse stretch reflex*** *or* ***autogenic inhibition***.

- This **inhibitory negative feedback lengthening reaction** prevents development of too much tension on the muscle and ***protects tearing of muscle or avulsion of tendon***[Q].
- Tendon organ *equalizes contractile forces of* different muscle fibers by inhibiting fibers exerting excess tension.

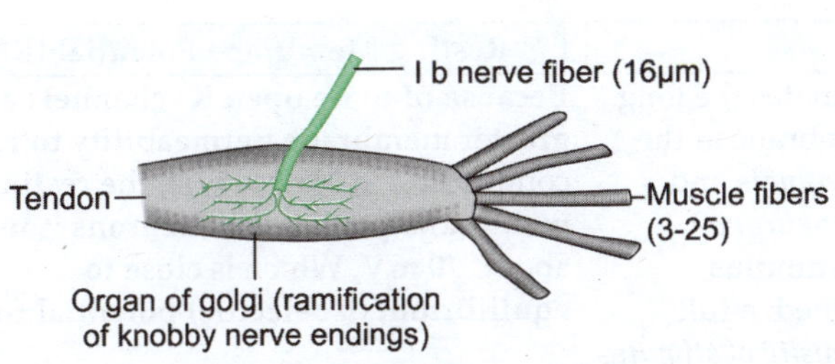

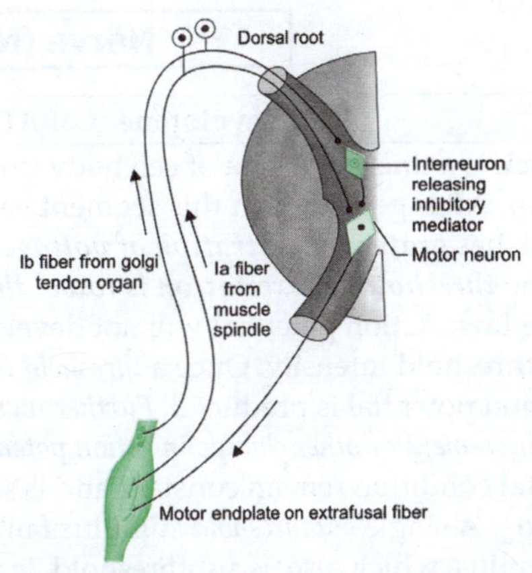

Withdrawal Reflex	Reciprocal Inhibition	Inverse Stretch Reflex
- Its a polysynaptic reflex occurring in response to noxious or painful stimuli - *The response is flexor muscle contraction & inhibition of extensor muscles*, so that the part stimulated is flexed & withdrawn from stimuli - On application of strong stumuli, about 0.2- 0.5 second after flexor & with drawl response in one limb, the opposite limb begins to extend, This is called ***cross extension reflex***Q. It is a part of withdrawal reflex as extension of the opposite limb can withdraw the entire body away from noxious stumuli.	- It is a phenomenon, in *which relaxation of antagonist muscles* occur, when a stretch reflex excites one muscle - Neuronal circuit which causes this reciprocal inhibition is called **reciprocal innervation.** - Ia fiber transmit impulse from protagonist muscle and cause inhibition of motor neuron to antagonist muscle. - *Bisynaptic* pathway, collateral from *Ia* fiber passing through **inhibitory Golgi bottle interneuron**	- It is *sudden relaxation of muscle* on development of high magnitude of tension. - It is ***autogenic inhibitory negative feed back lengthening reaction***Q, that protects against muscle tear. - ***Golgi tendon organ***Q is receptor for inverse stretch reflex.

Changes in Nerve Fiber after Injury

Degeneration of the distal part (Antegrade)	Degeneration of proximal part (Retrograde)	Stage of Regeneration
• Degeneration of distal part (distal to cut) is called *Wallerian degeneration.*Q • Within 24 hours histological and chemical changes occur • The ***axon cylinder swells up & breaks down into small rodlets.***Q • ***Myelin sheath breaks down into oily droplets, It occurs 8-32 days after injury.***Q • **Cells of the sheath of Schwann** – ***divide mitotically***Q & from cords of cells lying within the endoneurial tube (neurilemma) → macrophages remove the degenerating myelin & axis cylinder → thus schwann cell cytoplasm gradually fills the neurilemma, this process is *completed by 3 months.* • Hollow tube of neurilemma remains intact & K/a *ghost tube.*	• Same as distal generation but upto ***nearest node of ranvier (nearest collateral)***Q • **Changes in the cell body:** - Within 48 hours of injury the **nissl granules & rough endoplasmic reticulum** begins to disintegrate (K/a **chromatolysis**). - Golgi apparatus fragments - Cells swell - Neurofibril disappear & nucleus displaced to cell margin.	• *Axis cylinders from stumps grows & sprout out* (pseudopod like structure of fibril) • *After 2-3 weeks peripheral endoneural tube,* contain varying no of developing fibril • *Medullary sheath begins to develop in about 15 days &* completed within one year. • Repair of cell body (i.e. Nissl granules & golgi apparatus) → begins about 20 days after nerve section & is completed in 80 days.

Nerve (Neuron) Action Potential (AP)

Development of AP

- **Axon hillock** is a thickened area of cell body from which originates the long fibrous axon. AP is generated in this segment because the membrane at the axon hillock has ***grater concentration of voltage gated Na+ channels*** and therefore the ***threshold for excitation is lower than the rest of neurons***Q
- **All or none law**: Action potential will not develop unless the stimulus searches a threshold intensity. Once a *threshold intensity* is reached, a full fledged action potential is produced. *Further increase in the intensity of stimulus produce no increment or other change in action potential* as long as other experimental condition remain constant and is said to obey "all or none law".
- **Summation** – A single *subthreshold* stimulus fails to produce an AP. But if a second stimulus, which also, is subthreshold, is applied *sufficiently quickly* after the 1st one, the two stimuli are summated & excitation results.

Temporal	Spatial
- When summation is in relation to time	- Two subthreshold stimuli applied geographically closely but simultaneously

Propagation of AP

- An action potential once generated at a point on nerve depolarizes the adjacent areas &spreads in both direction, newly depolarized area producing action potential in their adjacent areas. Thus the nerve action potential ***travels with same amplitude*** Q
- ***As the AP propagates, the strength of AP remain undiminished.***Q
- ***An action potential is due to opening up Na^+ channels causing Na influx***Q.
- Any impulse conducted antidromically up the axons dies out ***because, post synaptical part of neurons lack chemical synaptic vesicles***Q that are needed for synaptic transmission. Therefore an impulse arriving at the post synaptic membrane cannot release synaptic mediator. **Axons** can conduct impulse in both direction. **Dendrites** are found on the axon's endings and so behave in the same way as the axons i.e. *bi-directional*.

Velocity of Conduction

- Conduction of nerve is an *active self propagating process* and impulse moves ***at a constant amplitude & velocity***Q. Conduction of nerve impulses, although rapid, ***is much slower than that of electricity.***Q
- Nerve fibers with a ***greater diameter & with the myelin sheath conduct faster.***Q
- New action potential is ***fastest in A type of fibers***Q (as it is myelinated & has a greater diameter).

Membrane Capacitance

- Myelination of nerve decreases membrane capacitance 50 folds & allow depolarization to occur very fast
- A ***decrease in capacitance increase the speed of action potential propagation***Q

Orthrodromic Conduction

Transmission at synapse is always in one direction (orthodromic) only because the neurotransmitter substance responsible for conduction is present in vesicles of presynaptic neurons onlyQ. ***The post synaptic neuron does not contain any neurotransmitter***Q. It has protein molecules embedded in it which serve as receptor for the neurotransmitter.

Susceptible to

The relative susceptibility of nerve fiber to

Hypoxia	Pressure	Local anaesthetics
*B> A> C*Q	*A> B> C*Q	*C > B >A* Q

Resting Membrane Potential (RMP)

Because of more open K^+ channels and greater membrane permeability to K^+(in comparison to Na^+) **at rest, the resting membrane potential in neurons** is usually about **-70 mV,** Which is **close to equilibrium (isoelectric) potential for K^+.**

Phases of AP

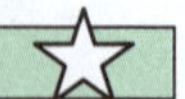

(i) **Depolarization of membrane** d/t Na^+ **influx**

(ii) **Firing level** – After initial 15 mv of depolarization, rate of depolarization increases. This is firing level.

(iii) **Upstroke phase** - rapid depolarization phase of membrane. It is due to rapid flow of Na^+ into the cell.

(iv) **Overshoot** – part of action potential during which membrane is positive.

(v) **Downstroke – Rapid return of membrane towards its resting potential** is the **repolarization phase** or downstroke. It is produced d/t (a) ***closing of Na^+ channels* (b) *opening of K^+ channels***

(vi) **Undershoot** – Membrane potential becomes more negative to form small but prolonged after hyperpolarization.

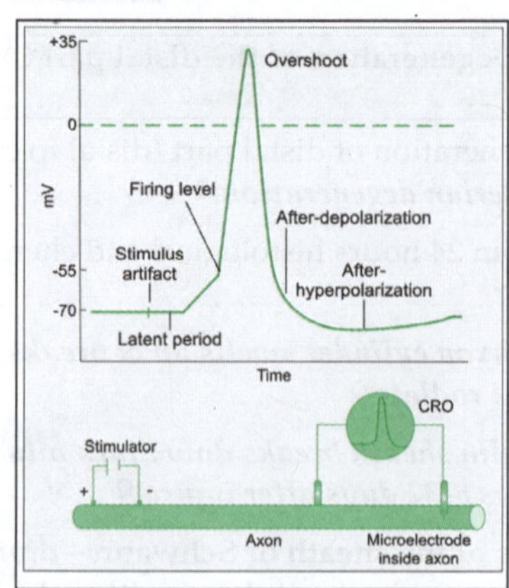

Action potential in a neuron recorded with one electrode inside the cell

Resting Membrane Potential (RMP)

- Neurons have **higher K^+** concentration **inside** whereas **higher Na^+ concentration outside the cell.** This concentration gradient is established by **Na^+K^+ATPase** which pumps Na+ ions out to exterior and take K+ ions inside (both against electrochemical & concentration gradient).
- Because of this concentratioin gradient, there is *passive diffusion of K^+ out of the cell and Na+ inside the cell.* Because of higher permeability, the **K^+ can cross the membrane about 100 times faster than Na^+.** So the amount of K^+ exiting out of the cell is much-much greater than the amount of Na^+ entering into the cell.
- So the **RMP** usually between -70mv (to -95mv) is **close to equilibrium (isoelectric) potential for K^+**[Q].
- During RMP The interior of cell is negatively and exterior is positively charged.

Accommodation

Only the current or stimulus which rises to its peak intensity rapidly causes the action potential to develop[Q]. The **current which rises to its peak very slowly does not produce AP**, although, at peak level, its strength may be adequate. This is called **accommodation** & occurs because the *activation or opening up of Na^+ channels do not develop with slowly rising current strength.*

Electrotonic potential (EP)

- **Electrotonus** is development of local, nonpropogating **electrotonic potential** due to application of subthreshold current to a nerve.
- A **cathode current** produces **hypo(de)polarization** (ie the *interior* of cell becomes *less negative or more positive)* called **catelectronic potential**. Conversely **anodal current** produces **hyperpolarization anelectronic potential** ie cell interior becomes more negative.
- At 7-15mv of depolarization (ie potential of minus -55mv) the **threshold firing potential** is reached and action potential develop.
  - ***If depolarization occurs rapidly,*** the opening of Na^+ channels overwhelms the repolarizing force and **action potential result** → nerve impulse generates.
  - ***If the induced depolarization is produced gradually slowly,*** the opening of K^+ channels balances the gradual opening of Na^+ channels and ***an action potential does not occur.***[Q]

Dendrite

Morphology

- The neuron has 5-7 process called **dendrites** that extends outwards from the cell body and arborise extensively
- Particularly in the *cerebral and cerebellar cortex*, the dendrites have small knobby projections called **dendrites spine**
- Neuron generally have 4 zones :
  1. *Receptor / dendritic zone,* where multiple local potential changes generated by synaptic connections are integrated.
  2. A site where propogated action potential are generated (the ***initial segment in spinal motor neuron, the initial node of Ranvier in cutaneous sensory neuron***[Q]**.)**
  3. Axonal process that transmits propagated impulse to nerve endings
  4. The nerve endings, where AP causes release of synaptic transmitters
- Most synapses are between terminal buttons (synaptic knobs) of pre synaptic cell & dendrites of post synaptic cell. *In cerebral cortex 98%* of synapses are on dendrites & only 2% are on cell bodies. In *spinal cord* the proportion of endings on dendrites is less in 80%

Receptor zone:
Graded electrogenesis

Site origin of
conducted impulses

Axon:
All or none
transmission

Nerve endings:
Secretion of
synaptic transmitter

Functional organization of neurons. Non-conducted local potentials are integrated in the receptor zone., and action potentials are initiated at a site close to the receptor zone (arrow). The action potentials are conducted along the axon to the nerve endings, where they cause release of synaptic transmitters.

Functions of dendrites

- The sites of current sources or sinks that electronically change the membrane potential at initial segment; i.e. they are merely *extensions of the soma that extends the area available for integration*. The effects of discharge at individual synaptic endings can be excitatory or inhibitory and *summation of all the excitatory and inhibitory effects* in dendrites determine whether an action potential is generated.
- *Very rarely propagated action potential may develop in dendrite* (It is important to know that *most dendrites can not generate and transmit action potential* because their membrane have relatively *few voltage gated Na+ channels*, so that their threshold for excitation is too high for AP to occur.
- Malleability of dendritic spine (i.e. appear, change & even disappear over a time scale of minutes & hours) and protein synthesis in dendritic

- On average, each neuron divides to form over 2000 synaptic endings and, since human CNS has *10'' neurons*, it follows that there are about 2×10^{14} synapse.
- Transmission in synapses may be very rarely *electrical* (low resistance bridge through which ions passes easily) e.g. in *lateral vestibular nucleus* or *chemical* (mostly).
- Synaptic cleft is ***20-40nm***[Q] wide. Across the cleft are many neurotransmitter receptors in postsynaptic membrane in thickened zone called **postsynaptic density**. Similarly **active zone** containing many proteins & rows of calcium channels is seen as thickened membrane in presynaptic membrane.
- Ca++ that triggers exocytosis of transmitter from synaptic vesicle enters the presynaptic neurons (active zone) and transmitter release occurs starts in *200-500μs*. The process by which synaptic vesicle fuse with the cell membrane involve **V-snare protein synaptobrevin in vesicle membrane** locking with the **t-snare protein syntaxin in the cell membrane.** The organization of synapses depends on **neurexins protein** bound to membrane of presynaptic neuron.

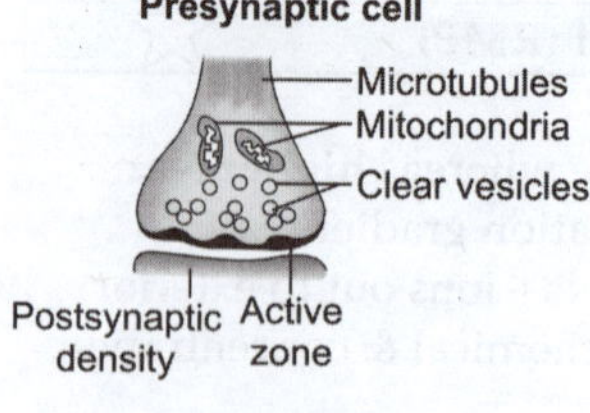

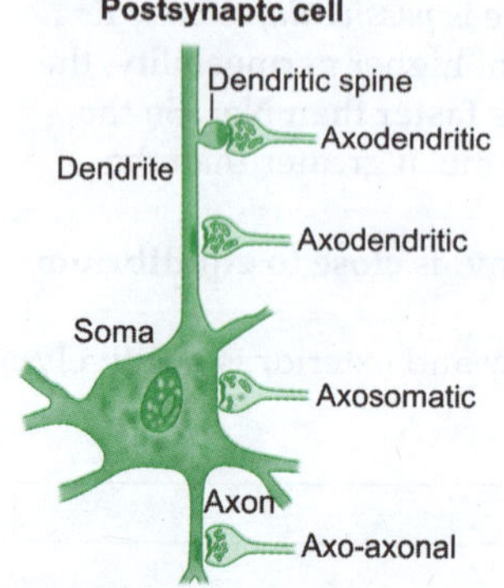

Axodendritic, axoaxonal, and axosomatic synapses. Many presynaptic neurons terminate on dendritic spines, as shown at the top, but some also end directly on the shafts of dendrites. Note the presence of clear and granulated synaptic vesicles in endings and clustering of clear vesicles at active zones.

spine alters the effects of input from individual glutaminergic synapses (NMDA & AMPA receptors) on the dendritic spine. These selective changes mediate ***learning and long term potentiation (LTP)***[Q].

- The AP is generated in the **initial segment** (***the portion of axon at and just beyond the axon hillock***[Q]). and its discharge is propagated in two directions : down the axon and back into soma. *Retrograde firing* of the soma in this fashion probably has value in *"wiping the slate clean"* for subsequent renewal of the interplay of excitatory & inhibitory activity on the cell.
- They can *transmit signals by electronic conduction* down the dendrite to soma but there is *decrement of postsynaptic potential* during transmission due to thin & permeable dendrite membrane that *leak K^+ & Cl^-*
- Current flow to & from the active synaptic knob on dendrites produce ***wave activity in EEG***[Q].

★ Several toxins which block neurotransmitter release are *zinc-endopeptidases* that cleave & hence inactivate proteins in the *fusion-exocytosis complex*. **Tetanus toxin & botulinum toxin- C, D, F, G** act on **syntobrevin & botulin toxin C** acts on *syntaxin*. **Botulinum toxin A & B** act on **SNAP-25**. Clinically, **tetanus toxin** causes spastic paralysis by blocking presynaptic transmitter release in CNS and botulism causes flaccid paralysis by blocking the release of acetyl choline (ACh) at neuromuscular junction.

Nissl Body (or Nissl Granule or Tigroid Body) 

- Named after Franz Nissl, a German neurologist **Nissl body** (or **Nissl granule** or **tigroid body**) is a large granular body found in the **soma, (or perikaryon , or cyton, or cell body, the bulbous end of a neuron, containing the cell nucleus)**[Q] and **<u>dendrites</u>** of neurons, **though not in the <u>axon</u> or <u>axon hillock</u>**.
- These granules are rough endoplasmic reticulum (with free ribosomes) and are the site of protein synthesis involved in the synthesis of neurotransmitters such as acetylcholine.
- Nissl bodies can be demonstrated by a method of selective staining developed by Nissl (Nissl staining), using an aniline stain to label extranuclear RNA granules. This staining method is useful to localize the perikaryon / cell body, and dendrites of neurons. Due to RNA's basophilic ("base-loving") properties it is stained blue by this method.
- Nissl bodies show changes under various physiological conditions and in pathological conditions they may dissolve and disappear (karyolysis).

Electric Events in Post Synaptic Neurons

Excitatory Post-Synaptic Potential (EPSP)

- **Excitatory post synaptic potential (EPSP)** or **generator (receptor) potential** (which is EPSP in Pacinian corpuscles) is a ***nonpropagating localized depolarizing potential, the magnitude of which is proportional to the intensity of stimulus (i.e. the amount of transmitters released by the pre synaptic neurons)***[Q]. So EPSP or GP(RP) are **graded potentials** rather than *"all or none" action potential.*
- Small **depolarization (hypopolarization)** changes in membrane of post synaptic cells are termed **excitatory (=EPSP),** If they increase the cell's excitability (ie probability of firing AP).
- EPSP begins about 0.5 ms after the afferent impulse reach the spinal cord; **peaks 11.5ms after** the stimulus and **declines exponeatially.**
- Produced by opening of ***Na^+ or Ca^{++} channels***[Q] producing an inward current. EPSP is **localized, nonpropogated**, inscribed and **summated.**
- EPSP's are directly ***proportional to the strength of initial stimuli (amount of transmitter released by the presynaptic neurons)***[Q].
- It does not obey all or none law. Stronger the stimulus greater will be EPSP. Strictly localized, that It ***is not self propagating***[Q] (unlike AP). It develops as a result of entry of all cations inside the cell, it is forerunner of an AP.

Inhibitory Post Synaptic Potential (IPSP)

- **Hyperpolarization** of postsynaptic membrane **makes it resistant to stimuli** (i.e. it **decreases the cell's excitability** or **probability of firing the AP)** and is k/a **inhibitory post synaptic potential (IPSP)**.
- Like EPSP, IPSP **peak 11.5ms after stimuli and decrease exponentially.**
- Produced by opening of *Cl^- channels*. Cl^- influx increases intracellular negativity and leads to hyperpolarization. Also produced by *K^+ efflux and closure of Na^+ or Ca^{++} channels.*
- Decreased excitability during IPSP (hyperpolarization) is *due to movement of membrane potential away from the firing level.* So more depolarization (excitatory) activity is required to reach firing level.
- The membrane potential, at which there is **no EPSP (or EPSC = excitatory post synaptic current),** or the postsynaptic potential disappears is k/a **reversal potential. When the membrane potential is at equilibrium potential for chloride E_{Cl}= -70 mV),** the EPSP disappears and at mores negative membrane potentials, it becomes positive **(=reversal potential**). This proves that IPSP is d/t Cl^-influx.

Synaptic Delay

- When an impulse reaches the presynaptic terminals, an interval of at least **0.5 ms,** occurs before a response is obtained in the postsynaptic neuron. It is because of time taken by synaptic mediators to be released & to act on receptors on membrane of post synaptic cell.
- Synaptic delay across one synapse is **0.5ms**; so it can determined that the reflex pathway is mono or poly-synaptic.

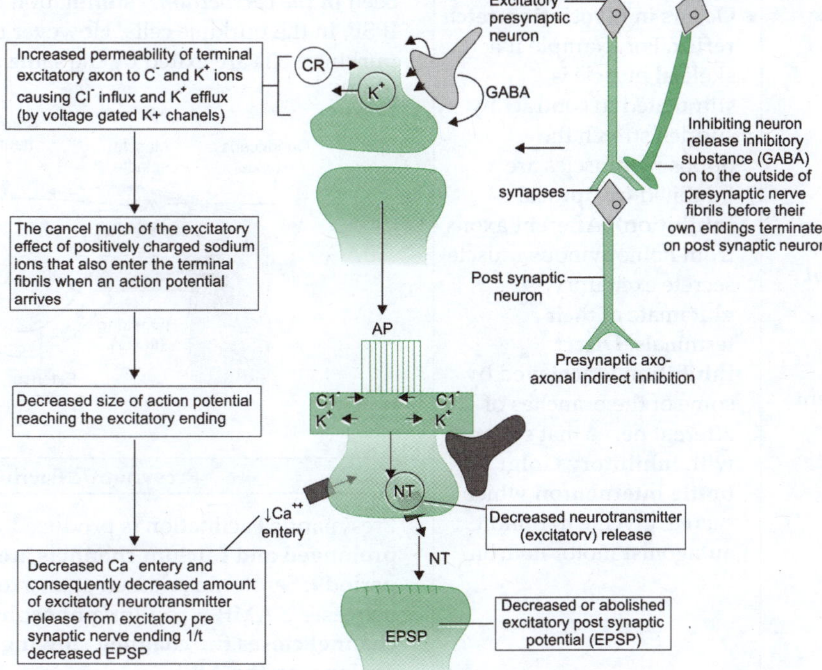

Synaptic Inhibition 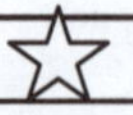

Presynaptic Inhibition

- This is also called *indirect inhibition.*
- ***It occurs d/t failure of presynaptic axon terminals to release the excitatory neurotransmitter substance***Q
- It occurs by ***axo – axonic transmission.***Q
- **Mechanism:**
  - GABA mediated increase in Cl^- conductance causing **Cl^- influx**
  - Opening of voltage gated K+ channels causing **K+ influx**
  - It causes ***decrease in EPSP***Q ***d/t decreased AP, decreased Ca++ entry & decreased neuro transmitter release.***Q
  - *Direct inhibition of voltage gated Ca++ channel opening* (necessary for exocytosis of neurotransmitter release)
  - *Direct inhibition of neurotransmitter* release (independent of Ca^{++} influx mechanism)
- **Antagonistic drug**:
  - ***Picrotoxin***Q inhibits presynaptic inhibition
  - ***Local anaesthetic do not affect presynaptic inhibition.***Q
- Occurs in **sensory pathways** where adjacent nerves often mutually inhibit one another which minimizes sideways spread & mixing of signals in sensory tracts.

Postsynaptic Inhibition

- This is also called ***direct (reciprocal) inhibition*** because it is not a consequence of previous discharge of post synaptic neuron. Where as **indirect inhibition** is d/t effects of previous post synaptic neuron discharge (eg. Postsynaptic cell can be refractory to excitation because it has just fired & is in refractory phase).
- It occurs ***d/t release of an inhibitory neuro-transmitter causing post-synaptic neuron to hyperpolarize (IPSP)***Q.
- **Mechanism:**
  - Inhibitory neurotransmitter
  - (GABA & Glycine) acts on postsynaptic membrane & *produce inhibitory post synaptic potential (IPSP)*
- **Antagonistic drug:** ***Strychnine***Q
- Occurs in **myotactic stretch reflex**. For example if a skeletal muscle is stimulated to contract by sudden stretch the opposing muscles are inhibited **(reciprocal inhibition).** Afferent axons from homonymous muscle secrete excitatory glutamate at their terminals. **Direct inhibition** is achieved by some of the branches of afferent nerve that synapse with **inhibitory Golgi bottle interneuron** which secrete glycine to inhibit antagonist motor neuron.

Renshaw Cell Inhibition 

- ***Negative – feed back inhibition of a spinal motor neuron via an inhibitory interneuron (Renshaw cell).***Q Interneuron releases glycine which is inhibitory in function.
- Renshaw Cell Inhibitory System is located in the ventral horns of the spinal cord in close association with the motor neurons. *Impulse generated in motor neuron activate the inhibitor interneurons (Renshaw cell) to secrete inhibitory mediator* & this slows / stops the discharge of motor neuron.

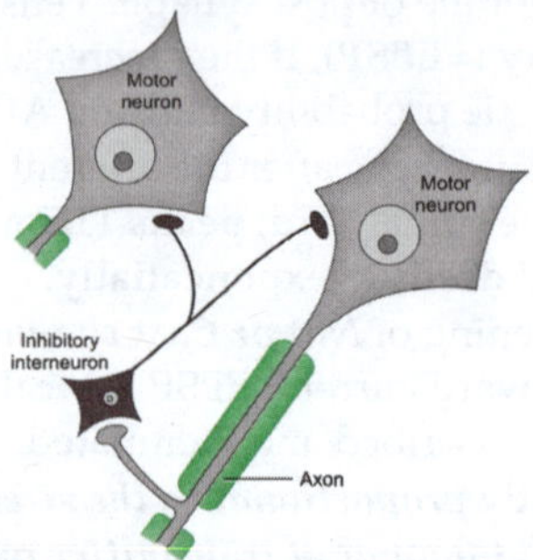

Negative feedback inhibition of a spinal motor neuron via an inhibitory neuron (Renshaw cell)

Feed Forward Inhibition

Seen ***in the cerebellum,***Q stimulation of basket cells produced IPSP, in the purkinje cells. However the basket cells & the purkinje cells are exited by the same parallel excitatory input.

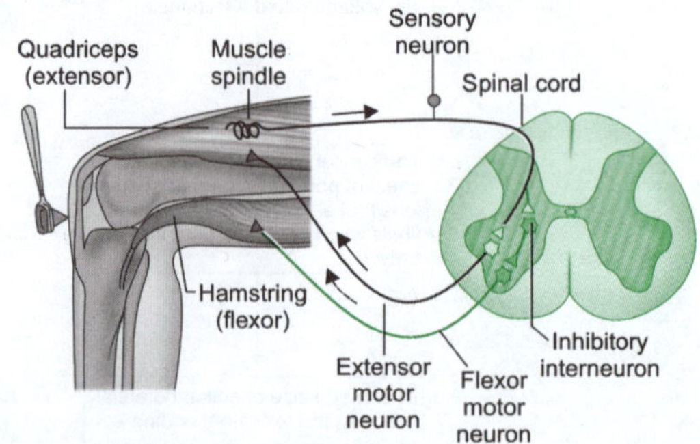

Presynaptic Facilitation 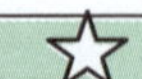

Presynaptic Facilitation is produced when the **AP is prolonged and calcium channels are open for a longer period**Q. Serotonin released at an axonaxonal ending increases c-AMP & resulting **phosphorylation of K^+ channel closes the channel, slowing repolarization & prolonging the AP.**

Transmission In Sympathetic Ganglia: Fast & Slow Responses of Postganglionic Neurons In Sympathetic Ganglia

Potential	Duration	Mediator	Receptor	Special features
Fast EPSP	30 ms	Acetylcholine	Nicotinic cholinergic	- Rapid depolarization that generates action potential
Slow IPSP	2 s	Dopamine	D_2	- *d/t increase in K^+ conductance.* - Dopamine is secreted by intensely fluorescent cells (SIF cells) in ganglia
Slow EPSP	30s	Acetylcholine	M_2 cholinergic	- d/t decrease in K^+ conductance
Late slow EPSP	4 min	Gn RH	Gn RH	Late slow EPSP has a latency of 1-5s and last for few minutes.

Sensory Information

Law of Projection

- States that, no matter where a particular sensory pathway is stimulated along its course to the cortex, the conscious sensation produced is referred to the location of the receptors.
- *Phantom limb* is an example of ***law of projection***[Q]. The patient complains of pain & proprioceptive sensation in the absent limbs, because the end of the nerves cut at the time of amputation are stimulated by pressure on them. The impulses generated in these nerve fibers came from sense organs in the amputated limb, thus the sensation felt are projected to where the receptors used to be.

Localization

- A single sensory axon & all its peripheral branches are termed **sensory units** . The **receptive field** of a **sensory unit** is the spatial distribution from which a stimulus produces a response in that unit.
- The size of **receptive field for light touch** can be measured y **two point threshold** test and it tests the integrity of **dorsal column (medial lemniscus) system,** the central ***pathway for touch and proprioception***[Q]. The minimum distance between the two caliper poins that can be perceived as separate points of stimulation is called **two points discrimination threshold** and is a mesure of **tactile acuity.**
- Information from sensory neurons whose receptors are at the peripheral edge of the stimulus is inhibited compared to information from the sensory neurons at the center of stimulus. This phenomenon is k/a **lateral inhibition** and it enhances the contrast between the center & periphery of a stimulated area and increases the ability of brain to localize a sensory input
- ***Lateral inhibition is responsible for localization of a stimulus site and two point discrimination***[Q].

Muller's Law of Specific Nerve energies

- The sensation evoked by specific sensory pathways are discrete from sense organ to cortex.
- States that , no matter how or where a particular sensory pathay for particular sense organ is stimulated along its course to the cortex, the sensation evoked is that for which the receptor is specialized.
- For example, if sensory nerve from a pacinian corpuscle in hand is stimulated by pressure at elbow or by irritation of tumor in brachial plexus or by stimulation of appropriate fibers of dorsal columns of spinal cord, thalamus or post central gyrus of cerebral cortex, the sensation produced would be touch.

Judgement of Stimulus Intensity

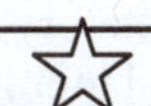

Weber – Fechner principle – Detection of ratio of stimulus strength

- It states that *gradation of stimulus strength are discriminated approximately in proportion to logarithm of stimulus strength.* In other words it emphasizes that *greater the background sensory intensity, the greater an additional change must be for the psyche to detect the change.* For example a person already holding 30gm weight can barely detect an additional 1 gm change and similarly when holding 300 gm can barely detect 10 gm change (the ratio remained same in both)
- **Weber-Fechner law:** states that the ***magnitude of the sensation felt is proportionate to the log of intensity of the stimulus***[Q]

Interpreted signal strength = Log x stimulus intensity + Constant

Power Law

- States that a person interprets changes in intensity of sensory stimuli approximately in proportion to a power function of the actual intensity.

Interpreted signal strength = K x $(\text{Stimulus} - k)^y$

- There are *three methods* by *which brain detects intensity* of a sensory stimulus (differentiates b/w two stimuli of different – intensities). If a greater or lesser pressure is applied to skin there will be variation (increase or decrease respectively) in
  - ***the receptor potential in the mechanoreceptor***[Q].
  - the ***frequency of the action potentials***[Q] generated by the stimulus in a given receptor.
  - the ***number of receptors activated by the stimulus***[Q].
- It now appears that a power function more accurately describes this ratio

  $R = KS^A$

  where R = senstion felt,

S = intensity of stimulus and K & A = Constants
- This is quantitatively accurate only for *higher intensities of visual, auditory & cutaneous sensory* experience & applies only poorly to most other types of sensory experiences.
- Frequency of action potential generated in sensory nerve fiber is also related to intensity of initiating stimulus by a power function.

(exponent y and the constant K & k are different for each type of sensation)

- When plotted on a graph using double logarithmic coordinates, *a linear relation can be attained between interpreted stimulus strength & actual stimulus strength* over a large range for almost any type of sensory perception.

Miniature End Plate Potential

- Miniature end plate potential does not result in firing of muscle fibre
- Its about 0.5 mv in amplitude.
- The size of *quanta of Ach released* varies *directly with Ca^{2+}* concentration & *inversely with Mg^{2+}* conc. At the end plate.

When a nerve impulse reaches the ending, the number of quanta released increases by several order of magnitude, and the result is the *large end plate potential* that exceeds the firing level of muscle fiber.

Generation of Action Potential in Postsynaptic Neuron

- The axon (devoid of Nissl granules) starts from a short pyramidal shaped part of cell body k/a **axon hillock**. In myelinated axons, the part of axon between axon hillock and beginning of myelination is k/a ***initial segment***. So initial segment is the *portion of axon at and just beyond the axon hillock.*
- In ***myelinated motor neurons, the unmylinated initial segment is the site of initiation of production of action potential (full fledged) and propogation of nerve impulse***[Q]. In **cutaneous sensory nerves**, the site of initiation of nerve impulse is **1st node of Ranvier.**
- Action potential begins in initial segment and not adjacent to excitatory synapses of soma because the initial segment membrane has *7 times greater concentration of voltage gated sodium channels* as does the soma. So the initial segment has ***lowest threshold of excitation***[Q]. The excitatory post synaptic potential (EPSP) that will elicit an action potential in initial segment is *+ 10 to + 20 milivolts* whereas > + 30 to + 40 mV is required for soma.
- When the *10 – 15 mV of depolarization* sufficient to reach firing level is reached and impulse is *propogated in two directions*: down the axon & back into the stoma. **Retrograde firing** of soma has *value in wiping the state clean for subsequent* renewal of interplay of excitatory & inhibitory synaptic knobs.

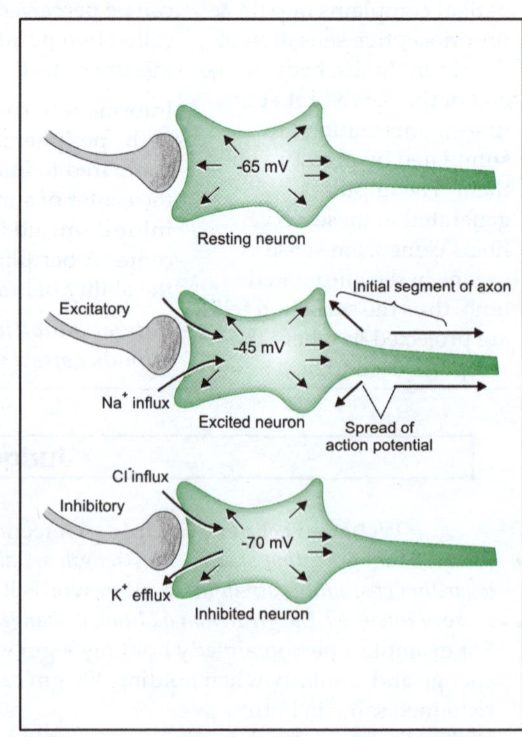

Transmission At Neuromuscular Junction ☆

Presynaptic Nerve Ending

Nerve impulse reach NM junction → **Increased Ca++ permeability of presynaptic neural membrane d/t opening of voltage gated Ca++ channels → Influx of calcium from synaptic space to interior of presynaptic nerve ending →** Calcium ion attracts acetyl choline (ACh) vesicles and draws /fuse them to neural membrane adjacent to dense bars leading to a ***marked increase in exocytosis/release of ACh in synaptic cleft***[Q]

↓

Synaptic Cleft

ACh diffuses through synaptic space and **binds to nicotinic cholinergic (Nm) receptors** in the **post synaptic motor end plate**. (ACh receptors are concentrated at the top of subneural clefts = junctional folds) → Binding of ACh to ACh receptors (which are ligand gated sodium channel) **increases Na+ and K+ conductance** of muscle cell membrane.

↓

In Post Synaptic Motor End Plate (Muscle Membrane)

Influx of positively charged Na+ ions into the muscle fibre creates a local positive potential change inside the muscle fiber i.e. **end plate potential (EPP) → Current sink** created between depolarized end plate (with EPP) and adjacent muscle plasma membrane **on (both sides) initiates an action potential** (ie depolarizes the adjacent muscle membrane to its firing level) → **Action potentials are generated on either side of end plate and are conducted away from end plate in both directions along the muscle fiber → AP (depolarization) spreads to all parts & to interior of muscle fibers by way of T (transverse) tubules** (communicate externally with ECF, contain ECF and are actually internal extension of cell membrane) → As AP reaches T-tubules, the **voltage change is sensed by DHPR (dihydro pyridine receptors)** on T tubule → DHPRs are physically linked to **calcium release (ryanodine receptor) channels in the adjacent sarcoplasmic reticular (SR) cisternae.** AP in T-tubule cause **conformational change in voltage sensing DHP receptors,** which **unlocks (opens) the Ca^{++} release channels in terminal cistern of SR** and permitting Ca^{++} to rapidly diffuse into the sarcoplasm (thick & thin filament). The calcium induced Ca^{++} release quickly amplifies the release of Ca^{++} → **Binding of Ca^{++} to troponin C, uncovering myosin binding sites on actin → Formation of cross linkage between actin and myosin** and sliding of thick on thin filaments producing movement.

↓

Acetyl choline degradation in synaptic cleft: ACh is rapidly removed by acetyl choline esterase, which is present in high concentration in synaptic space. **This prevents continued muscle re-excitation after muscle fiber has recovered from initial AP.**

Summary of Muscle Relaxation

Calcium ions are pumped back from sarcoplasm (myofibrillar fluid) into sarcoplasmic reticulum by an **ATP dependent Ca^{++} pump,** concentrating Ca^{++} ions about 10 thousand folds inside the tubules. **Calsequestrin protein** that can bind upto 40 times more Ca^{++} is found inside SR → **Decreased Ca^{++} ion concentration in sarcoplasm and release of Ca++ from troponin → Cessation of interaction between actin & myosin causing muscle relaxation**[Q].

Physiological Anatomy of NM Junction

Presynaptic Nerve Ending (End feet or Terminal Button)	Synaptic Cleft (Space)	Post synaptic Motor End Plate (Sarcolemma)
- Contains many **mitochondria** which provide ATP for synthesis of ACh in cytoplasm - Contain many small clear **synaptic vesicles** that rapidly absorb. ACh - Contain **voltage gated Ca^{++} channels**	- Contain large quantities of **actyline choline esterase enzyme** which destroys ACh	- Depress or invaginates to form **synaptic trough** or **synaptic gutter** in which nerve end feet fit in - **Subneural clefts** are neumerous small folds of muscle membrane increasing the surface area. - Contain **nicotinic (Nm) cholinergic receptors**

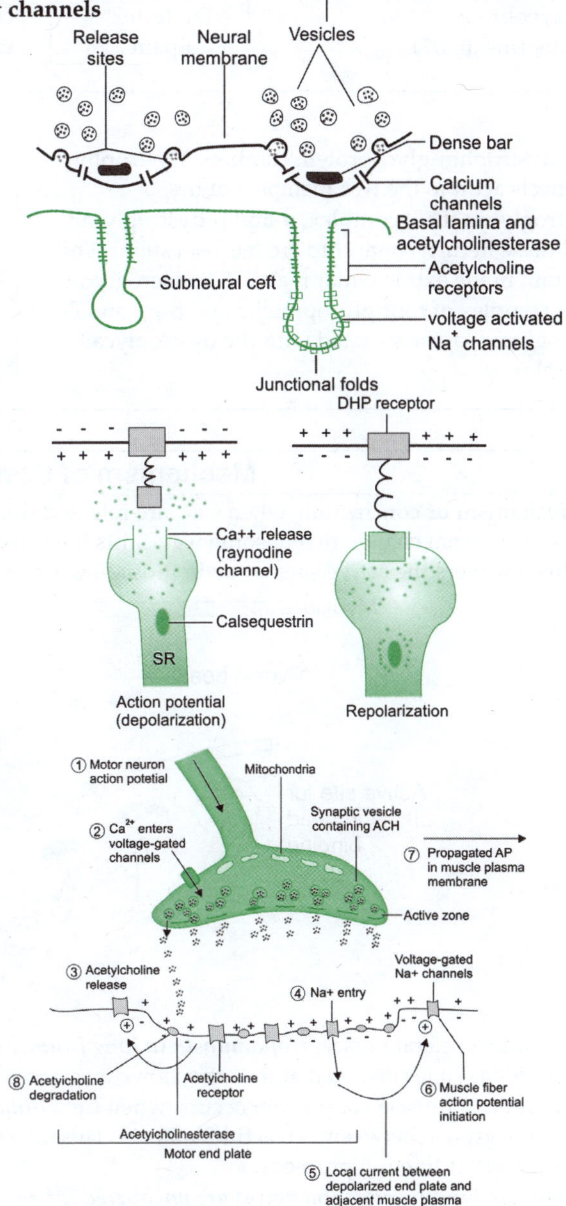

Sacrolemmal Proteins

Sarcolemma is the cell membrane of muscle fiber. It contains several integral (transmembrane) & peripheral proteins which form complexes. Defect of these proteins & complexes results in muscular dystrophies.

Proteins

Integral (Transmem-brane) protein
- *Dystroglycans (DG)*[Q] (β-dystroglycan)
- *Sarcoglycans (SG)*[Q] (α, β, γ, δ)
- Caveolin– 3
- Integrins (β, α7)

Peripheral proteins localizes to the cytoplasmic side
- *Dystrophin* [Q]
- Dysferlin
- Calpain

Proteins & glycoprotein complexes
- Integrin complex
- Dysferilin – caveolin complex
- **Dystrophin- dystroglycan – sarcoglycan complex** adds strength to muscle by providing a scaffolding for the fibrils & connecting them to extracellular environment.

The dystrophin-glycoprotein complex. Dystrophin connects actin to the two members of the dystroglycan (DG) complex, α-and β-dystroglycan, and these in turn connect to the merosin subunit of laminin in the extracellular matric. The sacroglycan (SG) complex of four glycoproteins, α-, β-, γ- and δ-sacroglycan, are associated with the dystroglycan complex.

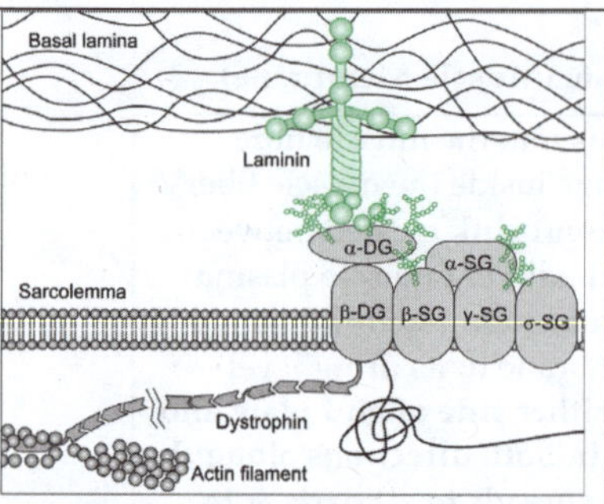

Perlecan

- Perlecan is a large multidomain proteoglycan, which is synthesized by both vascular endothelium & smooth muscle cells & deposited in extracellular matrix.
- It binds to & cross link many extracellular matrix components & cell surface molecules.
- It is a key component of vascular ECM. It promotes growth factor (FGF2) activity, stimulate endothelial growth & regeneration and maintain endothelial barrier function.
- In smooth muscle it is a potent inhibitor of cell proliferation and maintains vascular homeostasis.

Mechanism of Contraction of Skeletal Muscle

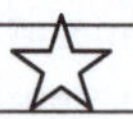

- **Mechanism of contraction**: when Ca^{2+} are released during the contraction process, the troponin complex undergoes a confirmational change that in some way shifts the tropomyosin molecules into the groove between the two actin strands. This uncovers the active sites on actin thus allowing myosin to bind the actin & contraction proceed.

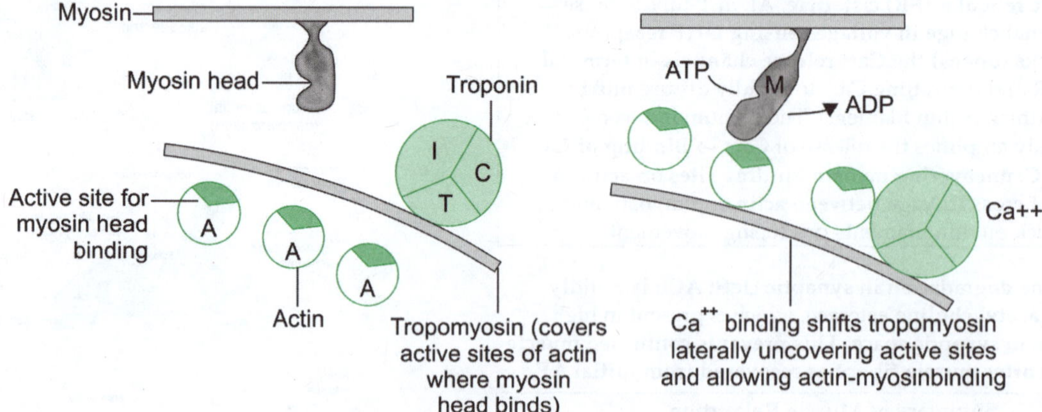

- In resting skeletal muscle ***tropomyosin (a long filamentous protein) covers the active sites of actin filament where myosin head binds to actin***[Q]. So that the attraction cannot occur between actin and myosin filaments to cause contraction.
- Initiation of muscle contraction occurs, when ***Ca^{++} binds toroponin C***[Q]. Binding causes lateral displacement of tropomyosin into the groove between two actin filaments. This uncovers active sites on actin thus allowing myosin head to bind the actin and contraction proceeds.
- ***7 myosin binding sites (on actin) are uncovered for each molecule of troponin that binds a calcium ion***[Q].

- An action potential (AP) develops on sarcolemma (cell membrane)→ AP proceeds & enters the T tubule → comes in contact with the cistern (dilated sarcoplasmic reticulum close to T tubules, store Ca++) → release of Ca^{2+} →*combine with troponin C→ this leads to loosening of tie between troponin & actin molecules → this causes release of tropomyosin from its fixed position* → myosin binding sites of actin are uncovered → myosin heads get attached with actin → contraction

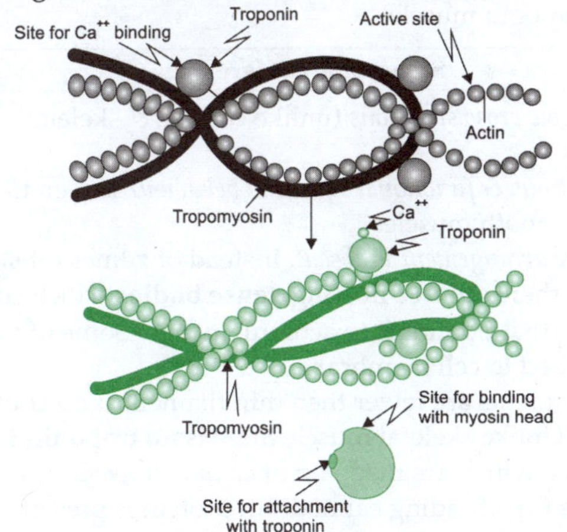

- **In the contracted state.**
  I) ***H zone is greatly narrowed or disappears***Q
  II) ***Width of I band is reduced.***Q
  III) ***Width of A band remains unchanged.***Q
  IV) The muscle fiber as a whole shortens.

A= Showing double helix of actin (resting state) polymer.
B = Changes seen with the onset of contraction
C = Actin monomer

Actinin	- Binds actin to Z line
Titin	- Connects Z line to M line and provides the scaffolding for sarcomere
Desmin	- Binds Z line to plasma membrane

★ Depolarization of T tubule membrane activates the sarcoplasmic reticulum via **dihydropyridine receptors** (named after drug which blocks them). They are voltage gated Ca++ channels in the *T-tubule membrane.* In cardiac muscle Ca++ influx via these channel triggers Ca++ release from sarcoplasmic reticulum. But in skeletal muscle, Ca++ entery by this route (from ECF) is not required for Ca++ release. Here these receptor serves as *voltage sensor & trigger* that unlocks Ca++ release from sarcoplasmic reticulum (SR). The Ca++ channels of SR are not voltage gated & k/a **ryanodine receptor** (locked in open position by plant alkaloid ryanodine).

Slow and Fast Twitch Fibers

- **Type I slow twitch red muscle fibers** are characterized by **smaller (lesser) diameter, number, force produced, velocity of contraction and fatigability**. It is innervated by smaller nerve fibers with lesser conduction velocity. Slow twitching muscle fibers **derive energy primarily from oxidative phosphorylation** and therefore their **mitochondrial content, capillary (vessel) density** and amount of myoglobin (responsible for red color) are **high**. Their **glycolytic capacity, calcium pumping capacity of sarcoplasmic reticulum and myosin ATPase activity (rate)** is lesser in comparison to fast twitch muscles.
- **Type II fast twitch white muscle fibers** are characterized by **large diameter and more number of fibers for higher force & velocity of contraction.** It derives energy primarily from **glycolytic pathway** and therefore they have large amount of glycolytic enzymes but have *less extensive blood supply, fewer mitochondria and deficit of red myoglobin (responsible for white color)* as oxidative metabolism is of secondary importance. Fast fibers have **extensive sarcoplasmic reticulum** for rapid release of calcium ions, **greater SERCA** 1 (than SERCA2) **activity**, and **higher & quicker calcium pumping & reuptake capacity** of **SR** (responsible for faster contraction & relaxation). Fast fibers **begin to develop tension at higher Ca++ concentration** (than slower fibers) because of **2 low affinity calcium binding sites in troponin C** (as compared to 1 in slow fibers)
  ★ SERCA 2 is greater in slow twitch & cardiac muscles

Smooth Muscles

Types: Two

- **Unitary (Visceral)** – Occur in large sheets, with *many low resistance gap junctional connections* between individual muscle cells
- Nerve fibers on fewer cells, with excitation spreading to other cells by gap junction i.e. it *functions in a syncytial fashion.*
- Found in wills of *hollow viscera* such as alimentary tract including gall bladder & ducts of digestive glands, ureter, urinary bladder, uterus and blood vessels.
- **Multiunit**: - Made up of individual units with *few (no) gap junctions.*

Mechanical Properties

- It can contract & relax continuously without any obvious stimulation, ***independent of its nerve supply***Q i.e. it has intrinsic rhythm.
- **Length tension relationship**
- Which is characteristic of skeletal & cardiac muscles **does not exist in visceral smooth muscles**Q**.**
- When stretched, smooth muscle initially contrast & exerts tension, but then it gradually relaxes & adopts the new length with no increase in tension; a phenomenon k/a **plasticity** or **stress relaxation** and is d/t **latch- bridges formation**.

- Each multiunit muscle cell has on passant endings of nerve fibers
- Found in *intrinsic muscles of eye (cliary body & iris), piloerector muscle and in precapillary sphincter*. So blood vessel has both type of smooth muscle.

Structural Differences

- *Lacks visible cross striations* (unlike cardiac & skeletal muscles)
- *Gap junctions & functional syncytial behaviour* is seen in unitary smooth muscles
- *Sarcomere arrangement is absent*. Instead of z lines (of skeletal muscle), there are free floating **dense bodies** which contain *α actinin* (that bounds it to actin filaments). Some of them are attached to cell membrane
- Thick filaments are fewer than thin filaments and contain myosin. Unlike skeletal muscle there is **no troponin in thin filaments**, which are made up of *actin & tropomyosin*. Instead a Ca^{++} binding calmodulin protein is present.
- *Sarcoplasmic reticulum* is present but *less extensive*. There are *no T tubules*, contain *few mitochondria* and depends, to a large extent, on *glycolysis* for their metabolic needs. Caveolae (small invaginations of cell membrane) are present.
- *No neuromuscular junction with motor end plates* (as in skeletal muscles); instead the terminal axon loose their myelin sheaths and branch into fine diffuse endings with enlargement along axon k/a *varicosities*, from which the neurotransmitter is released onto the interstitial fluid few nm away from cell membrane.

Electrical Properties

- *Less excitable (i.e. higher stimulation threshold and longer chronaxie)* than skeletal muscle
- A unique property of visceral smooth muscle is *depolarization* when it is suddenly stretched; the resulting action potential l/t contraction.
- **Variable RMP & shifting pacemakers**.
- Unitary muscle is characterized by *instability of its resting membrane potential* which is generally low ranging from *– 20 to – 60 mV*, and is unstable with no true resting value.
- Spontaneous discharge of impulse is organized into *basic slow wave rhythm* of membrane potential. (**slow sine wave like fluctuations**)
- Unlike cardiac muscle, there is *no fixed location of pacemaker* and several shifting pacemakers can exist at one time.
- Excitation may or may not be preceeded by AP
- **Variable types of action potentials**:
- AP is *generally low amplitude* about 60 mV (as compared with 120 mV) of skeletal muscle); there may be *no reversal of polarity (overshoot)*
- AP may take form of spikes (as in skeletal muscle) or *exhibit a prolonged platue* phase during repolarizaion as in cardiac muscle)
- ***Unlike skeletal muscles (which depolarize by opening voltage gated Na channel) smooth muscles have few Na channels and they open voltage gated Ca^{++} channels to let in Ca^{++} from ECF into cell to cause AP***[Q].

- On removing the stretching force, the muscle do not return to its previous size until active contraction is induced.
- **Slow & prolonged contractile response**:
- *Latent period (& therefore excitation contraction coupling)* is much *longer* than that of skeletal & cardiac muscle
- 500 ms delay in smooth muscles as compared to 10 ms delay in skeletal & cardiac muscles.

Mechanism of Contraction

- **Different source of calcium**
- As in skeletal & cardiac muscle, Ca^{++} plays a important role in initiation of contraction but the source of Ca^{++} increase is much different
- Unlike skeletal & like cardiac muscle ***most of the calcium which enters sarcoplasm comes from ECF and very little comes from sarcoplasmic reticulum***[Q]. So the source of Ca^{++} are:

1. Influx through voltage or ligand gated plasma membrane Ca^{++} channels[Q]
2. Efflux from intracellular stores through RyR
3. Efflux from intracellular sarcoplasmic stores through IP3 receptor Ca^{++} channels[Q]

- **Phosphorylation of myosin is essential for its binding to actin**
- Lack of troponin in smooth muscles prevents Ca^{++} activation via troponin binding. Rather Ca^{++} binds to calmodulin and resulting complex activates *calmodulin dependent* **myosin light chain kinase (MLCK).** This enzyme catalyzes the **phosphorylation of myosine light chain** on *serine at position 19*
- ***Myosin LC_{20} phosphorylation is a must and increases myosin ATPase activity***[Q] resulting in binding of myosin to actin and contraction . However, phosphorylation & dephosphorylation of myosin also occur in skeletal muscle but phosphorylation is not necessary for activation of ATPase
- **Dephosphorylation & Latch bridges**
- **Myosin LC is dephosphorylated** by **myosin light chain phosphatase** but it ***does not necessarily l/t relaxation & final detachment***[Q] of myosin cross bridges from actin until the intracellular concentration of Ca^{++} falls below a critical level.
- This continued attachment of myosin cross bridges to actin even after dephosphorylation creates **latch bridges**
- **Latch bridges *do not make significant cycles of attachment & detachment***[Q] between actin & myosin ***so do not require much ATP***[Q] and so maintain prolonged contractions without expenditure of much energy.
- If **epinephrine or NE** is added, the membrane potential becomes larger, the spikes decrease in frequency & muscle relaxes. Whereas **acetylcholine** addition l/t decreased membrane potential, spikes become more frequent, muscle becomes more active with an increase in tonic tension & number of rhythmic contractions.

Calmodulin

- It has 148 amino acid residues & 4 Ca++ binding domains. It's 115th aa. is trimethylated. It is extensively conserved & found in plants & animals both. Calmodulin is ***involved in contraction of smooth muscle.***Q It helps in initiation of contraction, not by, uncovering active site on actin molecule but by activating the myosin cross bridges.
- Is a ***Ca^{2+} binding protein***Q present in many cells notably ***in smooth muscles and brain cells***Q.
- Is a counterpart of Troponin. (Troponin is present in skeletal muscles)
- **Calmodulin binds with Ca^{2+} & capable of activating *5 different calmodulin- dependent kinases*** Q. They are:

(i) ***Myosine light chain kinase***Q – it phosphorylates myosin head conferring with the capability of binding with actin filament. This brings about contraction in smooth muscle.
(ii) Phosphorylase kinaseQ
(iii) **Ca^{2+}/ Calmodulin kinase I & II:** concerned with synaptic function
(iv) **Ca^{2+} / Calmodulin kinase III:** concerned with protein synthesis

Calcium Binding Proteins

- Troponin
- Calmodulin
- Calbindin

★ **Calcineurin**: is calmodulin activated protein, a phosphatase that inactivates Ca^{2+} channels by dephosphorylating them. It plays a role in activating T-cells.

Factors Responsible For Grading of Muscular Activity

Number of motor units (Recruitment)	With minimal voluntary activity only a few motor units discharge. With increasing voluntary effect more and more units are brought into play – 'Recruitment phenomenon'. With increasing motor units, force of muscle contraction increases
Frequency of Contraction (Summation)	Frequency of discharge in the individual fibre play a role. Tension developed during a tetanic contraction (with rapidly repeated stimulation) is greater than during individual twitches
Large motor units	Force of contraction depends on length of muscle – starling's law

Malignant Hyperthermia

This is a life threatening event characterized by ***uncontrolled release of Ca^{+2} ions from the sarcoplasmic reticulum***Q.

Association	Clinical features	Triggering agents	Treatment
With mutation in the gene $R_y – R_1$ gene encoding for the skeletal muscle **ryanodine receptor**	• ***Severe hyperthermia***Q • Contracture, rigidity • Tachycardia • Metabolic acidosis	• Succinyl choline • Halogenated anaesthetic - Halothane - Isoflurane - Sevoflurane	• Immediate cessation of anaesthesia • ***I.V. dantrolene***Q • Procainamide (because of possibility of VF) • Rapid cooling • 100% oxygen

Chapter 3. RESPIRATORY SYSTEM: REVIEW NOTES

Systemic Arteriole	Systemic Venule	Interpretation **What Happens in Systemic Capillaries**
Oxygenated blood with more PO_2	Deoxygenated blood with more PCO_2	- Decrease in O_2 & increase in CO_2 content - **O_2 dissociation curve shift to right**[Q] - **CO_2 dissociation curve shift to left**[Q]
- Less H^+ in RBC - Less HCO_3^- ion in plasma & RBC - Less Cl^- content of RBC - pH 7.40	- More H^+ ion in RBC - More HCO_3^- ion in plasma & RBC - More Cl^- content of RBC - pH 7.36	- Increase in HCO_3^- in plasma & RBC - **Increase H^+ & Cl^- content in RBC**[Q] - **PH decrease**[Q]
Small amount of fluid is filtered out and returns via lymphatics (which decreases its hematocrit)	- Because of more osmotically active ions (Cl^-, HCO_3^-) RBCs swell up by taking water (increases hematocrit)	- **Hematocrit increases by 3%**[Q] - **Protein concentration increases**[Q]

★ In lung all these effects are reversed in pulmonary capillaries.

P_{50}

- P_{50} is the index of affinity of hemoglobin for O_2. Higher the P_{50}, the lower the affinity of hemoglobin for O_2.
- Under normal condition when: 1) Hb is normal 2) $PaCO_2$ is 110 mm Hg 3) Temperature is 37°C and 4) 2,3 DPG is 15 µmol/gm of Hb. ***The value of P_{50} is 25 mm Hg ~ 3.6 KPa***[Q]. (1 mm Hg = 0.14 KPa)

Alveolar-Capillary Barrier (ACB)

- ACB is the structure through which the gases (like O_2 & CO_2) must diffuse from alveoli to reach pulmonary capillary blood. It includes

- Alveolar surfactant, alveolar epithelium and basement membrane - Capillary endothelium, plasma - RBC membrane, intra erythrocyte fluid and hemoglobin

- In healthy individuals, the distance b/w alveolar air and pulmonary capillary blood is about **0.3µm.**

Capillary Transit Time (CTT)

- It is the time that the **RBC spends in pulmonary capillary bed** (or time taken by blood **to flow from pulmonary artery to pulmonary vein.)**
- CTT is about **0.75 seconds,** whereas gas exchange (for O_2 & CO_2) between alveoli and blood is complete (i.e. equilibrium is attained) within **0.25** seconds, which means flow rate is adequate for full Oxygenation and CO_2 transfer. Thus O_2 & CO_2 transfer is normally **perfusion limited.**

CO Transfer Factor (T_{LCO}) and Diffusion Capacity of Lung (D_{LCO}) for CO

Carbon monoxide transfer factor (T_{LCO}) term is used for diffusion capacity of CO (D_{LCO}) because the measurement *does not solely reflect the diffusion properties of lung* (ie area and thickness of blood gas barrier). But it is **also dependent on volume of blood in pulmonary capillaries and alveolar volume.** T_{LCO} is product of (=) alveolar volume and (X) transfer coefficient (K_{CO}). **Diffusion capacity of O_2 (D_{LO2}) is 1.23 times of D_{LCO}.** The average D_{LCO} is 17 ml/min/mm Hg; so the D_{LO2} is 1.23 times of this i.e. 21 ml/min/mm Hg. Causes of

Increased T_{LCO} and K_{CO}	Decreased T_{LCO} and K_{CO}	Decreased T_{LCO} but increased K_{CO}
Factors which increase number of RBC that come in contact of CO such as ***polycythemia, left (L) to right (R) shunt***[Q], alveolar hemorrhage, alveolar inflammation, exercise & asthma.	Factors which decrease number of RBC that come in contact of CO such as **anemia, R→L shunt, pulmonary embolism,** primary pulmonary hypertension, interstitial lung disease, lymphangitis, obstructive airway disease.	Factors that cause increased density of blood per unit lung volume eg. extrapulmonary restriction like thoracic cage deformity, respiratory muscle weakness, pleural disease.

Oxygen Transport In Blood

Oxygen is carried in blood in 2 forms : dissolved in plasma and chemically combined with hemoglobin

O_2 Chemically Bound to Hemoglobin

- O_2 forms an easily reversible combination with hemoglobin (Hb) causing **conformational** change in deoxy Hb (tense /T state) to give **oxyhemoglobin (relaxed/R state). 97%** of O_2 in blood is transported in this chemical combination.
- The maximum amount of O_2 that can be combined with Hb is called **O_2 capacity**, indicating that all available O_2 binding sites of Hb are occupied by O_2.
- The amount of O_2 carried by Hb increases rapidly upto **P_{O2} of about 50 mmHg (83.5%)** but above that the curve becomes much flatter reaching **97.5% saturation at 100mgHg**. So the amount of O_2 bound to Hb does not increase (alter) in a person breathing 100% O_2 under hyperbaric conditions because the Hb has already become fully saturated at much lower P_{O2} (100mmHg).
- When the blood is equilibrated with 100% O_2 (at normobaric conditions ie P_{O2} 760mmHg), the normal Hb becomes 100% saturated. When fully saturated **each gram of normal Hb contains 1.39 ml of O_2**. However, normally some of the hemoglobin is in form of inactive Hb derivatives such as methemoglobin that cannot combine with O_2, This lowers the measured value (in vivo) to **1.34 ml of O_2 per gram of Hb** (practically).
- **O_2 saturation of Hb (Sat)** is the percentage of available binding sites that have O_2 attached and is given by

$$\mathbf{SaO_2 = Sat} = \frac{O_2 \text{ combined with Hb}}{O_2 \text{ Capacity}} \times 100$$

O_2 Dissolved in Plasma

- Only **3%** of O_2 is transported in dissolved state in water of plasma and cells. This obey's Henry's law i.e. **amount dissolved is proportional to partial pressure.**
- **Amount of O_2 dissolved in plasma** is the **linear function of P_{O2} (and = 0.003 ml O_2/dL blood/ mmHg P_{O2} = 0.003 ml O_2/100 ml blood / mmHg P_{O2}** i.e. for each mm Hg P_{O2}, there is 0.003 ml O_2 dissolved in 100ml or 1dL of blood). Because of its dependence on P_{O2}, this is the fraction of carried O_2 which alters with baricity (partial pressure) of inspired O_2 and **forms the basis of hyperbaric O_2 therapy.**
- Normal arterial blood with PO_2 of 100mmHg contains **0.3ml O_2 pr dl (100ml)**
- By utilizing this principle in hyperbaric (100%) O_2 therapy, **raising the inspired PO_2** to **3atm (=3 x 760 mmHg)** or **4atm (=4 x 760 mmHg)** increases the amount of plasma dissolved O_2 in arterial blood to about **6 ml/100ml** and **9ml/100ml** respectively.

Atmospheric pressure (atm) (P_{O2}) of inspired O_2	Amount of O_2 dissolved/ 100 ml in plasma
1 atm	0.003 x 760 = **2.28 mlQ** ≈ 2 ml
2 atm	0.003 x 760 x 2 = **4.56 mlQ** ≈ 4 ml
3 atm	0.003 x 760 x 3 = **6.84 mlQ** ≈ 7ml
4 atm	0.003 x 760 x 4 = **9.12 mlQ** ≈ 9 ml

- The total amount of O_2 bound to Hb is a **function of Hb concentration and percentage of Hb saturation (Sat).**

$$\mathbf{O_2 \text{ bound to Hb} = 1.39 \times Hb} \text{ (gm/100ml)} \times \frac{\text{Sat}}{100} \quad \text{(for pure Hb)}$$

$$\mathbf{= 1.34 \times Hb} \times \frac{\text{Sat}}{100} \quad \text{(practically invivo)}$$

- Because Hb is **100% saturated on breathing 100% O_2** in normobaric conditions (P_{O2} = 760mm Hg = 1atm) and normally blood has **15 gm Hb/100 ml**

$$\mathbf{O_2 \text{ capacity}} = O_2 \text{ bound to Hb} = 1.39 \times 15 \times \frac{100}{100} = \mathbf{20.8 ml\, O_2} / 100\text{ml blood}$$

$$\text{or } = 1.34 \times 15 \times \frac{100}{100} = \mathbf{20.1 ml\, O_2} / 100 \text{ml blood}$$

- The **O_2 saturation of arterial blood at the end of pulmonary capillaries** with **P_{O2} of 100 mm Hb** is **~97.5%** whereas that of **mixed venous blood** with P_{O2} of 40mm Hg is **~75%**. Due to physiological shunting the blood in **systemic arteries** is only **97% saturated.** Therefore arterial blood contains 19.8 mL of O_2/dL: 19.5 mL bound to Hb and 0.29 mL in solution And venous blood contains 15.2 ml of O_2 /dl : 15.1 mL bound to Hb and 0.12 mL in solution.

Gas content of blood

mL/dL of Blood containing 15g of Hemoglobin				
	Arterial Blood (PO_2 95 mmHg; PCO_2 40 mm Hg; Hb 97% saturated)		Venous Blood (PO_2 40 mm Hg; PCO_2 46 mm Hg; Hb 75% saturated)	
Gas	Dissolved	Combined	Dissolved	Combined
O_2	0.29	19.5	0.12	15.1
CO_2	2.62	46.4	2.98	49.7
N_2	0.98	0	0.98	0

PO_2 (mm/Hg)	% Sat of Hb (SaO_2)	Dissolved O_2 (mL/dL)
10	13.5	0.03
20	35	0.06
30	57	0.09
40	75	0.12
50	83.5	0.15
60	89	0.18
70	92.7	0.21
80	94.5	0.24
90	96.5	0.27
100	97.5	0.30

(PO_2: Difference of 10; Dissolved O_2: Table of 3)

★ For calculating the **total O_2 concentration of blood** (both in Hb & plasma)

Total O_2 content in blood = Hb bound O_2 + Plasma dissolved O_2

$$= \left[\mathbf{1.39 (or\ 1.34) \times Hb \times \frac{Sat}{100}}\right] + \mathbf{0.003\ P_{O2}}$$

Oxygen- Hemoglobin Dissociation Curve

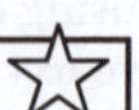

The relationship between partial pressure of O_2 and the percentage saturation of hemoglobin with O_2 can be explained graphically. And the graph is called O_2- hemoglobin dissociation Curve. It represents the affinity of hemoglobin for O_2.

Normal Curve

- ***S- shaped or sigmoid shaped***[Q] due to interconversion of hemoglobin from *low affinity tightly bound Tense configuration (T state) to high affinity released configuration (R state)* as more O_2 molecules are bound.
- Relaxed configuration exposes more oxygen binding sites & significantly increases O_2 affinity.
- Combination of the first heme with O_2 increase the affinity of second heme for O_2 (due to TR interconversion) and oxygenation of second increases the affinity of the third and so on.

★ ***P_{50} – The partial pressure of O_2 at which Hb saturation is 50%*** [Q]. The normal value is 26.6 mmHg

★ ***Myoglobin has hyperbolic O_2- binding curve.*** [Q]

Factors affecting affinity of Hb for O_2 and causing the curve to

Left Shift

- This means the **affinity of O_2 to Hb is increased and O_2 is bound more tightly to hemoglobin**[Q]**. So lower partial pressure of oxygen (PO_2) is required to bind a given amount of oxygen (i.e. P50 decreases)**[Q].
- This happens in lungs where O_2 is bound to Hb
- Factors leading to left shift are
  - **Alkalosis or ↑pH**[Q]
  - **↓ PCO_2**[Q] (CO_2 content of blood)
  - **↓ Temperature**[Q] **(Hypothermia)**
  - **↓ 2- 3 Biphosphoglycerate (2, 3 BPG)**

Right Shift

- This means the affinity of O_2 to Hb is decreased which favours release of oxygen to tissue[Q]. So higher PO_2 (partial pressure of O_2) is required to bind a given amount of oxygen (i.e. P_{50} rises).
- This happens in peripheral tissues and muscles where O_2 is delivered.
- Factors l/t right shift are
  - **Acidosis or ↓pH**[Q]
  - **↑ PCO_2**[Q] (CO_2 content of blood)
  - **↑ Tempeature**[Q] **(Hyperthermia**
  - **↑ 2- 3 BPG**[Q]

2, 3 Bisphosphoglycerate (2, 3- BPG) or 2, 3 Diphosphoglycerate 2, 3- DPG)

- It is *most abundant organic phosphate in RBC_5* where its concentration is approximately that of hemoglobin. It is synthesized from glycolytic intermediates *3-phosphoglyceraldehyde* by means of *Rapoport- leubering shunt*.
- It is *highly charged anion that binds to the β chains of deoxy hemoglobin*. One mole of deoxyhemoglobin binds to one mole of 2, 3 BPG. *A single molecule of 2, 3 – BPG binds to a positively charged pocket (cavity) formed by two β-chains*, in the centre of deoxyhemoglobin. Positively charged aminoacids of pocket form ionic bonds with negatively charged phosphate group of 2, 3- BPG.
- *It decreases O_2 affinity of hemoglobin* by binding to deoxyhemoglobin but not to oxyhemoglobin and stabilizing the taut conformation of deoxy hemoglobin.

$$\underset{(HbO_2)}{\text{Oxyhemoglobin}} + 2,3-\text{BPG} \rightleftharpoons \underset{(Hb-2,3-BPG)}{\text{Deoxyhemoglobin}} + O_2$$

- In this equilibrium, an increase in the concentration of 2, 3 – BPG shifts the reaction to right causing more oxygen to be released.
- Hemoglobin from which 2, 3 – BPG is removed has a high affinity for oxygen. However, *the presence of 2, 3 – BPG significantly reduces the affinity* of hemoglobin for oxygen, *shifting the oxygen dissociation curve to right*. This reduced affinity enable hemoglobin to releases oxygen efficiently at the partial pressure found in tissues.
- **Role of 2, 3 – BPG in stored & transfused blood:**
  Storing blood in acid- citrate – dextrose leads to a *decrease of 2, 3- BPG* in RBC. Hemoglobin deficient in 2, 3 – BPG displays an abnormally *high O_2 affinity & fails to unload its bound O_2* in tissues properly and thus acts as an **oxygen trap** rather than as oxygen transport system. However, transfused RBCs are able to restore their depleted supplies of 2, 3- BPG in *24-48 hours*; this may be a serius issue in critically ill patiens. ***This decrease in 2, 3 – BPG can be prevented by adding inosine (hypoxanthine – ribose) to the storage medium***[Q]. Uncharged inosine molecule enters RBC, releases its ribose moiety, gets phosphorylated and enters HMP pathway to become 2, 3-BPG. Hypoxanthine is formed during utilization of inosine to maintain or increase 2, 3 – BPG content. Thus ***while inosine increase / maintain 2, 3 – BPG content, hypoxanthine does not***[Q].
- In **chronic hypoxia & anemia** the concentration of 2, 3- BPG increases whereas, when pH falls (or is low), 2 3- BPG concentration falls because **acidosis** inhibits red cell glycolysis.

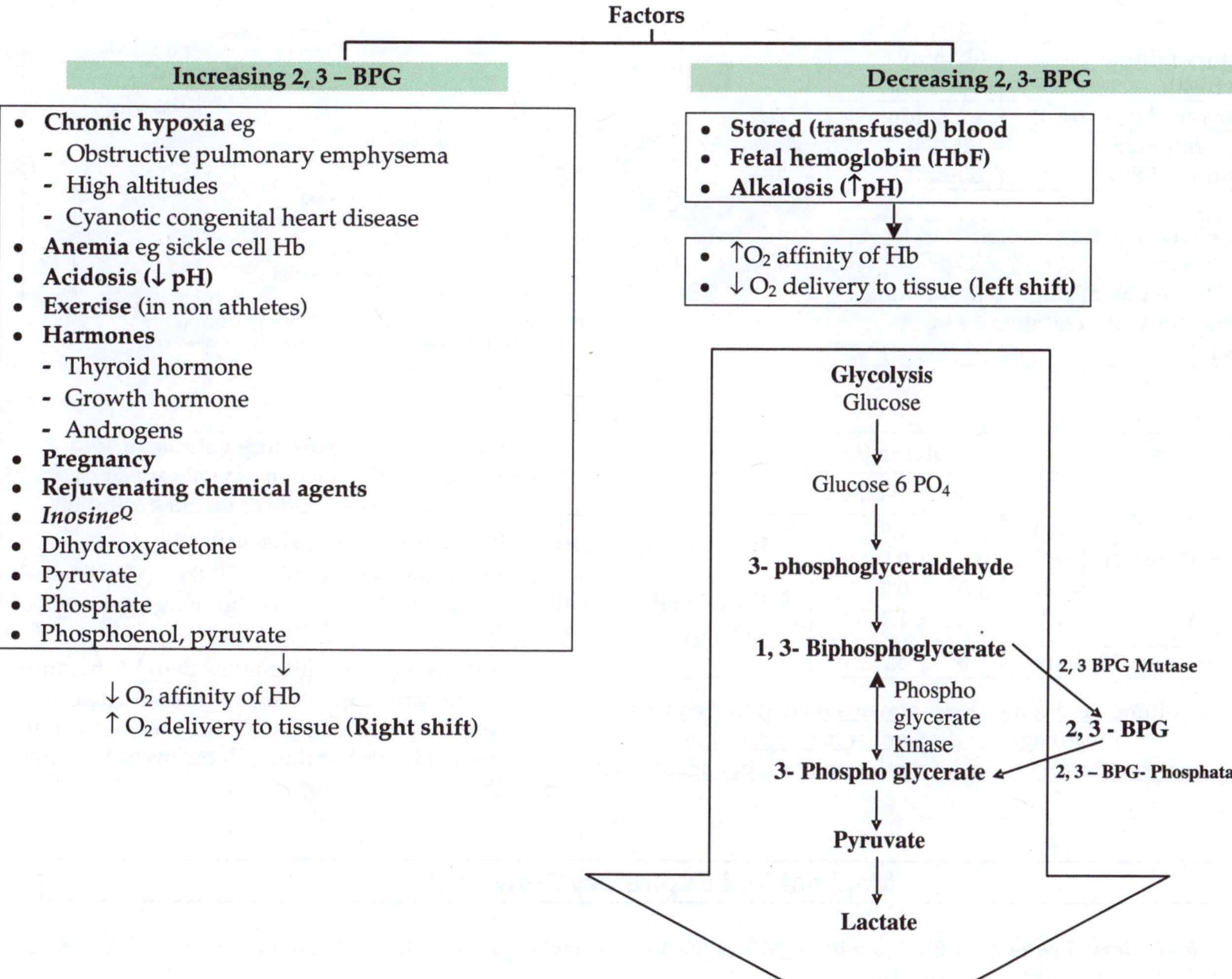

Lung Volume		
Tidal volume (T.V)	**500 ml**Q	Is the air that moves into the lung with each normal inspiration or the volume of air that moves out of lung with each expiration
Inspiratory reserve volume (IRV)	**3300 ml**Q	The air inspired with a maximal inspiratory effort in excess of tidal volume
Expiratory reserve volume (ERV)	**1000 ml**Q	The air expelled with a maximal expiratory effort in excess of tidal volume
Residual Volume (RV)	**1200 ml**Q	The amount of air remaining in the lungs even after forced expiration

Lung Capacities		
Inspiratory capacity I C=TV+ IRV	3800 ml.	Total amount of air that can be breathed in.
Vital capacity(VC) =TV+ IRV+ERV =IC + ERV	4800 ml.	Maximal amount of air that can be expelled out force fully after a maximal (deep) inspiration
Functional residual capacity FRC=ERV+RV	2200 ml.	It is the **volume of air remaining in the lung after normal expiration (after normal tidal expiration)**Q
Total lung capacity (TLC) =TV+IRV+ERV+RV =VC + RV =IC + FRC	**6000 ml. (4.2-6 lit**Q**)**	The amount of air present in the lung after a maximal inspiration. This **is the maximum volume to which the lungs can be expanded**Q

Respiratory minute volume (rest):	6L/min[Q]
Alveolar ventilation (rest):	4.2 L/min[Q]
Maximal voluntary ventilation (BTPS)	125-170 L/min[Q]

- Timed vital capacity: 83% of total in 1s; 97% in 3 s
- **Work of quiet breathing: 0.5 kg-m/min[Q]**
- **Maximal work of breathing: 10 kg-m/breath[Q]**

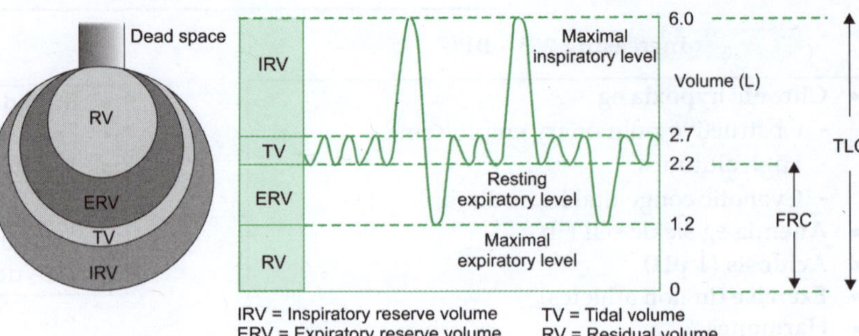

Volume (L)				
		Men	**Women**	
Vital Capacity	IRV	3.3	1.9	} **Inspiratory capacity** (IRV + TV)
	TV	0.5	0.5	
	ERV	1.0	0.7	} **Functional residual capacity** (ERV + RV)
	RV	1.2	1.1	
Total Lung Capacity		6.0	4.2	

Lung volumes and some measurements related to the mechanics of breathing. The diagram at the upper right represents the excursions of a spirometer plotter against time.

FEV_1[Q] : (Forced expiratory volume in 1st second) It is the fraction of vital capacity expired during the first second[Q] of forced expiration.

FEV_1 also **k/a timed vital capacity**.

- In normal person FEV_1 = 70-85% (70-85% of air is expelled in the 1st second of measurement of VC).
- FEV_1 is more sensitive index than VC because in the early stages of many chronic diseases (e.g. Emphysema), the VC may remain within normal limits but the FEV_1 begins to fall from the very beginning.

Maximal Mid Expiratory Flow Rate

The average expiratory flow rate during the middle 50% of the VC. [Forced expiratory flow (FEF) between 25 and 75% of the VC]. MMFR is also called **$FEF_{25\text{-}75\%}$**. Also know

Pulmonary Ventilation / Respiratory Minute Volume (RMV) **(RMV = TV x RR)**	***6000 ml***[Q] (6L) = 500x 12	The amount of air breathed in and out of lungs every minute. It is product of tidal volume (TV) and respiratory rate (RR). RMV = TVX RR
Maximal Voluntary Ventilation (MVV) **Maximal breathing capacity**	125-170L/min	The maximum amount of air which can be breathed in and out of lungs by forceful respiration in one minute.
Alveolar ventilation = (TV – Dead space volume) × RR.	4.2 liters	The amount of air utilized for gaseous exchange every minute.
Total dead space/ physiological dead space= Anatomical dead space + Alveolar dead space * In normal adult Physiological dead space = Anatomical dead space[Q]	• **Anatomical dead space** - The conducting part where gaseous exchange does not take place. It is volume of respiratory tract from nose up to terminal bronchiole. It is **150ml**. • **Alveolar dead space** - Those alveoli which are non functioning and those which do not receive adequate blood flow.	
Closing volume	The lung volume, at which, no further air can be expelled by expiratory effort.	

Closing Volume (CV) and Closing Capacity (CC)

- CV is volume below which the **terminal airway** connected to alveoli **gets closed** and hence the **gas cannot come in or out of alveoli.**
- In young subjects, the closing volume is about **10% of vital capacity (V C)**. It increases with age and becomes equal to about **40% of VC (i.e. = FRC)** at the age of 65 years.
- Relatively small amounts early **disease in the small airways** apparently **increases the closing volume.**
- **Closing capacity** is closing volume plus residual volume. CC = CV + RV. CC is higher in infants than in adults because of decreased elastic recoil, of lungs.

Single Breath N_2 Washout Test to measure CV

From mid inspiration, the subject takes a **deep breath (vital capacity single breath) of pure (100%) O_2** and then exhales steadily. The changes in **N_2 concentration of expired air (at lips)** is continuously measured during subsequent full exhalation.

4 phases of N_2 conc. can be recognized one after another.

1. **Phase I** or **initial gas exhaled** is the gas that filled the **pure dead space**. It contains **no** N_2 because inhaled gas is 100% O_2.
2. **Phase II: Mixture of dead space & alveolar gas** is exhaled (with increasing N_2 conc). The volume of dead space is volume of gas expired from peak inspiration to mid portion of phase II.
3. **Phase III: Pure alveolar gas** is exhaled (with constant N_2 conc). **Phase III terminates at (ie transition from phase III to IV) is closing volume (CV)**. The CV is the lung volume above RV (residual volume) at which the *airways in lower dependent parts of lungs begin to close off because* of the lesser transmural pressure in these areas. In most normal persons phase III also has a *slight positive slope* indicating a *gradual increase in the* proportion of expired gas coming from *relatively N_2 rich upper portions of lung*.
4. **Phase IV:** At the end of expiration, an abrupt increase in N_2 conc. is seen signaling closure of airways at the base of lung. This is caused by preferential emptying of apex, which has relatively high concentration of N_2. The gas in upper lung is richer in N_2 than lower dependent portions because the *upper lung alveoli are more distended at the start of inspiration* and therefore the N_2 in them is less diluted with 100% O_2 inspired from mid inspiration (because during a VC breath of 100% O_2, apex expands less and therefore previously occupied N_2 there is less diluted with O_2).

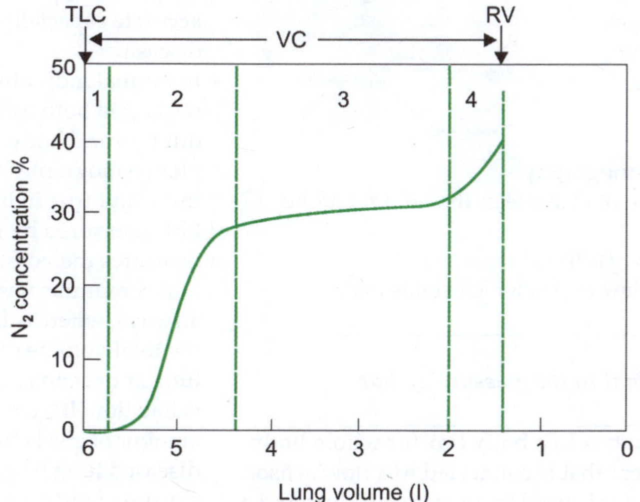

Functional Residual Capacity (FRC) or Relaxation Volume

- It is volume of **air remaining in lungs after normal (tidal) exhalation**. and is determined by the balance b/w the elastic recoil pressure generated by lung parenchyma to become smaller (**inward recoil**) and the pressure generated by chest wall to become larger (**outward recoil**). At FRC, transmural pressure across respiratory system (chest wall + lung) is zero (O). It is positive at greater & negative at smaller volumes.
- **FRC decreases** when the ***chest wall muscles are weak, (eg paralysis) or the elastic recoil of lung (i.e. tendency of alveoli to collapse) is more eg hyaline membrane disease***[Q] (i.e. lung elastic recoil > chest wall muscle force). Disease characterized by low FRC include ***pulmonary edema, pneumonitis & RDS/HMD. In hyaline membrane disease, FRC usually decreases below closing volume***[Q].
- When closing capacity exceeds FRC **(FRC < CC)**, some alveolar segments are collapsed during a portion of tidal breathing. This decreases V/P ratio and may cause hypoxia and hypercarbia. And when the **CC > FRC + TV**. (i.e. C C exceeds FRC plus tidal volume), lung segments will be collapsed during inspiration and expiration of tidal breathing. This further exaggerate V/P mismatch and l/t complete atelectasis. So respiratory therapy is designated to increase the lung volume towards normal FRC.
- Positive end expiratory pressure (**PEEP**) and continuous positive airway pressure (**CPAP**) raise FRC to a level above CV/CC in diseases associated with alveolar collapse; So the terminal airways remain open throughout the respiratory cycle.
- In presence of **airway obstruction**, **FRC increases** b/o premature airway closure, which traps air in the lung.

Pulmonary Function Test Measurements	Obstructive Lung Disease (OLD)	Restrictive Lung Disease (RLD)
Forced vital capacity (FVC) **FEV1** (Forced expiratory volume in 1 second) ***Vital capacity (VC)***	Decrease Decrease **Decrease**[Q]	Decrease Decrease **Decrease**[Q]
FEV1 / FVC	**Decrease**[Q](<72%)	**Normal to Increase**[Q]
FEF 25-75% (Forced expiratory flow rate from 25% to 75% of VC) or average mid maximal expiratory flow rate **(AMMEF)** **Slope of FV (flow-volume) loop**	Decrease Decrease	Normal to Increase Normal to Increase
PEFR (Peak expiratory flow rate i.e. greatest flow rate achieved during expiration in FV loop) **FEF_{50} (V_{max50})** and **FEF_{75} (V_{max75})** i.e. instantaneous flow rate in FV curve at which 50% & 75% of the VC remains to be exhaled respectively	Decrease Decrease	Normal Normal
Residual Volume (RV) **Diffusion capacity**	**Increase**[Q] Normal (↓ in emphysems)	**Decrease**[Q] **Decrease**[Q]
Total lung capacity (TLC)	**Normal to Increase**[Q]	**Decrease**[Q]

Examples

Obstructive lung disease
- Asthma[Q]
- Bronchiectasis[Q]
- Bronchiolitis
- Cystic fibrosis
- COPD i.e. chronic bronchitis[Q] & Emphysema[Q]

Mnemonic – **"ABCDE"**

Restrictive lung disease

I. Parenchymal
- Sarcoidosis
- Pneumo coniosis
- Idiopathic pulmonary fibrosis
- Drug / Radiation interstitial lung disease

II. Extraparenchymal

Neuromuscular	Chest wall
- ***Diaphragmatic palsy***[Q] - GB syndrome - Muscular dystrophy - Cervical spine injury	- ***Kyphoscoliosis***[Q] - Obesity - Ankylosing spondylitis

Tests for Pulmonary Compliance

Ptethysmography

- It is a technique to study the **varations in size or volume of a part of body** such as limb.
- **Plethysmograph** (a water tight chamber) is the instrument used and the limb (eg forearm) is sealed in it. Changes in the volume of forearm (because of changes in the amount of blood and interstial fluid it contains) change the volume of plethysmograph and displace water in it. This displacement is measured with a volume recorder.

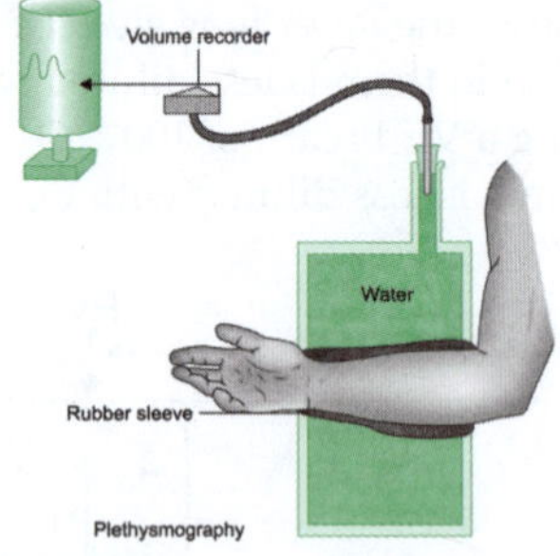

Venous Occlusion Plethysmography

- On occluding the venous drainage of a limb, the rate of increase in the volume of the limb is a funtion of *arterial blood flow*.

Body Plethysmography (BP)

- All types of plethysmograpy are based on Boyle's law of gas which states that at constant temperature

1. Pressure multiplied by volume is constant or
2. ***Volume of a sample of gas is inversely proportional to the pressure of that gas***[Q] i.e. $P_1 V_1 = P_2 V_2$

- In body plethyomography, subject sits in an air tight box k/a **body box (or whole body plephysmograph)** and breaths through a mouth piece that is connected to a flow sensor **(pneumotach /pneuotachograph)**; **pneumotachometer** is used to measure air flow and a mouth pressure transducer with shutter measures the alveolar pressure.
- Body plethysmography is used in measurement of thoracic (lung) volume including **total lung capacity (TLC) and residual volume (RV) and airflow resistance**.

Helium Dilution Technique (HDT)

- This technique to measure lung volumes **(RV, FRC and TLC)** is simpler, cheaper but often **less accurate** especially in lung disease.
- In normal individuals FRC measured both by helium dilution and body plethysmography are same. But this is not true in lung disease. FRC measured by HDT measures the volume of gas that communicates with the airways, whereas BP measures the total volume of gas in the lung at the end of normal exhalation. If a significant amount of gas is trapped in the diseased lung b/o premature closure of airways, the FRC determined by BP will be greater than that is measured by HDT.
- In HDT, a known concentration

Measurement of lung volumes

- The subject sits in a an airtight box and breaths normally through a mouth piece for few minutes and then subject makes panting respiratory efforts (i.e. breaths rapidly with maximum force) against a closed mouth piece (glottis).
- By measuring the volume (Δ V) and pressure changes in the box (P1 and P2 are pressure change of box at mouth), the volume of lungs is calculated (V = FRC). P1 x V = P2 x (V - ΔV)

During (Maximum) Expiration

Lung volume decreases (with **increase in pressure**) but the volume of gas in **chamber increases (with decreases in pressure)**

During Inspiration

Alveolar gas (volume) expands (increases) with decrease in pressure but the volume of gas in box decreases with increase in pressure

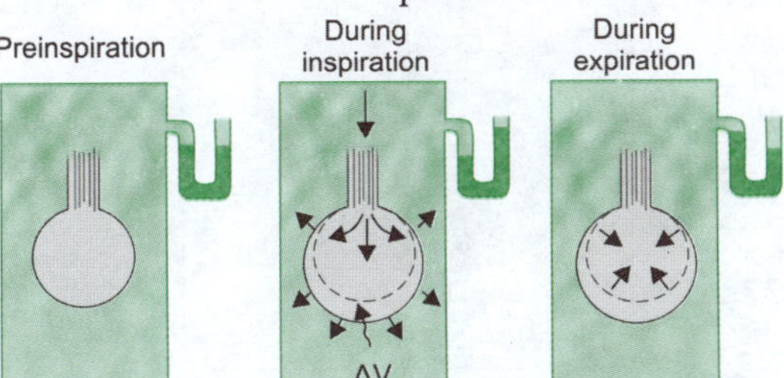

Measurement of airway resistance

- Airway resistance is the pressure difference between the alveoli and the mouth per unit of airflow.
- Using body plethysmography alveolar pressure is calculated by measuring change in volume of box (Δ V) (which is a reflection of change in alveolar volume).
- The difference b/w alveolar and mouth pressure divided by flow gives airway resistance.

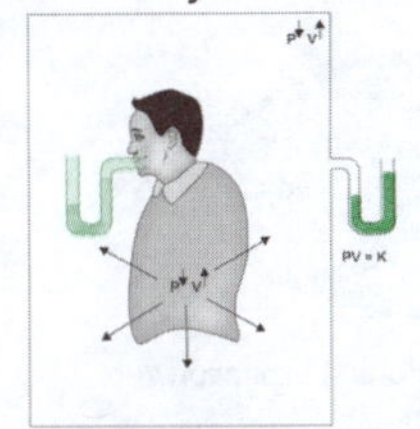

(C_1) of an inert gas like helium is added to a box of known volume (V_1). The box is then connected to an unknown (V_2) volume to be measured (in this case the lung volume). After adequate time for distribution of inert gas, the new concentration of inert gas in box (C_2) is measured

- The change in concentration of inert gas is used to determine the new volume ($V_1 + V_2$) in which the inspiration gas is distributed.

$$C_1 \times V_1 = C_2 \times (V_1 + V_2)$$

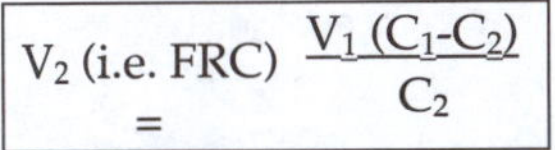

$$V_2 \text{ (i.e. FRC)} = \frac{V_1 (C_1 - C_2)}{C_2}$$

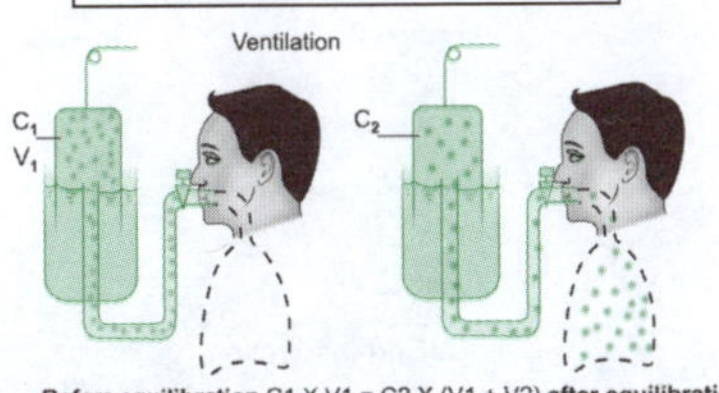

Pressures During the Breathing Cycle

- Simply stating, the pressure difference between alveolus and atmosphere is responsible for airflow into and out of alveolus (i.e. inspiratory & expiratory airflow). And pressure difference b/w alveolus (expanding lung) and intrapleural /or outside the lung (compressing the lung) is responsible for expansion & compression of lung.
- **Before inspiration begins, airway (alveolar) pressure** is everywhere **zero (0** i.e. equal to atmospheric pressure). In the absence of pressure gradient b/w atmosphere and airways, there is no airflow. But at the same time (before inspiration) **intrapleural pressure** is – **5cm H_2O** because of elastic recoil of lung- in other words there is a pressure of 5 cm of water holding the airway open. The negative pressure in pleural space relative to atmospheric pressure is created by **inward elastic recoil pressure of lung** and it acts to pull the lung away from the chest wall.
- Both the thoracic cage and the lungs are elastic structures. Being elastic structure they both tend to recoil, but in opposite direction:
  i. The thoracic cage has inherent tendency to expand, while trying to expand, it draws the parietal pleura with it (because parietal pleura is strongly attached to inner side of the chestwall)
  ii. The lungs have an inherent tendency to collapse because of their elasticity and surface tension of thin layer of fluid lining the alveoli.
- As the visceral pleura is strongly attached with the lungs, the pull in the opposite directions of the visceral and parietal pleura, creates a *negative intra- pleural pressure*. Normal intrapleural pressure = **- 4 to -5 mm Hg**[Q].; *stronger the* inspiration, more –ve is the intrapleural pressure
- Because of inherent elastic tendency of lungs to collapse, a negative force is always required on the outside of lungs to keep them expanded. And this is more so because in no airflow stage of breathing cycle the airway/alveolar pressure is '0' so only negative pressure outside the lung can prevent their collapse. Because the normal collapse tendency of lungs is about – 4 mmHg, the pleural fluid pressure must always be at least as negative as -4 mmHg to keep the lungs expanded. The ***basic cause of this negative intraleural pressure is lymphatic pumping of fluid***[Q].
- **As the inspiration starts,** the diaphragm and chest wall muscles contract and cause downward movement of diaphragm and upward & outward movement of rib cage. So with the onset of inspiration, **both intra pleural and alveolar pressure fall by 2 cm water** and flow of air begins. Because of pressure drop along the airway, the pressure inside is -2 cm of water (responsible for inward airflow), and there is -7cm of water intrapleural pressure holding the airway open. **So the intra pleural pressure also falls during inspiration and becomes more negative**. This decrease equals the lung elastic recoil, which increases as the lung inflates.

- Two reasons of intrapleural pressure fall during inspiration are – (1) as the *lung expands* its elastic recoil increases (2) and the *pressure drop along the airway* is a/w a further fall in intrapleural pressure. The extent of alveolar pressure fall depends on flow rate and the resistance of airways.
- At **end inspiration** air flow stops when alveolar pressure and atmosphere pressure become equal (O); but the airway transmural pressure (i.e. = airway pressure – pleural pressure) expanding the lung is 8 cm of water. In other words intrapleural pressure at end of inspiration is **-8cm of water**.
- On **expiration (exhalation)**, the diaphragm moves higher into the chest, **pleural pressure increases (i.e. becomes less negative**) and alveolar pressure becomes positive, the glottis opens and air again flows from alveolus (higher positive pressure) to lower atmospheric (O) pressure. The driving force for exhalation is the sum of elastic recoil of lung and pleural pressure.
- At the **onset of forced expiration**, both intrapleural pressure and alveolar pressure increases by **38 cm H_2O** and becomes positive.

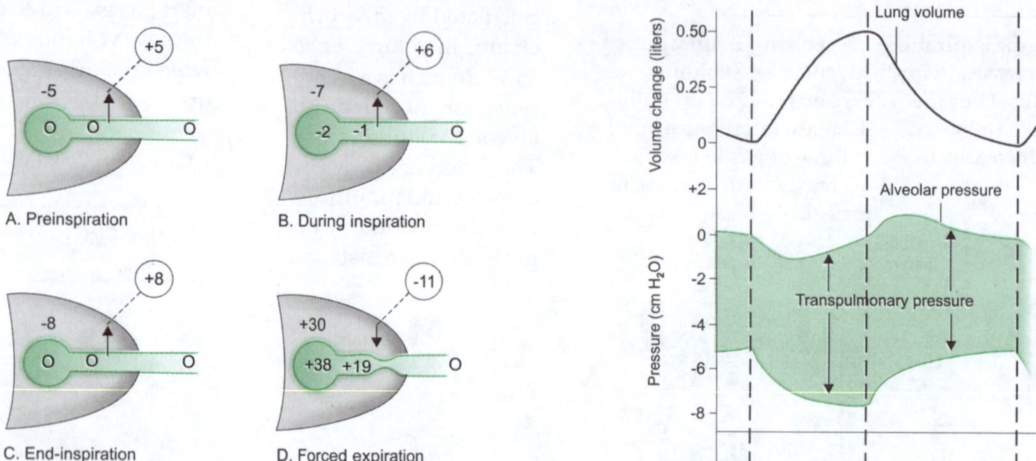

Pressures In & Around Lung ☆

- The pressure difference between the air spaces (**alveolar pressure = P_A**) and pressure surrounding the lung (i.e. **pleural pressure = P_{Pl}**) is called **transmural pressure across lung or transpulmonary /trans lung pressure** (P_L) $P_L = P_A - P_{PL}$ The lung requires positive transpulmonary pressure (i.e. relatively more alveolar or lesser pleural pressure) to increase its volume and the lung volume increases with increasing P_L. The lung has smallest size at P_L = O.
  Similarly the **transmural pressure across chest wall (P_W)** is difference b/w pleural pressure (P_{PL}) and pressure surrounding the chest wall (= body surface pressure; P_b) $P_W = P_{PL} - Pb$.
  The **pressure across respiratory system (Prs)** is sum of PL and PW.

  $P_{rs} = P_L + P_W = (P_A - P_{PL}) + (P_{PL} - P_b) = P_A - P_b$

- At **resting volume of lung (FRC)**, the elastic recoil of lung acts to decrease lung volume, but this inward recoil is offset (balanced) by the outward recil of chest wall, which acts to increase lung volume. At FRC, these forces are equal and opposite and the muscles are relaxed. When the chest is opened as in thoracotomy (surgery) the lung recoils until transpulmonary pressure is O and chest wall increases in size.
- The transmural pressure across respiratory system (Prs) at FRC is O. At TLC (total lung capacity) both lung pressure and chest wall pressure are positive and they both require positive transmural distending pressure. The **resting volume of chest wall** is volume at which transmural pressure for chest wall (P_w) is 0, and it is approximately 60% of TLC. So at volume > 60% of TLC, the chestwall is recoiling inwards and positive transmural pressure is needed, whereas at volumes < 60% of TLC, the chest wall tends to recoil outward.
- The intrapleural pressure is less negative at **base (-2.5 cm H_2O)** than at **apex (-10 cm H_2O)** at the **start of inspiration**. *More negative intrapleural pressure* at apex holds the lung in a *more expanded* position; and *so further increase* in volume per unit increase in intra pleural pressure are *smaller* than at the base because the already expanded lung is stiffer. *Ventilation is consequently lesser at* apex and greater at base. *Blood flow (perfusion) is also* greater at the base than apex. But the ***ventilation /perfusion ratio is low at base and high at apex*** because the relative change in perfusion is greater than the relative change in ventilation.

Examples

- For example at the start of expiration, pressure inside alveolus (P_A) is O (i.e. no air flow) and pleural pressure (P_{pl}) is – 30 cm H_2O. So transpulmonary pressure (P_L) of + 30 cm **($P_L = P_A - P_{pl}$** = O – (-30) = + 30) of water is holding the alveoli open. Because there is no flow , the pressure inside airways (P_{aw}) is also O and similarly + 30 cm H_2O of transairway pressure holds the airway open **($P_{ta} = P_{aw} - P_{pl}$)**.

With the contraction of expratory muscles both pleural and alveolar pressure rises + 90 cm each and becomes + 60 cm H_2O and + 90 cm H_2O respectively. So the P_L remains same but because of higher alveolar pressure (in comparison to atmosphere) airflow begins.

Because of gradual decrease in lung volume (decreasing driving pressure) and expiratory airflow resistance, there is gradual dissipation of airway pressure (P_{aw}). And at equal pressure point (i.e. the point at which the pressure inside the airways equals the pressure outside the airways) the airways become compressed **(dynamic airway compression).**

Forced Expiration, Equal Pressure Point & Dynamic Airway Compression

- **Alveolar pressure (P_A)** is the sum of pleural pressure (P_{PL}) and elastic recoil pressure (P_{el}). $P_A = P_{pl} + P_{el}$; and this is the **driving pressure** for expiratory gas flow. Because alveolar pressure exceeds atmospheric pressure (during expiration), gas begins to flow from alveolus to mouth, through open glottis. As gas flows out of alveoli the transmural pressure across the air way (P_{ta}) decreases. In otherwords, there is a gradual decrease in airway pressure (P_{aw}) from distal (alveoli) to proximal (trachea) respiratory tract. This **gradual pressure dissipation** is caused by
  i. **Expiratory airflow resistance (frictional pressure loss)**; the major site of resistance along bronchial tree is **large bronchi** (Berne & Levy) / **medium sized bronchi** (John West).
  ii. As the overall cross sectional area of the airways decreases towards the trachea, gas velocity increases. This acceleration of gas flow decreases the pressure (P_{aw}) and can make flow turbulent (increasing resistance).
  iii. As air moves out of lung, the *lung volume decreases*; which inturn *decreases the driving pressure* (alveolar pressure – intrapleural pressure) and the airways become narrower (increasing resistance).
- The **positive transpulmonary (P_L) and transairway pressure (P_{ta})** hold the alveoli and airway open. Because $P_L = P_A - P_{Pl}$ and $P_{ta} = P_{aw} - P_{Pl}$; it also means that alveolar pressure (P_A) or airway pressure (P_{aw}) greater than pleural pressure hold the alveoli or airways open. In other words, a negative intrapleural pressure (P_{pl}) is required to keep the airways stretched open.
- **Equal pressure point** is a point in respiratory tract between mouth and alveoli at which the pressure inside the airways equals the pressure that surrounds the airways. So the **airway proximal to equal pressure point** (towards mouth) become compressed because the pressure outside the airway exceeds the pressure inside the airway. This is called **dynamic compression of airways.**
- Just beyond the (proximal to) equal pressure point the transairway pressure (P_{ta}) becomes negative. Because **P_{ta} = Pressure in the airway** expanding it **(P_{aw}) – Pressure around the airway compressing it (i.e. pleural pressure P_{pl})** $P_{ta} = P_{aw} - P_{Pl}$. That is why no amount of expiratory effort will increase the flow further because the **higher pleural pressure** (which rises with increased expiratory effort) **also tends to collapse the airway at the equal pressure point (EPP)**, just as it tends to increase the gradient for expiratory gas flow (by increasing the pressure gradient b/w alveoli and atmosphere).
- That is how dynamic airway compression limits air flow in normal subjects during a forced expiration and the **airflow is independent of total driving pressure**. In other words during dynamic compression, **flow is determined by transpulmonary pressure ($P_L = P_A - P_{Pl}$) or alveolar pressure minus pleural pressure (not mouth pressure).** Hence the expiratory flow is **effort independent, flow limited and has greater airway resistance** (than during inspiration).
- Equal pressure point is **dynamic (not static)**. In normal lungs (without disease), the EPP occurs in airways that contain cartilage and thus they resist collapse. **As expiration progresses** (i.e. lung volume and elastic recoil pressure decreases), the **EPP moves distally**, deeper into the lung, closer to the alveoli. This occurs because the resistance of airways rises (d/t decrease in radius) as the lung volume falls, and therefore the pressure within airways fall more rapidly with distance from the alveoli. This resistive drop in airway pressure is greater in diseased lung (with airway obstruction secondary to mucus accumulation and inflammation). As a result EPP occurs in small airways that are devoid of cartilage causing them to collapse **(premature airway closure)**. The major site of increased resistance in patients with COPD is in airways ≤ 2mm dia.
- Dynamic airway compression may occur in diseased lung at relatively low expiratory flow rates, thus reducing exercise ability. DCA is exaggerated in emphysema because of reduced lung elastic recoil and loss of radial traction on airways.

Airway Resistance

- Highest airway resistance is in **medium sized /large bronchi**. The smallest airways contribute very little to overall total resistance because in smaller airways
  1. With increase in effective cross sectional area the airflow velocity decreases substantially and flow becomes laminar and
  2. The airway exist in parallel rather than in series. The resistance of airways in parallel is the inverse of sum of individual resistances $\left(\frac{1}{R_{total}} = \frac{1}{R_1} + \frac{1}{R_2} ....\right)$ whereas in series it is $R_{total} = R_1 + R_2 + ...R_n$
- **Normal airway resistance is 1 cm H2O/L. sec. It decreases as lung volume rises** because the airways are pulled open and similarly **resistance increases with decreasing lung volume. Density** and **viscosity** of **inspired gas** affect the airway resistance. In deep under water /Scuba diving the **increased pressure raises gas density and airway resistance. Whereas breathing a low density gas oxygen & helium mixture reduces air way resistance.**
- **Resistance of airways (R_{aw}) is low during laminar flow** and **higher during turbulent flow**. During laminar flow it can be calculated by Poiseuille's law ie is

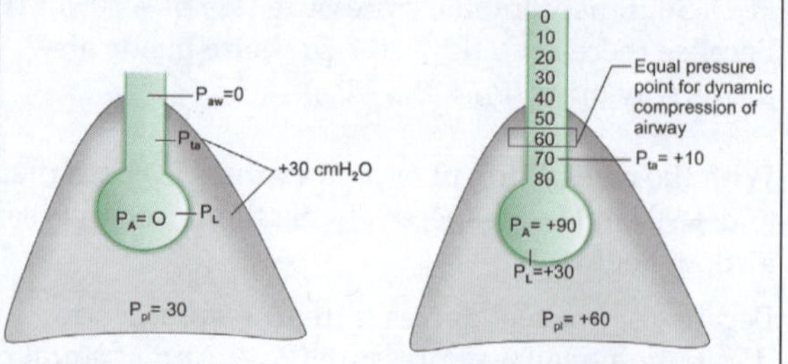

End inspiration / before start of exhalation = no flow, TLC

At start of expiration the EPP is higher up and in forced expiration on it moves distally at the end (later stages of exhalation) 1/t DCA

$$R_{aw} = \frac{8 \times \text{Length of tube (l)} \times \text{Gas viscosity } (\eta)}{\pi \times (\text{Radius of tube or r})^4}$$

Increased Raw	Decreased Raw
- **Low (decreased) lung volume**Q	- **High (increased) lung volume**Q
- **Forced expiration**Q	- During **inspiration & at TLC** (minimum)
- **More dense or viscous inspired gas**Q **eg when scuba diving**Q	- **Less dense /viscous inspired gas**Q eg the helium oxygen mixture
- **Turbulent airflow**	- **Luminar airflow**
- Airway in **series** (ie longer length)	- **Parallel airways** (smaller length)
- Less effective cross section (radius) eg medium & large bronchi	- Increased effective cross sectional area (radius) eg small airways

Work Load of Breathing

- It includes work done by respiratory muscles for
  - Stretching the elastic tissues of chest wall & lung (**Elastic work**, 65%) and
  - Moving inelastic tissues (**Viscous resistance**, 7%) and moving air through respiratory passage (**Airway resistance**, 28%) known as **non elastic work** (35%).
- Work of breathing can be calculated from relaxation pressure curve (by pressure X volume = $g/cm^2 \times cm^3 = g \times cm$).
- The elastic work required to inflate the whole respiratory system (ABCA) < the amount of elastic work required to inflate (increase volume of) lungs (ABCDEA) because part of work comes from elastic energy stored in thorax. The elastic energy (work) lost from thorax (AFGBA) is equal to gained by lungs (AEDCA)
- The pressure volume curves that the lung follows during inflation & deflation are different. This behaviour is k/a **hysteresis**. The lung volume at any given pressure during deflation is larger than during inflation. Pressure volume curve of lung is nonlinear, with the lung becoming stiffer at high volumes.
- In quiet breathing, when pressure is plotted against volume, it forms a **hysteresis loop** rather than a straight line because intrapuleural pressure changes l/t lung volume changes during inspiration & expiration. Area AXBYA represents non elastic work done required to over come lung viscosity & airway resistance

Work Capacity

- Capacity to do work (work capacity of all muscles skeletal & cardiac is greatly decreased in hypoxia & at high altitudes.
- **Work capacity is reduced in direct proportion to the decrease in maximum rate of O_2 uptake that the body can achieve**Q.
- Acclimatization increases work capacity

Person	Work capacity (% of normal)
Unacclimatized	50
Low lander acclimatized for 2 months	68
Naturally acclimatized native living at 1300 feet but working at 1700 feet	87

- **Resistance to air movement is relatively small during quiet breathing**[Q]. When air flow becomes turbulent during rapid breathing the energy required to move air is greater than when the flow is laminar. **Total work of quiet breathing is 0.3 – 0.8 kg- m /min, which rises markedly during exercise**[Q], and in diseases such as emphysema, asthma, & CHF.
- When over stretched, respiratory muscles contract with less strength, become fatique & fail (d/t length- tension relationship) leading to in adequate ventilation

- Naturally acclimatized native person can achieve a daily work output even at high altitude almost equal to that of low lander at sea level, but even well acclimatized low lander can almost never achieve this.

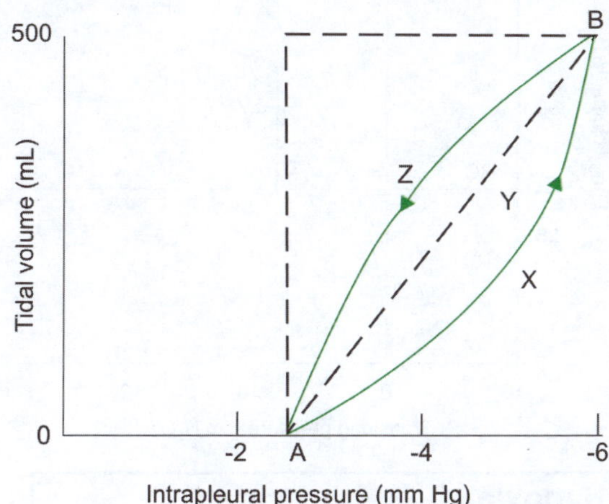

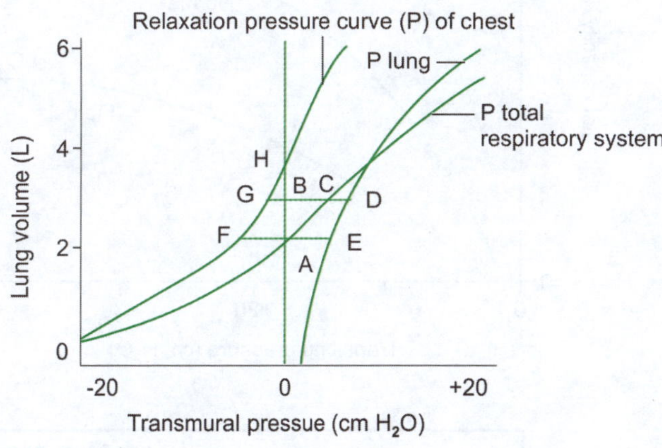

Compliance (Stretchability) / Elasticity

- Change in lung volume per unit change in distending (airway) pressure of lung (if enough time is allowed to reach equilibrium) is k/a lung compliance. So the **volume change per unit pressure change** or (volume change resulting from 1 cm H_2O change in pressure) or the **slope of pressure-volume curve** is k/a compliance.
- It is normally measured in the pressure range **where the relaxation pressure curve is steepest**. Because of hysteresis caused by surfactant, the **deflation P-V curve** is used for measurement. And lung compliance is the slope of line b/w any two points on deflation limb of pressure volume loop.

$$C_L = \frac{\Delta V}{\Delta P} = \frac{\Delta V}{\Delta P_{pl}}$$

- To measure pressure change (or pleural pressure change in lungs) **esophageal balloon** connected to pressure transducer is used, which is an excellent surrogate marker for pleural pressure. Esophageal pressure is not identical to intrapleural pressure but reflects its pressure change fairly well. However, the measurement **is not reliable in supine position** b/o interference by the weight of mediastinal structures.
- Unit of **compliance** (i.e. **stretchability or elasticity**) is mL (or liter) per cm H_2O. The compliance of normal human (both) lung is ***0.2L/cm H_2O (200 mL/Cm H_2O,)***[Q] which means every time the transpulmonary pressure increases 1 cm H_2O, the lung volume will expand 200 ml (0.2 L) after 10-20 seconds.
- Lung compliance (C_L) is *a measure of the elastic properties (or stretchability) of lung* and hence its *total capacity (TLC)*. It is a measure of how easily the lung is distended. High value refers to a lung that is *readily distended* and *low compliance* means a stiff lung that is *not easily distended*.
- Lung's elastic behaviour (i.e its tendency to return to its resting volume after distension) or compliance is due to geometrical (interwoven) arrangement of elastin and collagen fibers and elastic forces caused by surface tension. The compliance is a static measure of lung and chest recoil. Whereas **resistance** of lung & chest (i.e. pressure difference required for a unit of air flow) is a dynamic rather than static measurement that takes into account the resistance to airflow in airways.
- However, compliance also **depends on lung volume**; and patient with *one lung has approximately half compliance* of normal (i.e. half ΔV for a given ΔP). Expiratory compliance (measured during deflation) is slightly greater than inspiratory compliance (measured during inflation) . The compliance of respiratory system (combined lung & thorax) is exactly half of the compliance of lung alone (i.e. 110 ml/cm H_2O).

- Compliance of a lung depends on its **size (volume)**. Similarly lung is stiffer (less distensible or has smaller compliance) at high lung volumes (and high expanding pressures) as shown by the flatter slope of curve. For this reason **compliance per unit volume of lung (k/a specific compliance)** is measured to know intrinsic elastic properties of lung tissue.

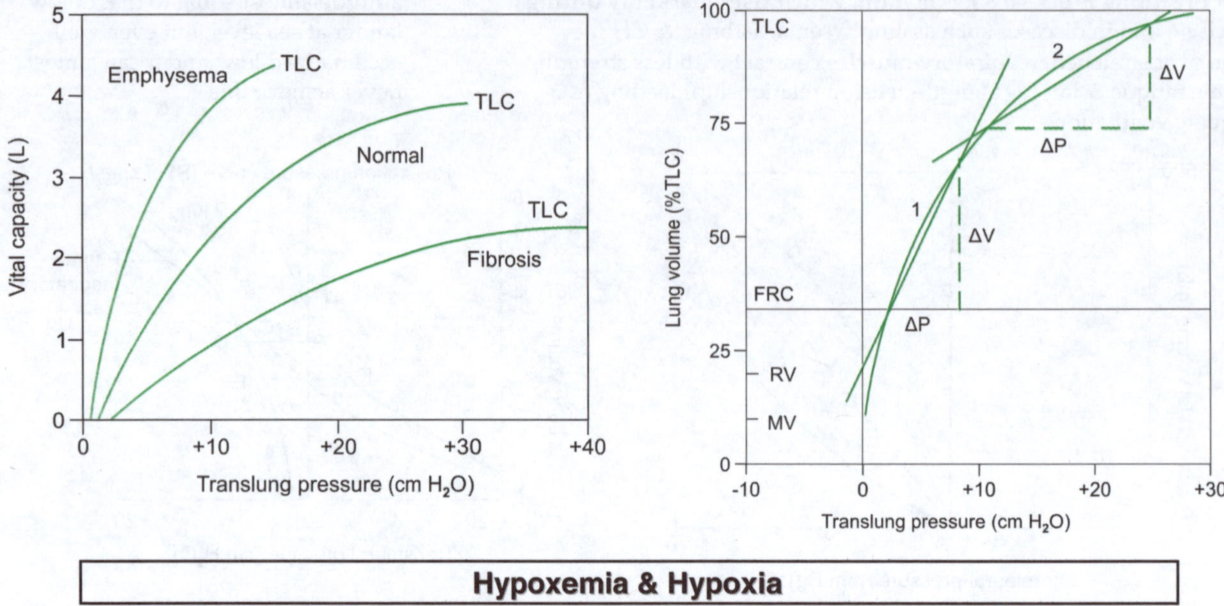

Hypoxemia & Hypoxia

- **Hypoxemia** means **low arterial oxygen tension** in blood (i.e. **low Pa_{O2}**). Arterial hypoxemia is defined as an arterial partial pressure of O_2 (i.e. Pa_{O2}) **< 80 mmHg** in an adult who is breathing room air at sea level.
- **Hypoxia** is O_2 deficiency at the tissue level to carry out normal metabolic functions and often occurs when Pa_{O2} is less than **60 mmHg**. **Anoxia** means no O_2 at all left in the tissue.
- **Hypercapnia** is an increase in partial pressure of arterial CO_2 (Pa_{CO2}) above the normal range (40 $\pm$ 2 mmHg) and **hypocapnia** is abnormally low Pa_{CO2} (< 35 mmHg).

4 Type of Hypoxia

- **Hypoxic hypoxia**, which occurs in high altitude & lung /respiratory diseases, is best diagnosed by measuring **partial pressure of arterial O_2 (PaO_2)**; and PaO_2 is **low (↓)** in it. In **anemic hypoxia**, there is decreased O_2 carrying capacity of blood d/t quantitative or qualitative deficiency of hemoglobin. So PaO_2 is normal but **O_2 content** is decreased.
- Both **stagnant and histotoxic hypoxia** are best diagnosed by arterio-venous O_2 difference, which increases in stagnant and decreases in histotoxic hypoxia. In stagnant (ischemic) hypoxia both PaO_2 and Hb are normal but the blood flow to the region is low so O_2 content is exhausted. Whereas in histoxic hypoxia tissue can not utilize available O_2.
- Each hemoglobin (Hb) molecule can **bind upto & $4O_2$ atoms** and each gram of Hb can bind upto **1.34 mL** of O_2 (= 100% saturation). **Oxygen saturation (S_{O2})** refers to the amount of O_2 bound to Hb relative to the maximum amount of O_2 that can bind to Hb. At 100% O_2 capacity 4 molecules of O_2 occupy the 4 heme groups of Hb; at 75% S_{O2} 3 of 4 heme grous are occupied.
- **O_2 content in blood** is **sum of dissolved O_2 and O_2 bound to Hb**. O_2 content is decreased in hypoxic and anemic hypoxia (i.e. in presence of CO_2, CO and anemia)
- Alveolar and arterial CO_2 are equal but alveolar & arterial O_2 are not. Normally alveolar O_2 (Pa_{O2}) is slightly greater than arterial O_2 (PaO_2). This difference is called **alveolar-arterial PO_2 difference ($AaDO_2$)**. It is not caused by imperfect gas exchange but is produced by small number of *veins that bypass the lung and empty deoxygenated blood directly into the arterial circulation.* Eg thebesian vessels of left ventricular myocardium drain into left ventricle (rather than into coronary sinus) and few bronchial & mediastinal veins drain into pulmonary veins. This **venous admixture (anatomic shunt)** decreases arterial P_{O2}. $AaDO_2$ is **< 15 mmHg** in normal individuals and rises ~ 3 mmHg per decade. Hence **< 25 mmHg** is the upper normal limit. An increased $AaDO_2$ is **hallmark of abnormal O_2 exchange.**

N = Normal, A = Alveolar, a = arterial, v = venous, A_aD_{O2} = Alveolar arterial O_2 partial pressure difference C_{aO2} / C_{VO2} = Concentration of O_2 in arterial & venous blood; S_{aO2} = Saturation of O_2 in arterial blood.

Type of Hypoxia	Causes	Amount of O_2: Continued	Amount of O_2: Delivered	Amount of O_2: Used	Arterio venous (Pao_2-P_{Vo2}) difference	Content/concentration: C_aO_2	Content/concentration: C_{VO2}	Saturation SaO_2	Partial Pressure (P) Alveolar: PAo_2	Alveolar: $PAco_2$	Arterial: Pao_2	Arterial: $PaCo_2$	$AaDo_2$ (P_{AO2}-Pao_2)	Venous: Pvo_2	P_{aO2} response to 100% O_2 administration	
Hypoxic/Anoxic Hypoxia or Hypoxemia (Level = Lung)	Hypoventilation	↓				↓	↓	↓	↓	↑	↓	↑	N	↓	↑	Helpful
	Decreased F_IO_2								↓	↑		↑	N		↑	
	Diffusion Impairment								N	N		N	↑		↑	
	Ventilation-Perfusion mismatch (V/Q low)		Low	N	-				V	↑/N		↑/N	↑		↑	
	Anatomic shunt								N	N		N	↑		LV	Limited value
	Physiological shunt								N	N		N	↑		LV	
Anemic Hypoxia (Level = Blood)	Anemia (Low Hb) CO Poisoning	↓	N	N	-	↓	↓	N	N	N	N	N	N	↓	LV	Limited value
Hypoperfusion/Ischemic/ Stagnant Hypoxia (Level=Circulation)	Vascular disease Cardiogenic shock	N	Low	N	↑	N	↓	N	N	N	N	N	N	↓	LV	Limited value
Histotoxic Hypoxia (Level = Tissue)	Cyanide poisoning Sodium azide Inhibition of cytochrome oxidase Beriberi	N	N	Low	↓	N	↑	N	N	N	N	N	N	↑	Of no value	

Effects of Hypoxia

- Hypoxia causes production of transcription factors (**hypoxia inducible factors; HIF_s**) made up of α and β subunits. In normally oxygenated tissues, the α subunit is rapidly ubiquitinated & destroyed. Where as in hypoxic cells α- subunit dimerizes with β subunit and activate genes that produce **angiogenic factors** & **erythropoietin**. The stimulus for secretion of erythropoietin is fall in O_2 tension in the tissues sensed by kidneys and liver.
- **Brain** is affected first. Less severe hypoxia l/t variety of mental aberrations like impaired judgement, drowsiness, dulled pain sensibility, excitement, disorientation, loss of time sense, headache, anorexia, nausea, vomiting, tachycardia (like those produced d/t alcohol intake). Whereas severe hypoxia l/t **hypertension, increased rate of ventilation** (b/o hypoxia of carotid chemoreceptor). And because **anemic hypoxia** do not stimulate peripheral chemoreceptor, **hyperventilation is not seen in it**
- Hypercapnia and to lesser extent hypoxia cause dyspnea.
- Cerebral blood flow :
  i. Increases if P_{aO2} decreases
  ii. *If ↓ P_{aO2} is associated with hyperventilation:* cerebral blood flow falls & hypoxia intensified
- Synpathetic discharge: Increases[Q] **by directly stimulating the vasomotor center.**
- Lactic acidosis[Q] : **In hypoxia a large proportion of pyruvate is reduced to lactic acid. (Glucose is broken down to pyruvate under anaerobic condition & generates ATP)**
- 2, 3 – DPG : Increases[Q], **which cause a right shift of O_2- dissociation curve.**
- Cardiac output[Q]: **Increases due to diffuse vasodilation (↓ P_{O2} cause vasodilation). Dilatation →↓BP→** *↑Heart rate.*[Q]

Cyanosis

- It is *bluish discolouration* of skin & mucous membranes resulting from an increased quantity of reduced (deoxygenated) hemoglobin. The deoxygenated hemoglobin has an intense dark blue purple color that is transmitted through the skin.
- In general cynosis becomes apparent when the mean capillary concentration of ***reduced Hb exceeds 4gm/dL (40gm/L)***[Q] *Harrison* ***/5gm per dl*** *(Ganong & Guyton)*. It is absolute rather than relative quantity of reduced hemoglobin that is important in producing cyanosis. Thus in a patient with severe anemia the relative amount of reduced Hb may be very high. However since the total conc. of Hb is reduced, the absolute quantity of reduced Hb may still be small, and ***therefore patients with severe anemia and even marked arterial desaturation may not display cyanosis***[Q]
- Definite cyanosis appears whenever the arteria blood contains **>5gms of deoxygenated Hb in each 100 milliliters of blood.** So a patient with **anemia** almost never becomes cyanotic because there is not enough hemoglobin for 5 grams to be deoxygenated in 100 ml of arterial blood. Conversely in patients with **polycythemia vera** (excess RBCs) the great excess of available Hb that can become deoxygenated leads frequently to cyanosis, even otherwise normal conditions.
- Cyanosis is **not a reliable sign of mild desaturation (i.e. early hypoxia)** because its recognizition depends on so many variables, such as lighting conditions and skin pigmentation. Cyanosis is **a late sign of hypoxia** and indicates the condition is **marked (profound)**. So it is never advisible to wait for cyanosis to appear to diagnose hypoxia. Similarly ***absence of cyanosis does not always indicate adequate airway and absence of hypoxia***[Q], because if the percentage saturation is high or in cases of anemia, cyanosis does not appear.
- A ***cherry red flush rather than cynosis is caused by COHb (carboxy hemoglobin)***[Q]

Central Cyanosis

- **Central cyanosis is caused by** inadequate oxygenation of systemic arterial blood due to decreased arterial oxygen saturation or hemoglobin abnormalities.
- *Central cyanosis is charachterized by cyanosis affective both mucous membranes and skin.*

Seen if

- ***Mean reduced (deoxygenated) hemoglobin >4/5gm/dl***[Q]
- ***O₂ saturation falls < 85%***[Q] *(In dark skinned detected when < 75%)*
- ***Methhemoglobin ≥ 1.5gm/dl***[Q]
- ***Sulfhemoglobin ≥ 0.5 gm/dl***[Q]

Causes

Decreased arterial O_2 saturation (SaO_2)

1.Decreased atmospheric pressure	- High altitude
2.Impaired pulmonary function	- Impaired O_2 diffusion - Alveolar hypoventilation - V/Q mismatch
3.Anatomic shunts	- Pulmonary A-V fistula - Congenital heart disease (some) - Multiple small intrapulmonary shunts
4.Hb abnormality (with low affinity for O_2)	- Methhemoglobinemia (hereditary acquired) - Sulfhemoglobinemia (acquired) - ***Carboxyhemoglobinemia (not true cyanosis)***[Q]

Peripheral Cyanosis

- It is caused by *slowing of blood flow & abnormaly great extraction of* O_2 from normally saturated blood.
- It results from vasoconstriction or decreased peripheral blood flow, reduced cardiac output or vascular occlusion.
- It is characterized by **cyanosis of skin alone & sparing of mucous membranes** (esp. oral cavity).
- Causes are-
  - ↓ Cardiac output
  - Arterial / Venous obstruction
  - Redistribution of blood flow from extremities
  - *Cold exposure*

Methemoglobinemia

- In **Methemoglobinemia**, iron within hemoglobin is oxidized from the ferrous (Fe^{++}) to ferric (Fe^{+++}) form, resulting in the inability to transport oxygen and carbon dioxide.
- It may result from exposure to oxidizing agents such as ***nitrites, nitrates***[Q], aniline dyes, and medication including local anesthetics benzocaine, lido caine, prilocaine, phenazopyridine hydrochloride, ***sulfonamides***[Q], chloroquin, inhalant in cyanide antidote kit, nitrogen oxide, nitro & nitroso – hydrocarbons, ***primaquine – type antimalarials***[Q], etc.
- Methemoglobinemia >*15%* causes symptoms of *cerebral ischemia*, and levels >60% are usually *fatal.*
- Congenital methemoglobinema arises from ***HbMI wata*** ($\alpha^{87\ His \rightarrow}$ ***Tyr) mutation***[Q] in globin or from mutation that impair enzyme that reduce methhemoglobin to hemoglobin ***(eg. methemoglobin reductase, NADP diaphorase)***[Q].
- ***IV methylene blue***[Q] (1mg/kg) is effective emergency therapy for >30% methemoglobinemia, symptomatic hypoxia or ischemia (but contraindicated in G6PD deficiency). Milder cases & follow up of severe cases are treated by ***oral methylene blue or ascorbic acid***[Q] (300 – 600 mg/day). Severe & refractory cases require ***exchange transfusion & hyperbaric oxygen***[Q].

Abnormal Respiratory Pattern ☆

Cheyne- Stokes respiration - Opium poisoning - Uremia - CCF - Hypoxia	*Rhythmic alteration of apnea and hyperapnea* due to anoxia. (c/b periods of waxing and waning tidal volume separated by period of apnea). It is a type of periodic breathing.
Biot's respiration - Meningitis (↑ICT)	Type of periodic breathing, that consists of one or more large tidal volumes separated by periods of apnea i.e. *irregularly irregular respiration*
Kussumal's respiration - Diabetic ketoacidosis - Uremia	*Rapid & deep breathing (Air hunger)*
Ondine's curse	Loss of automatic respiratory control with destruction of involuntary neural pathway.

Reduced Arterial O_2 Tension

Decreased inspiratory O_2 tension
- High altitude

Defect in oxygenation (VQ mismatch)=Type I failure
- **Defect in parenchyma**
  - **Pneumonia**
  - **ARDS**
- **Defect in lung vasculature**
  - Right to lung shunt

Defect in Ventilation = Type II failure
- **Obstruction**
  - COPD
- **Hypoventilation**
  - Decreased respiratory drive from CNS
  - Weakness of respiratory muscles

Carbon Monoxide (CO) Poisoning

Physiological Role of CO

- Small amounts of CO is formed in body and functions as ***gaseo transmitter vasodilator (along with NO and H_2S)***[Q].

Causes Anemic (not Histotoxic) Hypoxia

- CO is toxic because it reacts with hemoglobin (at the same point as does O_2) to form **carbon monoxyhemoglobin (carboxyhemoglobin** or **COHb**) and therefore displace O_2 from Hb thereby decreasing the O_2 carrying capacity of blood.
- CO poisoning causes **anemic hypoxia** because the *amount of Hb that can carry O_2 is reduced* but the total Hb amount of blood is unaffected by CO.

Left Shift of O_2 Dissociaton Curve

- COHb ***cannot take up O_2; liberates CO very slowly and shifts dissociation curve of remaining HbO_2 to left***[Q], decreasing the amount of O_2 released. This is why an anemic person who has 50% of normal amount o HbO_2 may be able to perform moderate work whereas an individual whose Hb is reduced to same levels because of COHb formation is seriously incapacitated.

High (250 times) Affinity for Hb

- The affinity of Hb for CO is **210 times** (Ganong) / **250 times** (Guyton) its affinity for O_2. So CO-Hb dissociation curve is almost identical to O_2 Hb dissociation curve except that partial pressure are at a level of 1/250. So a CO partial pressure of only **0.4 mm Hg** in alveoli (1/250 that of normal alveolar O_2 100 mm Hg PO_2), allows the CO to compete equally with O_2 for combination with the Hb and causes half the Hb in blood to become bound with CO instead of with O_2. Therefore CO pressure of only *0.6 mmHg can be lethal.*
- ***Transport and toxicity of carbon monoxide (CO) is limited to its diffusing capacity because hemoglobin combines with this gas so rapidly***[Q] that its partial pressure never has time to build up and is essentially *zero* in blood. The affinity of Hb for CO is **210 greater** than its affinity for O_2.

Reduced O_2 content but Normal PO_2

- Even though O_2 content of blood is greatly reduced in CO poisoning, the ***PO_2 of blood may be normal***[Q]. This makes it especially dangerous, because the blood is bright red and there are no obvious signs of hypoxemia (such as cynosis). Also, PO_2 is not reduced, and *feedback mechanism that usually stimulates increased respiration rate* in response to lack of O_2 (↓PO_2) is absent.

Clinica Toxicity

- Because the ***brain is the first organ affected***[Q], the person may become disoriented & unconscious before becoming aware of danger.
- The amount of COHb formed depends on *duration* of exposure to CO as well as *concentration* of CO in inspired air and alveolar ventilation. Death results when *70-80%* circulating Hb is converted to COHb. CO is also toxic to **cytochromes** in tissue but at 1000 times of lethal dose; so ***tissue toxicity plays no role in clinical CO poisoning***[Q].

Treatment

- The treatment is ***hyper baric pure oxygen and 5% CO_2***[Q]

Oxygen Toxicity (Poisoning)

Mechanism

- Once the alveolar PO_2 rises above a critical level (*>2 atmospheric PO_2) hemoglobin – oxygen buffer mechanism is no longer capable* of keeping the tissue PO_2 in normal safe range 20-60 mmHg, and tissue PO_2 can rise to hundreds or thousands of mm Hg.
- This results in *production of oxygen free radicals* (e.g. superoxide anion, singlet oxygen, & peroxide radical) in very high amount which completely swamp the enzyme system to remove them.
- Free radicals *oxidize poly unsaturated fatty acids* present in *cell membranes* (mainly) and some enzymes (proteins) of cellular metabolism.

Types

1) **Acute toxicity** results from *extremely high tissue PO_2* that occurs when O_2 *is breathed at very high alveolar* O_2 pressure for a short period. The *nervous tissue is most susceptible* because of its high lipid content.
2) **Chronic toxicity** results from breathing relatively lower concentration of O_2 but for prolonged periods. A person can be exposed to 1 atm pressure of O_2 for *indefinite period without developing CNS toxicity*. But it l/t **pulmonary toxicity** after only about *12 hours*

Effects

- **CNS (Bert) effect** is acute manifestation (minutes to an hour) of exposure to hyperbaric O_2, which results in
  - ***Hyperirritability f/b increased muscular twitching***Q
  - Ringing in ears
  - ***Conuilsions without warning***Q
  - ***Dizziness, irritability, disorientation***Q
  - Coma & death
- **Pulmonary (Smith) effects**, is usually d/t chronic exposure but may also be seen in acute.
  - ***Tracheobronchial irritation & pulmonary edema***Q are first presentations
  - *Lung passage congestion*
  - Atelectasis
- Retinal effects
  - ***Retrolental fibroplasia in neonates***Q
  - ***Ratinal damage***Q d/t angiogenesis causing disturbance of vision
- **Burnt out tissue** – i.e., d/t high metabolic rate and excess heat production, cytochrome system & finally tissue is damaged

Physiological & Pathological Effects of Smoking

Effect are related to number of cigarettes smoked, smoking duration, amount and type of smoke inhaled. The effects are produced by *nicotine & carbon monoxide*. It

Increases

- ***Glucose*** (from with in minute to an hour)
- ***Insulin*** (after an hour)
- ***Growth hormone*** (GH), within 30 minutes)
- ***Vasopressin, and IgE***
- Free fatty acid, cholesterol, Beta lipoprotein and , triglycerides
- Thrombogenic balance of prostacyclin & thromboxane A_2, **RBC**, hematocrit, leukocytes, & fibrinogen l/t alteration in platelet aggregation & survival that produce thrombosis.
- ***RBC, carboxyhemoglobin and hematocrit***Q
- ***Adrenaline & urinary catecholamines***Q & their metabolites (by stimulating adrenal medulla) → ***Increased heart rate (at rest & in exercise)***Q, cardiac out put, systemic BP (hypertension, vasoconstriction → Increased risk & extent of advanced **atherosclerotic vascular disease** in peripheral as well as coronary arteries causing *claudications, amputation, occlusive cerebro vascular disease (stroke), abdominal aortic aneurysm, myocardial infarction and failure of vascular reconstruction (graft occlusion)*.
- Endothelial (blood vessel) damage l/t increased permeability
- **Cancers** of lung, oral cavity, pharynx (naso/oro/hypo), larynx, naal cavity, paranasal sinuses, esophagus, stomach, pancreas, lieve, kidney (body and pelvis), ureter, urinary bladder, uterine cervix, and myeloid leukemia.
- Smoking may play a role in increasing *colorectal & premenopausal breast cancer*.
- COPD, chronic mucous hyper plasia, chronic productive cough, pulmonary emphysema.

Decreases

- ***HDL***Q
- Blood partial pressure of O2
- Immune response, IgA, IgG and IgM
- Uterine cancer among post menopausal women
- **Expiratory airflow**

No association

- Post menopausal breast cancer
- Endometrial cancer

Respiratory Failure

Respiratory failure is defined as a disorder wherein lung function is inadequate to meet the metabolic demands of the individual and is unable to maintain normal arterial gas level in the blood.

Type	Characteristic Features	Causes
RF-I	Represents **failure of oxygenation**, and is characterized by dysponea and secondary hyperventilation l/t - **Hypoxemia (P_{aO2} – decreased; < 60 mm Hg)** - **Increased alveolar – arterial Oxygen gradient**[Q] (P_{A-aO2} > 15 mm Hg) - **Normal** or **decreased P_{aCO2}** (≤ 40 mmHg) i.e. respiratory alkalosis	Results from failure in exchange of respiratory gases (mainly O_2) at the alveolar capillary junction (i.e. ***alveolar capillary block syndrome***) as a result of disease of **lung parenchyma**. There is **thickening of alveolar or capillary wall resulting in ventilation –perfusion (V-Q) mismatch.** Only O_2 transfers is affected because **CO_2 is 20 times more diffusible**. So causes are **I. Parenchymal (interstitial) lung diseases** - which thicken alveolar – capillary membrane eg. asbestosis, sarcoidosis, pneumoconiosis, beryllіosis, diffuse interstitial fibrosis, infiltrative lung disease like malignancy & granulomatosis. - Which separate A-C membrane like **pulmonary (interstial) edema** (in cardiac failure) and ***exudates (pneumonitis or pneumonia)***[Q] and (resultant) pulmonary fibrosis. II. Mixing of venous blood with arterial blood like ***right to left shunt*** [Q]. III. **Ventilation – Perfusion mismatch** [Q]**: In emphysema surface area for diffusion** decreases (i.e. poorly ventilated alveoli increase). Mn: **"RAPE-VIP"** = "Right to left shunt, Alveolar (pulmonary) edema, parenchymal disease (pneumonia), emphysema – ventilation perfusion mismatch".
RF II	Represents **failure (defect)** in **ventilation** and is characterized by **hypoventilation l/t** - **Hypoxemia** (P_{aO2} decreased; < 60 mmHg) - **Normal alveolar-arterial oxygen gradient** (P_{A-aO2} < 15 mmHg) - **Hypercapnia (P_{aCO2} > 40 mm Hg) i.e. respiratory acidosis** [Q]	**I. Decreased central respiratory drive to breathe** - Drug like morphine, sedative & anesthetics overdose. - Brain stem injury, ***bulbar poliomyelitis***[Q], hypothyroidism, sleep disordered breathing. **II. Respiratory muscle weakness** - Neuromuscular disorders like myasthenia gravis, GB syndrome, **bulbar poliomyelitis**, ALS. - Myopathy, polymyositis, electrolyte derangement. **III. Obstructive lung disease** - Acute obstruction like foreign body, laryngeal edema, bronchospasm, asthma - COPD (esp during acute exacerbation) like chronic bronchitis, emphysema, interstial lung disease. **IV. Increased load on respiratory system d/t** - Resistive load eg bronchospasm - **Reduced chest wall compliance** eg. pleural effusion, pneumo/fibro – thorax, abdominal distension (ascitis), ***rib cage disorder (kyphoscoliosis)***[Q], ankylosing spondylitis, flail chest. - Reduced lung compliance eg. atelectasis, **lung resection, alveolar edema (ARDS)**[Q]**, PEEP (positive end expiratory pressure).** - Increased minute ventilation requirements eg pulmonary embolism with increased dead space, sepsis.
RF III	Also called **peri-operative respiratory failure**	Occurs as a result of *atelectasis* and atelectasis is common in perioperative period
RF IV	Result of hypoperfusion of respiratory muscles	Occurs in patient with *shock*

Effects of Hypercarbia/ Hypercapnia (Increased CO_2 content of Blood)

Respiration	C.V.S	CNS	Eye
- Dyspnea	- **Tachycardia** - **Hypertension** (Due to sympathetic over activity)	- Headache - Dizziness - Loss of consciousness	**Mydriasis** (due to sympathetic activation)

Central (Neural) Control of Breathing 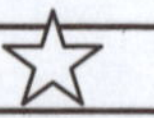

Medulary Respiratory Centers 

Main components of **respiratory control pattern generators responsible for automatic respiration** are located in medulla and inherent rhythmicity of breathing originates in medulla. Therefore periodic breathing is maintained in animals with brain transaction b/w pons & medulla. Medulla has.

1. Pre-Botzinger Complex (Pre-BOTC)

- **Spontaneous automatic rhythmic respiration is initiated by** a small group of synaptically coupled **pacemaker cells** in the **pre-Biotzinger complex (Pre-BOTC)** situated on either side of medulla between **nucleus ambiguous and lateral reticular nucleus.**
- Pre-BOTC neurons **discharge rhythmically**, producing rhythmic discharges in phrenic motor neurons, which can be abolished by section b/w the two (pre BOTC & phrenic motor neurons).
- Pre- Botzinger complex also *contact hypoglossal nuclei*, and the tongue is involved in the regulation of airway resistance.
- Pre-BOTC neurons discharge rhythmically even in in-vitro brain slices. However, hypoxia causes gasping and addition of cadmium causes occasional ***sigh-like discharge patterns.***
- Pre BOTC neurons have **NK1, μ-opioid and 5-HT4 receptors**; and in vivo substance P stimulates, opioids inhibit respiration and treatment with 5HT4 agonists block the inhibitory effect of opiates on respiration, with out inhibiting their analgesic effect.
- **Dorsal & ventral** group of respiratory neurons involved in **generation of respiratory pattern** (however, lesions of both do not abolish respiratory activity), project to pre-BOTC.

2. Dorsal respiratory group (DRG).

- DRG is composed of neurons located mostly in **nucleus tractus solitarius** and adjacent reticular substance in dorsomedial region in medulla.
- DRG constitute the initial intracranial processing station for afferent inputs from 9th & 10th cranial nerves, which originate from peripheral chemoreceptors, baroreceptors and several other receptors of airways and lungs.
- DRG is chiefly a/w **inspiration** and cause **rhythmic inspiratory discharge**. Action potential in inspiratory neurons begins weakly, and **increase steadily** in a **ramp like (crescendo) manner** for about 2 seconds. Then it ceases abruptly for 3 seconds, which turns off inspiratory muscles (diaphragm) and allows elastic **recoil of lung & chest wall** to cause expiration.

3. Ventral respiratory group (VRG)

- Located bilaterally about 5mm anterior & lateral to DRG, in ventrolateral region of medulla. It contains 3 group of both **expiratory and inspiratory neurons** (stimulating both).

(Rostral) **Nucleus retro fascialis**	Active during **expiration**
(Caudal) **Nucleus retroambiguus** (NRA)	Rostrally (cranially) located cells are active during **inspiration** and caudally located cells are active during **exhalation.**
Nucleus paraambiguus (NPA)	Has both **inspiratory & expiratory** neurons that travel in vagus nerve to laryngeal & pharyngeal muscles.

- VRG neurons remain almost totally *inactive during normal quiet respiration* but act as an over drive mechanism when ***high levels of ventilation*** are required esp during heavy exercise (when they especially provide powerful expiratory signals to abdominal muscles.)
- So, normal quiet breathing is caused only by repetitive inspiratory signals from DRG and VRG contributes extra respiratory drive for increased (greater than normal) pulmonary ventilation. Inspiration begins with abrupt increase in discharge from *NTS (DRG), NRA (Cranial cells) and NPA.*

★ The *fibers concerned with expiration* converge primarily on the internal intercostals motor neurons in the ***thoracic spinal cord.***Q

Pontine and Vagal Influence 

Spontaneous rhythmic discharge of medullary neurons is modified by neurons in pons and afferents in vagus (from receptor in airways & lungs). Pons has 2 centers.

1. Pneumotaxic center (PC)

- Located in **medial parabrachial & Kolliker-Fuse nuclei** of upper dorso-lateral pons, and contain neurons active during inspiration & neurons active during expiration. It transmit signals to inspiratory area.
- It may have a **role in switching between inspiration and expiration** and in **fine tuning of respiratory rhythm** (because normal rhythm can exist in the absence of this center)
- It controls the **switch off /(turn off point of inspiratory ramp** (of DRG), thus **inhibiting inspiration**. It regulates **inspiration volume** by controlling the **duration** of filling phase of lung cycle primarily, which has secondary effects on respiratory rate.

- Primary function of PC is to limit inspiration (volume) and secondarily increasing the rate of breathing. So stimulation or strong signal l/t **shallow & rapid breathing.**
- When pneumotaxic signal is weak (or damage to PC) causes **deep (greater tidal volume) and slower** respiration (in intact vagi animals); and **prolonged inspiratory spasms** resembling **breath holding (apneusis)** when the vagi are also cut. Stretching of lungs during inspiration initate impulses in afferent pulmonary vagi which inhibit inspiratory discharge. That's why depth of inspiration increases after vagotomy.

2. Apneustic Center

- Located in lower pons, **have an excitatory effect on inspiratory area of DRG**, tending to prolong the ramp action potential. It is normally inhibited by pneumotoxic center & vagus.
- Named so, because section just above this cause **apneusis *(prolonged inspiratory gasps) interrupted by transient expiratory effects*Q**.

Emotional-Limbic & Cortical-Voluntary Control.

- Cortex can override the functions of brain stem within limits if voluantry control is desired. eg by voluntary hyperventilation decreasing P_{CO2} and increasing arterior pH.
- **Ondines' curse is disruption of automatic control without loss of voluantry control of respiration. So respiration occurs only in awake state (not during sleep)Q.**
- **Limbic system & hypothalamus** alter pattern of breathing in emotional states such as fear & rage.

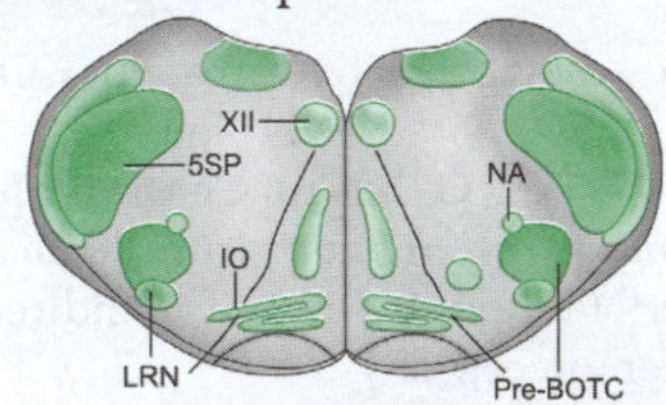

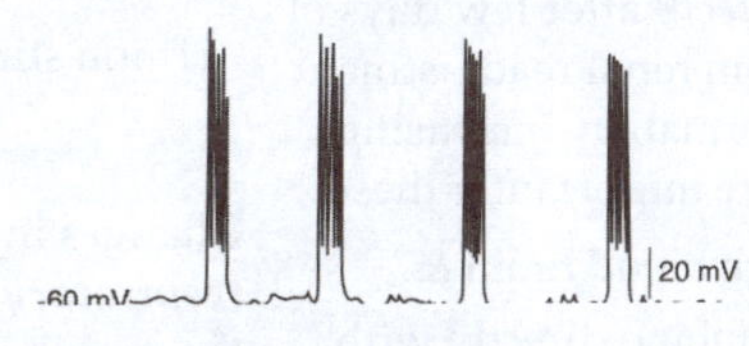

Chemical Control of Respiration

Central – Chemoreceptors

- Pneumotoxis
- *Pneumotaxic center, and dorsal & ventral respiratory group of neurons are not affected directly by changes in blood CO_2* concentration or H^+ ion concentration in CSF
- **A chemosenstive area**, located bilaterally, only 0.2 mm (Guyton)/200-400mm (John West) ***beneath the vental surface* of medullaQ, is highly sensitive to changes in either blood P_{CO2} or hydrogen ion concentration (in CSF and interstial fluid)**, and in turn excites other portions of respiratory center.
- **Central chemosensitive area** of respiratory center, that mediate hyperventilation produced by increase in arterial P_{CO2} after the peripheral chemoreceptors (carotid and aortic bodies) are denervated are located in **ventral surface of medulla oblongata** in the vicinity of exit of 9th & 10th CN (k/a **medullary chemoreceptor**). Additional chemoreceptors are located in vicinity of **nuclei of solitary tract, locus ceruleus and hypothalamus.**

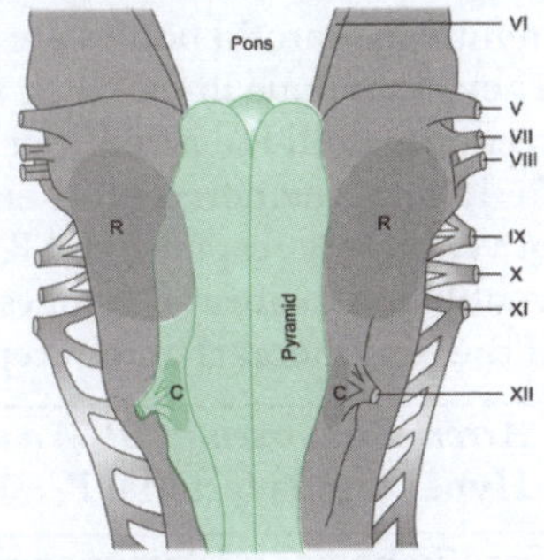

(R) Rostral & Caudal (C) Chemosensitive area in ventral surface of medulla

Primary Indirect Stimulus is CO_2 concentration (P_{CO2}) in Blood

- Although **CO_2** has very little direct effect in stimulating chemosensitive area, it does have a ***potent indirect effect*Q**.
- ***Carbon dioxide passes through blood brain barrier almost as if the barrier does not exist*Q**. So whenever, the blood PCO_2 increases, so does the PCO_2 of CSF and interstitial fluid of medulla. Here CO_2 reacts with water to form new hydrogen ions. Thus, paradoxically, *more H+ ions are released in respiratory chemosensitive sensory area of medulla when the blood CO_2 concentration increases than when the blood hydrogen ion concentration increases.*

Primary Direct Stimulus is H^+ ion concentration (or pH) in CSF and ECF.

- Central chemoreceptor is surrounded by **brain ECF (interstitial fluid) and CSF** and separated from blood by **BBB**, which is **relatively impermeable to H^+ and HCO_3^- (penetrate slowly)** although CO_2 diffuses across it easily.
- Blood brain barrier is not very permeable to H+ ion. So, ***changes in H^+ ion concentration in blood have very less effect in stimulating the chemosensitive neurons*Q** than do changes in blood CO_2, even though CO_2 is believed to stimulate these neurons secondarily by changing hydrogen ion concentration.
- ***H^+ ion concentration in CSF and interstitial fluid*Q** (not in blood) is the only important direct stimulus. An increase in H^+ ion concentration stimulates ventilation, whereas a decrease inhibits it.
- CSF with normal pH 7.32 has much lower buffering capacity than blood

- That's why, ***respiratory center is stimulated very strongly (but indirectly) by changes in blood CO_2 concentration***[Q]. Whereas, blood pH (H^+ ion concentration) has a little effect (b/o relative impermeability of BBB to H^+ ion)
- Changes in P_{CO2} of blood and CSF have only minor effects on respiration as long as H^+ ion concentration in CSF is held constant. Thus the effects of CO_2 on respiration are mainly d/t its movement into CSF and brain ECF, where it increases H^+ ion concentration and stimulates central chemoreceptors sensitive to H^+ ion. Thus **the CO_2 level in blood (P_{CO2}) indirectly regulates ventilation by its effet on pH (H+ ion concentration) of CSF**.
- A change in blood CO_2 concentration has a *potent acute effect* on controlling respiratory drive but ***only a weak chronic effect***[Q] after few days of adaptation. This results from renal readjustment of H+ ion conc. towards normal, by increasing blood bicarbonate. But more importantly these HCO_3^- ions diffuse through blood brain & blood – CSF barrier and combine directly with H+ near respiratory neurons.

b/o much less protein content. Therefore, the change in CSF pH for a given change in P_{CO2} is greater than in blood. Similarly, the CSF pH returns to its near normal value more promptly than does blood pH by renal compensation. That's **why CSF pH has more important effect on ventilation than blood P_{CO2}**. And for the same reason a person with long standing CO_2 retention (d/t chronic lung disease or exposure to 3% CO_2 for few days) has **nearly normal CSF pH** and, therefore, an abnormally low ventilation for his arterial P_{CO2}.

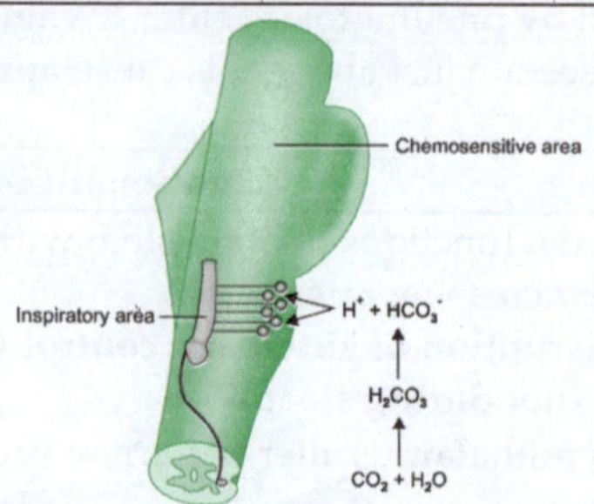

H^+ ion stimulates chemosensitive area, but CO_2 gives rise to most of the H^+ ion

O_2 has no Central role

Changes in ***O_2 concentration have virtually no direct effect on respiratory center***[Q] (although do have an indirect effect, acting through the peripheral chemoreceptor.)

Peripheral Chemoreceptors

- **Carotid bodies** (located at bifurcation of common carotid arteries) and **aortic bodies** (located above & below aortic arch) are the peripheral chemoreceptors; an these respond to **decrease in arterial P_{O2} and pH, and increase in arterial P_{CO2}.**
- In humans carotid bodies are most important; and the carotid but not the aortic bodies respond to a fall in arterial pH.
- They are unique in that their sensitivity to changes in arterial *P_{O2} begins around 500 mmHg*, have *non linear*; relatively little response until P_{O2} is reduced below 100 mmHg. Maximum response occurs below P_{O2} of **50 mmHg.**
- Peripheral chemoreceptors are responsible for all response to arterial hypoxemia (P_{O2}) and blood pH whereas, less than 20% of ventilatory response d/t P_{CO2} can be attributed to it. However, their response is more rapid and is useful in matching ventilation to **abrupt changes in P_{CO2}.**
- If **the peripheral chemo receptor** is denervated the response to

- ***Arterial hypoxemia (P_{O2}) and pH is completely abolished***[Q]
- **Hyper capnia (arterial P_{CO2}) is reduced by 30%.**

- Carotid bodies contain glomus cells of 2 types surrounded by fenestrated sinusoidal capillaries
- Intense fluorescent **type I or glomus cells** are closely associated with cup like endings of the *afferent nerves*. It resemble adrenal chromaffin cells & have dense core granules containing catecholamines that are released upon exposure to *hypoxia & cyanide*. The cells are excited by hyoxia & principle transmitter appears to be *dopamine* which excites the nerve endings by *D_2 receptors*
- The **type II cells** are *glial cells*, and each surrounds 4- 6type I cells. Their function is probably sustantecular
- Afferents from *carotid body* ascend to medulla via carotid sinus & *glossopharyngeal nerves* and fibers from *aortic bodies* ascend in the *vagi*
- Type I glomus cells have O_2 sensitive K^+ channels; whose conductance is reduced with hypoxia → l/t ↓ K^+ efflux →depolarizing the cell & causing Ca^{++} influx via L type Ca^{2+} channels → triggers AP & excitation of afferent nerve endings.

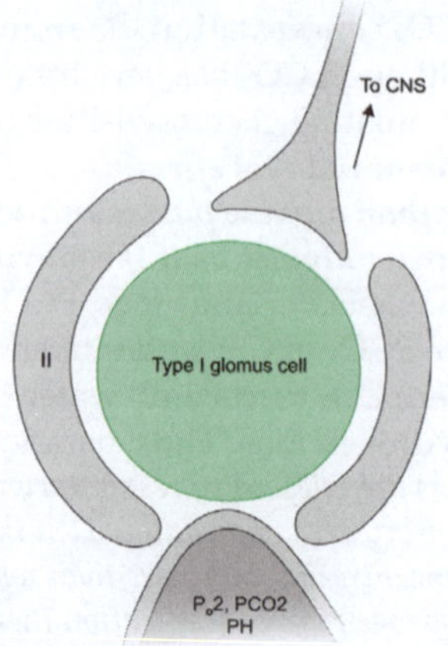

- The smooth muscles of **pulmonary arteries** contain similar *O_2 sensitive K^+ channels*, which mediate the ***vasoconstriction caused by hypoxia***[Q]. This is in contrast to *systemic arteries*, which contain *ATP dependent K^+ channels* that permit more K^+ efflux with hypoxia l/t vasodilation (instead of vasoconstriction)
- The blood flow in each 2mg carotid body is ~ *0.04 ML/min or 2000 ML/100gm/min*. Because of enormous blood flow the O_2 needs of the cells can be met largely by dissolved O_2 alone
- Therefore, the ***receptors are not stimulated in conditions such as anemia & carbon monoxide***

poisoningQ, in which amount of dissolved O_2 in the blood reaching the receptors is generally normal even though the combined O_2 in the blood is markedly decreased.

- The receptors are stimulated when the *arterial PO_2 is low or when, because of vascular stasis the amount of O_2 delivered to receptor per unit time is decreased.*
- ***Powerful stimulation is produced by cyanide***Q; which prevents O_2 utilization at the tissue level
- *Nicotine & lobeline* activate chemoreceptors.
- Infusion of K^+ increases the discharge rate in chemoreceptor afferents and since the plasma K^+ level is increased during exercise, the increase may contribute to exercise induced hyperpnea.

- The response of aortic bodies are similar but of lesser magnitude. In **humans** in whom **both carotid bodies** have been **removed but the aortic bodies left intact**, the response are essentially the same as those following **denervation of both carotid & aortic bodies in animals**: little change in ventilation at rest, but the ***ventilatory response to hypoxia is lost lost & ventilatory response to CO_2 is reduced by 30%***Q

Response of Chemoreceptors to hypoxemia

- The **peripheral chemoreceptors are sensitive to hypoxia but central chemoreceptors are not. These respond to P_{O2} rather than oxygen content** of arterial blood. For the same reason conditions with low O_2 content but normal P_{O2} like CO poisoning, anemia & methaemoglobin do not stimulate receptor (or cause reflex hyperpnoea)
- Body's mechanism for detecting O_2 lack is **relatively insensitive** (cause no significant hyperpnoea until O_2 conc < 8% or P_{O2} < 60 mmHg or Hb saturation < 70%) because reduced oxygenation of Hb causes it to bind H^+ and a fall in $[H^+]$ inhibits respiration, thereby countering the stimulatory effect of O_2 lack. The receptors are **non adapting** and continue to fire impulses as long as the P_{O2} is low, even after death of all tissues, and are responsible for last gasp of a dying man, hence they are called **ultimum moriens.**
- **If oxygen is administered to hypoxaemic patient**, who is unresponsive to high P_{CO2}, it could be dangerous, because the **rise in P_{O2} also removes the hypoxic stimulus** to respiration and the patient may die of CO_2 retention and coma (CO_2 narcosis).

Response to Hypercapnia

- **Both peripheral & central chemoreceptors are sensitive to CO_2 but peripheral receptors** are not (or less) important in control of respiration at physiological range. because they are **less sensitive** (have higher threshold).

However peripheral chemoreceptors **respond rapidly** within 1 second unlike central receptors which respond after a delay of some minutes (b/o time required for CO_2 to enter CSF and produce H_+).

Nonchemical Responses Mediated by Pulmonary Receptors and Reflexes

Receptor Type	Location	Impulse travel in (i.e. Vagal innervation)	Stimulus	Response / Reflex
Slowly adapting Stretch Receptor (pulmonary or bronchial stretch receptors)	**Airway smooth muscle** (?)	**Myelinated** vagal fibers	**Lung inflation**Q	- Inspiratory time shortening - **Hering-Breuer inflation & deflation reflexes**Q - Bronchodilation - Hyperpnea - Tachycardia
Rapidly adapting Irritant Receptors (type of stretch/mechano-receptor)	**Airway epithelial cells**	**Myelinated** vagal fibers	- **Lung Hyperinflation** Q - Exogenous & endogenous substances eg histamine and prostaglandins	- Increased airway resistance i.e. **broncho constriction** (eg asthama) - Mucus secretion - Cough - Hering-Breuer deflation reflex

- ★ **Bronchial C fiber receptors** located in the airways and innervated by *nonmyelinated fibers* are activated by **chemicals (notably bradykinin)** injected into bronchial artery. Their stimulation gives rise to *tachypnea, bronchoconstriction, and airway secretion*. Along with type *J (juxta pulmonary capillary) receptors, they contribute to air way defence reflexes.*
- ★ **Receptors in nose & upper airway** (nasopharynx, larynx & trachea) responding to mechanical & chemical stimulation l/t *sneezing, coughing, broncho constriction and aryngospasm.*
- ★ Impulses from **joint & muscle receptors of moving limb** stimulates ventilation during early exercise.
- ★ **Gamma system** or **muscle spindle of thoracic intercostal muscles and diaphragm** sense

J (Juxta-capillary/alveolar) Receptors (Juxta pulmonary capillary receptor or pulmonary C fiber receptor)	In pulmonary interstitial space close to blood capillaries of - **Pulmonary circulation** - **Bronchial circulation**	**Unmyelinated (pulmonary vagal) C fibers**	- **Lung Hyper inflation**Q **(large)** - Exogenous & endogenous agents eg capsaicin, bradykinin, serotonin, histamine, prostaglandins, phenyl diguanide - **Pulmonary edema, embolism & congestion**Q	- **Apnea** (d/t intense stimulation) **f/b** rapid, shallow breathing **(tachypnea) and dyspnea** - Broncho constriction - Mucus secretion - Brady cardia - Hypotension **(J-pulmonary chemoreflex)**

elongation of these muscles and reflexly control strength of contraction. For example *dyspnoea* is sensed by unusually large respiratory efforts required to move the lung.

★ **Pain** cause *apnea followed by hyperventilation*. **Heating of skin (or fever)** result in hyperventilation (partly d/t stimulation of hypothalamic thermoreceptor).

★ **Arterial (aortic & carotid sinus) baroreceptor stimulation by increased BP** causes reflex **hypoventilation or apnea;** whereas **decreased BP** l/t **hyperventilation** (thereby **enhancing venous return following severe hemorrhage**).

Respiratory Reflexes & Receptors

Head's Paradoxial Reflex

- Vigorous inflation of the lung reflexly induces a contraction of the diaphragm, further augmenting the size of breath. This activity is mediated by lung **irritant receptor.**Q
- **Rapidly adapting pulmonary stretch (mechano) receptor** also k/a irritant receptors lie between **airway epithelial cells of trachea & large airways**. They are stimulated by *noxious stimuli like gases, smoke, inhaled dust and cold air in the inspired air*. The impulses travel up in *myelinated fibers of vagus* and reflex effects include **broncho constriction** (increased airway resistance), coughing, mucus production and **hyperpnea** (John

Hering-Breuer Reflex & Stretch Receptors

- **Slowly adapting pulmonary stretch receptors** lie within airway smooth muscle. They discharge in response to lung distension and show little adaptation i.e. their activity is sustained with lung inflation. The impulse travels in large myeliated fibers of vagus nerve to DRG neurons and is responsible for Hering-Breur reflex.
- Their stimulation affects inspiration in much the same way as signals from *pneumotaxic center* i.e. when the lungs become over stretched (overly inflated), stretch receptors activate appropriate feed back response that **switches off the inspiratory ramp** and thus stops further inspiration. This is k/a Hering Breuer inflation reflex; and like pneumotaxic center, this reflex *increases rate of respiration*.
- Hering Breuer reflexes were once thought to play a major role in ventilation by determining the rate & depth of breathing by modulating the switch off mechanism in medulla. Eg **bilateral vagotomy**, which removes input from these receptors cause slow, deep breathing in most animals.
- However, more recent work indicates that H-B reflexes are **largely inactive in adult humans (not animals)** until tidal volume exceeds 1/1.5 liters, as in exercise. Eg transient bilateral vagal block by local anesthesia in awake human does not change either breathing volume or rate. Therefore this reflex **protect against excessive lung inflation rather than an important ingredient in normal control of ventilation, in adult humans.** Some evidence show that these reflexes may be more **important in newborn babies.**

H-B Inflation reflex

- When lung becomes overstretched, *the stretch receptors* located in the

H-B Deflation reflex

- Excessive deflation of lung causes reflex inhibition of expiration,

J-Receptor Reflex

- **J (juxta capillary) receptors**, are nerve **endings of unmyelinated C fibers** of vagus. They lie in alveolar walls close to pulmonary capillaries and are stimulated by **hyper inflation** of lungs, **intravenous or intracardiac** administration of chemicals such as **capsaicin, bradykinin & serotonin.**
- They are specially stimulated in **pathological states** when pulmonary capillaries become engorged with **emboli** (or blood) or when **pulmonary edema** or **pulmonary congestion** occurs in left heart failure, congestive cardiac failure and interstial lining disease.
- The impulse pass in vagus nerve and result in apnea (d/t intense stimulation) followed by rapid, shallow breathing and dyspnea (i.e. sensation of difficulty in breathing), bradycardia, hypotension, broncho constriction and mucus secretion (**pulmonary chemoreflex**). A similar response is produced by stimulation of receptors in heart ***(Bezold-Jarish reflex or coronary chemoreflex). The physiological role of this reflex is uncertain but probably occurs in pathological states like pulmonary congestion, pulmonary edema and pulmonary embolism***Q.

west)/ reflex apnea (Berne). They may have a possibl role in acute attack of asthma.

Protective Reflex

During swallowing, when food enters the oropharynx, there is a ***reflex inhibition of respiration***[Q] and closure of glottis, to prevent bolus from entering airways.

bronchi and bronchioles send signals to *respiratory neurons*. These signals switches off the inspiratory center and *stops further inspiration*. It is not activated until the tidal volume increases to 1.5 litres.

- Excessive inflation of lungs stimulate the stretch receptors, causing a **protective reflex nhibition of inspiration**. In other words, HB inflation reflex is an **increase in duration of expiration**, produced by steady lung inflation. The main reflex effect is slowing of respiratory frequency d/t an increase in expiratory time.

it may serve to protect against lung collapse (atelectasis). In other words, HB- deflation reflex is **decrease in duration of expiration** produced by marked deflation of lungs.

- If lungs are greatly deflated impulses from receptors, travel up via *vagus* to stimulate inspiration. It comes into play in conditions such as *atelectasis*.

Bronchial C-fiber Reflex

Similar reflex in response to chemicals injected into bronchial circulation.

Arterial-Baroreceptor Reflex

Fall in BP increases both vasomotor center (VMC) activity (↑ing BP) and pulmonary ventilation. Conversely increased BP cause reflex hypoventilation or apnea and ↓ BP through stimulation of aortic & carotid sinus baro receptor.

Pain & Temperature Reflex

Pain causes apnea f/b hyperventilation; and heating of skin may result in hyperventilation

Joint & Muscle receptor; Muscle spidle gamma system reflex

Surfactant

Production and Uptake

- Surfactant is produced by **type II alveolar epithelial cells (or pneumocytes)**, which develop to the end of **6th month (24th week)** of gestation.
- Synthesis of surfactant begins at 16-18/20/24 weeks (a/t various sources). It is stored in alveolar cells **until 26 weeks when** release on the alveolar surface occurs, and amount **peaks at 35 weeks of gestation** particularly during the **last 2 weeks before birth.**
- Type II pneumocytes are rich in mitochondria, ER, and **lamellar bodies** (i.e. membrane bound organelles containing whorls of phospholipids). Secretion of surfactant into the airways occur via **exocytosis of lamellar body**. Tubes of lipid called **tubular myelin** is formed from *extruded lamellar bodies* which inturn for phospholipids film. So tubular myelin is a precursor stage of surfactant as it is initially secreted from type II cells and has not yet spread.
- *β adrenergic agonist, purinergic agonists, activators of protein kinase C and leukotrienes* stimulate exocytosis of surfactant.
- Major routes of clearance of pulmonary surfactant are **reuptake** by type II cells, *absorption into lymphatics, and clearance by alveolar macrophages.*

Surface Tension

- When water forms a surface with air, there is a *strong attraction between its molecule on surface, which is always attempting to contract* the surface. This tight contractile membrane of surface holds the water drop together.
- On inner surface of alveoli, the water surface is also attempting to contract. This *attempts to force air out & cause alveoli to collapse*. This elastic contractile force of lung is called the surface tension elastic force.
- **Surface tension** is a force caused by water molecule at the air-liquid interface (in the alveoli) that tends to minimize surface area, thereby **making it more difficult to inflate the lung.** Higher pressure is required to inflate the lung with air than with saline because saline abolishes surface tension.
- Surface forces in a sphere attempt to reduced the area of surface and generate pressure with in sphere. According to **Laplace's law**, the amount of pressure generated in alveoli (P)

$$P = \frac{2\times \text{ surface tension } (T)}{\text{Radius of alveolus } (r)}$$

- P is inversely proportional to radius of sphere. So surface forces in smaller sphere generate higher pressure than those in larger sphere. As a result air moves from higher pressure (smaller sphere) to lower pressure (larger sphere) causing the small sphere to collapse and large sphere to become overdistended.

Effect of Surfactant

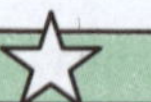

- **Surfactant** is a ***surface active agent which breaks this surface tension elastic force of water molecules in alveoli***Q. The reduction in surface tension is greater when the film is compressed because the molecules of DPPC are then crowded closer together and repel eachother more. **Surfactant lowers surface tension more in smaller spere than in larger sphere** (i.e. in lungs small surface area is a/w small surface tension). The net result is that **the pressure in small and large sphere (alveoli) is similar**, the tendency for small alveoli to empty into large alveoli is reduced and **alveoli are stabilized** (i.e. do not collapse).
- **Surface tension** of saline etc and its lowering by detergent etc is independent of area whereas **reduction of surface tension by surfactant is area dependent.** The surfactant thins out when alveoli are large and stretched during inspiration, but packs closely as the radius reduces during expiration. Because of surfactant small surface area is a/w small surface tension in lungs. Therefore the surface tension falls as the alveolus deflates.

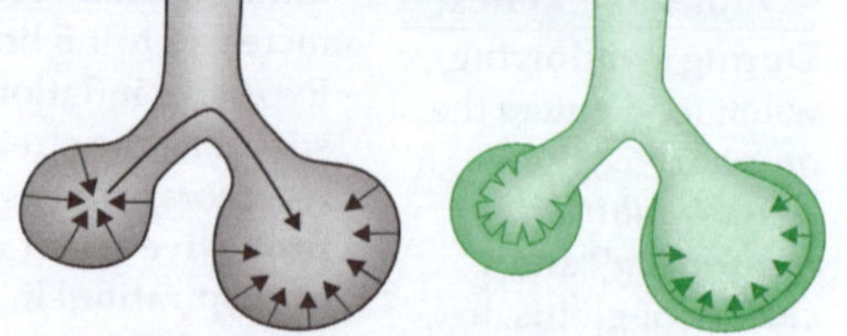

- B/O surfactant there is an increase in surface tension at high lung volumes and a decrease at low lung volumes. So lung can maintain alveoli at many different volumes. Otherwise, small alveoli would empty into large alveoli. As a result, the transmural pressure required to keep an alveolus inflated increases as lung volume (and transpulmonary pressure) increases and it decreases as lung volume decreases.
- ***Stability of alveoli is mainly the function of surfactant***Q which regulates the alveolar size by regulating surface tension and thus preventing their collapse at the end of expiration. As the alveoli increase in size (at the end of inspiration), the surfactant becomes more spread out over the surface of liquid allowing surface tension to increase. This effectively slows the rate of increase of alveoli preventing over expansion and helping all alveoli in lung to expand at the same time.
- ***Negative intrapulmonary pressure, residual air and compliance*** **mainly affect the inflation and deflation of lung**Q. They do have some effect on stability but most important factor remains surfactant as the maximum work of breathing is done to oppose surface tension.

Function

- **DPPC** is the **major component** and it **decreases surface tension.**
- Type II pneumocytes occupy only 5% of alveolar surface whereas surfactant must spread and form film over entire alveolar surface. **PG, SP-B, SP-C** and **calcium** have spreading properties, required for film formation. Mutation of SP-C gene is a/w *familial interstial lung disease.*
- SP-A is a large glycoprotein and has a collagen like domain in its structure. It is involved in *regulation of surfactant uptake by type II* pneumocytes. SP-A and SP-D (collection proteins) are involved in **innate immunity** in conducting airways and alveoli.
- **Reduces surface tension in alveoli**, which in turn *increases the compliance of lung*Q and reduces the work of expanding with each breath.
- Alveolar size regulation and **stability of alveoli is promoted**, which **prevents alveolar collapse (or alveolar atelectasis)** at the end of expiration.
- **Prevents transudation** of fluid (& **pulmonary edema) by keeping alveoli dry**. Because it counter 20 mmHg force of surface tension favouring transudation of fluid from blood into alveoli.

★ Knocking out GM-CSF gene l/t presence of excess surfactant proteins & lipids in mice (resembling pulmonary alveolo proteinosis of humans)

★ Mucin is a glycoprotein which is secreted by mucous secreting bronchoalveolar Ca.

Deficiency Occurs with

- ***Occlusion of main bronchus***Q
- ***Occlusion of one pulmonary artery***Q
- ***Cigarette smokers***Q
- Long term inhalation of 100% O_2.
- Cardiac surgery involving use of pump oxygenator.
- Deficiency of surfactant l/t **infant respiratory distress syndrome (IRDS) / hyaline membrane disease**, patchy atlectasis, and pulmonary alveolar proteinosis. **Exogenous bovine surfactant (beractant)** through endotracheal tube & mechanical ventilation is used for management in IRDS.
- RDS is common in **diabetic (↓ insulin) mothers, low thyroid harmone and low glucocorticoid levels** and in premature babies.

Mechanism of Decreasing Surface Tension

- ***Dipalmitoylphosphatidyl choline***, along with other phospholipids reduce surface tension ***by not dissolving uniformly in the fluid*** **lining the alveolar surface.** The hydrophilic head dissolves in fluid and 2 hydrophobic tails face the alveolar lumen. Instead, *part of molecule dissolve, while the remainder spreads over the surface of water.*
- The surface tension of this nonuniform surface containing surfactant is *5-30 dynes/cm*, which is ~ *1/12 to 1/2* of surface tension of pure water *(72 dynes/cm)*. Whereas, alveoli without surfactant produce *50 dyne /cm* surface tension.

Hyaline Membrane disease / Infant Respiratory Distress Syndrome (IRDS)

When surfactant is insufficienct, in premature infant, the air-water (blood) surface membrane tension becomes high, bringing great risk that alveoli will collapse during expiration. In RDS, the partially collapsed alveoli contain fluid **with high protein content, hyaline membranes** and lamellar bodies.

Alveolar collapse (atelectasis) d/t high surface tension

High surface tension in the alveoli makes it very difficult for the lungs to expand in child born deficienct in surfactant, because it would require intrapleural pressure as high as **-20 to -30** mm Hg to overcome the surface tension.

Prolonged immaturity of ENaCs (Epithelial Na^+ Channels) l/t retention of fluid in lungs

- During fetal life, Cl- is secreted with fluid by the pulmonary epithelial cells
- At birth there is a shift to Na^+ absorption by these cells Via ENa Cs and fluid is absorbed with Na+
- Immaturity of these channels l/t retention of fluid in lungs.

Pathophysiology

Decreased Alveolar surfactant[Q] ⟶ Increased alveolar surface tension ↓

- Hypoxemia
- CO_2 retention ⟵ Collapse / Atelectasis
- Acidosis

↓

Pulmonary hypoperfusion

↓

Endothelial damage — Epithelial damage

↓

Plasma leak into alveoli

↓

Fibrin + Necrotic cells[Q]

↓

Hyaline membrane.

Non-Respiratory – Metabolic Functions of Lungs ☆

Fate of biologically active substances metabolized in lungs

Synthesized & used in lungs	- *Surfactant*[Q] (DPPC) - Proteins collagen & elastin of framework - Carbohydrate mucopolysaccharide of mucous
Synthesized or stored & released into the blood. Mn-"**HAK**"	• **H**istamine • **A**rachidonic acid metabolites - **Prostaglandins & Thromboxane A_2** (by cyclooxygenase) - **Leukotrienes** including **SRSA** i.e. slow reacting substance of anaphylaxis (by enz. lipooxygenase) • **K**allikrien
Activated in lungs	- **Angiotensin I** is converted to **angiotensin II** by ACE.
Partially removed from the blood Mn-"**No-BAAPS**"	- **No**repinephrine (up to 30% is taken up by lungs) - **B**radykinin (80% inactivated by ACE) - **A**cetylcholine - **A**denine nucleotide - **P**rotaglandins E_1, E_2 and $F_2\alpha$ (almost completely inactivated) - **S**erotonin (almost completely removed by uptake & storage in platelets and released during anaphylaxis)
Passed through lungs without being metabolized (without significant gain or loss of activity) Mn-**"DOPA"**	- Angiotensin **II** - **A**drenaline (epinephrine) - **A**DH (Vasopressin) - **P**rostaglandin (**A_1**, **A_2**) - **P**rostacyclin (PGI_2) - **O**xytocin - **D**opamine & histamine

As Blood reservoir

Because lung is the only organ except the heart that **receives the whole circulation** and has uniquely remarkable ability to reduce its pulmonary vascular resistance by **recruitment and distension,** it acts as a reservoir for blood.

Blood filtration

Pulmonary capillary bed acts as a blood filter and remove small thrombi (clots), bubbles, detached cells and prevent them from entering systemic circulation.

Fibrinolysis and Anticoagulation

Lung is rich in mast cells, which **secrete anticoagulant heparin**. And pulmonary endothelium is rich in plasmin activator, which converts plasminogen into plasmin and promotes fibrinolysis. This is how lungs delay clotting and dissolve small clots (fibrinolysis).

Mucosal Immune System

Lungs contribute to defense against infection by **secreting immunoglobulin A (IgA)**. It also has other defense mechanism like- filtration, epithelial barrier, mucociliary clearance, MALT, innate & adaptive immune cells (like alveolar macrophage, NK cells, NK/T cells, dendrite cells, β lymphocytes, TCRαβ and TCR γδ lymphocytes providing humoral & cell mediated immunity)

Acid Base Balance, Sodium balance & cooling

Pulmonary Neuro-Endocrinal Cell (PNEC) System

It is more numerous in fetal/neonatal lung (than adults) and produce **amines (eg dopamine, 5 HT or serotonin)** and **neuropeptides (eg bombesin/GRP, CGRP and calcitonin)**. *Chromogranin A* immunohistochemical marker is most sensitive in identification. PNECS has **dual innervations from vagus and P/calcitonin gene related gene peptide IR nerve fibers.** It consists of

Solitary /Cluster PNECs

- PNECs (and their secretion) are involved in lung development like branching morphogenesis, direct mitogenic effects on epithelium and promote differentiation of adjacent epithelial cells.
- **Serotonin released from PNEC (eg Kultschitzky cells)/ PNEB** is involved in lung fluid production and clearance and help in transition form fetal to extrauterine life.
- PNEC/PNEB hyperplasia is seen in disorders like broncho pulmonary dysplasia, central hypoventilation syndrome, SIDS, NE hyperplasia of infancy, CF and pediatric asthma.

Pulmonary Neuro Endocrinal Bodies (PNEB)

- Because of membrane bound O_2 sensing complex (ie **O_2 sensing K^+ channels and protein NADPH oxidase)**, PNEB acts as airway O_2 sensor especially during adaptation to extrauterine life.
- Hypoxia (↓PO_2) activates O_2 sensor l/t Ca^{++} dependent *exocytosis of amines & peptides from dense core vesicles* (DCV=storage site).

Acid – Base Balance

- The pH of arterial plasma is **7.40** and that of venous plasma is slightly lower. A decreased pH below 7.4 is **acidosis** and an increase in pH above is k/a **alkalosis.** However, **0.05 pH variations** are without untoward effects. Normal pH range for adult is **7.35 – 7.45** and is maintained by **lung, kidney** and 3 main chemical **buffer systems in blood i.e. plasma proteins, hemoglobin and carbonic acid-bicarbonate system.**
- When acid-base disturbance develops, body uses same defence to compensate the pH change.
- First line of defence against acid-base disorder is instantaneous ECF & ICF buffering. Metabolite disorder are buffered in both ICF & ECF compartments whereas, all buffering in respiratory disorders occurs in ICF.
- Bicarbonate buffer system (main), Pi and plasma proteins are ECF buffers. Bone Ca^{++} is additional source of ECF buffering. Intracellular buffering involves movement of H^+ into & out of cell. The H_+ is titrated inside the cell by HCO_3^-, Pi and **histidine** group of hemoglobin (protein).
- **Lungs** are the second line of defence; **ventilation rate determines P_{CO_2}.** The lungs excrete over 10,000 mEq of carbonic acid per day compared to with < 100 mEq of fixed acids by kidneys.
- Third (final) line of defence is **kidneys**, which make appropriate adjustments in the excretion of HCO_3^- and net acid. However, this may take hours to days (time required to increase synthesis of PCT enzymes involved in synthesis of NH_4^+)
- **Compensation of respiratory acidosis /alkalosis:**
  - **10 mmHg increase in P_{CO_2}**, increases HCO_3^- level **1 mmol/L** in acute and **4 mmol/L** in chronic (>24hrs) stage. However, HCO_3^- does not increase above 38 mmol/L
  - **10 mmHg decrease in P_{CO_2}** decrease **2 mmol/L** HCO_3^- level and **7 mmol/L H+** or increase **0.1 pH** in acute stage. Whereas in chronic stage 10 mmHg decrease in P_{CO_2} cause **4-5 mmol/L** drop in HCO_3^- and **3 mmol/L** drop in HCO_3^- and 3mol/L fall in H^+ or **0.03** rise in pH
- **Compensation of metabolic acidosis / alkalosis:**

  1 meq/L decrease/increase in HCO_3^- cause 1.2 mmHg decrease/0.7 mmHg increase in P_{CO_2} rspectively.

Calculation of pH: Handerson – Hasselbach Equation showing effect of CO_2 & HCO_3^- concentration

$$pH = pK_A + \log \frac{[HCO_3^-]}{[CO_2]}$$

- Because CO_2 follows Henry law, its concentration (in mmol/lit) can be replaced by solubility (α) × partialpressure (P_{CO_2}). And at body temperature (37°C), α = 0.03 and pK_A= 6.1; so

$$pH = 6.1 + \log \frac{[HCO_3^-]}{0.03 \times P_{CO_2}}$$

- Because normal HCO_3^- concentration in arterial blood is 24 mmol/lit and P_{CO_2} = 40 mmHg.

$$pH = 6.1 + \log \frac{24}{0.03 \times 40} = 6.1 + \log 20 = 6.1 + 1.3 = 7.4$$

- This shows the **effect of P_{CO_2}** (which is **determined by lungs)** and **HCO_3^- concentration** (determined by chiefly by **kidney.)**

4 Types of Acid-Base Disturbances

The ratio of bcarbonate/P_{CO_2} can be altered in 4 ways: both HCO_3^- and P_{CO_2} can be lowered or increased

I. **Respiratory Acidosis** is caused by **↑ed P_{CO_2} (hypercapnia caused by hypoventilation)**, which *decreases HCO_3^-/P_{CO_2} ratio and thus pH.* It is compensated by intracellular **(ICF) buffers** and **increased net acid excretion (NAE) by kidney** i.e. kidney excreting a more acid urine by secreting H^+ ions in form of NH_4^+ or $H_2PO_4^-$; and reabsorbing HCO_3^- **(conserving bicarbonate).**

II. **Respiratory Alkalosis** is caused by **↓P_{CO_2} (hypocapnia)**, which **increases HCO_3^- /P_{CO_2} ratio and thus elevate pH.** A ↓ P_{CO_2} is caused by **hyperventilation** (eg at high altitudes). It is compensated by ICF buffer and **↓NAE (or increased HCO_3^- excretion)** by kidney.

III. **Metabolic Acidosis** is caused by **↓HCO_3^-** (d/t accumulation of acids as in diabetic ketoacidosis, or tissue hypoxia l/t lactic acidosis). The **ratio of HCO_3^-/P_{CO_2} and so pH falls.** It is compensated by ICF & extracellular (ECF) buffers, lungs (hyperventilation that ↓ P_{CO_2}) and ↑ renal NAE.

IV. **Metabolic Alkalosis** is caused by **↑HCO_3^-** (d/t alkali ingestion or prolonged vomitting) and thus raising **HCO_3^-/P_{CO_2} ratio and pH.** It is compensated by ICF & ECF buffers, lung (hypoventilation) and ↓ renal NAE.

High Altitude

The composition of air stays the same, but the ***total barometric pressure falls***Q with increasing altitude, therefore ***PO_2 also falls***Q. Hypoxic hypoxia is a problem in normal individuals at high attitude.

Mountain sickness

- Condition characterized by the ill effects of hypoxia at high altitude. **This syndrome develops 8-24 hours after arrival and lasts 4-8 days**Q.
- ***Low PO_2 stimulates the arterial chemoreceptors***Q leading to an immediate *increase in pulmonary ventilation* → This blows off CO_2 (↓PCO_2 & ↑pH) → Inhibits the brain stem respiratory center → ***Respiratory distress***Q

Pathophysiology	Symptom
- Expansion of gases in the git-	- **Nausea, vomiting**
- **Pulmonary**Q **edema -** ***(d/t ↑ed pulmonary capillary permeability and normal left atrial pressure)***Q	- ***Breathlessness Pulmonary hypertenson***Q
- **Cerebral edema**Q **-** [low PO_2 causes *vasodilation* in brain & if cerebral auto regulation does not compensate, ↑ in capillary pressure favours ↑ ed transduation of fluid into brain tissue]	- Headache - Irritability - Insomnia - Weakness

Acclimatization

An acclimatized person is a person who has developed compensatory mechanism so that hypoxia causes lesser effects on the body.

1. **Increased pulmonary ventilation (Hyper ventilation)**
   - Hypoxic stimulation of *central chemoreceptor (carotid and aortic)* increases alveolar ventilation
   - **Increase in pulmonary ventilation blows off CO_2, ↓ PCO_2 and there by increases pH** & inhibits central chemoreceptors (respiratory center). However with **acclimatization over 2-5 days**, CSF begins to expel HCO_3^- & pH↓ es, this stimulates central chemoreceptors of respiratory center
2. **Polycythemia and ↑ed Hb**
3. **↑ed diffusion capacity**
4. Circulatory system show
   - *Increased cardiac output (30%) immediately*, which becomes normal with in few weeks as *blood hematocrit increases.*
   - *Increased (systemic) tissue capillarity* (or angiogenesis) and capillary permeability.
5. **Cellular** - Increased mitochondrial oxidative enzymes
6. ***2-3 DPG rises within RBC, shifts the O_2^- dissociation curve to the right.***Q So O_2 unloading to tissue becomes easier.

Compensatory Mechanism Involved In Acclimatization

Ventilatory Response

- The initial ventilatory response is small as alkalosis tends to counteract effect of hypoxia. However **ventilation increases** over next 4days (d/t ↓ CSF PH). After 4 days, ventilatory response begins to decline slowly but it takes years of residence at higher altitudes for it to decline to the initial levels.
- The ***respiratory alkalosis*** produced by hyper ventilation ***shifts O_2-Hb dissociation curve to the left***Q, but a concomitant ***increase in RBC 2, 3, BPG*** tends to ***decrease the O_2 affinity of hemoglobin***Q
- The net effect is a small **increase in P_{50}**. The decrease in O_2 affinity makes more O_2 available to tissue. However the value of increase in P_{50} is limited because when the arterial PO_2 is markedly reduced, the decreased O_2 affinity also interferes with O_2 uptake by Hb in lung.
- Hyperventilation cause respiratory alkalosis d/t CO_2 washout.

Blood Response

- *Erythropoietin* secretion increases & then falls after 4 days when ventilatory response increases & arterial PO_2 rises
- *Increase in RBC* begins in 2-3 days and is sustained as long as the individuals remain at high altitude

Compensatory Changes In Tissue

- *Mitochondria* increase in number
- *Myoglobin* increases, which facilitates the movement of O_2 in tissue
- *Cytochrome oxidase* content increases

Decompression Sickness

(Compressed Air Sickness, Dysbarism, Air Sickness, Bends, Diver's Paralysis, Caisson's Disease)

The disorder occur when a *person returns rapidly* to normal surroundings (atmospheric pressure) *after exposure to high atmospheric pressure*, as in deep sea.

- Because of ↑ed barometric pressure at deep sea, compression occurs. This compression reduces the volume of gases in the body.
- Due to sudden return to atmospheric pressure, the N_2 is decompressed and escapes from the tissue. Being a gas it forms bubbles, the bubbles obstruct the blood flow producing air embolism.
- **Aviators**Q may develop decompression sickness if they are suddenly decompressed at very high altitudes as a result of cabin failure.
- It manifest as bends (joint pain most commonly in knee), staggers (vertigo d/t formation of bubbles in vestibular apparatus), chocking sensation, paresthesias accompanied by rashes & itching.

★ *Mountaineer* suffer from mountain sickness due to decreased *barometric pressure.*

Effects of High partial pressure of gases on body

N_2 Narcosis

- At high tissue concentrations, **N_2 and other rare gases** such as helium & argon behave as anesthetic gases
- Mild N2 narcosis sets in at round 120 feet below sea surface and individual feels *like one intoxicated with alcohol & is in high spirits* exhibit a joviality & loses his cares a phenomenon referred as **raptures of death.** Manual dexterity is maintained but intellectual function is impaired.
- At 150-200 feet, diver becomes drowsy; at 200-250 feet strength decreases & becomes too clumsy to perform required work. Beyond 250 feet (8.5 Atm. Pressure) becomes almost useless.
- At high concentrations, nitrogen behaves as anesthetic gases and show ***increased solubility in lipid (fatty) substances of neuronal membrane and makes them less excitable by altering ionic conductance***Q.

Oxygen Toxicity

- **Breathing high concentration (or very high alveolar O_2** pressure) causes lung damage, nausea, muscle twitching, dizziness, irritability, disorientation, disturbances of vision and brain seizure followed by coma.
- *Above a critical alveolar PO_2 (> 2 atmP)*, the hemoglobin – O_2 buffering mechanism fails & tissue PO_2 rises to hundreds or thousands of millimeters of mercury
- At these high levels amount of **toxic oxidizing free radicals** (such as *superoxide free radical O_2 & peroxide free radical in form of hydrogen peroxide)* swamp the *enzyme systems (peroxidases, catalses, and superoxide dismutases)* designed to remove them
- In excess, free radicals **oxidize the poly unsaturated, fatty acids of cell membrane and some cell enzymes.** The *nervous tissues with its high lipid content is particularly vulnerable.* There fore acute lethal O_2 toxicity is caused by brain dysfunction.

Chapter 4. CARDIOVASCULAR SYSTEM: REVIEW NOTES

Conducting System of Heart

Anatomy

- **S.A node** is located at the ***junction of superior venacave with right atrium***Q just deep to the epicardium, near the superior end of sulcus terminalis
- **AV node** is located in the *right postero-inferior region of interatrial septum* near the opening of coronary sinus
- There are three bundles of atrial fibers that contain purkinje type fibers and connect the SA node to AV node
  - *Anterior* internodal tract of *Bachman*
  - *Middle* internodal tract of *Wenckebach*
  - *Posterior* internodal tract of *Thorel*
- Conduction also occurs through atrial myocyte but it is more rapid in these bundles
- *AV node is the only conducting pathway* between atria & ventricles
- Bundle of His gives off a left bundle branch (LBB) and continues as right bundle branch (RBB). The LBB divides into an anterior and posterior fascicle
- The *branches & fascicles run subendocardially* and come into contact with purkinje system whose fibers spread to all parts of ventricular myocordium

Blood supply

Part	Artery
SA Node	Atrial branches of - ***Right coronary artery (65%)***Q - Left coronary artery (35%)
AV Node	- ***Right coronary artery***Q
Bundle of His	- ***Right coronary artery***Q
RBB	- ***Left coronary artery***Q
LBB	- Left coronary artery (mostly) - Right coronary artery (rarely)

Histology

- It is composed for the most part of ***modified cardiac muscle***Q that has fewer striations and indistinct boundaries.
- The SA node and to a lesser extent AV node also contain small round cells with few organelles which are connected by gap junctions. These are actual **Pacemaker cells** also called **P cells**
- The atrial muscle fibers are separated from those of ventricles by a fibrous tissue ring, and normally the only conducting tissue between the atria and ventricle is the bundle of His.

Innervation

- **SA node** develop from structures on the *right* side of embryo *AV node* from structures on *left side*. This is why
  - SA node is supplied by right vagus & rt. Sympathetics
  - AV node is supplied by left vagus & lt. Sympathetics
- On each side, most **sympathetic fibers come** from the stellate ganglion.
- *Noradrenergic fibers are epicardial* whereas *vagal* fibers are endocardial
- Reciprocal inhibitory effect occurs b/w sympathetic & parasympathetic system.
  - Neuropeptide Y secreted from noradrenergic endings inhibit acetyl choline release.
  - Ach inhibit norepinephrine release.

Action Potential in Cardiac Ventricular Muscles

- **Resting membrane potential** is much more negative i.e. **-90 mili volts** in ventricular muscle fibers instead of **-55 milivolts** in the **nodal fibers.**
- **Action potential in cardiac muscle** fibers averages about **105 mili volts** i.e. the intracellular potential rises form a very negative *-90 mV between beats* to slightly positive *+20 mV during each beat*.

☆ Difference b/w AP of Cardiac & Skeletal Muscles

Cardiac muscles have prolonged AP (Action potential) and a platue phase, whereas skeletal muscles do not because

1. AP of skeletal muscle is caused and almost entirely by sudden opening of fast Na^+ channels for a very short period. At the end of this abrupt closure, repolarization occurs and AP is over in another thousandth of a second. Whereas AP in **cardiac muscle** is caused by same **fast Na^+ channels** as well as **slow Ca^+ (Na^+ - Ca^{++}) channels** which are slower to open and more importantly *remain*

- **3 type of membrane ion channels** in cardiac muscles responsible for causing the voltage changes include

Channel	Effect
Fast Na^+ Channel	Rapidly opening of fast sodium channels for 10,000 ths of a second) causes **rapid influx of positive sodium ion (Na^+)** to the interior of cardiac muscle fiber (**Na^+current, I_{Na}**). It is responsible for **rapid upstroke spike of action potential** or **rapid depolarization phase O**.
	Initial rapid repolarization phase 1is caused by inactivation of Na^+ channels.
Slow Ca^{++} (Na^+ - Ca^{++}) Channels	**Slower opening** of slow calcium (or sodium-calcium) channels for about 0.3 second (i.e **longer duration**) causes large **influx of both Ca^{++} and Na^+** positive ions to interior of cardiac muscle fibre. This **(Ca^{++} current/influx, Ica mainly)** is responsible for **maintenance of prolonged period of depolarization or platue phase (2)** of ventricular AP.
Potassium (K^+) Channels	Rapid diffusion of large amounts of **positive K^+ ions** in outward direction **(efflux)** from the cardiac muscle fibre (Ek^+, K^+ current) immediately **returns the membrane potential to its resting levels**, thus ending the AP

open for several tenths of a second (i.e prolonged duration) thereby maintaining **prolonged period of depolarization**, causing the **platue phase**.

2. In *skeletal muscles*, Ca^{++} ions for contraction is derived from *intracellular sacroplasmic reticulum*. Whereas, in *cardiac muscles the Ca^{++} that enters during plate phase* activate the muscle contractile process.

3. Immediately after the onset of AP, the **permeability of cardiac muscle fiber for K^+ decreases about 5 folds** as a result of excess Ca^{++} influx through Ca^{++} channels. Therefore, **greatly decreased outflux of positively charged K^+ ions** during AP platue in cardiac muscles prevents early return of AP voltage to its resting levels. This greatly decreased K^+ permeability is not seen in skeletal muscles.

Difference b/w AP of Cardiac Muscle & Sinus Nodal Fibers

- AT the less negative (- 55 mV) RMP of nodal fibers the **fast Na^+ channels** mainly have already **become inactivated (or blocked).** Therefore only **the slow Na^+ channels can become activated (open) and cause AP.**
- So *AP is slower to develop in nodal fibers than ventricular fibers.* Similarly return of potential to its negative resting state occurs slowly as well rather than the abrupt return that occurs in ventricular muscles.

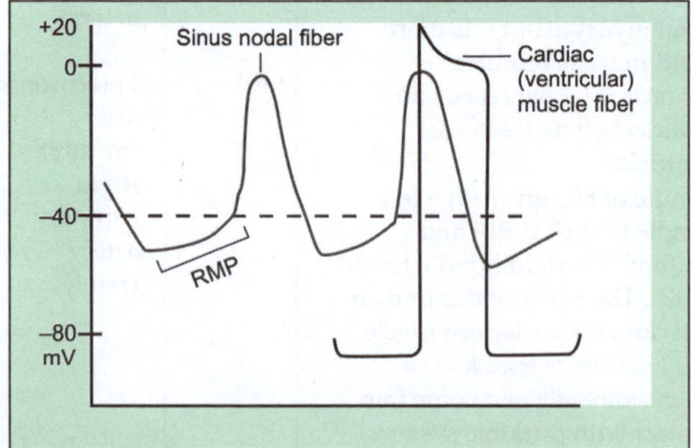

Mechanical Events in Cardiac Cycle (= 0.80 sec)

Both (left & right) sides of heart have *similar but slightly asynchronous* events. Right atrial systole and right ventricular ejection begins before that of left. Whereas, right ventricular contraction starts after that of left. Events include

Ventricular Systole = 0.27 sec

It has 2 phases which are

1. Isovolumetric (Isovolumic, Isometric) Contraction = 0.05 sec

Both ***AV (atrioventricular) valves ie mitral (bicuspid) and tricuspid valves aswell as aortic and pulmonary valves' are closed***[Q] **during this phase.** Ventricle contracts as a closed chamber with both the semilunar & AV valve closed until the pressure in left and right ventricle exceeds the pressure in the aorta

2. Ventricular Ejection=0.22 sec

When ***aortic and pulmonary valves open***[Q], the blood flows out of ventricle and ventricle ejection begins. Because the **end diastolic ventricular volume is 130ml** and end **systolic ventricular volume** is **50 ml. The ejection fraction** (or %of EDVV that is ejected with each stroke) is **~65%** .EF is a useful measure of ventricular function.

Diastole = 0.53 sec duration

It has 3 phases which are

1. **Early diastole** = 0.12 sec

In **0.04 sec** of **protodiastole** the ejection stops and **aortic & pulmonary valves close.**

In **0.08 sec** of **isovolumetric ventricular relaxatioin,** ventricle relax as closed cavity with both the semilunar & AV valve closed until the pressure in ventricles falls below the pressure in the atria.

2. **Late Diastolic Ventricular Filling**
3. **Atrial Systole (Contraction) Ventricular Filling.**

In both of these pheses **AV valves** are **open** and **semilunar (aortic & pulmonary) valves are closed.**

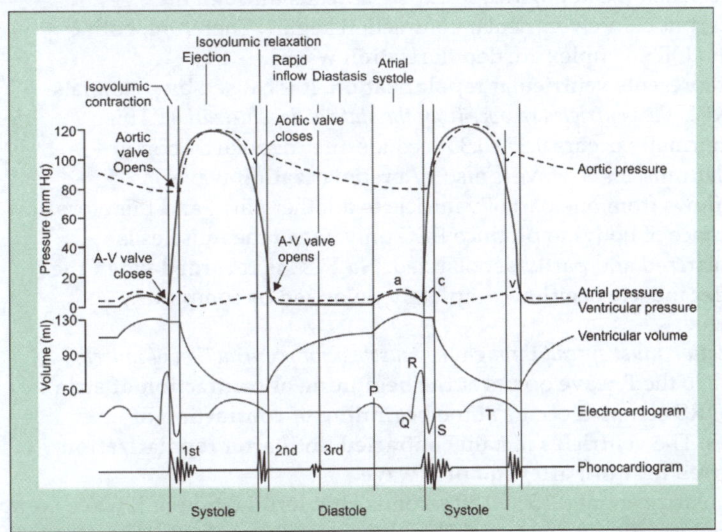

Vector Analysis of ECG

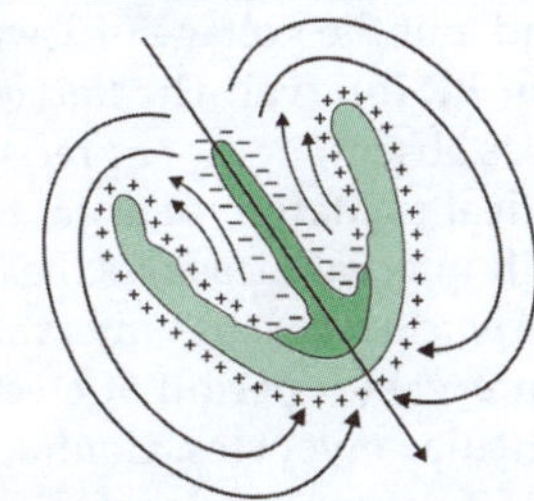

Instantaneous Mean Vector through the partially depolarized ventricles

- At a given time (instant) during the cardiac cycle, heart current flows in a particular direction. A **vector (arrow)** *points in direction of the electrical potential* generated by the current flow, with the **arrowhead in the positive direction**. The length of arrow is drawn proportional to the voltage of the potential. This is called **resultant vector** in the heart **at a given instant.**
- At the instant of **partial depolarization of ventricles** (septum & apical endocardial walls shown by negative signs and shaded area), the electrical current flows between the depolarized areas inside the heart and non-depolarized areas on the outside of heart (shown by *long elliptical arrows*). Overall, *far more current flows downward from the base of ventricle toward the apex* than in upward direction. So **instantaneous mean vector** (i.e.) the **summated vector of generated potential at this particular instant) during septal depolarization is** represented by the **long black arrow** drawn ***through the centre of the ventricles in a direction from base toward apex***[Q].
- **Directions of vector: When a vector is exactly horizontal and directed towards the person's left side,** the vector is said to extend in the direction of **0 degree** . From this 0° reference point, the scale of vector direction rotates **clockwise**. So when the vector extends **from above to vertically straight downward,** it is in the direction of **90°**. When it extends from person's **left to right** the direction is **180°**; and when it extends **straight upwards**, it has a direction of **–90° (or + 270°).**
- **Mean QRS vector:** is the average direction of the vector during spread of the depolarization wave through ventricles. In a normal heart it is about **+59°** which means that **during most of depolarization the apex of heat remains positive with respect to the base of heart.**

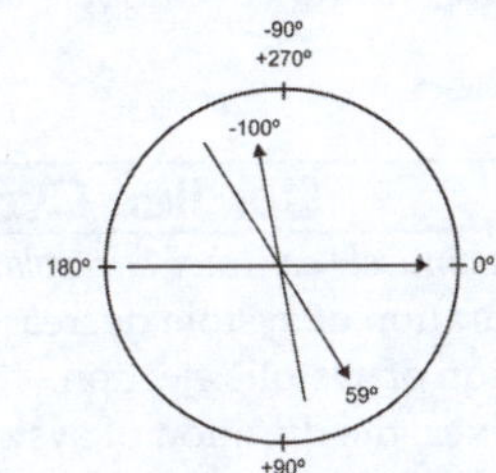

Direction of Vector

- If it is assumed that three ECG electrode locations form the points of an **equilateral triangle (Einthoven's triangle)** and the heart lies in the centre of this triangle; the vector at any given movement in two dimensions of frontal plane can be calculated from any two standard limb leads.
- **Mean QRS vector (electrical axis of heat)** is plotted by using the average QRS deflection in each lead (or by measuring the net differences between the positive of negative peaks of QRS). The normal direction of mean QRS vector is **–30° to +110°. Left axis deviation** is present if calculated axis **falls to left of –30°** and may be d/t **left ventricular hypertrophy. Right axis deviation** is present if axis **falls to the right of +110°** and suggests **right ventricular hypertrophy**.

Normal Electrocardiogram (ECG)

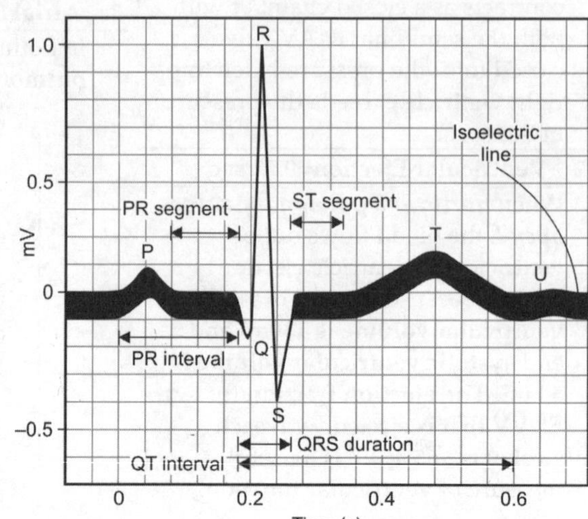

- **P wave** reflects **atrial depolarization** before atrial contraction begins. **QRS complex (wave)** reflects **ventricular depolarization** before contraction. In other words, QRS complex is caused by potentials generated when the depolarization wave spreads through the ventricles, but before ventricular contraction begins. Therefore, both P waves and QRS complex are **depolarization waves.**
- **T wave** represents **ventricular repolarization.** It is caused by potentials generated *as the ventricles recover from the state of depolarization.* This process normally occurs 0.25– 0.35 seconds after depolarization in ventricular muscles. T wave is also k/a **repolarization wave.**
- Current flows from one part of ventricle to another part (and therefore to the surface of body) to produce ECG only when the muscles is partly polarized and partly depolarized. **No ECG is recorded when the ventricular muscle is either completely polarized or completely depolarized.**
- *Depolarization must spread through the muscle before contraction of muscle can occur.* So the **P wave** occurs **at the beginning of contraction of atria** and the **QRS complex** occurs at the **beginning of contraction of ventricles.** The **ventricles remain contracted until after repolarization has occurred i.e. until after end of T wave.**
- Atria repolarize about 0.15 to 0.20 seconds after termination of P wave i.e. approximately during QRS complex. Therefore **atrial repolarization wave (atrial T wave)** is usually *masked by much larger QRS complex (of ventricular depolarization).*
- Ventricular repolarization begins about 0.20 seconds after the beginning of depolarization (QRS complex) in some fibers and takes as long as 0.35 seconds in others. Thus, ventricular repolarization (T wave) is prolonged process extending over 0.15 second, but the voltage of T wave is lesser than the voltage of QRS complex, partly b/o its prolonged length.
- **P-Q or PR interval:** The *time between the beginning of P wave and the beginning of QRS complex* is called PR interval (when Q wave is absent) or more precisely P-Q interval. It is a measure of the time from the **onset of atrial activation (ie beginning of electrical excitation of atria) to the onset of ventricular activation (or excitation).**
- The PR interval measures the *time between the atrial and ventricular depolarization, including the physiological delay imposed by cells in AV junction area.* PR interval is normally 0.16 second (0.12 – 0.20 second). It shortens as the heart rate increases.
- **QT interval** (or **period of electrical systole of ventricles**) is closely correlated with the **mean action potential duration of ventricular myocytes.** Contraction of ventricles lasts from the **beginning of Q wave** (or **R wave**, if Q wave is absent) **to the end of T wave**: an interval k/a QT interval. Normally QT interval is 0.4 second, but is *inversely related with the heart rate* because the duration of myocardial cell action potential varies inversely with the heart rate. A **heart rate related (corrected) QT interval (QTc)** can be calculated as $QT\sqrt{R} - R$ and normally is **≤ 0.44 second.**

Cardiac Cycle : Pecualirities

- *Cardiac muscle contract & repolarize faster at higher heart rates (HR)* and the duration of systole decreases mainly d/t a decrease in the duration of systolic ejection.
- However, the duration of systole is much more fixed and the **diastole is shortened to a much greater degree**
- **Only during diastole, coronary blood flows to the endocardial portion of left ventricle and heart muscles rest.** Most of the ventricular filling occurs in diastole. So at very high heart rates (>180/min) filling may be compromised decreasing cardiac output per minute.

Duration (in seconds) of	In Cardiac Muscle at HR		Skeletal Muscle
	75/min	200/min	
Cardiac cycle	0.80	0.30	-
Systole	0.27	0.16	-
Action potential	0.25	0.15	0.007
Absolute refractory period	0.20	0.13	0.004
Diastole	0.53	0.14	-

- **Because of prolonged action potential,** cardiac muscles cannot contract in response to a second stimulus until near the end of initial contraction. That's why **cardiac muscles cannot be tetanized like skeletal muscles.** The highest rate at which heart can contract is **400/min (theoretically)** but AV node will **not conduct >230 impulses/min** b/o its long refractory period. Hence ventricular rate > 230/min is only seen in **paroxysmal ventricular tachycardia.**
- Exact clinical measurement of **isovolumetric ventricular contraction** is difficult but **simultaneous recordings of ECG, phonocardiogram and carotid pulse can easily measure**

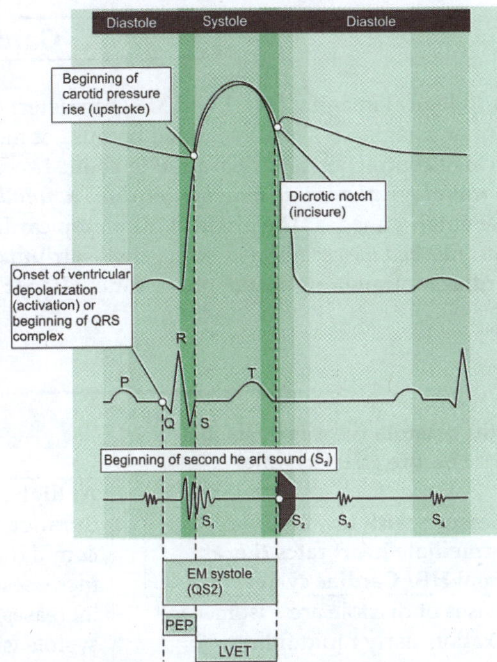

1. **Total Electromechanical systole (Q-S2 interval)**
   It is period **from onset of ventricular depolarization (activation) or QRS complex to the closure of aortic valves, as determined by the onset on second heart sound (S2)**
2. **Pre-ejection Period (PEP)**
   It is difference between QS2 and LVET and represents the **electrical and mechanical events preceding systolic ejection**
3. **Left Ventricular Ejection Time (LVET)**
   It is the period between the **begining of carotid pressure rise to dicrotic notch (incisura)**

- **Normal PEP / LVET ratio** is **0.35;** which increases without change in QS2 when left ventricular function is compromized

Period	Definition	Measured by
Electromechanical systole **(QS_2)**Q	Period from the beginning of QRS complex to the closure of aortic valve (2nd heart sound).	Electrocardiogram (for QRS complex) Phonocardiogram (show the 2nd heart sound.
Left ventricular ejection time (LEVT)	Period from carotid pressure rise to the dichrotic notch	***Carotid transducer***Q (measures carotid pressure rise & dichrotic notch)
Pre- ejection period (PEP)	Time for electrical as well as mechanical events that precede systolic ejection	Is the ***difference between QS_2 and LVET.***Q

❖ PEP/LVET is normally 0.35 seconds. *When left ventricular performance is compromised it increases without a change in QS_2.*

Fourth (Atrial) Heart Sound (S_4)

- It is a ***low pitched presystolic sound which can almost never be heard with a stethoscope (& ear) because of its weakness and very low frequency – usually ≤20 cycles/ second (H_z)***Q. It is caused by ***in thrushing of blood into ventricles (ventricular filling***Q, which initiates vibration) ***when the atria contracts***Q.
- S_4, sometime becomes audible, when atrial pressure is very high or ventricle is stiff (diminished ventricular compliance) increasing the resistance to normal filling. When audible it is best heard *with bell of stethescope, at left ventricular apex in left lateral position* and accentuated by exercise (isotonic or isometric) in the supine position.
- Pathologically S_4 may be seen in
  - Pulmonary stenosis & hypertension (right S_4)
  - Aortic stenosis & systemic hypertension
  - Ischemic heart disease – HOCM – Mitral regurgitation
  - Advanced age (physiological)

Ventricular Extrasystole/ Premature Beat

In abnormal conditions, the His- Purkinje fibers or the myocardial fibers may discharge spontaneously, that result in a beat that occurs before the expected next normal beat & transiently interrupts the cardiac rhythm.

- They have ***bizarrely shaped prolonged QRS***Q because of slow spread of impulse from focus to rest of the ventricle
- The P wave is usually buried in the QRS complex-
- Tendency to be followed by ***compensatory pause***Q because when the normal impulse (of SA node) reaches ventricle, they are still in the refractory period following depolarization from the ectopic focus.
- They do not interrupt the regular discharge of SA node (whereas atrial premature beats interrupt normal rhythm)
- They are ***not strong enough to produce radial pulse.***Q
- Ventricular premature beats, ***in the absence of ischemic heart disease, is usually benign.***Q

Cardiac Motion and Imaging

- Radiological imaging by CT and MRI can detect coronary artery disease in early stage. However, the use of these tools to cardiac imaging is severely limited because of motion artifacts produced by constantly in motion heart completing an entire cycle of contraction and relaxation in about 1 second.
- *So **radiological cardiac imaging*** **requires a *'window'* of *minimum cardiac motion to reduce motion artifacts*** and achieve meaningful images. The phase of minimum cardiac motion is although variable and depends on several factors especially *heart rate and the chamber* (i.e. right /left – atrium or ventricle) *to be specifically imaged*. However, the **phase of minimum cardiac motion (= optimum phase for cardiac & coronary vessel imaging).**

Mid diastole (i.e. diastasis just before atrial systole)

In persons with low / intermediate heart rates (i.e. at normal HR/ Cardiac cycles)

4 phases of diastole are – isometric relaxation, early rapid filling, diastasis and atrial systole.

Late Systole

At high heart rates; because the duration of diastole is shortened & mid diastolic cardiac motion increases as the heart rate increases, whereas the duration of systole is less affected by changes in heart rates.

Phase of Relatively	
Rapid Cardiac Motion	**Minimum Cardiac Motion**
- Early systole - Mid systole - Early diastole (during rapid filling) - Late diastole (atrial systole)	- **Mid diastole (diastasis**[Q]**)** - **Early diastole** (during isovolumetric relaxation) - **Late systole**

Measurement of Cardiac Output

Direct Fick Method

- **Direct Fick method** for measuring cardiac output is based on **oxygen Fick principle** which states that the amount of a substance taken up by any organ (or whole body) per unit of time is equal to arterial level of substance minus the venous level (A-V difference) times of blood flow. However, the arterial blood should be the sole source of substance taken up.
- Cardiac output is determined by measuring the **amount of O_2 consumed by the body in a given period** (such as **O_2 absorbed per minute by lungs in ml/mn) and dividing this by A-V difference (ie arterio-venous O_2 difference) across the lungs** (in ml/lit)

$$\text{Cardiac output (L/min)} = \frac{O_2 \text{ Consumption ml/min}}{\text{Ateriovenous } O_2 \text{ difference } (A_{O_2}\text{-}V_{O_2})} = \frac{O_2 \text{ absorbed/min by lungs (ml/min)}}{\text{Ateriovenous } O_2 \text{ difference across lungs (ml/L of blood)}}$$

- Rate of O_2 absorption is measured by **oxygen meter** measuring the rate of disappearance of O_2 from respired air. A_{O_2} can be measured **from any systemic arterial blood**, where V_{O_2} is measured from **pulmonary artery** (or right ventricle)

Indicator Dilution Method

- **Indicator (dye) dilution method** is based on **Stewart – Hamilton principle** which states that when an innocuous (harmless) dye (indicator or radioactive isotope) that stays in blood stream during the test, is injected into venous system (eg arm vein); the cardiac output is equal to **amount of dye injected divided by its average concentration in arterial blood** after a single heart circulation (determined after extrapolation).
- **Cardiogreen dye** is usually injected as bolus in arm vein. The **log of indicator concentration** in serial arterial samples is plotted against time as the **concentration rises, falls and the rise again indicating recirculation** of dye. Therefore it is necessary to **extrapolate the early down slope of curve to zero point (abscissa)**, giving the time for first passage of indicator through the circulation (**Extrapolated time – concentration curve**). The cardiac output for that period is calculated & then converted to output per minute.
- In **thermodilution technique, cold saline** is used as an indicator because of 2 important advantages (1) *complete innocuous nature of saline, (2) recirculation is not an issue* since cold is dissipated in tissue making repeated determinations easy.
- Through a **double lumen catheter**, *saline is injected into the right atrium* (via smaller arm of catheter) and *temperature change is measured in pulmonary artery*, using a thermistor (via longer side of catheter). The *temperature change is inversely proportional to the extent that the cold saline is diluted by blood* ie the amount of blood flowing through the pulmonary artery.

$$\textbf{Cardiac Flow (F)} = \frac{\text{Amount of indicator injeced(E)}}{\text{Instananeous concentration of indicator in arterial blood i.e. } \int_0^{\alpha} C\,dt}$$

Myocardial (Heart) Contractility

Myocardial contractility has major influence on stoke volume. The relationship between *ventricular stroke volume and end diastolic volume* is called **Frank-Starling curve**. This (length-tension)**curve shifts upwards and to the left** as **contractility** is **increased** (eg in sympathetic stimulation). Wheareas, the curve shifts **downwards and to right when contractility decreases** eg in vagal (parasympathetic stimulation).

Intrinsic Factor	Extrinsic Factor
Length of activation[Q] **= Length – Tension relation in cardiac muscle.** - Most important factor - **Frank- starling law**: "Energy of contraction is proportional to initial **length of cardiac muscle fiber." Length of muscle fiber (preload) is proportionate to end diastolic blood volume (preload)**[Q].	• **Adrenergc neural stimulation / Sympathetic stimulation**[Q] - Inotropic effect is smaller, maximum in atria. It becomes important when the heart is increased as it permits adequate diastolic filling. • **Cardiac rate and rhythm** changes (**force- frequency** relation) eg post extra systolic potentiation d/t increased availability of intracellular Ca^{++}. • **Sympathetic & parasympathetic impulses**[Q]. • Circulating catecholamines • Hypoxia, hypercarbia, acidosis • Digitalis & other inotropic agents

Medullary Centres regulating Blood Pressure

Vasomotor Centre (VMC)

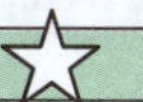

- Collection of glutaminergic *neurons in superficial medullary reticular formation*, known as **C_1 neurons**, serves as pressure area of VMC. Cell bodies of C1 cells lie in *ventrolateral region of upper half of medulla.*
- These neurons are ***spontaneously active day & night, tonically discharging impulses (in rhythmic manner)***[Q] to the heart and blood vessels through **lateral reticulospinal tract**
- These reticulospinal tracts synapse with **preganglionic** neurons of **sympathetic** nervous system located in **intermediolateral grey column** of spinal cord (thoraco lumbar sympathetic out flow)
- **Post ganglionic** sympathetic neuron secrete **nor adrenaline** thereby increasing sympathetic activity and causing *tonic vasoconstrictor & cardioaccelerator activity* resulting in →
  - Vasoconstriction
  - ↑BP
  - ↑Cardiac output
  - ↑Stroke volume
- **Regulation of VMC activity**

1. Baroreceptor reflexes:

Baroreceptors are *stretch receptors* located in *walls of aortic arch & carotid sinus*, they are tonically active & ***exert tonic inhibition of VMC and facilitation of CVC***[Q].

Cardiovagal Centre (CVC)

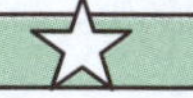

- It refers to **nucleus ambiguous** which lies lateral to VMC (medulary reticular neurons)
- It receives afferents via **Nucleus tractus solitarus (NTS)** & in turn sends parasympathetic impulses to heart via the **vagus**, so cardiovagal centre
- The neurons in CVC ***do not discharge rhythmically (i.e. are not tonically active)***[Q]
- The discharge increases parasympathetic activity there by resulting in →
  - Vasodilation
  - ↓BP
  - ↓Cardiac output
  - ↓ Heart rate

★ A pecularity of sympathetic system, which is not found in parasympathetic system, is the fact that entire thoraco lumbar outflow is always activated as a unit, whereas the parasympathetic stimulation is very discrete, affecting specific muscles or glands.

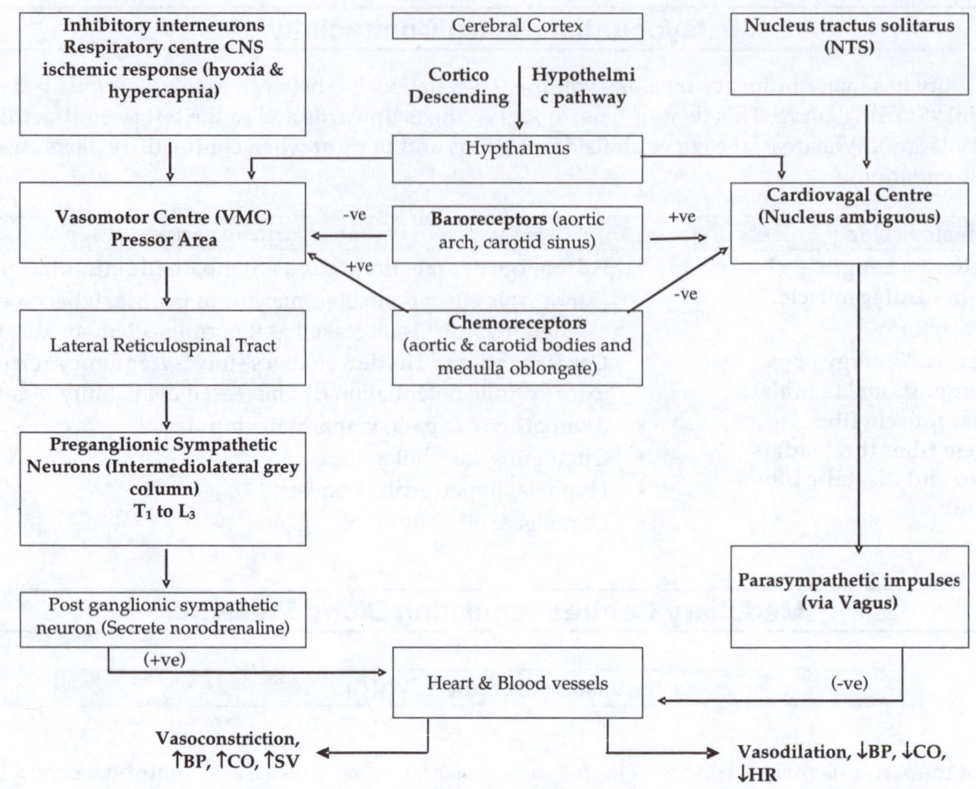

Vasomotor Control ☆

Main control of BP is exerted by a group of neurons in medulla oblongata K/a ***Vasomotor area (center).***

Afferents to vasomotor area

Direct Stimulation
CO_2 Hypoxia
Excitatory inputs
From cortex via hypothalamus From pain pathways and muscles From carotid and aortic chemoreceptors
Inhibitory inputs
From cortex via hypothalamus From lungs From carotid, aortic, and cardiopulmonary baroreceptors

- **Baroreceptors** are *stretch receptors* in the walls of heart & vessels eg *carotid sinus & aortic arch*, walls of atria, pulmonary veins & pulmonary circulation. **Carotid sinus is a small dilation of internal carotid artery** just above the bifurcation of common carotid.
- Receptor are also located in **walls of right and left atrium at the entrance of SVC and IVC** and **pulmonary veins** as well as in **pulmonary circulation**. In **low pressure part of circulation**, these are K/a **Cardiopulmonary receptors**. These are **stimulated by** ***distension or pressure rise in structure*** **(total cardiovascular output)**[Q].

Efferents from vasomotor area

- **Sympathetic outflow:**
  - Neurons that mediate increased sympathetic discharge project to sympathetic preganglionic neurons in *intermedio lateral gray column (IML) of spinal cord*. Cell bodies of these neurons are locate in *rostral ventrolateral medulla (RVLM)!* The excitatory transmitter is glutamate.
  - It causes increase in heart rate (chronotropic effect) & force of cardiac contraction (ionotropic effect), Vasoconstriction, ↑ BP, ↑HR, ↑stroke volume and ↑ cardiac output
- **Parasympathetic outflow:**
  - Neurons of vagal fibers arise in dorsal motor nucleus of vagus & nucleus ambiguous.
  - It causes ***vasodilation, fall in BP, and increase in storage of blood in venous reservoirs, decrease in heart rate and cardiac output***[Q]

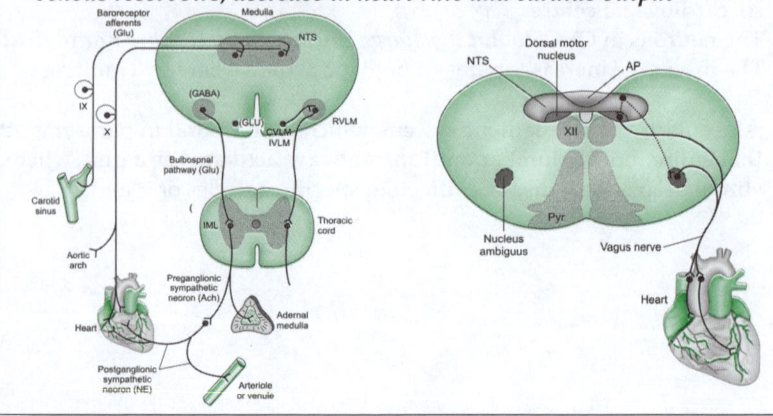

- The afferent from *carotid body* pass through *carotid sinus branch of glossopharyngeal (9th) nerve* and from *aortic arch* through *vagus nerve*. Both are called **buffer nerves.** Most of them end in *nucleus tractus solitarius (NTS)*. Excitatory glutaminergic projections extends from
- NTS to *caudal & intermediate ventrolateral medulla (CVLM & IVLM)*, where they stimulate GABA secreting inhibitory neurons that projects to *rostral ventrolateral medulla (RVLM)*
- NTS to vagal motor neurons in the *dorsal motor nucleus & ambiguous*
- Thus increased baroreceptor discharge inhibits tonic discharge of vasoconstrictor nerves & ***excites vagal innervation, producing – vasodilation, venodilation, a drop in BP, brady cardia and a decrease in cardiac output***[Q].

Cushing's Reflex (Phenomenon)

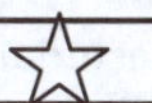

Etiology

- It is a special **CNS ischemic response** that results from **increased intracranial tension** (or increased CSF pressure around the brain in cranial vault).
- Causes of increased ICT may be space occupying lesions such as

1. ***Brain tumor***[Q]
2. Cerebral abscess
3. ***Head trauma***[Q] with associated intra cranial bleeding eg epidural/ subdural/ cerebral-haemorrhage

Pathophysiology

- When the ICT or CSF pressure rises to equal the arterial pressure, it compresses the whole brain as well as the arteries in the brain and cuts off the blood supply to the brain, thereby activating the CNS ischemic response
- Compromized blood supply, local hypoxia & hypercapnia of **RVLM (rostral ventro lateral medulla) neurons or vasomotor area** increases their discharge and evoke Cushing's reaction raising systemic arterial pressure.
- The resultant **rise in systemic arterial pressure** (d/t ischemic stimulation of vasomotor regions in mdeulla) tend to restore the blood flow to medulla, thereby protecting the vital centers of brain from loss of nutrition if ICT rises enough to compress cerebral arteries.
- The rise in BP is **proportional** to increase in intracranial tension (over a considerable range) and causes a **reflex decrease in heart rate via the arterial baroreceptors**. This is why bradycardia rather than tachycardia is characteristically seen in patients with increased ICP (intra cranial pressure)

Effects on Heart

Sympathetic & Parasympathetic Innervation

- ***Vagal (parasympathetic)*** *fibres are mainly distributed to atria* & not much to ventricles. This explains the fact that the *main effect of vagal stimulation is to decrease heart rate* rather than to decrease the strength of heart contraction greatly (which is dependent on ventricle)
- **Sympathetic (noradrenergic)** fibres are distributed to *both atria & ventricle*. So its stimulation has a strong effect on *both heart rate (chronotropic) & force of contraction (ionotropic)*

Denervation

- At rest, there is a moderate amount of tonic discharge in cardiac sympathetic nerves, whereas vagal tone (tonic discharge) is of good amount.
- So when **vagi are cut** (or *parasympatholytic drug eg atropine is given)* the normal resting ***heart rate rises (from 70) to 150-180 beats/min due to unopposed sympathetic tone.***[Q]
- If both noradrenergic & cholinergic systems are blocked, the heart rate is ~100 beats / min.

Exercise

- Cardiac muscle has the unique property of contracting & repolarizing faster when the heart rate is high
- Cardiac muscle cannot be tetanized as it has prolonged action potential during which muscle is refractory & will not contract in response to second stimulus until near the end of initial contraction.
- The duration ***of systole is much more fixed than that of diastole and when the heart rate is increased (eg. in exercise), diastole is shortened to a much greater degree.***[Q]

Duration of	At HR 75/min	At HR 200/min
Cardiac cycle	0.80	0.30
Systole	0.27	0.16
Diastole	0.53	0.14
Action potential	0.25	0.15
Absolute refractory period	0.20	0.13
Relative refractory period	0.05	0.02

Effects of Assuming Supine (Lying down) Posture

Cerebral blood flow

Auto regulated extremely well & **maintained at normal levels** between arterial pressure limits of 60-140 mmHg

Pulmonary blood flow

- In **standing** posture ***apex is less perfused than base***[Q]
- **On lying down** blood ***flow to lung apex increases***[Q]

Cardiovascular system

	Onlying	On standing
- **Stroke volume** **Cardiac output** - **Venous return** - Central blood pool - **Central venous pressure** - **Arterial BP** - Abdominal & limb flow	Increase	Decrease
- **Heart rate** - Peripheral venous pooling - **Total peripheral resistance** - Abdominal & limb resistance - Small vein pressure	Decrease	Increase

★ Gravity has marked effect on pulmonary circulation. In **upright** position in ***upper parts of lung (apex) the blood flow is lesser than the base***[Q]. In middle portion & upper lung blood flow is determined by *pulmonary artery – alveolar pressure difference,* and pulmonary veins whatever amount of blood the constrictions (produced by alveolar pressure) lets flow into them (**Water fall effect**). In lower lung alveolar pressure is lower than pressure in all parts of pulmonary circulation, so blood flow is determined by *pulmonary artery – pulmonary vein pressure.* On lying down blood flow to lung apex increases

★ On standing, at head level arterial and jugular venous pressure falls 20-40 mmHg and 5-8 mmHg respectively reducing the drop in perfusion pressure (arterial – venous pressure). Cerebral vascular resistance is reduced (d/t ↓JVP l/t ↓ICP that presses the vessels). There is only ***20% decrease in cerebral blood flow***[Q] d/t autoregulatory mechanism activated by ↑PCO_2 (partial pressure of CO_2), and ↓in pH and PO_2. However, the amount of O_2 extracted increases and so the cerebral O_2 consumption is about the same in supine & upright position. (Ganong).

★ Venous return must equal cardiac output overtime as vascular system is a closed circuit.

★ ***Cerebral blood flow is autoregulated extremely well without significant change in cerebral blood flow between mean, arterial pressure limits of 60- 140 mmHg***[Q] (Guyton).

Sequence of events on Assumption of Erect Posture
Pooling of blood in lower extremity ↓ Insufficient return of blood through inferior venacava (↓ ***in central venous pressure***)[Q] ↓ Reduced preload ↓ ↓Stroke volume ↓ ↓Cardiac output

Effect on Cardiovascular system	
Arterial blood pressure	↓ es
Central venous pressure	↓es[Q]
Abdominal & limb flow	↓ es by 25%
Cardiac output	↓es by 25%[Q]
Stroke volume	***↓es by 40%***[Q]
Heart rate	↑ es

Compensatory Mechanism

The reduced C.O together with decreased arterial pressure in the brain (d/t force of gravity) can cause cerebral ischemia. This can cause syncope. This is prevented by the following mechanism

As the C.O falls

BP falls

↓

Stretching on the baroreceptor of Aortic sinus decreases

↓

Vosomotor center active (Normally firing from Aortic & carotid baroreceptor keeps the V.M.C inhibited)

↓

Sympathetic system activated

↓

Tachycardia + Vasoconstriction
(***↑Heart rate & ↑peripheral resistance***)[Q]

↓

B.P restored (syncope avoided)

Diastolic Pressure

- **Systolic pressure** is peak pressure reached during systole, similarly, **diastolic pressure** refers to lowest pressure during diastole
- ***Elsticity of aorta and large arteries is mainly responsible for origin & maintenance of diastolic pressure (by wind kessel elastic recoil effect)***[Q]. Because the elasticity is

Higher in younger subjects	**Lower in old persons**
- Diastolic pressure is maintained - Pulse pressure is narrow	- Diastolic pressure is decreased - Pulse pressure is widened

Measures of Venous Return & Degree of Filling of Veins

Mean Circulatory Filling Pressure (MCFP)

- It is the ***pressure that would exist every where in the circulation if the heart pumping is stopped***[Q] (by shocking with electricity to cause VF or in any other way), and the pressure is allowed to equilibrate through out the system.
- The normal value is **7 mm Hg** at (5 lit **blood volume)**. An increase in **Blood volume** increases the MCFP, while hypovolaemia (as in dehydration & haemorrhage) decreases it
- At **4 litre** blood volume, the MCFP is close to 'O' and this volume is k/a **unstressed volume of circulation**. The MCFP increases almost linearly with increase in volumes
- **Strong sympathetic stimulation** constricts all systemic blood vessels, larger pulmonary vessels & even chambers of heart, therefore, decreasing the capacity of system. So that at each level of blood volume MCFP is increased. At normal blood volume maximal sympathetic *stimulation & inhibition* cause MCFP to rise / decrease to *17 mm Hg & 4 mm Hg* respectively.

Mean Systemic Filling Pressure (MSFP)

- It is slightly different from the MCFP. It is the *pressure measured every where in the systemic circulation after blood flow has been stopped by* **clamping the large blood vessels at the heart**, so that the pressure in the systemic circulation can be measured **indepently from** those in **pulmonary circulation**.
- It is *almost impossible to measure* in living animals. Although it is ***important pressure for determining venous return***[Q]
- ***It is almost always nearly equal to MCFP***[Q] because the pulmonary circulation has only 1/10 as much blood & < 1/8 as much capacitance as the systemic circulation.
- The normal MSFP is **7 mmHg** venous return curves demonstrate that *greater the MSFP* (eg 14), the *greater the tightness* with which circulatory system is filled & the more the venous return curve shifts *upward & to the right*. And vice versa. In other words, the greater the system is filled the easier it is for blood to flow into the heart. The less the filling, the more difficult it is for blood to flow into heart.

Blood Pressure

Spurious high

Conditions where more pressure is required in the cuff to obliterate the artery

- ***Small cuff***[Q]
- ***Obesity***[Q]
- ***Thick calcified vessels***[Q]

Falsely low

Auscultatory gap: During measuring of BP (in hypertensive individuals) the *sound of Korotkoff* sometimes disappear at pressure well above the diastolic pressure, then reappears at lower pressure *(Auscultatory gap)* to again disappear at the diastole.

To avoid it, palpatory method of cuff is used until the radial pulse is obliterated.

Methods of Measurement of BP

Direct Intraarterial method

- The *artery is catheterized* & connected to a mercury manometer or pressure transducer.
- ***Measures accurate BP***[Q]

Indirect

- By **sphygnomanometer** (External pressure required to cause occlusion of blood flow, indicates the pressure inside the vessels)
- Giver ***falsely high reading***[Q]: the pressure induced in the cuff, is dissipated in the tissue of arm (or thigh), so at a pressure equal to arterial pressure, the arteries fail to close. Thus pressure has to be raised further for that.

★ ***Korotkoff sound is d/t arterial turbulence.***[Q]

BP & VR Measurement

The overall blood flow in circulation of adult at rest is about 5 liter/min which equals to cardiac output because it is the amount of blood pumped by heart per unit time. So

Blood pressure = Cardiac output × peripheral resistance[Q] or Blood flow (Q) × resistance (R)	
Venous return[Q] **=** $\frac{MSFP - RAP}{RVR}$	MSFP = Mean systemic filling pressure RAP = Right atrial pressure RVR = Resistance to venous return

Baroreceptors

Stretch receptors in the walls of the heart & blood vessels (in adventitia)

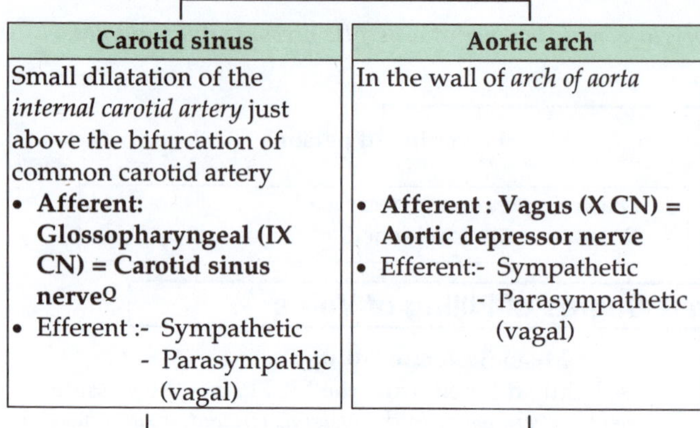

Carotid sinus	Aortic arch
Small dilatation of the *internal carotid artery* just above the bifurcation of common carotid artery • **Afferent: Glossopharyngeal (IX CN) = Carotid sinus nerve**[Q] • Efferent :- Sympathetic - Parasympathetic (vagal)	In the wall of *arch of aorta* • **Afferent : Vagus (X CN) = Aortic depressor nerve** • Efferent:- Sympathetic - Parasympathetic (vagal)

Most afferent fibers reach **nucleus of tractus solitarius (NTS)** and secrete excitatory neurotransmitter **glutamate. Excitatory** (glutamate) projections from NTS extend to **vagal motor neurons** in **nucleus ambiguus** and **dorsal motor nucleus.** Excitatory projections from NTS also reach to **CVLM (caudal ventrolateral medulla)** where they stimulate GABA secreting inhibitory neurons inhibiting **RVLM** (rostral ventrolateral medulla) and **ultimately sympathetic activity**. So ***baroreceptor stimulation, stimulates parasympathetic and decreases sympathetic activity***[Q].

Stimulation of Baroreceptors

↑BP → Baroreceptors stimulated

Inhibits Vasomotor center (↓ Sympathetic activity) | **Vagal (Parasympathetic) stimulation**

✶ Reverse occurs when BP decreases

- Vasodilation - **↓BP (Hypotension)**[Q]
- Venodilation - ***Bradycardia***[Q]
- ↓CO (cardiac output)

- **When carotid sinus nerve is sectioned.** Loss of inhibitory impulse from carotid sinus nerve → *Medullary vasomotor center activated* → ↑ sympathetic discharge → Vasoconstriction (↑BP), ↑HR & ↑ CO.
- The baroreceptors do not fire when mean BP *is below 30 mm Hg* (fire maximally at mean BP of *150 mm Hg*). Carotid sinus nerve and vagal fibres from aortic arch commonly called ***Buffer nerves.***
- *Severing only carotid sinus nerve will not lead to decrease in BP because aortic arch baroreceptors are still functional. If both are severed the BP rise to more than 200-300 mm Hg.*

Effects of Acceleration

- The effects of gravity on the circulation are multiplied during acceleration or deceleration.
- Force acting on the body as a result of acceleration is commonly expressed in 'g' units, 1'g' being the force of gravity on the earth's surface.

Positive 'g' (Black outs)	Negative 'g' (Red outs)
• Is the force due to acceleration acting in the long axis of body from head to foot • During exposure to positive 'g' blood is thrown into lower part of the body, and consequently there is decrease in cerebral arterial pressure.	• Is the force due to acceleration acting in the long axis of body in opposite direction. • During exposure to negative 'g' blood pools into the upper part of the body, and consequently there is an increase in cerebral arterial pressure.
Positive 'g' creates a tendency for	**Negative 'g' creates a tendency for**
• Decreased cardiac output • Decreased cerebral arterial pressure • Black out and unconsciousness	• Increased cardiac output • Increased cerebral arterial pressure - intense congestion of head / neck vessels - echymosis around eyes - severe throbbing head ache • 'Red out' and mental confusion

During Exposure to Positive 'G'

- Arterial pressure in the head is reduced, but so are venous pressure and intracranial pressure and this reduces the decrease in arterial blood flow that would otherwise occur.
- Cardiac output is maintained for a time because blood is drawn from the pulmonary venous reservoir and because the force of cardiac contractions is increased.
- At accelerations more than '5g' however vision fails (black outs) and unconsciousness follows almost immediately.

Effects of Gravity (G)

Positive G	Negative G
- ***Blood is centrifuged toward the lower limbs***[Q] so the pressure in the lower limbs increases - Cardiac output decreases - ***Black out of vision*** [Q] occurs	- ***Blood is centrifuged towards the head***[Q] so cerebral blood pressure rises. - ***Cardiac out put increases***[Q] - *Red out occurs*

Negative G: is a state of weightlessness, it occurs when airplane descends very rapidly

Endothelins

- This 21 aminoacid polypeptide structurally resembles sarafotoxins (b) found in venom of Israeli burrowing asp, snake. It is of 3 types endothelin 1 (ET1), endothelin 2 (ET2), & endothelin 3 (ET3); all encoded by a different gene.
- **Endothelin 1 *produced in endothelial cells is one of the most potent vasoconstrictor*[Q].**

Endothelin 1 gene ⟶ Big endothelin 1 (39 aminoacid prohormone of only 1% activity) $\xrightarrow[Trp-Val\ bond\ clevage]{endothelin\ converting\ enzyme\ (ECE)} E.T.1$

- 2 types of endothelin receptors, both of which are coupled to *phosphotipase* C via G proteins are ET_A an ET_B. The *ET_A receptor* is specific for endothelin 1 and mediates vasoconstriction
- *ET_B receptor* responds to all *three endothelins* & is coupled to Gi. It may mediate *vasodilation and developmental effects.*

Secretion

Big ET 1 & ET1 are secreted in blood only in small amounts, and mostly they are secreted into the media of blood vessels and act in a paracrine fashion to regulate vascular tone. ET1 is not stored in secretory granules. Factors regulating its secretion are

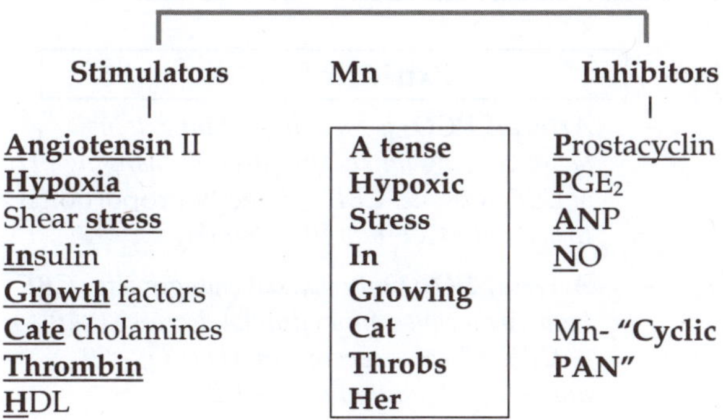

Function

- *ET1 is found in* endothelial cells, brain & kidney. *ET –2 is mainly produced in* kidney & intestine. *ET3 is found in* brain (high conc), blood, kidney and gastrointestinal tract.
- *Endothelins produced by both* astrocytes & neuron *are abundant in brain* in early life. *They are found dorsal root ganglia, ventral horn cell, cortex, hypothalmus, & cerebellar purkinje cells. They* **regulate transport across blood brain barrier**[Q].
- *Endothelin produces* **mesengial cell mediated decrease in GFR (glomerular filteration rate)**[Q].
- *It plays a role in* closing ductus arteriosus at birth.
- ***ET1** is primarily a* **paracrine regulator of vascular tone**[Q]. *It is* **vasoconstrictor, bronchoconstictor, ionotroic (cardiac stimulant)**[Q], *which stimulates aldosterone secretion & atrial natriuretic peptide release.*
- *ET1 is implicated in pathogenesis of* congestive heart failure, myocardial infarction, coronary vasospasm and hypertension. *Deletion of both alleles of ET1 gene results in craniofacial abnormalities, Hirschsprung's disease (megacolon) & death d/t respiratory failure at birth.*

Fluid Filtration Across Capillaries

Rate of filtration along a capillary depends on *starling forces. i.e.,*

- **Hydrostatic pressure gradient** (hydrostatic pressure in capillary minus hydrostatic pressure in interstitial fluid)
- **Capillary (hydrostatic) pressure (Pc)** tends to force fluid *outward* through capillary membrane
- **Interstitial fluid (hydrostatic) pressure (Pi)** tends to force fluid *inwards* through capillary membrane when Pi is *positive* but *outward* when Pi is *negative*

- **Osmotic pressure gradient** (colloid osmotic pressure of plasma minus colloid osmotic pressure of interstitial fluid.)
- **Capilary plasma colloid osmotic pressure (π_C)** tends to cause osmosis of fluid *inward* through capillary membrane
- **Interstitial fluid colloid osmotic pressure (π_i)** tends to cause osmosis of fluid *outward* through the capillary membrane.

If the sum of these forces, the **net filtration pressure (NFP) is positive (+),** there will be *fluid filtration (outward movement)* from capillaries. And if NFP is *negative (-ve),* there will be net fluid absorption from interstitial space into capillaries (inward movement). At arteriolar end of capillary, NFP is +ve & at venular end, it is –ve.

NFP = Hydrostatic pressure gradient – Osmotic pressure gradient
NFP = (Pc – Pi) – $(\pi_c - \pi_i)$
NFP = $P_c - P_i - \pi_c + \pi_i$

↓

Rate of fluid filteration is also dependent on number & size of pore in each capillary as well as number of capillaries in which blood is flowing. These factors are expressed as **capillary filteration coefficient (K_f).**
Fluid movement / Filteration = $K_f \times NFP$

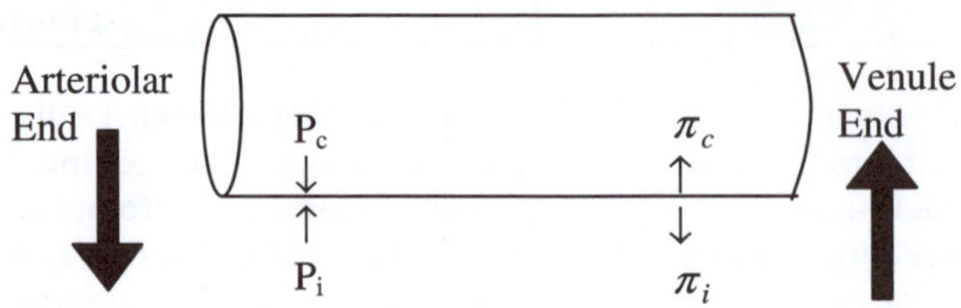

Factors Regulating Cerebral Blood Flow (CBF)

Intrinsic factors

- **Cerebral metabolism rate**[Q] *proportionally increase CBF*
- ***Cerebral perfusion pressure (CPP)***
  CPP = Mean arterial pressure (MAP) – Intracranial pressure (ICP) or central venous pressure (CVP), which ever is greater. CPP is primarily dependant on MAP (or BP) as ICP is usually <10 mmHg. CPP is normally 80-100 mmHg. Autoregulation maintains a steady CBP as CPP may vary between 60-160 mmHg. Decrease in CPP cause cerebral vasodilation, & elevation results in vasoconstriction.
- *Blood viscosity fall l/t rise in CBF & vice versa*
- ***Blood viscosity** fall l/t rise in CBF & vice versa*
- ***Autonomic system***
- ***Substance released from astrocytes***

Extrinsic factors

- ***Arterial PCO_2** is most important extrinsic factor causing immediate effect by changing pH of CSF & tissue. CBF is* directly proportional *to arterial PCO_2 b/w 20-80 mmHg.*
- ***Arterial PO_2**: Only marked changes alter CBF Hyperoxia cause only minimal decrease (~10%) in CBP, whereas severe hypoxia (PO_2 <50 mmHg) profoundly increase CBF*
- ***Temperature:** Hypothermia of 1°C decreases CBF 5-7% whereas pyrexia has reverse effect.*

Arteriovenous Anastomosis (Shunt Vessels)

- Shunt vessels are ***short muscular vessels that connect arterioles and venules, by passing the capillaries***[Q].
- Like other vascular smooth muscles the ***shunt vessels are under the control of sympathetic nervous system (& receive sympathetic innervation)***[Q]
- **Uneven distribution** : shunt vessels are mainly concentrated in tissue with a small surface area / volume ratio eg fingers, toes, ears, & nose.
- Shunt vessels are found in skin and nasal mucosa especially in
  - Hands : Palm & fingers
  - Feet : Sole & toes
  - Face : Ear, Nose & lips
- **No nutritive only thermoregulatory function**: Nutrition is provided by capillaries since capillaries deliver O_2 to tissues. Because shunt vessels bypass capillaries, these have **no nutritive function**.
  However shunt vessel have **important role in thermoregulation**. These provide an important *site of body heat transfer* between skin & blood stream. By dilating in cold conditions and directing large volumes of blood through these vessels, it provides a ***valuble mechanism to prevent tissue freezing and cold damage to the extermilies***[Q]

Laminar (Streamline) Flow

- A **streamline flow** is also K/a **laminar flow** because it moves in layers (or lamina). So a dye carefully introduced into a given lamina (layer) remain in that lamina as the fluid moves longitudinally along the tube.
- In laminar flow the layer touching the wall of tube adheres to it and hardly moves b/o friction, while the concentric layer or lamina next to it shear/slide against this motionless layer with less friction. In this way the inner lamina moves faster than laminae on their outside with the result that the portion of **fluid at the center moves fastest**. This is why the shape of progressing front is **parabola.**
- The **velocity at the center** of stream (in stream line flow) **is maximal** and equal to twice the mean velocity of flow across the entire cross section of the tube. Flow of blood in vessels is normally **laminar (stream line),** which means the layer in the center of stream has highest velocity & peripheral layer (near blood vessel wall) has lowest. Streamline flow is silent. Therefore no sounds are heard with stethoscope in normal arteries.
- **Average velocity of flow** is inversely proportional to the total cross section area of that vessel. Therefore the average velocity of blood is high (33 cm/s) in aorta (CS 2.5 cm^2), **declines steadily in smaller vessels** and is lowest in the capillaries (0.3 mm/s), which have 1000 times the total cross sectional area of aorta (i.e. 2500 cm^2).
- The average velocity of blood flow increases again in veins and is relatively high in venacava, although not so high as in the aorta. ***So the cause of laminar flow in small vessels is large area of cross section and less average velocity***[Q].

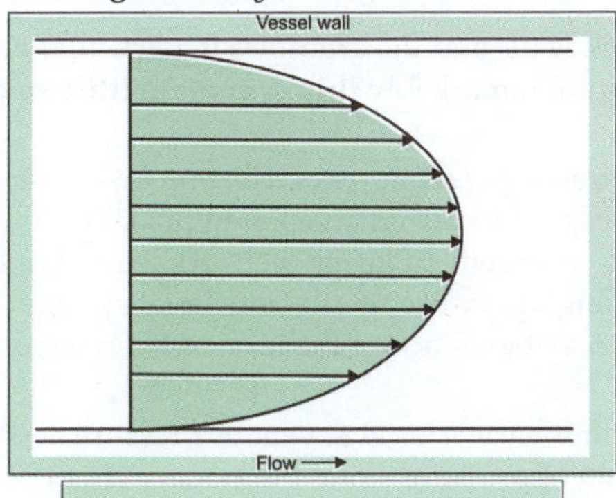

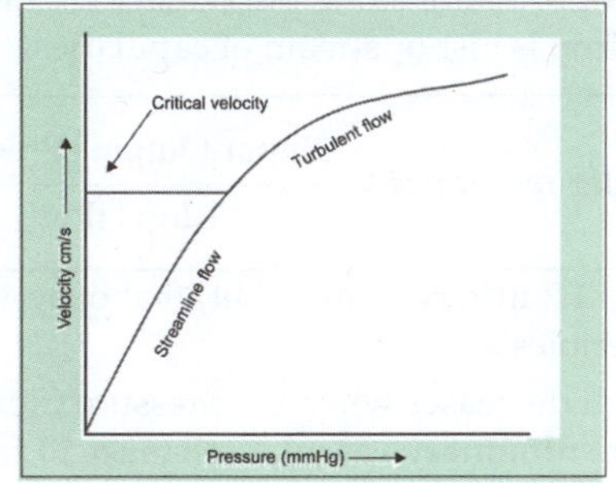

Turbulence

- **Turbulent flow** is a *chaotic flow* with *irregular motions* and *flows in all directions;* it forms *eddies or whirlpools* and fluid elements *do not remain confined to definite lamina,* but *rapid, radial mixing occurs.*
- Turbulent flow offers more resistance than laminar flow; so greater pressure is required to force a given flow of fluid through the same tube when the flow is turbulent than when it is laminar. In turbulent flow, pressure drop is approximately proportional to the square of flow rate whereas in laminar flow, the pressure drop is proportional to the square of flow rate whereas in laminar flow, the pressure drop is proportional to the first power of the flow rate. So to produce same flow a pump like heart must do considerably more work if turbulence develops.
- Laminar flow occurs at velocities upto *critical velocity,* at or above which the flow becomes turbulent, and creates sound. Turbulent flow accounts for development of **heart sounds, murmurs** a/w valvular heart disease, **Korotkov sounds** heard during the measurement of arterial blood pressure, **bruits** heard over arteries constricted by atherosclerotic phaque and **functional cardiac murmurs** heard in patients with *hyper dynamic circulation (as thyrotoxicosis & severe chronic anemia).*
- Turbulence is more common in anemia because of **reduced viscosity** and **high flow velocities** a/w high cardiac output.
- Turbulence is usually accompanied by **audible vibrations. Blood clots** and **thrombi** are more likely to develop in turbulent flow than in **laminarflow.**

Critical Velocity

Critical Velocity (Vc) at which turbulence occurs is **proportional** to the **viscosity** (η) of fluid, but **inversely proportional** to the **density** of fluid (ρ) and **radius** of tube (r) i.e

$$Vc = \frac{K\eta}{\rho r}$$

Probability of Turbulence 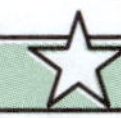

- Probability of turbulence is expressed by **Reynolds number** (i.e. ratio of inertia to viscous forces)

$$\text{Reynolds number (Re)} = \frac{\rho DV}{\eta}$$

ρ = density of fluid ; D = diameter of vessel
V = velocity of flow ; η = Viscosity of fluid

- ***The higher the value of Re, the greater the probability of turbulence***[Q]***. If Re is < 2000, the flow is usually not turbulent. When Re > 3000, turbulence is almost always present***[Q]. For RE / NR between 2000 and 3000, the flow will be transitional between laminar and turbulent.
- So ***high fluid densities, large tube diameters, high flow velocities and low fluid viscosity predispose to turbulence***[Q]. Constriction of arteries increases velocity of blood flow and thus produces turbulence. In addition to these, ***abrupt variations in tube dimensions or irregularties*** in the tube walls may produce turbulence.
- Re for most biological fluids including blood is **1000.** Laminar flow is disturbed at branching of arteries and turbulence may be produced because at the sites of branching Re > 200-400 (instead of >3000) can cause turbulence.

Pulmonary Circulation

- Pulmonary circulation begins with **main pulmonary artery**, which receives the **mixed venous (deoxygenated) blood** pumped by the *right ventricle*. Pulmonary arteries branch and accompany the airways as far as terminal bronchioles. Beyond that they break up to supply the ***capillary bed*** which lies in walls of alveoli, oxygenate blood and convey this oxygenated blood to small **pulmonary veins** that run *between the lobules* and eventually unite to form the **4 large veins** which drain into the **left atrium**. Vessels can be divided into.

Alveolar vessels (i.e. **pulmonary capillaries** & slightly larger vessels in the corner of alveolar walls) are exposed to alveolar pressure (i.e. very close to atmospheric pressure) as they are virtually surrounded be gas. The pressure difference b/w inside & outside of capillary is called **transmural pressure**. When alveolar (out side) pressure rises above the pressure inside, the capillaries collapse.

Extra-alveolar vessels (i.e. all the arteries and veins that run through the lung parenchyma) are exposed to pressure *considerably less than alveolar pressure* (even less than intraplural pressure). Their caliber is remarkably affected by lung volume because this determines the expanding pull of parenchyma on their walls; and are *pulled open by radial traction of surrounding parenchyma*. The very large vessels near the hilum that are outside the lung parenchyma are exposed to intrapleural pressure.

- With a surface area of 70-80 m^2 which is nearly as large as alveolar surface area, the **pulmonary capillary bed** is the **largest** vascular bed in body. The network of capillary is so rich that it is considered as *a sheet of flowing blood interrupted* in places *by small vertical posts*, rather like an under ground parking.
- The **pressures in the pulmonary circulation is very pulsatile and remarkably low (mean, systolic & diastolic pressures** in main pulmonary artery are **15, 25 & 8 mmHg**, respectively) whereas the mean pressure in aorta is 100 mmHg – about **6 times** more than in the pulmonary artery. The pressures in the right & left atriums are 2 and 5 mmHg that are not very dissimilar. So the pressure differences, from inlet to outlet in circulations are

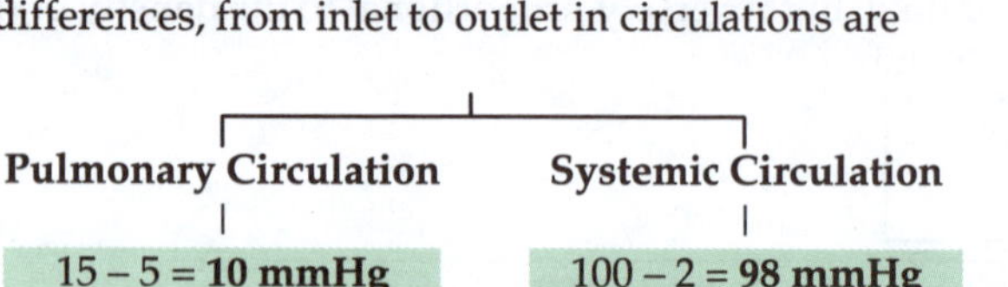

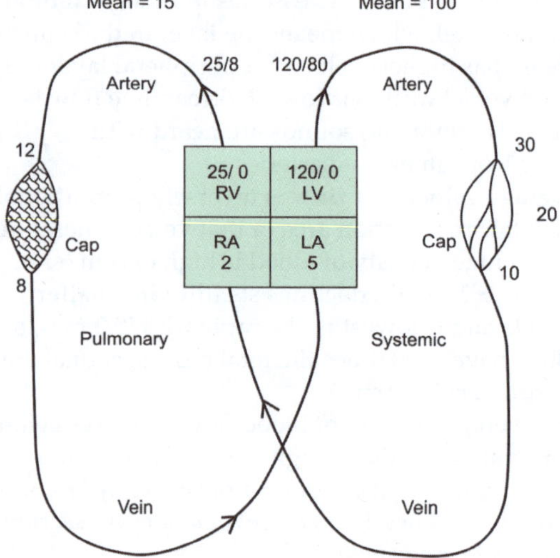

- In striking contrast to the systemic circulation, where the arteries have thick walls and the arterioles in particular have abundant smooth muscles, the walls of **pulmonary artery** and its branches are remarkably **thin** & **contain little** smooth muscle (so that they are easily mistaken for veins)
- The *lung has to accept whole of the cardiac output at all times*, therefore it requires *stretchable arteries with thin (less muscular) walls*. Whereas, it is *not concerned with directing blood from one region to another* (except in localized alveolar hypoxia) so its *arterial pressure is as low as is consistent with lifting blood to the top of lung (only)*. This arrangement keeps the work load of right heart as little as is feasible for efficient gas exchange to occur in the lung. Similarly high pressure muscular arterial systemic circulation help to regulate the adequate supply of blood to organs which may be for above the level of heart (eg outstretched arm).
- The pressure within pulmonary capillaries lies about half way between pulmonary arterial & venous pressure and *varies considerably throughut the lung d/t hydrostatic effects*. However the distribution of pressure along pulmonary circulation is far **more symmetrical** than in systemic circulation, where most of the pressure drop is just upstream of capillaries.

$$\text{Vascular resistance} = \frac{(\text{Input-Output})\,\text{Pressure}}{\text{Blood flow}}$$

- The total pressure drop in pulmonary circulation from pulmonary artery to left atrium is only **10 mmHg**, against about **100 mmHg** for systemic circulation (b/w aorta & right atrium). As the blood flow through the two circulations is virtually same (~ 6 liters / min), ***so the pulmonary vascular resistance is only one tenth***Q = [(15 – 5) /6 = 1.7 mm Hg x min / lit] that of systemic circulation, where the high resistance is largely caused by very muscular arterioles.
- Extraordinarily **(10 times) smaller** normal pulmonary vascular resistance even decreases when the pressure (flow) within it rises i.e. **an increase in either pulmonary venous or arterial pressure causes pulmonary vascular rsistance to fall**. This decrease in pulmonary vascular resistance eg during exercise occurs d/t passive process of

Recruitment	Distension
- Under normal resting conditions of cardiac output, some pulmonary capillaries are either closed or open but with no blood flow (i.e. they remain unperfused). - As the cardiac output is increased and pulmonary blood flow & pressure begins to rise, these previously closed / unperfused capillaries begins to open. - This recruitment establishes new parallel pathways for blood flow, thus **lowering the overall pulmonary vascular resistance.** - Recruitment is a passive process of increasing the number of open parallel capillaries that were previously not utilized in the resting state. This is the chief mechanism of fall in pulmonary vascular resistance that occur as the **pulmonary artery pressure is raised from low levels.**	- Under normal resting conditions of cardiac output, perfused pulmonary capillaries are not distended to their maximum caliber /diameter. - As the cardiac output & pulmonary blood flow increases to much higher level or when the lungs fill with blood, as it does in left heart failure, which is a/w elevated left atrial pressure the internal pressure the internal pressure or transmural pressure gradient of already perfused/open pulmonary blood vessel increases causing distension of vessels. - **Distension** is chiefly a **passive** change in shape of capillaries from near flattened to more circular. This **increase in caliber, widening** or distension causes fall in pulmonary vascular resistance and is the predominant mechanism at relatively **high vascular pressure.**

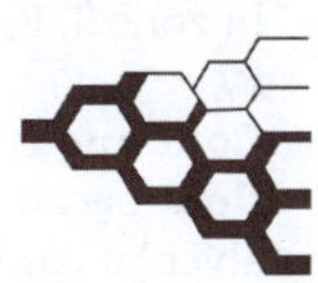

Normal

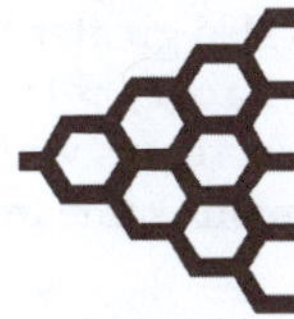

Recruitment

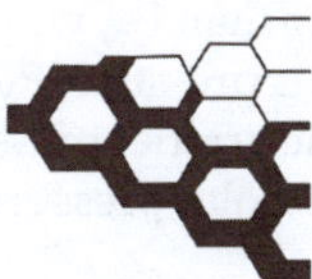

Distension

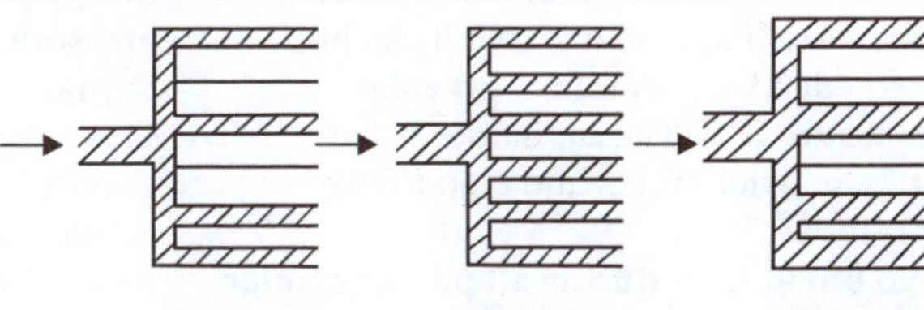

- Passive processes of recruitment and distension lower pulmonary vascular resistance (and maintain pulmonary artery pressure) over a wide range of cardiac output. **Lung volume** also determine the **pulmonary vascular resistance** (which **increases both at high and low lung volumes**). Lung collapse (low lung volume) increases pulmonary vascular resistance b/o reduced caliber/collapse of extra alveolar vessels. Whereas, vascular resistance increases with large lung inflations (large lung volumes) because of reduced caliber of capillaries d/t stretching and thinning of alveolar walls.
- Pulmonary vascular resistance increases with **alveolar hypoxia** (d/t constriction of small pulmonary arteries) and **drugs causing contractionof smooth muscle of extra alveolar vessels** (eg serotonin, histamine and norepinephrine). Whereas acetylcholine & isoproterenol relax smooth muscle in pulmonary circulation.
- Because pulmonary circulation is **low pressure, low resistance system**, it is **influenced by gravity much more** dramatically than the systemic circulation is. For every **1 cm** increase in height above the heart, there is **0.74 mmHg** decrease in hydrostatic pressure. This effect of gravity on blood flow affects **arteries and veins equally**. This is why in upright position blood flow increases from apex of lung to the base, where it is greatest. And in supine position it is less in anterior (upper most) and greater in posterior (lower) regions.
- **The blood volume in the lungs is *about 450 ml, 9% of total blood volume.* 70ml in pulmonary capillaries & remainder is divided equally b/w arteries and veins.** *Blood flowing to the lungs through bronchial arteries* is 1-2% of total cardiac output. Pulmonary resistance is *about one- seventh* of systemic vascular resistance. In the lung the **capillary volume** at rest is **70ml** which may approach 200ml during exercise.
- Pulmonary capillary pressure is ~ *10 mmHg* & oncotic pressure is *25 mHg*, so an ***inward – directed pressure gradient of about 15 mmHg***[Q] keeps the alveoli free of all but a thin film of fluid. Mean pressure is *about 15 mm* Hg (in systemic 90 mm Hg)
- ***Ventilation / perfusion ratio for whole lung at rest is 0.8***[Q] ***(4.2 L/min ventilation/ 5.5 L/min blood flow). Ventilation as well as perfusion declines in a linear fashion from the base to apex of the lungs***[Q] ***in upright position. So, ventilation as well as perfusion is more in lower lobes***[Q]***. However, ventilation / perfusion ratios are high in upper portions of lung (highest at apex)***[Q], which accounts for the predilection of tuberculosis in this area.
- On lying down, pulmonary blood volume increases by upto 400 ml, which is discharged into general circulation when the person stands up. This shift ***decreases vital capacity in supine position***[Q] & is responsible for the occurrence of orthopenia in heart failure.
- ***Pulmonary small arteries & arterioles constrict in response to hypoxia***[Q] (especially when O2 conc. falls below 70% of normal or <73 mm Hg PO_2). This is ***opposite to the effect observed in systemic vessels***[Q], which dilate rather than constrict in response to low O_2 levels. This distributes blood flow where it is most effective (i.e., in most aerated areas). So the pulmonary blood is distributed in proportion to their alveolar oxygen pressures. The vasoconstriction occur *d/t*

presence of K^+ gated channels in pulmonary vessels.

- Gravity has a marked effect. So at **apex there** is ***lower intravascular pressure, less blood flow, less ventilation and perfusion***Q and greater transmural pressure, more negative intrapleural pressure and larger alveoli as compared to base
- ***Pulmonary veins are collapsed in the upper & middle lung lobes. They are distended in the lower lobes.***Q This is because of effect of gravity. There is marked pressure gradient in the pulmonary arteries (/veins) from the top to the bottom of lungs (maximum arterial pressure in the base of lung). In the upper & middle lobes the pressure in the pulmonary veins is below the atmospheric pressure in the alveoli, this causes these veins to collapse. And pressure in the basal lobes is high enough to keep them distended.
- 30 cm of lung height l/t *23 mm Hg pressure* difference b/w highest & lowest points of lung, about *15 mmHg* of which is *above* the heart and *8 below i.e.*, pulmonary artery pressure is 15 mm Hg lower in uppermost & *8 mmHg* higher in lowermost portions of lung than the PAP at level of heart
- The capillaries in alveolar wall are distended by blood pressure inside them and compressed by alveolar air pressure on their out sides. This results in three lung zones

Zone 1 : No Blood flow

- It is a zone where **pulmonary arterial pressure (Pa)** is so low that it can be **exceeded by pulmonary alveolar pressure (P_A)**. The capillaries collapse b/o greater external P_A, and blood flow ceases.
- **No blood flow during all part of cardiac cycle** because capillary pressure is < alveolar air pressure during whole cardiac cycle.
- No gas exchange takes place and become ***part of physiological (alveolar) dead space***Q
- Under normal conditions this zone does not exist; however during **positive pressure mechanical ventilation** (when P_A increases) and in **severe blood loss** (when Pa decreases sufficiently) zone 1 can be established.

Zone 2 : Intermittent Blood flow

- In **upper third of lung** (or zone 2), pulmonary arterial pressure is greater than P_A, which is also greater than pulmonary venous pressure (P_V) i.e. **Pa > P_A > P_V**. This is because the arterial pressure increases with gravity but the alveolar pressure remains same in whole lung.
- **Intermittent blood flow** occurring only during pulmonary arterial pressure peaks in systole
- Systolic arterial pressure > alveolar air pressure; but diastolic arterial pressure < alveolar air pressure
- So the blood flow is determined by the difference b/w arterial and alveolar pressure not the usual arterial venous pressure difference. Indeed venous pressure has no influence on flow unless it exceeds P_A.
- Because P_A > P_V, it partically collapses capillaries causing **damming / Starling resistor /Sluice or water fall effect.**

Zone 3 : Continuous Blood flow

- In zone 3, **P_a >P_v> P_A**.
- **Continuous blood flow** because the alveolar capillary pressure remains greater than alveolar air pressure during the entire cardiac cycle
- Found in lower areas of lung

Bronchial Circulation

- Bronchial arteries arise directly from aorta and ***provide nourishment / oxygenated blood to lung parenchyma***Q. Bronchial arteries are usually 3 in number, accompany the bronchial tree and divide with it.
- The main function of bronchial artery is to provide oxygenated systemic blood & nutrition to lungs i.e. walls of conducting airways (bronchi, bronchioles) down to and including respiratory bronchioles, blood vessels (eg pulmonary arteries), nerves, lymph nodes and most of the visceral pleura.
- Bronchial circulation receives **1-2%** of total cardiac output, which increases as much as 10 to 20% (of CO) in cystic fibrosis. Approximately 1/3 of blood returns to right atrium via bronchial veins; whereas the **remainder drains into the left atrium via pulmonary veins**. The erosion of inflamed tissue into these vessels secondary to bacterial infection is responsible for hemoptysis.
- ***Bronchial circulation causes venous admixing***Q (i.e. **mixing of un-oxygenated** bronchial venous **blood directly into oxygenated** pulmonary venous **blood**) as its 2/3rd blood returns through pulmonary veins.
- **Gaseous exchange** (i.e. removal of CO_2 from deoxygenated blood and mixing of O_2 = oxygenation) takes place in **pulmonary circulation of lung.**

Myocardial Oxygen Consumption

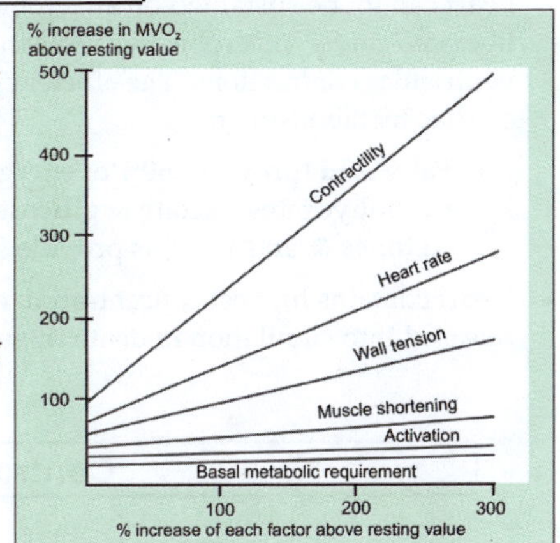

- **Basal O_2 consumption** (determined by stopping the heart and artificially maintaining coronary circulation) is *2 mL/100 gm /min,* which is ***considerably higher than that of skeletal muscle***[Q]. O_2 consumption by beating heart is *9 mL/100 gm /min at rest,* which is the ***highest per unit mass consumption of O_2***[Q].
- Due to very high O_2 extraction, the *arterio – venous O_2 difference (ML/L) is also maximum in heart.* So increase in O_2 demand requires increase in coronary blood flow otherwise ischemia develops.
- Factors that enhance *magnitude & /or rate of tension* development will increase myocardial O_2 demand. So ***increasing heart rate increases O_2 demand by increasing rate (number of tension cycles developed/minute); whereas increasing inotropy (contractility) by increasing both magnitude & rate of tension developed***[Q].
- So myocardial O_2 consumption is ***primarily determined by intramyocardial tension, contractile state & heart rate***[Q].

Myocardial O_2 consumption	α	***Heart rate, Contratility, Intramyocardial tension***[Q].
	α	Venticle work/ beat
	α	***Stroke volume*** x ***Mean arterial pressure***[Q]

- *Left ventricular stroke work is 7 times greater than that of right ventricle* since the aortic pressure is 7 times greater than the pulmonary artery pressure. Theoratically, a 20% increase in stroke volume without a change in arterial pressure and a 20% increase in arterial pressure without a change in stroke volume should produce the same increase in O_2 consumption But because of **La plac relationship**, ***pressure work (i.e, increase in after load or mean arterial pressure) produces a greater increase in O_2 consumption than volume work (i.e., increase in preload***[Q] or stroke volume). This is why angina is more common in AS than AR (aortic regurgitation). According to **La place law**

Intramyocardial tension (T) α Intraventricular pressure (P) x ventricular radius (r)

- **Factors determining (directly proportional to) myocardial oxygen demand**

Heart Rate	**Contractility of ventricles (Inotropy)**	**Intramyocardial wall Tension**
Demand increases & decreases with HR. (i.e. **MOC ∝ HR**)	Demand increases & decreases with contractility. (i.e. **MOC ∝ Contractility and ionotropy**)	• Wall tension is **directly proportional to** - **Intracavitatory pressure (P i.e. after load)** & - **Ventricular Radius (R i.e. preload)** • It is **inversely proportional to wall thickness (h)** **Intramyocardial wall Tension** $= \frac{PR}{2h}$

- **Energy (ATP or O_2) expandature: Basal metabolism** of heart tissue normally accounts for ~ 25% of myocardial ATP use (and therefore *same is the myocardial oxygen demand in resting individual*). In basal metabolism *energy is consumed in cellular processes other than contraction* eg energy dependent ion pumping. The energy spent during **isovolemetric contraction (internal cardiac work) phase** of the cardiac cycle accounts for **maximum portion (~50%)** of total myocardial oxygen (or ATP) consumption despite the fact that heart does no external work during this period. It is during the **ejection phase** of the cardiac cycle that the heart actually perform **external cardiac work** but the energy (ATP) or O2 consumed is only **25%**

Myocardial O_2 / Energy (ATP) consumption (Demand)

- **Basal Metabolism**
  - **Basal metabolism (cellular process other than muscle contraction in resting individuals)** — **25%**
- **Muscle Contraction**
  - **External cardiac work (during ejection phase)** — **25%**
  - **Internal Cardiac work** (during **isovolemetric contraction)** — **50%**

- Energy required for cardiac contractions derives **almost entirely from aerobic metabolism**, and unlike skeletal muscle the heart cannot be sustained on anaerobic metabolism for any length of time, & cannot incur an O2 debt. This is because energy liberated under anaerobic metabolism, constitutes an insignificant 1% of total energy need & is not adequate to sustain ventricular contractions. The efficiency (i.e. work done to energy expenditure) of normal heart is **20- 25%**. The substrates for cardiac metabolism are:
  - **Fatty acid** (provides 60% of energy)
  - **Carbohydrates (lactate & glucose)** provide 35% of energy
  - **Ketones & amino acids** provide 5% of energy
- Heart contains highest concentration of **aspartate amino transferase (AST)** then any other tissue in body & this enzyme is released into circulation in death of any part of myocardiam.

Control of Blood Flow in Splanchinic Circulation

Splanchnic circulation – The whole amount of blood that passes through the liver and open into the inferior venacava via hepatic veins. ***Splanchnic vessels contain 20-30% of total blood volume***[Q].

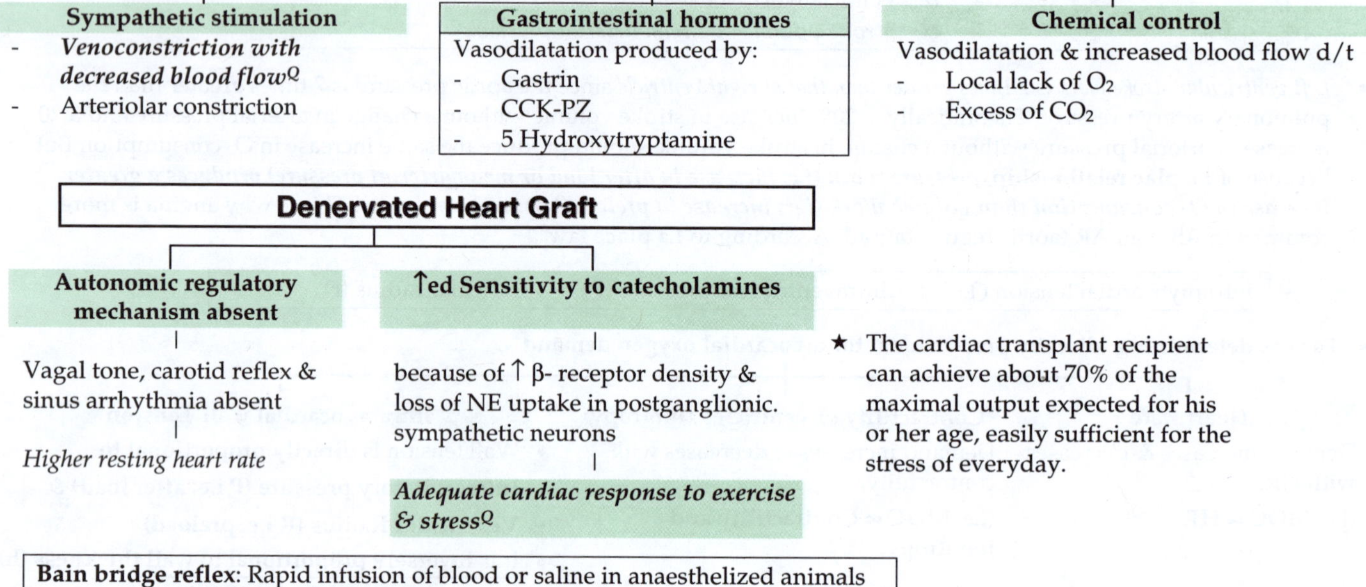

Bain bridge reflex: Rapid infusion of blood or saline in anaesthelized animals produces a rise in heart if the initial heart rate is low.
Infusion of fluids in person with transplanted heart increases the rate of recipient's atrial remant but fails to affect the rate of the transplanted heart.

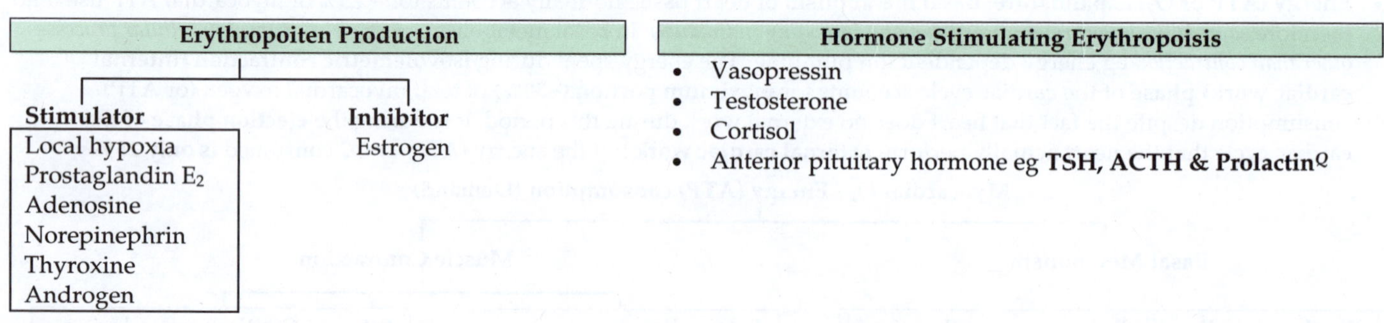

2,3 DPG & Hemoglobin

- 2,3 DPG is present in high concentration in erythrocytes (HbA> HbA_2)
- ***2,3 DPG greatly reduces the affinity of Hb to O_2*** Q (shifts O_2-dissociation curve to right)
- ***Fetus Hb (HbF) consists of α2Y2, this tetramer has much lower affinity for 2-3 DPG than adult Hb***Q & Corresponding a higher affinity for O_2.

Viscosity of Blood Depends on

Hematocrit

Percentage of the volume, of blood occupied by red blood cells. Viscosity is directly proportional to hematocrit.

- *Increased* — Polycythemia
- *Decreased* — Anemia

Composition of the plasma

Depends upon the presence of plasma proteins such as immuno globulins & the resistance of the cells to deformation. (viscosity is disectly proportional to composition of the plasma)

- *Increased* — Multiple myeloma
- *Decreased* — Hereditary spherocytosis

Neutrophils

Biochemical Features
- Active glycolysis - Active pentose phosphate pathway - Moderate oxidative phosphorylation - Rich in lysosomes and their degradative enzymes - Contain certain unique enzymes (e.g. myeloperoxidase and NADPH-oxidase) and proteins - Contain CD 11/CD 18 integrins in plasma membrane

Neutrophils

Primary granules	Secondary granules
• Appears at *promyelocytic stage* • Cotain following enzymes - ***Myeloperoxidase***Q - Hydroxylase - ***Lysozyme***Q - Elastase - ***Cathepsin G***Q - Defensin - Phospholipase A_2	• Appears at *myelocytic stage* • Contain following enzymes - Lactoferrin - Lysozyme - Alkaline phosphatase - Plasminogen activator - Phospholipase A_2

- Arneth count: counting of lobes in the neutrophils.

Some important enzymes and proteins of neutrophils

Enzyme or Protein	Reaction Catalyzed or Function	Comment
Myeloperoxidase (MPO)	$H_2O_2 + X^-$ (halide) + $H^+ \rightarrow$ HOX + H_2O (where $X^- = Cl^-$, HOX = hypochlorous acid)	Responsible for the green color pus Genetic deficiency can cause recurrent infections H_2O_2-MPO-Halide. System is most efficient bactericidal system in neutrophils
NADPH-odixase	$2O_2$ + NADPH $\rightarrow 2O^-$ + NADP + H^+	Key component of the respiratory burst Deficient in chromic granulomatous disease
Lysozyme	Hyrolyzes link between N-acetylmuamic acid and N-acetyl-D-glucosamine found in certain bacterial cell walls	Abundant in macrophages
Defensins	Basic antibiotic peptides of 20-33 aminoacids	Apparently kill bacteria by causing membrane damage
Lactoferrin	Iron-binding protein	May inhibit growth of certain bacteria by binding iron and may be involved in regulation of proliferation of myeloid cells
CD11a/CD18, CD11b/CD18, CD11c/CD18[2]	Adhesion molecules (members of the integrin family)	Deficient in leukocyte adhesion deficiency type I (MIM 116920)
Receptors for Fc fragments of IgGs	Bind Fc fragments of IgG molecules	Target antigen-antibody complexes to myeloid and lymphoid cells, eliciting phagocytosis and other responses

★ Lysome is not found in *erythrocytes, prokaryotes & virus*. PH inside the lysosome is lower than that of cytoplasm. ***Acid phosphatase***Q is the marker enzyme of lysosome.

Natural Killer (NK) Cells

- **Natural Killer (NK) cells** are ***large, granular lymphocytes, which kill virus infected cells and cancer cells by cell mediated immunity***[Q]. They release **perforin** (perforates cell membrane) and **granzyme** (cause apoptosis). NK cells differ from cytotoxic T cells in that they **lyse sensitive cell targets on first contact (without a prior antigen sensitization).** They ***do not require thymic processing***[Q] and do not express surface T cells antigen receptors.
- NK cells make 10-15% of leukocytes in blood. NK cells also play important role in **antibody dependent cellular cytotoxicity (ADCC).** In ADCC, Fc receptor of NK cell bind to antibody attached to target cell. This provides NK cell another opportunity to inhibit the replication of viruses and intracellular bacteria.
- NK cells have 2 types of cell receptors: (1) **lectin like NK cell receptor** that binds to protein not carbohydrate and (2) **KIRs** (killer immunoglobin like receptors which recognize MHC class I molecules HLA-B or HLA-C. NK cells turn into **lymphokine activated killer cells** (which is more efficient in killing) on exposure to lymphocytic secretions like IL2 and IFNγ.

Coagulation Pathway ☆

Factor 10 can be activated by either of intrinsic or extrinsic system

Intrinsic pathway

First step in **intrinsic system** is *activation of factor 12* which is catalyzed by *high molecular weight kininogen (HMW K) and Kallikrein*. It occurs in *vivo* (body) when *blood is exposed to collagen fibers* underlying the endothelium in blood exposed to collagen fibers underlying the endothelium in blood vessels and can be brought about in *vitro (test tube)* by exposing the blood to electronegative charged wettable surface such as glass & collagen fibers.

Extrinsic pathway

Extrinsic system is triggered by release of *tissue factor or tissue thromboplastin* (TPL) a *lipoprotein – phospholipid mixture* from traumatized tissue, which is a proteolytic enzyme & activates factor 7. Extrinsic pathway is *inhibitor by tissue factor pathway inhibitor*, which forms a quarternary structure with *TPL, factor 7a & factor 10a*

HMWK
Kallikrein

TPL (Tissue thromboplastin)=(3)
TFI (Tissue factor pathway inhibitor)

(12)
(11)
(9) ← - - - (7)
PL, Ca^{++}
PL, Ca^{++}
(8)
TPL
(10)
Prothrombin activator
(5) PL, Ca^{++}
Prothrombin (2) → **Thrombin**[Q]
Fibrinogen (1) → **Fibrin**
(13)
Stable cross linked fibrin
Common Pathway

Clotting Factors ☆

Factor	Names	Clinical Syndrome
I	**Fibrinogen**[Q]	**Afibrinogen**
II	**Prothrombin**[Q]	Hypoprothombinemia (hemorrhagic tendency in liver disease)
III	Thromboplastin	
IV	Calcium	
V	Proaccelerin, labile factor, accelerator globulin	Parahemophilia
VII	Proconvertin, SPCA, stable factor	Hypoconvertinemia
VIII	Antihemophilic factor (AHF), antihemophilic factor A, antihemophilic globulin (AHG)	Hemophilia A (classic hemophilia)
IX	Plasma thromboplastic component (PTC), Christmas factor, antihemophilic factor B	Hemophilia B (Christmas disease)
X	Stuart–Prower factor	Stuart-Prower factor deficiency
XI	Plasma thromboplastin antecedent (PTA), antihemophilic factor C	PTA deficiency
XII	Hageman factor, glass factor	Hageman trait
XIII	***Fibrin stabilizing factor, Laki-Lorand factor***[Q]	
HMW-K	High-molecular-weight kininogen, Fitzgerald factor	
Pre-K_a	Prekallikrein, Fletcher factor	
Ka	Kallikrein	
PL	Platelet phospholipid	

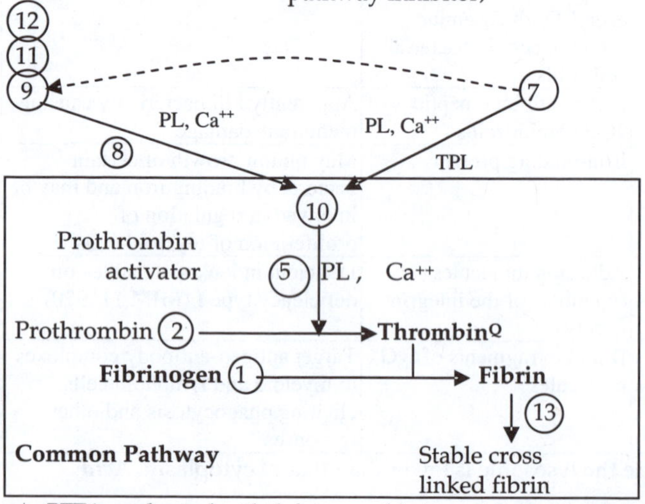

★ PTT is **prolonged** with deficiency of factors : ***8, 9, 11, 12, 2, 1, Prothrombin***[Q]
★ PT is **prolonged** with deficiency of : ***5, 7, 2, 1, Prothrombin***[Q]
★ Except for the first two steps in intrinsic pathway, calcium ions are required for promotion or acceleration of all blood clotting reactions

Features	Hemophilia A (Classical hemophilia)	Hemophilia B (Christmas disease)
Defect	Deficiency of coagulant subunit of factor VIII i.e. VIIIC **factor VIII=VIIIC + VWF**	***Deficiency of factor IX***[Q]
Pathway of coagulation affected	Instrinsic pathway	Intrinsic pathway
Clotting Time	↑	↑
PTT	↑	↑
PT	N	N
BT	N	N

Clotting Factors Involved in

Intrinsic Pathway Only	Common Pathway	Extrinsic Pathway Only
- 12 (XII) - 11 (XI) - 9 (IX) - 8 VIII - Prekalle krein - HMW Kininogen	- **10** (X) - **5** (V) - **2** (II) - **1** (I) - **13** (XIII)	- **7** (VII) - Tissue thromboplastin (III)

APTT

- Measures time required to generate thrombin & fibrin polymer via **intrinsic & common pathway**
- Reflects activity of

12, 11, 9, 8 + 10, 5, 2, 1

PTT

- Measures time required to generate thrombin & fibrin polymer via extrinsic **& common pathway**
- Reflects activity of

7 + 10, 5, 2, 1

Anticlotting Mechanisms in Normal Vascular System 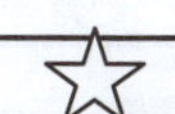

Prevention of Clotting

Endothelial Surface Factor

- **Smoothness of Endothelial cell surface** *prevents contact activation of intrinsic clotting system*
- **Glycocalyx (Mucopoly sacchride) layer on Endothelium** (mucopolysaccharide) layer repels clotting factor & plateletts
- **Thrombomodulin**, a thrombin binding protein, ***expressed in all endothelial cells, except those in crebral microcirculation***[Q]. It prevents clotting in 3 ways
  - By *removing thrombin* (activator of factor 5 & 8)
  - *Thrombin- thrombomodulin* complex activates *protein C* that acts as an anti coagulant by *inactivating activated factor V & VIII*
  - **Activated protein C (APC)** also inactivates inhibitor of tissue plasminogen activator, *increasing the formation of plasmin*

Circulating Anticoagulants in Blood

- **Antithrombin action of Fibrin and Antithrombin III (AT III)**
  - Most important anticoagulants in blood are those that remove thrombin viz *fibrin and anti thrombin III or antithrombin- heparin cofactor*
  - During clot formation, **85-90% of thrombin** (formed from prothrombin) **becomes adsorbed to the fibrin fibers**. This prevents spread of thrombin into remaining blood &, hence prevents excessive spread of clot.
  - **Antithrombin III**, a circulting *protease inhibitor* that binds to *serine protease,* combines with the remaining thrombin that does not adsorb to fibrin (in *12-20 minutes*)
- **Heparin**, is a mixture of *highly negative sulfate polysaccharides* with molecular wt. ~ 15-18 thousand. It is produced in large quantities by **basophilic mast cells** located in pericapillary connective tissue. (Basophils also secret small amounts). However, its *concentration in blood is low* and by itself it has *little or no anticoagulant property* . But
  - Its binding with antithrombin III, increases effectiveness of antithrombin III 100 – 1000 times. As a result **heparin – antithrombin III complex** removes free thrombin from blood almost *instataneously*
  - Heparin- antithrombin III ***also removes (inhibits) activated clotting factors IX, X, XI, XII***[Q].

Lysis of Blood Clot

- **Plasmninogen (Fibrinolytic) System**
  - **Activated proein C (APC)** inactivates inhibitors of t-PA, increasing the formation of **plasmin (fibrinogen)** from plasminogen.
  - Large amounts of plasminogen is trapped in the clot, which is activated after few days by **tissue plasminogen activator (t-PA)** a very power full activator which is very slowly released by injured tissue & endothelium. Other activators are **urokinase type plasminogen activator (U-PA)** and *thrombin.*
  - Plasminogen (profibrinolysin), when activated becomes **plasmin (fibrinolysin)**. Plasmin is a proteolytic enzyme (like trypsin), which *digest fibrin & fibrinogen* with the production of *fibrinogen degradation products (FDP) that inhibit* thrombin. It also lyses *prothrombin, factor V, VIII and XII.*
- **Recombinant t-PA (Altepase) and Streptokinase** (bacterial enzyme) are used as fibrinolytic agents in MI.
- **Annexin II**, forms a *platform on endothelial cells* on which components of fibrinolytic system interact, producing fibrinolysis. **Annexin V** forms a *shield around phospholipids* involved in coagulation has an anti thrombotic effect.

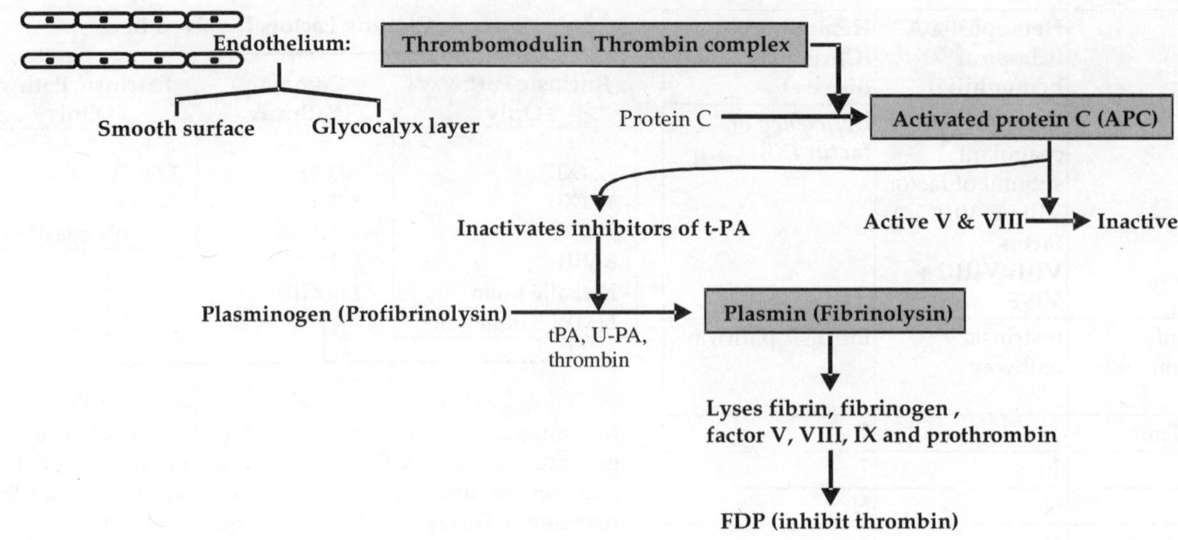

ABO Blood Group system

- **Highly immunogenic ABO blood group antigen** is due to **complex oligosaccharide (glycoprotein) found on RBC membrane.** It is inherited as **medelian autosomal dominants**[Q].
- Alleles of ABO gene are located on long arm of **chromosome 9** (and of **Rh genes** on chromosome **1)**. One of the 3 gene types (A, B, O) determines blood group.
- Individuals can be divided into 4 major blood group types on the basis of **antigens** (or **agglutinogens**) present on **membrane of RBC**. They are called agglutinogens as they are responsible for blood cell agglutination in transfusion reactions. **Type A individuals have A antigen, type B have B, type AB have both A & B, and blood group type O have neither antigen.**
- **A and B antigens are complex oligosaccharides that differ in their terminal sugar moiety**[Q]. **H antigen** is present in all blood types. H gene coding fucose transferase that adds a terminal fucose, forms H antigen. Individuals with **type A** express a second transferase that catalyzes placement of a terminal **N-acetylgalactosamine** on H antigen, whereas **type B** (individuals) express a second transferase that places a **terminal galactose**. Individuals **with AB blood group have both** and **with O blood have neither transferases** (i.e only H antigen persists in O group).
- **Plasma antibodies** against RBC agglutinogens are called **agglutinins**. Antigens very similar to A and B are very common in **intestinal bacteria** and possibly **food** to which new borns are exposed. These substances initiate the development of Anti A & Anti B antibodies. Therefore, infants rapidly develop antibodies against the antigens not present in their own cells. So type A blood group individual develop anti B, type B develop anti A, type O develop both, and type AB individual develop neither.
- Immediately after birth, the quantity of agglutinins in the plasma is almost zero. An infant begins to produce agglutinins, 2 to 8 months after birth and maximum titre is reached at 8 to 10 yrs. of age. Then it gradually declines throughout the remaining years of life.
- Anti A and anti B antibodies are **isohaemagglutinins (iso antibodies)** as they are produced by an individual against antigens

Geno type	Blood Type	Frequency (%) in US	Aglutino-gens (Antigens)	Agglutinins (antibody) in plasma	Plasma agglutinates RBC types
OO	**O**	47	-	**Anti A** **Anti B**	A,B, AB
OA/ AA	**A**	40	**A**	**Anti B**	B, AB
OB/ BB	**B**	10	**B**	**Anti A**	A, AB
AB	**AB**	3	**A&B**	-	None

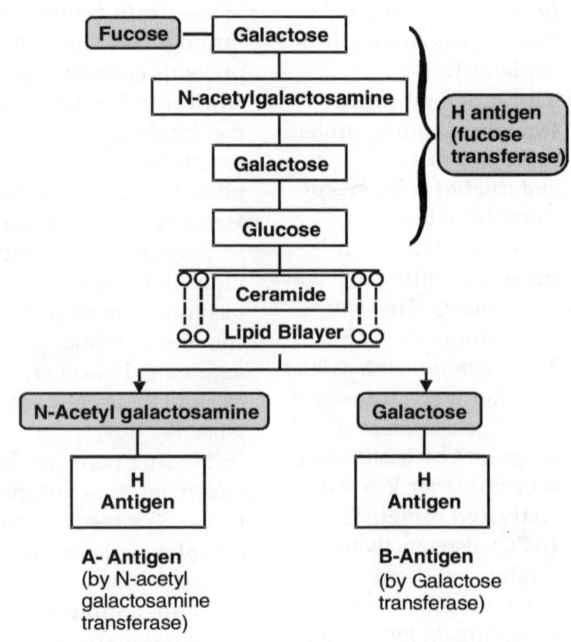

produced by members of same species (isoantigens).

- Antibodies are usually lgM type and cannot cross placenta. O type individual can produce IgG type antibodies.
- The basic difference between ABO blood group system and other blood group systems (such as Rh, Kell, Duffy, MNSs blood groups), which makes the ABO group so important is that - **preformed ABO antibodies** are present in persons serum when his RBCs lack the corresponding antigen (ie. *anti B antibody would be present in a person of type A and type O blood groups. These two blood groups do not have the 'B' antigen on the RBCs*). This is not the case with other blood groups. Preformed antibodies are not present.
  They are formed only after an exposure to the antigen, for example ***Rh negative person do not have anti- Rh antibodies****, these antibodies are formed only after an exposure to Rh positive blood (by a blood transfusion, i.e. this makes the first blood transfusion safe even if mismatched)*. These preformed antibodies, rapidly destroy the RBCs of any mismatched blood transfusion.
- *"In clinical transfusion practice, the ABO blood groups are the most important and can never be ignored in red cell transfusion, because individuals who genetically lack any antigen, have antibodies against the red cell types that they have not inherited. These antibodies can destroy red cells rapidly in circulation"*. But the question arises – why are these agglutinins (antibodies against AB antigen) produced in people who do not have the respective agglutinogens (A or B antigens) on their RBCs? The answer is that - Small amounts of group A and B antigens enter the body in food, in bacteria, and in other ways, and these substances initiate the development of the anti-A and anti-B agglutinins

Landsteiners Law in relation to agglutinogen (antigens) and agglutinins (antibodies)
- If an **antigen** is **present on RBC membrane** the **corresponding antibody (agglutitin)** must be **absent in plasma.** - If an **antigen** is **absent on RBC** membrane, the **corresponding antibody (agglutinin)** must be **present in the plasma.**

Chapter 5. DIGESTIVE SYSTEM: REVIEW NOTES

Body Fluid	K+ ion conc (meq/L)	Total secretion (L/day)	pH
Saliva	25-30 (low flow) 15-20 (high flow)	1 (-1.5)	6 – 7
Stomach	10 (may be upto 32)	1.5 (-2.5)	**1 -3.5**
Pancreatic	4.5 (same as plasma	1	**8 – 8.3**
Bile	5- 6 (in liver bile) 12 (in gall bladder bile)	1	7.8
Small intestine	10-12 (in ileum)	1.8	7.5-8
Large intestine	*75 (rectum)*[Q]	0.2	7.5-8
Brunner's gland secretion	-	0.2	8-8.3

Digestive Enzymes

Activator	Proenzyme/ Enzyme
Trypsin (activates only pancreatic enzymes)	- ***Chymotrypsinogens /chymotrypsin***[Q]. - Pro carboxypeptidase A/ carboxypeptidase A - Procarboxypeptidase B/ carboxy peptidase B - Pro-colipase/colipase - Pro-elastase/elastase - Pro-phospholipase A_2/phospholipase A_2
Enteroeptidase	- ***Trypsinogen/Trypsin***[Q]
HCl	- ***Pepsinogens / pepsin***[Q]
Cl-	- Salivary and pancreatic α amylase

★ Amino / Carboxy / **endo** – peptidases cleave amino terminal / carboxy terminal / *mid portion* of polypeptides respectively.

Source

- **Salivary gland** - α amylase
- **Lingual glands** – lipase
- **Stomach**
  - ***Pepsinogen***[Q]
  - Lipase
- **Cytoplasm of mucosal cells**
  - Peptidases
- **Intestinal mucosa**
  - Enteropeptidase
  - Aminopeptidase
  - Carboxypeptidase
  - Endopeptidase
  - Dipeptidase
  - Maltase, lactase
  - Sucrase, α dextrinase
  - Trehalase
  - Nuclease
- **Exocrine pancreas**
  - ***Trypsin***[Q]
  - ***Chymotrypsin***[Q]
  - Elastase
  - ***Pancreatic lipase***[Q]
  - Bile salt-acid lipase
  - Colipase
  - Cholestery ester hydrolase
  - Pancreatic α amylase
  - Carboxy peptidase A and B
  - Phospholipase A_2
  - Ribonuclease
  - Deoxyribonuclease.

Proproteins (Proenzymes or Zymogens)

- **Zymogen is an inactive precursor of enzyme / protein that require selective proteolysis for activation.** Selective proteolysis involves one or more highly specific proteolytic clips that may or may not be accompanied by separation of resulting peptide. So selective proteolysis often result in **conformational changes** that *create the catalytic site of an enzyme* or it **unmasks the active site of an enzyme** by removing small region of peptide chain (by hydrolysis of specific peptide bond).
- Enzymes needed **intermittently but rapidly** often are secreted in an initially inactive form since new synthesis and secretion of required proteins might be insufficiently rapid to respond to a pressing pathophysiological demand such as clot formation, clot dissolution, tissue repair etc. So proenzymes **facilitate rapid mobilization of activity** in response to physiological need.
- Proteolytic digestive enzymes are known as **proteases**. These are secreted as inactive **zymogens**. The *synthesis of enzymes as Zymogens protects the cell from being digested by its own product* **(autodigestion)**. Proteases are of two types

Exopeptidase	Endopeptidase
Hydrolyse peptide bonds one at a time from the **ends** of polypeptide chain	Hydrolyse peptide bonds in *midportion* between specific aminoacids. eg. are Pepsin, Elastase, Trypsin, Chymotrypsin

Carboxypeptidase	Aminopeptidase
(in pancreatic huice)	(in small intestine)
Cleaves aminoacid from carboxy terminal	Cleaves aminoacid from amino terminal

Pepsinogen (zymogen) —*HCl*[Q]→ **Pepsin** (in stomach)

Trypsinogen (zymogen) —*Enterokinase*[Q]→ **Trypsin** (in small intestine)

Trypsin can activate several proenzymes

1. **Chymotrypsinogen** to chymotrypsin
2. **Procarboxypeptidase** A/B to carboxypeptidase A/B
3. **Proaminopeptidase** to aminopetidase
4. **Proelastate** to elastase

- Most of clotting factors (**factor 2, 7, 9, 10, 11, 12) are zymogens of serine proteases**. Similarly **tissue plasminogen activator (t-PA) and angiotensinogen** are also screted as zymogens.

Trypsin

It is a proteolytic enzyme (proserine-proteinase) involved in digestion of proteins – chymotrypsinogen, procarboxypeptidase A & B, procolipase, prophospholipase A2, and proelastase. It is secreted in inactive form trypsinogen

Activators of trypsin

Active site which is histidylserine residue is unmasked in the process of activation. It is brought about by –

- ***Enterokinase***[Q], a glycoprotein enzyme of intestinal juice at a pH of 5.5
- **Autocatalytically by trypsin** once it is formed at a pH of 7.9
- Ca++ is also required.

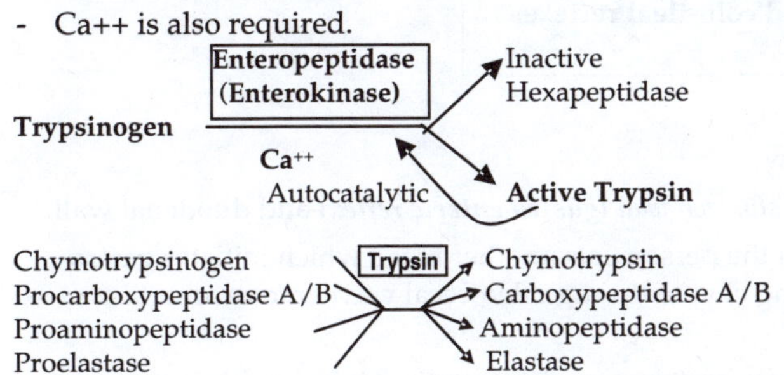

Inhibitors of trypsin

- ***Alpha (α) 1 antiproteinase or Alpha (α) 1 antitrypsin***[Q]
- Di isopropyl fluro phosphate (DFP)
- Egg white (containing water soluble mucoprotein)
- Human and bovine colostrums
- Raw syoabean

★ α1 antitrypsin is synthesized by hepatocytes and macrophages & is *principal serine protease inhibitor* that inhibits trypsin, elastase etc by forming complexes with them. Its deficiency has role in *emphysema* mainly in subjects with *zz genotype*. Methionie (residue-358) of α_1 antitrypsin is involved in its binding to proteases. *Smoking inactivates* it by converting it to methionine sulfoxide. So it cannot neutralize proteases, This is particularly devastating in Pizz phenotype who already have low levels of α1 antitrypsin.

Regulation (Phases) of Gastric Secretion

Gastric secretion & motality are regulated by *neural & humoral mechanism and has 3 phases*

- **Neural components** are ***local autonomic reflexes involving cholinergic neurons and parasympathetic impulses from CNS (by vagus nerve)***[Q]. Vagal stimulation increase gastrin secretion by release of GRP.
- **Humoral components** are hormones such as *gastrin, GRP and acetylcholine*

Cephalic Phase

- **Mainly mediated by vagal (parasympathetic) inputs** originating from the **dorsal vagal complex** in brain. Vagal outflow to stomach cause *GRP & acetylcholine* release, there by initiating secretion.
- It results from *sight, smell, thought, or taste* of food even before food enters stomach

Gastric Phase

- Once the food enters the stomach it excites
  - **Gastrin mechanism (predominantly** responsible for secretion) because of meal constituents
  - **Lung vago-vagal reflex** (form stomach to brain to stomach) and **local enteric reflexes** are activated by distension of stomach & stretch receptor activation. These further amplify secretion.

Intestinal Phase

- Once the food enters upper portion of small intestine (esp duodenum) it causes small amounts of gastric juice secretion because of ***gastrin released from duodenal mucosa***[Q] (Guyton)
- Although small intestine has gastrin containing cells

- Neurogenic signals of gastric secretion arise in cerebral cortex, & in *appetite centers of amygdala and hypothalmus. The efferent fibers travel through vagus nerve*Q (dorsal motor nuclei).
- This *parasymathetically (vagally)* mediated phase can be *conditioned.* Tension, anger & hostality increase gastric secretion whereas fear & depression decrease it.
- **It accounts for 20% of gastric secretion**Q (Guyton) / $\frac{1}{3}$ to $\frac{1}{2}$ of acid secretion (Ganong)

- **Meal buffers gastric acidity** which otherwise is a inhibitory feed back signal to shut off secretion secondary to release of **somatostatin** (which inhibits G, ECL cells and parietal cells).
- Receptors for **local enteric reflex** are in wall of stomach & mucosa and *respond to **stretch and chemical stimuli mainly amino acids & products of protein digestion.*** The fibers from receptor reach submucosal plexus, which synapse on postaganglionic parasympathetic neurons that end on parietal cell & increase acid secretion
- It accounts for ***most (70%) of gastric secretion***Q (~ 1500ml)

instillation of amino acids directly into duodenum *does not increase circulating gastrin levels.*

- Fats, carbohydrates & acid in duodenum inhibit gastric motality, acid and pepsin secretion via **neural & hormonal (peptide YY)** mechanisms. That's why gastric acid secretion is increased proportionately to the amount of small intestine removed.

Factors Affecting Intestinal Motality

Hormonal	Neural	Physical & chemical
- **Gastrin, CCK, insulin, motilin, substance P and serotonin enhance intestinal motality**Q. Whereas, **secretin, neurotensin and glucagon inhibits small intestinal motality**Q. - *Stomach emptying (motality) is inhibited* by cholecystokinin (CCK), secretin & gastric inhibitory peptide (GIP) whereas gastrin increase stomach motality.	- **Parasympathetic (cholinergic) stimulation (Ach) enhances gastric & intestinal motality**Q - Sympathetic stimulation inhibit gastric & intestinal motality. - **Gastro-enteric, gastro-colic, duodeno-colic reflexes increase motality, while entero-gastric and colo-ileal reflexes inhibit motality**Q**.**	- ***Distension of gut increases motality***Q - Chemical stimulation by acid, protein products & fatty acids alter motality by increasing secretin and CCK secretion.

Intestinal motality is dependent of gastric motality; as explained below

- Peristalitic activity of small intestine is *greatly increased by distension of stomach wall* ***(gastro enteric reflex)*** and duodenal wall.
- Chyme is sometimes blocked at ileocecal valve for several hours, until the person eats another meal, which initiates **gastro-ileal reflex**. This intensifies perstalsis in ileum and forces the remaining chyme through ileo-cecal valve into cecum (large intestine)
- **Gastro- colic & duodeno- colic autonomic reflexes** result from *distension of stomach and duodenum.* ***These facilitate appearance of propulsive mass movements after meals, in large intestine***Q**.**
- **Entero- gastric reflex** *inhibits stomach secretions and motality* (by inhibiting pyloric pump propulsive contractions & increasing tone of pyloric sphincter) based on the signals from small intestine and colon.
- Reflexes from colon inhibit emptying of ileal content into the colon via **colono-ileal reflex.**

Gastrin

Gastrin is a hormone which is ***produced by G-cells in the lateral wall of glands in the antral portion of gastric mucosa***Q**.** It is also found in ***pancreatic islets in fetal life, gastrinomas of pancreas,*** and ***pituitary gland***Q, hypothalamus, medulla oblongata and in vagus & sciatic nerves.

Actions
• Stimulation of ***gastric acid and pepsin secretion***[Q]
• Stimulates growth of mucosa of stomach, small & large intestine **(trophic action).**
• ***Promotes gastric emptying***[Q]
• Stimulation of *Insulin secretion.*

★ ***Total acid secretion*** depends upon the ***functional parietal cell mass***[Q].

★ Acid secretion is stimulated by
- ***Histamine Via H_2 receptor***[Q].
- Acetylcholine via M_3 receptor.

★ **H_2 blocker** eg ranitidine *decreases gastric acid secretion;* But *proton pump inhibitor* like omeprazole blocks gastric acid secretion.

Factors affecting Gastrin Secretion

Any stimuli that *affect gastrin* seretion also *affects acid secretion* from the stomach

Stimuli that increase gastrin (& HCl) secretion		Stimuli that inhibit gastrin secretion
- Oligo-Peptides and amino acids in gastric lumen - ***Distention***[Q]	Luminal	- ***Acid***[Q] - ***Somatostatin***[Q]
- ***Ca^{2+}***[Q] - Epinephrine	Blood borne	- ***Secretin***[Q], GIP, ***VIP***[Q], ***glucagons, Calcitonin***[Q]
- ***Increased vagal discharge*** via bombesin **GRP** [Gastrin Releasing Polypeptide - Noncholinergic]	Neural	-

Factors Regulationg Gastric Emptying

Increase Emptying (Gastric Factors)

- **Gastric food volume distending (stretching) the stomach wall** elicit local myentric reflexes thereby accentuating pyloric pump & inhibiting pyloric sphincter. Distension by water quickens emptying more then distension by solids
- **Gastrin** mild to moderately enhances pyloric pump.

Decrease Emptying (Duodenal Factors) 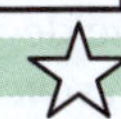

- Enterogastric nervous reflexes
- **Hyperosmolarily** of duodenal content (chyme) decreases, whereas hypoosmolarity increases emptying of gastric content
- Hormonal feed backs involving **cholecystokinin (CCK;** mainly **d/t protein & fat entering duodenum)**[Q]**, secretin (b/o acidic chyme)**[Q]**, gastric inhibitory peptide**(GIP; weak), **peptide YY** (messenger) and somatostatin (±)
- Carbohydrate rich food leaves stomach in few hours. Protein rich food leaves more slowly & ***emptying is slowest after fat rich meal***[Q]. **Carbohydrate (fastest) → protein → Fat (slowest emptying)**

Amphipathic Bile Acids: Micelles

- Bile acids are synthesized from cholesterol and bile salts are sodium & potassium salts of bile acid.
- Bile salts have ***amphipathic nature***[Q]. i.e. they have both hydrophilic and hydrophobic domains. Therefore they tend to form cylindrical disk called *micelles*, with the hydrophilic surface facing out and the hydrophobic surfaces facing in.
- ***Lipids collect within the micelles. Bile acids have detergent action on lipids d/t amphipathic nature***[Q].
- The micelles play are important role in keeping lipids in solution & transporting them to the brush border, where they absorb.

Proteins Synthesized by Liver

Protein	Function
Albumin	*Ormotic regulator; and carrier protein* binding hormone, aminoacids, sterioids, vitamins, & fatty acids
α-fetoprotein	*Osmotic regulator; binding and carrier protein for hormones,* amino acids (although functions are uncertain but because of its structural homology to albumin these functions are assigned)
α_1-antiprotease	*Trypsin & general (serum & tissue) protease inhibitor*
α_2- macroglobulin	*Serum endoprotease inhibitor*
Antithrombin III	Protease inhibitor of intrinsic coagulation system (1:1 binding)
Angiotensinogen	Precursor to pressure peptide angiotensin II
Apolipoprotein B	Lipid carrier assembly of lipoprotein particles
Antithrombin C, Protein C	Inhibition of blood clotting
Coagulation factors II, VII, IX, X	Blood clotting
Ceruloplasmin	Transport copper (6 atoms Cu/mol)
C- reactive protein[Q]	Uncertain, tissue inflammation, bind complement C1q
Fibrinogen	Precursor to fibrin in hemostasis
Haptoglobin[Q]	Bind & transport cell free hemoglobin (1:1 binding)

Hemopexin	Binds to prophyrin, particularly heme for heme recycling.
Insulin like growth factor I	Mediator of anabolic effects of growth hormone (binds to IGF-1 receptor)
Orosomucoid	Uncertain, ± role in inflammation
Sterioid hormone binding globulin	Carrier protein for steroid in blood
Thyroxine binding globulin	Carrier protein for thyroid hormone in blood
Trans- thyretin (Thyroid binding pre albumin)	Carrier protein for thyroid hormone in blood
Transferrin	Transport of iron

★ ***Most of other plasma proteins except antibodies (γglobulins or immunoglobins) are synthesized in liver*Q.**

Enterogastric Reflex

When the chyme enters the intestine, the gastric muscle is inhibited and the motility stops leading to **stoppage of gastric emptying – enterogastric reflex**. This reflex involves the **vagus nerve**. Factors that stimulate enterogastric reflex

1. Degree of ***distention of duodenum*Q**
2. Any degree of irritition of duodenal mucosa
3. The degree of ***acidity of duodenal chyme*Q.**
4. The degree of (high) ***osmolarity of chyme*Q**
5. ***Presence of breakdown products of protein and fat*Q.**

★ **Chyme** – Peristaltic movements of stomach mix the food bolus with gastric juice and convert it into semisolid material.

Postvagotomy Diarrhoea

- Truncal vagotomy is associated with climically significant diarrhoea in 5-10% of patient.
- Factors responsible for diarrhoea are:
  - Intestinal dysmotility ***(Irregular peristalsis)*Q.**
  - ***Rapid gastric emptying*Q.**
  - Bile acid malabsorption
  - Bacterial over growth due to ***decreased gastric acid secretion*Q.**
  - Fat malabsorption
  - Exaggerated gastrointestinal peptide response.

Motality of Colon

Mixing & Retarding Movements

Consistent with its primary function (of water & electrolyte absorption), the **two predominant motality patterns of large intestine are directed** not to propulsion of colonic content but rather to **retarding (slowing) their movement and mixing of contents.** Both originate in response to local conditions eg distension. Two types include

Short Duration (8 sec) Stationary Pressure Waves or Segmentation Contractions

Originating in **circular muscles**

Long Duration (20-60 sec) Peristalitic waves

Produced by **teniae coli** and may *propogate over short distances* **in both directions ie orally as well as aborally.**

High Amplitude (Intensity) Propagating Contractions or Mass Action Contraction

- In healthy individuals colon engages in high intensity (amplitude) motality pattern that *sweesps along the length of large intestine from cecum to rectum*
- It occurs about **10 times per day and occurs only in the colon**
- As a result of both local influences & long reflex arcs, there is *simultaneous contraction of smooth muscles over large confluent areas.* They move exclusively in **aboral direction** and are designed to clear the colon of its contents.
- It moves colonic content from one portion to another and then into rectum – and rectal distension initiates defecation reflex. Although can be associated with defecation *it does not necessarily result in defecation.*

Primary Fuction of Large Bowel

- Large intestine (colon) works as a reservoir for the residual meal that cannot be digested or absorbed. The major primary role of colonic epithelium is to either absorb or secrete electrolytes & water rather than nutrients. Secetion (confined to crypts) maintains the sterility of crypts.
- By absorbing 90% of fluid, it converts 2L of isotonic chyme that enters colon to 250 ml of semisolid feces. However, colon has 3 times more **(4 to 6L) reserve capacity for fluid absorption;** and diarrhea results only after exceeding this.

BER of Colon

- Basal electrical rhythm that governs the rate & origin sites of smooth muscle contraction in small intestine does not cross the ileocecal valve to continue into the colon. So the movements of colon are cordnated by the BER of colon.
- The frequency of BER/wave, unlike in small intestine, increases along the colon, from about **2/min at the ileocecal valve to 6/min at the sigmoid colon.**

Transit Time In Small & Large Intestine

Test meal / undigested food reaches	Transit time
1st part of test meal reach **cecum**	4 hr
Colon entery of all undigested portion	8-9 hr
Traverse the **first third (ascending)** colon	6 hr
Traverse the second third of colon (ie transverse colon)	9 hr
Reach the **terminal part of colon (sigmoid colon)**	12 hr
From sigmoid colon to anus	Much slower

* 70% matter reach stool in 72 hrs but total passage takes >1 week

Defecation Reflex

- There are two types of defecation reflex.
  1. *Intrinsic reflex* mediated by local enteric nervous system
  2. *Parasympathetic defecation reflex* mediated by *sacral segment* of the spinal cord.
- In both these types, the reflex is initiated by distention of the rectum by the feces and causes *increased peristalsis* in the *descending* colon, *sigmoid colon* and *rectum*. This forces the feces toward the anus.

In a similar way, when the *rectum is inflated with gas* (CO_2) *in* ***sigmoidoscopy****, nerves are stimulated* and causes increased *peristalsis in* the descending colon, sigmoid ***(distal colon)***Q and rectum.

Water Regulation in Intestine

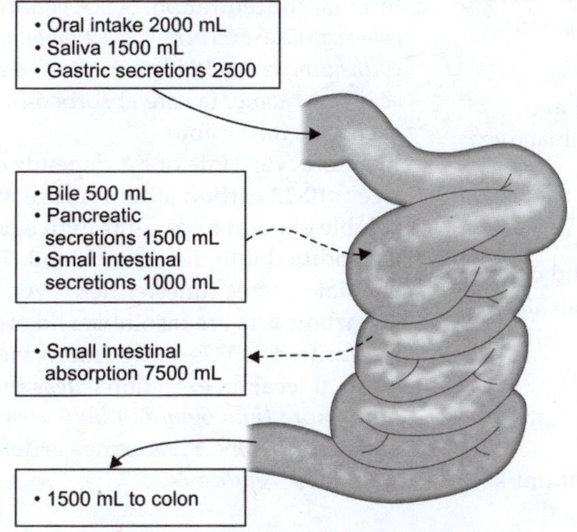

Small-intestinal water transport. Typical quantities (in volume per day) of fluid entering and leaving the small intestinal lumen in healthy adult are given

Agents that stimulate absorption or inhibit secretion of water
• Adrenal Hormones - Cate cholamines i.e. Epinephrine, Norepinephrine, Dopamine - Aldosterone - Glucocorticoids • Angiotensin • ***Somatostatin (D- Cell)***Q • Enkephalin • Neuropeptide Y & peptide YY- (L-cell)

★ Secretion of regulatory peptides – *somatostatin* by ***D-cell***Q, *Colecystokinin* by ***I–cell****, peptide YY & glucagons like peptide –2* by ***L-cell****,* secretin by **S-** cell, motilin by **M-** cell and Neurotensin by **N-** cell.

Substance Absorbed	Site: Small intestine			Colon
	Upper (Proximal Jejumum mainly duodenum in most cases except NaCl & HCO_3^-)	Mid	Lower (distal ileum)	
1. Na+	3+	2+	3+	3+
2. Cl-	3+	2+	+	+
3. Ca++	3+	2+	+	?
4. Long chain fatty acid (absorption & conversion to triglycerides)	3+	2+	+	0
5. Water soluble & fat soluble vitamins except B_{12}	3+	2+	0	0
6. Iron (Fe++)	3+	+	+	?
7. SO_4^{-}	2+	+	0	?
8. Pyrimidines (thymine & uracil)	+	+	?	?
9. K+	+	+	+	Secretion
10. Sugars (glucose, galactose etc).	2+	3+	2+	0
11. Aminoacids	2+	3+	2+	0
12. Antibodies (in newborn)	+	2+	3+	?
13. Bile salts	+	+	3+	
14. Vitamin B_{12}	0	+	3+	0
15. Betaine, Dimethylglycine, sacrosine	+	2+	2+	?

Lipid (Fat) Digestion 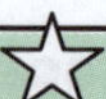

In Stomach: By Lingual & Gastric Lipase

- **Lingual & gastric lipases are of little quantitative significance for fat digestion**Q except in cases of pancreatic insufficiency. However, they may produce *FFAs that causes release of CCK* by singaling to most distal parts of GI tracts.
- **Lingual lipase:**
  - Secreted by **Ebner's glands** on the dorsal surface of the tongue.
  - It is an acid- stable lipase.
  - It is active in stomach & can digest as much as 30% of dietary triglyceride

Role of Bile Salts: Formation of Micelles

- Fats are finely ***emulsified*** in the small intestine by the ***detergent action of bile salts***Q, lecithin, monoglycerides and phosphatidylcholine.
- Lipids & bile salts interact spontaneously to *form micelles.*
- Micellar formation solubilize the lipid & provides a mechanism for their transport to the enterocytes.

In Small Intestine: By Pancreatic Lipase, Colipase & Bile Salts

- Most fat digestion begins in the *duodenum.* Enzyme involved are:

1. Pancreatic Lipase

   It acts on fats that have been emulsified. It hydrolyzes **1 and 3 bonds of TG (triglycerides)** with ease but bond 2 at a very low rate, so producing *FFA (free fatty acids) and 2-monoglycerides (2-monoacylglycerol).*

2. Pancreatic-Colipase

   A protein, which is secreted in pancreatic juice. Secreted in inactive form & activated by **trypsin**.

   It facilitates the activity of lipase by binding to – COOH terminal and opening (benting back) the lid covering the active site of lipase. It also allows lipase to remain associated with droplets of dietary lipids

3. Bile Salt Activated Lipase: Cholesterol Esterase

   It is *10-60 times less active*, but unlike pancreatic lipase, it catalyzes the hydrolysis of cholesterol esters, eastrers of fat soluble vitamins & phospholipids as well as triglycerides.

Fat Absorption 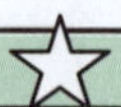

- Major fat absorption takes place ***in upper small intestine (mainly jejunum & duodenum) except short chain fatty acids which is absorbed in colon***Q.
- **Short chain FAs (SCFAs)** are 2-5 carbon weak acids produced in colon by action of colonic bacteria on complex carbohydrates, resistant starches & dietary fibers that escape digestion in upper gitract. ***60% of SCFAs is acetate, 25% propionate & 15% butyrate***Q withan average 80 mmol/1 luminal concentration. SCFAs contribute to *caloric intake, exert trophic action on coloic epithelium, combat inflammation and maintain acid-base balance* (as are absorbed in exchange for H^+ ion).
- In enterocytes, fate of FA depends on their size. **<10-12 carbon atom FAs** are water soluble enough to pass through enterocytes unmodified into the portal blood. They circulate as free (unesterified) FAs. But **>10-12 carbon FAs** are insoluble and are reesterified to TGs in the enterocytes.
- Normal fecal fat excretion is ***less than 6gm /day, more than 6gm/day indicates malabsorption***Q. **Steatorrhea** is defined as stool fat **>** ***7gm/day***Q.

Vitamin B / Cyanocobalamine

Absorption

- Vitamin B_{12} normally binds to ***intrinsic factor***Q ***(secreted by parietal or oxyntic cells of gastric mucosa)***Q
- Complex is taken up by ***cubilin***Q. (High affinity apolipoprotein) in the ***distal ileum***Q.
- This triggers absorption of complex by endocytosis.
- In ileal enterocytes, B_{12} is transferred to ***transcobalamine II (transporter protein)***Q.

Causes of Deficiency

- Due to inadequate dietary intake is *very rare.*
- Produced by ***Gastrectomy***Q, with removal of intrinsic factor producing tissue
- ***In pernicious anemia***Q.

★ Deficiency causes ***megaloblastic anemia***Q.

Iron Absorption

Almost all iron absorption occurs in ***duodenum and upper jejunum (proximal small intestine)***Q.
Most of the iron in diet is in ferric form (Fe^{3+}) but it is ***ferrous*** ***(Fe^{+2}) that is absorbed***Q. Transport of Fe^{2+} into enterocyte occurs via ***DMT1.***

Increased by		Decreased by
• Acids • ***Ascorbic acid (Vit C)***Q • Amino acid containing SH – group • Meat	*Reduces* Fe^{3+} into Fe^{2+}	• Alkalies • ***Phosphates***Q • ***Phytates***Q (in maize, wheat) • Tetracyclin • Presence of other food in stomach

Role of Colonic Microflora (Enteric Bacterial Ecosystem)

Large intestine contains a unique biological ecosystem consisting of trillions of commensal (non pathogenic) bacteria that engage in a life long symbiotic relationship with their human host. This colonic ecosystem is established shortly after birth and remains remarkably stable unless disturbed by antibiotics. It is highly unusual relationship as other body compartments are largely sterile. It is involved in

Fermentation & Digestion of Complex Carbohydrate

- Colonic bacteria **metabolize meal components that are not digested by host enzymes** and make their products available to the body via **fermentation**. It provides advantage to the host in that the colonic bacteria are capable of performing metabolic reactions that do not take place in mammalian cells.
- Carbohydrates that humans cannot digest without bacterial help include **complex carbohydrate, resistant starches, dietary fibers, mucin (moucous)** produced by gut and oligosaccharides / sugars that the body failed to digest /absorb d/t some pathology eg lactose in lactose intolerance

Formation of Short Chain Fatty Acids (SCFAs)

- Colonic bacteria form SCFAs by femanting carbohydrates (starches, fibers). SCFAs are 2-5 carbon weak acids with 80mmol/L average normal concentration in lumen. About 60% of this is **acetate**, 25% **propionate** and 15% **butyrate**.
- SCFAs are absorbed & metabolized to make a significant contribution to total calory intake – **butyrate is a critical energy source for colonocytes.**
- **SCFAs excert a trophic effect on colonic epithelium cells.** The colonic epithelium turns over rapidly even in health, limiting the genetic damage that might otherwise be caused by exposure to toxins in lumen. However, this also increases the risk of malignancy. The colonic flora (via SCFAs) is involved in **promoting development of normal colonic epithelium and in stimulating its differentiated functions.** Butyrate regulates the expression of specific gene in colonic epithelial cells and may **suppress the development of a malignant phenotype**. Expression of SMCT1 (sodium monocarboxylate transporters 1) eg SLC5A8 may be reduced in colon cancers, thereby reducing butyrate uptake – which may contribute to malignant transformation. So SCFAs *increase the growth of intestinal epithelial cells and control their proliferation & differentiation* (ie **promoting normal development & stimulating differentiation**)
- **SCFAs combat inflammation** (prevent inflammatory bowel disease) *maintain acid –base equilibrium* (absorbed in part by exchange for H+) and promote absorption of Na+, Mg^{++}, Ca^{++} and Fe^{++}

Metabolism of Exogenous & Endogenous Substances

- Gut flora forms **secondary bile acids** and deconjugate any bile acids that have escaped uptake in terminal ileum
- Contribute to formation of **intestinal gas**.

Detoxification

- *Detoxify xenobiotics (eg drugs) & dietary carcinogen* (but may also generate toxic or carcinogenic compounds from dietary substrates.

Antimicrobial

- Gut flora **limits the growth & invasion of pathogenic microorganisms** by
1) Functioning as a physical barrier to prevent attachment of pathogens.
2) Forming microbicidal substances,
3) Triggering gene expression in epithelium that counteracts the adverse effects of pathogens

Prevent Allergy & Provide Immunity

- Gut flora is not essential for life as animals raised in germ free conditions apparently develop normally. However, in these animals the ***mucosal immunity is immature and intestinal epithelial cells differentiate more slowly***Q
- Colonic microflora trains immune system preventing allergy & providing immunity.

Synthesis of Vitamin K & Biotin

Substrate	Enzymes	Products	Disposition
Endogenous Substrates			
Urea	Urease	Ammonia	Passive absorption or excretion as ammonium
Bilirubin	Reductases	Urobilinogen Stercobilins	Passive reabsorption Excreted
Primary bile acids	Dehydroxylases	Secondary bile acids	Passive reabsorption
Conjugated bile acids (primary or secondary)	Deconjugases	Unconjugated bile acids	Passive reabsorption
Exogenous Substrate			
Fiber	Glycosidases	Short-chain fatty acids Hydrogen, CO_2 and methane	Active absorption Excreted in breath or flatus
Amino acids	Decarboxylases and deaminases	Ammonia and bicarbonate	Reabsorbed or excreted (ammonia) as ammonium
Cysteine, methionine	Sulfatases	Hydrogen sulfide	Excreted in flatu

Diet

Estimated Average Requirement (EAR)

It is an average daily nutrient intake estimated to **meet the requirement of 50% of healthy** individuals in particular life stage & gender.

Recommended Dietry Allowance (RDA)

- It is the average daily dietry intake that is sufficient to meet the nutrient requirement of **nearly all (97-98%)** individuals in a life stage & gender group.
- ***RDA is based on EAR and is statistically set at 2 standard deviations above EAR***Q
- ***RDA is neither equal to AI nor to recommended minimum requirement***Q for healthy individuals. Rather, it is intentially set to provide a margin of safety for most individuals. In fact for many individuals RDA would be in excess (but not injurious) of their needs.

Adequate Intake (AI)

- It is based on estimates of nutrient intake, by a group (or groups) of apperantly healthy individuals, that are assumed to be adequate
- At is set instead of RDA *if* sufficient scientific evidence is *not available to calculate the EAR on RDA*

Transit Time in Small Intestine & Colon

- The first part of a test meal reaches the caecum in about 4 hours, all of the undigested portions have entered the colon in 8-9 hours.
- On average, the first remnants of the meal reach the hepatic flexure in 6 hours, the splenic flexure in 9 hours & the pelvic colon in 12 hours.
- ***From the pelvic colon to the anus, transport in much slower***Q.
- As much as 25% of the residue of a test meal still be in the rectum in 72 hours.

So, the ***transit time of colon is the longest***Q.

Dietary Fibre

Defined as all ingested food that *reaches the large intestine* in an essentially *unchanged form*.

Advantage

- **Contributes bulk by absorbing water 10-15 times of its own weight** (provides a larger volume of indigestible material to the colon) and thus *hastens passage through the gut*, ***decreasing the transit time***Q. High fiber diet aids water retention during passage of food along the gut, producing larger & softer feaces; there by reducing stool – transit time.
- ***Reduces incidence of***Q:
  - Diverticulitis, constipation hemorrhoids
  - *Cancer of colon*Q
  - DM (diabetes mellitus)
  - Coronary artery disease
- ***Soluble fiber lower total blood cholesterol levels by lowering LDL or bad cholesterol level***Q. It also ***slows the absorption of sugar and reduce the risk of developing type II diabetes***Q. Soluble fibers found in legumes & fruits eg gums & pectin, *lower blood cholesterol level*; and *slow stomach emptying* and thus *delay the post prandial rise in blood glucose* so it is beneficial in diabetes.

Components

Consist of all plant cell wall components that cannot be digested by animals own enzymes. These include

- **Cannot be hydrolysed or digested** (by endogenous enzymes) but is fermented by GI bacteria
  - **Cellulose**
  - **Hemicellulose**
  - **Pectin**
  - **Pentosans**
  - **Gums & aliginates**
- **Neither digested nor fermented**
  - *Lignin*Q

Category

It is of two types

Insoluble fiber

- It promotes movement of material through digestive system & increase stool bulk
- Whole wheat flour, wheat bran, nuts, & vegetables are good source
- **Cellulose, hemicellulose & lignin are insoluble**

Soluble fiber

- It is dissolved in water to form a gel like material
- Oat, flax seeds, peas, beans, apple, cirtus fruits, carrots, barley & psyllium are good source.
- *Pectins; gums and oliginates* are soluble

Glycemic Index

***Glycemic index** is a measure of a food's ability to elevate blood sugar level*. The indexing is done by comparing a foodstuffs digestion rate to that of glucose, with a glycemic index of 100. The higher the glycemic index, the faster will it enter the blood and increase the blood sugar level.

Glycemic index is used to lable the food as good and evil. Foods with a **high glycemic index of 60 and above** are considered unhealthy as they break down quickly and spike blood sugar level. **Low glycemic foods** enter the blood stream slowly and provide sustained long term energy (maintain stable blood sugar levels)

High glycemic food	
Glucose	**100**
Baked potato	85
Corn flakes	**84**
Honey	73
Watermelon	72
White bread	70-72
Table sugar	65
Ice Cream	**61**

Moderately Glycemic food	
Orange Papaya	58
White rice	58
Brown rice	55
Popcorn	55
Sweet potato	54
Mango	55
Banana	50
Carrots	49
Orange	44

Low Glycemic food	
Apple	37
Yoghurt	33
Skimmed milk	32
Kidney beans	27
Peanuts	14

Adipose Tissue

- ***Fatty acid stored in adipose tissue in form of neutral TAG, serve as the body's major fuel storage reserve[Q].*** It is highly concentrate source of energy as it is highly reduced, largely anhydrous and yield *9 k cal/gm energy* (as compared to 4 k cal/g of protein & carbohydrate).
- *Fat stores constitute 75% of energy reserve and protein stores 25%.* Glycogen is the smallest resource of stored energy. Metabolic fuel stores in 70 kg man are

Fat : 15 kg = 135,000 K cal > Protein : 6 kg = 24,000 k cal > Glycogen : 0.2 kg = 800 k cal.

Acceptable Macronutrients Distribution Ranges (AMDR)

- ***Main source of energy in humans is carbohydrate. The primary role of dietary carbohydrate is to provide enegy[Q].***
- The carbohydrates are not essential nutrient, because the carbon skeletons of amino acids can be converted into glucose by gluconeogenesis. However the absence of dietary carbohydrates l/t ketone body production, protein degradation & gluconeogenesis.
- Recommended dietary allowance (RDA) for carbohydrate is set at **130 gm/day** for adults & children, based on the amount of glucose used by carbohydrate dependent tissues, such as *brain and RBC.*
- Adults should consume **45-60%** of their total calories from carbohydrate and added sugars represent no more than 25% of total energy.
- *Very low carbohydrate diets,* providing only 20 gm/day, but permitting unlimited consumption of fat and protein *promote weight loss because of high energy (ATP) cost of gluconeogenesis.* Since there is a continual demand for glucose, there will be a considerable amount of gluconegenesis from amino acids; the associated high ATP cost must then be met by oxidation of fatty acids.
- Glycogen is the only carbohydrate in options

Macronutrient	Range (% of energy)	KCl gm
Carbohydrate (No less than 130 gm/day)	45 – 65	
Protein	10-35	4
Fat - n-6 only unsaturated FA - n-3 Polyunsaturated FA	20-25 5- 10 0.6–1.2	9
Carbohydrate No less than 130 gm/day - Added sugars - Fiber in men : 38 gm - in women: 25gm	45-65	4

Quality of protein : Protein digestibility corrected aminoacid Scoring (PDCAAS)

Source		PDCAAS value
Aninial protein	Egg	1
	Milk	1
	Beef / Poultry /Fish	0.82- 0.92
	Gelatin	0.08
Plant protein	Soyabean	1
	Kidney beans	0.68
	Whole wheat bread	0.40

Chapter 6. EXCRETORY SYSTEM: REVIEW NOTES

Renal Medullary and Cortical Structures

- Renal corpuscle (Bowmen's capsule & glomerulus), convoluted proximal part of proximal tubule, distal part of thick ascending limb of loop of Henle, ***juxta glomerular apparatus (i.e. macula densa of DCT, JG cells of afferent arterioles & lacis cells)***[Q], distal convoluted tubule (DCT), collecting segment and cortica collecting ducts as well as interlobar, arcuate, interlobular vessels, afferent arteriole, glomerular capillaries, efferent arteriole and peritubular capillaries are found in **renal cortex**.
- Whereas, straight part of proximal tubule, ***thin descending & ascending limb and proximal part of thick ascending limb of loop of Henle; medullary collecting duct as well as ascending & descending vasa recta***[Q] lie **in renal medulla (pyramid)**

Difference

	Cortical Nephron	Juxtamedullary Nephron
Over all %	85% nephrons	15% nephrons
Loop of Henle	Short	Long
Peritubular capillary network	Short	Long & form hair pin loops (vasa recta)
O_2 extraction	Very less	Large
PO_2	50 mm Hg	15 mm Hg
Blood flow	Large	Less

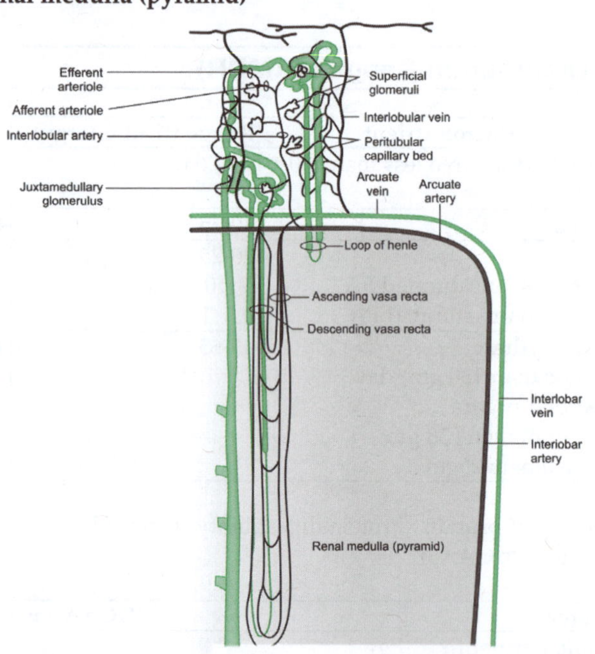

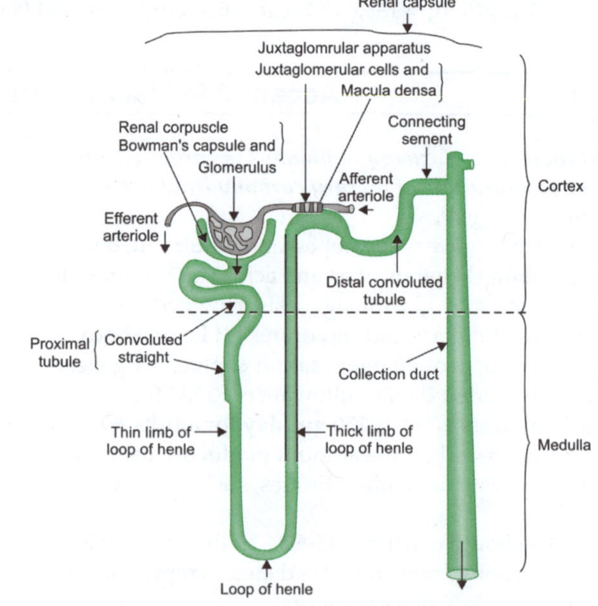

Schematic drawing of a juxtamedullary nephrons, the loops of Henle are short, and reach only the outer medulla.

Nephron & Glomerular Filtration

- Each human kidney has about ***1 – 1.3 millin nephrons***[Q]. The length of nephron including collecting ducts ranges from *45-65mm*. The human **PCT** is about ***15 mm long***[Q] & 55 μm diameter; **DCT** is about ***5 mm long***[Q] and collecting ducts are 20 mm long.
- The nephrons with glomeruli in outer portions of renal cortex have short loops of Henle (**cortical nephrons**). Whereas, about ***15%***[Q] (Ganong) / ***20- 30%*** [Q] (Guyton) nephrons have glomeruli in the renal cortex near the medulla **(Juxta-medullary nephrons).** These have long loops of Henle extending down into medullary pyramids.
- Total area of glomerular capillary endothelium across which filtration takes place is *0.8m²*. *Pore size* of endothelium of glomerular capillary is *70-90nm diameter*. *Filtration slits* formed by pseudopodia of podocytes (epithelial cells) is *25 nm*. Functionally glomerular membrane permits neutral substance upto *4 nm diameter* freely and *excludes substance > 8nm totally*.

Measurement of Renal Plasma Flow (RPF)

To measure renal plasma flow, a substance, which is *filtered and secreted* but *not reabsorbed*, should be used. **Para aminohippuric acid** is such a substance and its clearance indicates renal plasma flow.

$$\textit{Renal plasma flow}^{Q} = \frac{U_{PAH}\,V}{P^{PAH}}$$

U_{PAH} - conc of PAH in urine
P_{PAH} - conc of PAH in plasma
V - urine flow

- **At low plasma concentration of PAH**, it is almost completely cleared from the plasma by a combination of glomerular filtration and tubular secretion and indicates renal plasma flow.
- **When plasma concentration of** ***PAH are elevated beyond 30mg /dl; the secretary mechanism*** **becomes saturated**, and the transport maximum (TM) is reached, so the clearance of PAH from plasma is decreased **giving a false low value of RPF.**

Renal Blood Flow

- ***Kidney receives 1.2 – 1.3 liters of blood / minute or 25% of cardiac output at rest***[Q].
- **Glomerulus receives capillaries from afferent arterioles**
- Afferent arterioles are short straight branches of inter lobar arteries originating from renal artery.
- Each afferent arteriole divides into multiple capillary branches. 20 -50 such fenestrated capillary loops form **glomerulus** (glomerular vessels)
- The loops rejoin to form another efferent arteriol, which then supplies the tubular part of nephron before emptying into renal veins.
- As the afferent arteriole enters glomerulus, the cells of tunica media (smooth muscle layer) become more numerous & contin rennin granules. These are called **juxta (i.e. next to) glomerular cells**. At the site of origin of distal convoluted tubule (DCT), which is in close contact with the juxta glomerular cells of afferent arteriole, the cells of DCT become taller & larger, with more prominent nuclei than the other cells lining the tubule, and are called **macula densa**. The macula densa functions together with ' JGC, hence they are jointly referred to as the **juxta glomerular apparatus.** By **tubuloglomerular feed back** macula densa stimulate JGC to release rennin. The mediator is NO.

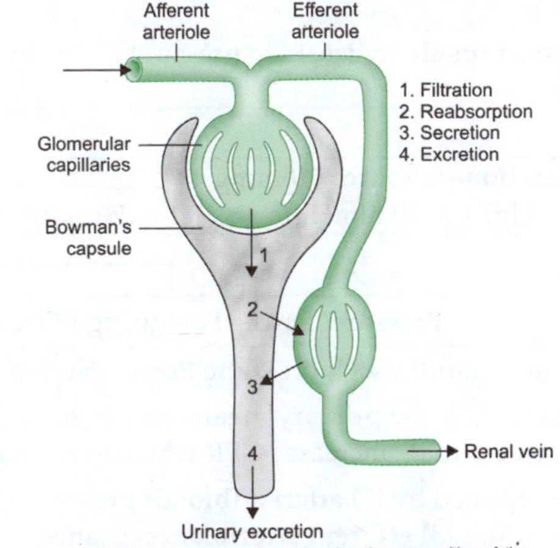

Basic kidney processes that determine the composition of the urine. Urinary excretion rate of a substance is equal to the rate at which the substance is filtered minus its reabsorption rate plus the rate at which it is secreted from the peritubular capillary blood into the tubules.

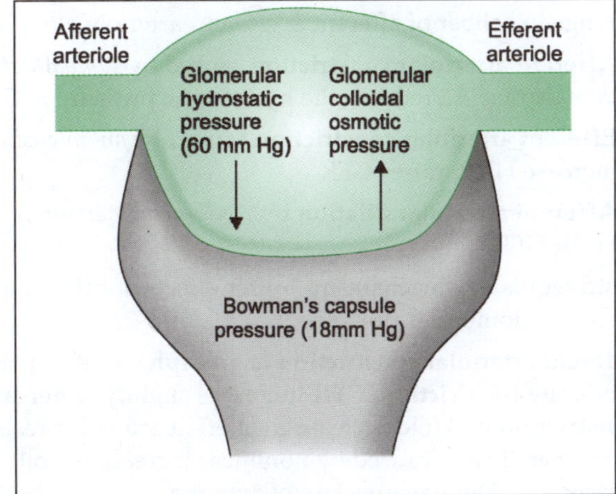

Determination & Regulation of GFR

GFR, like renal blood flow, remains constant over a wide range of perfusing pressure, from *80 – 180 mmHg* d/t autoregulation. **Factors affecting GFR** are those affecting fluid exchange across capillaries & are governed by Starting's force. **GFR is determined by changes in**

Net Filtration Pressure

- It is sum of hydrostatic and colloid osmotic pressures (forces) across glomerular capillary membrane. The forcing

Glomerular Capillary Filtration Coefficient (Kf)

- **Glomerular capillary filtration coefficient (Kf)** is a product of **(1) hydraulic conductivity or permeability and (2) filtering surface area of glomerular capillaries**
- It can be measured indirectly (not directly) by this equation

$$K_f = \frac{\text{GFR}}{\text{Net filtration pressure}} = \frac{125\,\text{ml/min}}{10\,\text{mmHg}} = 12.5\,\text{ml/min/mmHg}$$

1. Favouring filtration

- **Glomerular hydrostatic pressure** (P_G) inside glomerular capillaries **(60 mmHg)**
- **Bowman's capsule colloid osmotic pressure** (π_B) of proteins outside glomerular capillaries **(OmmHg)**

- **Kf / 100 gms weight for kidney is 4.2ml/min/mmHg (about 400 times higher)** than average (0.01) of other capillary system of body. This extremely high Kf value of glomerular capillaries is **responsible for their rapid rate of fluid filtration**
- **GFR is increased by raising Kf and decreased by reducing Kf, but changes in Kf** donot provide a primary day to day mechanism for regulation of GFR
- *Chronic uncontrolled hypertension and DM* gradually decrease Kf by increasing the glomerular capillary basement membrane thickness.

2. Opposing filtration

- **Glomerular osmotic pressure (π_G)** ie colloidal osmotic or oncotic pressure of glomerular capillary plasma proteins **(32 mmHg)**
- **Bowman's capsule hydrostatic pressure** (P_B) ie hydrostatic pressure outside the glomerular capillaries in Bowman's capsule

So **net filtration pressure = 10mmg =**
P_G (60 mmHg) + π_B (0 mmHg) – P_B (18mmHg)- π_G (32mmHg)

Pressure /Forces Favouring Filtration

1. Glomerular Capillary Hydrostatic Pressure (P_G)

- Changes in P_G is the **primary means for physiological regulation of GFR**. Increase in P_G increases GFR whereas, decrease in P_G reduces GFR.
- P_G is determined by (1) **arterial (blood) pressure (2) afferent arteriolar resistance** and (3) **efferent arteriolar resistance**
- Increase in BP increases hydrostatic pressure & GFR whereas decrease in blood pressure decreases HP & GFR
- Change in caliber of afferent & efferent arteriole alter GFR as follows
  - **Afferent arteriolar constriction** caused by *sympathetic stimulation or thromboxane* A2 reduces the hydrostatic pressure & GFR
  - **Efferent arteriolar constriction** caused by *angiotensin II or ANP* increase HP & raises GFR
  - **Afferent arteriolar dilation** by *ANP (atrial natriuretic peptide)* increase HP & GFR
- Auto regulatory mechanisms buffer effects of BP and maintain relatively constant glomerular pressure
- **Efferent arteriolar constriction** has a **biphasic effect** on **GFR** ie at **moderate constriction, GFR increases** slightly, whereas with **severe constriction** (> 3 fold increase in efferent arteriolar resistance) **GFR decreases.** This is caused by nonlinear increase in colloid osmotic pressure by Donnan effect exceeding the P_G.

2. Bowman's capsule Colloid Osmotic Pressure (π_B)

Glomerular filtrate in Bowman's capsule has nil proteins & so almost zero pressure.

Pressure / Forces Opposing Filtration

1. Bowman's Capsule Hydrostatic Pressure (P_B)

Increased P_B i.e. **intra (Bowman's) capsular pressure (m.c. d/t ureteric obstruction) oppose hydrostatic filtering pressure & filtration** thereby decreasing GFR.

2. Glomerular Capillary Colloid Osmotic Pressure (π_G)

- **Glomerular capillary colloid osmotic pressure** or **glomerular oncotic pressure** (plasma oncotic /osmotic pressure) is exerted by proteins in blood plasma and tries to pull water into the circulation (ie capillary). It is *unimportant* and normally *opposes filtration.*
- **Glomerular filtrate is** essentially **protein free** because glomerular capillaries are relatively impermeable to proteins. This results in ***almost zero (or very low) colloidal osmotic pressure of glomerular filtrate***[Q]. Therefore ***glomerular oncotic pressure is much higher than that of glomerular filtrate***[Q] ***in Bowan's capsule***[Q].
- Conditions causing *fall in plasma protein concentration* such as **nephrotic syndrome** and **cirrhosis** decrease glomerular plasma osmotic pressure.

★ **Fluid emerging from loop of Henle and entering the distal tubule is always hypotonic**. This is because of two factors
- Ascending loop of Henle & initial part of DCT are impermeable to water
- Ascending loop of Henle & DCT actively transport solutes out of tubule into interstitum.

Filterability

- As the *plasma volume* is *3 liters* and *GFR is 180 L/day* (7.5L/h or 125 mL/min) the entire plasma is filltered & processed about *60 times each day*.
- **Filterability** of **1** means that the substance is filtered as freely as water. ***Electrolytes such as sodium (Na^+), and small organic compounds such as glucose, inulin are freely filtered***[Q] (filterability = 1).
- Filterability of solutes is *inversely related to their size*. As the molecular weight of molecule approaches that of *albumin*, the filterability rapidly decreases, approaching zero
- 0.75 filterability means that the substance is filtered only 75% as rapid as water. ***Myoglobin (F = 0.75) and albumin (F = 0.005) are not freely filtered***[Q].
- **Glomerular filtrate** is ***protein free, and devoid of any cellular element, including RBC***[Q]. The concentration of other constituents including *most salts & organic molecules*, are similar to the concentration in plasma (i.e., are freely filtered). ***Exception to this generalization are few low molecular weight substances, such as calcium & fatty acid***[Q], which are partially bound to plasma proteins and thus not filtered freely.
- **Neutral substances** with molecular diameter of **< 4 nanometers** are *filtered freely* and filtration of substance **> 8 nm** approaches *zero*, as the pores of glomerular membrane are of ~ *8 nm (80 angstroms)* size. Between 4 – 8 nm, filtration is inversely proportional to diameter. ***However, negatively charged large molecules are filtered less easily than positively charged molecules of equal molecular size***[Q], and even neutral molecule are filtered much more easily than negatively charged molecules of same size. This is because, the **negative charges of basement membrane & podocytes restrict and repel large negatively charged and attract positively charged molecules**[Q]. This explains, only 0.2% filtrability of negatively charged albumin with an effective diameter of ~ 7 nm.
- **Inulin** (a polymer of fructose found in dahalia tubers, MW 5200) that is freely filtered, neither reabsorbed nor secreted in tubules, and **creatinine** (that is freely filtered, secreted & reabsorbed in some amount) are used to measure glomerular filtration rate (GFR).

Measurement of GFR

GFR can be measured ***by measuring the excretion & plasma level of a substance that is freely filtered through glomeruli and neither secreted not reabsorbed by the tubules***[Q].

Requirement of substances used to measure GFR	Substances used
- Filtered freely - Neither reabsorbed, nor secreted by tubules - Nontoxic - Not metabolized by body.	- ***Inulin (standard)***[Q] - Creatinine

Clearance of Substance, Tubular Secretion & Reabsorption

- **Renal plasma clearance** is the volume of plasma from which a substance is completely removed by kidney in a given amount of time. Therefore **clearance (GFR) of substance X =**

$$\frac{\textbf{Ux (concentration of X in urine) multiplied by V (urine flow per unit of time)}}{\textbf{Px (arterial plasma level of X)}}$$

- If a **clearance of a substance is greater than GFR**, then an additional *tubular secretion* (of substance from blood into tubule) ***must be present***[Q] but it *doesn't mean* that if there is tubular secretion, the clearance of a substance will always be more than GFR, as there may also be tubular reabsorption of substance.
- **Clearance or amount of substance excreted** (depends on)

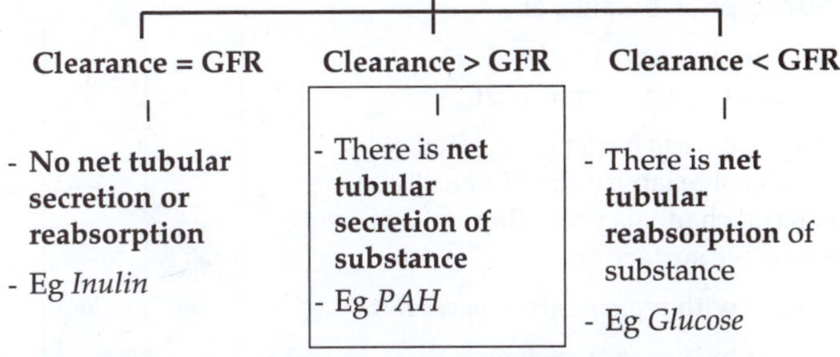

- The tubular fluid is ***hyper tonic in descending limb and hypotonic in ascending limb of loop of Henel***[Q] because
  - **Thin descending limb** is highly permeable to water, so water is reabsorbed (moved out) making tubular fluid *hypertonic*.
  - **Thin ascending limb** is *permeable to Na^+ & Cl^-* which is moved out of tubular lumen making tubular fluid *hypotonic*.

Transport Maximum (T_m) 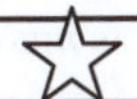

For most ***substance that are actively reabsorbed or secreted there is a maximum rate at which the solute can be transported***[Q] after k/a transport maximum. This limit is d/t saturation of specific transport system.

Tm for kidney in practice is less than calculated value (i.e.,threshold of substance is less than its Tm) because, not all nephrons have the same Tm and some of the nephron excrete substance before others have reached their Tm[Q]. It is important to know that overall Tm of substance for kidney is reached when all nephrons have reached their capacity to reabsorb or secrete that substance.

Tm for glucose in normal adult is ~***375 mg/min***[Q], whereas its filtered load is only 125mg/min (GFR × Plasma glucose = 125 ml/min × 1 mg/ml). With large increase in plasma glucose &/or GFR, which increase the filtered load above 375 mg/min, the excess glucose filtered is not reabsorbed & passes into urine. However, even when the plasma glucose concentration rises above **200 mg/100ml** (2mg/ml) (so filtered load is 250 mg/min, which is less than Tm), a small amount of glucose appears in urine. This is known as **threshold** of glucose. So **renal threshold** of substance is the plasma level at which it first appears in urine in more than the normal minute volumes (amount).

Predicted renal threshold for glucose would be 300mg/dl (i.e. 375 mg/min T_{mG} divided by 125 ml/min GFR). However, the **actual renal threshold** is about 200 mg/dl (of arterial plasma) or 180 mg/dL (of venous). This deviation between ideal & actual curves is k/a **splay**. This (less than predicted) actual renal threshold is obtained as not all nephrons have identical T_m.

Tm for substanes that are actively reabsorbed

Glucose[Q]	375 mg/min
Lactate	75 mg/min
Plasma protein	**30 mg/min**
Urate[Q]	15 mg/min
Amino acids[Q]	1.5 mM/min
Phosphate[Q]	0.10 mM/min
Sulfate[Q]	0.06 mM/min

Tm for substances that are actively secreted

Para-amino hippuric acid	80 mg/min
Creatinine	16 mg/min

Substances that do not exhibit Tm

- **Substances that are passively reabsorbed** do not demonstrate Tm, because their rate is determined by *electrochemical gradient, permeability*, & time that solute remains within tubule eg. are ***urea, chloride***[Q], water
- Some actively transported substance also have *electrochemical gradient- time transport*. e.g. is ***Na reabsorption in PCT***[Q]. *However in DCT* (where epithelium has much tighter junction & so transporting only small amounts of Na^+) *sodium reabsorption exhibits Tm.*

Proximal Tubular Reabsorption

- PCT epithelial cells favour reabsorption because of
  - large number of *mitochondria* supporting active transport.
  - *extensive brush border* on luminal side & extensive labyrinth of intercellular & basal channels providing extensive surface area
  - loaded with *protein carrier molecules*
- In **first half** of PCT, *sodium* is reabsorbed by cotransport along *with glucose, amino acid, bicarbonate & other organic ions*, leaving behind a solution that has a higher concentration of Cl^-
- But in **second half of PCT**, little glucose & amino acid remains to be absorbed. So *Na^+ is now reabsorbed with Cl^-* ions.

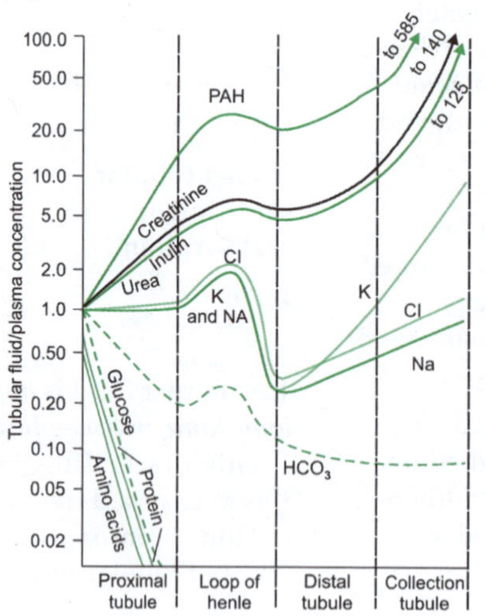

Changes in Concentrations

The total solute concentration (i.e., osmolarity) remains same all along PCT, but

- Concentrations of few organic solutes such as *glucose, amino acids, and bicarbonate decrease* markedly along the length of PCT because these are more avidly reabsorbed than water.
- Concentration of *Na^+* remains relatively **constant**, (despite of its high reabsorption) throughout PCT because water permeability keeps pace with high Na^+ reabsorption.
- Concentration of K^+, & Cl^- also remain constant
- Solutes that are less permeant & also not actively reabsorbed such as *PAH > creatinine > Inulin > urea* **increase** in concentration along PCT.

Reabsorption of Water

Obligatory Reabsorption

- Absorption of water in ***proximal tubules secondary to Na⁺ reabsorption***Q
- Absorption of water in renal tubules independent of plasma osmolality (irrespective of water balance)
- Filtered water is reabsorbed isoosmotically & is *independent of ADH levels.*

Facultative Reabsorption

- Absorption of water in distal ***tubules and collecting duct in presence of ADH***Q
- Absorption of water depends on *variation in plasma osmolality*
- Normally DCT and collecting ducts are not permeable to water but in presence of ADH, these segments become permeable.

★ ***Thick ascending limb of Henle & early distal tubule are both impermeable to water***Q & no reabsorption occurs irrespective of water balance.

Role of Vasopressin (ADH)

- ***ADH or vasopressin is key regulator of water output***Q. Vasopressin acts on the collecting ducts and enhances their permeability to water. When vasopressin is absent the collecting duct epithelium is relatively impermeable to water and only 2% of water is reabsorbed. However by the time water reaches collecting duct, a maximum of *60-70% has already been re- absorbed in the proximal tubules.*

Feature	% of water reabsorbed in absence of vasopressin	% of water reabsorbed in presence of vasopressin
Proximal tubule	***60-70%***Q	***60-70%***Q
Loop of Henle	15%	15%
Distal tubule	5%	5%
Collecting duct	2%	***10%***Q

- Thus the ***greatest fraction of filtered water (60-70%) is reabsorbed in proximal tubule irrespective of presence or absence of vasopressin***Q.

Alteration in Water Metabolism by Vasopressin

	GFR (ml/min)	% of filtered water reabsorbed	Urine volume (L/d)	Urine concentration (mosm /kg H_2O)	Gain /Loss of water in excess of solute (L/d)
Urine isotonic to plasma	125	98.7	2.4	***290***	...
Vasopressin present	125	99.7	0.5	***1400***Q (almost 5 time of plasma)	1.9 gain
No vasopressin (Diabetes insipidus)	125	87.1	23.3	30	20.9 loss

Sodium Reabsorption

Percentage	Site
60%	***Proximal tubule***Q (by Na^+ - H^+ exchange)
30%	Thick ascending limb (by Na^+ - $2Cl^+$ - K^+ cotransport)
7%	Distal convoluted tubule (by Na^+ - Cl^- cotransport)
3%	Collecting duct. (via ENaC channels)

Bicarbonate (HCO_3^-) Reabsorption

Segment	% HCO_3 reabsorbed	% Na^+ reabsorbed
Proximal tubule	***80-90%***Q	***60%***Q
Loop of Henle (thick)	10%	30%
Distal tubule & collecting duct.	Remainder	10%

Permeability and Transport In Various Segments of Nephron

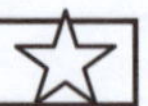

Segments	Permeability			Active transport of Na^+	Osmolality
	H_2O	Urea	NaCl		
• **Proximal tubule**	Permeable	Permeable	Permeable	Present	*Isosmotic*Q
• **Loop of Henle**					
- Thin descending limb	4+	+	±	0	***Hypertonic***Q
- Thin ascending limb	0	+	4+	0	Hypotonic
- Thick ascending limb	0	±	±	4+	Hypotonic
• **Distal convoluted tubule**	±	±	±	3+	***Hypotonic***Q
• **Collecting tubule**					
- Corticle tubule	3+*	0	±	2+	Isotonic
- Outer medullary portion	3+*	0	±	1+	
- Inner medullary portion	3+*	3+	±	1+	Hypertonic

* ***Indicates presence of vasopressin***Q.

- ***At the end of proximal tubule 60-70% of filtered solute is reabsorbed & also 60-70% of filtered water is reabsorbed***Q. Thus in the proximal tubule, water moves passively out of the tubule, along osmotic gradients set up by active transport of solutes and ***Isotonicity is maintained***Q.
- ***Intratubular content in DCT is Hypotonic***Q This is because of two factors:
  a) The distal tubule, particularly its first part, is relatively impermeable to water.
  b) The ascending limb of loop of Henle and the DCT have a strong & active system of reabsorption of solutes. Active transport of Na^+, co- transport of K^+ /Cl^- occurs out of thick ascending limb, thereby diluting the contents of DCT.

Thus while most of the solutes are reabsorbed, water remains behind, causing dilution of tubular fluid.

- The segments of nephron that are **impermeable to water: *Thin ascending limb*Q*, *Thick ascending limb*Q*, *Ist part of distal tubule (DCT)*Q**

Sodium Dependent Glucose Transporter (Symport)

- Since the intracellular Na^+ concentration is low in intestinal & renal cells, Na^+ moves into the cells along its concentration gradient.
- *Glucose moves with the Na^+* & released into the cell.
- The Na+ is then transported to lateral intercellular spaces & the glucose is transported by GLUT-2 into the interstitium & then into capillaries.
- This is an example of *secondary active transport* i.e. the energy for glucose transport is provided by the *active transport of Na^+ out of cells*.

Na^+ Transport

Sodium dependent glucose transporter (symport) in intestine

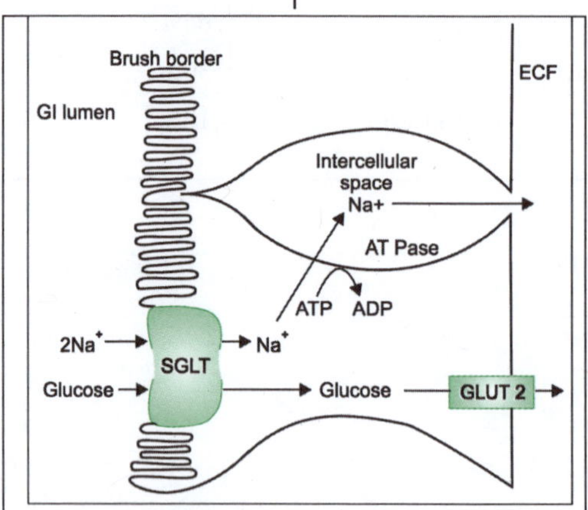

Transport proteins involved in the movement of Na+ & Cl- across renal tubular cells

Site	Apical Transporter	Fuction
Proximal Tubule	Na+/glucose CT Na+/Pi CT Na+ amino acid CT Na+/lactate CT Na+/H+ exchanger Cl-/base exchanger	Na+ uptake, glucose uptake Na+ uptake, Pi uptake Na+ uptake, amino acid uptake Na+ uptake, lactate uptake Na+ uptake, H extrusion Cl- uptake
Thick ascending limb	Na+-K+-2Cl- Na+/H+ exchanger K+ channels	Na+ uptake, Cl- uptake , K+ uptake Na+ uptake, H+ extrusion K+ extrusion (recycling)
Distal convoluted tubule	NaCl CT	Na+ uptake, Cl- uptake
Collecting duct	Na+ channel (ENac)	Na+ uptake

Also know:

- Glucose mechanism also transport ***glactose***Q.
- Fructose utilizes different mechanism, it is transported by ***facilitated diffusion***Q.
- Glucose is incorporated in ORS to ***facilitate Na^+ absorption***Q.

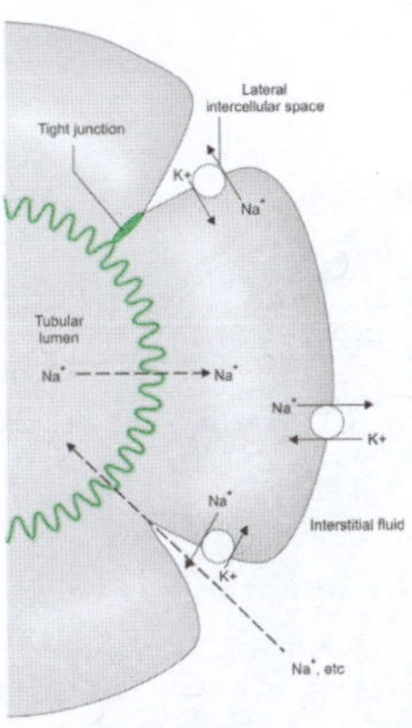

Mechanism of Na+ absorption in the Proximal Tubule

Loop of Henle

Thin descending limb

- This segment is ***highly permeable to water.***Q
- As this segment passes through inner medullary interstitium (which is increasingly hypertonic) more water is reabsorbed ***making tubular fluid hypertonic***Q

Thin ascending limb

Fluid becomes more **dilute in this segment because of movement** of ***Na^+ and Cl^-*** out of tubular lumen.

Thick ascending limb

- In this segment, a carrier co- transports ***one Na^+, one K^+ and 2 Cl^-***Q from the tubular lumen into the tubular cells.
- This is an example of **secondary active transport *; the Na^+ is actively transported***Q from the cells into interstitium by *Na^+ - K^+ AT pase* in the basolateral membrane, keeping intracellular Na^+ low.
- ***The K^+ diffuses back***Q into tubular lumen via ROMK.
- The ***Cl^- moves into interstitium***Q ***via ClC – Kb channels***Q. *(Barttin)*

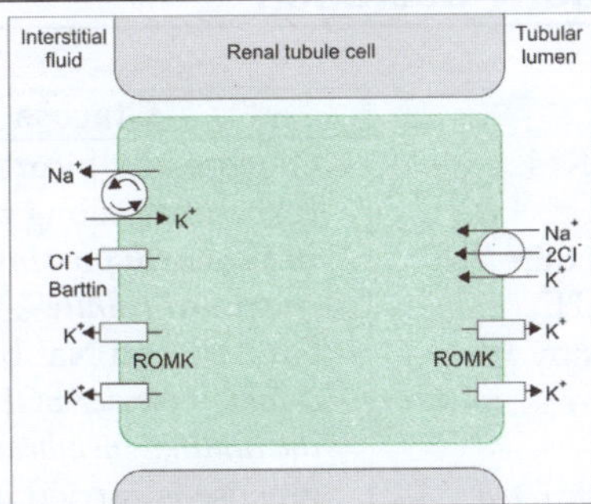

NaCl transport in the thick ascending limb of the loop of Henle. The Na+ - K+-2Cl- cotransporter moves these ions into the tubular cells by seconday active transport. Na+ is transported out of the cell into the interstitium by Na+-K+ ATPase in the basolateral membrane of the cell. Cl- exits in basolateral ClCKb Cl- channels. Bartin, a protein in the cell membrane, is essential for normal ClC-Kb function. K+ moves from the cell to the interstitium and the tubular lumen by ROMK and other K+ channels.

Tubulo Glomerular Feedback

- It is a feedback from the renal tubules, to the glomerulus to regulate the GFR, in an attempt to ensure constant sodium chloride delivery to the distal tubule.
- The sensor for this response is macula densa
- ***The macula densa senses the changes in sodium chloride concentration.***
- The Na+ and Cl- enter the macula densa cells via the Na+ - K+ - 2Cl- cotransporter.

Macula Densa

- It is ***specialized group of epithelial cells in the distal tubule***Q ***tht comes in contact with the efferent and particularly afferent arteriole***Q.
- Macula densa cells contain golgi apparatus which are intra cellular secretory organelle directed towards the arterioles.
- It is the short segment of renal tubule *at the end of thick ascending limb & continues into distal tubule.* It is located at the joint where afferent arteriole enters glomerulus and efferent arteriole leaves, and thus at this location the tubule is in contact with both the afferent and efferent arterioles (as depicted in figure)
- Juxta glomerular apparatus consists of macula densa (in DCT) & JG cells in afferent & efferent arterioles

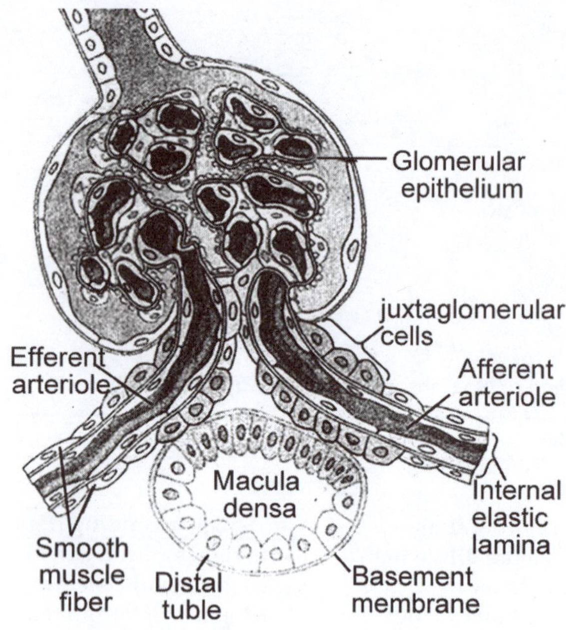

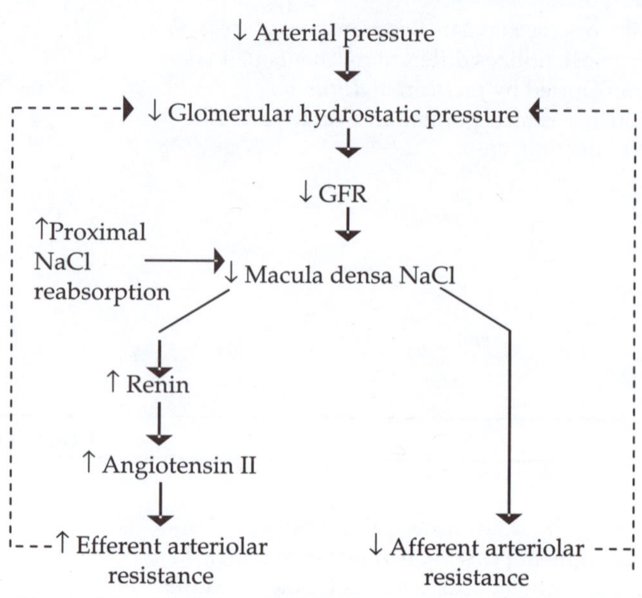

Macula densa feedback mechanism for autoregulation of glomerular hydrostatic pressure and glomerular titration rate (GFR)

Reabsorption / Secretion

Na^+	K^+	Glucose	Aminoacids
• ***Na^+ resorption occurs in all segments of nephron excepting descending limb of loop of Henle*Q.** • Na^+ is *actively transported* into interstitium by Na^+ K^+ ATPase • **Reabsorption** - ***PCT – 60% (Major portion)*Q** - Thick ascending limb LH –30% - ***DCT – 7%*Q** - CT – 3%	• **Much** of the filtered K^+ is ***reabsorbed in PCT*Q**. • Some *K^+ is secreted* in thin descending limb of LH. • Again *K^+ is reabsorbed* by *thick ascending limb of LH* by Na^+- K^+ - $2Cl^-$ cotransporter. • In *Distal tubule K^+ is secreted* [In exchange of each Na^+ reabsorbed either one K^+ or H^+ are secreted]	• Glucose and bicarbonate are reabsorbed along ***with Na^+ in the early portion of proximal tubule*Q.** • Glucose and Na^+ bind to the *common carrier SGLT – 2 in the luminal membrane* and glucose is carried into the cell as Na+ moves down its electro chemical gradient	• Amino acid reabsorption is **most marked in the early portion of PCT.** • The main carrier in the luminal membrane *co – transport Na^+*

Acidification of Urine

Removal of H^+ ions (generated by metabolism) is done by renal tubules, therefore kidney failure produces *renal or metabolic acidosis.* H^+ ions are extruded by renal tubules by *H^+ ion secretion* or *proton secretion*, this occurs in two sites:

Proximal tubule (PT) | **Collecting duct**

In both PT & distal tubule within *the lining cells* of tubules, CO_2 & H_2O in presence of ***carbonic anhydrase*Q**, produce H_2CO_3 which splits into H^+ & HCO_3^-

Proximal tubule (PT)	Collecting duct
• *In PT*, H+ ion is secreted into the lumen on exchange • of one Na^+ by help of *Na^+ H^+ exchanger*. • The H+ ions *within the lumen* are utilized to produce • H_2CO_3 which subsequently breaks down into H_2O & CO_2. So *very little free H^+ ions* appear. Therefore the ***pH of the fluid in PT*** does not fallQ.	• In CD, H+ ion is secreted *actively* by the help of *proton pump.* • *Within the lumen* of CD, H+ ion react with Na_2HPO_4 (alkaline sodium phosphate, because virtually all HCO_3^- are reabsorbed in PT) & NaH_2PO_4 (acidic sodium phosphate) is produced and one Na^+ is released which is reabsorbed. ***Acid sodium phosphate makes the urine acid*Q.** • H^+ concentration can be ↑ed as much as 900 folds in CD

Syndrome of Inappropriate ADH Secretion (SIADH)

- **Syndrome of inappropriate ADH secretion (SIADH) is characterized by relatively excessive ADH levels or plasma ADH levels** that are elevated above what would be **expected on the basis of body fluid osmolality, blood volume and blood pressure** – hence named inappropriate ADH secretion. Patients with SIADH **retain water** and their **body fluids (eg serum) becomes progressively hypoosmotic.** In other words, decreased excretion of excess water results in **reduced (low) plasma osmolality (ie hypoosmotic body fluids), hyponatremia (reduced plasma Na^+) but the urine is hyper-osmotic (more concentrated) and contain increased urinary Na^+** than would be expected on the basis of low body fluid osmolality.
- SIADH is characterized by **low plasma osmolality, hyponatremia (decreased plasma / serum Na^+), inappropriately high urine osmolality and significant amounts of sodium in urine (↑urinary Na^+)**
- In SIADH, *restricted wate intake* is necessary to prevent cellular overhydration. **Declomycin** , an *agent causing reversible nephrogenic diabetes insipidus* (ie ADH deficiency l/t dehydration, polyduria & polydipsia), may also be useful.
- Bartter & Schwartz clinical criteria for diagnosis of SIADH include

1. SIADH is most common cause of **euvolemic-hypoosmolality.** Euvolemia is defined clinically on the basis of **absence of signs of hypovolemia (ie tachycardia, orthostatic or postural hypotension** decreased skin turgor & dry mucous membranes) or **hypervolemia** (generalized edema, ascites etc). Other causes of euvolemic hypoosmolality such as hypothyroidism, hypocortisolism (pituitary ACTH deficiency or Addison's disease) and diuretics must be excluded.
2. **Hypoosmolality (decreased effective osmolality) of ECF or serum** (<275 mOsm/ kg H_2O) and **hyponatremia (reduced plasma Na^+)**; however, pseudo hyponatremia or hyper glycemia must be excluded.
3. **Inappropriately high urine osmolality (concentration)** ie > 100 mOsm/kg H_2O. It does not mean that urine osmolality is greater than that of plasma. It only means that the urine is less than maximally diluted. And urine osmolality is not necessarily elevated inappropriately at all levels of plasma osmolality.
4. **Elevated urinary sodium excretion (↑urinary Na^+)** on a normal salt & water intake. It is present in most patients but is neither 100% diagnostic nor its absence rules out the diagnosis.

Nephrogenic Syndrome of Inappropriate Antidiuresis

Nephrogenic syndrome of inappropriate antidiuresis (NSIA) occurs d/t *gain of function (activating) mutations is* ***V_2 receptor gene*** resulting in its *constitutive activation even in the absence of ADH.* It present with same laboratory findings as those of SIADH including **hypoosmolar serum, hyponatremia (↓serum Na^+), hyperosmolar urine and ↑urine Na^+.** But **unlike SIADH** (where **high ADH levels** are responsible for water retention by kidneys) **patients with NSIA have undertrevels levels of ADH** in their plasma.

Concentration & Dilution of Urine

When the urine is concentrated, solute are excreted in excess of water. Conversely, when the urine is dilute, water is excreted in excess of solutes. Renal clearance is the rate at which plasma is' cleared of solutes (osmotic clearance) & water (free water clearance).

Osmolar Clearance (Cosm)

- It is the volume of plasma cleared of solutes each minute i.e., the rate at which plasma is cleared of solute.
- It is calculated by

$$C_{osm} = \frac{Rate\ of\ osmolar\ clearance}{Plasma\ osmalarity\ (P_{osm})}$$

$$C_{osm} = \frac{Urine\ osmolarity (U_{osm}) \times Urine\ flow\ rate\ (V)}{P_{osm}}$$

★ Diluting / concentrating ability of kidney may be impaired d/t
- inappropriate ADH secretion
- inability of distal tubule, collecting tubule, and collecting ducts to respond to ADH (nephrogenic diabetes insipidus) and / or
- impairment of counter – current mechanism, which depends on hyper osmotic medullary interstitium.

★ Furosamide, like other loop diuretics, act by inhibiting Na^+ - K^+ -2Cl^- symporter in thick ascending loop of Henle. It abolishes the corticomedullary osmotic gradient and blocks negative as well as positive free water clearance.

Free Water Clearance (C_{H_2O})

- It is the *volume of plasma cleared of solute free water* each minute (per unit time).
- Rate of free water clearance represents the rate at which solute free water is excreted by kidney.
- It is calculated as the difference between water excretion (urine flow rate) and osmolar clearance

$$C_{H2O} = V - C_{osm}$$

$$C_{H2O} = V - \frac{(U_{osm} X V)}{(P_{osm})}$$

- It can be

Positive

It means *urine osmolarity < plasma osmolarity* indicating.
- Kidneys are forming dilute urine
- Water is being removed from plasma by kidneys in excess of solutes
- Water free of solutes (= free water) is being lost from body
- Plasma is being concentrated

Zero

Kidney is producing *urine isosmotic to plasma*

Negative

Urine osmolarity is greater than plasma osmolarity indicating *water conservation*

Differential Diagnosis of ECF Hyponatremia

Findings	Type I Hypervolemic	Type II Hypervolemic	Type IIIA-Euvolemic	Type IIB Euvolemic (SIADH)
History / Cause	CHF, Cirrhosis, Nephrosis	Salt & Water loss	**ACTH-cortisol deficiency**, Nause & vomiting	Infections & neoplasms of brain, antitumor drugs, pulmonary diseases & carcinoma of lung (esp small cell type)
Hypervolemia (edema, ascitus)	Present	Absent	Absent	**Absent**
Hypovolemia (postural hypotension)	∓	±	±	**Absent**
BUN, Creatinine, Uric acid	**High- normal**		**Low-normal**	
Serum K+	Low –normal		Normal	
Plasma Renin activity	High		Low	
Urinary Na+	**Low**		***High***Q	
Serum albumin	Low normal	High normal	Normal	
Serum cortisol	Normal – high		Low	Normal

Actions of ADH (on Kidney)

- Primary action of ADH on kidneys is to **increase the permeability of collecting duct to water** and to increase permeability of **medullary portion of collecting duct to urea.** It stimulates **reabsorption of NaCl** by thick ascending limb of Henle's loop, distal tubule & collecting duct
- ADH exerts its antidiuretic effect by binding & **activating V2 (vasopressin 2) receptors on basolateral membrane** of **principal cell** of late distal tubule & collecting duct. V2 receptor is coupled to adenyl cyclase via stimulatory G protein (Gs). So ADH binding to V2 receptor increases intracellular c-AMP → activates protein kinase A (PKA) ultimately resulting in **insertion of vesicles containing aquaparin 2 (AQP 2) water channels into the apical membrane of cell**, as well as synthesis of more AQ P2. With the removal of ADH, AQP2 water channels are reinternalized into the cell and apical membrane again becomes impermeable to water. This **shuttling (translocation) of water channels** into & out of apical membrane controls its permeability to water. Because the *basolateral membrane is freely permeable to water (d/t AQP3 & 4 channels)*, any water that enters the cell through apical membrane thereby results in net absorption of water from tubule lumen.

★ ADH exerts its antidiuretic effect by activating V_2 receptors and involves rapid translocation of aquaporins (protein water channels) from endosomes (where they are stored inside the cell) to luminal membranes of principle cells of collecting tubules and duct. It is important to mention that V_{1A} receptors mediate vasoconstriction by ADH. And V_{1B} (V_3) receptors are unique to pituitary, where they mediate increased ACTH secretion from corticotropes.

★ **V1 receptor** is present on **vascular smooth muscle** and mediates **vasoconstrictor** response to ADH (accounting for its **vasopressin** name).

Potassium (K^+)

K^+ concentration

- **Potassium** is the main *intracellular cation*Q.
- ***About 98% of total body potassium is contained inside***Q the cell (150mg) & only 2% in the extracellular fluid.
- This ECF/ ICF gradient of potassium is responsible for neuro- muscular function and made possible by activity of *Na^+ K^+ pump on the cell membrane*Q.
- ***About 3/4 th (109mg) of total body potassium (150mg) is present in skeletal muscle)***Q

Factors affecting K^+ concentration

Shift K^+ into cells *(Decrease extracellular K^+)*Q	**Shift K^+ out of cells** *(Increase extracellular K^+)*Q
• *Insulin*Q • *Aldosterone*Q • *β-adrenergic stimulation*Q • *Alkalosis*Q • *Diarrhoiea*Q Mn: **"In A BAD"**	• Insulin deficiency (DM) • Aldosterone deficiency • *Acidosis*Q • *β- blocker*Q • *Tissue injury*Q (cell lysis) • *Strenuous excercise*Q

Hyperkalemia In Metabolic Acidosis

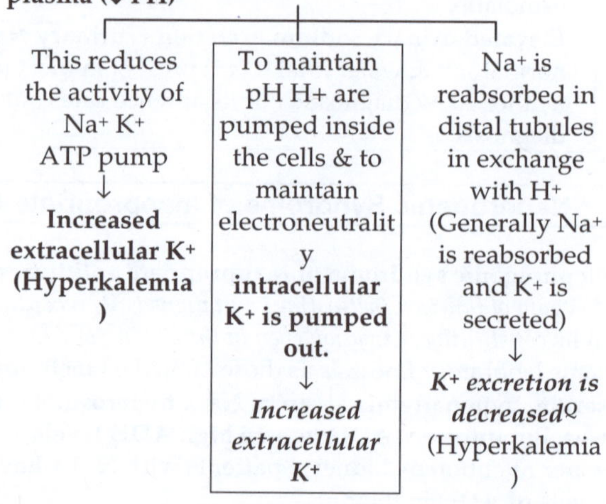

Buffer in Blood

1) **Plasma proteins**
   In the blood, ***proteins***[Q] are *effective buffers* because *both their free carboxyl and amino groups dissociate*
2) **Hemoglobin**
   Imidazole group of histidine residue in ***hemoglobin***[Q] provides an important buffer system
3) **Carbonic acid – bicarbonate system**
   Handerson – Hasselbach equation for this system is
   $pH = pK + \log \frac{[HCO_3^-]}{H_2CO_3}$

Principal Buffers in Body Fluids

Blood	H_2CO_3 HProt HHb	⇌ ⇌ ⇌	H^+ +***HCO_3^-***[Q] H^++ ***Prot*** ⊖[Q] H^++ ***Hb^-***[Q]
Interstitial fluid	H_2CO_3	⇌	H^++ HCO_3^-
Intracellular fluid	Hprot H_2PO_4	⇌ ⇌	H^++ Prot ⊖ H^++ ***HPO_4^{2-}***[Q]

★ **Phosphate buffer** is mainly present in ***intracellular fluid***[Q]. Phosphate concentration is too low in plasma for this system to be a quantitatively important buffer.

Siggard – Anderson Curve Nomogram

- **Siggard – Anderson curve nomogram** is used to plot the acid –base characteristic of arterial blood and is helpful in clinical situation. *PCO_2* is plotted on the vertical axis and *pH* on the horizontal axis.
- **Vertical line through pH 7.40:**
  - Any point to left of this line indicates acidosis
  - Any point to right indicates alkalosis
- **Horizontal line through PCO_2 of 40 mmHg:**

  Position of point above or below this horizontal line defines the effective degree of hypoventilation or hyperventilation.

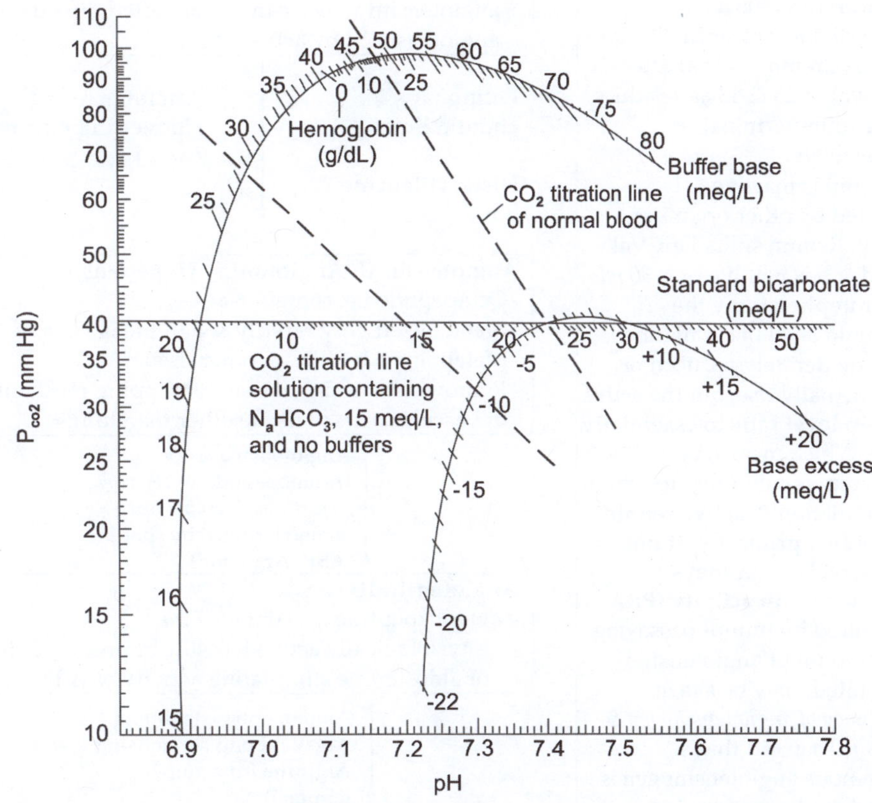

Siggard-Anderson curve nomogram

Renin Angiotensin System ☆

- A fall in BP is sensed by **intra renal baroreceptor (juxtaglomerular /JG) cells in afferent arterioles of renal glomeruli**
- JG cells release *a glycol protein hormone renin, with enzyme function* (mol wt 37, 326)
- Renin is an **aspartyl (acid) protease**. The molecule is made up of *2 lobes (domains)* between which the active site (containing **2 aspartic acid residues** at positions 104 & 292) is located in deep cleft.
- **Preprorenin** (406 aa) is converted to **prorenin** (383aa) to active renin (340 aa) after removal of 23 & 43 aa residues from aminoterminal respectively.
- Prorenin is inactive & is secreted by other organs eg ovary. Rennin splits **Leu-Val bond** & has helf life of < *80 min*.
- After **nephrectomy** the prorenin level in circulation is only moderately reduced or may actually rise, but the **active rennin level falls to essentially zero**. Which means, very little prorenin, is converted to rennin in circulation **& active rennin is product primarily, if not exclusively of kidneys**
- **Plasma rennin activity (PRA)** measured by immunoassaying the amount of angiotensin I generated, may be *low in deficiency of angio tensinogen & rennin*. To avoid this, exogenous angiotensinogen is added & **plasma rennin concentration (PRC)** rather than PRA is measured.

Angiotensinogen / Renin substrate
- Glycoprotein with 453 amino ac (aa)
- ***Synthesized in liver***[Q] with a 32 aa sequence that is removed in ER.
- ↑ed by angiotensin II, cytokines, estrogen, thyroid hormone& glucocorticoids

⇨ **Renin** ↓ **Renal** **Leucine- valine bond**

Angiotensin I
- Decapeptide i.e. contain **10 aa**.
- No established action (i.e. **physiologically inactive**
- Aminopeptiase act on it to produce (des- Asp) angiotensinI which can be converted directly to angiotensin III by action of ACE

Pulmonary endothelium ↓ **Angiotensin Converting enzyme (ACE)** ⇦

Histidyl-leucine bond

Angiotensin II/ Angiotonin / Hypertensin
- Octapeptide i.e. contain **8 aa**
- Metabolized very rapidly & half life is *1-2 min*
- Metabolized by RBC & other tissues
- Removed from circulation by trapping mechanism in vascular beds of tissue other than lungs

↓ **Angiotensinase** (Aminopeptidase *removing aspartic acid residue* from amino terminal by splitting **ASP- Arg bond)**

Angiotensin III
- Hepta peptide i.e. contain ***7 aa***
- Physiologically active has 40% of pressor & 100% of aldosterone stimulating activity of A II

↓ Aminopeptiase (splitting **Arg-Val bond** & removing **Arginine** from amino terminal)

Angiotensin IV
- Hexapeptide i.e. contain **6 aa**
- Has some activity

- ACE is *dipeptidyl carboxy peptidase* that split off **histidyl- leucine** bond from angiotensin I forming angiotensin II
- It inactivates **bradykinin**. So increased tissue bradykinin produced by ACE inhibition acts on β2 receptor to produce the **cough** that is an annoying side effect
- ACE is located in **endothelial cells of pulmonary (lung) capillaries** (& partly in kidneys and other organs).
- It is an **ectoenzyme** existing in 2 forms: **somatic** (found throughout the body) & **germinal** (found solely in spermatozoa & postmeiotic spermatogonic cells)
- Both forms have single transmembrne domain & a short cytoplasmic tail. However somatic ACE is 170 KDa protein with **2 homologous extracellular doman & catalytic sites** (containing **Zn**$^{++}$)
- Germinal ACE is 90 kDa protein with **1 extra cellular domain & active site (Zn++)**
- Both forms are formed from a single gene. Knocking out ACE gene lowers BP & fertility in males but not in females.

Actions of Angiotensin II 

Blood Vessels (AT_{1A} receptors)

- ***Potent arteriolar (Vaso) constrictor***[Q] causing
  - Rise in systolic & diastolic BP
  - Rise in total peripheral resistance
- Its pressor activity is decreased in *cirrhosis* & in *Na^+ depleted individuals*. Because circulating angiotensiin II is increased in those conditions, whch down regulates angiotension receptors in vscular smooth muscle

Brain (AT_{1A} receptors)

It *does not penetrate blood brain barrier*, but triggers responses by acting on circum ventricular organs (out side BBB)

- *Area postrema* is primarily responsible for *pressure potentiation*. Angiotensin II acts here *to decrease the sensitivity of baro reflex*
- **Dipsogenic effect** (ie. **Increase thirst or water intake**) is d/t action of *subfornical organ (SFO) & organum vasculosum of lamina terminalis (OVLT)*.

★ Angiotensin sensitive thirst centre is in anterior hypothalus (periventricular optic recess) whereas osmometeric thirst centre is in median anterior hypothalamus.

- **↑Antidiuretic hormone (ADH) or vasopressin)** from *posterior pituitary*
- **↑ACTH**

Adrenal Cortex (AT_{1B} receptors)

Increase secretion of aldosterone[Q] which

- ***Promotes Na+ & water reabsorption***[Q]
- Expands ECF (l/t ↑CO)
- Facilitates K^+ excretion

Other actions

- Direct effect on **PCT** to *increase Na+ reabsorption* by increasing Na+ - H+ exchange
- **Contraction of mesangial cells** with resultant ***decrease in GFR***[Q]
- Direct action on **post ganglionic sympathetic neurons** facilitates *release of norepinephrine*

Chapter 7. ENDOCRINE SYSTEM: REVIEW NOTES

Receptors and Second Messengers

Receptors

Group II: Cell membrane

- Membrane receptors are specific to protein, peptides & catecholamines
- ***Involved in molecular transport***Q e.g. large molecule by endocytosis or exocytosis.
- Binding of molecule to receptor gives ***specificity to process.***Q
- Involved in transduction of signal (after binding of ligand with receptors) that influences intracellular process.
  - Activation of intracellular enzymes
  - Alteration of permeability of membrane result in opening of ion channels.

Group I (Lipophilic) Hormones that bind to Intracellular Receptors

- Hormone diffuses through plasma membrane of all cells but only encounter their specific, high affinity intracellular receptors in target cells.
- **Steroid receptor superfamily**: are soluble DNA binding proteins that regulate the trancription of specific genes. Hormone receptor complex first undergoes an **activation reaction** and is the signal for group I hormones
- ligand – receptor complex directly provides the signal to specific genes whose rate of transcription is there by affected.

Receptors with Intrinsic Ion Channels

These cell surface receptors enclose ion selective channels (Na^+, K^+, Ca^{2+}, Cl^-) within their molecule. *Agonist binding opens the channels & causes depolarization / hyperpolarization* depending on the ion that flows through.

This includes:

- ***Nicotinic cholinergic receptor***Q
- Glutamate receptor
- Glycine receptor
- ***$GABA_A$ receptor***Q
- $5HT_3$ receptor

Receptor	Acts Through
- Muscarinic receptor, opioid and $GABA_B$	- G- protein coupled receptor
- M1, M3 (muscarinic)	- IP3-DAG
	- CAMP
- M2 muscarinic, Opioid μ ,δ	- ↑K^+, Ca^{+2}↓
- $GABA_B$	

At Cytoplasmic Receptors

Hydrophobic (lipophilic) steroid hormones eg **glucocorticoid** diffuse across plasma membrane and encounter their **cognate receptor in the cytoplasm of target cells**. Hormone (ligand)-receptor binding activates receptor by resulting in conformational change in the receptor leading to dissociation of heat shock protein (hsp) 90 (from receptor). This activated receptor hormone complex moves (translocates) from cytoplasm to nucleus and the **nuclear localization sequence** of receptor binds with high affinity to a specific DNA sequence called **hormone response element (HRE)**. The DNA bound-hormone-receptor serves as a high affinity binding site for **co-activator proteins** enhancing transcription. Example includes **Steroidal hormones** like

- ***Glucocorticoids & mineralocorticoids***Q
- ***Androgens (testosterone), estrogen & progestins***Q
- ***Retinoic acid (retinoids)*** Q
- **Vit D_3 (1, 25-$(OH)_2$ D_3)** Q

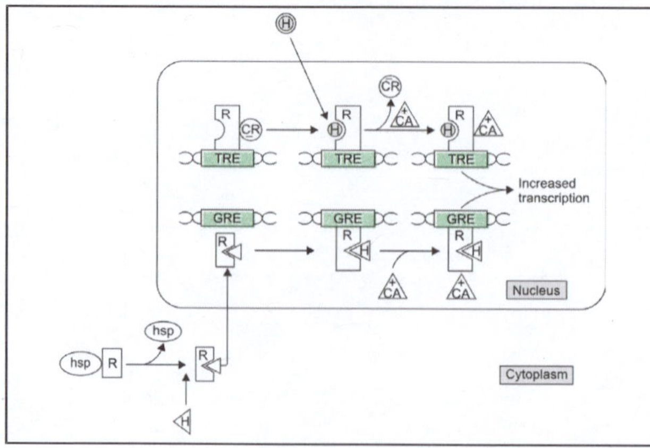

At Nuclear Receptors

Thyroid hormones & retinoic acid directly enter the nucleus where their cognate (hetero dimeric) receptors are already bound to appropriate hormone response element (HRE). However this **DNA bound receptor fails to activate transcription because it exists in a complex with a co repressor.** The association of hormone (ligand) with receptor results in dissociation of the co-repressor (s). The liganded receptor is now capable of binding co-activators resulting in recruitment of RNAP II & GTFs and activation of gene transcription.

Includes ***Thyroid*** (T_3 & T_4) ***hormones***Q

Classification of Hormones by Lipid/Water Solubility

Group I Hormones	Feature	Group II Hormones
Are *lipophilic (i.e. lipid or steroid soluble)*[Q]	**Solubility**	Are **hydrophilic** (i.e. **water soluble**)
Being insoluble in water, they are **transported in blood bound to a plasma protein**; their association with carrier protein (commonly globulin) circumvents the problem of solubility	**Transport (Carrier) protein**	Carrier protein is **not required** as they themselves are water soluble
They are **not stored** & secreted on demand (**except thyroid** hormones; thyroxine stores can last for several weeks)	**Synthesis & storage**	They are synthesized in **endoplasmic reticulum (ER)**, like all proteins and stoed in granules or vesicles.
Prolonged (hours-days) d/t transport protein	**Plasma half life** ($t_{1/2}$)	**Short** (minutes)
In target cells, they easily penetrate lipophilic plasma membrane to act **intracellularly in cytosol or nucleus**	**Site of action & Receptor**	Being lipid in soluble, they ***act on plasma membrane receptors***[Q], and **do not enter the cell** to act.
Slower in onset and **prolonged** in duration. Their actions are terminated in liver.	**Action**	Rapid in onset and shorter in duration (bcoz cell entery is not required)
Hormone –receptor complex undergoes activation reaction and moves into the nucleus to bind with high affinity to a specific DNA sequence k/a **hormone response element (HRE).**	**Mediator** or **Intra cellular messenger**	Use intracellular **second messengers like c-AMP, c-GMP, IP3-DAG, calcium –calmodulin and kinases** etc.
All **steroid hormones** & ***thyroid (T3, T4) hormones***[Q] (see HRE table below)	**Examples**	- **Catecholamines** (adrenaline & noradrenaline) - Protein (glycoprotein) and poly peptide hormones which includes all hormones of 1. Hypothalamus (except PIF) 2. Anterior & posterior pituitary 3. Pancreatic & parathyroid hormones 4. Gastro intestinal hormones 5. Calcitonin (from thyroid,) *renin*[Q], & **erythropoietin**, (kidney), **angiotensin, atrial natriuretic peptide/ANP** (heart), **leptin** (from adipocyte)

Hormone	HRE	DNA sequence
Glucocorticoids **Mineralocorticoids** **Progestins** **Androgens**	GRE MRE PRE ARE	GGTACA NNN TGTTCT ← →
Estrogens	ERE	AGGTCA - - - TGA/TCCT ← →
Thyroid hormones **Retinoic acid (retinoids)** **Vitamin D**	TRE RARE VDRE	AGGTCA N3,4,5 AGGTCA → →
cAMP★	CRE	TGACGYTCA

★ Not of group I

Adenyl Cyclase – Cyclic-AMP Pathway

- 5 components are involved in the mechanism by which ligands bring about changes in the intracellular concentration of C- AMP
  - *Catalytic unit* ***adenyl cyclase*** (a trans membrane protein crossing membrane *12 times*) which ***catalyzes the conversion of ATP to CAMP***[Q]
  - *Stimulatory & Inhibitory receptors*
  - *Stimulatory (Gs) & Inhibitory (Gi) – G proteins* that link the receptor to the catalytic unit
- Ligand binding to stimulatory receptor (Gs α)- subunit stimulates; whereas binding to inhibitory receptor (Gi -α subunit) inhibits adenyl cyclase.
- 2nd messenger of this pathway is **C- AMP** (cyclic adenosine 3′, 5′ – monophosphate) formed from ATP by action of enzyme *adenyl cyclase* & converted to physiological inactive form (5¹ AMP) by *phosphodiesterase*. *Methyl xanthines* such as *theophylline & caffeine* inhibit phosphodiesterases hence

Toxin	Mode of Action
Pertussis Toxin	Inhibits adenyl cyclase (through Gi α subunit)
Heat stable enterotoxin (ST) by enterotoxigenic E.Coli	Persistent activation of *gaunylate cyclase* & elevation of intracellular *Cyclic -GMP*
- **Cholera Toxin** - **Heat labile enterotoxin (LT)** produced by enterotoxigenic strains of E.Coli	**ADP ribosylation (activation) of Gsα subunit** l/t persistant chronic activation of adenyl cyclase → **elevated c-AMP → activates PKA → Phosphorylation of CFTR & Na⁺ - H⁺ exchanger – ↓ Na⁺ absorption & ↑Cl⁻ secretion → watery diarrhoea**

augment hormonal effect mediated by C-AMP.

- ***C- AMP activates protein kinase A (PKA) which phosphorylates protein, changing their conformation & altering their activity***[Q]. In addition active catalytic subunit of PKA moves to nucleus & phosphrylates **C-AMP responsive element binding protein (CREB).** This transcription factor then binds to DNA & alter transcription.

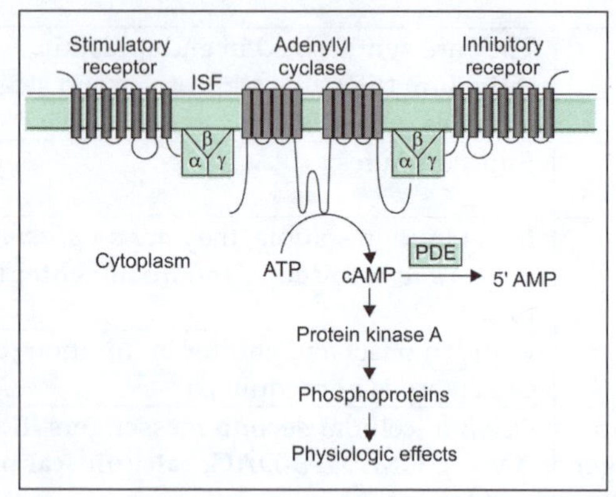

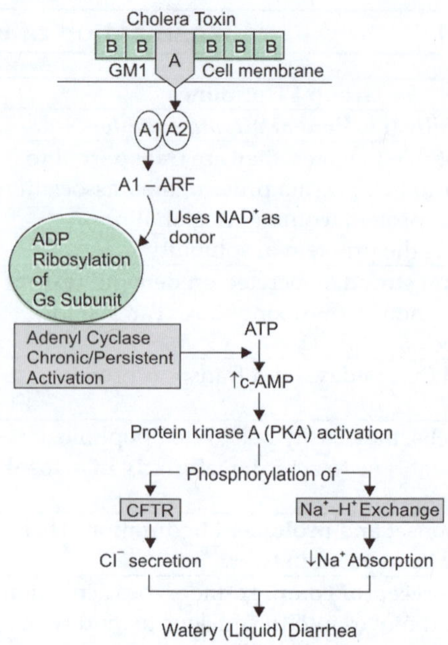

Nuclear Receptor

- Steroid hormone receptors are *monomeric phosphoproteins*. Each receptor has *6 codomains (A to F)*.
- All have centrally located **DNA – binding domain (DBD)** or **C- domain** containing **2 *zinc finger binding motifs***[Q] that allows receptor to bind with high affinity to a DNA sequence called *hormone response element (HRE)*, either *as homodimer, as heterodimer (retnoid X receptor, RXR* or as monomer.
- Multifunctional **ligand binding domain (LBD)** in carboxy terminal half (*E domain*) of receptor. It ***binds to hormones (steroid), or metabolites***[Q] and also mediate binding of *heat shock proteins (hsp), dimerization, nuclear localization, and transactivation*.
- At **carboxy (C) terminal**, transcription activation function (**AF_2**) of *F domain* interacts with *coactivators and facilitate trans activation*.
- Hightly variable **hinge region** (*domain D*) *seperates DBD from LBD* and provides flexibility to receptor to *assume different DNA binding* conformations.
- Highly variable **amino (N) terminal** contain another transactivation domain – **AF_1** (*at domain A/B*). It is also k/a *modulator* region as it is involved in activating transcription. It is *responsible for receptor isoforms* that share same DBD & LBD but exert different response because of association of various *coregulators*.

Receptor	Steroid class	Retnoid X receptor	Orphan
Binding	Homodiners ○○	Heterodimer ○□	Homodimer △△
Ligand	Steroid	9-Cis Retinoic acid + (X)	Not known
DNA element	Inverted repeat → ←	Direct repeat → →	Direct repeat → →
Example Hormone receptor for	**Glucocorticoids, mineralocorticoids, estrogen, androgen, & progestin**	**Thyroid hormone, retinoic acid, vitamin D, &** metabolite ligands eg. PPAR α, β & γ, F X R, PXR/ SXR, LXR, and CAR	COUP – TF; TR-2, GEN 8, HNF-4, TLX

- Group I lipophilic hormones cross plasma membrane of all cells but encounter intracellular receptor in target cells.
- Hormone (ligand) receptor complex first undergoes an activation reaction in 2 ways

Glucocorticosteroid encounters their receptor in cytoplasm ↓ Its binding with receptor results in *dissociationof heat shock protein 90* (hsp 90) from the receptor ↓ This activated receptor – ligand complex moves into nucleus and binds *to hormone response element* (HRE), eg glucocorticoid / steroid etc. response element depending on ligand ↓ DNA bound- ligand receptor complex serves as binding site for *transcriptional co regulatos (coactivators)* that enhance gene transcription.	*Retinoids, & thyroid hormone* go directly into nucleus ↓ In this case the receptor is already bound to HRE (here thyroid hormone response element = TRE or retinoic acid response element = RARE) but fails to activate transcription b/o ***presence of co repressor***[Q]. ↓ Binding of ligand with this receptor results in dissociation of co-repressor ↓ Activated ligand receptor complex binds coactivators resulting in activation of gene transcription.

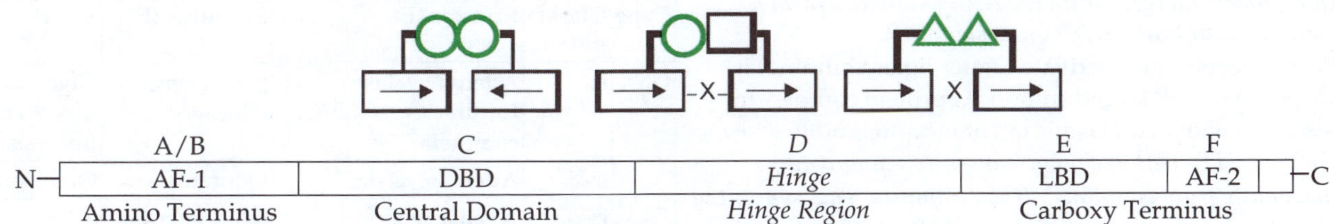

Structure of Nuclear (Androgen) Receptor

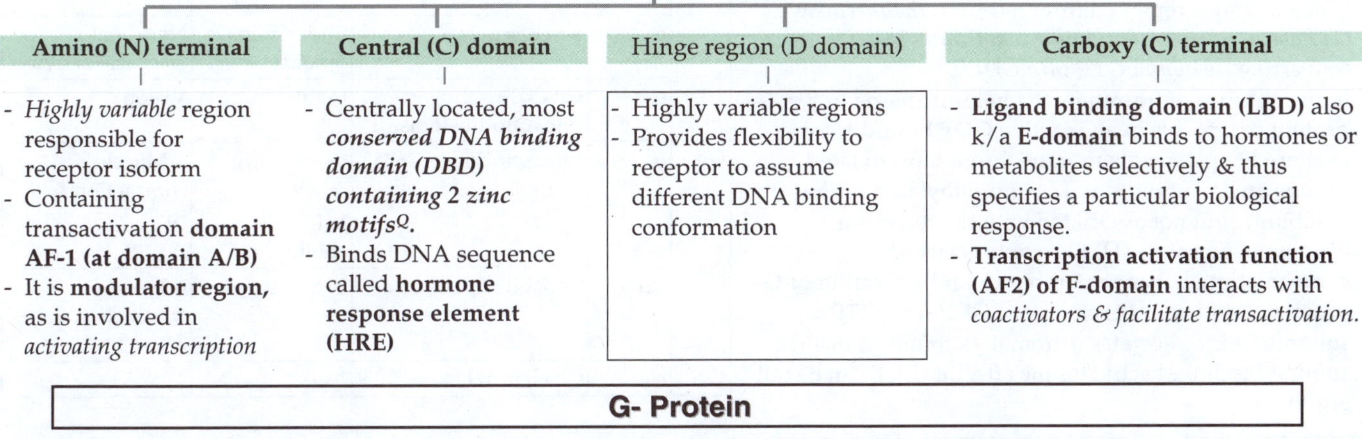

G- Protein

G- Protein is nucleotide regulatory protein that bind GTP and translate a signal to a biological effect inside the cells.

Small G Protein	Large Heterotrimeric G proteins
Involved in many cellular function. ***They are related to product of ras proto-oncogene***Q - **Rab family :** *regulates rate of vesicle traffic* between endoplasmic reticulum, golgi apparatus, lysosome, endosomes & cell membrane - **Rho / Rac family :** mediates interaction b/w cytoskeleton & cell membrane - **Ras family :** *regulates growth* by transmitting signals from the cell membrane to nucleus	• These couple cell surface receptors to catalytic unit, that catalyze the intracellular formation of second messengers or couple the receptor to ion channels. • Are made up of ***3 subunits – α, β, and γ***Q. The α unit is bound to GDP and it separates from βγ subunit, when a ligand binds to G protein coupled receptor. The ***intrinsic GTPase activity of α subunit converts GTP to GDP***Q and this leads to reassociation of α with the βγ subunit. • All the hetrotrimeric G-protein coupled receptors are proteins that ***span the cell membrane seven times (serpentine receptors)***Q • Can be divided into 5 families – Gs, Gi, Gt, Gq and G_{13} • *Cholera toxin* stimulates binds Gs α subunit and adenyl cyclase; whereas *pertusis* toxin bind *Gi α subunit* and inhibit adenyl cyclase. • There are three major effector pathway through which G- protein coupled receptor function: i) ***Adenyl cyclase : c-AMP pathway (Via Gs & Gi)*** Q ii) ***Phospholipase C : IP_3 – DAG pathway (Via Gq)***Q iii) Channel regulation:

G Protein Coupled (Linked) Receptor (GPCRs)

- These ***cell surface receptors bind to the ligand at the cell surface***Q. And have ***7 transmembrane segments that loop in and out of the cell membrane***Q. So the receptor is also k/a **seven transmembrane domain (7TM) receptors, heptahelical or serpentine receptor**.
- Part of receptor that protudes into cytoplasm (cytoplasmic tail of receptor) is coupled to G protein that has 3 different subunits (hetrotrimeric) - α, β, γ. This G protein has an ability to bind guanosine nucleotides.

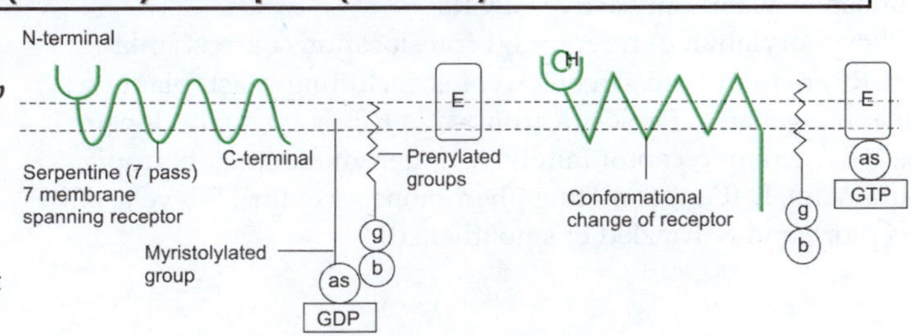

- *In resting (inactive) state the α, β, γ subunits form a complex that binds GDP on α subunit*[Q]. When receptor gets **activated** (after ligand binding) it causes this GDP bound trimeric G protein complex to associate with cytoplasmic tail of receptor and to *exchange GDP by GTP*. ***This exchange causes α subunit to dissociate from combined β & γ subunits. This separated α subunit brings about biological effect***[Q]. The β & γ subunits do not separate from each other and activates variety of effectors. (So dissociation of subunits l/t action).
- When ligand is removed from receptor, ***the intrinsic GTPase activity of α subunit inactivates itself by converting its bound GTP into GDP***[Q].

Type/Class of G protein		Effector (E)	Stimulus (H)	Effect
GS	α_s	**Adenyl cyclase↑ Cardiac $Ca^{++}/Na^{+}/Cl^{-}$ channels↑**	β-adrenergic & Glucagon	Glyconeogenesis, glycogenolysis, lipolysis
	α_{-olf}	**Adenyl cyclese ↑**	Odorant	Olfaction
Gi	$\alpha_{-i-1,2,3}$	**K^+ channels ↑ Adenyl cyclase↓**	α_2 adrenergics & acetylcholine	Decreased heart rate
		Ca^{++} channels ↓	M_2 Cholinergics	
	α_0	**K^+ channels ↑**	Endorphins, opioids	Neuronal electrical activity
	α_t	**C-GMP-phosphodiesterase ↑**	Light	Vision
Gq	α_q	**Phospholipase C6β1↑**	α_1 adrenergics & M1 cholinergics	↓ Muscle contraction & ↓ BP
	α_{11}	**Phospholipase Cβ2↑**	α_1 adrenergics	↓ Muscle contraction & ↓BP
G_{12}	α_{12}	Cl^- channel	?	?

- In the **absence of hormone, the heterotrimeric (α,β,γ) G protein** complex is in an **inactive GDP bound form** anchored to plasma membrane through **prenylated** groups on β γ subunits and by **myristoylated groups** on α-subunit , but not associated with the receptor. Binding of hormone (H) to receptor causes **conformational change** of receptor and **activation of G protein complex** d/t exchange of GDP with GTP on α subunit. This dissociates α-from β,γ subunit so that α-subunit binds and activates the effector (E). E can be (all are ↑)

> - **↑adenyl cyclase, $Ca^{++}/Na^{+}/Cl^{-}$ channels** for **α-s**
> - **↑K^+ channels for α_I and α_0**
> - **↑ Phospholipase $C\beta_1$** for α_q and phospholipase **$C\beta_2$ for α_{11}**
> - **↑ C GMP phosphodiesterases** for **α_t** and **Cl^-** channel for **α_{12}**

- Depending on the coupling of ligand (hormone) to inhibitory G protein(Gi) or stimulatory G protein (Gs) receptors, these can either decrease or increase the activity of intracellular enzyme. (so it is not dependent on α subunit).
- Mechanism of action: Ligand (photon, protein, amine hormone, & neurotransmitter) binding → conformation change & activation of G protein → exchange of GDP for GTP and dissociation between α- and β γ subunits which interact with **effectors**.
- α - subunit act on Na, Ca, K- channels and phospholipse – C (PLC). β γ subunit acts on adenyl cyclase, phospholipase A2, DLC, Ca – ATPase etc.
  - **Adenyl cyclase – cAMP pathway activation (i.e. adenyl cyclase activation l/t ↑ cAMP)** causes stimulatin of cAMP dependent prtein kinase *(protein kinase A) which phosphorylates the receptor*[Q].
  - G protein coupled receptor kinase are protein kinase that phosphorylates only active GPCRs
  - Phosphorylation of receptor l/t translocation & arrest linking.
- GPCRs are found **only in eukaryotes**, including yeast, plants & choanoflagellates. These are grouped in 6 classes: A (rhodopsin like); B (secretin receptor family); C (pheromone/metabotropic glutamate); D (Fungal mating pheromone receptor); E (cyclic AMP receptor); and F (frizzled or smoothened).

Ligands for GPCRs

Neurotransmitters	Tachykinins	Arachidonic Acid derivatives
- *Adrenaline*[Q] - *Noradrenaline*[Q] - *Dopamine*[Q] - 5-Hydroxytryptamine - Histamine - Acetylcholine (ACH) - Adenosine - Opioids	- Neurokinin A - Neuropeptide K - Substance P	- Thromboxane A2
	Peptides	**Other Ligands**
	- Angiotensis II - Arginine vasopressin - Oxytocin - VIP, PTH, GRP, TRH	- **Endothelins** - **Platelet activating factor** - Cannabinoids - Odorants - Light - Tastants
Glycoprotein - Hormones		
- LH, FSH, hCG - TSH		

- Catecholamines (adrenaline, noradrenaline & dopamine) act through G protein coupled receptors. **α_1 adrenargic catecholamine use phospholipid C(IP_3 – DAG) and α_2 & β adrenergic catecholamines** use **C-AMP (adenyl cyclase)** second messenger system.
- Hetrotrimeric GTP binding proteins (G- proteins) are cell membrane proteins that have ***seven transmembrane segments that loop (pass) in & out of cell membrane***[Q]. **(serpentine protein)**
- Cytoplasmic tail is coupled to GTP that has 3 part (trimeric) - α, β, γ subunits.

Second Messenger

- Binding of 1st messenger (ligand) to cell surface receptors l/t a short lived increase (or decrease) in concentration of low molecular weight intracellular signaling molecules which relay & amplify the strength of signal received. These are k/a second massengers.
- **Second messengers** (concept proposed by E.W. **Sutherland**) are **intracellular signaling molecules** mediating intracellular hormone/ ligand (1st messenger) function.
- *Hormones or drugs require receptors for their action.* Some receptors are directly attached to effector molecules and *some receptors are coupled to effector by second messengers.* **Second messenger** are intermediary molecule that intervene between the original message (Hormonal signal) and the ultimate effect on the cell (intracellular metabolic process).
- Hormone combines with receptor → Receptor changes shape → Combines with Gs protein → Gs protein release GDP & binds GTP → Adenylcyclase activates → ATP converted to c-AMP → ↑cAMP (2nd messenger) → Activates proteinkinase → Phosphorylates proteins → Inactivate or activates enzyme.
- Thus, the only direct effect that a ligand / hormone / drug (1st messenger) has on cell is to activate a single type of membrane receptor. The intracellular signaling molecule ie second messenger does the rest.
- Second messangers respond differentially to a hormone or drug because of receptors but ***cells respond to second messangers differentially because of different enzymatic composition***Q. *Cell respond differentially to second messenger because the enzyme present in cells respond differentially* to increase or decrease in cAMP.
- Second messengers like cAMP, cell membrane phospholipids (DAG) **regulate activity of protein kinase enzyme (which phosphorylates substrate protein), thereby modifying enzyme activity. The diversity of protein kinases** present within a cell provides for complex regulatory circuits which control numerous growth & metabolic processes.
- Types & examples of second messengers include

1) Cyclic neucleotides eg **C- AMP and C- GMP**
2) **Diacyl glycerol (DAG) & Inositol 1, 4, 5- triphosphate (IP_3)**
3) Calcium & calmodulin
4) **Protein kinase** such as PKA, PKC, and Ca^{++} - Calmodulin (CaM) – Kinase
5) Gases eg NO (nitric oxide),CO & H_2S

★ **DAG** & **phosphatidylinositols** are **hydrophobic (water insoluble),** whereas **IP3, Ca^{++}, cAMP & cGMP are hydrophilic (water soluble).**

Classification of Hormone (Ligand = 1st Messenger) by Mechanism of Action

Bind to Intra-cellular Receptors

- **Nuclear Receptors: Thyroid hormones (T_3 & T_4)**Q
- **Cytoplasmic Receptors**

- ***Thyroid Hormone***Q
- Retinoic acid
- Androgen
- ***Estrogen***Q
- Progesterone
- ***Glucocorticoid***Q
- ***Mineralo-corticoid***Q
- **Vitamin D_3 (1, 25 $(OH)_2$ D_3**

Bind to Cell Surface Receptor and Act via Second Messengers

Adenylyl cyclase cAMP (2nd messenger) system

- **ACTH, Angiotensin II** (epithelial cells), **ADH**
- **Calcitonin, Catecholamines** (Beta-receptors), **CRH**
- **Glucagon, FSH, HCG, LH**
- **PTH** (parathyroid hormone), **TSH, Vasopressin** (V2 receptor epithelial cells)
- **Secretin, Somatostatin**

Guanylate Cyclase-cGMP (2nd messenger) System

- **ANP** (atrial natriuretic peptide)
- **NO**
- Muscarinic cholinergic agents & oxytocin (Tayler)

Cell Membrane Phospholipid Second Messenger System

- Hormones activate transmembrane receptors that activate **phospholipase C**. It catabolizes breakdown of cell membrane phospholipids esp **PIP_2, (phosphatidyl inositol biphosphate)** into **2 second messengers IP3 (inositol triphosphate) & DAG (diacyl glycerol)**. IP3 mobilizes calcium ions from mitochondria & ER which has its own 2nd messenger effects. Whereas **DAG activates protein kinase C (PKC) enzyme** which phosphorylates proteins. In addition lipid portion of DAG is arachidonic acid (a precursor of prostaglandin).
- Hormones using phospholipase C: **IP3 / DAG or IP3- calcium & DAG – PKC 2nd messengers** include
  - **Acetyl choline, α1 Adrenergic, Angiotensin II (vascular smooth muscle)**
  - Oxytocin Gn RH. GHRH. TRH, Vasopressin (V1 receptor vascular smooth muscle)

Protein Tyrosine Kinase

- Insulin, **Insulin like growth factors (IGF)-1 & II**
- **EGF, PDGF, NGF, FGF, MCSF**

Calcium – Calmodulin 2nd Messenger system

Normal calcium ion concentration in cells (10^{-8} to 10^{-7} mol/L) when **rises to 10^{-6} to 10^{-5} mol/L** because of entery of Ca^{++} into cells activate calmodulin system. It activates **myosin light chain kinase** to stimulate contraction in smooth muscle & other cells.

★ The ***insulin, epidermal growth factor (EGF) and IGF-1 receptors have intrinsic protein tyrosine kinase activities***Q located in their cytoplasmic domains.

★ Role of cGMP in insulin: ***insulin action in certain tissue may be mediated through cGMP***Q which activates protein kinase, which in turn phosphorylates certain enzymes to modulate their activities. *[Shinde Chatterjea 5th/P-200]*

Calmodulin

Calmodulin is the *most widely* distributed small *calcium binding protein.*

Calmodulin has 4 calcium binding sites and full occupancy of these sites induces marked conformation changes that allow calmodulin to activate enzymes & ion channels.

Calmodulin + Ca^{+2} → activated calmodulin → *Activation of enzymes & ion channels.*

Calcium Calmodulin Complex

Activates Calmodulin – dependent protein kinase

a. Myosine light chain kinaseQ
b. phosphorylase kinaseQ
c. Ca^{2+} / calmodulin kinase I
d. Ca^{2+} / calmodulin kinase II, III

Regulate various microfilament mediated process in non contractile cells including

- Cell motility
- Cell conformation changes
- Mitosis
- Endocytosis

Parathyroid Hormone (PTH)

Regulation of Synthesis & Secretion

- Synthesis & secretion of parathyroid hormone (PTH) are regulated primarily by **serum ionized calcium concentration** sensed by ***calcium sensing receptor (CaSR) located on chief cell of parathyroid gland***. When ionized **serum Ca^{++} levels decrease below 1.3mM** (eg d/t prolonged low calcium diet), **PTH synthesis and secretion increases** (to restore Ca^{++} levels). Whereas when extracellular serum Ca++ increases above 1.3 mM, PTH decreases & serum calcium diminishes. Even with very high levels of serum calcium a low rate of PTH synthesis & secretion persist.
- When **hypocalcemia** results from *PTH deficiency, PTH levels are low*, whereas in hypocalcemia d/t *vitamin D deficiency, PTH levels are increased* as a compensatory response to hypocalcemia. In ***hypercalcemia*** *due to malignancy & vitamin D intoxication, PTH concentrations are low*, whereas in primary hyper parathyroidism (adenomatous or hyperplastic parathyroid glands), PTH levels are elevated even though hypercalcemia persists.
- PTH synthesis is stimulated by **β-adrenergic agonists & magnesium** (minor) whereas phosphate has no affect. PTH synthesis is impaired in severe hypomagnesemia.

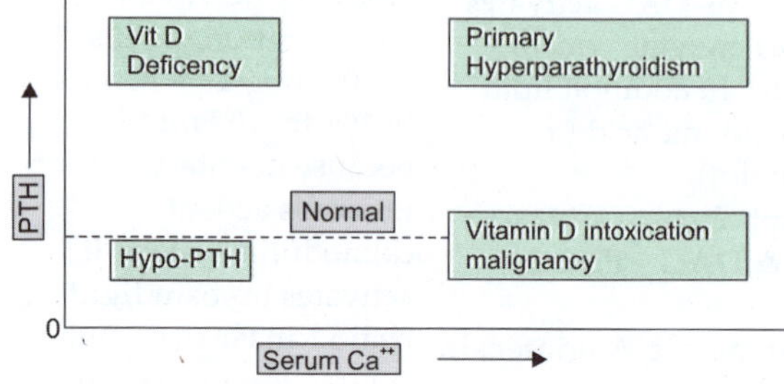

Biological Effects

PTH is a ***84 aminoacid linear polypeptide hormone***Q. **Bone and kidneys** are two main target for organs affected by PTH. PTH cell surface receptors are coupled to adenyl cyclase & **c-AMP** is the intracellular mediator of PTH action.

1. **Bone**: PTH acts directly on bone to **increase bone resorption** (↑ calcium & phosphate release in plasma).

- PTH has a rapid and a slow phase of bone resorption.

I. **Rapid phase** *begins in minutes & increases progressively for several hours*. It results from activation of *already existing bone cells (mainly osteocytes & osteoblasts)* to promote calcium & phosphate absorption (bone osteolysis) in 2 areas: (1) From bone matrix in vicinity of osteocytes and (2) From bone surface in vicinity of osteoblasts. **Osteoblasts & osteocytes have receptor** proteins on cell membrane for **binding PTH**. Long processes of osteocytes & osteoblasts form extensive **osteocytic membrane system** containing osteocytic membrane pumps that pumps calcium from bone fluid to ECF (when activated by PTH).

II. **Slower phase** requires several **days to weeks** to become fully developed. It results from proliferation of **osteoclasts**, followed by greatly increased osteoclastic resorption of bone itself, not only absorption of calcium phosphate salts from bone. **PTH stimulates osteoclastic activity through an indirect mechanism because osteoclasts do not have membrane receptor proteins for PTH**. PTH binds to receptors on osteoblasts (& osteocytes) & cause them to release **secondary signals (cytokines) including osteoprotegerin ligand (OPGL) = RANKL (receptor activator of nuclear factor kB ligand)**. OPGL transforms proosteoclastic cells into mature osteoclasts. The stimulation of osteoclastogenesis requires **M-CSF** (macrophage colony stimulating factor) and **RANK ligand** surface proteins on osteoblasts.

Bone Resorption	Rapid Phase	Slow Phase
Begins	**Minutes to hours**	**Days to weeks**
Results from	Direct activation of **preexisting osteoblasts & osteocytes (osteocytic membrane system)** by PTH	PTH **indirectly stimulates osteoclastogenesis** (transformation of prosteoclast into mature osteoclasts) through **OPGL (RANK ligand)** & M. CSF cytokines released by osteoblasts.

Hormone Involved in Calcium Metaboism

Features	PTH	Vitamin D	Calcitonin
Stimulus for secretion	↓ serum Ca^{2+}	↓serum Ca^{2+} ↓serum P ↑ PTH	**↑ serum Ca^{2+}**Q
Action on: - Bone	↑ **resorption** Q	↑ resorption	↓ **resorption**Q
- Kidney	-↓**P reabsorption** Q (↑ urinary CAMP) -↑ Ca^{2+} reabsorption	-↑ P reabsorption -↑ Ca^{2+} reabsorption	
- Intestine	↑ Ca^{2+} absorption (via activation of vit D)	-↑ Ca^{2+} absorption (calbindin D- 28k) -↑ P absorption	
Overall effect on: - Serum Ca^{2+}	↑ Q	↑	↓
- Serum P	↓Q	↑	

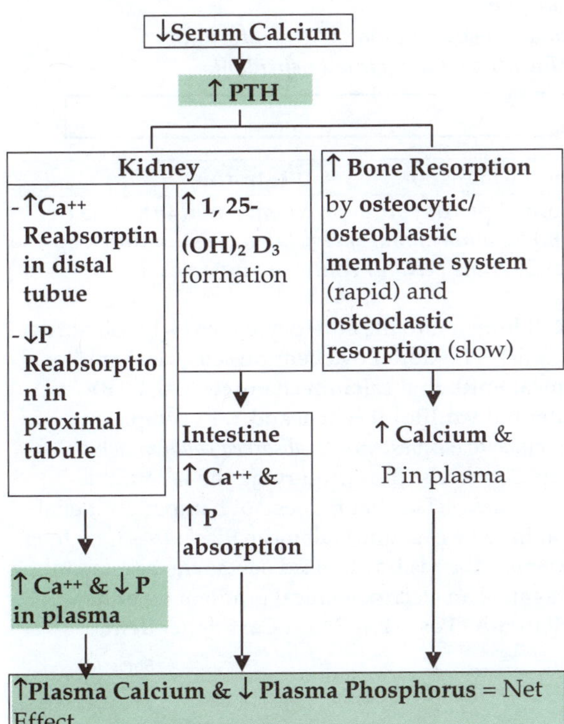

Mechanism	**Absorption of calcium phosphate salts** from bone matrix **near osteocytes & bone surface near osteoblasts**	**Osteoclastic resorption of bone**

- **Estrogen stimulate osteoblasts** to produce **osteoprotegerin (OPG)** or **osteoclastogenesis inhibitory factor (OCIF),** a cytokine which acts as a decoy (fake) receptor binding to OPGL & preventing OPGL from binding its receptor, thereby inhibiting osteoclastogenesis and bone resorption. Vitamin D and PTH stimulate osteoclastogenesis (production of mature osteoclasts) by dual action of inhibiting OPG production and stimulating OPGL formation.

2. Kidney: PTH **decrease calcium excretion (or increase absorption) in late distal tubule** and **increase excretion (or decrease reabsorption) of phosphasphate in proximal tubule**

- Normally **98-99%** of filtered Ca^{++} is reabsorbed in kidneys: about **60% from proximal tubule, 25% from ascending loop of Henle** and small extent in **distal tubule.**
- **Distal tubular reabsorption of calcium** depends on **TRPV5** (transient receptor potential vanniloid type 5) channels, whose expression is regulated by **PTH**. The increased Ca^{++} absorption due to **PTH** occurs mainly in **late distal tubules, collecting tubules**, early collecting ducts & ascending loop of Henle (±) . Although Ca^{2+} excretion is increased in hyper parathyroidism because increase in amount filtered overwhelms the effect on reabsorption. **PTH increases plasma Ca^{++} levels.**
- Normally 85- 90% of filtered phosphate (Pi) is reabsorbed mainly through **active transport in proximal tubule** involving 2 sodium dependent phosphate cotransporters Na- Pi II a & Na Pi II c. **PTH decreases phosphate reabsorption in proximal tubule by powerfully inhibiting Na – Pi IIa** causing it to internalize & degrade. So PTH **decreases plasma phosphate leve by this phosphaturic action.**
- PTH also **increases** rate of **reabsorption of Mg^{++} (magnesium)** and **hydrogen ions (H^{+})** while **decreases reabsorption of sodium (Na^{+}), potassium (K^{+}) and aminoacids** and result in mild metabolic acidosis

3. Intestine : PTH increases absorption of Ca^{++} (mainly) & phosphorus (±) indirectly via vitamin D_3 (1, 25 dihydroxycholecalciferol)

- Calcium is primarily absorbed from **upper small intestine.** Ca^{++} absorption is *facilitated by proteins and inhibited by phosphates & oxalates.*
- **Both PTH and hypophosphatemia** (produced d/t phosphaturic action of PTH) **stimulate 1 α-hydroxylase activity in kidney to increase formation of 1, 25, $(OH)_2$ D_3.** This active vitamin D then increases gastrointestinal absorption of calcium (mainly) and phosphorus. So PTH indirectly promotes intestinal absorption via activation of vitamin D.
- Ca^{++} is transported across brush border of intestinal epithelium via **TRPV 6 channels** and binds to intracellular **calbindin D 9K** protein, which sequesters the absorbed calcium so that it does not disturb epithelial signaling processes that involve calcium, thereby delivering it to basolateral membrane of epithelial cells. From here Ca^{++} is transported into blood stream by **NC X 1 (Na^{+} / Ca^{++} exchanger)** or **Ca^{++} dependent ATPase.** Normally phosphate (Pi) is absorbed, in *duodenum & small intestine* ***by NaPi IIb transporter*** that takes advantage of low intracellular Na^{+} concentration established by NaKATPase on baso lateral membrane of intestinal epithelial cells to load Pi against its concentration gradient. Intestinal absorption of Ca^{++} & phosphate is increased by 1, 25 vitamin D_3.

Calcium Metabolism

- **Vit D** *is really a hormone,* since skin is the major source of Vitamin D. And only when sun exposure is inadequate a dietary source is required. The adequate intake recommended for adults it ***200 IU (5μg) if sun exposure is adequate, and 400 – 800 IU/day in the absence of sunlight***Q. Osteomalacia is associated with intakes <100 IU/day. Maximum (upper) limit of dietary intake of vit D is 2000 IU (50μg) /day in adults is now recommended d/t concerns about potential toxic effects.
- Vitamin D from **plant** source is in form of *vitamin D2,* whereas from *animal* source is *vitamin D3.* Both have equivalent biological activity and fate. Vit D enters circulation, whether absorbed from intestine or synthesized cutaneously, bound to vitamin D binding protein, an *α-globulin* synthesized in liver.
- **In Skin** – Vitamin D_3 (Cholecalciferol) is formed as a result of irradiation of 7 dehydroxy cholesterol by UV rays from sun.
- **In Liver** – Conversion of cholecalciferol to ***25- hydroxy cholecalciferol***Q occurs. 25(OH)vitamin D is the major circulating and storage form of vitamin D. 88% of 25(OH)D circulates bound to vitamin D binding protein, 0.03% is free and rest circulates bound to albumin. The half life of 25(OH)D is 2-3 weeks, which is greatly reduced when vitamin D binding protein levels are reduced as in nephritic syndrome.

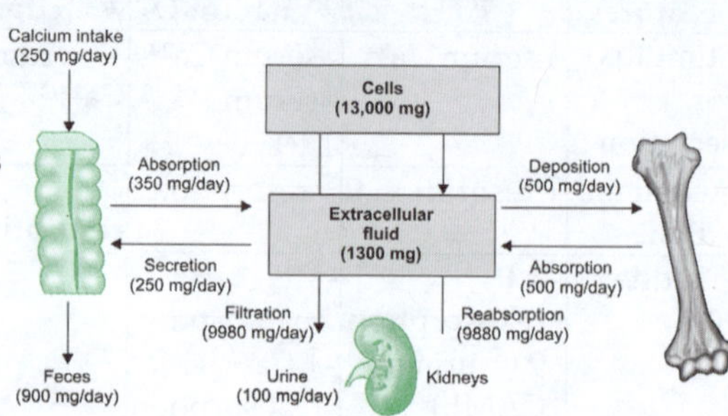

Overview of calcium exchange between different tissue compartments in a person ingesting 1000 mg of calcium per day. Note that most of the ingested calcium is normally eliminated in the feces, although the kidneys have the capacity to excrete large amounts by reducing tubular reabsorption of calcium.

- **In Kidney** – Formation of ***1, 25 – dihydroxy cholecalciferol takes place in proximal tubules of kidney***Q which is the active form of vitamin – D.
- 1α hydroxylase is also present, so 1,25 $(OH)_2$ D_3 also formed ***in placenta, in Keratinocytes of Skin & macrophages and granulomas of sarcoidosis, tuberculosis, berylliosis as well as lymphomas***Q. *But in these pathological granulomas, interferon γ and TNF induce enzyme activity and these are not regulated by calcium and 1,25 $(OH)_2$ D feed back. Therefore hypercalcemia may occur b/o elevated 1,25 (OH)2D, which is treated by glucocorticoids, ketoconazole or chloroquin.*

★ **In sarcoidosis** ***pulmonary macrophage***Q produces 1, 25 $(OH)_2$ D_3 due to apparent stimulation of 'Y' – interferon.

★ **In Ca lung** plasma Ca^{2+} level increased d/t ***ectopic production of PTHrP (Parathormone related peptide)***Q.

Calcium (Ca^{++})

- The body of young adult contains ~ *1100gm (27.5mol)* of Ca; *90%* of it is in skeleton. The plasma calcium, is normally about ***10gm /dL (5meq / L, 2.5 mmol / L)***Q, of which *50%* is ionized. The remainder is bound ionically to negative charged proteins (predominantly albumin & immunoglobins) or loosely complexed with phosphate, citrate, sulphate. ***It is the free ionized calcium, that is a vital second messenger***Q and necessary for ***blood coagulation, nerve conduction and muscle contraction***Q. The level of plasma calcium at which fatal tetany occurs is still above the level at which clotting defect would occur.
- Since the extent of calcium binding by plasma protein is proportionate to the plasma protein level, it is important to know the plasma protein level when evaluating the total plasma calcium. An algorithm to correct for protein changes adjusts the total *serum calcium (in mg / dL) upward by 0.8 times the defecit in serum albumin (in gm/dl) or by 0.5 times the defect in serum immunoglobin* (in g/dl). So corrected calcium concentration

Ca^{++} and Pi Transport in Small Intestine

- 200 mg calcium is absorbed per day form ***proximal small intestine (ie duodenum and jejunum) by a hormonally regulated (ie stimulated by 1,2, dihydroxy vitamin D) trans cellular route and by a passive paracellular route***Q.
- Ca^{++} movement from GI lumen into the enterocyte (across brush border of intestinal epithelial cells) is favoured by chemical/electrical gradients and is facilitated by **apical epithelial calcium channels** k/a **TRPV (transient receptor potential vanilloid) type 6 and 5.** In cytoplasm, **calbindin D_{9k}** protein *binds to (sequesters) the absorbed calcium, which maintains low cytoplasmic Ca^{++} levels* (thus preserving the favourable lumen to enterocyte Ca^{++} *gradient)* so that it does not hamper epithelial signaling processes that involve calcium. Calbindin 9k *shuttles Ca^{++} from apical to basolateral membrane.* Ca^{++} is transported across the basolateral membrane into blood against an electrochemical gradient by **either plasma membrane calcium ATPase (PMCA),** a **Ca^{++} dependent ATPase or sodium/calcium exchanger ($3Na^+/1Ca^{++}$ antiporter = NCX1)**. 1, 25 dihydroxy vitamin D stimulates all components of Ca^{++} **absorption in intestine.**

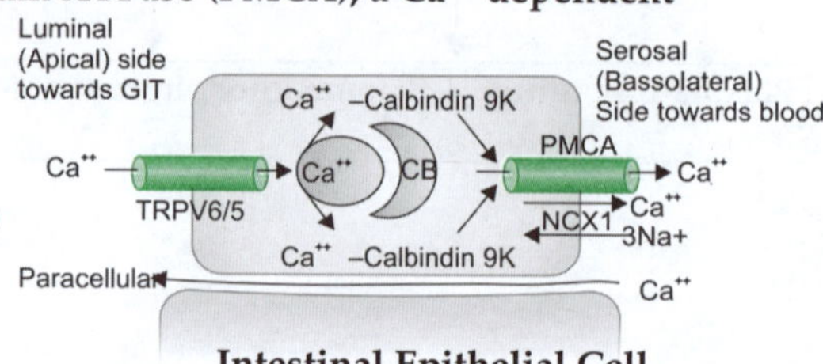

Intestinal Epithelial Cell

= **Total calcium level (mg/dL) + 0.8 mg/dL (0.2MM)** for every decrement in serum albumin of 1.0 gm/dL (below the reference value of 4.1 gm/dL of albumin).

= **Total calcium level (mg/dL) + 0.5 mg/dL** for every decrement in serum immunoglobulin of 1gm/dL.

- *PH affects* the calcium level, for example tetany appear at much higher total Ca^{++} levels, if patient hyperventilates, increasing plasma pH. Plasma proteins are more ionized when the pH is high, providing more protein anion to bind with calcium thus reducing effective amount of ionized calcium. In same way ***acidosis increases ionized Ca^{++} levels***[Q].
- Intestinal absorption of calcium involves both active (transcellular) and passive (paracellular) mechanism. Passive absorption is nonsaturable & approximates 5% of intake, whereas active mechanism controlled by 1, 25, $(OH)_2$ D, normally ranges from 20- 70%. ***Active absorption occurs mainly in proximal small bowel (duodenum & proximal jejunum)***[Q]. ***Optical rates of Ca^{++} absorption requires gastric acid***[Q]. This is especially true for weakly dissociable calcium supplements as $CaCO_3$.
- Calcium interchange between plasma and rapidly exchangeable reservoir of bone is 500mmol per day. Whereas between plasma and stable pool of bone is only 7.5mmol/day. A large amount of calcium is filtered in kidney but 98-99% of filtered calcium is reabsorbed – **60% of which occurs in PCT** and remainder in **ascending loop of Henle** (25%) and **distal tubule** (small extent).

Total diffusible calcium	**1.34**
- Ionized (Ca^{++})	1.18
- Complexed to HCO_3^-, citrate etc	0.16
Total nondiffusible (protein bound) calcium	**1.16**
- Bound to albumin	0.92
- Bound to globulin	0.24
Total plasma calcium	**2.50**

- Phosphate (Pi) absorption by jejunum remains constant at 70% and is under control of 1, 25 dihydroxy vitamin D. Transcellular Pi absorption across apical bursh border mediated by **Na^+ -Pi cotransporter (NPT2)** is the limiting step.

Calcium Transport Along Nephron

- **99% of filtered Ca^{++} is reabsorbed by nephron**. About 1% ie 200 mg/day is excreted in urine which is equal to net amount daily absorbed in git.

Part of Nephron	% of Ca^{++} Reabsorbed	Mechanism
PCT	**60-70%** of total	- **Passive paracellular** path between cells across tight junction accounts for **80% reabsorption**. It occurs via *solvent drag* in entire PCT and *by positive luminal voltage* (i.e. diffusion) in distal half PCT. - Active transcellular path accounts for 20% of total PCT reabsorption.
Loop of Henle (cortical thick ascending limb)	20%	- Via both paracellular and trans cellular paths by same mechanism as of PCT but with one difference i.e. *Ca^{++} is not reabsorbed by solvent drag as TAL is impermeable to water.*
DCT **Collecting duct**	9% <1%	- **Exclusively active transcellular** because the tubule lumen (DCT) is electrically negative with respect to blood so the Ca^{++} is reabsorbed against electrochemical gradient.

- Mutations in **claudin 16**, a protein component of tight junction in **TAL** (thick ascending limb of Henle's loop) **cells**, causes **familial hypomagnesemic hypercalciuria** b/o enhanced excretion of Ca^{++} & Mg^{++} (d/t fall of passive paracellular absorption of these ions).

Calcium Sensing Receptors (CaSR)

Calcium sensing receptors (CaSRs) are present in **PTH secreting cells of parathyroid glands, calcitonin secreting parafollicular cells in thyroid gland** and **calcitriol (Vit D) producing cells of proximal tubules** (i.e. in the cells producing **hormone involved in regulation of serum calcium).** CaSRs are also present in ***thick ascending limb of loop of Henle and distal tubule (DCT)***[Q] to directly regulate Ca^{++} homeostasis. **Small intestine cells lack CaSRs**

Feature	AD **Familial Hypocalciuric Hypercalcemia (FHH)**	**Autosomal Dominant Hypocalcemia**
Cause	Inactivating mutation in CaSR	*Activating* mutation in CaSR
Clinic Features	- **Hypercalcemia** d/t deranged Ca^{++} regulated PTH secretion (i.e. **PTH is elevated at all plasma Ca^{++} levels**). - **Hypocalciuria** d/t enhanced Ca^{++} reabsorption in TAL and DCT as a result of elevated PTH and defective CaSR	- **Hypocalcemia** d/t deranged Ca^{++} regulated PTH secretion (i.e. **PTH level is decreased at any level of plasma Ca^{++})** - **Hypercalciuria** d/t decreased PTH levels and defective CaSR.

Parathyroid Related Peptide and Hypercalcemia

- *Humoral hypercalcemia of malignancy* is most often associated with *overproduction of PTHrP*.
- PTHrP is structurally related to PTH & binds to the PTH receptor producing features similar to hyperparathyroidism (hyper cacemia)
- Mutation in *Ras oncogene* stimulates PTHrP production.
- HHM occurs in about 5% of patient with cancer.
- HHM is most common in cancers of ***lung***[Q], ***breast***[Q], *head & neck, genitourinary tract,* esophagus, ***multiple myeloma***[Q] & lymphoma.
- Many bone metastasis eg breast, multiple myeloma produce PTHrP leading to local osteolysis and hyper calcemia.

Features of Hypocalcemia

Symptoms	Signs
1) ***Numbness and tingling of circumoral region & the tips of fingers and toes***[Q].	1) ***Chovstek's***[Q]: Contraction of facial muscles in response to tapping the facial nerve anterior to the ear.
2) ***Extensive spasm of skeletal muscle causes cramps & tetany***[Q].	2) ***Trousseau's sign***[Q]- Capal spasm occurring after occlusion of brachial artrery with a blood pressure cuff for 3 minutes.
3) ***Carpopedal spasm***[Q] occurs.	3) ***Erb's sign***[Q]- Muscle contraction can be produced by application of sub threshold electrical stimulation.
4) *Laryngospasm with stridor.*	4) ***Peroneal sign***[Q] – Tapping over the peroneal nerve at the neck of fibula will produce planter flexion & adduction of the foot (pedal spasm).
5) ***Hyperactive tendon reflex***[Q]	
6) ***Prolongation of QT interval***[Q].	
7) *Increased intracranial pressure* occurs in some patient with long standing hypocalcemia. *Papilloedema* is associated with these cases	

Calcium Metabolism in Mammalian Cells

- Concentration of *intracellular* Ca^{2+} is 100 nmol/L and it is ***about 12000 times less than that in extracellular fluid.***[Q]
- Ca^{2+} is stored in *endoplasmic reticulum* and *mitochondria* & can be released from them to replenish cytoplasmic Ca^{2+}
- Calcium binding proteins bind cytoplasmic Ca^{2+} and when activated in this fashion, bring about a variety of physiological effect.
- Ca^{2+} enter cell via (i) Voltage gated Ca^{2+} channels (ii) Ligand gated Ca^{2+} channels (T & L types) (iii) Store operated Ca^{2+} channels (SOCCs)
- It is transport out of cell by *(Active transport)*[Q]
  - *(i)* ***Ca^{2+} H^+ ATPase antiport***[Q]: cause ***$2H^+$ inside & Ca^{2+} outside***[Q] of membrane at the cost of hydrolysis of ATP.
  - *(ii)* ***Na^+ Ca^{2+} antiport***[Q]: It is a counter transport causes ***3 Na^+ inside & $2Ca^{2+}$ outside***[Q] of membrane.
  - *(iii)* *Ca* – Mg ATPase
- Calcium movement into the internal stores is through the action of **sarcoplasmic or endoplasmic reticulum Ca++ ATP ase (SERCA pump)**[Q].
- Calmodulin is Ca^{2+} binding protein involved in contraction of smooth muscle.

★ **Passive transport** is when molecules traverse membrane by electro mechanical gradient (Passively). **Uniport** is form of transport where only one substance is transported. **Symport** is binding of more than one substance to transport protein & substances are transported across the membrane together. **Antiport** is the transport exchange one substance for another.

IP_3 & Ca^{++}

- ***Inositol triphosphate (IP_3) diffuses to the endoplasmic reticulum, where it triggers the release of calcium into cytoplasm***[Q]. **IP_3** is the major second messenger that causes release of Ca++ from ER through the IP_3 receptor activation (a ligand gated channel). So **one second messenger (IP_3) causes release of another second messenger (Ca^{++})**[Q].
- Inositol triphosphate and diacylglycerol (DAG) both of which are second messengers, are associated with Gq subset of G protein mediated receptors.

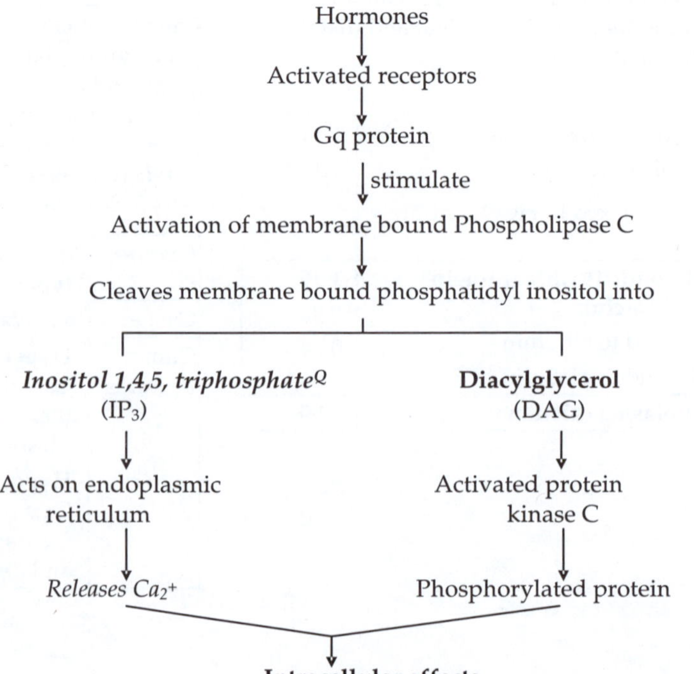

Endocrine Pancreas

- Although scattered through-out the pancreas, islets are more plentiful in **tail**. All 1-2 million human islets have copious blood supply. Blood from islets, like that from gastrointestinal tract (but unlike that from any other endocrine organs) drain into **hepatic portal vein**.
- On the basis of staining & morphological properties islets cells can be divided into at least 4 types

Islets cell type		Secretion	% of total endocrine volume
A cells	**Alpha (α)**	*Glucagon*[Q]	10 -20%
B cells	**Beta (β)**	*Insulin*[Q] *& amylin*	**60 -75%** (most abundant)
D cells	**Delta (δ)**	*Somatostatin*[Q]	5%
F cells	**PP cells**	*Pancreatic polypeptide*[Q]	< 5% overall, but ~ 80% in posterior head & uncinate process
D1 cells		**VIP**	-

- Most abundant **B (β) cells** are usually located in **center** of each islet, which tend to be surrounded mainly by many A (α) cells and few if any F cells in outer rim in ***tail, body, and anterior & superior part of head of pancreas***. Whereas, **posterior part of head** (including **uncinate process**) of pancreas have **large number of F cells** & few A cells.
- **A cell (glucagon) rich islets** arise embryologically from **dorsal** pancreatic bud whereas, **F cell (pancreatic polypeptide) rich islets** arise from **ventral** pancreatic bud.
- In B cells granules, insulin forms different size & shape polymers or **zinc (Zn) aggregates** / complexes (so these are **heterogenous**) in different species. A cell and D cell granules are relatively homogenous (uniform).

Exocrine Pancreas

- Pancreas secretes its exocrine products as ***enzymatically inert proenzymes*** both ***to prevent self digestion***[Q] & *to efficiently utilize the enzymes* within the lumen of duodenum. **Trypsin** is a powerful *pancreatic proteolytic enzyme* which would digest the pancreatic cells, if not produce as ***proenzyme (inactive form) – trypsinogen***[Q]. Trypsimogen is activated in the intestinal tract by enzyme called ***enterokinase***[Q].
- **The self digestion of pancreas is prevented by:**

1) The *majority of the enzymes* are ***synthesized as inactive proenzymes***[Q] (with the exception of amylase & lipase)
2) The enzymes are sequestered in membrane – bound zymogen granules in the acinar cells.
3) Activation of proenzymes requires conversion of inactive trypsinogen to active trypsin by duodenal enteropeptidase (enterokinase)
4) ***Trypsin inhibitors including serine protease inhibitor Kazal type 1 are present within acinar and ductal secretion***[Q]
5) Trypsin contains a critical self- recognition cleavage site that allows trypsin to inactivate itself.
6) Lysosomal hydrolases are capable of degrading zymogen granules when normal acinar secretion is blocked.
7) Acinar cells are remarkably resistant to the action of trypsin, chymotrypsin & phospholipase A_2.

★ ***Pancreatic enzymes require alkaline medium for their activity so bicarbonate secretion will help in their activity***[Q].

Pancreatic Juice (Exocrine Juice)

Features

- ***Isoosmotic with blood plasma***[Q]
- **Volume** = *~1500ml/day*[Q]
- **PH** = ~ 8 (alkaline)
- ***Rich in enzymes***[Q] (about 20 different enzymes are secreted by pancreas)

Stimulant For Secretion

Secretin	- Produced *by duodenal mucosa*[Q] - ***Stimulated by acidity***[Q] of chyme - Stimulates a ***bicarbonate***[Q] rich pancreatic secretion.
Cholecystokinin (CCK)	- Produced by ***jejunal***[Q] mucosa. - Stimulated by ***fat***[Q] in chyme - Stimulates ***enzyme rich***[Q] pancreatic secretion
Acetylcholine	- Acts on acinar cells via phopholipase C. - Causes discharge of zymogen granules
Vagal stimulation	- Stimulates ***enzyme rich***[Q] secretion

Starvation/Fasting

Effects on Carbohydrate Metabolism

- During first few days – *Glycogenolysis*[Q] provides the major & immediate source of glucose, after which glucose level begins to fall.
- Hypoglycemia ***depresses insulin***[Q] secretion & thus ***increase gluconeogenesis***[Q].
- Gluconeogenesis maintains blood sugar but at subnormal level. Thus ***glucose tolerance is decreased***[Q].
- ***Antagonistic hormones are increased***[Q]:
  - ***Glucagon increases***[Q] (tend to increase blood glucose)
  - ***GH level increases***[Q] (tend to increase blood glucose)
- *After 2 days of fasting*, the major substrate for energy product will be ***stored fat***[Q]. (as *glycogen reserve is exhausted in first 2 days*).
- Catabolism of fat will load to ***increase in FFA in blood***[Q].

Hormone Changes

Insulin	- Decreased
Glucagon	- ***Increases***[Q]
Growth hormone	- ***Increase***[Q]

Insulin

Nobel Prizes

- Nobel prize for isolation of insulin was given to **Frederick G. Banting and J.J.R. MacLeod** in 1923. Banting immediately announced that he would share his prize with **Charles Best**; Macleod shared his with **J.B. Collip**.
- **Fredrick G Sanger** got Nobel prize in 1958 **for sequencing insulin structure** (ie for ***determining the complete aminoacid sequence of both polypeptide chains of bovine insulin)***[Q]
- Fredrick Sanger again with Walter Gilbert got Nobel prize in 1980 for sequencing of large nucleic acid (DNA) molecule.

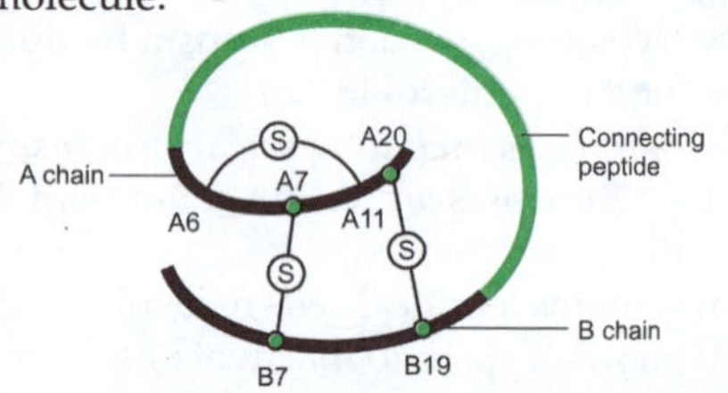

Structure and Synthesis

- Insulin has ***two interchain (A7 – B7, & A20 – B19) and one intrachain (A6 – A11) disulfide bridges with in AB hetrodimeric structure***[Q].
- Insulin is synthesized as pre-pro-hormone (MW 11, 500), which makes it difficult to synthesize insulin in laboratory even after synthesizing A, B chains. This pre prohormone is directed by *hydrophobic 23 aminoacid pre or leader sequence* into cisternae of endoplasmic retinaculum, which is then removed to form *9000 MW proinsulin*.
- Starting from amino terminal, the chain sequenc of proinsulin is.

B chain——— Connecting (C) peptide ——A chain

- Proinsulin molecule undergoes on initial cleavage by *trypsin like enzyme* followed by serries of several cleavages by ***carboxypeptidase like enzyme resulting in formation of equimolar amounts of mature hetrodimeric (AB) insulin and C – peptide***[Q]. ***(1 : 1 ratio)***[Q].
- **Pork insulin differs** from human insulin ***by only one amino acid residue***[Q]. It also has low antigenicity.
- Human insulin produced in bacteria by recombinant DNA technology is used to avoid antibody formation.

Factors Affecting Insulin Secretion

- **Plasma glucose concentration** is the **most important** regulator of insulin secretion, and glucose acts directly on pancreatic B cells. The response to hyper glycemia is **biphasic** i.e. a *rapid but short lived initil spike* followed by more *slowly developing prolonged increase (second phase)*. Glucose enters β-cells via GLUT-2 transporters and is phosphorylated by glucokinase then metabolized to pyruvate in cytoplasm. Pyruvate enters mitochondria form ATP by oxidative phosphorylation and also cause increase in intracellular glutamate (via TCA cycle).

Regulation of Insulin Secretion by plasma glucose

Rapid short lived increase in secretion

*ATP **enters cytoplasm,*** **inhibiting ATP sensitive K+ channels & reducing K+ efflux.** ***This depolarize B cells and Ca++ influx via voltage gated Ca++ channels cause exocytosis of readily releasable pool of insulin containing secretory granules,* producing initial spike of insulin secretion.**

Slow, Prolonged increase in secretion

***Glutamate** act as intracellular 2nd messenger on second pool of secretory granules. It* primes secretory granules *for secretion,* maturing them by decreasing their pH. *This commits granules to the releasable form producing prolonged 2nd phase of insulin release.*

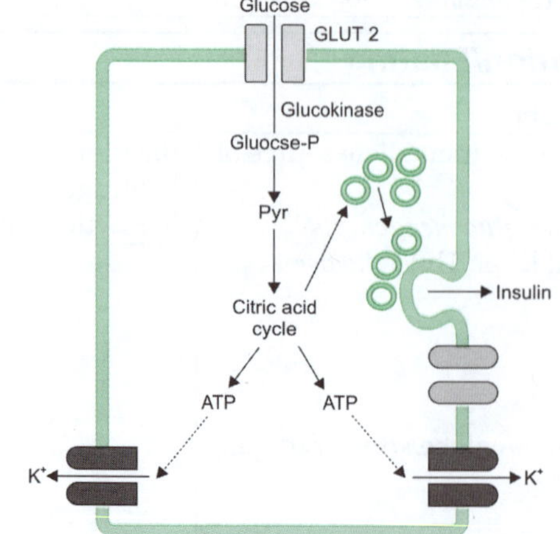

Stimulators (↑ Insulin serection)	Inhibitors (↓ Insulin secretion)
- Increased blood levels of **glucose**, mannose, **amino acids** (esp **leucine & arginine**), free fatty acids, **β-keto acids** (eg aceto-acetic acid). - Obesity, insulin resistance - Intestine (gut) hormones (**GIP**=gastrointestinal peptide, **GLP**=glucagons like peptide 1 [17-36], **gastrin, secretin, cholecystocynin = CCK**) - ***Glucagon, GH (growth hormone) and glucocorticoids***[Q] - Parasympathetic stimulation and acetyl choline **(Ach)** - **Cyclic AMP** and various substances generating c-AMP - **β-Adrenergic** stimulation (fors) - Sulfonylureas (glyburide, tolbutamide) - Theophylline	- Fasting and decreased blood glucose levels - **2 deoxyglucose** and **mannoheptulose** - **Somatostatin** - **Leptin**, Galanin - Insulin - **α Adrenergic stimulators *(epinephrine, norepinephrine)***[Q] - β-Adrenergic blockers (propranolol) - K+ depletion - Diazoxide - Thiazide diuretics - Phenytoin - Alloxan - Microtubule inhibitors

- **Glucose, mannose, amino acids** (esp **arginine & leucine**) and **β-keto acids (eg acetoactic acid)** provoke greater insulin secretion, when administered orally (than that by parenteral /iv route). This is b/o **gut /gastrointestinal hormones – gastric inhibitory peptide (GIP), glucagons like peptide (GLP)-1 (7-36)/entero glucagons, secretin, gastrin & CCK.**
- Glucagon, growth hormone (GH), glucocorticoids, β-adrenergic stimulation, parasympathetic stimulation (acetylcholine) and C-AMP increase insulin secretion. Whereas, ***α-adrenergic stimulation (by epinephrine & norepineprine), somatostatin***[Q], leptin & galanin **decrease insulin secretion.**
- So **catecholamines** (epinephrine & nor epinephrine) have a dual effect on insulin secretion. They decrease it via α2 adrenergic receptors and increase it via β-adrenergic receptors. But the **net effect is inhibitory**. However, if catecholamine are administered after α-blockage, it stimulates insulin secretion d/t unopposed β-action.

Effect of Insulin on K^+ and PO_4^{3-}

- Insulin **increases** the **transport of potassium (K+) from plasma into cells** by stimulating the **Na^+-K^+ - ATPase pumps** in cell membranes of *muscle, liver and adipocytes*. This results in ***lowering of plasma (extracellular) K+ concentration i.e. hypokalemia***[Q].
- Infusions of insulin (and glucose) significantly lower the plasma K+ levels in normal individuals and are used for temporaty relief of hyperkalemia in patients with renal failure, waiting for dialysis.
- Hypokalemia often develops when patients with diabetic acidosis are treated with insulin.
- Insulin *induces rapid entery of glucose into cells*, a process which is followed by *phosphorylation reaction in glycolytic pathway, lowering the intracellular concentration of inorganic phosphate*, and therefore promotes phosphate ($PO^{3-}{}_4$) entry into cells. This is how insulin l/t hypophosphatemia (decrease plasma /ECF PO_4^{3-})

Factors Influencing K+ Distribution

Shift K^+ into cells (decreae extra cellular potassium) = Cause Hypokalemia	***Shift K^+ out of cells (increase extracellular potassium) =Cause Hyper kalemia***
- ***Alkalosis***[Q] - Aldosterone - β-adrenergic stimulation - ***Insulin***[Q]	- ***Acidosis***[Q] - Aldosterone deficiency (Addion's disease) - β adrenergic blockade - Insulin deficiency (diabetiese mellitus) - Cell lysis - Sternuous exercise - Increased extracellular fluid osmolarity

Insulin: Summary

Embryology

Insulin containing granules can be identified in the human fetal pancreas by 9 to 10 weeks and ***detectable in fetal plasma by 12 weeks***[Q]. **Glucagon** secretion begins by *8th week.* **Thyroxin** secretion begins by *10th to 12th week.*

Substance with Insulin like Activity

- Insulin
- Proinsulin
- Nonsuppressible insulin-like activity (NSILA)
- Low-molecular-weight fraction
  - IGF-I
  - IGF-II
- High molecular-weight fraction (mostly IGF bound to protein)

Principal Actions

Rapid (seconds)
- ***Increased transport of glucose, amino acids, and K+ into insulin-sensitive cells***[Q]

Intermediate (minutes)
- Stimulation of protein synthesis
- Inhibition of protein degradation
- ***Activation of glycolytic enzymes and glycogen synthase***[Q]
- ***Inhibition of phosphorylase and gluconeogenic enzymes***[Q]

Delayed (hours)
- Increased in mRNAs for lipogenic and other enzymes

Insulin Stimulates lipogenesis by

- ***Increasing acetyl – Co A carboxylase activity***[Q], (most important enzyme in regulation of lipogenesis). This allosteric enzyme is activated by citrate, which increases in concentration in well fed state and is an indicator of a plentiful supply of acetyl CoA.

Effects on Various Tissue

Effects on Various Tissue
Adipose tissue - Increased glucose entry - ***Increased fatty acid synthesis and lipogenesis***[Q] - Increased glycerol phosphate synthesis - Increased triglyceride deposition - ***Activation of lipoprotein lipase***[Q] *increased clearance of VLDL & chylomicron.* - ***Inhibition of hormone-sensitive lipase***[Q] *inhibits lipolysis* - Increased K^+ uptake
Muscle - Increased glucose entry - Increased glycogen synthesis - ***Increased amino acid uptake***[Q] - ***Increased protein synthesis in ribosomes***[Q] - Decreased protein catabolism - Decreased release of gluconeogenic amino acids - Increased ketone uptake - ***Increased K+ uptake***[Q]

Insulin causes **hypoglycemia. Hormones** causing hyperglycemia (**opposite action**)

- ***Catecholamines***[Q] (epinephrine, norepinephrine)
- ***Glucagon***[Q]
- ***Growth hormone***[Q], ACTH
- Glucocorticoids
- ***Thyroid hormones***[Q]

- ***Increasing transport of glucose into cells***[Q] like adipose tissue.
- ***Increasing availability of pyruvate for fatty acid synthesis and glycerol 3 phosphate for easterification***[Q] of newly formed fatty acids.
- ***Activates pyruvate dehydrogenase in adipose tissue but not in liver***[Q].
- ***Decreases intracellular C- AMP level***[Q] – thus **inhibitibiting lipolysis** in adipose tissue and thereby ***reducing concentration of plasma free fatty acid and thus long chain acetyl CoA***[Q], an inhibitor of lipogenesis.

Liver

- ***Decreased ketogenesis***[Q]
- ***Increased protein synthesis***[Q]
- Increased lipid synthesis
- Decreased glucose output due to decreased gluconeogenesis; ***increased glycogen synthesis; and increased***
- ***Glycolysis***[Q]
- Inhibits glycogenolysis & glucose uptake.

General

- Increased cell growth

★ Vagal stimulation causes stimulation of insulin secretion but only when blood sugar level is high.

★ **Glucagon**: In the liver, it acts via Gs to activate adenyl cyclase & ***increase intracellular cAMP. An increase in ratio of insulin to glucagons*** implies a decreased concentration of glucagons & hence ***decreased ratio of c AMP***[Q].

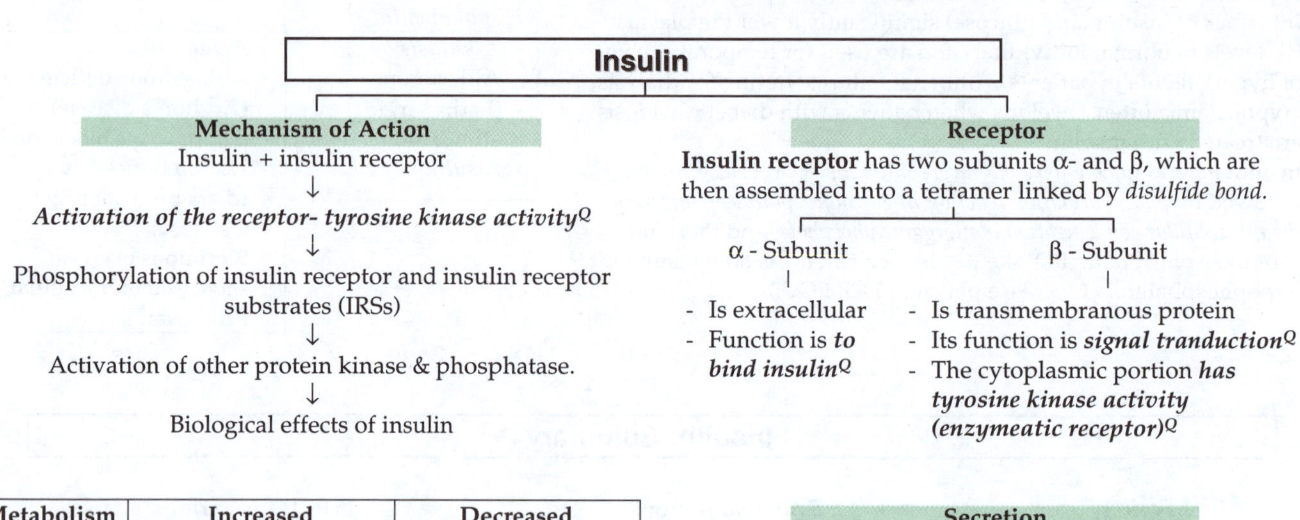

Metabolism	Increased	Decreased
Carbohydrate	- **Glycolysis** **Glycogenesis** (glycogen synthesis) - **Glucose uptake** - **HMP shunt**	**Gluconeogenesis** **Glycogenolysis** (glycogen degradation)
Protein	Protein synthesis	Protein degradation
Fat	**Lipogenesis** (fat synthesis)	**Lipolysis** **ketogenesis**

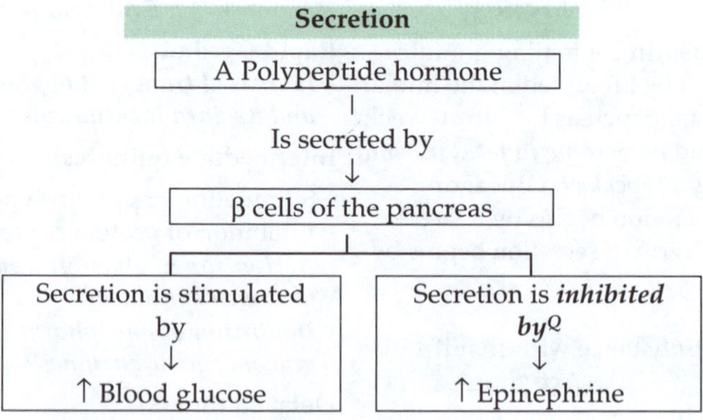

Effect of Insulin On Metabolism of

Carbohydrate

Net effects is – To ↓*blood glucose level* ↑*glycogen storage*[Q]

Increases

- **Glycogenesis in liver & muscle** by *activating* enzyme ***glycogen synthetase***[Q]
- **Glycolysis**: ↑Utilization of glucose for providing energy, by inducing the synthesis of following enzymes
  - ***Phosphofuctokinase***[Q]
  - ***Pyruvate kinase***[Q]
  - Glucokinase
- **HMP shunt**: by *inducing:*
  - Glucose –6 PO_4 dehydrogenase
  - 6 Phosphogluconate dehydrogenase

Decreases

- ***Gluconeogenesis*** in liver by *inactivating* following enzymes:
  - ***Pyruvte carboxylase***[Q]
  - Phosphoenol pyruvate carboxykinase
  - Fructose 1, 6, biphosphatase
  - Glucose – 6 – phosphatase
- **Glycogenolysis in liver** by *inactivating* following enzyme
  - Glycogen phosphorylase

Glucose- 6 phosphatase

Protein

Increase protein synthesis by increasing **RNA polymerase**

Decrease protein degradation by decreasing transaminases & deaminases

Lipids

- ***Enhanced uptake of glucose in adipose cells via GLUT 4 transporter and increased K⁺ uptake***[Q]
- Insulin **increases lipogenesis** (i.e. *fatty acid glycerol phosphate and triglyceride synthesis*[Q]) and **decreases lipolysis** (and so ↓*TG degradation,* ↓*glycerol,* ↓*free fatty acid level and* ↓*ketogenesis*[Q])
- **Fatty acid synthesis is increased by activating** following enzymes
  - ***Acetyl COA carboxylase***[Q] (rate limiting enzyme)
  - ATP citrate lyase (↑ acetyl COA synthesis from citrate)
  - Pyruvate dehydrogenase complex (↑ availability of acetyl COA from pyruvate)
  - Fatty acid synthase
  - Malic enzyme
- **Triglyceride synthesis is increased** by
  - ***Activating lipoprotein lipase***[Q] which hydrolyses TG from VLDL & chylomicrons and release FFA (pool 2) used for TG synthesis.
  - Increased FA synthesis provide acyl CoA (pool 1)
- **Lipolysis is decreased** by
  - *Activating phosphoprotein phosphatase and phosphodiesterase* (both inactivate TG lipase)
  - Inhibiting hormone sensitive lipase
- ***Inhibiting hormone sensitive lipase***[Q] (principal action of insulin in adipose tissue, which reduces release of FFA & glycerol)
- **Decreased β oxidation, cholesterol synthesis and ketogenesis** d/t decrease plasma FFA levels by decreasing HMG CoA synthetase

Glucose Transport In Various Tissue

	Active transport Energy requiring process that transport glucose 'against' concentration gradient	**Facilitated transport** Glucose movement follows a conc. gradient, i.e. from high glucose conc. to a lower one.
Insulin sensitive	-	- Muscle: ***skeletal & cardiac muscle***[Q] - ***Adipose tissue***[Q]
Insulin insensitive	Epithelia of - Intestine - ***Renal tubules***[Q] - Choroids plexus	- ***Erythrocytes***[Q] - Leukocytes - Lens of eye - Cornea - Liver - Brain

❖ **Insulin increases entry of glucose *into liver cells,* but *by an indirect mechanism*[Q].**

Inhibitors & Toxins

- **Sodium dependent glucose transporter (SGLT or Na+ glucose co transporter)** ***is inhibited by phlorizin***[Q] whereas, **phloretin** inhibits ***sodium (Na+) independent glucose transporter (GLUT 2) in intestine***[Q].
- Fish **neurotoxin tetrodotoxin** (applied externally) ***block*** Na^+ ***channels***[Q] (esp early membrane voltage dependent *Na^+ current;* hence 'm' gates controlling Na^+ channels externally) where as **enzyme pronase** (applied internally) block voltage dependent *inactivation of Na^+ current (hence 'h' gates* controlling Na^+ channels from inside).
- **Tetraethyl ammonium** or **4 aminopyridine** block ***potassium channel***[Q] (esp delyed voltage dependent increase in K^+ permeability and hence 'n' gate).
- **Ouabain** that comes from ***adrenal glands is a digitalis like steroid and a Na+ - K+ ATPase inhibiting factor***[Q]. It causes
  - *Natriuresis and raises* rather than lowers blood pressure
  - *Inhibition of iodide trapping* (active transport of iodide in follicular cells) in thyroid
  - Black most of calorigenic action of thyroid hormone
- **Vandate** inhibits Na^+ - K^+ - ATPase pump when present inside the cell.
- **Azide, Cyanide** and **H_2S** block site III (complete IV) of electron transport chain and inhibit terminal transfer of electrons to molecular O_2

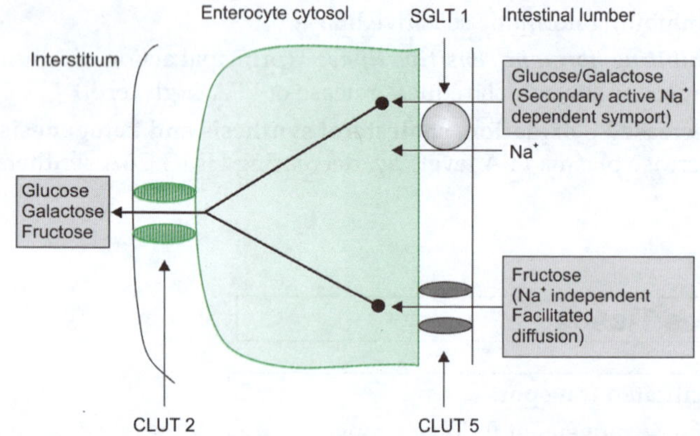

Absorption of Hexose in Intestine

- Hexoses are *rapidly and completely* absorbed before the meal reach terminal ileum
- Transport of most hexoses (glucose & galactose) is *dependent on Na^+ ions* in intestinal lumen; a high Na^+ concentration facilitates and a low concenteration inhibits sugar influx into the epithelial cells.
- This is because Na^+ & glucose share a same **cotransporter or symport, the sodium dependent glucose transmporter** (SGLT), Na^+ glucose cntransporter). These (SGLT 1 & 2) resemble glucose transporters responsible for facilitated diffusion in that they cross cell membrane 12 times and have their – COOH & - NH2 terminals on cytoplasmic side of membrane. However , there is no homology to glucose transporter (GLUT). **SGLT- 1** is *responsible for uptake of dietary glucose from gut* where as **SGLT-2** is *responsible for glucose transport out of renal tubules.*
- As the intracellular Na+ conc. is low in intestinal cells (as it is in other cells), *Na^+ moves into the cell along conc. gradient and glucose is contransported with it. From here glucose is transported by* ***GLUT -2*** *into interstitium* (& thence to capillaries), and Na+ into the lateral intercellular space.
- So glucose transport is a **secondary active transport** i.e. the *energy* for glucose transport is *indirectly provided by active transport of Na^+ out of cell,* which maintans the concentration gradent (so more Na^+ & consequently more glucose enter)
- **SGLT – 1** transports glucose & galactose. But fructose utilizes Na^+ independent **GLUT -5** for its facilitated diffusion from intestinal lumen into enterocytes and **GLUT- 2** for transport outside enterocytes into interstitium
- ***Like glucose reabsorption in PCT of kidney, insulin has no (little) effect on intestinal absorption (transport) of sugars***[Q]. Neither process require phosphorylation, and ***both, are normal in diabetes but depressed by drug phlorizin***[Q].

Insulin Resistance in Obesity

It is caused by **decreased ability or inability of insulin to**

1. Increase GLUT-4 Mediated Uptake of Glucose by Skeletal Muscle	2. Repress Hepatic Glucose Production by Glycogenolysis & Gluconeogenesis	3. Repress Hormone Sensitive Lipase (HSL) or Increase LPL in Adipose Tissue
- Increased burden of glucose in skeletal muscle with decrease uptake promote lipogenesis and **excessive TG accumulation (lipotoxicity).** - By products of FA & TG synthesis like diacylglycerol and ceramide accumulate and stimulate signaling pathways **(eg protein kinase C-dependent pathway) that antagonize signaling** from the insulin receptor (IR) or IRS (insulin receptor substrate) protein.	- Decreased repression of these pathways r/i increased burden of intrahepatic glucose that is converted to FFAs & TG. The influx of glucose and FFAs exceed the ability of liver to pakage lipids into VLDL for secretion & transport to adipose tissue. So it **stores increasing amounts of TG causing hepatic steatosis (fatty liver or lipotoxicity)** that progress to **nonalcoholic steatotic hepatitis (NASH).** - **Cytokine TNFα** produced by adipose tissue antagonize insulin signaling pathway.	- **High HSL & low LPL** are major factors in dyslipidemias a/w insulin resistance & diabetes. - Increased paracrine diabetogenic factors in adipose tissue like **TNFα**, resist the actions of insulin.

Stress Syndrome: CRH – ACTH – Cortisol Axis

- In **maintenance of internal homeostasis (ie avoiding stress) and reproduction** processes, multiple hormones cooperate to bring about organized biochemical & physiological responses.
- The **primitive signal of glucose (substrate) lack** is expanded to a broder **signal of fright or stress** and evokes a coordinated neural and endocrine response. Any stressful event eg. *surgery, infection, burn* triggers a hypermetabolic state in which a resting energy expenditure is increased alongwith body temperature.
- **CRH-ACTH – cortisol axis is central** to this integrated response to stress.

Features of Stress Syndrome

- **Corticotropin releasing hormone (CRH) is increased in response to noxious environmental stimuli like pain, trauma, hypoglycemia, infection, surgery, hypovolemia**. Various nervous impulses using several neuro transmitters (NTs) like norepinephrine, serotonin, acetylcholine, dopamine, and GABA reach CRH neurosecretory cells and cause release of CRH
- In response to CRH, both ACTH and **β endorphins** (secreted β-LPH & mature β-endorphin) are released in equimolar quantities β-endorphin produce **central analgesic response**.
- **Glucagon & catecholamines (epinephrine & norepinephrine) are increased, stimulating glycogenolysis (glucose production in liver**) for immediate use by critical organs such as the brain.
- **Cortisol** production is increased in adrenal cortex which induces **gluconeogenesis** (glucose production from noncarbohydrate source like muscles & other body proteins)
- **Glucogon, epinephrine, ACTH** and **growth hormone (GH)** stimulate **lipolysis** and **free fatty acids (FFA) & ketones are released** into the circulation to be used as an alternative metabolic fuel.
- ***Insulin is suppressed***[Q] that results in **decrease in glucose utilization.**
- One form of stress that is cold, specially in neonate causes increased **TRH** secretion due to depressed metabolism of neurons in pre- optic area by cooling which release inhibitory discharge, permitting TRH secretion.
- **ADH (vasopressin), angiotensin & aldosterone synthesis is increased enhancing salt water retention**
- So increased glucose production (by glycogenolysis & gluconeogenesis) and decreased utilization of glucose results in **hyperglycemia**. There is marked increase in release of aminoacids from tissue protein, particularly from skeletal muscle for gluconeogenesis. However, synthesis of specific proteins may increase
- These metabolic changes are coordinated with **increased sympathetic nervous system activity causing peripheral vasoconstriction and increased blood pressure**.

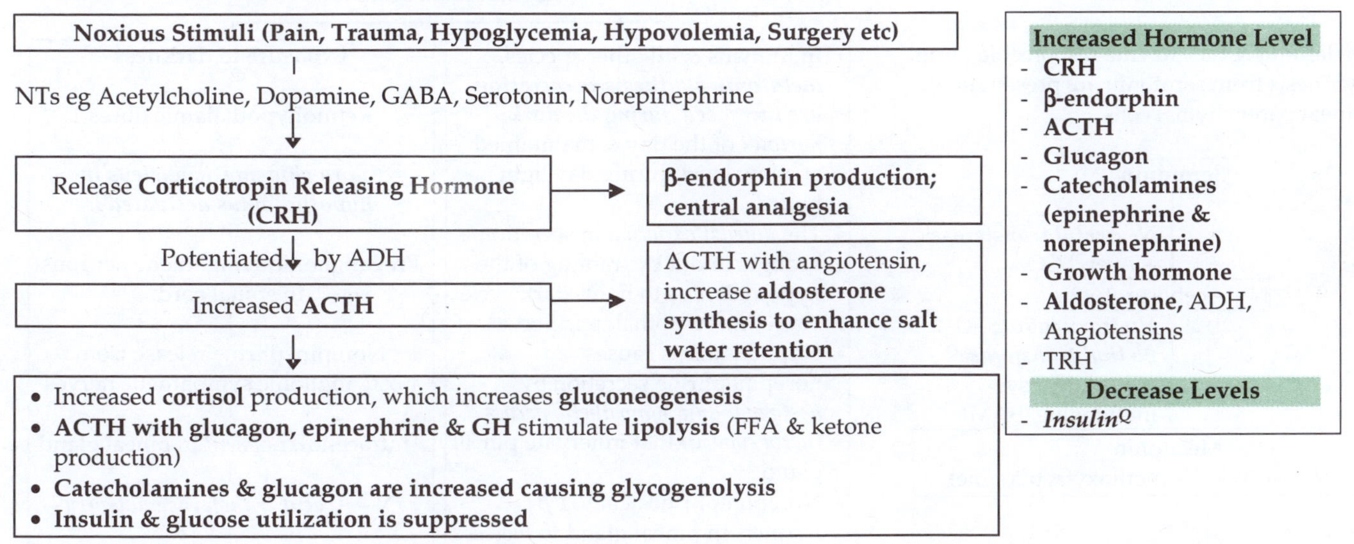

Increased Hormone Level
- **CRH**
- **β-endorphin**
- **ACTH**
- **Glucagon**
- **Catecholamines (epinephrine & norepinephrine)**
- **Growth hormone**
- **Aldosterone,** ADH, Angiotensins
- TRH

Decrease Levels
- *Insulin*[Q]

Stress

Any change in the environment that changes or threatens to change an existing optimal steady state.

↑ACTH l/t↑ glucocorticoids; which acts by
- Maintenance of vascular reactivity to catecholamines
- Also necessary for catecholamines to exert their full FFA – mobilizing action, and FFA are important emergency energy supply

- **Activate sympathetic system** l/t **↑Catecholamines**
- **Increase glucagon** and decrease anabolic hormones e.g. insulin & testosterone

Gluconeogenesis & Lipolysis

★ *Hypophysectomized* animals or *adrenalectomized* animals treated *with maintenance dose of glucocorticoids, die* when exposed to the same stress. However sympathectomized animals tolerate stress with relative impunity.

★ Increase in ACTH secretion to meet emergency situation are mediated almost exclusively through hypothalamus via release of *CRH* (a polypeptide produced by neurons in *paraventricular nuclei*, secreted in *median eminence* & transported in portal- hypophyseal vessels to anterior pituitary where it stimulates ACTH secretion. Inputs from ***suprachiasmatic nuclei* provides the drive for *diurnal rhythm***[Q]

System	Other effects of stress
Endocrinal	- ***↑catabolic hormones eg catacholamines, cortisol & glucagon***[Q] - ↓ anabolic hormones eg insulin & testosterone
CVS	Hypertension, tachycardia,↑ CO (↓ in LVF) &↑TPR
Hematology	Hypercoagulability, ↑platelet adhesiveness,↓ fibrinolysis
Immunology	Leukocytosis, Lymhopenia

Melatonin

Synthesis

Melatonin & the enzyme responsible for its synthesis from serotonin are present in pineal parenchymal cells.

Serotonin
↓ ***N- Acetyl transferase***[Q] + Acetyl COA
N – Acetylserotonin
↓ ***Hydroxy indole –O- methyl transferase***[Q] + S – Adenosyl methionine (SAM)
Melatonin (N – Acetyl –5 – methoxytryptamine)

Regulation of secretion

- In humans & all other species, ***melatonin synthesis & secretion are increased during the dark period***[Q] of the day & maintained at a low level during day light hours.
- The *diurnal variation* in secretion is brought about by training of the hypothalamus to light- dark cycle via retino-hypothalamic nerves.
- Hypothalamus causes norepinephrine secretion by *postganglionic sympathetic nerves (nervi conarii)* that innervate pineal gland.
- Norepinephrine acts Via *β- receptors* in pineal gland to *increase intracellular c AMP*. cAMP increases N-acetyltranferase activity. Thus increases melatonin synthesis & secretion.

Exposure to darkness
|
Retinohypothalamic fibres
|
Supra chiasmatic nucleus in hypothalamus activated[Q].
|
Preganglionic sympathetic neurons in spinal cord
|
Norepinephrine release from postganglionic sympathetic nerves
|
↑intracellular cAMP in pineal gland
|
↑N – Acetyl transferase activity[Q]
|
↑Hydroxyindole – O – methyl transferase[Q]
↓
↑Melatonin

Somatomedins

- Somatomedins are **polypeptide growth factors**, *secreted by liver* and other tissues, which *mediate the effects of growth hormone (somatotropin or STH)* on growth, cartilage and protein metabolism.
- **Liver** (and to a much lesser extent, other tissues) form somatomedins, *when stimulated by somatotropin (or growth hormone).* That is why gwoth hormone supplied directly to cartilage chondrocytes cultured outside the body fails to produce proliferation & enlargement of chondrocytes whereas, growth hormone injections into intact living animal does cause it.
- Somatomedins are also k/a **insulin like growth factors (IGFs)** because many of its effects on growth are similar to effects of insulin on growth.
- At least 4 types have been isolated 3 of which are
  - *Somatomedin A* or insulin like growth factor 2 *(IGF2)* or multiplication stimulating activity *(MSA)*
  - *Somatomedin B* derived from *vitronectin*
  - *Somatomedin C* or *IGF 1* is the most important type & its concentration closely follows the rate of growth hormone secretion
- The principal & in humns probably the only circulating somatomedins are *IGF1 & IGF-2*. these factors *closely relate to insulin,* except that their *C chains are not separated* and they have *an extension of A chain called the D domain.*
- The activity that is not suppressed by antiinsulin antibodies is called **non suppressible insulin like activity (NSILA)**. Most, if not all, of this *activity persists after pancreatectomy* and is d/t IGF1and IGF II. However because of 100 fold weaker binding to insulin receptor the insulin like activity of IGF 1 & 2 is *weak enough* to prevent diabetes mellitus after pancreatectomy. Insulin also binds to IGF 1 receptors whereas IGFI & II bind to all 3 i.e. insulin, IGFI & IGF II receptor

Comparison of insulin & IGF

	Insulin	IGF-I	IGF-II
Name	-	**Somatomedin C**	Multiplication stimulating activity (MSA)
No. of amino acids	51	70	67
Source	Pancreatic β cells	**Liver,** & other tissues	Diverse tissue
Level regulated by	Glucose	Growth hormone after birth, nutritional status	-
Plasma levels	0.3-2 ng/mL	10-700 ng/mL peas at puberty	300 -800 ng/ml
Plasma binding proteins	Absent	Present	Present
Role	Metabolism control	Skeletal & cartilage growth	Growth during fetal development

Characteristics of IGF- II

- Hormone relaxin (both isoforms) resemble IGF-II
- Largely *independent of GH* & plays a role in *growth of fetus before birth.*
- If over expressed in fetus, growth of organs esp tongue other muscles, kidney, heart & liver is disproportionate.
- In adults IGF II gene is expressed only in *choroids plexus & meninges*
- IGF II receptor has distinct structure & is involved in the intracellular targeting of acid hydrolyses & other proteins to intracellular organelles

Substances with insulin like activity in plasma

- Insulin
- Proinsulin
- Non suppressible insulin like activity (NSIL) d/t
  1. **Low molecular weight fraction** i.e. small amounts of *free plasma IGF 1 and IGF2*
  2. **High molecular weight fraction** i.e. large amounts of IGFs bound to proteins

5 characteristic features of somatomedin

- Secretion is independent of growth hormone before birth but is stimulated by growth hormone after birth. Its concentration rises during childhood, peaks at puberty & then declines to low levels in old age.
- It has pronounced growth stimulating activity (epiphyseal growth & protein synthesis)
- ***Stimulates sulfate incorporation into cartilage proteoglycan chondroitin sulfate***[Q]
- Insulin like effects on adipose tissue (antilipolytic) and muscles
- Mitogenicity for fibroblasts
- IGI- 1 receptor is similar to insulin receptor & uses same intra cellular signaling pathways.

- **Pygmies of Africa & Levi-lorian dwarf** have a – congenital inability to synthesize somatomedin C in adequate amount. Therefore, even though their plasma concentration of GH is either normal or high, they have diminished amounts of somatomedin C l/t small statures.

- IGF I & II are tightly bound to proteins (*IGF binding protein 3 or IGFBP3* accounts for *95% binding*) in plasma, at least for IGF I this prolongs their half life in circulation to about 20 hours. Whereas the growth hormone weakly binds to protein & has a short half life of 20 minutes.
- It seems that GH & somatomedins can act both in cooperation & independently to stimulate pathways that l/t growth. **GH** promote growth of muscle & bone. Its metabolic actions are *counter regulatory to insulin as it induces glycogenolysis & gluconeogenesis in liver to increase blood glucose* and mobilizes free fatty acids (i.e. *lipolysis*). It inhibits glucose uptake by muscle & fat cells, so more glucose is provided to brain & heart. Simultaneously, GH stimulates lipolysis in fat cells providing free fatty acids to heart & active skeletal muscle. But **IGFI** structurally similar to insulin is capable of *increasing glucose utilization & decreasing lipolysis*. These effects are opposite to those of acute, antiinsulin actions of GH.

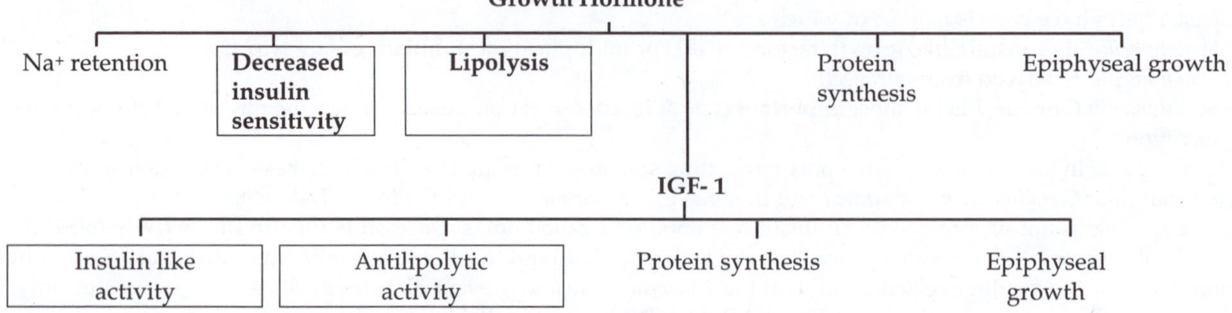

Posterior Pituitary Hormones: ADH & Oxytocin

- Posterior pituitary gland (or **neurohyophysis**) is composed mainly of *supporting, non (hormone) secreting glial like cells* k/a **pituicytes** which act simply as a supporting structure *for terminal nerve fibers (& nerve endings)* from nerve tracts that originate in the **supraoptic** and **paraventricular nuclei of hypothalamus**. These tracts pass to posterior pituitary through the pituitary stalk (**hypophysial stalk**).
- Hormones of neurohypophysis are actually synthesized in **cell bodies (soma) of magnocellular (large) neurons** in the **supraoptic** and **paraventricular nuclei of hypothalamus**
- **ADH (vasopressin)** is formed primarily (5/6th part) in ***supraoptic nuclei***[Q] and **oxytocin** is formed mainly (5/6th part) in ***paraventricular nuclei***[Q]. However, *each of these nuclei can synthesize about 1/6th as much of the second hormone* as of its primary hormone. In other words hypothalamus contains 2 types of magnocellular neurons – some making ADH (predominantly found in supraoptic nuclei) and others making oxytocin (mainly found in paraventricular nuclei); however *both types of neuron (cells) found in both nuclei*.
- Like other peptide hormones, neurohypophyseal hormones are also synthesized as part of larger precursor molecules. The precursor for oxytocin, **prepro-oxyphysin** contains a 19 aminoacid (aa) signal /leader sequence f/b oxytocin (9 aa) and **neurophysin** I (93 aa). **Prepro-pressophysin**, the precursor for arginine vasopressin is similar but larger molecule that contains 19 aa signal (leader) sequence f/b vasopressin (9 aa), **neurophysin II** and a 39 aa **glycopeptide**. The precursor molecules are synthesized in ribosomes of cell bodies of magnoneurons. Their *leader sequence is removed in endoplasmic reticulum*, packaged into **secretory granules (or Herring bodies)** in the golgi-apparatus and then are transported down the axon in these granules **in combination with carrier protein (neurophysins)** by axoplasmic flow to the nerve endings in posterior pituitary, *requiring several days to reach the gland*.
- During transport, cleavage of precursor molecules occur and the **storage granule** in the nerve endings ***contain free vasopressin or oxytocin***[Q] and corresponding neurophysin (+ glycopeptide in case of vasopressin). All these products are secreted in blood (Ganong)/Both neurophysin & hormone are secreted together, but because they are only loosely bound to each other, the hormone separates almost immediately (Guyton). So vasopressin & oxytocin are typical **neural hormones** i.e. hormones secreted into the circulation by nerve cells (**neurosecretion**)
- Oxytocin & vasopressin secreting neurons *also generate & conduct action potentials*, which on reaching to their endings trigger release of hormones from storage granules by *Ca^{++} dependent exocytosis*. At rest these neurons are *silent or discharge at low, irregular rates* (0.1-3 spikes/s)
- If the **pituitary stalk (Containing axons** of magnocellular neurons) is **cut above gland** but the entire hypothalamus is left intact, the posterior pituitary hormones continue to be *secreted normally, after a transient decrease for a few days*; however they are then secreted by cut ends of fibers *within the hypothalamus and not by nerve endings in posterior pituitary* (Guyton-928). (Transient) Decrease of ADH l/t **polyuria & diabetes insipidus**. And similarly decrease of **hypothalamic prolactin inhibiting hormone (PIH)**, dopamine leads to an increase in circulating prolactin causing ***galactorrhea***[Q].

- Stimulation of vasopressin secreting neurons causes an *initial steady increase* in firing rate f/b a prolonged pattern of **phasic discharge /phasic bursting**, in which periods of high frequency discharge alternate with periods of electrical quiescence. In different neurons this phasic bursting is **non-synchronous**, well suited to maintain a prolonged increase in the output of vasopressin.

- Stimulation of oxytocin secreting neuron causes a **synchronous, relatively short, high frequency discharge** causing release *a pulse of oxytocin* and consequent milk ejection in post partum females.

- Both ADH & oxytocin are polypeptides, each containing 9 amino acid with almost identical sequences except that in vasopressin, phenylalanine, & arginine replace isoleucine and leucine of oxytocin in 3rd & 8th positions respectively. Vasopressin is **arginine vasopressin (AVP)** in most mammals, **lysine vasopressin** in hippopotami & most pigs (in it arginine is replaced by lysine) and mixture of both arginine & lysine vasopressin in some pidgs & marsupials.

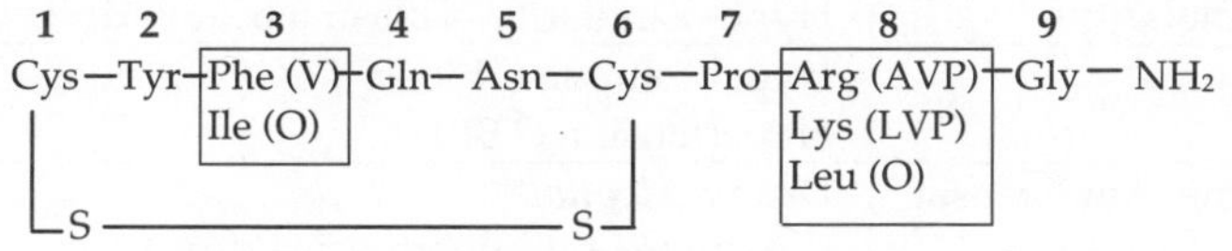

```
 1     2      3          4      5      6      7        8          9
Cys—Tyr—[Phe (V)]—Gln—Asn—Cys—Pro—[Arg (AVP)]—Gly—NH2
 |       [Ile (O)]               |      [Lys (LVP)]
 |                               |      [Leu (O)]
 └S ——————————————————————————— S┘
```

★ Vasopressin plays important role in BP regulation *in hemorrhage & dehydration.* **Conivaptan (YM O87)**, a drug with both V_{1a} & V_2 antagonist action is approved for treatment of hyponatremia.

- Vasopressin & oxytocin are also synthesized in the gonads & adrenal cortex and oxytocin is present in thymus. Circulating vasopressin is rapidly inactivated (t ½ = 18 min) mainly in liver & kidney.

• Control of vasopressin (ADH) secretion

- **Hyperosmolarity** or **increased effective osmotic pressure** of plasma (> **285** mOsm/kg) is the most sensitive & important stimulator of ADH secretion. At 285 mOsm /kg effective osmotic pressure of plasma, vasopressin is at or near the limits of detection but below this is undetectable and when pressure is increased above 285, vasopressin secretion increases. So osmolality of plasma is maintained very close to 285 mOsm/L in normal individuals.
- Vasopressin secretion is regulated by *Osmoreceptors located in anterior hypothalamus.* They are outside the BBB in circumventricular organs primarily the **organum vasculosum** of **lamina terminalis (OVLT)**. Osmotic *threshold for thirst is same or slightly greater than the threshold of ADH secretion* (Ganong) Osmoreceptors (neurons) are located *in the vicinity of AV3V (antero-ventral region of 3rd ventricle) region and supraoptic nuclei.* ***Subfornical organ*** **(SFO)** is a structure at the upper part and **OVLT** is a structure at the inferior part of AV3V. Between these two organs is **median preoptic neucleus**, which has multiple nerve connections with SFO, OVLT, supraoptic nuclei and blood pressure control centers in medulla. Electrical stimulation or stimulation by angiotensin II of AV3V region can alter ADH secretion, thirst & sodium appetite (Guyton).

All 3 types of vasopressin receptors are G protein coupled

ADH Receptor	Site of action	Function	2nd messenger
V_{1A}	***Vascular smooth muscle***[Q]	Potent **vasoconstrictor** (invitro), relatively large amount is needed to raise BP in vivo (b/o ↓CO caused by action in brain)	**Phosphatidyl-inositol** hydrolysis to increase the intracellular **Ca++ concentration**
	Area postream of brain	**Decrease in cardiac output** (CO)	
	Brain stem & spinal cord	Neurotransmitter & involved in cardiovascular (↓ CO) control	
	Liver	Cause **glycogenolysis**	
$V_{1B} = V_3$	**Anterior pituitary**	Increased **ACTH** secretion by corticotropes	
V_2	***Principal cells of collecting duct***[Q]	Exerts ***antidiuretic effect***[Q] by insertion of **water channels**, a protein k/a **aquaporin-2** into the apical (luminal) membranes of principle cells of collecting ducts. These channels are stored in *endosomes* inside the cells and ADH causes their rapid translocation to luminal membranes. The movement of water across membranes by simple diffusion is augmented by aquaporins (13 i.e. AQPO to AQ P12 channels in almost all tissues have been identified.)	Activation of adenyl cyclase; acts through ***Gs to increase C-Amp***[Q]

- ADH secretion is stimulated by *either an increase is ECF* ***osmolarity or decrease in effective blood volume.*** **However,** ***ADH secretion is considerably more sensitive to small changes in osmolarity***Q than to similar changes in blood volume. For example, 1% ↑in osmolarity or 10% ↓in blood volume is required to ↑ADH level.
- With severe decrease (>10%) in blood volume, cardiovascular reflexes (i.e., arterial baro receptor reflex & cardio pulmonary reflex) play a major role in stimulating ADH secretion.
- ***The usual day to day regulation of ADH secretion during simple dehydration is effected mainly by changes in plasma osmolarity***Q. However, decreased blood volume greatly enhances response.

Factors Affecting ADH Secretion

Increasing ADH (Vasopressin) Secretion	Decreasing ADH (Vasopressin) Secretion
- ***Hyper osmolarity***Q (↑plasma osmolarity)	- Hypo-osmolarity (↓plasma osmolarity)
- Hypovolumia (↓blood /ECF volume) - Hypotension (↓BP)	- Hypervolumia (↑blood / ECF volume) - Hypertension (↑BP)
- Drugs : Clofibrate, Carbamazepine, Angiotensin II	- Drugs: ***Alcohol***Q Clonidine (antihypertensive drug) Haloperidol (dopamine blocker)
- Nausea (100 times increase in ADH) - Vomiting - **Surgery, exercise**Q,emotion, stress, **pain**	

Relationship between T_4 & T_3

T4	T3
- Thyroid secretes more T_4 than T_3. - T_4 is major circulating hormone. - T_4 is ***more tightly bound to plasma protein (15 times)***Q - ***Half life of T_4 (6-7 days) is more***Q than T_3 (1-2 days).	- T_3 is 5 times more potent than T_4 - T_3 acts faster than T_4. - ***T_3 is more avidly bound to nuclear receptors***Q than T_4. - About 1/3 of T_4 is converted to T_3 in peripheral tissue.

It is believed that T_3 is active hormone & T_4 is only transport form.

Effects of Thyroxine on

Oxidative metabolism	- T_3 stimulates ***increase in O_2 uptake of all tissue***Q, *excepting brain & testis.* - Metabolism of all tissues (except brain & testis) is increased i.e. ***↑BMR***Q. - T_4 & T_3 causes *calorigenesis* (excessive colory production)
Carbohydrate metabolism	- T_3 increases gluconeogenesis - T_3 increase glycogenolysis - These two factors causes *elevation of blood sugar level.*
Lipid metabolism	- T_3 reduces serum cholesterol by increasing its metabolism. - ***T_3 increase lipolysis***Q (adrenaline mediated) - Lipolysis result in increase FFA.
Protein metabolism	T_3 enhances both catabolism & anabolism of proteins. But under physiological condition anabolism> catabolism.
Skeletal system	- T_3 help *growth of the bone*, it does not act directly on bone cells. - T_3 potentiate effect of a) *GH*,b) insulin like grow factor (*IGF*) on bone → Bone growth - T_3 helps in bone maturation also.
CNS	- Required for growth & development of brain during fetal & post natal period - T_3 is required for *myelination of nerve fibers in brain*
CVS	- T_3 ***increases mycocardial contractility and heart rate***Q. (β1sympathetic receptor increase under the influence of T_3)
Temperature regulation	- T3 causes calorigenesis →↑ heat production

Thyroxine Releasing Hormone

TRH (hypothalamic tripeptide) stimulates release of:	**TRH stimulation testing** – is useful in diagnosis of:
- TSH - Prolactin - ***GH***Q	- Hyperthyroidism - ***Recurrent acromegaly***Q - Gonadotropin secreting tumour - Cases where documentation of prolactin deficiency is necessary.

Na^+ / I^- Symporter (NIS)

The thyroid cell membrane facing the capillaries contain a symporter that transports Na^+ & I^- into the cells against the electro chemical gradient for I^-.

NIS is also present in:

- ***Salivary gland***Q
- ***Mammary gland***Q
- *Ciliary body of eye*
- *Gastric mucosa*
- *Placenta*
- *Choroids plexus*

but their uptake is not affected by TSH.

Actions of Glucocorticosteroids (GC)

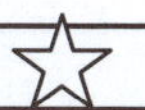

Metabolic Actions

It is an *anti-insulin hormone* that is *catabolic to peripheral* tissue & *anabolic to liver.*

Carbohydrate Metabolism

- It causes **hyperglycemia** (i.e. plasma glucose level is increased and that is why it is called glucocorticoid) and *makes diabetes worse* by

1. **Increased gluconeogenesis** in liver
   - as a result of enhanced hepatic catabolism of aminoacids (d/t induction of aminotransferases, trypthophan dioxygenases / pyrrolase alanine / tyrosine transaminase) which make more substrate available
   - induction of key enzymes of gluconeogenesis e.g. *pyruvate carboxylase, PEP carboxykinase, fructose 1-6 biphosphatase & glucose 6 phosphosphatase*
2. **Decreased glucose uptake & utilization in peripheral tissue,** except the brain and heart.
3. **Decreased glycolysis** in peripheral tissue

- **Glycogen deposition (or increased glycogen synthesis) in liver**
  - as a result of increased glucose formation from amino acids & glycerol (i.e. gluconeogenesis) and
  - Stimulation of glycogen synthase & protein phosphatase 1 enzyme

Lipid metabolism

- **Increase lipohysis** and liberate *free fatty acids* (FFA) and *glycerol*, both of which are increased in plasma
- Decrease esterifcation, ↓ triglyceride formation and ↓ α glycogen P.
- GC & thyroid hormones are facilitatory or permissive to other lipolytic hormones eg. *epinephrine, norepinephrine, glucagons, ACTH, TSH, GH, α and β melanocyte stimulating hormone* (MSH) and *vasopressin*. Many of these activate *hormone sensitive lipase.*

Protein metabolism

- Overall it causes *negative mitrogen balance.*
- In extrahepatic tissue (esp. muscles) **proteolysis** (protein breakdown) is increased l/t increased availability of amino acids in plasma.
- It *promotes amino acid uptake by liver* enhancing gluconeogenesis & protein synthesis here.
- Inhibits amino acid uptake & ↓ protein synthesis in peripheral tissue.

Permissive action on catecholamines

- Despite no direct bronchodilator or vasoactive property, GC *is necessary for bronchodilation & vasoconstrictor action of catecholamine* (in maintaining BP). It inhibits enzyme *COMT (catecholamine-o-methyl transferase)* which inactivates catecholamines.
- Similarly GC is necessary for *calorigenic effects of catecholamines and glucagons.*
- ***Osteoporosis***[Q]
- **Facilitate renal excretion of water**[Q]
- **Glucocorticoids inhibit intestinal absorption & enhance renal excretion of Ca^{++}**[Q]
- Antiinflammatory action is d/t decreased
  - permeability of capillary
  - release of lysosomal hydrolase (d/t stabilized lysosomal membrane) & interleukin 1 from granulocytes.
  - Formation of bradykinin, PGs, PGI2, Tx & leukotrienes (by **inhibiting phospholipase A2)**[Q]
- **GC decrease number of eosinophils** (by increasing their sequestration in spleen and lung), basophils and lymphocyte; reduce the size of lymph node & thymus; and reduce secretion of cytokines. It increases number of RBC, platelet & neutrophils.

Metabolic Actions Of Glucocorticoid ☆

It is a catabolic hormone. Their function appears to be oriented to maintain blood glucose levels during starvation – so that brain continues to get its nutrients.

Carbohydrate metabolism

- *Promote glycogen deposition* in liver and promote ***gluconeogenesis***[Q]
- They ***inhibit glucose utilization by peripheral tissue***[Q], resulting in hyper glycemia, resistance to insulin and a diabetes like state

Protein metabolism

- Cause ***protein breakdown***[Q] & aminoacid mobilization from peripheral tissues causing muscle wasting, lympholysis, loss of osteoid from bone and thinning of skin
- The amino acids are used up in gluconeogenesis → excess urea is produced → negative nitrogen balance

Fat metabolism

- ***Promote lipolysis***[Q] (d/t glucagons, GH, adrenaline & thyroxine) and C-AMP induced break down of triglycerides i.e.is **ketogenic**
- **Redistribution of body fat occurs.** Subcutaneous tissue over extremities loses fat which is deposited over face, neck & shoulder – *moon face, fish mouth, buffalo hump* This is because peripheral adipocytes are less sensitive to insulin

★ In stress *vasopressin*[Q] also increases Glucocorticoids

★ In adrenal insufficiency, the blood glucose is normal as long as food intake is maintained, but fasting precipitates hypoglycemia & collapse. This is because glucocorticoids are necessary for glucagons to exert its gluconeogenic action during fasting.

Circadian (Diurnal) Rhythm of ACTH, Cortisol & Eosinophil

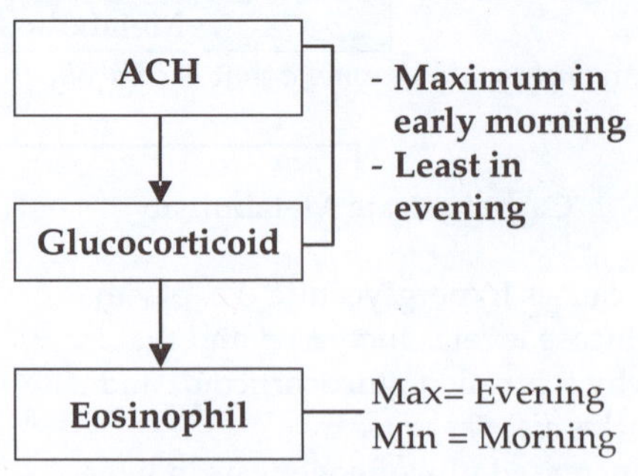

- **Suprachiasmatic nuclei (SCN) of hypothalamus** is the **biological clock** responsible for **diurnal (circadian) rhythm of ACTH**, which intum leads to **diurnal rhythm of cortisol (glucocorticoid) secretion**. In humans, **ACTH irregular bursts** (episodes of high secretion) are **most frequent in early morning and least frequent in the evening**. Increased ACTH secretion is not d/t stress of getting up in the morning as these bursts occur before waking up. Even if the length of day is experimentally lengthened to >24 hrs ie if the person is isolated and day's activities are spread over more than 24h, the adrenal cycle also lengthens, but the ACTH burst *still occurs during period of sleep*. The circadian rhythm of ACTH secretion is present in patients with adrenal insufficiency receiving constant dose of glucocorticoids.
- **Cortisol decrease the number of circulating eosinophils by increasing their sequestration in the spleen & lung.** So the ***diurnal variations in blood eosinophilic counts is inversely related to the circadian cortisol levels***Q. The eosinophilic concentration in blood is < 450 / mL usually. A reciprocal relationship to plasma cortisol, causes the diurnal eosinophilic concentrations to vary ~ 2 fold (40%) with **eosinophilic count lowest in morning and peaking in evening.**

Aldosterone

Actions

- **Increase the *reabsorption of Na$^+$*** from the urine, sweat, saliva & the contents of the colon.
- Retention of Na+ in ECF **expands ECF volume.**
- **Facilitation of *K$^+$ extrusion*** by the renal tubular cells.
  [aldosterone causes ***Na conservation + K$^+$ excretion***]
- In the kidney aldosterone act primarily on *principal cell (P cells)* of *collecting duct*.

Secretagogue	Intracellular mediator
ACTH	Cyclic AMP, protein kinase A
Angiotensin II	Diacylglycerol, protein kinase C
K^+	Ca^{2+} via voltage-gated Ca_{2+} channels

Regulation of secretion

- **Increased Renin – angiotensin system is the principal regulator & greatly increase aldosterone secretions.**
  - Renin is secreted from *juxtaglomerular cells* that surround afferent arteriole. Angiotensin II, is formed by the action of rennin, and it stimulates aldosterone secretion
  - Factors (↓ ECF volume, hypotension) that increase renin secretion & angiotension II formation that stimulates aldosterone secretion
- **Increased K+** (not Na+) **ion concentration** in ECF greatly increase & by far most important electrolyte in regulation of aldosterone secretion.
- Increased Na+ ion concentration in ECF *very slightly* decrease aldosterone secretion.
- **ACTH** is necessary for aldosterone secretion but has little effect in controlling the rate. A small amount of ACTH secreted is enough to produce normal amount of aldosterone but total absence can significantly reduce aldosterone secretion.
- ***Endothein***Q & also epinephrine, nor epinephrine cause vosoconstriction of efferent & afferent arteriole →↓ GFR & ↓ renal blood flow. It causes ***↑ed level of plasm ANP, rennin & aldosterone***Q.
- **Stimuli that increase aldosterone secretion and**

Glucocorticoid secretion also increased	Glucocorticoid secretion unaffected
- Surgery - Anxiety - Physical trauma - Hemorrhage	- High potassium intake - Low sodium intake - Constriction of inferior vena cava in thorax - Standing - Secondary hyperaldosteronism (in some cases of congestive heart failure, cirrhosis, and nephrosis)

Excess Mineralocorticosteroid (Aldosterone)

Increased ECF and arterial pressure but very small effect on plasma Na^+ concentration

- Although aldosterone has a potent effect in decreasing rate of Na+ ion excretion, ***but plasma Na^+ level is elevated only slightly if at all because water is retained with osmolically active Na+ ions***[Q]
- ***Consequently ECF volume is expanded and blood pressure rises***[Q]
- When ECF expansion (& ↑BP) passes a certain point, Na+ and water excretion is usually increased (called **pressure natriuresis & pressure diuresis** respectively) inspite of continued action of mineralocorticoids on renal tubules. This **aldosterone escape phenomenon** is due to *increased secretion of ANP.*
- Because of this escape, mineralocorticoids do not produce edema in normal individuals & in hyper aldosteronism

Hypokalemia, Muscle weakness & alkalosis (Mild)

- Aldosterone cause **K^+ secretion** into tubules inexchange for sodium reabsorption in **principal cells of renal collecting tubules**
- Aldosterone causes **hypokalemia** not only by causing *loss of K^+ ions* from ECF *into urine* but also stimulating transport of K^+ from ECF *into cells.*
- Severe **muscle weakness** develops (at K+ < 2) because of altered electrical excitability of nerve & muscle fiber membrane
- Aldosterone also causes **secretion of H^+ ions** in exchange for Na^+ in **intercalated cells of cortical collecting tubules.** This leads to decreased H+ ion concentration in ECF causing **mild alkalosis.**

So excess mineralocorticoid leads to *hypokalemic (K^+ depletion) alkalosis with weakness* & tetany and *Na^+ & water retention usually with out edema but with hypertension & polyuria.* It may be d/t

Primary hyperaldosteronism: Conn syndrome

- D/t primary adrenal disease such as adrenal hyperplasia (u/l or b/l), adenoma of zone glomerulosa, adrenal carcinoma or GRA
- ***Renin secretion is depressed***[Q]

Secondary hyperaldosteronism

- Caused by cirrhosis, heart failure, nephrosis
- ***High plasma rennin activity***[Q]

AME Syndrome & 11 β HSD type 2

- Invitro (in lab), the mineralocorticoid receptor has much higher affinity for glucocorticoids than the glucocorticoid receptor does, & glucocorticoids are present in large amount in body (vivo). But binding of glucocorticoids to mineralocorticoid receptor (& so production of mineralcorticoid effects by glucocorticoids) is prevented by presence of **11 β hydroxyl steroid dehydrogenase tye 2** enzyme in mineralocorticoid sensitive tissues. This enzyme leaves aldosterone untouched, but converts cortisol to cortisone & corticosterone to its 11 oxy derivatives. These 11 oxy derivatives do not bind to receptor.
- If **11 β hydroxysteroid dehydrogenase type 2** is congenitally **absent or inhibited by prolonged ingestion of licorice (containing glycyrrhetinic)**, cortisol has marked mineralocorticoid effects resulting in **apparent mineralocorticoid excess (AME syndrome**.
- Patient with AME have clinical picture of hyper aldosteronism because **cortisol** is acting on their mineralo corticoid receptors, & their *plasma aldosterone levels and plasma rennin activity is low.*

Ovarian Reserve

- It refers to the *size of resting / nongrowing /primordial follicle population,* which reflects the *quantity (no) of growing follicles and quality of oocytes within it.* So ovarian reserve determines the *functional reproductive potential of ovary.*
- Under the influence of FSH and LH, there is rapid growth of several follicles in ovary, during first few days of each menstrual cycle. But after a week only 1 follicle begins to outgrow all the others /which involute by a process called **atresia** and thus preventing more than one child from developing with each pregnancy).
- Ovarian reserve (& capacity of ovary to produce eggs) decline with *advancing age.* Best predictor of ovarian reserve is age. **Tests that can determine ovarian reserve** include

FSH level on day 3

- FSH levels are elevated in an attempt to force the aging ovary to respond. Cycle **day 3 FSH levels** are used for assessment because at this time *follicles produce low levels of estrogen (& inhibin B)* which has negative feedback on FSH
- High FSH indicates poor ovarian reserve and < 10 IU/mL FSH on day 3 predict adequate ovarian oocyte reserve.

FSH level on day 10 after clomifene citrate (antiestrogen) challenge test

- It is a provocative test *2-3 times more sensitive* than day 3 FSH level. So it is the **best screening test** which **unmask patients** which might be missed with a day 3 FSH level test.
- In this test after measuring FSH & estrogen levels on cycle day 3 (following the onset of menses), an **antiestrogen clomiphene citrate** 100 mg is given *from day 5 to 9* and repeat estimation of FSH and estrogen levels are done on **day 10**.
- Being antiestrogen, clomiphene inhibits negative feedback of estrogen on hypothalamus, thus hypothalamus perceives false signals that patient does not have enough estrogen. This induces pituitary to rise FSH & LH which inturn initiates follicular growth to produce more estrogen. Clomiphene *can exert this effect only when ovarian reserve or estrogen level is low.*
- Positive test indicate low ovarian reserve & poor chance to conceive.

FSH level	Result
< 15	Good
> 15 < 20	Border line
> 20.	Poor

Serum-Inhibin B levels

- Inhibin B is secreted by **granulosa cells of ovary** predominantly during *follicular phase* (i.e. by follicles) *to inhibit FSH secretion by pituitary.*
- So ovary with decreased reserve will secrete less inhibin B (i.e. **decreased serum inhibin B levels**) and thus leading to higher FSH levels.
- It is less sensitive than FSH level tests.
- **Ultrasound** scanning to **count** number of **antral follicles** is more accurate than estimating ovarian volume.

Estrogens

Structure and Synthesis

- The naturally occurring estrogens are 17- β - estradiol, estrone & estriol
- They are **secreted primarily by granulose cells of ovarian follicles, corpus luteum and the placenta**[Q]
- Their biosynthesis depends on ***aromatase enzyme***[Q] which converts testosterone to estradiol.
- They are also formed from aromatization of androstenedione in the circulation.

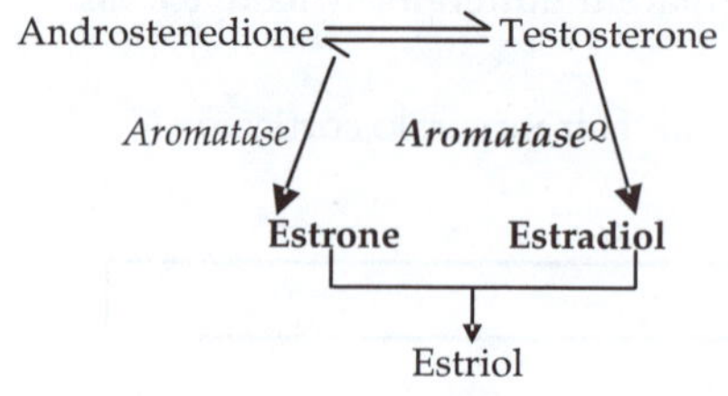

Effects

- Estrogen induced growth requires continuous replenishment of energy, *mainly generated by glycolysis*
- It regulates *GLUT 1 expression* and ***induction of glycolytic enzymes***[Q]
- It promotes energetic capacity of mitochondria by ***maximizing aerobic glycolysis***[Q].
- *Increased HDL* and *plasma triglyceride level* (d/t lipolysis & increased TG synthesis)
- Reduced cholesterol & LDL
- Estrogen causes ***fat to be stored in buttocks, thighs & hips in women.***[Q] In post menopausal women with decreased estrogen production, fat migrates to abdomen (central obesity). Men store fat in abdomen d/t sex hormone difference.
- Many studies show that hormone replacement therapy (HRT) has *no highly deleterious effect in patients with NIDDM or with impaired glucose tolerance test.* Infact HRT significantly *lowers HbA_{1C}* levels in NIDDM.
- It was *progesterone component* of OCP (with higher doses) that *produces abnormal glucose tolerance tests* with elevated insulin level or *worsening of NIDDM.*
- ***At physiological levels, estrogen and testosterone apparaently increase the insulin sensitivity***[Q] and increase insulin dependent metabolic processes eg tissue glucose uptake & lipid synthesis (where as progesterone has the opposite effect). However ***outside the physiological window these steroids may promote insulin resistance.***[Q]
- Post menopausal women who take estrogen replacement therapy (ERT) are less likely to develop diabetes; and if they do have disease, are able to maintain good blood sugar control.

Sertoli Cells (S C)

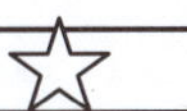

- SC are *large, complex glycogen containing cells* that lines the wall of seminiferous tubules (of testis) along with primitive germ cell. They all *contact basal lamina* and stretch all the way to lumen i.e. they *extend from basal lamina to lumen* where their apical plasma membranes form complex recesses which envelop spermatids & spermatozoa until the latter are mature enough for release.
- SC form a major cellular component of tubule before puberty & in elderly. They are ***supporting, non spermatogenic cells***[Q] of seminiferous tubules.
- Long cell process of SC extends between spermatogonia in **basal** compartment (near basal lamina) and between spermatocytes in **adluminal** (near lumen) compartment
- Its nucleus is *euchromatic, irregular or pear shaped*, contains 1-2 prominent nuclei, & is usually aligned perpendicularly to the basal lamina. The cytoplasm *is rich in lysosome*, consistent with its phagocytic action
- SC have high affinity ***FSH receptors***[Q] that bind FSH & stimulates production of ABP which concentrates testosterone. Spermatogenesis requires presence of FSH & high intertesticular levels of testosterone.
- **Functions of sertoli cells** are

Role in spermato & Spermiogenesis

- ***Germ cells must stay in contact with SC to survive***[Q] & this contact is maintained by **cytoplasmic bridges**
- SC provide **trophic mechanical support** to germ cells through out the stages of spermatogenesis
- **Maintenance or Nourishment**: SC are rich in *glycogen* and provide a source of nourishment to spermatogenic series
- **Phagocytosis** of excess cytoplasmic fragments (residual body) during spermiogenesis
- **Release of spermatozoa**: SC participate in release of sperm by extruding axial components of spermatid while holding & phagocytizing lobules of their cytoplasm
- ***Play important role in controlling spermatocyte & spermatid differentiation & maturation***[Q] (Gray's – 1267)

Form Blood Testes Barrier (BTB)

- Occluding **tight junctions between sertoli cells forms the BTB**[Q]
- BTB *protects the developing spermatogenic cells from blood borne noxious agents & immunological attack.*
- *Steroids (eg androgen* from interstitial cells of Leydig) and *maturing germ cells* can penetrate this barrier with ease while passively diffusing macromolecule & small ions, are prevented from passing from the blood into lumen

Endocrine Functions

- **Mullerian Inhibiting (Regression) Factor / Substance (MTS).** SC secrete MIS which cause ***regression of Mullerian (paramesonephric) ducts in males during fetal life***[Q].
- **Inhibin : SC are under control of FSH** from anterior pituitary; and in turn secrete inhibin **which by negative feed back *inhibits FSH release***[Q]
- Contain **Enzyme Aromatase (CYP- 19)** which *converts androgens into oestrogens*

Exocrine functions

- ***Synthesis & seretion of Androgen Binding protein (ABP): ABP binds and concentrates the androgens (testosterone)***[Q] secreted by Leydig cells. It causes great concentration of testosterone in seminferous tubules. A high concentration of androgens is essential for the production & maturation of spermatozoa
- **Secretion of seminal fluid**: SC secrete a fluid into seminiferous lumen *rich in K+ , HCO_3^-, androgen, oestrogen, inositol & glutamic and aspartic acid but low Na+, Cl- (like ICF)*, -- protein, glucose. It contains androgen binding protein, steroids (testosterone) and inhibin. Maintenance of its composition depends on BTB and it is necessary for onward transport of spermatozoa
- **Secretion of H-Y antigen**

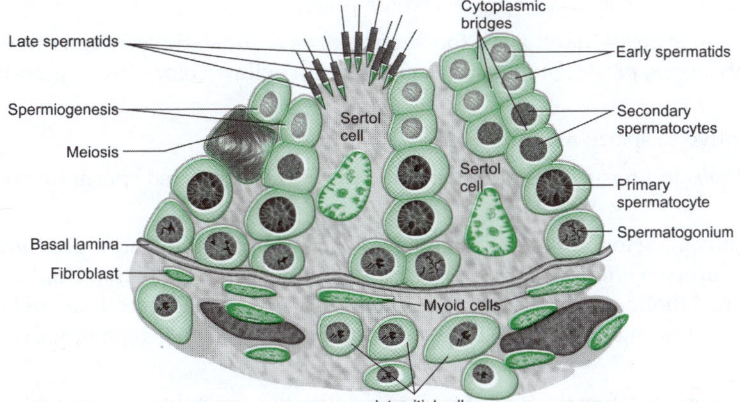

★ Sertoli cells have ***receptors for FSH, and testosterone***[Q]. After combining with FSH, sertoli cells stimulates the ***first half of spermatogenesis***[Q]. Subsequently *testosterone – sertoli cell* binding causes development of last half of spermatogenesis. Testosterone is converted to 5α dihydrotestosterone by sertoli cells.

★ **Interstitial cells of Leydig** are lipid containing cells present in between the seminiferous tubules in testis. ***Leydig cells secrete testosterone***[Q] into the bloodstreem.

Onset of Puberty

- Puberty begins earlier in girls. Because both sexes show a similar *increase in GnRH and LH* at the onset of puberty, whereas *FSH secretion shows sexual diamorphism* i.e., its secretion varies between both sexes in childhood & early puberty. It has been suggested that ***differences in the timing of onset of puberty b/w both sexes is due to differences in FSH seretion***[Q].
- FSH secretion is under regulation of ***FSH regulatory peptides (& GnRH). So the FSH regulatory peptides which stimulate FSH secretion cause early onset of puberty whereas puberty is delayed by peptides that inhibit FSH secretion***[Q]. **FSH – regulatory peptide**

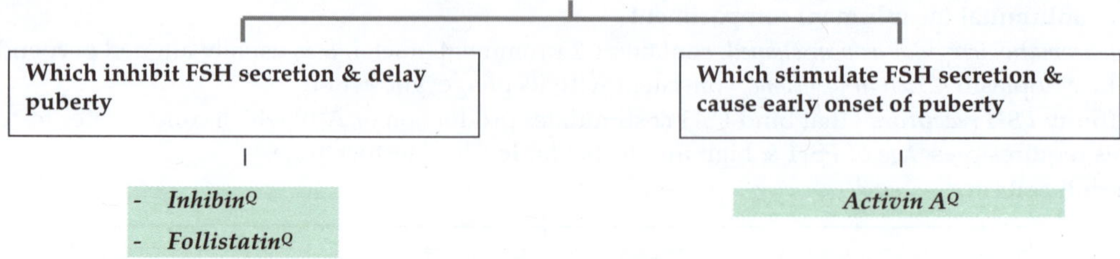

★ So ↑ activin – A causes early puberty and ↑ inhibin & ↑ follistatin delay puberty.

Spermatogenesis

- **Spermatogenesis** occurs in ***germinal epithelium of seminiferous tubules***[Q]
- ***Epididymis reabsorbs 99% of testicular fluid and concentrates and stores spermatozoa***[Q]. After a 18-24 hour stay in epididymis sperms develop the ***capability of motility***[Q] which is important for fertilization in vivo. But fertilization occurs in vitro even if an immotile spermatozoa from head of epiddymis is microinjected directly into an ovum.
- Out of 120 million sperms formed each day by both testes, ***only a small quantity can be stored in epididymis but most are stored in vas deferens***[Q].
- **Progressive motality** (i.e. ability to move forward) is acquired in epididymis by activation of **Cat sper protein** localized to *principal piece of sperm tail*. This protein is a *Ca++ ion channel* that permits *cAMP generalized Ca^{++} influx*.
- Ejaculation involves **P2 x receptor** ligand gated cation channels (that respond to ATP) mediated contraction of vas deferens
- Normal motile, fertile sperms are capable of *flagellated movement* at *1- 4 mm/min* velocity. Its activity is greatly enhanced in a neutral & slightly alkaline medium and with increasing temperature (which also increases metabolism rate & so decreases life span). Mildly acidic medium decreases activity & strongly acidic medium causes rapid death.
- Although sperm can live for *many weeks in male genital ducts*, once ejaculated their maximum life is ***1-2 days in female genetal tract***[Q]. When frozen at temperatures below – 100°c, sperms can be preserved for years.
- **Seminal vesicle** ***provide the bulk (60%) volume of semen***[Q] that flushes the spermatozoa & prostatic secretion out of urethra. It is rich in *fructose, vitamin C (citric acid), K^+, fibrinogen, prostaglandins and flavins* (giving yellow color). Prostaglandins aid fertilization by
  - Making female cervical mucus more receptive to sperm movement
  - Causing *backward reverse peristaltic contractions* in uterus & fallopian tubes to move the ejaculated sperm towards the ovaries.
- **Prostatic fluid** is rich in calcium, citrate ion, phosphate ion, a clotting enzyme and a profibrinolysin and it ***provides slightly alkaline medium by neutralizing the acidity of other seminal fluids & vogina***[Q]. It is important to note that fluid of vas deferens is acidic d/t presence of citric acid & metabolic end products of sperm and so are vaginal secretions (pH 3.5- 4). Sperms are not optimally motile until pH of surrounding fluid is 6- 6.5 *Spermatozoa express olfactory receptors* & ovaries produce odorant molecules (chemotaxis)
- After ejaculation spermatozoa undergo two processes in female genital tract to acquire the capability of fertilization.

Capacitation

- It is a period of ***conditioning of sperms in female reproductive tract particularly in isthmus of uterine tubes***[Q]
- It normally requires *1- 10 hours* and l/t some changes that are
1. Uterine & fallopian tube fluids *wash away the inhibitory factors* that suppress sperm activity in male genital ducts
2. Sperm *gradually lose much of their excess cholesterol* that has been continually added to the cell membrane covering the sperm acrosome, toughening this membrane & preventing release of its enzymes. So loss of cholesterol weakens the membrane at the head of sperm.
3. *Increased entery of Ca^{++}* ions d/t increased membrane permeability, changes the activity of flagellum, giving it a powerful **whiplash movements** in contrast to its previously weak undulating motions.
4. Ca^{++} ions change acrosomal cell membrane, so that it can release its enzyme rapidly & easily during acrosomal reaction.

Acrosome Reaction

- When ovum is released , it still carries with it multiple layer of granulose cells. Before a sperm can fertilize the ovum, it must dissolute *the granulose cell layer* and thick covering of ovum *zone pellucida.*
- *Hyaluronidase* stored in acrosome of sperm depolymerizes the hyaluronic acid polymers in intercellular cement that hold ovarian granulose cell together.
- When sperm reaches zona pellucida, its anterior membrane binds with receptor proteins and then rapidly the entire acrosome dissolves releasing all the acrosomal enzymes. Within minutes, these enzymes open a penetrating pathway through zona pellucida to inside the ovum

Hormones Stimulating Spermatogenesis

Testosterone (Androgen)

- Secreted by *Leydig cells* located in interstitiumof testis is essential for *growth & division of testicular germinal cells*, which is the first stage in forming sperm
- The stages from *spermatogonia to spermatids* appear to be androgen dependent
- *Maturation of spermatids to spermatozoa* depends on angrogen acting on sertoli cells in which the developing spermatozoa are embedded.

Follicle stimulating Hormone (FSH)

- Secreted by anterior pituitary gland and acts on sertoli cells to facilitate the *last stages of spermatid maturation* i.e. the conversion of spermatids to sperm (the process *of spermiognesis*)
- Promotes the *production of androgen binding protein (ABP)*

FSH & androgens maintain the *gametogenic function of testis*

Estrogens

- Formed from *testosterone* by sertoli cells when they are stimulated by FSH
- Is probably essential for spermiogenesis
- Estrogen content of fluid in *rete testis* is high & the walls of rete contain numerous ER α esterogen receptors, In this region, fluid is reabsorbed & spermatozoa are concentrated. If this does not occur, the sperm entering the epididymis are diluted in large volume of fluid, & infertility results.

Leuteinizing Hormone (LH)

- Secreted by anterior pituitary gland & stimulates leydig cells to secrete *testosterone*
- After hypophysectomy, injection of LH produces a high local concentration of angdrogen in testes, & this maintains spermatogenesis.

Growth Hormone (GH)

- Promotes early division of spermatogonia
- In its absence, as in pituitary dwarts, spermatogenesis is severely deficient or absent, thus causing infertility.

Testosterone & Male Sterility

- The fact that **intratesticular levels of testosterone** need to be greater than **100 folds higher than circulating** levels of hormone **to maintain normal** rates of **spermatogenesis**; however, it is the circulating levels of testosterone that provide the negative feedback to pituitary & hypothalamus is an important loophole in male reproductive axis.
- This means that **exogenous testosterone** (T) administration can raise circulating levels of T. sufficient to **inhibit LH** but not sufficient to accumulate in testis at required concentration for normal spermatogenesis. However, decreased LH levels will further **diminish intratesticular production of testosterone** by Leydig cells resulting in **reduced spermatogenesis**.
- This is the cause for **sterility in** cases of prolonged ***testosterone administration or steroid abuse in men***[Q]. And this loophole is recently being researched as a possible strategy for developing **male oral contraceptives**.

Contraction Stress Test (or Oxytocin Challenge Test)

It is an *invasive method* to assess fetal well being during pregnancy, when there is alteration in FHR in response to uterine contraction. It *suggests fetal hypoxia.*

❑ Procedure

Oxytocin is infused and the alteration in FHR during uterine contraction are noted.

❑ Interpretation

*Positive*Q - ***Persistent late deceleration of FHR***Q
- It is associated with ↑ed incidence of IUD, fetal distress & low Apgar score.

*Negative*Q - No late deceleration or significant variable deceleration
- associated with good fetal outcome.

Indication
- **IUGR**Q
- **Postmaturity**Q
- **Hypertensive disorder of pregnancy**Q
- **Diabetes**Q

Contraindication
- **Compromised fetus**Q
- Previous history of **caesarean section**Q
- **Complication likely to produce preterm labour**Q.
- **APH**Q

Congenital Adrenal Hyperplasia

Types	Main function of enzyme	Mineralo cortcoid (M)	Gluco corticoid (G)	Androgen	Features
21- OH-deficiency	Glucocorticoid & Mineralocorticoid production	↓	↓↓	↑	• **Hypotension**Q (salt losing virilization) • **Virilization**Q in females • **Precocious puberty in females**Q.
11 hydroxylase-deficiency	Glucocorticoid production	↑	↓↓	↑	• **Hypertension**Q • **Virilization**Q in females • **Precocious puberty in females**Q.
17-hydroxylase deficiency	Glucocorticoid & Androgen production	↑	↓	↓↓	• **Male hermaphrodite**Q • **Primary amenorrhea in females**Q. • **Hypertension**Q
3 - β-hydroxylase deficiency	Mineralcorticoid & glucocorticoid production.	↓	↓	↑	• Male hermaphrodite.

Summary

Hypertension (is seen in)
- 17 hydroxylase deficiency
- 11 Hydroxylase deficiency

Male Pseudohermaphroditism (present in)
- 17 hydroxylase deficiency
- 3 – hydroxylase deficiency

Female Pseudohermaphroditism (present in)
- 21 hydroxylase deficiency
- 11 hydroxylase deficiency

Amniotic Fluid: Composition & Volume

- **Liquor amnii** is derived from *filtration (from maternal vessels) across amniotic membrane* (most important in early stages so AF resembles blood plasma), filtration from *fetal vessels via umbilical cord*, secretion from amniotic epithetiun, *fetal urine & fetal lung secretions*
- Anount of AF increases *upto 6-7 months* and then diminishes slightly to become <1 lit at the end of pregnancy. Deficiency of AF is **oligohydroamnios** and usually result from premature rupture of membrane, uteroplacental insufficiency or urinary track malformations like renal agenesis. Absent AF is **ahydroamnios.** Oligohydroamnios at < 20 weeks may cause **pulmonary hypoplasia.**
- **Polyhydroamnios** is > 2 lit AF. It may occur d/t reduced fetal swallowing (owing to anencephaly, **oesophegeal / upper gi atresia**, compression d/t cong. diaphragmatic hernia) or decreased AF absorption and **increased fetal urination.**

Water = 98-99%
Solid = 1-2%
- Organic solids include lipids (50mg%), NPN (30mg%), **glucose** (20mg%), uric acid (4mg%), protein (0.3 mg%), hormones (eg prolactin, insulin & renin), IGF-BP1, fibronectin and urea.
- Inorganic solids like Na^+, Cl^- and K^+.

Placentral Hormones and Pregnancy

- Endocrine function begins with the onset of implantation, when syncytiotrophoblasts start secreting the LH like protein **hCG (human chorionic gonadotropin),** which *prevents luteolysis* (i.e. maintains the viability of corpus luteum) and thus maintains a high level of luteal derived progesterone production during the *first 10 weeks*. By this time (8-10 weeks), the syncytiotropholasts aquire the ability to make progesterone at sufficient levels to maintain pregnancy independently of corpus luteum (- referred to as **luteal – placental shift**).
- hCG has a α glycoprotein subunit (α-GSU) and a hormone specific β-sub unit (β-hCG). Antibody used to detect hCG in pregnancy tests and laboratory assay ***detect the β subunit***Q. Being similar to LH, hCG binds with high affinity to LH receptors. But the β subunit of hCG is longer than that of LH & contains more sites for glycosylation, which greatly increase the stability ($t_{1/2}$ = 24-30 hours) allowing it to rapidly accumulate in maternal circulation such that the hCG is **detectable within maternal serum within 24 hours of implantation.**
- Maternal serum hCG level doubles every 2 days for first 6 weeks & peak at about 10 weeks, then decline to a constant level at about 50% of the peak value. This ***rapid increase is responsible for the nausea of morning sickness***Q a/w early pregnancy.
- Small (1-10%) amount of hCG enters fetal circulation and *stimulate fetal leydig cells* (to produce testosterone before fetal gonadotropic axis is fully mature) and *fetal adrenal cortex*.
- **Human placental lactogen (hPL)** also k/a **human chorionic somato mammotrophin (hCS)** is a protein hormone (structurally similar to GH and prolactin /PRL) that is produced in syncytiotrophoblast. It can be detected within syncytiotrophoblast by 10 days after conception & in maternal serum by 3 weeks of gestation. Maternal level rises progressively during gestation (related to size of placenta). It is protein anabolic & lipolytic (like GH) and stimulates mammary gland growth & development (like PRL). Its antagonistic action to insulin is the major basis for **diabetogenicity (insulin resistant state** or accelerated starvation) of pregnancy. Mammary gland development in pregnancy results from action of hPL, PRL, estrogen & progestins. Both hPL & PRL act as fetal GHs & stimulate production of fetal growth promoting hormones insulin like growth factors (IGF) I & II.
- Placenta (syncytiotrophoblast) also produce progesterone, estrogen and corticotropin releasing hormone (CRH). Progestore production by placenta is largely unregulated (i.e. produces as much as the supply of cholesterol & levels of CYP 11 A1 & 3β-HSD allow). Placental steroidogenesis differes from that in adrenal, cortex , ovaries & testis in that cholesterol is transported into the placental mitochondria by mechanism that is **independent of St AR protein**. This first step of steroidogenesis is not regulated, rate limiting step in placenta as it is in other steroidogenic glands. So fetus with inactivating mutation in StAR protein will develop hypogonadism, lipoid congenital adrenal hyperplasia but will produce normal progesterone levels by their placenta. ***Progesterone production by placenta does not require fetal tissue and are largely independent of fetal health***Q ***(i.e. cannot be used as a measure of feta health)***Q.

Nitric Oxide (NO) / Endothelium Derived Relaxing Factor (EDRF)

Synthesis and Metabolism

- Nitric oxide (NO) is synthesized from **L-arginine**[Q] in a reaction ***catabolized by cytosolic enzyme nitric oxide synthase (NOS)***[Q]. Details of the reaction are as following.

Substrates	Coenzymes	Enzyme	Mechanism	Products
L-Arginine[Q] Oxygen (O_2) **NADPH**	**FMN** **FAD** **Thiol** (Ganong) **BH_4 (tetra hydro biopterin)** **NADPH,Heme (Lippincot).**	Cytosolic NOS **(e/n/i) isoform.**	**5e- oxidation of amide nitrogen of arginine**	**Citrulline** **NO**

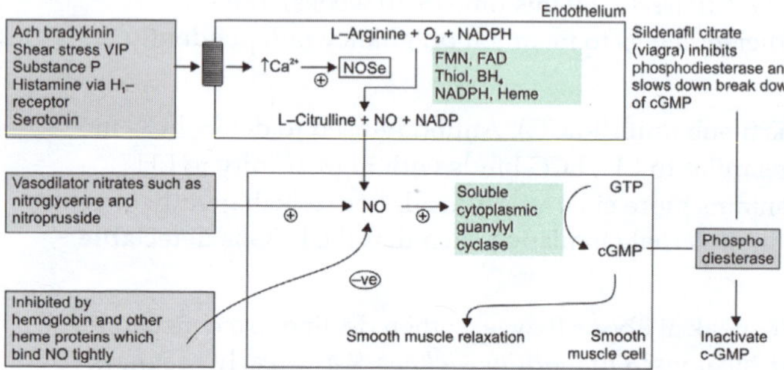

- NO is inhibited by hemoglobin and other heme proteins, which bind it tightly
- NO has **very short half life** ($t_{1/2}$) in tissues **(3-10 seconds)** because it reacts with oxygen and superoxide and then converted into nitrates and nitrites including **peroxynitrite ($ONOO^-$)**, a reactive nitrogen species (RNS), which decomposes to form **highly reactive OH• radical**.

- 3- isoforms or subtypes of NOS are

NOS-Subtype	Found in	Activated by	Feature	Result of gene Knock out in Mice
NOS-1 = n-NOS (Constitutive calcium dependent, neuronal-NOS)	***Nervous (neural) tissue***	**↑ed (increased) intracellular calcium** concentration activate NOS n & e. So vasodilator agents like *acetyl choline (ACh), bradykinin, Shear stress, VIP, substance P and histamine via H_1 receptors* which act via endothelium activate NOS by ↑ calcium	Ca^{2+}-calmodulin dependent, **constitutive enzyme** (i.e *synthesized at a constant rate* regardless of demand). NOS- n & e *constantly prodce low levels of NO.*	**Pyloric stenosis,** resistance to vascular stroke, aggressive sexual behaviour (males) indicating its role in **smooth muscle relaxation.**
NOS-3 = e-NOS (Constitutive, calcium dependent, **endothelial** NOS)	**Endothelial cells**			**Elevated mean blood pressure** (hypertension) indicating its role in maintaining normal BP in vivo.
NOS-2 = i-NOS (Inducible, calcium independent, immune NOS)	**Immune cells** including **macrophage, monocytes, neutrophils & hepatocytes**	Not activated by Ca^{2+} (i.e. calcium independent enzyme) but is induced by inflammatory cytokines, tumor necrosis factor α- (TNFα), *γ-interferon, bacterial lipopolysaccharide and bacterial endotoxins* (inducer vary with cell type). **Induction results in large amount of NO** being produced over hours or days.		More susceptible to certain types of **infection.**

Functions

- **Smooth Muscle relaxation (of vessels & gi tract mainly).**

- NO synthesized by e NOS in endothelial cells, diffuses to **vascular smooth muscle** and activate cytosolic guanylate (guanylyl) cyclase (catalytic action), resulting in rise of c-GMP levels. Cyclic GMP activates protein kinase G, which phosphorylates Ca^{++} channels, causing decreased enetry of Ca2+ into smooth muscle cells. This decreases the calcium – calmodulin activation of myosin – light chain kinase, thereby decreasing smooth muscle contraction and favouring **relaxation.**
- **Acetyl choline (Ach), bradykinin, vasoactive intestinal peptide (VIP), substance P, serotonin, histamine** via **H_1** receptors and **shear stress** (d/t rapid blood flow in arteries & arterioles) act indirectly via endothelium cells to produce endothelium derived relaxing factor (EDRF) or NO (by increasing Ca^{++} concentration) and causing vasodilation. That is why vasodilation caused by Ach etc can be abolished if endothelium cells are stripped from underlying smooth muscle. However, **adenosine, atrial natriuretic peptide (ANP), and histamine via H2 receptors** produce relaxation of vascular smooth muscle that is independent of endothelium.
- When flow to a tissue is suddenly increased by small arteries and arteriolar dilation (d/t local mechanism like O_2 deficiency),

the large arteries to tissue also dilate d/t **shear stress** or **viscous drag** of blood against the vascular walls of arterioles relasing NO.

- Vasodilator nitrates like **nitroglycerine** & **nitroprusside are metabolized** to produce **NO (endogenous nitrovasodilator)**, causing vascular smooth muscle relaxation and lowering BP.
- **Resistance vessels (small arteries & arterioles)** are in continous state of No mediated vasodilation. NO also controls resting vasodilator tone of in central veins but not in peripheral veins.
- Inhibitors of NO synthase l/t vasoconstriction and elevation of BP, indicating its importance in maintaining BP in vivo.
- Inhibitors of NO synthase l/t vasoconstriction and elevation of BP, indicating its importance in maintaining BP in vivo.
- Release of NO with consequent vasodilation and engorgement of corpora cavernosa l/t **penile erection**. This accounts for efficacy of **sildenafl citrate (viagra)** which slows the break down of cGMP by inhibiting phosphodiesterase (used for erectile dysfunction)
- **NO, VIP, PACAP and ATP** are inhibitory neurotransmitters of enteric motor neurons that mediate **gastrointestinal smooth muscle relaxation**. Low level of NO is involved in causation of ***pylorospasm in infantile hypertrophic pyloric stenosis***[Q].

• **Inhibits adhesion, activation and aggregation of platelets**

- Products of platelet aggregation cause NO release and resulting vasodilation keeps blood vessels with intact endothelium patent. Whereas endothelial damage produces vasoconstricton and platelet aggregation.
- NO is involved in vascular remodeling, angiogenesis and pathogenesis of atherosclerosis. It is seen that some patients of heart transplant develop an acclerated form of atherosclerosis in the vessels o transplant.

• Constitute part of **primitive immune system** by mediating **macrophage bactericidal activity**

- Induced by inflammatory mediators i-NOS produce NO in large amounts which decomposes to, **highly bactericidal $OH^{\bullet}$ radical**.
- Mediates tumoricidal & cytotoxic actions

• **Gaseous neurotransmitter in brain & peripheral autonomic system.**

- NO is produced by nerve terminals in granular cell layer of cerebellum and hippocampus and seem to be involved in long term behaviour and potentiation of memory.
- Gaseous neurotransmitter NO differs from other small molecule transmitters in that it is *neither preformed & packaged /stored into synaptic vesicles in pre synaptic terminals nor released by exocytosis*. Instead, it is *synthesized almost instantly as needed*, is **highly permeant** & simply diffuses out of presynaptic terminals to neighbouring cells (eg post synaptic neurons) over period of secons. Their synthesis is triggered by depolarization of nerve terminal (Ca^{++} influx).
- There are *no specific reuptake mechanisms nor do they undergo enzymatic destruction*, so their action appears to be ended by diffusion or binding to superoxide anions or scavenger proteins,
- NO usually does not alter greatly membrane potential but instead changes intracellular metabolic functions that modify neuronal excitability for seconds/minutes / or longer in post synaptic neuron.
- NO is a neurotransmitter at synapse b/w **inhibitory motor neurons of enteric nervous system and gastrointestinal smooth muscle cells** – causing ***smooth muscle relaxation in gitract***[Q].
- NO has role in **neurotoxicity**.

• **May have role in skeletal muscle relaxation**

Chapter 8. GENERAL PHYSIOLOGY: REVIEW NOTES

Resting Energy Expenditure (REE) or Resting Metabolic Rate (RMR)

- It is amount of energy required to maintain essential physiological functions of body to maintain life.
- REE is energy expanded by body *during resting state without fasting*, whereas, BMR is the energy expanded *during resting & fasting state*
- So REE is *slightly higher than BMR* but the factors that influence REE are *essentially the same factors* that influence the BMR.

REE = BMR + Energy used in digestion of food

- Recently ingested food increase the metabolic rate because of their **specific dynamic action (SDA).** The SDA of a food is the obligatory energy expenditure that occurs during its assimilation into the body as a result of different chemical reactions associated with digestion, absorption & storage of food in body. This is called **thermogenic effect of food** because these processes require energy & generate heat. It accounts for **8%** of total daily energy SDA is *5% fat, 6% for carbohydrate and 30% for proteins* (i.e. it takes 30 K cal to assimilate amount of protein sufficient to raise metabolic rate 100 K cal.
- **The primary factor affecting REE & BMR** is ***fat free lean body mass***Q (i.e. metabolically active muscle & internal organs). Fat (adipose tissue) is metabolically inert & does not contribute to BMR or REE. **Body surface area** is a reasonable determinant of lean body mass.
- In determining metabolic rate, O_2 consumption is measured & then converted to energy production by multiplying *4.82 Kcal/ L of O_2 consumed.*

Basal Metabolic Rate (BMR) 

- The metabolic rate determined at rest, at least 12 hours after the last meal after a night of restful sleep, at an ambient temperature of about 25°C (68°-80°F) and the subject is free from any illness (physical or psychic factors that cause excitement). It represents the energy required for normal body function. No sternous activity is performed for at least 1 hour before test & no physical activity is permitted during the test. BMR is expressed as ***K cal energy consumed per m^2 body surface area per hour***Q. ***BMR is directly proportional to total body surface area***Q:
- From 50% to 70% of daily energy expenditure in sedentary individual is attributable to BMR until very old age. **Factor affecting BMR**

- **Primary factor** affecting (and most closely related to) BMR & REE is **lean (fat-free) body mass**, which gives an estimate of *metabolically active tissue* (i.e. muscle & internal organ). **Body surface area** is a reasonable determinant of lean body mass. **Katch – Mc Ardle formula** is used to calculate BMR is

BMR = 370 + (21.6 X Lean body mass in kg)

- Other factors affecting BMR & REE are

Factor	Increasing (↑) BMR & REE	Decreasing (↓) BMR & REE
Age	**Early age** (i.e. neonates & children)	Most of the decline in BMR with **increasing age** (i.e. adults & old age) is related to replacement of metabolically active muscle mass with adipose tissue, which has a lower rate of metabolism.
Sex	**Males**	**Females** (b/o lower percentage of mucscle mass & higher percentage of adipose tissue).
Growth	**Pregnancy, lactation, growing age** & reproduction.	
Feeding	Recent **ingestion of food** esp diet containing proteins.	***Fasting, starvation, malnutrition (↓upto 40% during prolonged starvation)***Q
Environmental temperature	Cold or very hot (uncomfortable) temperature. Curve relating BMR to temperature i.e. **'U' shaped** i.e. BMR rises when environmental temperature is both below or higher (above) body temperature	Hot comfortable climate
Body temperature	**Fever** raises BMR (**14%** for each degree celsium clevation).	
Hormones	**Thyroxine** (key regulator), catecholamines (epinephrine & norepinephrine), Growth hormone, male sex hormones. Eg ***hyper thyroidism or thyrotoxicosis***Q.	
Others	Smoking, Caffeine, **muscular exercise (exertion)** during or just before measurement, emotiona hyperactivity & stress.	Sleep (falls ~ 10%), ***Obesity***Q (d/t high fat / muscle ratio). **Skeletal muscles** even under resting conditions, account for 20-30% of BMR
Height, weight, BMI	Tall thin	Short obese
	Body surface area (BSA) can be similar in both but BMR differs. **BMR has highest correlation with lean body mass (LBM) > Body mass > BSA > Body weight > BMI > Height** (r is 0.95, 0.85, 0.84, 0.80, 0.64 & 0.57 respectively) BMR = 3.52 $W^{0.75}$ is higher than it would be if it was due solely to body area that is BMR = 3.5 $W^{0.67}$	

Age Related Physiological Changes

1. General 2. Respiratory 3. CVS	Proportion of body fat increases ***Compliance decreases***[Q] ***BP increases***[Q] as arterial elasticity decreases.
4. Endocrine	- ***Glucose tolerance decreases***[Q] - *ADH secretion increases*
5. GIT	- ***Gastric acidity decreases***[Q] - ***Colonic motility decreases***[Q] - Increased chances of constipation

6. Hematological	- T- lymphocyte function deteriorates - Immune mechanism deteriorates
7. Renal	- ***GFR decreases***[Q] - ***Clearance decreases***
8. Genital	- ***Prostate enlargement***[Q] - ***Vaginal mucosal atrophy***[Q]
9. Bone 10. Brain	***Osteoporosis***[Q] (particularly in females) Brain atrophy leading to amnesia

Exercise

Muscle blood flow

- ***Sometimes increases at or even before the start of exercise probably d/t neurally mediated sympathetic vasodilation***[Q].
- When a muscle contracts, if it develops >10% of its maximal tension, the blood *vessels in it are compressed*. And if tension *>70% blood flow is completely stoped*. However, b/w contractions blood flow is increased as much as *30 folds*
- Once exercise has started local mechanism maintaining high blood flow include ***fall in tissue PO_2, and a rise in tissue PCO_2, temperature & K^{+}***[Q]
- K^+ depleted individuals show a lesser increase in flow during early phase of exercise and a greater tendency of ***exertional disintegration (rhabdomyolysis) of muscles***[Q].
- Dilation of arteriole cause *increase in number of open capillaries, & increased cross sectional area* of vascular bed but the flow *velocity & overage distance between blood and active cells (i.e., the distance O_2 & metabolites must diffuse) is greatly reduced*.
- ***O_2 dissociation curve shifts to the right***[Q] d/t ↑ temperature & ↓ pH, so that more O_2 is given up by blood. ***2-3 DPG in RBC is***

Circulatory changes

- *Heart rate rises* with just the thought of performing muscle contraction even if muscle contraction is prevented by local infusion of neuromuscular blocker) and is probably d/t *psychic stimulation of medulla oblongata.*
- Cardiovascular response depends on type of muscle contraction

Feature	Isometric	Isotonic
Heart rate	Increase (less)	Prompt increase
Cardiacout put	Increase (less)	Increase
Systolic BP **Diastolic BP**	Sharp rise in both	Rise moderately Unchanged or decrease
Stroke volume	Little change	Marked increase
Peripheral resistance	Increased d/t compression of blood vessels & reduced blood flow in contracting muscles	Decreases d/t vasodilation in exercising muscle.
Cardiac work load	More	Less

- *Maximum heart rate increase during exercise decreases with age.*
- Lymph flow and venous return is

Ventilation

- With the **onset** of exercise, ventilation ***increases abruptly followed after a brief pause by a gradual increase***[Q]. When exercise ceases, it decreases abruptly followed after a brief pause by a gradual decline. With *moderate* exercise the *depth of respiration* is mostly increased, which is accompanied by an increase in *respiratory* rate when the exercise is more *strenuous*

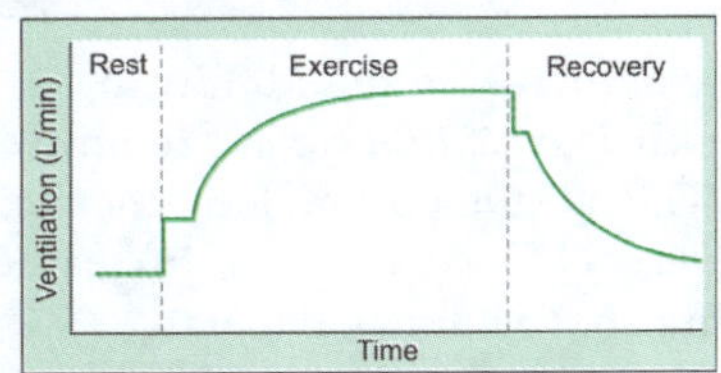

- **Abrupt increase** ***at start is d/t psychic stumuli & afferent impulses from proprioceptors in muscles, tendons, & joints***[Q].
- **Gradual increase** is humoral even though ***arterial PCO_2, PO_2 and pH remain constant during moderate exercise***[Q]. ***Increase body temperature, ↑ ed plasma K^+ levels, increased neuronal sensitivity to CO_2***[Q] (that detect fluctuations) and probably O_2 may play role.
- **Gradual decrease** after exercise does not reach basal levels until O_2 debt is repaid. And the stimulus to ventilation is *elevated arterial H^+ concentration* d/t lactic acidemia. (It is neither arterial PCO_2 which is normal or low, or arterial PO_2 which is normal or high).
- In vigorous exercise, more *lactic acid* is produced causing *metabolic acidosis*,

Temperature

- ***Body temperature rises***[Q] & hypothalmic centers that control heat dissipating mechanism are activated
- *Increased sweat production* & its vaporization is the major path for heat loss
- Some heat is radiated from skin and increased ventilation cause heat loss in expired air.

increased[Q] and this further decreases O_2 affinity of hemoglobin.

- ***Artero – venous O_2 difference, O_2 consumption, energy output is increased***[Q].

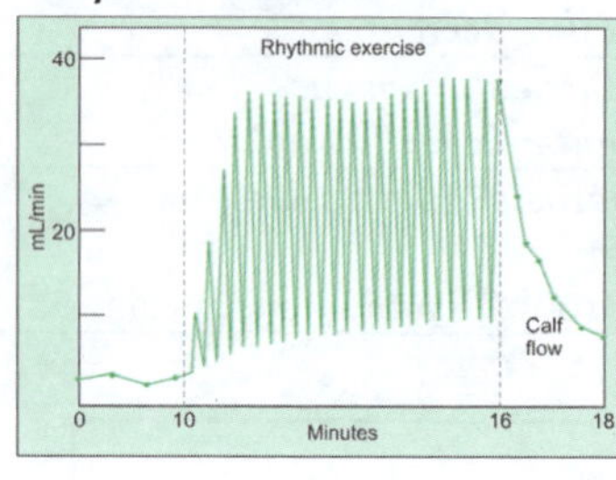

greatly increased

- After exercise *BP may transiently drop* to subnormal levels because accumulated metabolites keep vessels dilated for a short period. However, BP soon returns to normal pre exercise levels. *Heart rate returns to normal more slowly.*
- Cardiac output may exceed upto 35 L/min during isotonic exercise, which is proportional to O_2 consumption. And the *regional blood flow* is

which is buffered by *more production of CO_2 & hyperventilation*. Alveolar and arterial CO_2 change relatively little (**iso capnic buffering**) and *alveolar PO_2 increase.* With further lactic acidosis & hyper ventilation alveolar & arterial PCO_2 falls.

- The PO_2 of blood flowing into pulmonary *capillary falls*, so that *alveolar – capillary PO_2 is increased* and more O_2 enters the blood. The amount of CO_2 removed from blood is increased.

Decreased in	Maintained in	Increased in
- Inactive skeletal muscle	- ***Brain***[Q] (750 ml/min)	- Active skeletal muscle
- Kidney	- Skin (500 ml/min)	- Heart (coronary blood flow)
- Liver		- Lung
- Gastrointestinal etc.		

Control of Blood Flow through Skeletal Muscles

The tremendous increase in muscle blood flow that occur during exercise (muscle activity) is ***caused primarily by local metabolites (chemical effects) acting directly on muscle arterioles to cause vasodilation***[Q]

- The main cause of **increased blood flow to exercising muscle** is ***vasodilation due to local metabolites***[Q]. The most important local chemical effect is *reduction of O_2 in muscle tissue.* **Increased arterial pressure** above normal, **β (beta) adrenergic receptor mediated vasodilation in exercising muscle** and **α (alpha) adrenergic receptor mediated vasoconstriction** in resting muscles are other factors responsible for increased blood supply in muscles during exercise.
- **Increased (not decreased) β_2 adrenergic stimulation** (in humans) and **cholinergic stimulation** (in some animals like dogs, cats) are responsible for **skeletal muscle vasodilation** whereas, **α_1 adrenergic** stimulation cause skeletal muscle **vasoconstriction.** Epinephrine excites more of β receptors (=vasodilation), whereas α vasoconstrictor receptors are excited especially by norepinephrine.

Primary Regulation: Local Metabolites (Chemical Effects)

Reduction of oxygen in muscle tissue is most important local chemical effect. O_2 deficiency causes release of **vasodilator substances** eg.

- Adenosine (most important but experiments have shown that it has decreased effect on vasodilation in exercising muscles)
- Potassium (K^+) ion
- Adenosine triphosphate (ATP)
- Lactic acid
- Carbon dioxide (CO_2)

Associated Regulatory Factor: Increased Sympathetic Tone

It is responsible for circulatory changes that support increased blood flow to muscle eg.

- ↑ Heart rate and BP
- Vasoconstriction of peripheral vessels (other than vessels in active muscle that are dilated d/t local metabolites)
- Venoconstriction of veins & capacitance vessels to increase filling pressure.

Physiological Changes in Exercise

- With the onset of exercise, there is an ***abrupt increase in ventilation***[Q]; followed after a brief pause by further more gradual increase. The increased stimulation is presumably due to *psychic stimuli* and ***afferent impulses from proprioceptors***[Q] in muscles, tendons and joints.
- During muscular exercise, increase in O_2 consumption is proportionate to the energy expended, and *all the energy needs are met by aerobic process.* With more muscular exertion, aerobic resynthesis of energy stores cannot keep pace with their utilization and *lactate is produced* (d/t *anerobic breakdown of glucose*):

- **With vigeourous exercise** buffering of increased amount of lactic acid, liberates CO_2 and this further increases ventilation. With further accumulation of lactic acid, the ↑in ventilation outstrip CO_2 production and **alveolar P_{CO2} falls as does arterial P_{CO2}**[Q]. The decline in P_{CO2} provides respiratory compensation for metabolic acidosis
- **Arterial pH and HCO_3^- decrease**[Q] with severe exercise due to lactic acidosis
- Strenuous exercise can cause **Hyperkalemia**[Q] by releasing K^+ from skeletal muscle.

Respiratory
- **↑ed O_2 uptake & Consumption**[Q]
- ↑ed ventilation
- ↑ ed alveolar – capillary PO_2 gradient
- **↑ ed CO_2 excretion**[Q]
- **↓ P_{aCO2}**[Q]
- **↑ P_{aO2}**[Q]
- **↓ ed pH, HCO_3^-**[Q]

CVS
- **HR↑ ed**[Q]
- **Stroke volume↑ ed**[Q]
- BP↑ ed
- Muscle blood flow –↑ed in isotonic exercise –↓ed in isometric exercise

Metaboic
- ↑ ed glucose uptake
- ↑ ed insulin sensitivity
- **↑ ed K^+**[Q]

During Exercise
- The contractile muscles **need more O_2**[Q] for energy production.
- This need is meet by increasing the blood supply to the muscles. Cardiac activity increases to **increase the stroke volume**[Q]. Capillary bed of the contracting muscle dilate and many previously closed capillaries open up.
- In contracting muscle the amount of O_2 extracted from blood increases **(3 fold increase in O_2 extraction from each unit of blood)**[Q]. This is because of right shift of Hb – O_2 dissociation curve.

Energy Sources & Metabolism During Muscle Contraction

Energy derived anaerobically in 100 meter race of (10s) is 85% whereas in long distance run (of 1 hour) is 5% only. After exercise, extra O_2 is consumed to remove the excess lactate, replenish **phosphocreatine and ATP stores** and replace O_2 that was released by myoglobin. This **O_2 debt** is measured by determining O_2 consumption after exercise until a conslant basal consumption is reached and substeracting the basal consumption from total. It may be 6 times of basal consumption. **At rest and during light exercise**, muscle utilizes lipids in the form of **free fatty acid**[Q] as their energy source. As **intensity of exercise increases carbohydrate**[Q] becomes the predominant component in muscle fuel mixture. There are three important metabolic system that supply energy for muscle contraction.

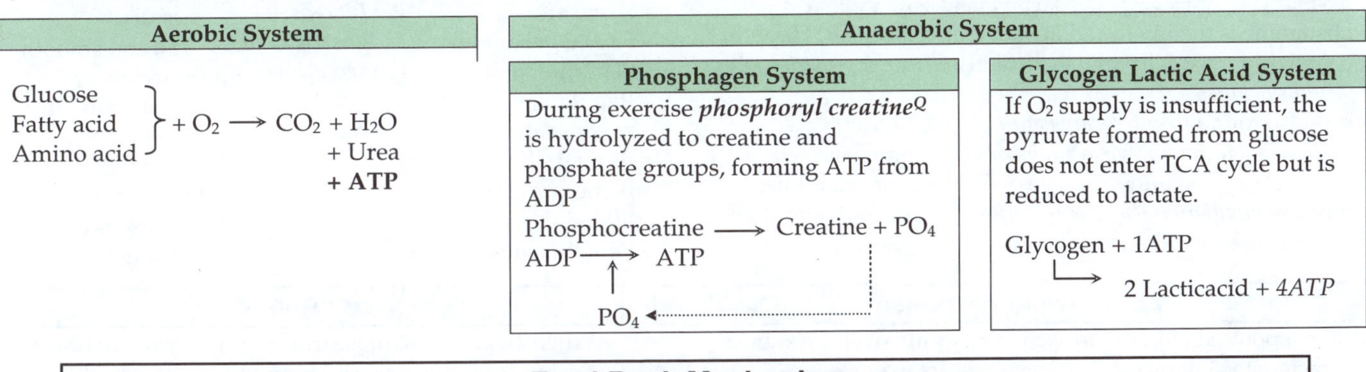

Feed Back Mechanism

There are 2 type of feedback mechanisms:

Positive feedback mechanism
- Better known as 'Vicious cycle'
- It is often of a milder degree & can therefore be overcome by stronger negative feed back control of the body and vicious cycle fails to develop.
- Examples are : [Mnemonic : **CLASP**]

C	- **Clotting blood**[Q] - **Ca^{2+} entry into sarcoplasmic reticulum**[Q]
L	- **LH surge during ovulation**[Q]
A	- **Action Potential**[Q]
S	- **Shock**[Q]
P	- **Parturition**[Q]

Negative feed back mechanism
- In this if some factor become excessive, a control system initates negative feedback, which consist of series of changes that return the factor towards a certain mean value.
- Examples are
  - **ACTH secretion**[Q]
  - Aldosterone – K^+ secretion
  - Glucose regulation
  - **GH secretion**[Q]
  - **BP regulation**[Q]

Haptoglobin

- It is a plasma glycoprotein that binds extracapsular hemoglobin (Hb) in a tight non-covalent complex. Its amount ranges from 40mg- 180 mg of hemoglobin binding capacity / deciliter.
- Only 10% of degraded hemoglobin is released in circulation (i.e. extra corpuscular) the remaining 90% is present in old damaged RBCs, which are degraded by histiocytic system.
- Free Hb (molecular mass 65KDa) passes through glomerulus and precipitate in tubules. However, after binding with haptoglobin (90 KDa) the Hb-Hp complex (155KDa) becomes too large to pass through glomerulus. So the function of haptoglobin is to prevent loss of free hemoglobin into kidney and conserve the valuable iron present in hemoglobin, which would otherwise be lost to the body.
- Humans have 3 polymorphic forms, k/a Hp 1-1, Hp 2-1, Hp 2-2. Low levels of haptoglobins are found in patients with **hemolytic anemia**. This is explained by the fact that where the life of Hp is 5 days, the t½ of Hb-Hp complex is 90 minutes, the complex being rapidly removed by **hepatocytes**. So when the hepatoglobin is bound to Hb, it is cleared from plasma about 80 times faster than normally.
- Hb is an acute phase protein & is elevated in variety of inflammatory states.

★ **Haptoglobin related protein** binds hemoglobin; **hemopexin** binds free heme; and **albumin** binds metheme (ferric heme)

Histamine

Synthesis & Catabolism

- Histamine is formed by decarboxylation of aminoacid histidine.

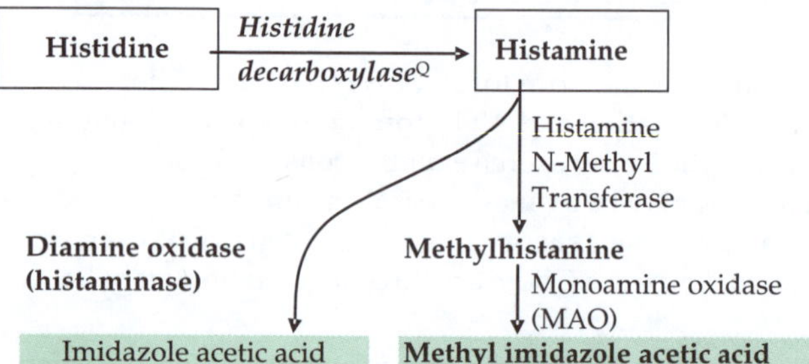

- Histamine is mainly found in *mast cells* & *basophils*. Heparin containing mast cells are plentiful in *anterior & posterior lobes of pituitary glands.*
- It is also found in *enterochromaffin like (ECL) cells of gastric mucosa and histaminergic neurons* of brain (non mast cell histamine). Histaminergic neurons have their cell bodies in *tuberomammillary nucleus of posterior hypothalamus*, and their axons project in all parts of brain.

Receptors and Functions

- It has three types of receptor – H1, H2 and H3. The H1 receptor activate phospholipase C, & H2 receptors increase intracellular C-AMP. Most, if not all of the H3 receptors are presynaptic and they mediate inhibition of release of histamine & other neurotransmitter via G protein
- Its major actions are

CNS

- ***Arousal***[Q]
- Sexual behaviour
- Sensation of itch
- Regulation of secretion of some anterior pituitary hormone
- Blood pressure
- Drinking
- Pain threshold

Gastric mucosa

Increased gastric acid secretion[Q] (via H2 receptor)

- **Marked vasodilation** of small blood vessels
- **Visceral smooth muscle constriction** in airway, (broncho-constriction) uterus and intestine

Lewis Triple Response

When a pointed object is stroked very firmly over the skin, a characteristic 3 part response develops. Its features are-

1. ***Red reaction (red line)***[Q] is due to transient ***capillary engorgement (vasodilation) caused by histamine***[Q] released from damaged tissue. Histamine relaxes precapillary sphincter thus l/t capillary dilation.
2. ***Flush or flare***[Q] is spreading of redness beyond the injury (red line). It is ***due to arteriolar dilation mediated by axon reflex***[Q] (may be a indirect effect of histamine)
3. ***Wheal***[Q] is local edema and elevation of skin due to ***increased permeability of capillaries & post capillary venules with consequent extravasation of fluid***[Q]. Capillary permeability is increased due to *histamine* & other mediators.

- ***Triple response is present after total sympathectomy***[Q]. The *flare is absent in locally anesthetized or denervated skin* after sensory nerves have degenerated; but it is present immediately after nerve block or section above the site of injury.

Axon Reflex

- When an area of skin is stroked, sensory nerve fibres arising from the area are stimulated and carry the impulse to respective spinal cord segment as usual. However durig this journey a branch of this nerve gets activated and the impulse returns back to cutaneous arteriole (without reaching the spinal cord) *causing this arteriole to dilate*. This is one of the few reflex in out body which *does not involve CNS*.
- So it is a response in which impulses initiated in sensory nerves by the injury are, conducted antidromically down other branches of sensory nerve fibers.
- **Substance P** is the transmitter released at central termination of sensory C fiber neurons. And *substance P & CGRP* are present in all parts of neuron. Both *dilate arteriole* (produce *flare*) and substance P causes *extravasation of fluid* (wheal) also.

Kinin System

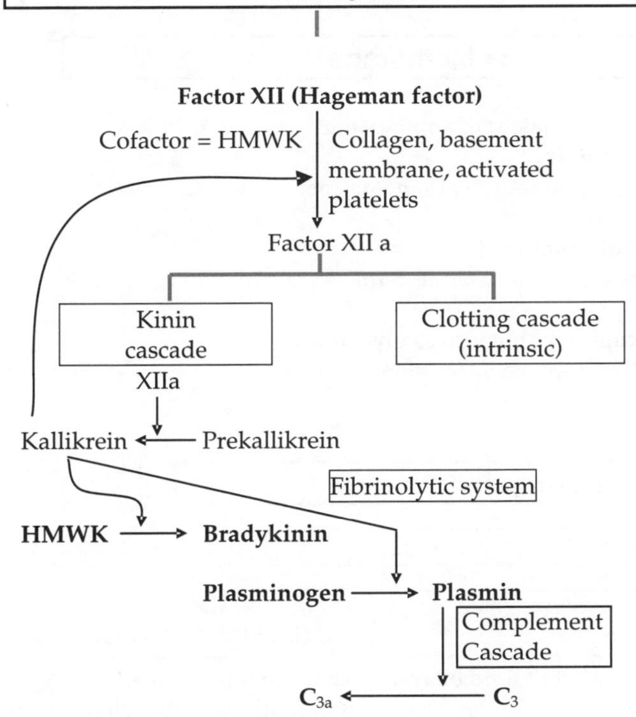

Factor XII (Hageman factor)

Cofactor = HMWK → Collagen, basement membrane, activated platelets

Factor XII a

- Kinin cascade
- Clotting cascade (intrinsic)

XIIa

Kallikrein ← Prekallikrein

Fibrinolytic system

HMWK → **Bradykinin**

Plasminogen → **Plasmin**

Complement Cascade

C_{3a} ← C_3

Roles of Inflammatory Mediators

Vasodilation **Mn-"No pH"**	- NO (nitric oxide) - Prostaglandins E1, E2, D2, I2 - Histamine
Vascular leakage (increased permeability) Mn-**"in, ine & ene + P"**	- Vasoactive amines (histamine, serotonin) - Bradykinin - Araphylatoxins (C3a & C5a) through liberating amines - Leukotrienes C4, D4, E4 - Substance **P** - PAF
Chemotaxis, leukocyte recruitment & activation	- C5a - Leukotrienes B4 - Chemokines - IL-1, TNF - Bacterial products - HETE, lipoxins
Fever	- IL-1, TNF - Prostaglandins
Pain	- Prostaglandins - Bradykinin
Tissue damage	- Neutrophil & macrophage lysosomal enzymes - NO - Oxygen metabolites
Vasoconstriction	- Thromboxane - Leukotrienes C4, D4, E4

Chapter 9. CELL PHYSIOLOGY: REVIEW NOTES

Composition of Cell Membrane / Plasma Membrane

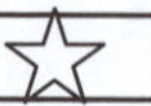

- Cell membrane is **composed of proteins > lipids > carbohydrate**Q. It has 3 classes of amphipathic lipids: **phospholipids > cholesterol (steroid or sterol) > glycol (sphingo) lipid**Q.
- Major membrane **phospholipids** are: **lecithin (phasphatidylcholine), phosphatidyl ethanolamine, phosphatidyl inositol, phosphatidyl serine and sphingomyelin**Q.
- **Glycolipids** include **cerebrosides** (galactosyl & glucosyl ceramide) and **ganglioside**.
- **Oleic acid** is most abundant unsaturated fatty acid. **Triglycerides are absent**Q and **cholesterol** confers a stiffening & strengthening effect.
- Carbohydrate in plasma membrane is predominantly present as **glycoprotein** but also as **glycolipids** in small amount. These oligosacchrides give cell an **identity** (and so are responsible for blood groups & transplant rejection).

Function of Cell Membrane Components

Phospholipid

Along with cholesterol	Membrane Lipid Rafts	Caveolae (Lipid raft + Caveolin-1)
Maintains fluidity of membraneQ As membrane fluidity increases, its permeability to water & small hydrophilic molecule increases.	- Are **speciatized dynamic areas of exoplasmic (outer) leaflet** of lipid bilayer **enriched in cholesterol, sphingolipids (sphingomyelin), glycosphingolipids (ganglioside, GM_1), saturated phospholipid** and certain integral proteins like **GPI (glycosylphosphatidyl inositol) anchored proteins** (in outer leaflet) and **acylated/prenylated proteins** (inner leaflet). - Membrane lipid raft microdomains are some what thicker, more ordered & tightly packed than the remainder of bilayer membrane but float freely in the membrane. **Lipid rafts contain 3 to 5 times more cholesterol and 50% more sphingolipids** compared to surrounding plasma membrane - They compartmentalize (or cluster) certain components of **signal transduction** and other cellular processes by serving as **organizing centers**; close clustering may increase the efficiency. They also influence membrane fluidity, protein trafficking, receptor trafficking, neurotransmission, G protein signaling, endocytosis & binding of viral pathogens. Defective GPI anchors cause paroxysmal nocturnal hemoglobinuria (PNH).	- They are **flask shaped indentations** of the cell membrane **facing the cytosol** in the region of **lipid raft**. Mostly **caveolin-1** protein is involved in their formation form lipid raft. - Proteins detected in coveolae form various component of signal transduction system eg **insulin receptor**, & some G proteins, **folate receptor**, endothelial nitric oxide synthase **(eNOS).** - Caveolin protein is a dimer; each monomer is anchored to the inner leaflet of plasma membrane by 3 palmitoyl molecules. - Caveolae mediates transcytosis of macromolecules (IgA) from luminal side, **endocytosis** of cholesterol containing lipoproteins and fusion & budding of viral particles.

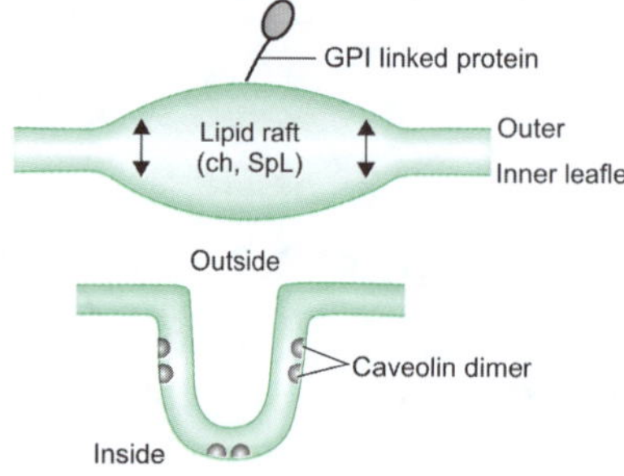

Protein

Every membrane possesses a different complement of protein. [Cell to cell variation of membrane protein]

Integral/Transmembrane Proteins

- They interact with the phospholipids and require the use of detergents for their solubilization.
- ***generally span the lipid bilayer***[Q]
- ***distributed asymmetrically across the lipid bilayer***[Q]
- ***are usually globular proteins*** [Q]
- they are amphipathic in nature
- Integral proteins are amphipathic in nature and contain both hydrophobic and hydrophilic regions.
- ***Hydrophillic regions are located at the ends while the transmembrane region i.e. the region that traverses the core of the bilayer is composed of a stretch of hydrophobic amino acids.***[Q]
- Integral protein are in **Vander Walls** contact with hydrophobic region of membrane.

Peripheral (Extrinsic) Proteins

- Peripheral proteins present embedded in either the inner or outer leaflet of the lipid bilayer.
- They do not interact directly with the phospholipids in the bilayer and do not require use of detergents for their release
- They are weakly bound to the hydrophilic region of specific integral proteins ***by ionic interaction or hydrogen bonds.***[Q]

Lipid Content Of Membranes

Phospholipid	Glycosphingolipid	Sterols
- **Phosphoglycerides** are more common and consist of *glycerol + fatty acid* (usually even numbered mostly 16, 18 – are unbranched. & canbe saturated or unsaturated) + *phosphate* (phosphoric acid) + nitrogenous or nonnitrogenous base (choline, ethanolamine, serine & inositol) - **Sphingomyelin** : glycerol is replaced by sphingsine.	Are ***sugar containing lipid***[Q] built on a back bone of ceramide. They include ***galactosyl – and glucosyl ceramide (cerebrosides) and ganglosides***[Q]	Mainly cholesterol

Fluidity of Membranes & Transition Temperature (Tm)

The ***fluidity of membranes****, are highly dependant upon the* ***lipid composition of the membrane****. In a lipid bilayer, the* **hydrophobic chains of the fatty acids can be highly aligned or ordered** *to provide a rather* **stiff structure**. *As the temperature increases, the hydrophobic side chains undergo a transition from the ordered state (more gel-like or crystalline phase) to a disordered one, taking on a more liquid like or fluid arrangement. The temperature at which the structure undergoes the transition from ordered to disordered (i.e melts) is called the* ***transition temperature*** *(Tm).*

Higher values of Tm is caused by (i.e. *higher temperatures are required to increase the fluidity of membrane*)

Longer & more saturated Fatty acid chains[Q] (as these interact more strongly with each other via longer hydrocarbon chains. Saturated FAS have straight tail)

- **Unsaturated fatty acids**, which generally exist in Cis form in membrane, *make kinked tails*. As more kinks are inserted, the ***membrane becomes less tightly packed and therefore more fluid***[Q]
- Therefore UFA,s increase fluidity by decreasing the compactness of the side chain packing with out diminishing hydrophobicity
- The phospholipid of cell membrane generally contain at least one unsaturated fatty acid with at least one Cis double bond.

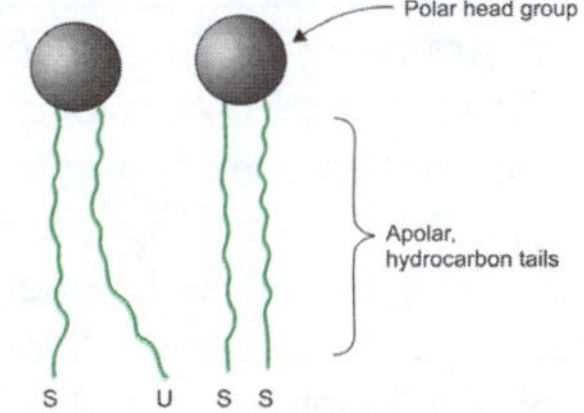

Diagrammatic representation of a phospholipid or other membrane lipid. The polar head group is hydrophilic, and the hydrocarbon tails are hydrophobic. The fatty acids in the tails are saturated (S) or unsaturated (U); the former are usually attached to carbon 1 of glycerol and the latter to carbon 2. Note the kink in the tail of the unsaturated fatty acid (U), which is important in conferring increased membrane fluidity.

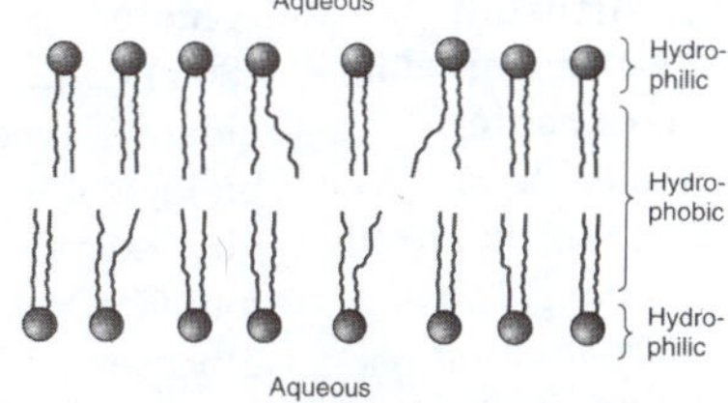

Diagram of a section of a bilayer membrane formed from phospholipid molecules. The unsaturated fatty acid tails are kinked and lead to more spacing between the polar head groups; hence to more room for movement. This in turn results in increased membrane fluidity.

Cholesterol modifies the fluidity of membranes. At temperature

Blow Tm	**Above Tm**
It interferes with the interaction of hydrocarbon tails of fatty acids and thus *increases fluidity*	It limits disorder because it is more rigid than the hydrocarbon tails of the fatty acids and cannot move in the membrane to the same extent, thus *limiting fluidity*.

- At high cholesterol : phospholipid ratio, Tm are altogether indistinguishable
- The fluidity affects the membrane functions. It increases *permeability to water* and other small *hydrophilic molecules*, and *lateral mobility of integral proteins*.
- The fluidity of the plasma membrane is highly dependant upon the lipid composition of the membrane.
- **Saturated fatty acids:** *Increase the transition temperature and hence* ***decrease the fluidity***.
- **Unsaturated fatty acids (PUFA)** : *Decrease the transition temperature and hence* ***increase the fluidity of membrane***.

Properties of Cell Membrane

- Membranes are ***asymmetrical***[Q] sheet like enclosed structure with distinct out and inner surfaces. This asymmetry is attributed to
  - irregular distribution of protein with in the cell membranes
  - external location of carbohydrate attached to membrane protein. (inside – outside asymmetry)
  - specific enzymes are located exclusively on the outside or inside of membranes, (inside – outside asymmetry)
  - gap junction synapses and tight junctions occupy only smaller regions of membrane and generate *local (regional) asymmetry* there is *inside – outside (transverse) asymmetry of the phospholipids*
- The choline- containing phospholipids **(phosphotidylcholine or lecithin & sphingomyelin)** are located mainly in the outer molecular layer; the aminophospholipids **(phosphotidyl serine & phosphotidylethanolamine)** are preferentially located in inner leaflet. There must be limited transverse mobility (flip- flop) of the membrane phospholipid to maintain this transverse asymmetry. Phospholipids exhibit an extraordinarily slow rate of flip flop. When certain membrane proteins such as *erythrocyte protein glycophorin are inserted artificially* into synthetic bilayers, the frequency of phospholipid fillip –flop increases as much as 100 folds.
- **Membranes are composed of – lipids, proteins and carbohydrates** and membranes are *dyanic structure*
  - Major lipids in mammalian membranes are ***phospholipids (phosphoglycerides > sphingomyelin), glycolipids & cholesterol.***
  - Membrane lipids are ***amphipathetic i.e. contain both hydrophobic & hydrophilic regions***[Q].
  - Membrane lipids are bilayer
  - Proteins are associated with lipid bilayer (± covalent linkage) and may be integral or peripheral in location.
  - Ion channels are transmembrane proteins that allow selective entry of various ions; ionophores are molecules that act as membrane shuttle for various ions and aquaporins are proteins that form water channels in certain molecules.
- **Oleic acid** is most abundant unsaturated fatty acid in animal membrane lipids. Sphingolipids are found in membranes specifically in tissues of nervous system. Degree of unsaturation determines fluidity of membrane and cholesterol helps to regulate it.

Osmosis, Osmolarity, Osmolality, Osmotic Pressure, Tonicity & Oncotic Pressure

Osmosis

- **Osmosis** is the **diffusion /movement of water (solvent)** through a **semiermeable membrane** (permeable to solvent, but not to solute) from an area of *high water potential /activity/concentration to low water potential /thermodynamic activity/concentration* (i.e. from lower solute concentration to higher solute concentration). So **osmosis** is net diffusion of water across a selectively

Mole and Osmole

- A **mole** is molecular weight of a substance in grams eg MW of glucose is 180; its mole is 180 gm and NaCl is 58.5gm. An **Osmole** (Osm) is *gram MW (mole) of substance divided by numer of osmotically active freely moving particles* that each molecule liberates in solution. For biological solutions, the **milliosmol** (mOsm i.e. 1/1000 of 1 Osm) is used. A molecule of glucose (nonionizing) compound gives only one active particle whereas 1 molecule of ionizing NaCl yields 2 and $CaCl_2$ or Na_2SO_4 yields 3 molecules. Therefore 1 mole of glucose yields 1 osmole of glucose; 1 mole of NaCl yields 2 osmoles (Na^+ and Cl^-); and 1 mole of $CaCl_2/Na_2SO_4$ yields 3 osmoles. (Ca^{2+} & $2Cl^-$ /$2Na^+$ & SO_4^{2-})
- Osmole (in place of grams) unit is used to express concentration of solution in terms of number of particles. **1 Osmole = 1 gram molecular weight of osmotically active solute**. So for glucose 180 grams = 1 gram MW = 1 Osmole whereas, for sodium chloride 58.5 grams = 1 gram MW = 2 Osmoles (as NaCl dissociates into 2 osmotically active particles).

permeable membrane down their **concentration (chemical) gradient**. Because presence of solute decreases the concentration of water on that side (when compred to equal volume of pure water). Hence in osmosis water moves from solution of lower solute concentration (which also means higher water concentration) to higher solute concentration (= lower water concentration).

- Osmosis can be opposed by *applying a pressure in the opposite direction of osmosis* (i.e. on solution containing lower water / higher solute concentration). The precise amount of hydrostatic pressure necessary to prevent the osmosis or osmotic flow of solvent (water in most cases) is called **osmotic pressure**. It is an indirect measure of solute and water concentration of a solution. The higher the osmotic pressure of a solution, the higher the solute and lower the water concentration of that solution (and viceversa)

Osmotic Effectiveness

- Although a homogenous solution contains osmotically active particles and can be said to have an osmotic pressure, it can exert an osmotic pressure *only when it is in contact wit another solution across a membrane permeable to the solvent but not to the solute.*
- For a molecule (substance) to exert and maintain a stable osmotic pressure, it *must be effectively confined to one side of the membrane (i.e. must not cross the membrane)*. For a molecule that can **freely cross the cell membranes**, like **urea**, can not sustain a stable osmotic effect. Such a substance causes only transient osmotic effects and is said to be **osmotically ineffective (ineffective osmole)**. Similarly a substance like **glucose** that is **metabolized**

Osmolarity & Osmolality

- **Osmolarity** is numbers of **osmoles per liter** (in **1 liter**) of solution (plasma), whereas **osmolality** is numer of **osmoles per kilogram** of solvent (water). (Mn "Both Osmolar and liter end in r")[Q]. For dilute solutions such as body fluids the difference between osmolality and osmaolrity is insignificant. Although, strictly speaking, it is osmolality (Osmoles per kg of water) that determines osmotic pressure. However, because of difficulty of measuring kgs of water in a solution, osmolarity (i.e. osmoles per liter) is used. Measurement of **osmolarity** are **dependent on temperature** because the volume of solvent varies with temperature while osmolality is not. For this reason osmolality is preferred term for biological systems.
- Like **vapour pressure lowering, freezing point depression and boiling point elevation**, the **osmotic pressure** depends solely on **number of molecules** in that solution. It is **not dependent on type or size** of molecule, their **mass or chemical nature (eg valence)**- i.e. it is *fundamental colligative property of solutions*. The reason for this is that each particle in a solution, regardless of its mass, exerts, on average, the equal amount of pressure against the membrane (i.e. large particle with greater mass have slower velocities & smaller particles have higher velocities in a way that both have almost equal kinetic energies).
- A solution that has 1 osmole of solute dissolved in each kilogram of solvent is said to have an osmolality of 1 osmole/kg. In body fluids solvent is water and the density of water is 1, so osmolal concentration can be expressed as osmoles/kg of water. 1 milliosmole /kg means 1/1000 osmoles dissolved in 1 kg of solvent. Similarly 1 osmole of solute dissolved in each liter of solution is said to have osmolarity of 1 osmole/lit. Total osmolarity (osmolality) of each of the three compartments of body fluid is **300 milli osmoles per liter (or kilogram of H_2O)** with the plasma being about *1 mOsm/L greater than that of interstitial and intercellular fluids.*
- However, the corrected osmolar activity of body fluids is **281** (Guyton) /**290** (Ganong) mOsm/L with plasma being about 1 mOsm/L greater. The reason for the difference is that many of the ions in body fluids eg Nacl are *highly attracted to one another* consequently, they *cannot more entirely unrestrained* in fluids and contribute some what less than 2 mOsm of osmotically active particles per liter.
- **Na^+** and its accompanying anions esp Cl^- & HCO_3^- contribute all but 20 osmoles per liter in ECF. Although concentration of plasma proteins is large when expressed in grams per liter, they usually contribute < 2mOsm/L b/o their high molecular weight. The major non electrolytes of plasma – glucose & urea are in equilibrium with cells and contribute to 5mOsm/L of osmolarity each.

Substance	Concentration (Osmolarity in mOsm/L H_2O)		
	ECF		Intracellular Fluid (ICF)
	Plasma	Interstitial	
Na^+	142	139	14
K^+	4.2	4	140
Mg^{++}	0.8	0.7	20
Cl^-	108	108	4
HCO_3^-	24	28.3	10
Phosphocreatine	-	-	45
Carnosine	-	-	14
Protein	1.2	0.2	4
Glucose	5.6	5.6	-
Urea	4	4	4
Total	301.8	300.8	301.2
Corvated	282	281	281
Total Osmotic pressure (mmHg) at 37°C	5443	5423	5423

is also osmotically ineffective because its concentration is not sustained (d/t metabolism). Although glucose is not freely diffusible b/o large size.

- So **osmotically effective** substances are neither freely permeable nor metabolized eg *plasma proteins* and various complex *polysaccharides like dextrean*, sucrose. Sodium chloride is osmotically effective because even though Na+ & Cl- ions can diffuse through cell membranes Na+ is maintained extracellularly b/o sodium pumps in cell membrane.
- The clinical significance of osmotic effectiveness (in management of hypovolemia) is that a solution used to restore and maintain circulating blood volume must be one whose active constituents remain within the circulation or at least, ECF (i.e. neither metabolized nor diffuses into cells). Hence although **5% glucose** solution is *isotonic (isomotic) with plasma when initially infused intravenously*, but cannot be used to treat hypvolemia because glucose is metabolized, so the net effect is that of infusing a hypotonic solution. But **0.9% saline solution (NaCl)** can be used as it remains isotonic because there is no net movement of osmotically active particles into cells and the particles are not metabolized.
- Similarly **300 mmol/L solution of sucrose & urea** both are isosmotic (i.e. have same osmolality) to intracellular fluid **(i.e. 300 m Osm/ Kg H_2O)** but cells (eg RBCs) placed in urea solution swell & burst and those in sucrose solution maintain their nomal volume. So *effectively sucrose solution is isotonic but urea solution is hypotonic* b/o high permeability of urea (d/t urea uniporters in cell membrane) and impermeability of sucrose.

Tonicity

- **Tonicity** is used to describe *osmolality* of a solution *relative to plasma* and its *effect on volume of cell*. The tonicity depends on concentration of impermeant solutes. Solutions that have the same osmolality as plasma are said to be **isotonic**, and these solutions do not change the volume of a cell (Osmolarity = 282 m Osm/L or osmolality = 282 mOsm/kg of H_2O). Solutions with **greater osmolality** (>282) are called **hypertonic** and water will diffuse out of cell into ECF, concentrating the ICF, **shrinking the cell** and diluting ECF. Solutions with **lesser osmolality** (< 282) are **hypotonic** and water will diffuse into cell causing dilution of intra cellular fluid and **cell swelling** while ECF is concentrated until both solutions have about the same osmolality. Similarly solutions with same, higher or lower osmolarity respectively, compared with normal ECF, without regard for whether the solute permeates the cell membrane are called **isosmotic, hyperosmotic** and **hyposmotic**.

Measurement of Osmotic Pressure (π)

1. By measuring pressure that must be applied to prevent water from entering the solution with higher solute concentration.
2. By **freezing point depression**: **1 mol per liter** of an ideal solution depresses the freezing point of water by **1.86°C**. So the numer of milliosmoles per liter in a solution equals the freezing point depression divided by **0.00186**.
The average freezing point for human plasma is **– 0.54°C**, which corresponds to an osmolality of **290 mOsm/kg**. This is equivalent to an osmotic pressure of **7.3** atm against pure water.
3. **By Van't Hoff's equation (Law)**
$\pi = \sigma\ (\eta\ CRT)$ where π = osmotic pressure; σ = reflection or osmotic coeffieicnt which is O for freely permeable substance like urea and 1 for totally impermeable like sucrose; η = number of dissociable particles per molecule eg 1 for glucose & 2 for **NaCl; C** or **ΔC** = total (or difference in) solute concentration (mol/L); R = natural gas constant (62 mm Hg x l/mmol x °K or 0.082 atmL/mol °K) and T = absolute temperature (°K) for body fluid it is 37°C (= 273+37 = 310° Kelvin). In few books π = CRT where C is solute concentration in osmoles/L (i.e. it includes both n & C of this formula).
So somotic pressure (π) for totally impermeable (σ = 1), non-dissociable (n = 1) molecule at 1 mol/L concentration in body fluids (i.e. T = 310°K) is
π = 1(1x 1 x 0.082 x 310) = **25.4 atm = 19300 mm Hg** Because **1 atm = 760 mmHg**
And similarly for 1 milimole /L solute concentration which is equal to 1/1000 mole/L. The π would be **2.54 x 10^{-2} atm** or **19.3 mmHg**. This means, ***for each miliosmole concentration gradient across the cell membrane 19.3 mmHg or 0.0254 atm osmotic pressure is exerted***[Q]. Or in other words, at normal body temperature (37°C) a concentration of **1 osmole per liter** will cause **19300 mmHg (or 25.4 atm)** osmotic pressure in solution.
Because concentration of body fluid is 300 mili Osmole/liter so the (π) should be = 19.3 x 300 = 5790 mmHg. However, actually it is **5500 mmHg** (0.93 times of calculated value) because due to attraction between few ions the corrected effected osmolarity is about 280 mOsm/L (0.93 times of calculated value).

- **0.9% (=0.9grams/100 mililiters = 9gm/L) NaCl** is isotonic to plasma. Because the MW of NaCl is 58.5, the molarity of 0.9% solution is 9g/L ÷ 58.5 g/mol = 0.154 mol/L; and the osmolarity is 0.154 x 2 = 0.308 Osm/L = 308 mOsm/L (because 1 molecule provides 2 particles). Now because **each mOsm/L of body fluid exerts 19.3 mmHg of osmotic pressure** (at 37°c); the osmotic pressure of 0.9% NaCl would be 308 mOsm/L x 19.3 mmHg/mosm/L = 5944 mmHg. However this value is higher than the actual because the **osmotic reflection coefficient** of NaCl is 0.93. Therefore the actual osmolarity of 0.9% Nacl is 0.93 x 308 = 286 mOsm/L

Oncotic Pressure

- **Oncotic pressure** is the osmotic pressure (π) generated by large molecules (esp proteins) in solution. It does not conform to van't Hoff's law most probably because of size & shape of protein molecule. Proteins exert 26-28 mm Hg of oncotic pressure in human plasma, which although appears to be small (28 mm Hg ~ 1.4 mOsm/kg H_2O) is an important force involved in fluid movement across capillaries.

Fick's Law of Diffusion

Fick's law of diffusion explains *passive diffusion along concentration gradient*^Q. The magnitude of diffusing tendency is directly proportionate to the **cross sectional area** across which diffusion is taking place and the **concentration gradient or chemical gradient**, which is the difference in concentration of the diffusing substance divided by the thickness of boundary. Thus

Net rate of diffusion (J) = α Area (A) and concentration gradient $\left(\frac{\Delta C}{\Delta X}\right)$

$$J = -DA\frac{\Delta C}{\Delta X}$$

$$Flux = -PA\,\Delta C.$$

$$Flux = -PA(C_i - C_o)$$

- Where D = Diffusion coefficient and
- Minus (-) sign = Indicates the direction of diffusion when molecules move from higher to lower concentration, $\left(\frac{\Delta C}{\Delta X}\right)$ is negative, so multiplying it with – DA gives a positive value.
- Δ C = Concentration inside (Ci) – Concentration outside
- Since thickness of biological membrane (Δ x) is constant at 10^{-6} cm, D/x simplifies to permeability coefficient (P).

The net flux of solute is from high to low concentration. And the time required for equilibrium by diffusion is proportionate to the *square of diffusion distance.*

Resting Membrane Potential (RMP) Established by ☆

Selective permeability of cell membrane

K⁺ diffusion potential

- K^+ is highly permeable at resting condition (all the K^+ leak channels are opened in resting condition).
- ***K^+ efflux is much greater than Na^+ influx***^Q ***because it is 100 times more permeable.***
- ***Net outward diffusion of K+ make interior of cell more negative and is believed to be the main mechanism responsible for RMP***^Q. This is supported by effects of

Na^+ diffusion potential

Most of Na^+ channels are closed at rest, so only very little amount of Na^+ diffuses into cells.

Concentration (mmol/L)

Ion	Intracellular Fluid	Extracellular Fluid	Equilibrium Potential (mV)
Na+	12	145	+65
K+	155	4	**-95**^Q
H+	13×10^{-5}	3.8×10^{-5}	-32
Cl-	3.8	120	**-90**^Q
HCO3-	8	27	-32
A	155	0	…

Membrane potential = *-90 mv*^Q

Sodium-Potassium Pump

- Sodium & potassium ions are *activately transport* in opposite direction across the cell membrane by electrogenic pump called Na^+ K^+ - pump.
- It pumps ***$3Na^+$ outside for each $2K^+$ pumped to inside of membrane.***^Q i.e. pump creates some **negativity inside and positivity outside i.e. it is electrogenic**
- But Na^+ - K^+ pump contributes no more than **-5mv** to RMP.

Increasing Extracellular K+ concentration

- ***Lowers RMP and negatively of membrane***^Q because increase in [K+] reduces the concentration gradient which causes the net outward diffusion of K+
- It depolarizes the cell

Decreasing Extracellular K+ concentration

- ***Increases magnitude of RMP and negativity of membrane***^Q by increasing concentration gradient
- It **hyperpolarize** the cell

- Changes in *internal concentration* of K^+ cause change in RMP as predicted by *Nernst equations*
- Alteration in Na^+ & Cl^- concentrations do not produce comparable results.

K⁺ Balance

- K+ is the ***major intracellular cation***Q. The normal plasma K+ conc. is ***3.5- 5 mmol/L***Q, whereas that inside the cell is ~ *150 m mol/L*. Therefore the amount of K+ in the ECF *(30-70 mmol)* constitukes < 2% of total body K+ content *(2500- 4500mmol)*. The ratio of ICF to ECF-K+ conc. (normally 38:1) is the principal ***result of the resting membrane potential***Q and is crucial for ***neuromuscular function***Q.
- The passive outward diffusion of K+ is quantitatively the most important factor that generates the resting membrane potential. ***Na+ K+- ATP ase pump actively transports K+ in & Na+ out of the cell in a 2:3 ratio***Q. The activity of pump is stimulated by *increased intracellular Na+ conc* and inhibited by *digoxin toxicity, CHF, CRF*

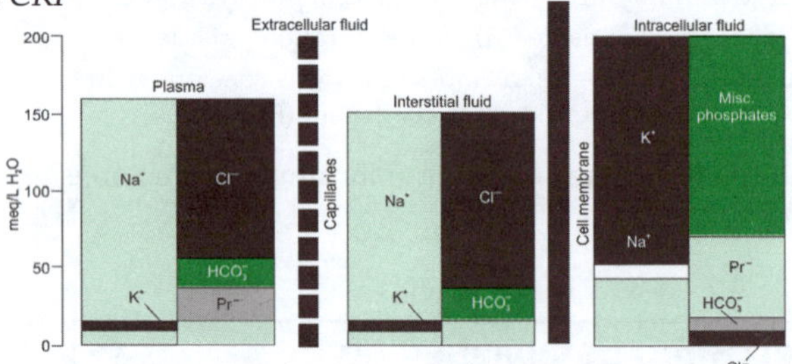

Electrolyte compostion of human body fluids. Note that the values are in meq/L of water, not of body fluid.

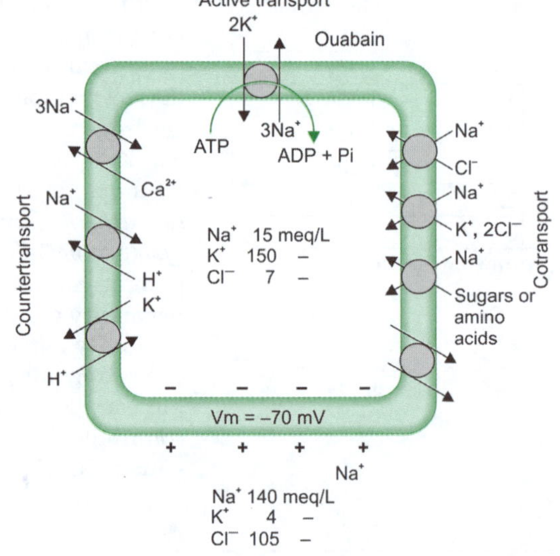

K⁺ Excretion

- Renal excretion is the major route of elimination. The filtered load of K+ (GFR x Plasma conc. = 180 L/d x 4mmol /L = 720 mmol /d) is 10 –20 folds greater than the ECF K+ content
- Some 90% of filtered K+ is reabsorbed by proximal convoluted tubule & loop of Henle. *Proximally* the K+ is *reabsorbed passively with Na+ & water*, whereas the luminal *Na+- K+ - 2Cl- cotransporter* mediates K+ uptake in the *thick ascending limb of loop of Henle*
- There fore K+ delivery to distal nephron [distal convoluted tubule & cortical collecting duct (CCD)] approximates dietary intake
- Net distal K+ secretion or reabsorption occurs in the setting of K+ excess or depletion respectively. The cell responsible for K+ secretion in late distal convoluted tubule (or connecting tubule) & **CCD is the principal cell**. Virtually ***all regulation of renal K+ excretion and total body K+ balance occurs in distal nephron***Q
- The rate of *K+ secretion is proportionate to the rate of flow of tubular fluid* through the distal portion of nephron, because with rapid flow there is less opportunity for the tubular K+ conc to rise to a value that stops further secretion. In collecting duct Na+ is generally reabsorbed & K+ is secreted. There is no rigid one for one exchange & ***much of the movement of K+ is passive***Q, However there is electrical coupling in the sense that intracellular migration of Na+ tends to lower the potential difference across tubular cell & this favours movement of K+ into the tubular lumen. Since Na+ is also reabsorbed in association with H+ secretion, there is competition for the Na+ in the tubular fluid. And *K+ excretion is decreased* when amount of *Na+ reaching distal tubule is small* & when *H+ secretion is increased.*
- Potassium secretion is regulated by two physiological stimuli – aldosterone & hyperkalemia

Diffusion & Active Transport

Process in which solute particles move from a more concentrated environment to a less concentrated one in order to bring a uniform concentration throughout.

Simple Diffusion

- Molecules can passively traverse the bilayer down electro chemical gradient.
- Energy is not required

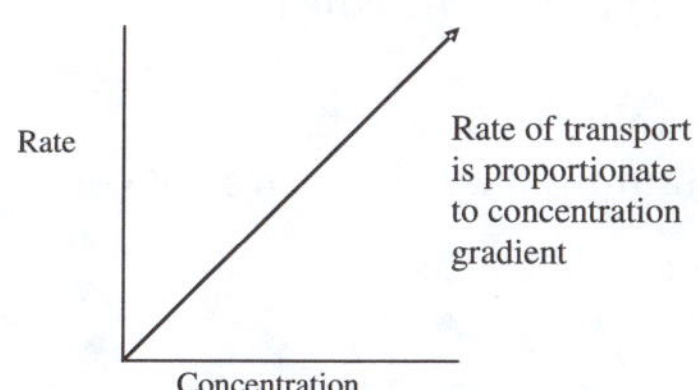

Simple Diffusion

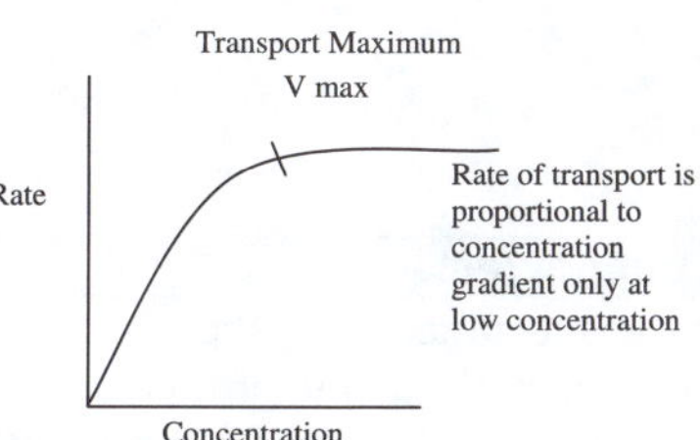

Facilitated Diffusion

Facilitated Diffusion

- When carrier protein (transporter protein) move substance ***in the direction of their chemical or electrical gradient***[Q] ***without any energy expenditure (energy is not required)***[Q].
- ***Facilitated diffusion is a form of passive (no energy) transport that occurs along an electro chemical gradient and requires no energy***[Q]***. The rate of transport is not always proportionate to the concentration gradient because it is mediated through carrier proteins***[Q].
- **At lower concentrations** before the carrier protein becomes saturated (or before V_{max} is reached), the rate of facilitated diffusion is *proportionate to concentration* gradient whereas, at higher concentrations when carrier protein becomes saturated (V_{max} is reached) the rate of facilitated diffusion becomes constant.
- *Hormones* regulate facilitated diffusion by changing the number of transporter available. e.g :- ***Insulin increases glucose transport in fat & muscle***[Q].
  - Glucocorticoids increases transport of amino acid into liver.

Active Transport

When carrier proteins move substances ***against their chemical or electrical gradient by expenditure of energy.***[Q]
eg. ***Na^+ - K^+ pump***[Q]

Type of Carrier Protein

a) **Uniport**: when they transmit only one substance
b) **Symport** : binding of more than one substance to the transport protein & the substances are transported across the membrane together e.g. ***Na^+ glucose symport in intestine.***[Q]
c) **Antiport:** transport protein exchange one substance for another. e.g.in Na^+ K^+ Atpase.

Saturation Kinetics

- While in other transport mechanism, the rate of diffusion approaches a maximum, called **Vmax**, as the concentration of substance increases and then pleateu's off i.e. attains saturation at a particular level. This is called ***saturation kinetics mechanism***[Q].
- **Saturation kinetics** will be seen in any transport process which *involves carrier proteins* eg. ***facilitated diffusion and active transport***[Q]***.***
- The rate at which a substance can be transported by these mechanism depends upon the rate at which the carrier protein can undergo conformational change between its active state & inactive state.
- So the rate at which molecules can be transported by this mechanism can never be greater than the rate at which the carrier protein undergoes conformational change.
- This limits the rate of transport in these process.

Ionophores

Certain microbes synthesize small organic molecules called *ionophores*, that function as shuttle for the movement of ions across membrane.

Structure

Ionophores contain ***hydrophilic centers*** that bind specific ions & are *surrounded by* ***peripheral hydrophobic regions.***

Types

a) **Mobile ion carriers**: Like *valinomycin* (refer uncoupler of oxidative phosphorylation)
b) **Channel formers**: Like gramicidin, Nigericin
Nigricin: acts as an ionophore for K^+ but in exchange for H^+, therefore abolishes *pH gradient* across the membrane.
Valinomycin & Nigricin: If present, both membrane potential & pH gradient are abolished & phosphorylation is completely inhibited i.e. ***conversion of ADP to ATP is inhibited***[Q]

Characters

- Ionophores are termed because of their ability to complex specification & facilitate their transport through biological membrane.
- The properties are d/t their ***lipophilic character***[Q] which allow penetration of lipid membranes.

Transport Across Membrane

Small uncharged (neutral) molecules

Pass freely by simple passive diffusion down an electrochemical gradient[Q]***.***

★ **Active transport** is *against electrochemical gradient* and requires energy; whereas **passive diffusion** is always *down electrochemical gradient* and does *not require energy.*

- **Charged molecules**
- **Larger uncharged (neutral) molecules**
- **Some small uncharged (neutral) molecules,** through

- *Channel proteins or prions*[Q] (are transmembranous beta barrel proteins that act as pores through which molecules can diffuse, by simple passive diffusion)
- *Carrier proteins* allow *fecilitated passive diffusion* as well as *active transport.*

Transport Across Cell Membrane

Exocytosis

- Vesicles containing material for export are ticketed to the cell membrane, where they bound via the v- *SNARE / t- SNARE arrangement*
- The area of fusion then breaks down, leaving the content of vesicle outside & cell membrane intact. This is Ca^{++} dependent process.
- In exocytosis, ***cytoplasmic sides of two membranes fuse***[Q] and there is net *increase in surface area of cell* (d/t adding of extra membrane)

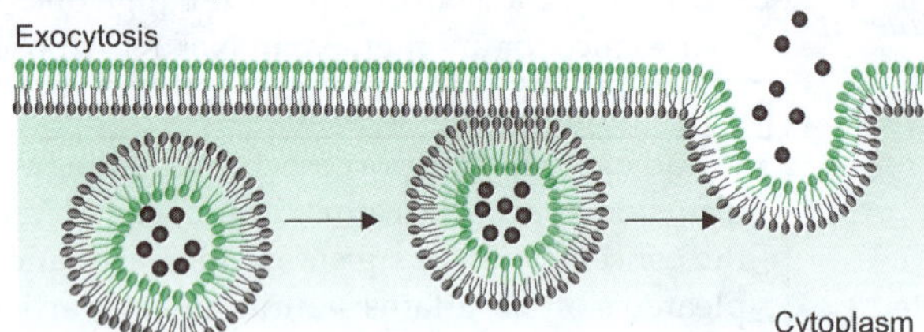

Endocytosis

- It is the reverse of exocytosis and may be *phagocytosis (cell eating) & pinocytosis (cell drinking)*
- ***In endocytosis two non cytoplasmic side of membranes fuse***[Q]
- It l/t removal of cell membrane preventing cell to enlarge and thus maintaining the surface area of cell.

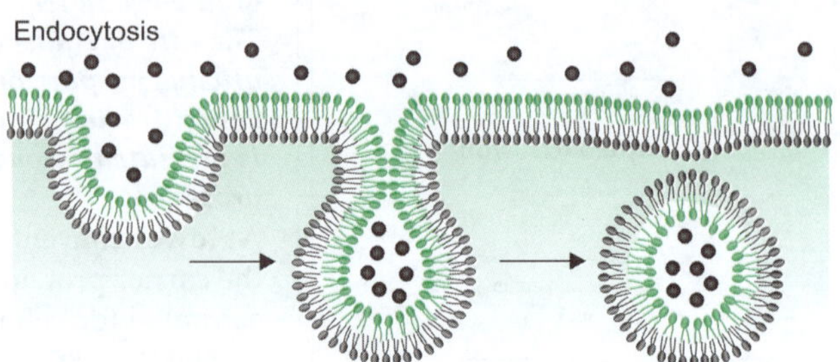

Features	Exocytosis	Endocytosis
Definition	The process by which the substances are expelled from the cell. It is the *extrusion of cell bound vesicles, and* ***requires Ca^{2+} and energy***[Q]	The process by which the substance enter the cell without actually passing through the membrane. ***It requires: Energy, Ca^{2+} & contractile element in the cell***[Q].
Mechanism	The inner membrane of vesicle fuses with the outer plasma membrane, while cytoplasmic side of vesicle fuses with the cytoplasmic side of plasma membrane. Thus the contents of vesicles are externalized.	When segment of plasma membrane invaginates enclosing a minute volume of ECF & its contents. The invagination is pinched off, leaving the engulfed material in the membrane- enclosed vacuole & the cell membrane intact.
Types	Secretion from the cell occurs Via two pathway **Constitutive**: Prompt transport of proteins to cell membrane in vesicles with no processing. **Nonconstitutive**: Protein from the golgi apparatus initially enters secretory granules, where processing occurs.	**Endocytosis** → **Phagocytosis** → **Pinocytosis**: Fluid phase pinocytosis; Receptor mediated absorptive pinocytosis

Endocytosis

Pinocytosis

- It is a property of all cell.
- It is cellular uptake of fluid & fluid contents.[Q]

Fluid phase pinocytosis

Is a *nonselective process* in which the uptake of solute is simply *proportionate to its concentration* in the surrounding extracellular fluid.

Absorptive pinocytosis

- Is a *receptor mediated selective process* primarily responsible for the uptake of macromolecules. The vesicles formed during absorptive pinocytosis are derived from invaginations (pits) that are coated on the cytoplasmic side with a ***filamentous material called clathrin.***[Q]
- The protein *dynamin* which binds & *Hydrolysis GTP*, is necessary for the pinching off of clathrin coated vesicles from the cell surface (also called *pinchase)*

Phagocytosis

- Occurs only in specialized cell such as macrophage & granulocyte.
- Involves ingestion of large particles such as viruses, bacteria, cells or debris

Fate: Most endocytic vesicles fuse with primary lysosomes (early endosome) to form secondary lysosomes which contain hydrolytic enzymes. & therefore are specialized orgenelle for intracellular disposal.

★ *Clathrin*[Q]: Clathrin molecules have the shape of triskelion (three legs radiating from central hub). As endocytosis progresses, the clathrin molecule form a geometric array that surrounds the endolytic vesicle. Once complete vesicle is formed, it falls off & recycle to form another vesicle.

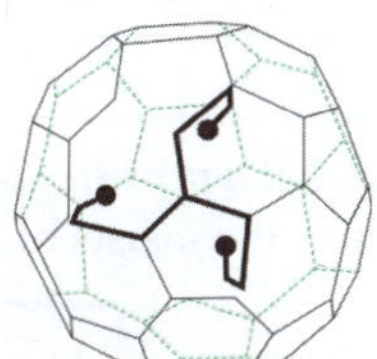

Clathrin molecule on the surface of an endocytotic vesicle. Note the characteristic triskelion shape and the fact that with other clathrin molecules it forms a net supporting the vesicle.

Intercellular Communication

(Transmission of regulatory signals or chemical messenger between cells)

Without entering ECF (extra cellular fluid)

Gap Junction

- At gap junction, the intercellular space narrows from *25 nm to 3 nm.*
- Its unit **connexons** (an aqueous hemi channel) is made up of **6** transmembrane protein subunits called **connexins**. Each connexin has 4 membrne spanning regions.
- Connexon surround a channel, which when lined up with the channel of corresponding connexon in adjacent cell, ***permits the substance to pass between the cells without entering extracellular fluid***[Q].
- Diameter of channel is 2 nm, which permits the passage of ions. Sugars, amino acids & other solutes with molecular wt upto 1000. These pores are much larger than those formed by ligand or voltage gated channels & thus permit rapid propogation of chemical messenger & electrical activity from cell to cell.
- The connexons keep the adjacent cell membranes at a fixed gap of 2-4 nm, hence the name gap junction.
- X linked *Charcot Marie Tooth disease* (peripheral neuropathy) is a/w mutation of connexin gene.
- By means of gap junction myocardial & visceral smooth muscle cells have a *syncitial behaviour* and conduct impulse from cell to cell.

Through ECF

- **Neural synaptic signaling**
  Neurotransmitter released from presynaptic neuron cross a narrow *synaptic cleft (ECF)* to act on post synaptic neuron
- **Paracrine & autocrine signaling** products of cell diffuse in the ECF to affect nearby neighbouring cell (paracrine) or the same all (autocrine).
- **Endocrine signaling**
  - Hormones secreted by endocrine organs reach target cells via *circulating body fluid (i.e. blood or ECF)*
  - Hormones bind on target cell to intracellular receptors or extracellular receptor (present in ECF). And G protein coupled receptors are extracellular receptor.

Endosomes and their role in receptor mediated Absorptive Pinocytosis

- These are transient cellular structures involved in the transport of macromolecules from the exterior of cells to its interior.
- They do not contain hydrolytic enzymes, are less dense than lysosomes and have an internal pH of 5.0.
- Endosomes receive the receptor-ligand complex by fusing with the 'coated vesicles'
  (Coated vesicles consist of Receptors, Ligand (macromolecule) and a layer of clathrin protein)
- On fusion, the coated vesicles discharge their macromolecules into the interior of endosomes.
- ***The low pH within the endosome, breaks the linkage between receptor-macromolecule complex and releases the receptor, the macromolecule, clathrin, and membrane fragments***[Q].

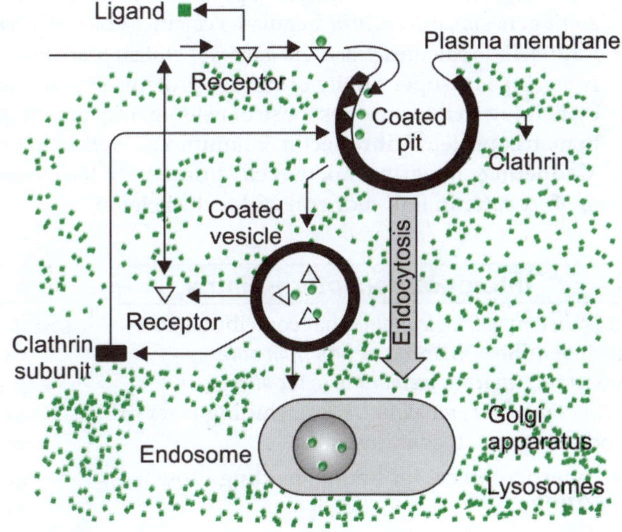

Extracellular Matrix

Cells are surrounded by *extracellular matrix* often referred to as *connective tissue.* It can be organized into 2 forms: interstitial matrix & basement membrane. It consists of 3 major classes of molecules

Structural Fibrous Proteins

- **Collagen**
  - *Fibrillar (type 1, 2, 3, 5, & 11) collagens are most abundant and found in interstitial matrix* (which also contain non fibrillar collagens)
  - ***Basement membrane contains non fibrillar (mainly type 4) collagen*** Q
  - ***Provide tensile strength. Scurvy affects its triple helical structure*** Q.
  - Deficiency l/t *Ehler Danlos synsrome, Alport syndrome, epidermolysis bullosa, osteogenisis imperfecta, chondrodysplasia and Menke's disease*
  - Scurvy affects structure of collagen
- **Elastin**
  - Confers ***extensibility and recoil*** Q to tissues such as *skin, blood vessels, lung, ligament & uterus.*
  - Deficiency l/t **William's Beuren syndrome and supravalvular aortic stenosis**
- **Fibrillin**
  - In elastic fibers, central core of elastin is surrounded by *peripheral* network of *microfibrils, that consists of 350 KD glycoprotein – fibrillin*
  - Serves as *scaffold for deposition of elastin* & assembly of elastic fibers.
  - Defects results in *abnormal elastic fibers in Marfan's syndrome.* Mutation in **fibrillin 1 gene** present in Microfibrils cause **Marfan syndrome** whereas, mutation in **fibrillin 2** cause *congenital contractural arachnodactyly* but not Marfan syndrome.

Gel of Proteoglycans & glycosaminoglycans (GAGs)

- Hyaluronic acid
- Chondratin sulfate
- Keratin sulfate
- Heparin
- Heparan sulfate
- Dermatan sulfate

Specialized Glycoproteins

- **Fibronectin** is an important *glycoprotein of extracllular interstial matrix,* also found in soluble form in plasma, which is involved in cell adhesion & migration.
- **Laminin** is a ***most abundant glycoprotein of glomerular & other basal lamine*** Q that has binding sites for type IV collagen, heparin & integrins

Cell Adhesion Molecule (CAM)

- Stored in cytoplasm or located in cell membrane as receptor and priovide interaction between the same cells (**homotypic interaction**) or different cells types (**hetrotypic interaction**).
- Classified into 4 main families *immunoglobulin family CAMs, cadherins, integrins & selectins.* Some other secreted adhesion molecules are – *SPARC* (secreted protein acidic, and rich in cysteine or *osteonectin*), *thrombospondins* (both inhibiting angiogenesis), *osteopontin* (regulates calcification) and ***tenacin***
- **Cadherin** is calcium *dependent adhesion protein providing homotypic interaction* and forming *zonula adherens & desmosomes.* **Integrins is a** super family of surface proteins present on wide variety of cells that *links the outside of cells to their inside* there by helping to integrate response of cells eg. movement, phagocytosis. It provide adhesion both b/w cell & ECM (by binding to matrix proteins **fibronectin** & **laminin** as well as to other cells.
- Cadherin & integrins link the cell surface with the cytoskeleton (inside of cells) through their binding to actin. β & α **catenin** link cadherin with cytoskeleton.

Interphotoreceptor – Matrix

It is viscous *biological glue* that contributes to retinal adhesion and extends *from outer (external) limiting membrane to the surface of retinal pigment epithelium.* (i.e. including layer of rods & cones). It contains.

- Interphotoreceptor Retinal Binding Protein (IRBP)
- Proteoglycans – Glycosaminoglycans
  - Sulphated / Non sulphated chondroitin
  - Hyaluronic Acid

Mimecaine/Osteoglycin/Osteo inductive Factors

- It is a *small leucine rich proteoglycans (SLEPs)* that is abundant in extracellular *matrix of bone, cartilage and connective tissue.*
- It is important for collagen fibrillogenesis, cellular growth, differentiation and migration and can induce ectopic bone formation,
- BMP-1 converts mimecan from precursor to mature form & potentiates it to modulate the formation of type 1 collagen fibrillogenesis
- In atherosclerotic lesions, mimecan mRNA is downregulated in media & upregulated in activated endothelium and neointima, whereas protein is accumulated in front edge of migrating smooth muscle.

- Fibronectin
- ***Sialoprotein associated with rods and cones (SPARC)***
  (SPARC / Osteonectin / BM – 40)
- Intercellular Adhesion Molecule I (ICAM- 1)
- Hyaluronic Acid Receptor (CD44 antigen)
- Lysosomal enzymes
  - ***Matrix metalloproteinases***
  - ***Tissue Inhibitors of Metalloproteinases (TIMP)***

Matrix Metalloproteinases (MMP)

A family of enzyme, having more than 20 members. These are involved in *degradation of basement membrane & ECM.*

Gelatinases / Collagenases (MMP2 & 9)
Degrade amorphous collagen & fibronectin (of basement membrane)

Stromelysins (MMP 3, 10 & 11)
Degrade amorphous collagen, fibronectin, laminin & proteoglycan (found in basement membrane)

Collagen

It is the ***most abundant & important protein***Q in animal world providing extracellular framework for multicellular organisms. In addition a number of proteins eg. *C1q complement, pulmonary surfactant* proteins SP- A and SP-D have collagen like domains in their structure and sometimes referred to as non collagen collagens

Types Of Collagen Based on

Structure

Class	Type
Fibril-formin	I, II, III, V and XI
Network-like	IV, VIII, X
FACITs	IX, XII, XIV, XVI, XIX
Beaded filaments	VI
Anchoring fibrils	VII
Transmembrane domain	XIII, XVII
Others	XV, XVIII

★ Just go through this chart and don't get confused by the genes & types as both are usually similar (i.e. type 1=gene 1)
★ Only remember those points which are dark & bold

Location

Type	Genes	Tissue
I	COL1A1	Most connective tissues, including **bone**
II	COL2A1	**Cartilage, invertebral disc vitreous humor**
III	COL3A1	**Extensible connective tissues** such as **skin, lung**, and the **vascular system (hollow organ)**
IV	COL4A1-COL4A6	*Basement membranes*Q
V	COL5A1-COL5A3	Minor components in tissues containing collagen I
VI	COL6A1-COL6A3	Most connective tissues
VII	COL7A1	**Anchoring fibrils at dermo-epidermal junction**
VIII	COL8A1-COL8A2	**Endothelium**, other tissues
IX	COL9A1-COL9A3	Tissues containing collagen II
X	COL10A1	**Hypertrophic cartilage**
XI	COL11A1, COL11A2, COL2A1	Tissues containing collagen II
XII	COL12A1	Tissues containing collagen I
XIII	COL13A1	Many Tissues
XIV	COL14A1	Tissues containing collagen I
XV	COL15A1	Many Tissues
XVI	COL16A1	Many Tissues
XVII	COL17A1	**Skin hemidesmosomes**
XVIII	COL18A1	Many Tissues (eg **Liver, Kidney**)
XIX	COL19A1	**Rhabdomyosarcoma cells**

Endostatin forming collagen, *in endothelial cells.* (XV, XVIII)

Structure

- All collagens have triple ***helical structure***Q
- A striking feature is occurrence of *glycine at every 3rd position* of triple helical portion of α- chain.
- This repeating structure ***(Gly- X-Y)n***Q is an absolute requirement for the formation of triple helix
- ***Proline and hydroxyproline***Q (formed by hydroxylation of proline by prolyl hydroxylase whose cofactors are vit C & α ketoglutarate) *confirrigidity to collagen*. These acquire 100 of X & 100 of Y positions.
- Lysine in Y position is also modified to hydroxy lysine through the action of lysyl hydroxylase and similar cofactors.
- Galactose or galactosyl glucose is added to hydroxylysines through an ***O- glycosidic linkage, a glycosylat ion site that is unque to collagen***Q.
- It is further stabilized by formation of *covalent cross links* both within and between the triple helical units through the action of ***lysyl oxidase***Q, a *Cu dependent enzyme* that oxidatively deaminates the E- amino groups of lysine & hydroxy- lysine yielding reactive aldehydes.
- Several *collages (eg. Type IV)* are characterized by interruptions of triple helix with stretches of protein *lacking Gly-X-Y repeats*. This results in areas of globular structure interspersed in triple helical structure.

Post translational modifications

- Collagen is synthesized on ***ribosome***Q in precursor form- *pre procollagen*, which contains a *leader or signal sequence* that directs it into the lumen of ***endoplasmic reticulum***Q
- In ER leader sequence is removed, hydroxylation of proline & lysine and glycosylation of hydroxytysine in procollagen takes place
- Procollagen contains ***extension peptides***Q (Polypetides of 20- 35 Kda) at its carboxy & amino terminal ends (not present in mature collagen)
- Extension peptide contain *cysteine residue*. While *amino terminal* forms only *intra chain disulfide* bonds, the *carboxy terminal* form *both intra chain & inter chain* disulfide bond. These assist in triple helix formation.
- After formation of triple helix, no further hydroxylation or glycosylation take place
- Following secretion by the way of ***golgiapparatus***Q and packed into ***secretory vesicles***Q, extracellular enzymes called *procollagen aminoproteinase* and *procollagen carboxy proteinase* remove extension peptides at the amino and carboxy terminal ends respectively, resulting in formation of collagen.

Diseases

Disease	Gene /Enzyme
Ehler danlos SyndromeQ	
- type IV	CoL- 3A1
- type VI	**Lysyl hydroxylase**
- type VII AR	**Procollagen –N proteinase**
- type VII AD	COL- 1A1 & 1A2
- ***Osteogenesis imperfecta***Q (type 1) - **Osteoporosis**	COL – 1A1& 1A2
- Severe **chondrodysplasia** - **Osteo arthritis**	COL 2A1
- Schmid metaphysical chondrodysplasia	COL- 10A1
- **Alport Syndrome** (AR & X- linked)	COL –4A3 & 4A6
- **Epidermolysis bullosa dystrophic**	COL –7A 1
- **Menkes disease**	**Lysyl hydrxylase**

★ **Scurvy** also affects the structure of collagen

★ **Marfan syndrome** is d/t mutation in the gene for *fibrillin*, a protein present in microfibrils

★ **Hunter syndrome** is a mucopoly saccharidosis d/t def. Of enzyme *iduronidase* that is involved in degradation of glycosaminoglycans

Proteoglycans & Glycosaminoglycans

- **Proteoglycans** are *protein* that contain *covalently linked glycosaminoglycans*. Examples are syndecan, betaglycan, serglycan, perlecan, aggrecan, versican, decorin, biglycan & firomodulin.
- The protein of PG that bound covalently to glycosaminoglycans are called *core proteins*. It is synthesized in *endoplasmic reticulum* and few GAG linkage also form here. Most of later GAG chains & modification occur in *golgi apparatus*.
- An O- glycosidic bond between xylose (Xyl) & ser is unique to proteoglycans.
- The amount of *carbohydrate* in PG is usually much greater than found in glycoproteins & may be *upto 95%*
- ***Aggrecan is found in cartilage***Q
- **Glycosaminoglycans (GAG)** is an *unbranched polysacehride made up of repeating disaccharides*, one component of which is always an *amino sugar*, either *D- glucosamine (Glc-N), or D- galactosamine (Gal–N)*. The other component (except in case of keratan sulfate) is uronic acid either *L-glucronic acid* (Glc-UA) or its 5′epimer, *L- iduronic acid* (Id- UA)
- 7 types of GAGs are – *hyaluronic acid, chondroitin sulfate, keratan sulfates I & II, heparin, heparan sulfate & dermatan sulfate*
- With exception of hyaluronic acid, all GAGs contain sulfate groups, either as O- esters or N- sulfate (in heparin & heparan sulfate). Hyaluronic acid affords another exception because there is no clear evidence that it is attached covalently to protein

Major proteins of Glycosaminoglycans

GAG	Sugars	Sulfate	Linkage of protein	Location
HA	GlcNAc, GlcUA	Nil	No firm evidence	Synovial fluid, vitreous humor, loose connective tissue
CS	GalNAc, GlcUA	GalNAc	Xyl-ser; assoiated with HA via link proteins	Cartilage, bone, cornea
KS I	GlcNAc, Gal	GlcNAc	GlcNAc-Asn	Cornea
KS II	GlcNAc, Gal	Same as KS I	GalNAc-Thr	Loose connective tissue
Heparin	GlcN, IdUA	GlcN GlcN IdUA	Ser	Mast cell
Heparan sulfate	GlcN, GlcUA	GlcN	Xyl-Ser	Skin fibroblasta, aortic wall
Dermatan sulfate	GalNAc, IdUA, (Glc.UA)	GalNAc IdUa	Xyl-Ser	Wide distribution

Mucopolysaccharidoses (MPS)

Etiopathogenesis

- Degradation of GAGs is carried out by a battery of lysosomal hydrolases. These include- endoglycosides, exoglycosidases, & sulfatase
- Deficiency of one of the lysomal hydrolases involved in degradation of one or more of GAGs l/t mucopolysaccharidoses.
- This results in accumulation of GAGs in various tissues including liver, spleen, bone, skin & CNS.
- GAGs are composed of repeating disaccharide unit with either
  - amino sugar = d – glucosamine or
or D- galoctosamine
  - acid sugar = D- glucoronic acid
L- iduronic acid
- There is ***increased excretion of accumulated GAG, D- glucronic acid or L- iduronic acid in urine***[Q].

Type of MPS

Type	Syndrome	Enzymatic Defect	Accumulated / Urinary metabolite
I	**Hurler** or **Scheie**	***α- L- Iduronidase***[Q]	- ***Dermatan sulfate***[Q] - ***Hepran sulfate***[Q]
II	**Hunter**	*Iduronate sulfatase*	
III A	**Sanfilippo A**	*Heparan sulfate N- sulfatase (sulfamidase)*	***Heparan sulfate***[Q]
III B	**Sanfilippo B**	*α-N- Acetyl glucosaminidase*	
III C	**Sanfilippo C**	*Acetyl transferase*	
III D	**Sanfilippo D**	*N- Acetylglucosamine 6 sulfatase*	
IV A	**Moriquio- A**	*Galactosamine –6- sulfatase*	- Keratan sulfate - Chondroitin –6 sulfate
IV B	**Morquio -B**	*β- Galactosidase*	- Keratan sulfate
VI	**Maroteauxlamy**	*N- acetyl galactosamine 4- sulfatase (aryl sulfatase β*	Dermatan sulfate
VII	**Sly**	*β- Glucronidase*	- Dermatan sulfate - Heparan sulfate - Chondroitin 4/6- sulfate

Mucolipidosis (MLS)

I	**Sialidosis**	*Sialidase (neuraminidase)*	Glycoprotein fragments
II	**I- Cell disease**	UDP- N- acetyl glucosamine: glucoprotein- N- acetylgluco samininylphospho transferase (Acid hydrolases thus lack phosphomannosyl residues)	Glycoprotein fragments
III	**Pseudo Hurler Polydystrophy**	As with ML-II but deficiency is incomplete	Glycoprotein fragments

★ **Mucolipidosis (MLS)** denote diseases that combine features common to both *mucopolysaccharidoses & sphingolipidoses*.

Keratins

Are fibrous insoluble proteins of animals derived from ectodermal (skin) cells. They include the structural protein elements of skin (leather is almost pure keratin) as well as the biological derivatives of ectoderm, such as hair, wool, scale, nails, quills, hoofs, horn & silk. There are two classes of keratins.

α- Keratins	β- Keratins
- Are relatively rich in cystine residues and thus contain many disulfide cross bridges - They contain most of the common amino acids - Include ***hard & brittle proteins containing high content of cystine (~22%) and so higher number of disulfide bonds. Eg- nails and horn***[Q]; as well as the ***softer, more flexible keratins of skin, hair and wool, which contain about 10- 14% of cystine (lesser disulfide bonds)***[Q].	- Contain *no cysteine or cystine* but are rich in aminoacids with small side chains particularly *glycine, alanine, and serine* - Are found in the fibers spun by spiders and silkworins and in scales, claws and beaks of reptiles and birds. - An important difference is that the *α- keratins stretch when heated*; hair for example stretches when exposed to moist heat but contracts to its normal length on cooling. The *β- Keratins do not stretch under these conditions.*

Molecular Motors

Molecular motors are ATPase that move proteins, organelles, and other cell parts (their cargo) to all parts of the cells.

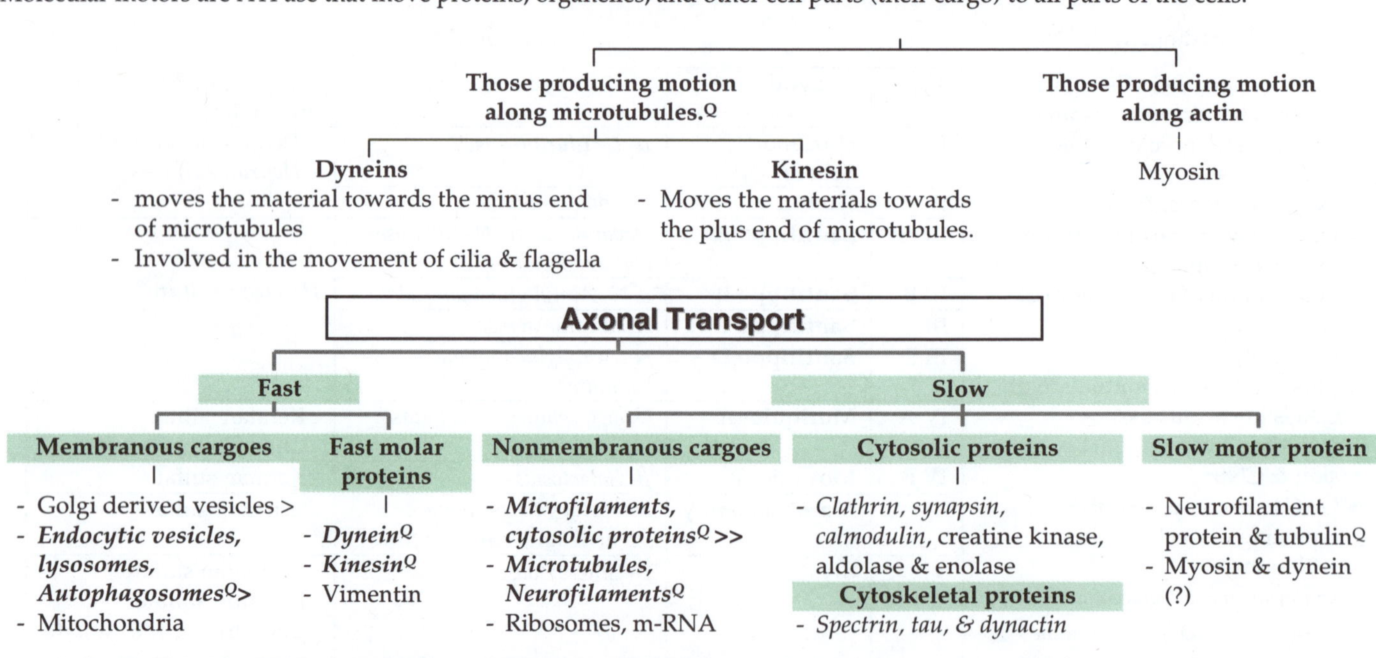

Axonal Transport of Membranous & Non membranous Cargoes

- It is now known that intracellular transport is coordinate by **molecular motor proteins** that bind cargoes and convey them in a particular direction along cytoskeletal polymer tracks. This includes every type of membranous organelle and transport vesicle (**membranous cargoes**), as well as **nonmembranous cargoes** such as cytoskeletal polymers, cytosolic protein complexes, ribosomes, and messenger RNAs.
- **Membranous organelles move most rapidly**, in the fast components of axonal transport, whereas **nonmembranous cytoskeletal polymers and cytosolic protein complexes move more slowly**, in the slow components. Recent studies suggest that slow axonal transport is generated by fast motors and that the slow rate is due to rapid movements interrupted by prolonged pauses.
- Materials destined for the axon are transported **anterogradely**, toward the axon tip, and materials destined to return are transported **retrogradely**, toward the cell body. This **bidirectional transport** process, known as **axonal transport**, is not fundamentally different from the pathways of macromolecular and membrane traffic that occur in all eukaryotic cells, but it is remarkable for its scale

- Membranous organelles are the principal cargoes of fast axonal transport. The many proteins, lipids, and polysaccharides that move along the axon at fast rates do so by virtue of their association with one or more subclasses of organelle or vesicle, either because they are sequestered within its lumen, embedded in its membrane, or bound to its surface.
- Both **neurofilaments and microtubules move at fast rates**, approaching the rate of movement of membranous organelles, **but the average rate of movement is slow** because the movements are both infrequent and bidirectional. Thus, the overall speed and direction of neurofilament and microtubule movement is a temporal summation of anterograde and retrograde movements and pauses, perhaps not fundamentally dissimilar from the behavior of mitochondria in axons described above. As is the case for mitochondria, the slow overall rate of movement of neurofilaments and microtubules suggests that these structures move with a low duty ratio, spending most of their time not moving.
- The **rapid rate of movement** of neurofilaments and microtubules in axons indicates that they are transported by fast motors, perhaps similar or identical to motors that move membranous organelles. Several lines of evidence suggest that **dynein** may transport axonal microtubules anterogradely, perhaps relative to the microfilament matrix, and that **dynein and kinesin** may transport axonal neurofilaments bidirectionally along microtubules by the same mechanism that is thought to move **vimentin** along microtubules in nonneuronal cells
- **Cytoskeletal proteins** have been the exclusive focus of studies on **slow axonal transport** in recent years, but it is important to remember that several hundred other proteins also move in this rate group, representing the entire spectrum of cytosolic proteins that comprise axoplasm. Some examples include proteins involved in vesicle dynamics such as clathrin and synapsin; regulatory proteins such as calmodulin; metabolic enzymes such as creatine kinase, aldolase, and enolase; cytoskeletal proteins such as **spectrin, tau, and dynactin**; and motor proteins such as dynein and myosin
- Cytoskeletal polymer tracks are made up of intracellular network of filamentous structure. All eukeryotic cells have 3 types of filaments - Microfilaments (actin filaments)
    - Microtubules (tubulin filaments)
    - Intermediate filaments has 4 classes: keratins, neurofilaments, lamins and vimentin like proteins

Golgi Complex (Apparatus) / Dictyosome

- It is a collection of smooth membrane enclosed sacs (*cisterns*) that are stalked like dinner plates, usually near the nucleus. It has membrane similar to those of smooth ER. It is usually composed of ≥4 stalked layers of ≥6 sacs in each apparatus
- It is a **polarized structure** with a ***cis (proximal) and trans (distal) sides***[Q].

Cis side of GC receives or ***transpost endoplasmic reticulum (ER) vesicles***[Q] containing newly synthesized proteins	In **median part** of golgi lumen, post translational modification takes place to form *glycoprotein & lipoprtein* by adding carbohydrate & lipid moeity respectively	**Trans side** of GC release proteins in ***secretory vesicle***[Q], which shuttle to *cell surface & lysosome*

★ Presence of **SNAREs (Soluble N-ethylmalemite – sensitive factor attachment receptor)** *protein* determine, where inside the cell vesicle would go. V (for vesicle) SNAREs interact with t (for target) SNAREs. In this way vesicles are ticketed for specific loci (eg cell membrane , GC, lysosome) by particular molecule such as mannose- 6 – phosphate.

★ ***Initial glycosylation of proteins occurs in ER***[Q] by attachment of preformed oligosaccharides but these oligosaccharides *undergo modifications to form variety of different carbohydrate moieties in golgi apparatus.*

★ Lysosome is present in all animal cells ***except RBC***[Q]. It has pH (~5) lower than that of cytosol. Acid phosphatase is its marker

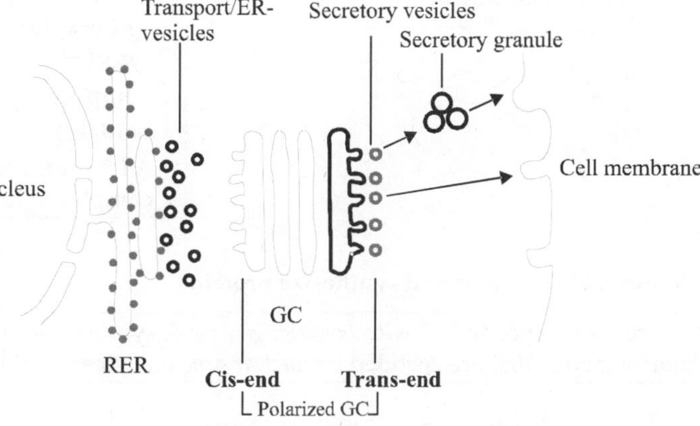

Enzymes & Metabolic Functions of Mitochondria

Outer Membrane

- For activation & transport of fatty acids (FA)
  - **Acyl Co A synthetase (thiokinase)** activates free FA
  - **Carnitine palmitoyl transferase 1** (transports longchain FA as carnitine derivatives)
- Biosynthesis of triacyglycerol & phospholipids
  - **Glycerol phosphate acyl transferase**
- **Monoamine oxidase (MAO)** for neurotransmitter metabolism
- *Kynureninase* (tryptophan metabolism)
- Phospholipase A_2
- Nucleoside di phosphokinase
- Cytochrome b_5 & cytochrome b_5 reductase
- Uncoupling proteins
- Dihydrorotate dehydrogenase (of pyrimidine metabolism)

Inter membrane space (b/w outer & inner membrane)

- *Creatine kinase*[Q] (of creatine phosphate shuttle facilitating transport of high energy phosphate from mitochondria) in active tissues such as heart & skeletal muscle
- Adenyl (adenylate kinase)
- Nucleoside diphosphokina se
- Sulfite oxidase

Inner Membrane

- Relative impermeability of inner **membrane** necessitates **exchange transporters**
  - Phosphate & adenine nucleotide transporter
  - Dicarboxylate & tricarboxylate transporter
  - Pyruvate symport
  - α-ketoglutarate and glutamate/aspartate transporter (of *Mallae shuttle*)
  - Glycerol 3 phosphate dehydrogenase (of *Glycerophosphate shuttle*) on outer surface
  - Energy linked proton tranlocating transhydrogenase
  - **Carnitine palmitoyl transferase 2** and **carnitine acyl carnitine translocase** (in transport of long chain of FA)
- Ketone body formation
  - D (-) -3- hydroxybutyrate dehydrogenase
- Enzymes of oxidative phosphorylation or respiratory chain which include
  - Electron transferring **flavoproteins eg complex I (NADH dehydrogenase complex II (Succinate dehydrogenase)**
  - CoenzymeQ (ubiquinone)
  - Electron transferring cytochromes eg **Complex III (cytochrome b c_1)** cytochrome c
    Complex IV(Cytochrome aa_3 or oxidase)
  - **ATP synthase (F1/F0 ATPase or complex V** for *ATP synthesis*)

Soluble Matrix

- **Pyruvate dehydrogenase**
- **Enzymes of TCA (citric acid cycle)**
  - Citrate synthase
  - Aconitase
  - Isocitrate dehydrogenase
  - α-Ketoglutarate (α-oxaloglutarate) dehydrogenase
  - Succinate thiokinase (succinyl Co A synthatase)
  - Fumarase
  - Malate dehydrogenase
- Anplerotic reactions (by which cycle intermediates are siphoned off in other pathways or replenished)
  - ***Aspartate amino transferase (SGOT)***[Q]
  - ***Glutamate dehydrogenase***[Q]

★Both in urea cycle

- **Urea cycle enzyme**
  - ***Carbamoyl phosphate synthetase 1***[Q]
  - N-acetylglutamate synthase
  - ***Ornithine transcarbamoylase***[Q]
- Alcohol metabolism
  - ALDH2
- **Glutaminase**
- **Enzymes of β oxidation**
- Heme synthesis (part)
  - ALA (aminolevulinate) synthase

Mitochondria both import and synthesize proteins

- 13 proteins are encoded by *mitochondrial genome* & synthesized in that organelle using its own protein synthesizing system
- Majority (about 100) are encoded by *nuclear gene* on cytosolic polyribosome and imported to mitochondria

Location of Liver Enzymes

Plasma (cell) membrane (bound)	Cytosolic or Cytoplasmic	Mitochondrial Matrix
- ***5[1] Nucleotidase (or Nucleotide phosphatase, NTP)***[Q] - Gamma Glutamyl Transferase (or Transpeptidase = GGT) - Alkaline phosphatase (ALP)	- Lactate dehydrogenase (LDH) - SGPT (Serum glutamate **pyruvate transaminase**) or **ALT** (alanine amino transferase) - SGOT (AST) cytosolic isoenzyme	- ***Glutamate dehydrogenase (GDH)***[Q] - SGOT (serum glutamate oxaloacetate transaminase) or AST (**aspartate** aminotransferase) – ***mitochondrial isoenzyme***[Q]

Major Proteins of

Cartilage		Bone	
Collagen Protein	**Non Collagen protein Mn-"ACP"**	**Collagen protein**	**Non Collagen Protein**
• ***Collagen type*** 2[Q] (90-98% of all articular cartilage collagen) • Collagen – 5, 6, 9, 10, 11	• Anchorin C-2 • Chondronectin • Proteoglycans - ***Aggrecan***[Q] (major proteoglycan) - Non – aggregating large proteoglycan - DS – PG1 (biglycan) - DS – PG2 (decorin)	• ***Collagen type 1***[Q] (90% of total bone protein) • **Collagen type-5**	• **Bone specific** - *Osteocalcin* - *Bone sialoprotein* - *CSPG III* • Non specific - Bone morphogenetic proteins (BMPS) - Osteopontin - Osteonectin (Bone SPARC Protein) - Proteoglycans C S-PG1 (biglycan) & CS – PG2 (decorin) - Plasma proteins

Cytoskeleton

The cell cytoplasm is not a sac of fluid. Essentially all eukaryotic cells contain three types of filamentous structures (responsible for ***cell shape change)***[Q].

Actin (Micro) Filaments (*7- 9.5 nm* in diameter)	**Inter mediate Filaments** (*10-12 nm* in diameter)	**Microtubules** (*25 nm* in diameter)
- G – actin (present in most cells) spontaneously polymerizes to form a double helical F- actin filaments in appropriate conc. of *Mg^{++} and KCl* - F actin form microfilaments that exists as bundles of tangled appearing meshwork underlying plasma	Most are relatively stable components of cytoskeleton not under going rapid assembly & disassembly and not disappearing during mitosis, as do actin and many microtubular filaments. As important exception is laminin, which subsequent to phosphorylation, disassemble at mitosis and reappear when it terminates.	- ***Are necessary for formation and function of the mitotic spindle***[Q] ***and thus are present in all eukaryotic cells.*** - Involved in ***intracellular movements of endocytic & exocytic vesicles***[Q], and form the major structural component of *cilia & flagella.* - In *axons & dendrites* they maintain structure & participate in *axoplasmic flow* of material. - Microtubule consists of *13* longitudinally arranged profilaments, each consisting of *dimers of α & β tubulin.* + *Organizing center,* located around a pair of centriole, **γ-tubulin, GTP and MAPs**[Q] (microtubule associated proteins eg. tau) play important role in assembly & stabilization

membrane referred to as *stress fibers.*

- Stress fibers disappear as cell motality increases or upon malignant transformation of cells by chemical or onchogenic viruses.

Proteins	Distributions
Keratins	
Type I (acidic) Type II (basic)	Epithelial cells, hair, nails
Vimentin-like	
Vimentin	Various mesenchymal cells
Desmin	Muscle
Glial fibrillary acid protein	Glial cells
Peripherin	Neurons
Neurofilaments	
Low (L), medium (M), and high (H)	Neurons
Lamins	
A, B and C	Nuclear lamina

- Microtubules are in ***state of dynamic instability***Q constantly assembling and disassembling. They *exhibit polarity* ***(plus & minus ends)***Q this is important in their growth & their ability to direct intracellular movements.
- Some drugs eg ***colchicines, vinblastin, paclitaxel & griseofulvin***Q bind to micro tubule and interfere with their assembly or disassembly

Protein	Function
Dynamin (use GTP)	Involved in *endocytosis*
Kinesin (use ATP)	In *Axonal transport to move* vesicle down the axon to wards the +ve end of microtubule formation
Cytosolic Dynein (use ATP)	In axonal transport flow of material towards negative end
Axonemal Dyneins	Power ciliary flagellar movement

Cell Cycle

- Cell cycle is the period of time between the birth of a cell and its own division to produce two daughter cells. It can be divided into **4 distinct phases**, which are **G1, S, G2, M.** The combination of **G1, S & G2** phases is k/a **interphase** and **M phase** is the **mitotic phase**.
- The duration of cell cycle and its stages varies greatly between cell types. The ***time taken for S, G_2 and M phases are similar for most cell types***Q, occupying about 6-8, 2-4 and 1-2 hours respectively whereas the duration of ***G_1 shows considerable variation***Q as *short as 2 hours* in rapidly dividing cells i.e. embryonic tissue or *longer than 12 hours* in some adult tissue.
- **G_1 phase** – ***is most variable***Q because, in this phase cells are not committed to DNA replication, *can enter resting state or progress to next cell division.* In mammals because of the time required for a cell to progress of S – phase through mitosis from beginning is typically 12-24 hours irrespective of duration of G_1 phase; almost all the ***variation in proliferating rates are attributable to the amount of time spent in G_1/Go state***Q.

Phase		State	Description
G0	Gap 0	**Quiescent (Senescent or Resting) Phase**	Cells that retain the capacity for proliferation, but which are no longer dividing have entered resting (quiescent) phase, even though they may be quite active physiologically. Growth factors can stimulate quiescent cell to leave Go and re enter the cell cycle.
G1	Gap 1	**Presynthetic phase**	In this phase *cell responds to growth factors, irreversibly directing cells to start another cell cycle.* During G1, most of the molecular, machinery required to complete another cell cycle is generated. Proteins encoded by certain tumor suppressor genes (eg Rb) block the cell cycle in G1 check point.
S	**Synthesis**	**DNA synthesis (replication)**	***DNA synthesis (or replication of genome)***Q occurs during S phase, at the end of which the DNA content of cell has doubled.
G2	Gap 2	**Premitotic**	During G2, cell prepares for division; cytoplasmic enlargement & DNA repair can occur; phase ends with onset of chromosome condensation and breakdown of nuclear membrane
M	**Mitosis**	Cell division (mitosis)	Cell growth stops and cell divides into 2 daughter cells with identical copies of parent cell genome

NOTES

BIOCHEMISTRY

MCQs with Answers and Explanations

Chapter -1 CARBOHYDRATE METABOLISM

QUESTIONS

Glycolysis

1. **Enzyme catalyzing reversible step in glycolysis is /are:** *(PGI 14,10)*
   A. Phosphofructokinase ☐
   B. Enolase ☐
   C. Pyruvate kinase ☐
   D. Phospho-glyceromutase ☐
   E. Glyceraldehyde-3-phosphate-dehydrogenase ☐
2. **Enzyme responsible for complete oxidation of glucose to CO_2 to water is present in** *(AIIMS 15,07)*
   A. Cytosol ☐
   B. Mitochondria ☐
   C. Lysosomes ☐
   D. Endoplasmic reticulum ☐
3. **About glycolysis true is:** *(PGI 09)*
   A. Occurs in mitochondria ☐
   B. Complete breakdown of glucose ☐
   C. Conversion of glucose to 3C units ☐
   D. 3 ATP's are used in anaerobic pathway ☐
4. **Fluroide ions act by inhibiting -** *(PGI 05)*
   A. Enolase ☐
   B. Hexokinase ☐
   C. Cytochrome oxidase ☐
   D. Carbonic anydrase ☐
5. **In glycolytic pathway, products formed are**
   A. Fructose-2, 6-Biphosphate *(AIIMS 12)* ☐
   B. Fructose-1, 6-Biphosphate ☐
   C. Glyceraldehyde-3-Phosphate ☐
   D. All of the above ☐
6. **Compound that joints glycolysis with glycogenesis & glycogenolysis** *(Jipmer 04, WB-03, Assam 05)*
   A. Glucose 1, 6 bi phosphate ☐
   B. Glucose 1 PO_4 ☐
   C. Glucose 6 PO_4 ☐
   D. Fructose 1, 6 bi phosphate ☐
7. **Peroxidase enzyme is used in estimating**
   A. Haemoglobin *(AIIMS 07)* ☐
   B. Ammonia ☐
   C. Creatinine ☐
   D. Glucose ☐
8. **Which of the following enzymes catalyze the irreversible steps of glycolysis?** *(AIIMS 13)*
   A. Glucokinase, phosphofructokinase, pyruvate carboxylase ☐
   B. Hexokinase, fructose1, 6 biphosphatese, pyruvate kinase ☐
   C. Glucokinase, phosphofructokinase, pyruvate kinase ☐
   D. Enolase, fructose 1,6 biphospahatase, phosphofructokinase ☐
9. **Key glycolytic enzymes for irreversible step (s) in glycolysis is/are:** *(PGI 12, 08)*
   A. Enolase ☐
   B. Phosphofructokinase ☐
   C. Pyruvate kinase ☐
   D. Glyceraldehyde-3-phosphate dehydrogenase ☐
   E. Hexokinase ☐
10. **In glycolysis, the first commited step is catalysed by** :
   A. 2 ,3 DPG *(AIIMS 07)* ☐
   B. Glucokinase ☐
   C. Hexokinase ☐
   D. Phosphofructokinase. ☐
11. **The rate-limiting enzyme in Glycolysis is** : *(AI 02)*
   A. Phosphofructokinase ☐
   B. Glucose-6-dehydrogenase ☐
   C. Glucokinase ☐
   D. Pyruvate kinase ☐
12. **Glycolytic enzymes (s) inhibited by fluoride:**
   A. Hexokinase *(PGI 08)* ☐
   B. Aldolase ☐
   C. Enolase ☐
   D. Pyruvate Kinase ☐
   E. Phosphofructokinase ☐
13. **Fluoride, used in the collection of blood samples for glucose estimation, inhibits the enzyme**: *(AI 05)*
   A. Glucokinase. ☐
   B. Hexokinase. ☐
   C. Enolase. ☐
   D. Glucose-6-phosphatase. ☐
14. **Fluoride inhibits which enzyme** *(AI 03)*
   A. Pyruvate kinase ☐
   B. Succinyl dehydrogenase ☐
   C. Enolase ☐
   D. Aldolase ☐
15. **Anticoagulant used to estimate glucose from a sample sent from PHC is:** *(AIIMS 11, 06)*
   A. EDTA ☐
   B. Calcium oxalate ☐
   C. Potassium oxalate + NaF ☐
   D. Sodium citrate ☐
16. **Which of the following anticoagutant used in estimating blood glucose prevents glycolysis -**
   A. Oxalate *(DNB 06)* ☐
   B. Citrate ☐
   C. NaF ☐
   D. Heparin ☐
17. **Cancer cells derive nutrition from** *(AIIMS 01)*
   A. Glycolysis ☐
   B. Oxidative phosphorylation ☐
   C. Increase in mitochondria ☐
   D. From a fast food joint ☐
18. **Insulin acts on which enzyme in glycoysis-** *(AI 03)*
   A. Glucokinase ☐
   B. Hexokinase ☐

C. Glucose 6-Phosphatase ☐
D. Adenylate kinase ☐

19. **True statements about Glucokinase is/are:** *(PGI 03)*
A. Km value is higher than normal blood sugar ☐
B. Found in liver ☐
C. G-6P inhibit it. ☐
D. Has both Glucose 6 Phosphatase and Kinase activity ☐
E. Glucose enter into cells through GLUT-2 ☐

20. **After overnight fasting, levels of Glucose transporters are reduced in** *(AIIMS 10, AI 09)*
A. Brain cells ☐
B. Hepatocytes ☐
C. Adipocytes ☐
D. RBCs ☐

21. **Insulin dependent entry of glucose is seen in-**
A. Liver *(NBE P 15)* ☐
B. Brain ☐
C. Heart ☐
D. Kidney ☐

22. **Glucose is transported in pancreas through which receptor-** *(NBE P 15)*
A. GLUT 1 ☐
B. GLUT 2 ☐
C. GLUT 3 ☐
D. GLUT4 ☐

23. **Within the RBC, hypoxia stimulates glycolysis by which of the following regulating pathways?** *(AI 07)*
A. Hypoxia Stimulates pyruvate dehydrogenase by increased 2,3 DPG ☐
B. Hypoxia inhibits hexokinase ☐
C. Hypoxia stimulates release of all Glycolytic enzymes from Band 3 on RBC membrane ☐
D. Activation of the regulatory enzymes by high PH ☐

24. **TCA cycle does not take place in -** *(JIPMER 02, AI 05)*
A. Hepatocyte ☐
B. Osteocyte ☐
C. Neuron ☐
D. Erythrocyte ☐

25. **Mature RBC contains all except -** *(AIIMS 04)*
A. Enzyme of HMP shunt pathway ☐
B. Enzyme of TCA cycle ☐
C. Glycoytic enzymes ☐
D. Pyridine nubleotides ☐

26. **The end product of one stage fermentation is -**
A. Formic acid *(JIPMER 05, PGI 04)* ☐
B. Pyruvate ☐
C. Lactate ☐
D. Ethanol ☐

Shuttle Systems

27. **During gluconeogensis reducing equivalents from mitochondria to cytosol are transported by**
A. Malate *(AIIMS 02)* ☐
B. Aspartate ☐
C. Glutamate ☐
D. Oxaloacetate ☐

28. **Malate shuttle is important in** *(AIIMS 04, AI 08)*
A. Glycogenolysis ☐
B. Glycolysis ☐
C. Gluconeogenesis ☐
D. HMP shunt ☐

PDH Complex

29. **Congenital lactic acidosis may occur d/t defect in**
A. Pyruvate decarboxylase *(AI 10)* ☐
B. PDH complex ☐
C. Transketolase ☐
D. α-ketoglutarate dehydrogenase ☐

30. **First substrate of Kreb's cycle is:** *(AIIMS 07)*
A. Pyruvate ☐
B. Glycine ☐
C. HCl ☐
D. Lipoprotein ☐

31. **Coenzymes for pyruvate dehydrogenase are A/E**
A. TPP *(Jipmer 03, WB 02, KA 01)* ☐
B. CoA ☐
C. Lipoic acid ☐
D. FAD ☐
E. NADPH ☐

32. **Pyruvate dehydrogenase complex has all enzyme components except** *(SGPGI 04, AMU 05, UP 05)*
A. Decarboxylase ☐
B. Transacetylase ☐
C. Dehydrogenase ☐
D. Phosphatase ☐

33. **Pyruvate dehydrogenase contains all except -**
A. Biotin *(NBE P 13,14)* ☐
B. NAD ☐
C. FAD ☐
D. CoA ☐

34. **Which of the following vitamins does not pariciate in oxidative decarboxylation of pyruvate to acetyl CoA-**
A. Thiamine *(NBE P 15)* ☐
B. Niacin ☐
C. Riboflavin ☐
D. Biotin ☐

35. **Pyruvate can be converted directly into all the following except:** *(AI 02)*
A. Phosphoenol pyruvate ☐
B. Alanine ☐
C. Acetyl CoA ☐
D. Lactate ☐

36. **Arsenic inhibits all except** *(AI 009, UP 10)*
A. PDH ☐
B. Lipoic acid ☐
C. α-KG dehydrogenase ☐
D. Enolase ☐

37. **Thiamine deficiency causes decreased energy production because** *(AI 11, AIIMS 08)*
A. It is required for the process of transamination ☐
B. It is co-factor in oxidative reduction ☐
C. It is co-enzyme for transketolase in pentose phosphate pathway ☐
D. It is co-enzyme for pyruvate dehydrogenase. ☐

Citric Acid Cycle

38. Oxaloacetate + Acetyl CoA → Citrate + CoASH This reaction is: *(AIIMS 04)*
A. Reversible ☐
B. Irreversible ☐
C. Can be reversed by catalase ☐
D. Competitive ☐

39. In TCA cycle of tricarboxylic acid, which is first formed *(Assam 04, WB 01, Bihar 02)*
A. Isocitrate ☐
B. Citrate ☐
C. Succinate ☐
D. Fumarate ☐

40. In TCA cycle, citrate is converted into, after losing a molecule of H_2O - *(DNB 09, UP 01)*
A. Isocitrate ☐
B. Cis-aconitate ☐
C. Oxaloacelate ☐
D. Glutarate ☐

41. Which of following inhibitor in TCA cycle acts by blocking citrate - *(KA 03, TN 02)*
A. Fluroacetate ☐
B. Arsenite ☐
C. Malonate ☐
D. None of the above ☐

42. Fluroacetate inhibits - *(AP 01, CMC 09, JIPMER 08)*
A. Citrate synthetase ☐
B. Aconitase ☐
C. Succinate dehydrogenase ☐
D. Alphaketoglutarate dehydrogenase ☐

43. Which one of the following is the correct sequential order in which the given enzymes of Kreb's cycle are formed after a molecule of acetyl CoA enters the cycle-
A. Citrate, Oxaloacetate, Ketoglutarate *(DNB 11)* ☐
B. Ketoglutarate, Oxaloacetate, Citrate ☐
C. Citrate, Ketoglutarate, Oxalocetate ☐
D. Oxaloacetate, Ketoglutarate, Citrate ☐

44. Specific poison for succinate dehydrogenase is -
A. Cyanide *(Delhi 03, Raj 04, Rohtak 04)* ☐
B. Malonate ☐
C. Arsenite ☐
D. Fluoride ☐
E. Malate ☐

45. What is the substrate for the only physiologically irreversible reaction in the Kreb's Citric acid cycle-
A. Citrate *(NBE P 13)* ☐
B. Alpha ketoglutarate ☐
C. Succinate ☐
D. Malate ☐

46. Intermediate metabolite in TCA cycle are A/E:
A. Pyruvate *(PGI 06)* ☐
B. Isocitrate ☐
C. Oxaloacetate ☐
D. Malonate ☐
E. Nitric oxide ☐

47. Which of the following substance binds to acetyl CoA and condenses OAA, inhibiting the TCA cycle:
A. Arsenite *(AIIMS 10)* ☐
B. Fluoroacetate ☐
C. Malonate ☐
D. Fumararte ☐

48. Malonate competetively inhibits- *(AIIMS 05)*
A. Fumarate dehydrogenase ☐
B. Succinate thiokinase ☐
C. Aconitase ☐
D. Succinate dehydrogenase ☐

49. Number of ATPs produced from adipose tissue from 1 NADH (NAD+/NADH) through respiratory *(PGI 11)*
A. 0 ATP ☐
B. 1 ATP ☐
C. 2 ATP ☐
D. 2.6 ATP ☐
E. 3 ATP ☐

50. ATP'S are formed in the following steps of kreb's cycle: *(PGI 06)*
A. Isocitrate dehydrogenase ☐
B. Succinate dehydrogenase ☐
C. Succinate thiokinase ☐
D. Malate dehydrogenase ☐

51. In TCA cycle, CO_2 is released from: *(PGI 08)*
A. Thiokinase ☐
B. Isocitrate dehydrogenase ☐
C. Citrate dehydrogenase ☐
D. Alpha ketoglutrate ☐

52. Proper functioning of Kreb cycle does not occur with deficiency of: *(PGI 2K)*
A. Thiamane ☐
B. Riboflavin ☐
C. Vitamin E ☐
D. Vit K ☐

53. Which among the following controls is an allosteric inhibitor of TCA cycle: *(PGI 09)*
A. Pyruvate dehydrogenase ☐
B. Keto glutarate dehydrogenase ☐
C. Isocitrate dehydrogenase ☐
D. Malate dehydrogenase ☐

54. In vivo control of citric acid cycle is effected by:
A. Acetyl CoA *(PGI 01)* ☐
B. Coenzyme A ☐
C. ATP ☐
D. Citrate ☐
E. NADH ☐

55. Of the following groups of amino acids produce common component of the TCA cycle is:
A. Alaine, isoleucine, leucine, lysine *(PGI 09)* ☐
B. Serine, asparagines, glycine, glutamate ☐
C. Isoleucine, valine, methionine ☐
D. Prolone, leucine, tryptophan ☐

56. Substrate level phosphorylation is catalysed by : *(AIIMS 10,14; NBE P 15,14)*
A. Succinate dehydrogenase ☐
B. Succinate Thiokinase ☐

C. Malate dehydrogenase
D. Hexokinase

57. Substrate level phosphorylation is seen in the conversion of: *(NBE P 15, 14; AI 09)*
A. Acetoacetate to a-keto glutarate
B. Succinyl CoA to Succinate
C. Fumarate to malate
D. Succinate to fumarate

58. Substrate-level phosphorylation seen in reaction catalysed in: *(PGI 15,13,08)*
A. Succinate dehydrogenase
B. Alfa-ketoglutarate dehydrogenase
C. Succinyl CoA thiokinase
D. Malate dehydrogenase
E. Cis-aconitase

High Energy Compounds

59. Immediate energy supply for muscle contraction- *(NBE P 15)*
A. GTP
B. ATP
C. Creatine phosphate
D. Fatty acid

60. Immediate source of energy is- *(NBE P 15)*
A. Cori's cycle
B. HMP
C. ATP
D. TCA cycle

61. Which energy molecule gives 10.5 kcal/molecule- *(NBE P 15)*
A. ATP
B. GTP
C. Creatine phosphate
D. Glucose-6=phosphate

62. Which of the following is high energy phosphate bond (produce ATP on hydrolysis): *(NBE P 15,13;PGI 15,11)*
A. F-6-phosphate
B. Creatine phosphate & Carbamoyl phosphate
C. Glucose-1-phosphate
D. Glucose-6-phosphate

63. High energy phosphate compounds are: *(PGI 12, 10)*
A. ATP
B. ADP
C. Creatinine phosphate
D. Acetyl CoA
E. Glucose 1 phosphate & glucose 3 phosphate

Respiratory Chain and Oxidative Phosphorylation

64. Among the following, the maximum redox potential is for: *(PGI 08, 05)*
A. NADH/NAD
B. Succinate/Fumarate
C. Ubiquinone
D. Fe^{+3}/ Fe^{+2}

65. Which vitamin is involved in Redox reactions- *(NBE P 15)*
A. Pyridoxin
B. Biotin
C. Folic acid
D. Riboflavin

66. Riboflavin is a constituent of- *(NBE P 15)*
A. FMN
B. NAD
C. PLP
D. THF

67. In oxidative phosphorylation, the ATP production and respiratory chain are linked by: *(AI 02)*
A. Chemical methods
B. Physical methods
C. Chemiosmotic methods
D. Conformational changes

68. About oxidative phosphorylation true is: *(PGI 07)*
A. Generation of ATP's
B. Generation of ADP's
C. Utilization of ATP's
D. Utilization of NADP

69. ATP is generated in ETC by- *(NBE P 15)*
A. Na + k+ ATPase
B. Na + CI-ATPase
C. Fo F_1 ATPase
D. ADP Kinase

70. Which component transfers four protons: *(PGI 10, 09)*
A. NADH-Q Oxidoreductase
B. Cytochrome –C oxidase
C. Cytochrome C - Q oxidoredictase
D. Isocitrate Dehydrogenase
E. Succinate Q Reductase

71. In ETC, Oxidative phosphylartion (ATP formation) is regulated by: *(PGI 11)*
A. NADH Co-Q reductase
B. Cytochrome C oxidase
C. Glutathione reductase
D. Isocitrate dehydrogenase
E. Co-Q-Cytochrome C reductase

72. True about ATP synthase is all except: *(PGI 05)*
A. One rotation produce 3 ATP
B. Fo unit functions as proton channel
C. α and β subunits rotate
D. Bent axle is formed by ε and γ subunits

73. Internal respiration are: *(PGI 03)*
A. Exergonic and anabolic
B. Exergonic and catabolic
C. Endergonic and anabolic
D. Endergonic and catabolic
E. Cytochrome-C reductase involved

74. Mitochondrial membrane protein contain transporter of: *(PGI 03)*
A. NADH
B. Acetyl COA
C. NADPH
D. ATP

75. Inernal respiration are: *(PGI 03)*
A. Exergonic and anabolic
B. Exergonic and catabolic
C. Endergonic and anabolic
D. Endergonic and catabolic
E. Cytochrome-C reductase involved

76. Cyanide is toxic because it - *(DNB 14, PGI 04)*
A. Inhibits cytochrome oxidase ☐
B. Forms cyan meth Hb ☐
C. Inhibits ATP carrier in mitochondria ☐
D. Inhibits Na-K-ATP ase ☐

77. Cytochrome oxidase in oxidative phosphorylation is inhibited by: *(PGI 06, 02, 14)*
A. CO ☐
B. H_2S ☐
C. Cyanide ☐
D. Amobarbital ☐
E. Rotenone ☐

78. Cyanide affects respiratory chain by- *(NBE P 15)*
A. Non-competitive reversible inhibition ☐
B. Competitive reversible inhibition ☐
C. Suicide irreversible inhibition ☐
D. Non-competitive irreversible inhibition ☐

79. The electron flow in Cytochrome C oxidase can be blocked by: *(AIIMS 14, 06)*
A. Rotenone ☐
B. Antimycin-A ☐
C. Cyanide ☐
D. Actinomycin ☐

80. Cellular oxidation is inhibited by : *(AI 09; NBE P 13)*
A. Cyanide ☐
B. Carbon dioxide ☐
C. Chocolate ☐
D. Carbonated beverages ☐

81. The specialized mammalian tissue/organ in which fuel oxidation serves not to produce ATP but to generate heat is: *(AI 06)*
A. Adrenal gland ☐
B. Skeletal muscle ☐
C. Brown adipose tissue ☐
D. Heart ☐

82. Dinitrophenol causes: *(AI 07)*
A. Inhibition of ATP synthase ☐
B. Inhibition of electron transport ☐
C. Uncoupling of oxidation and phosphorylation ☐
D. Accumulation of ATP ☐

83. Which of following prevent formation of ATP by blocking movement of ADP across mitochondrial membrane: *(AIIMS 10)*
A. Atractyloside ☐
B. Rotenone ☐
C. Oligomycin ☐
D. Ouabain ☐

84. Atractiloside act as- *(NBE P 15)*
A. Uncoupler ☐
B. Inhibitor of oxidative phosphorylation ☐
C. Inhibitor of complex 1 OF ETC ☐
D. Inhibitor of complex III of ETC ☐

85. Natural uncoupler is- *(NBE P 15)*
A. Thermogonin ☐
B. 2,4 nitrophenol ☐
C. 2,4 Dinitrophenol ☐
D. Oligomycin ☐

86. During phagocytosis, the metabolic process called respiratory burst involves the activation of: *(AI 06)*
A. Oxidase ☐
B. Hydrolase ☐
C. Peroxidase ☐
D. Dehydrogenase ☐

87. Cytosolic Cytochrome C mediates *(AIIMS 06)*
A. Apoptosis ☐
B. Electron transport ☐
C. Krebs cycle ☐
D. Glycolysis ☐

88. RQ of a person on pure carbohydrate diet will be: *(AIIMS 16)*
A. 1 ☐
B. 0.7 ☐
C. 1.2 ☐
D. 1.5 ☐

Glycogen Metabolism & Storage Disease

89. Branching enzyme is found in- *(NBE P 15,13)*
A. Glycogenesis ☐
B. Glucogenesis ☐
C. Glycogenolysis ☐
D. Glycolysis ☐

90. Main enzyme for glycogen metabolism- *(NBE P 15,14)*
A. Glucose-6- phosphatase ☐
B. Glycogen synthase ☐
C. PFK-1 ☐
D. None of the above ☐

91. In glycogen metabolism, some metabolically important enzymes found in the liver are converted from their inactive dephosphorylated state to active phosphorylated state. Which of the following is true? *(AIIMS 12)*
A. Always activated by c AMP dependent protein kinase ☐
B. Commonly seen in fasting state than in fed state ☐
C. Catecholamines directly cause their phosphorylation ☐
D. ATP activates phosphorylase ☐

92. Adrenaline acts on which enzyme in glycogenolysis- *(AI 09)*
A. Glucokinase ☐
B. Hexokinase ☐
C. Phosphorylase ☐
D. Gluc diphosphatase ☐

93. The major fate of glucose-6 Phosphate in tissue in a well fed state is: *(AI 07)*
A. Hydrolysis to glucose ☐
B. Conversion to glycogen ☐
C. Isomerization to fructose 6 phosphate ☐
D. Conversion to ribulose 5 phosphate ☐

94. In the fed state, major fate of Glucose 6-PO_4 in tissues is *(AIIMS 03)*
A. Storage as Fructose ☐
B. Storage as Glyceraldehyde 3-PO_4 ☐
C. Enters HMP shunt via Ribulose 5-PO_4 ☐
D. Storage as glycogen ☐

95. **In muscle, phosphorylase b is inactivated by:**
A. cAMP *(AIIMS 08)* □
B. Ca ions □
C. Glucose □
D. ATP □

96. **True regarding glylcogenolysis is /are A/E** *(PGI 08)*
A. PP_1 is a dephosphorylating enzyme □
B. Vasopressin increases it □
C. Oxytocin decreases it □
D. Ca^{++} is a synchronizer and allosteric activator □
E. δ subunit is catalytic □

97. **Phosphorylase b is maintained in an inactivated state by** *(AI 08)*
A. ATP □
B. c AMP □
C. Calcium □
D. Insulin □

98. **Which of the following is a debranching enzyme -**
A. Glycogen synthetase *(AIIMS 15,14,10)* □
B. Glucose-6-phosphatase □
C. Amylo (1,6) glucosidase □
D. Amylo 1,4, - 1 , 6 transglycosylase □

99. **Sequence of events in glycogenolysis?** □
A. Phosphorylase, Glucan transferase , Debranching, Phosphorylase *(PGI 14,08)* □
B. Debranching, Phosphorylase, transferase, phosphorylase □
C. Transferase , phosphorylase, Debranching, phosphorylase □
D. Any of the above. □

100. **In which of the following tissues, is glycogen incapable of contributing directly to blood glucose?**
A. Liver *(AI 08)* □
B. Muscle □
C. Both □
D. None □

101. **The enzyme not present in the skeletal muscles OR Muscle cannot make use of glycogen for energy because of deficiency of** *(AIIMS 08, 15; PGI 14,12,06)*
A. Creatinine phosphokinase □
B. Hexokinase □
C. Phosphofructokinase □
D. Glucose 6 phosphatase. □

102. **Which of the following does not cross the cell membrane**
A. Glucose-6-phosphate *(AIIMS 02)* □
B. Glucose □
C. Nitrous oxide □
D. Carbon monoxide □

103. **Muscles are not involved in which glycogen storage disease:**
A. I *(PGI 12, 07)* □
B. II □
C. III □
D. IV □

104. **G_6 phosphatase deficiency seen in:** *(PGI 06, 09)*
A. Von Gierke's disease □
B. Taysach's disease □
C. Pompe's disease □
D. Anderson's disease □
E. Fabry's disease □

105. **An infant has hepatorenomegaly, hypoglycemia hyperlipidemia, acidosis & normal structured glycogen deposition in liver. What is the diagnosis:**
A. Her's disease *(PGI 01)* □
B. Von Gerke's ds □
C. Cori's ds □
D. Anderson's ds □
E. Pompe's ds □

106. **A person with von Gierke's disease has ketosis. All are true for ketosis in this patient except:** *(AIIMS 13)*
A. Lactic acidosis □
B. Hypoglycemia □
C. Fat mobilization is less □
D. Hypertriglyceridemia □

107. **The cause of hyperuricemia and gout in glucose-6-phosphatase deficiency is :** *(AIIMS 01)*
A. More formation of pentose □
B. Decreased availability of glucose to tissues □
C. Increased accumulation of sorbitol □
D. Impaired degradation of free radicals □

108. **Glycogen storage diseases include all the following except:**
A. Von Gierke's disease *(PGI 06)* □
B. Fabry's disease □
C. Mc Ardle's disease □
D. Fragile syndrome □
E. Krabbe's disease □

109. **Coris disease is due to defect in-** *(NBE P 15)*
A. Branching enzyme □
B. Debrandhing enzyme □
C. Myophosphorylase □
D. Hepatic phosphorylase □

110. **Which among the following is not a cause of fasting hypoglycemia?** *(AI 11)*
A. Glucagon excess □
B. Glucose 6 phospatase deficiency □
C. Uremia □
D. Glycogen synthase deficiency □

111. **Metabolites in HMP shunt are all except**
A. Glycerol-3 phosphate *(AI 05)* □
B. Sedoheptulose-7 phosphate □
C. Glyceraldehyde-3 phosphate □
D. Xylulose-5 phosphate □

112. **NADPH is produced by OR The major source of NADPH for fatty acid synthesis:**
A. Glycolysis *(AIIMS16,13,08; NBE P 14,13)* □
B. Citric acid cycle □
C. Hexose monophosphate shunt □
D. Glycogenesis □

113. **Which is NOT a product of Pentose phos-phate pathway** *(AIIMS 13,10)*
A. Glyceraldehyde 3-PO_4 □
B. NADPH □
C. Sedoheptulose PO_4 □
D. CO_2 □

114. NADPH is generated by the action of *(DNB 13,10)*
- A. Glucose 6 Phosphate dehydrogenase ☐
- B. Glucose 1 phosphate dehydrogenase ☐
- C. Glucose 1.6 diphosphate dehydrogenase ☐
- D. All of the above ☐

115. HMP shunt is of great importance in cellular metabolism because it produces -
- A. ATP *(NBE P 15; UP 04, WB 05)* ☐
- B. ADP ☐
- C. Acetyl CoA ☐
- D. NADPH ☐

116. Dehydrogenases of HMP shunt are specific for -
- A. FAD *(AIIMS 14; DNB 15)* ☐
- B. NAD ☐
- C. NADPH ☐
- D. FMN ☐

117. Which one of the following enzymes use NADP as coenzyme- *(DNB 14, 12)*
- A. Glyceraldehyde-3-phosphate dehydrogenase ☐
- B. Lactate dehydrogenase ☐
- C. Glucose-6-phosphate dehydrogenase ☐
- D. Beta hydroxy acyl CoA dehydrogenase ☐
- E. Mitochondrial isocitrate dehydrogenase ☐

118. Step in HMP pathway requiring TPP
- A. G6 PD *(AP 02, TN 01,KA 09)* ☐
- B. 6 Phoshogluconate dehydrogenase ☐
- C. Transketolase ☐
- D. Transaldolase ☐

119. The main products of HMP shunt are all except -
- A. 6-NADPH *(Raj 02, Delhi 03, Punjab 03)* ☐
- B. 2-Fructose-6-PO4 ☐
- C. 1-Glyceraldehyde-3-po4 ☐
- D. 1-CO_2 ☐

120. Which of the following enzyme is a constituent of HMP shunt- *(UP 04, BHU 05)*
- A. Glucose-6-phosphatase ☐
- B. Hexokinase ☐
- C. G-6-P dehydrogenase ☐
- D. Phosphorylase ☐

121. Sites where HMP shunts can occur include - *(PGI 05)*
- A. Liver ☐
- B. WBC ☐
- C. Lactating mammary gland ☐
- D. Testes ☐
- E. All ☐

122. Which of the following metabolic pathways does not generate ATP: *(AI 08)*
- A. Glycolysis ☐
- B. TCA Cycle ☐
- C. Fatty Acid Oxidation ☐
- D. HMP Pathway ☐

123. The most common enzyme deficiency in man is -
- A. Glucose-6-phosphate dehydrogenase ☐
- B. Glucose-6-phosphatase *(AP 08, AI 06)* ☐
- C. Hexokinase ☐
- D. Glucose-1.6-diphosphatse ☐

124. Regarding HMP shunt all of the following are true except: *(AI 07)*
- A. Occurs in the cytosol ☐
- B. No ATP is produced in the cycle ☐
- C. It is active in Adipose tissue, Liver and Gonads. ☐
- D. The oxidative phase generates NADPH and the Non oxidative phase generates pyruvate. ☐

125. In G-6PD deficient patient haemolysis is due to decrease in
- A. H^+ *(AIIMS 05)* ☐
- B. TPP ☐
- C. NADH ☐
- D. NADPH ☐

Calvin Cycle, Cori & Cahill Cycle

126. Enzymes of Calvin cycle are: *(PGI 10)*
- A. G-6-PD ☐
- B. Sedoheptulose- 1-7- bisphosphatase ☐
- C. Glyceraldehyde 3 PO_4 dehydrogenase ☐
- D. Phosphoribulose kinase ☐

127. Increased levels of alanine in serum after fasting suggest: *(AIIMS 11)*
- A. Increased release of alanine from muscle ☐
- B. Reduced amino acid utilization for gluconeogenesis ☐
- C. Break in continuity of plasma membrane resulting in leakage of amino acids ☐
- D. Decreased uptake of alanine by liver ☐

128. During prolonged starvation, the rate of gluconeogenesis depends on *(AIIMS 11)*
- A. Increased alanine levels in liver ☐
- B. Decreased cGMP in liver ☐
- C. ADP in liver ☐
- D. Decreased essential fatty acids in liver ☐

129. Transamination reaction is *(PGI 10)*
- A. Net deamination with splitting of NH_3 ☐
- B. α-ketoglutarate is NH_2 donor ☐
- C. Transaminase enzyme & pyridoxial PO_4 binding is covalent ☐
- D. Glutamate is formed ☐
- E. Non reversible pingpong reaction ☐

130. True about amino group of amino acid is *(PGI 09)*
- A. Accepted by α-ketoglutarate ☐
- B. Funneled to L- Glutamate ☐
- C. Prevents oxidative breakdown ☐
- D. Oxidative deamination is the 1st step to remove it ☐
- E. SGPT / SGOT transfer it ☐

131. True about glutamate dehydrogenase is A/E
- A. Liver mitochondrial enzyme *(AMU 09, UP 10)* ☐
- B. Use both NAD^+ or $NADP^+$ coenzyme ☐
- C. Inhibited by ADP & activated by GTP ☐
- D. Reversible oxidative deamination ☐

132. Gluconeogenesis from lactate needs all except-
- A. Transport oflactate from muscle to liver ☐
- B. Conversion of lactate to pyruvate *(NBE P 15)* ☐
- C. Transamination of pyruvate to alanine ☐
- D. None of the above ☐

133. During starvation, muscle uses- *(NBE P 15)*
A. Fatty acids ☐
B. Ketone bodies ☐
C. Glucose ☐
D. Proteins ☐

Gluconeogenesis

134. Glucose can be synthesized (by gluconeogenesis) from all except *(AIIMS 15,14,12; AI 10; NBE P 15,14, PGI 14,13)*
A. Aminoacids eg alanine ☐
B. Glycerol from adipose tissue ☐
C. Acetoacetate / Fatty acids/Palmitate /GH ☐
D. Lactate/Lactic acid/ Pyruvate ☐

135. Which is not ketogenic- *(NBE P 15)*
A. Leucine ☐
B. Lysine ☐
C. Methionine ☐
D. Tryptophan ☐

136. Which is not Glucogenic- *(NBE P 15)*
A. Arginine ☐
B. Histidine ☐
C. Glycine ☐
D. Lysine ☐

137. All are used in gluconeogenesis except- *(NBE P 15)*
A. Oleate ☐
B. Succinate ☐
C. Glutamate ☐
D. Aspartate ☐

138. True about Acetyl CoA: *(PGI 15,11)*
A. Precursor for synthesis of cholesterol and other steroids. ☐
B. Form ketone bodies ☐
C. Starting material for synthesis of fatty acid ☐
D. Arise from glycolysis ☐

139. Acetyl Co-A acts as a substrate for all the enzymes except:
A. HMG-Co A synthetase *(AIIMS 03)* ☐
B. Malic enzyme ☐
C. Malonyl CoA synthetase ☐
D. Fatty acid synthetase ☐

140. Acetyl CoA can be converted into all of the following, Except *(AI 09, AIIMS 11, 10)*
A. Glucose ☐
B. Fatty Acids ☐
C. Cholesterol ☐
D. Ketone bodies ☐

141. True about gluconeogenesis: *(PGI 13)*
A. Prevent hypoglycemia during prolonged fasting ☐
B. Occur in both muscle and liver ☐
C. Fructose 2,6-biphosphate stimulate it ☐
D. Excess of acetyl co A cause stimulation ☐
E. Carbon skeleton of amino acid is involved in gluconeogenesis ☐

142. True about gluconeogenesis- *(NBE P 15)*
A. Occurs mainly in muscle ☐
B. It is reverse of glycolysis ☐
C. Alanine & lactate both can serve as substrate ☐
D. Glycerol is not a substrate ☐

143. Which of the following enzymes is/are involved in neoglucogenesis except: *(PGI 15,13,08)*
A. Phosphoglycerate kinase ☐
B. Fructose 1, 6-biphosphatase ☐
C. Phosphoglucomutase ☐
D. Pyruvate carboxylase ☐
E. Isomerase

144. Enzyme to both common in gluconegenesis and glycolysis pathway is : *(NBE P 13; AI 08)*
A. Phosphofructokinase ☐
B. Fructose 2,6-biphosphatase ☐
C. Hexokinase ☐
D. Glucose 6 phosphatase ☐

145. Which of the enzyme of glycolysis is used in gluconeogenesis- *(AIIMS 13; NBE P 15,14)*
A. Glucokinase ☐
B. PFK ☐
C. Pyruvate kinase ☐
D. Phosphotriose isomerase ☐

146. Products formed from alcohol and not intermediates of TCA cycle/glycolysis: *(PGI 06)*
A. Acetaldehyde ☐
B. Pyruvate ☐
C. Lactate ☐
D. Oxalate ☐
E. Malate ☐

147. In well fed state gluconeogenesis in liver is inhibited by *(AIIMS 11, DNB 12)*
A. Protein breakdown in muscle ☐
B. Alanine content in liver ☐
C. ADP level ☐
D. cGMP ☐

148. Which of these is most effective for gluconeogenesis?
A. Citrate stimulation of acetyl carboxylase *(AIIMS16)* ☐
B. Acetyl-CoA stimulation of pyruvate carboxylase ☐
C. Fructose-2,6-biphosphate stimulation of phosphofructokinase-2 ☐
D. Fructose-1,6-biphosphate stimulation of phosphofructokinase-1 ☐

149. Gluconeogenesis in Fasting state is indicated by *(AIIMS 12)*
A. Citrate activation by acetyl Co-A carboxylase ☐
B. Pyruvate Carboxylase activation by Acetyl CoA ☐
C. Fructose 1,6 bisphosphate activates Pyruvate Kinase ☐
D. Fructose 2, 6 bisphosphate activates PFK-1 ☐

150. A genetic disorder renders fructose 1,6 – biphosphatase in liver less sensitive to regulation by fructose 2,6 – biphosphate. All of the following metabolic changes are observed in this disorder except: *(AI 04)*
A. Level of fructose 1,6-biphosphate is higher than normal ☐
B. Level of fructose 1,6 – biphosphate is lower than normal ☐
C. Less pyruvate is formed ☐
D. Less ATP is generated ☐

151. Phospho-dephosphorylation of phosphofructokinase and fructose 1, 6, biphosphatase by fructose 2, 6, Biphosphate regulation is seen in: *(PGI 03)*
- A. Brain
- B. Liver
- C. Adrenal Cortex
- D. RBC
- E. Muscle

152. Glyconeogenic capability of cell is determined by the presence of: *(PGI 05)*
- A. Pyruvate dehydrogenase
- B. Glucose 6 phosphatase
- C. Pyruvate carboxylase
- D. Fructose 1-6 biphosphatase
- E. Pyruvate carboxykinase

153. Which of the following events does not occur when concentration of glucose in the liver decreases: *(AI 12)*
- A. Inactivation of phosphofructokinase-2 (PFK-2)
- B. Activation of Fructose Bisphosphatase-2 (Fructose 2, 6 Bisphosphatase)
- C. Increased levels of Fructose 2, 6 – Bisphosphate
- D. Increased levels of Glucagon

154. After 50 gm of glucose is feed orally: *(PGI 08)*
- A. Decrease ketone body production
- B. Increased lactate production upon exercise
- C. Decreased gluconeogenesis
- D. Increased gluconeogenesis

155. PFK-1 inhibitor- *(NBE P 15)*
- A. AMP
- B. Citrate
- C. Glucose 6 phosphate
- D. Insulin

Fructose Metabolism

156. False about hereditary fructose intolerance is: *(AIIMS 08)*
- A. Deficiency of fructose 1- phosphate aldolase.
- B. Accumulation of fructose 1 - phosphate in tissues
- C. Hyperglycemia
- D. Liver & kidneys are involved.

157. Fructokinase is necessary for: *(PGI 08)*
- A. Fructose-1-PO_4
- B. Ructose 1,6 diphosphate
- C. Fructose 6 phosphate
- D. Glyceraldehyde

158. An enzyme involved in the catabolism of fructose to pyruvate in the liver is: *(AI 03)*
- A. Glyceraldehyde-3-phosphate Dehydrogenase
- B. Phosphoglucomutase
- C. Lactate-dehydrogenase
- D. Glucokinase

Galactose Metabolism & Intolerance

159. Enzyme defect in galactosemia- *(NBE P 15)*
- A. Uridyl transferase
- B. Galactokinase
- C. Epimerase
- D. All of the above

160. A few days after birth, a child becomes lethargic, refuses feeds and vomits during breast feeding. On examination he is pot bellied. Benedict's test is positive in urine. What is the likely reducing sybstance present in urine: *(AIIMS 10)*
- A. Glucose
- B. Fructose
- C. Sucrose
- D. Galactose

161. Galactosaemia commonly is due to deficiency of-
- A. Galactose-1 phosphate uridyl transferase
- B. Galactose-1 phosphatase *(PGI 05)*
- C. Glucose-1 phosphatase
- D. Glucose-6 phosphatase

162. A newborn infant refuses breast milk since the 2nd day of birth, vomits on force-feeding but accepts glucose-water, develops diarrhea on the third day, by 5th day she is jaundiced with liver enlargement and eyes show signs of cataract. Urinary reducing sugar was positive but blood glucose estimated by glucose oxidation method was found low. The most likely cause is deficiency of : *(AIIMS 03)*
- A. Galactose-1-phosphate uridyl transferase.
- B. Beta galactosidase.
- C. Glucose-6-phosphatase.
- D. Galactokinase

163. True regarding galactosemia: *(PGI 01)*
- A. Mental retardation occurs
- B. Absent disaccharidase in intestine
- C. Defect in epimerase
- D. Defect in galactose 1 PO_4 uridyl transferase

164. Reducing sugar in urine is seen in: *(PGI 15,13)*
- A. Fanconi anemia
- B. Lactose intolerance
- C. Galactosemia
- D. Phenylketonuria
- E. Salicylate poisoning

165. A patient has normal blood glucose level as estimated by Glucose –Oxidase Peroxidase method, shows positive Benedicts test in urine. Which of the following is likely cause?" *(AIIMS 16)*
- A. Fructosemia
- B. Galactosemia
- C. Denaturation of glucose
- D. Faulty tests

166. The molecule, which is the intiator of cataract formation in the eye lens and whose 1- phosphate derivative is responsible for liver failure, is: *(AIIMS 05)*
- A. Sorbitol
- B. Mannitol
- C. Inositol
- D. Galacticol

167. A child presents with hepatomegaly and bilateral lenticular opacities. Deficiency of which of the following enzymes will not cause such features.
- A. Galactose-1-phosphate uridyl transferase
- B. UDP-galactose-4-epimerase *(AIIMS 11)*
- C. Galactosekinase
- D. Lactase

168. A young man finds that every time he eats dairy products he feels very uncomfortable. His stomach becomes distended. He develops gas and diarrhea frequently. These symptoms do not appears when he eats foods other than dairy products. Which of the following is the most likely enzyme in which this young man is deficient? *(AI 04)*

A. α-amylase ☐
B. β-galactosidase ☐
C. α-glucosidase ☐
D. Sucrase ☐

Alcohol Metabolism

169. In chronic alcoholism the rate limiting component for alcohol metabolism excluding enzymes is / are:

A. NADP *(PGI 08)* ☐
B. NAD ☐
C. NADPH ☐
D. FADH ☐
E. FAD ☐

170. All are used in the diagnosis of diabetes mellitus except: *(AI 11, AIIMS 10)*

A. FBS ☐
B. HbA1c ☐
C. D-xylose absorption test ☐
D. OGTT ☐

Carbohydrate Classification

171. Which of the following are enantiomers:

A. D-Galactose & L-Glucose *(PGI 11, DNB 12)* ☐
B. d-Galactose & 1-Glucose ☐
C. D-Mannose & L-Mannose ☐
D. d-Mannose & l-Mannose ☐
E. D-glucose and L glucose ☐

172. Epimer combination (s) is /are

A. D-glucose & D-fructose *(PGI 14,10,09)* ☐
B. D-mannose & D-talose ☐
C. D-glucose & D-mannose ☐
D. D-glucose & D-gulose ☐
E. D- galactose & D-glucose ☐

173. Epimers of glucose- *(NBE P 15)*

A. Mannose ☐
B. Glyceraldehydes ☐
C. Fructose ☐
D. None ☐

174. Inulin like fructans are used as prebiotics as they are non digestible. Resistance to digestion in the upper GI tract results from: *(AI 10)*

A. Absence of digestive enzyme in the upper GIT ☐
B. Beta configuration of anomeric C2 ☐
C. Low pH of the stomach ☐
D. Presence of alpha-osidic linkages ☐

ANSWERS & EXPLANATIONS:

Glycolysis

1. **B, D, E i.e. Enolase, Phospho-glyceromutase, Glyceraldehyde-3-phosphate-dehydrogenase**
2. **B i.e. Mitochondria** *[Ref: Harper's 28/e P-149-53; Lippincott 5/e p. 96-103; Vasudevan 6/e p. 93-97; Chatterjea 7/e P-306-10]*
3. **C i.e. Conversion of glucose to 3 C units**

- **Enzymes of glycolysis** – a process which **converts 6 carbon glucose to 3 carbon unit pyruvate & lactate**Q – are present in **cytoplasm**. Whereas complete oxidation of glucose (to CO_2 & H_2O) requires **mitochondrial enzymes (of TCA cycle).**
- Out of total 9 enzymes used in glycolysis
- 3 enzymes – **hexokinase, phosphofructokinase (PFK-1) and Pyruvate kinase** are used in **irreversible steps.**
- 6 enzymes – **phosphohexose isomerase, aldolase, glyceraldehydes 3 phosphate dehydrogenase, 1, 3- biphospho glycerate kinase, phosphoglyceromutase and enolase** are used in **reversible steps**Q.
- 2 enzymes used in **energy utilizing steps** are – **hexokinase** (using **1 ATP**) and **phosphofructokinase / PFK-1** (using **1 ATP**). This energy consumption is for 1 molecule of glucose.
- 3 enzymes used in **energy producing steps** are – **glyceraldehydes 3phosphate dehydrogenase** (producing **2 NADH = 5 ATP), 1, 3 – biphospho glycerate kinase** (producing **2 ATP**), and **pyruvate kinase** (producing **2 ATP**). This energy production is for 1 molecule of glucose or 2 molecules of glyceraldehyde 3-P.

4. **A i.e. Enolase** 5. **D i.e. All of the above** 6. **C i.e. Glucose 6 PO_4**
[Ref: Harper's 28/e P-149-50, 583; Lehninger 5/e p. 150-53, 582-84; Vasudevan 6/e p. 93; Chatterjea 7/e p. 306-9]

Glucose 6 phosphate is an important compound that **joins several metabolic pathways viz. glycolysis, glycogenolysis, glycogenesis, gluconeogenesis and pentose phosphate pathway**Q.

7. **D i.e. Glucose** [Ref: Enzymes in industry & medicine Arnold: New studies in biology; http://www.ncbe.reading.ac.uk/ncbe/protocols /pracbiotech/ pdf/glucdet.pdf]

Oxidase – peroxidase enzyme system is used to determine glucose in urine & bloodQ.

8. **C i.e. Glucokinase, phosphofructokinase, pyruvate kinase**
9. **B i.e. Phosphofructokinase; C i.e. Pyruvate kinase; E i.e. Hexokinase**
10. **D i.e. Phosphofructokinase** [Ref: Harper's 29/e P-170-77; Lehinger 3/e P-541]

- **The irreversible reaction catalysed by PFK –1 (Phosphofructokinase) is the step that commits a cell to channel glucose into glycolysis**Q.

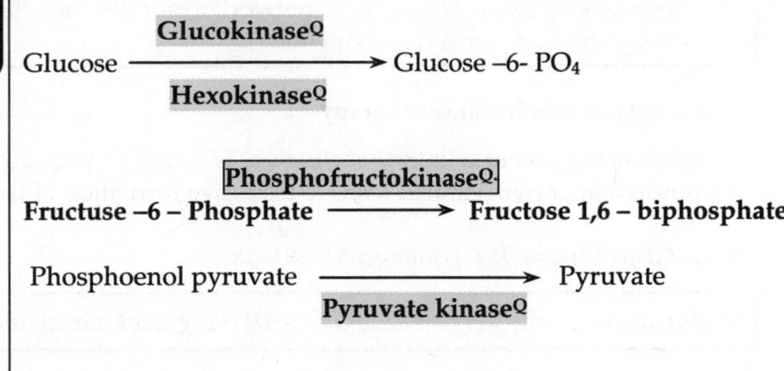

- A **Committed step** is an irreversible reaction which commits the product for a particular metabolism. There are three steps in glycolysis that are physiologically irreversible.
- Thus here the reaction Glucose → Glucose 6 PO_4 appears to be the 1st committed step
  But the product formed (i.e. Glucose – 6- PO_4) is not particularly committed for glycolysis. It is only committed for metabolism inside the cell (can enter into many pathways, glycolysis being one of them), so its not the Ist committed step.
- The next irreversible reaction is fructose → Fructose 1, 6- biphosphate **This reaction commits the cell to channel glucose into glycolytic pathway**Q. Thus this reaction is Ist committed step of glycolytic pathway.
- Glucose 6 PO_4 can flow either into glycolysis or through alternative oxidative pathways. The irreversible reaction catalysed by PFK-1 is the step that commits a cell to channel glucose into glycolysis.
- 3 enzymes – **hexokinase (glucokinase), phosphofructokinase (PFK-1) and Pyruvate kinase** are used in **irreversible steps.**

11. **C i.e. Glucokinase > A i.e. Phosphofructokinase** *[Ref: Harper's 28/e p. 150, 152, 166-65; Lehninger 5th/e p.578-81]*

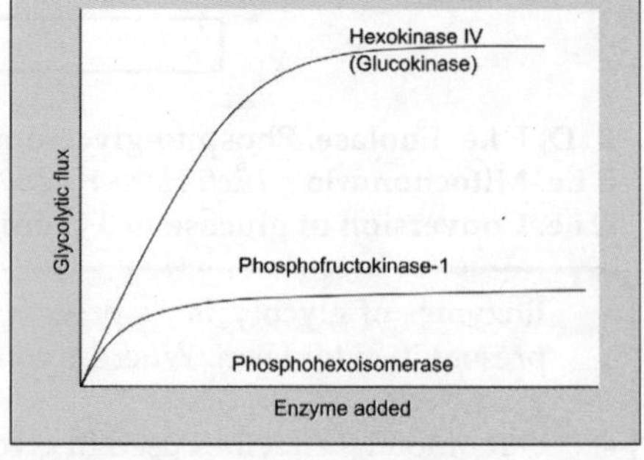

- Glycolysis is regulated at 3 steps *involving irreversible exergonic* reactions i.e. the reaction catalyzed by: **hexokinase (or glucokinase), phosphofructokinase (PFK-1)** and **pyruvate kinase**. The phosphofructo kinase reaction may be considered to be functionally irreversible under physiological conditions; it is both inducible & subject to allosteric regulation and *has a major role in regulation of rate of glycolysis - Harper*
- For glycolysis, PFK – 1 was considered the rate limiting enzyme, because it was know to be closely regulated by fructose 2, 6 biphosphate & other allosteric effectors. But experiments suggest that henokinase IV (glucokinase) & PFK-1 both contribute to setting the flux (rate) through pathway (hexokinase more than PFK-1). Flux control coefficient contradicted the conventional wisdom; it showed that ***hexokinase, not PFK-1 is most influential in setting the flux (rate) through glycolysis***Q. - *Lehninger*

12. **C i.e. Enolase** 13. **C i.e. Enolase** 14. **C i.e. Enolase**

[Ref: Harper's 27/e P-152-53; Chatterjea 7/e P-308-10]

For blood glucose estimation in the laboratory, fluoride is added to the blood to prevent glycolysis by the cells by inhibiting 'enolase' so that blood glucose is correctly estimated.Q

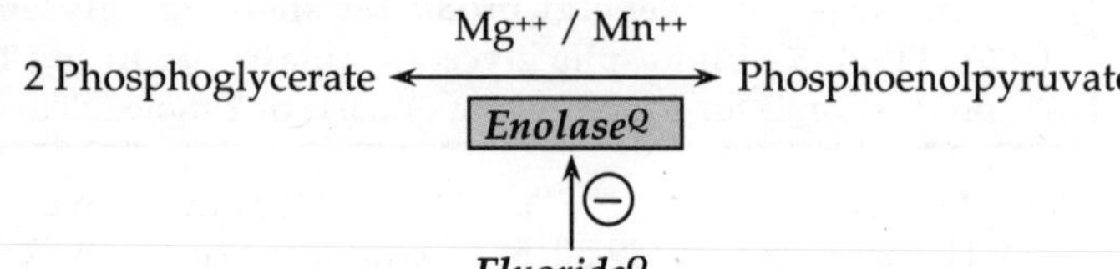

15. **C i.e. Potassium oxalate + NaF** 16. **C i.e. NaF** *[Ref: Chattergea & Shinde 7/e p. 308-10; Harper's 27/e p. 152-53]*

The anticoagulant mixture used to estimate blood glucose from a sample contains anticoagulant & glycolytic inhibitor as there is loss of 1-2% of glucose /hour due to glycolysis of RBCs.

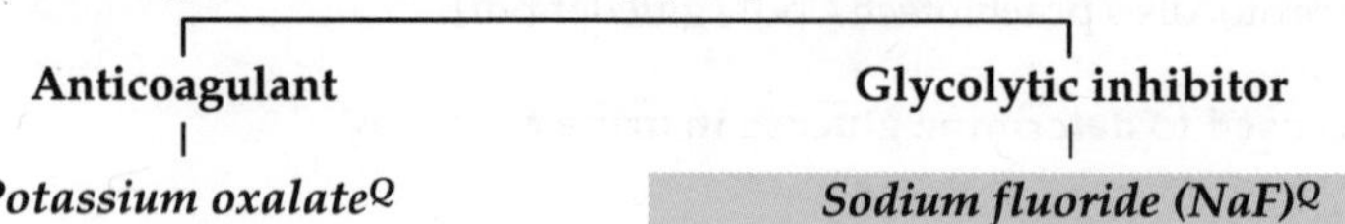

17. **A i.e. Glycolysis** *[Ref: Harper's 27/e P-151; 26/e P-136, Lehinger 3/e P541]*

Cancer cells ***derive nutrition from glycolysis***Q. Cancer cells are multiplying at a rapid rate for which they need energy. But they lack an extensive capillary network to supply the cells with O_2. So the tumor cells have to depend on anaerobic process – *Glycolysis* for ATP production

Role of glycolysis in cancer therapy

In fast growing cancer cells, *rate of glycolysis is very high*, produces more pyruvic acid (PA) than TCA cycle can handle. Accumulation of pyruvic acid leads to excessive formation of lactic acid producing *Lactic acidosis.*

18. **A i.e. Glucokinase** *Ref: Lehninger 5/e 591, 583*

In **glycolysis** insulin ***acts on hexokinase IV (i.e. glucokinase) and hexokinase II***Q but not on other (I & III) hexokinase

19. **A i.e. Km value is higher than normal blood sugar; B i.e. Found in liver; E i.e. Glucose enter into cells through GLUT-2**
20. **C i.e. Adipocytes** 21. **C i.e. Heart** 22. **B i.e. GLUT 2**

[Ref: Lippincott 4th/ed pg-312; Lehninger 5th/ed pg-391-93, 608, 441-42, 583-85; Chatterjea 6/e P-271; Vasudevan 3/e 73, 74]

Insulin sensitive (dependent) glucose transporter, GLUT- 4 that are found in ***adipose tissue***Q and **skeletal muscles** are *reduced in fasting state, when the insulin levels are low.*

Glucose Transporters

Insulin dependent (sensitive)
Facilitated transport

- *Adipose tissue*Q - **Skeletal Muscle** - **Heart**	**GLUT-4**

↓
Decrease in fasting

Insulin insensitive (not dependent)

Active transport
- Intestine epithelium
- Renal tubules
- Choroid plexus

Facilitated transport

RBC, Placenta, BBBQ, Colon, Kidney	**GLUT-1**
Pancreas (β-cells)Q, Liver, Small intestine, Kidney	**GLUT 2**
Brain, Placenta, Kidney	GLUT 3
Intestine, Testis, Kidney, Sperm **(fructose transport)**	GLUT 5
Leukocyte, Spleen	GLUT6
Lens Cornea	
Liver	GLUT7

23. **C i.e. Hypoxia stimulates release of all glycolytic enzymes from Band 3 on RBC membrane.** *[Ref: Ganong 533, 670, 720, 733, 14f; http://www.jbc.org/cgi/content/abstract/266/7/4106; http://www.pnas.org/cgi/content/full/102/7/2402]*

- RBC membrane cytoskeletal protein **spectrin** is anchored to **transmembrane anion exchanger protein Band 3** by protein **ankyrin & protein 4.2**. Another cytoskeletal protein **actin** is attached to transmembrane **glycophorin C** by **protein 4.1**. Tropomyosin, tropomodulin, adducin and 4.9 are other proteins.
- **Band 3**, is a multifunction RBC transmembrane protein, which is important for its ***cytoskeletal structure, cell shape, anion exchange activity and glycolysis*Q*. Band 3 is responsible for chloride shift in RBC*Q*. Hypoxic deoxygenation of hemoglobin causes Band 3 tyrosine phosphorylation and thereby stimulates glycolysis by releasing glycolytic enzymes from band 3 on RBC membrane*Q**.
- **In** *kidney*, **I cells** contain *Band 3, an anion exchange protein* in their basolateral cell membrane, which may function as a $Cl^- - HCO_3^-$ exchanger for the transport of HCO_3^- to interstitial fluid.
- In animal cells, *principal regulators of intracellular pH* are HCO_3^- *transporters* such as Band 3 $Cl^- - HCO_3^-$ exchanger, $3Na^+ - HCO_3^-$ cotransporters and a $K^+ - HCO_3^-$ cotransporter.

24. **D i.e. Erythrocytes** 25. **B i.e. Enzymes of TCA cycle**

Erythrocytes (RBC) lack mitochondria (so TCA cycle enzymes) and completely rely on glucose as their metabolic fuel. They metabolize it by anaerobic glycolysisQ.

26. **D i.e. Ethanol** *[Ref: Harper's 27/e p. 151, Lippincott's 4/e p. 96]*

Aerobic glycolysis in cells with mitochondria & adequate oxygen supply	**Anaerobic glycolysis** in cells that **lack mitochondria (eg RBCs) or deprived of sufficient O_2**	**Fermentation** in yeast & some other microorganisms
PyruvateQ is the end product and NADH enters oxidative phosphorylation for ATP production	***Lactate***Q is the end product as NADH formed in glycolysis is reoxidized by reducing pyruvate to lactate.	***Ethanol***Q is the end product as pyruvate is decarboxylated & reduced into it

Shuttle Systems

27. **A i.e. Malate** 28. **B i.e. Glycolysis**
[Ref: Harper's 28/e P-155; Vasudevan 6/e p. 228; Chatterjea 7/e P-321-22]

Mallate shuttle is a system by which ***reducing equivalents (NADH) produced in glycolysis***Q are transferred from cytosol to mitochondria to yield energy.

NADH produced ***in the glycolysis***Q, *is extramitochondrial* where as the *electron transport chain, where NADH has to be oxidized to NAD+ is in the mitochondria* (Oxidation of 1 NADH yields 3 ATP/2.5 ATP). NADH is impermeable to mitochondrial membrane, so to enable *transfer of NADH inside mitochondria Shuttle system is utilized.*

PDH- Complex

29. **B i.e. PDH complex** 30. **A i.e. Pyruvate** 31. **E i.e. NADPH**
32. **D i.e. Phosphatase** 33. **A i.e. Biotin** 34. **D i.e. Biotin** *[Ref: Lippincott's 5/e p. 109-12]*

Pyruvate, the end product of *aerobic glycolysis* is transported into mitochondria by specific pyruvate transporter, where it is converted to ***acetyl CoA by pyruvate dehydrogenase (PDH) complex***Q. It uses **niacin (as NAD), riboflavin (as FAD) and thiamin (as TPP)**Q.

Pyruvate Dehydrogenase (PDH) Complex

It is not the part of TCA cycle, but is the *major source of acetyl CoA – a 2 carbon substrate for cycle*. The **irreversibility** of PDH reaction precludes the formation of pyruvate from acetyl CoA, and explains why glucose cannot be formed from acetyl CoA by gluconeogenesis. PDH complex is a multimolecular aggregate of 3 enzymes components and 2 regulatory enzymes.

Component enzyme	Coenzyme
E_1 = **Pyruvate dehydrogenase (decarboxylase)**	***Thiamine pyrophosphate (TPP)***Q
E_2 = **Dihydrolipoyl trans acetylase**	***Lipoic acid & CoA***Q
E_3 = **Dihydrolipoyl dehydrogenase**	***FAD, & NAD+***Q

Regulatory enzyme	Activator of enzyme	Action
PDH kinase (c-AMP-independent)	ATP, Acetyl CoA, NADH	Phosphorylates & inhibits (turn.off) E1
PDH phosphatase	Ca^{++}	Dephosphorylates or activates (turn on) E_1

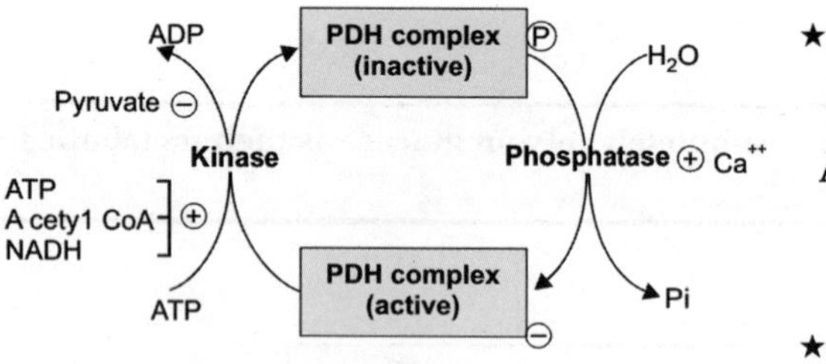

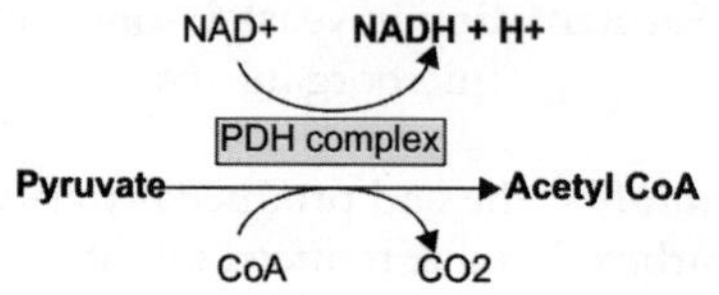

★ Pyruvate is a potent inhibitor of *PDH kinase* therefore it activates E1.

★ Acety CoA & NADH formed in this reaction allosterically inhibit active form of E_1

★ **So energy produced in complete aerobic oxidation of 1 glucose molecule is 30-32 ATP** (new concept)

Aerobic glycolysis	**PDH complex reaction**	**Cirtic Acid Cycle**
5-7 ATPQ	2NADPH or **5 ATP**	**10 ATP** x 2 i.e. **20 ATP**

★ Each glucose molecule gives rise to 2 pyruvate molecules & so 2 TCA cycles occur.

- *X-linked dominant deficiency in E1 component of PDH complex*, although rare, is the most common cause of ***congenital lacticacidosis***Q. This enzyme deficiency results in inability to convert pyruvate to acetal CoA, causing pyruvate to be converted to lactic acid via lactate dehydrogenase. This mainly affects *brain which relies on TCA cycle for most its energy* & is particularly sensitive to acidosis.
- **Leigh syndrome** *(subacute necrotizing encephalomyelopathy)* occurs d/t defects in mitochondrial ATP production as a result of mutation of *PHD complex, electron transport chain or ATP synthase.* It can affect both nuclear & mitochondrial DNA.

35. **A i.e. Phosphoenol Pyruvate** *[Ref: Harper's 28/e P-155, 165-67; Lippincott 5/e p. 105-103, 118; Shinde & Chatterjea 6/e P-305]*

Pyruvate can be directly converted to **acetyl CoA** (by oxidative decarboxylation), **oxaloacetate** (by carboxylation), **alanine** (transamination); and **lactate** (in anaerobic conditions). ***But pyruvate can not be directly converted to phosphoenol pyruvate (a reaction of gluconeogenesis)[Q]. However, phosphoenol pyruvate can be directly converted to pyruvate (in glycolysis)[Q].***

36. **D i.e. Enolase**

Arsenite (trivalent form of arsenic) forms a stable complex with thiol (-SH) group of **lipoic acid**, making it unavailable to serve as a coenzyme. So arsenic poisoning is primarily d/t ***inhibition of enzymes that require lipoic acid (lipoate) as a coenzyme including E2 of PDH complex, α-Ketoglutarate dehydrogenase and branched chain α-ketoacid dehydrogenase[Q].***

37. **D i.e. It is coenzyme for pyruvate dehydrogenase**

Thiamin (vit B_1) has central role in energy yielding metabolism especially of carbohydrates. So ***thiamin requirement increases in excess intake of carbohydrates and its deficiency leads to decreased energy production[Q]***. Hampered or **decreased function of pyruvate dehydrogenase enzyme** (which forms acetyl CoA from pyruvate) and **α-ketoglutarate dehydrogenase enzyme** (of TCA cycle) in which thiamin acts as coenzyme is the main cause of this decreased energy production. Decreased PDH function also ***l/t pyruvic and lactic acidiosis[Q]***.

Citric Acid Cycle

38. **B i.e. Irreversible**

Formation of Citric Acid from Acetyl –COA and Oxaloacetate (OAA) is 1st and irreversible step of TCA, giving 7.8 K cal (exergonic reaction[Q])

Acetyl COA + OAA + H_2O —*Citrate synthase*→ **Citric acid[Q]** + COA – SH

1st step of TCA cycle.
An *irreversible* reaction, gives 7.8 K cal (exergonic reaction)

39. **B i.e. Citrate**
40. **B i.e. Cis aconitate**
41. **A i.e. Fluroacetate**
42. **B i.e. Aconitase**
43. **C i.e. Citrate, ketoglutarate, oxaloacetate**
44. **B i.e. Malonate**
45. **B i.e. Alphaketoglutarate**
46. **A i.e. Pyruvate, D i.e. Malonate, E i.e. Nitric oxide**
47. **B i.e. Fluoroacetate**
48. **D i.e. Succinate dehydrogenase**
49. **D i.e. 2.6 ATP**
50. **A i.e. Isocitrate dehydrogenase; B i.e. Succinate dehydrogenase; C i.e. Succinate thiokinase; D i.e. Malate dehydrogenase**
[Ref: Lehninger 5th/e p. 630; Harper's 28/e P-143-46; Chatterjea 7/e p. 316-19; Lippincott's 5/e p. 109-13; Vasudevan 6/e p. 219]

- **Energy producing enzymes** in Kreb's (TCA) cycle are - α **-**ketoglutarate dehydrogenase, Malate dehydrogenase, Isocitrate dehydrogenase, Succinate **dehydrogenase** and Succinate thiokinase.
  Mn – **A KG MIS** (- dehydrogenase) is **ST** (successful teacher)
- **One NADH** may produce **2.5 ATP** and **1 FADH** may produce *1.5 ATP through respiratory chain[Q]*.

51. **B i.e. Isocitrate dehydrogenase**

2 molecules of carbon dioxide are released in TCA cycle. One before and one after α - ketoglatarate. Enzymes used are – ***isocitrate dehydrogenase and α ketoglutarate dehydrogenase[Q]*** respectively.

52. **A i.e. Thiamine; B i.e. Riboflavin** *[Ref: Harper's 28/e P-146]*
53. **C i.e. Isocitrate dehydrogenase** *[Ref: Debajyoti Das 101]*

> The enzyme of TCA cycle having allosteric inhibitor is ***isocitrate dehydrogenase***[Q].
> The *allosteric activator* is *ADP* and **allosteric inhibitor** *is ATP and long chain aceyl COA*

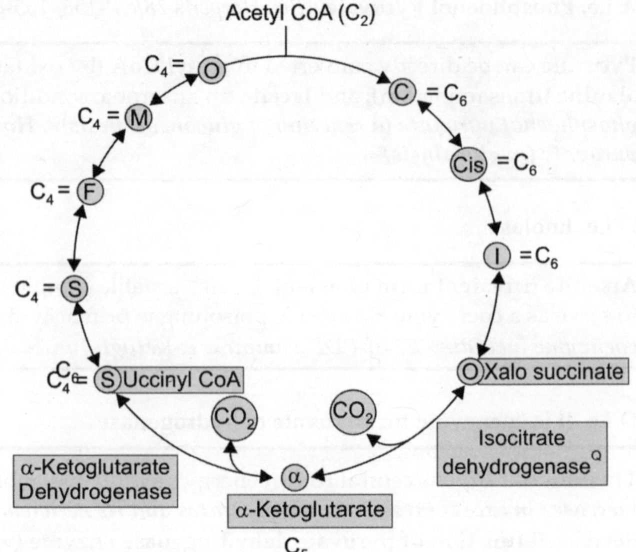

54. **C i.e. ATP, E i.e. NADH**
55. **C i.e. Isoleucine, Valine, methionine**
[Ref: Harper's 28/e P-147, 248; Lehninger 5/e p. 861]

> Valine, Isoleucine and Methionine[Q] produce ***succinyl COA*** which is an important component of TCA cycle. [Mn: **Successful VIM**]

56. **B i.e. Succinate Thiokinase**
57. **B i.e. Succinyl CoA to succinate**
58. **C i.e. Succinyl CoA thiokinase**

Substrate & Oxidative Phosphorylation

There are *two types of phosphorylation of ADP to ATP*

Substrate level phosphorylation

- Is production of ATP 'at the substrate' without the participation of electron transport chain
- Formation of ATP does not require ATP
- Respiratory chain does not participate
- It is not affected by dinitrophenole

- In TCA cycle

Succinyl CoA —(***Succinate thiokinase***[Q])→ Succinate

- In Glycolysis

1, 3- biphos-Phoglycerate —(***Phosphoglycerate Kinase***[Q])→ 3 phospho glycerate

Phosphoenol Pyruvate —(***Pyruvate Kinase***[Q])→ (Enol) pyruvate

Oxidative Phosphorylation at Respiratory Chain Level

Generation of High Energy Phosphate In Catabolism of Glucose			Number of (P) Formed per Mole of Glucose
Pathway	**Reaction Catalyzed by**	**Method of ~ Production**	
Glycolysis	Glyceraldehyde-3-phosphate dehydrogenase	Respiratory chain oxidation of 2 NADH	6*
	Phosphoglycerate kinase	Phosphorylation at substrate level	2
	Pyruvate kinase	Phosphorylation at substrate level	2
			10
Allow for consumption of ATP by reactions catalyzed by hexokinase and phosphofructokinase			-2
		Net	8
	Pyruvate dehydrogease	Respiratory chain oxidation of 2 NADH	6
Citric acid cycle	Isocitrate dehydrogenase	Respiratory chain oxidation of 2 NADH	6
	α-ketoglutarate dehydrogenase	Respiratory chain oxidation of 2 NADH	6
	Succinate thiokinase	Phosphorylation at substrate level	2
	Succinate dehydrogenase	Respiratory chain oxidation of 2 $FADH_2$	4
	Malate dehydrogenase	Respiratory chain oxidation of 2 NADH	6
		Net	30
Total per mole of glucose under **aerobic conditions**			38
Total per mole of glucose under **anaerobic conditions**			2

★ It is assumed that NADH formed in glycolysis is transported into mitochondria via the malate shuttle. If the glycerophosphate shuttle is used, only 2 ~ (P) would be formed per mole of NADH, the total net production being 26 instead of 38. The calculation ignores the small loss of ATP due to a transported of H^+ into the mitochondrion with pyruvate and a similar transport of H+ in the operation of the malate shuttle, totaling about 1 mol of ATP. Note that there is a substantial benefit under anaerobic conditions if glycogen is the starting point, since the net production of high-energy phosphate in glycosis is increased from 2 to 3, as ATP is no longer required by the hexokinase reaction.

High Energy Compounds

59. **C i.e. Creatine phosphate** 60. **C i.e. ATP** 61. **C i.e. Creatine phosphate** 62. **B i.e. Creatine phosphate & Carbamoyl..**
63. **A, C, D i.e. ATP, Creatinine phosphate, Acetyl CoA** *[Ref: Vasudevan 6/e p. 225-26; Harper 29/e p. 530-40; Satyanaran 3/e 222-23]*

- **ATP, GTP, UTP, creatine phosphate and CoA derivatives (like acetyl/succinyl /fatty acyl / HMG-CoA)**Q and **carbamoyl phosphate** are **high energy compounds**. Wherease, ADP, glucose 1 or 6 phosphate, fructose 6 PO4 and glycerol 3 PO4 are **low energy compounds.**
- **Creatinine phosphate gives 10.5 KCal/molecule**Q.

Respiratory Chain & Oxidative Phosphorylation

64. **D i.e. Fe^{2+}** 65. **D i.e. Riboflavin** 66. **A i.e. FMN**
[Ref: Lippincott 5/e p. 76-77; Harper 28/e p. 99, 103-5; Chatterjea 7/e p. 133-129; Lehninger 5/e p. 708-18-515]

- Because electrons tend to flow spontaneously from carries of lower redox potential (E°) to carries of higher redox potential. The **order (sequence) of electron carriers in ETC of mitochondria** (and so the ***increasing order of redox potential)*** is

Substrate → **$NADP^+$ / NADPH** → NAD^+/NADH → NADH dehydrogenase **(FMN)** / NADH dehydrogenase ($FMNH_2$) → FAD/$FADH_2$ → Ubiquinone or Coenzyme **Q** → **Fe^{3+}** / Fe^{2+} in cytochromes **b** → **C_1** → **C** → **a** → **a_3** → **O_2**

(Mn: "**NFQ b C_1 c a a_3 O_2**")

- **Riboflavin (vitamin B2) in form of FAD / FMN**Q **and niacin in form of NAD^+/$NADP^+$ function as coenzymes in Redox (oxidation & reduction) reactions**Q.

67. **C i.e. Chemiosmotic methods** 68. **A i.e. Generation of ATPs** 69. **C i.e. Fo F_1 ATPase**
70. **A i.e. NADH-Q Oxidoreductase; C i.e. Cytochrome C-Q oxidoreductase**
71. **A, B, E i.e. (NADH Co-Q reductase, Cytochrome C oxidase, Co-Q-Cytochrome C reductase)**

- **Mitchell's chemiosmotic hypothesis links the respiratory (i.e. electron transport) chain to ATP production (i.e. oxidative phosphorylation)**Q. It explains how the free energy generated by the transport of electrons from NADH to molecular oxygen (in respiratory chain) is used to produce ATP from ADP + Fi (from proton pumps).
- For each NADH oxidized (pair of electron), **complex I (NADH –Q- oxido reductase)** and **complex III (ubiquinone /Q-cytochrome C- oxidoreductase) pump (translocate) 4 protons (H+) each, whereas complex IV (Cytochrome C-oxidase) translocates only 2 protons (H+).** In ETC. **oxidative phosphorylation (ATP formation)** occurs at these sites (ie complex I, III & IV)
- **In ETC, ATP is generated by F0-F1 ATPase (=ATP synthase)**Q. **F_0 subunit** forms **proton channel** and **(F1 sububit generate ATP (3ATPs per rotation)**Q.

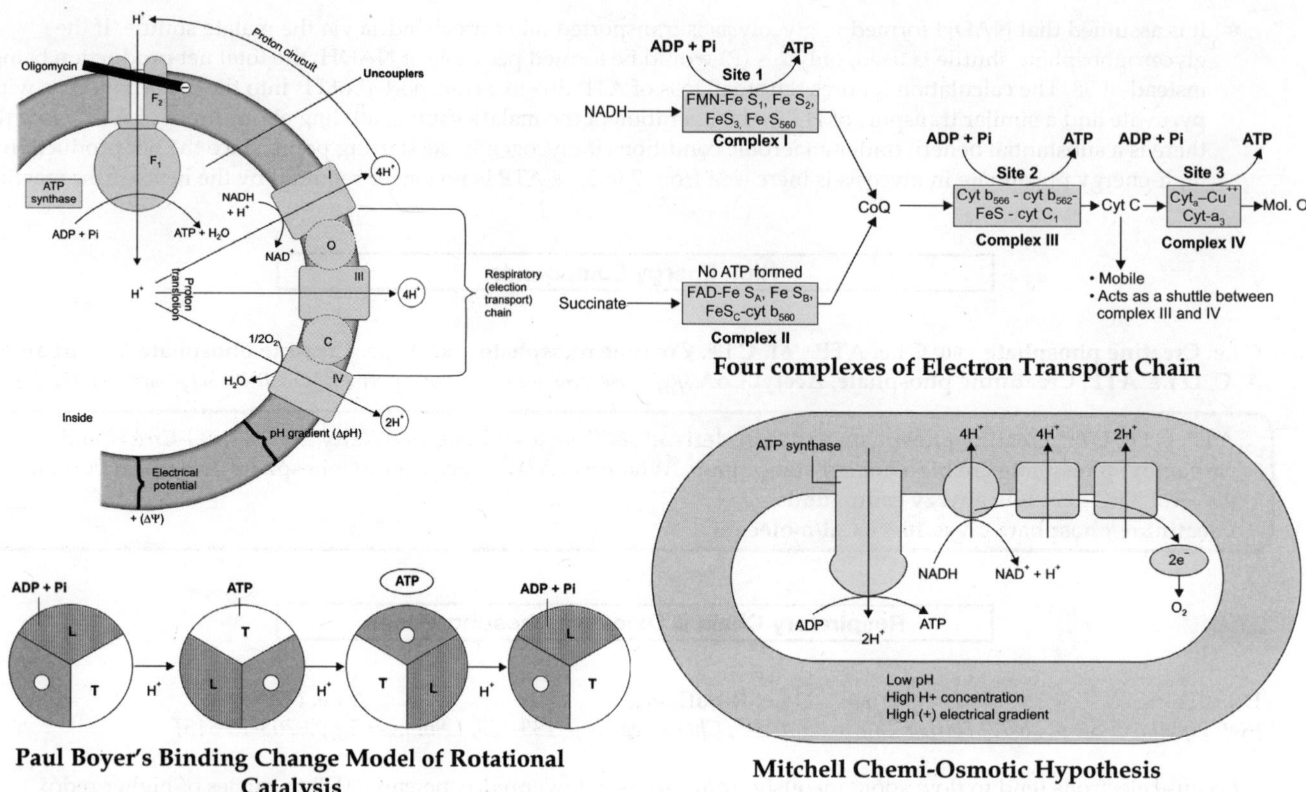

Four complexes of Electron Transport Chain

Paul Boyer's Binding Change Model of Rotational Catalysis

Mitchell Chemi-Osmotic Hypothesis

72. **C i.e. α and β subunits rotate** 73. **B i.e. Exergonic & Catabolic; E i.e. Cytochrome – C reductase involved**
[Ref: Chatterjea 6/e P-120-130; Lehninger 3/e P- 661- 72]

> **Internal respiration** is ***exergonic and catabolic***[Q] and it uses ***cytochromes b, c_1, c, a, a_3***[Q].

- In biological oxidations the term exothermic & endothermic are replaced by exergonic and endergonic. Thus in **exergonic** and **endergonic** reactions, *free energy is released or absorbed respectively.*
- **Internal respiration** is utilization of O_2 and production of CO_2 by cells. It involves oxidative phosphorylation & generation of ATP through respiratory chain. The respiratory chain collects, transports and oxidizes reducing equivalents (-H or electrons). The energy of electron transfer is sufficiently conserved in proton gradient and these reactions are highly ***exergonic***[Q]. Most of the e- arise from action of dehydrogenases that collect electron from ***catabolic pathway***[Q] and funnel them into universal electon acceptor – NAD, or $NADP^+$ or FAD or FMN.

74. **A i.e. NADH, C i.e. NADPH; D i.e. ATP***[Ref: Harper's 28/e P-109-110; Lippincott 5/e p. 79-80; Lehninger 3/e P-660; Vasudevan 6/e p. 234]*

> **Inner mitochondrial transporter contains specific transporter that carry** cytosolic ***NADH /NADPH***[Q]***, ADP & ATP***[Q].

75. **B i.e. Exergonic & Catabolic; E i.e. Cytochrome C reductase involved** 76. **A i.e. Inhibits Cytochrome oxidase**
77. **A i.e. CO; B i.e. H_2S; C i.e. Cyanide** 78. **D i.e. Non-competitive irreversible inhibition**
79. **C i.e. Cyanide** 80. **A i.e. Cyanide** 81. **C i.e. Brown adipose tissue**
82. **C i.e. Uncoupling of oxidation & phosphorylation** 83. **A i.e. Atractyloside**
84. **B i.e. Inhibitor of oxidative phosphorylation** 85. **A i.e. Thermogonin**
[Ref: Harper 28/e p. 108-10; Chatterjea 7/136-37; Vasudevan 6/e p. 234; Lehninger 5/e p 714; Lippincott 5/e p. 77-79]

- Electron transport in **complex IV – Cytochrome c oxidase (Cytochrome a, a_3)** is inhibited by ***cyanide (CN^-), carbon monoxide (CO), hydrogen sulfide (H_2S) and azide***[Q].

- **Brown adipose tissue** is the specialized mammalian tissue in which ***fuel oxidation serves not to produce ATP but to generate heat***[Q]. (i.e. oxidation is not coupled with phosphorylation). This **uncoupling of oxidative phosphorylation** is due to presence of **thermogenin (or UCP1/uncoupling protein 1)** a **natural physiological uncoupler**. So brown fat is used for heat generation (not ATP production) *in new born and during hibernation in animals.*
- **2-4-Dinitophenol**, dicoumarol (vitamin K analogue), calcium, CCCP (Chloro carbonyl cyanide phenyl hydrazone), FCCP (trifluoro carbonyl cyanide phenyl hydrazone),- valinomycin, aspirin are **synthetic uncouplers.**
- **Atractyloside (glycoside) inhibits oxidative phosphorylation (i.e. ATP synthesis)**[Q] by ***blocking transporters (translocases) responsible for movement of ADP (into) & ATP (out) across the inner mitochondrial membrane***[Q]. Whereas **oligomycin** binds to *ATP synthase* (**F_o** domain so name starts with O) closing the ***proton channel and blocking the flow of protons***[Q].

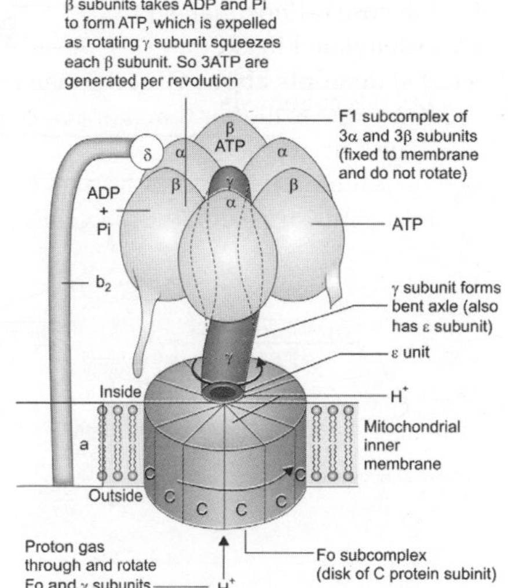

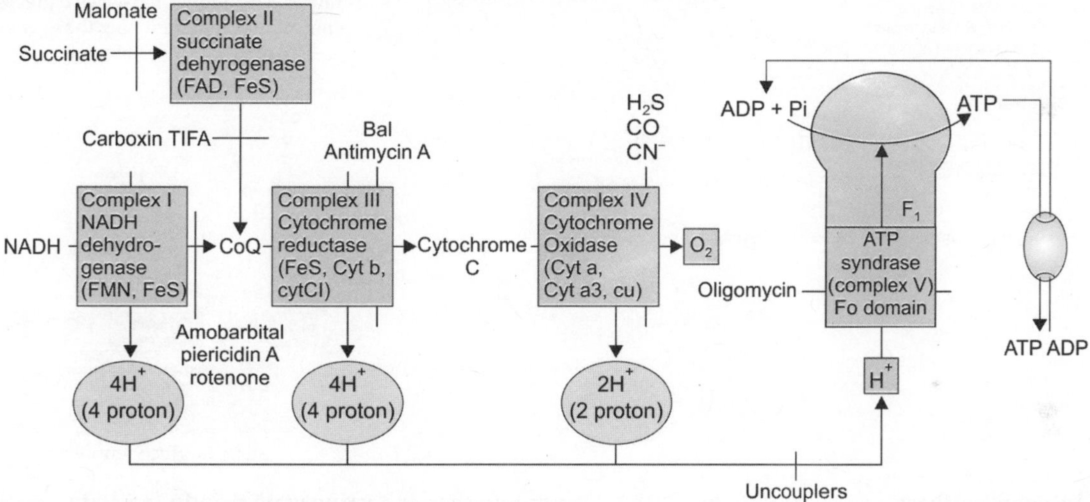

86. A i.e. Oxidase *[Ref: Robbins 7th/60; Chatterjea 6/e P-18]*

The electron transport chain system responsible for the respiratory burst is 'NADPH oxidase' (on oxidase enzyme)

The biochemical mechanism of microbial killing and degradation following phogocytosis is called 'respiratory burst'.
This is accomplished largely by oxygen dependent mechanisms.
'The generation of reactive oxygen intermediates is due to rapid activation of an oxidase (NADPH oxidase)'.

87. A i.e. Apoptosis *[Ref: Robbins 7/e p-29-30]*

Cytochrome C has *two very opposite roles.* **Within the mitochondrial membrane** it serves as *electron carrier in oxidative phosphorylation.* But when it leaks out into cytosol it ***combines with Apaf I and activates caspase-9 to mediate apoptosis***[Q]. This dual functioning is known as **moonlighting.**

88. A i.e. 1 *[Ref: Harper 30/e p. 148]*

Fuel	O_2 Consumed (L/g)=A	CO_2 produced (L/g)=B	RQ (=B/A)
Carbohydrate	0.83	0.83	1[Q]
Protein	0.97	0.78	0.8
Fat	2.02	1.4	0.7
Alcohol	1.43	0.97	0.66

Respiratory Quotient (R/Q) is the ratio of volume of CO_2 produced and O_2 consumed. It **increases from pure fat (0.7) to pure protein (0.8) to pure carbohydrate** (1= in fasting state)

Glycogen Metabolism & Storage Diseases

89. A i.e. Glycogenesis

Glycogenesis and Glycogenolysis

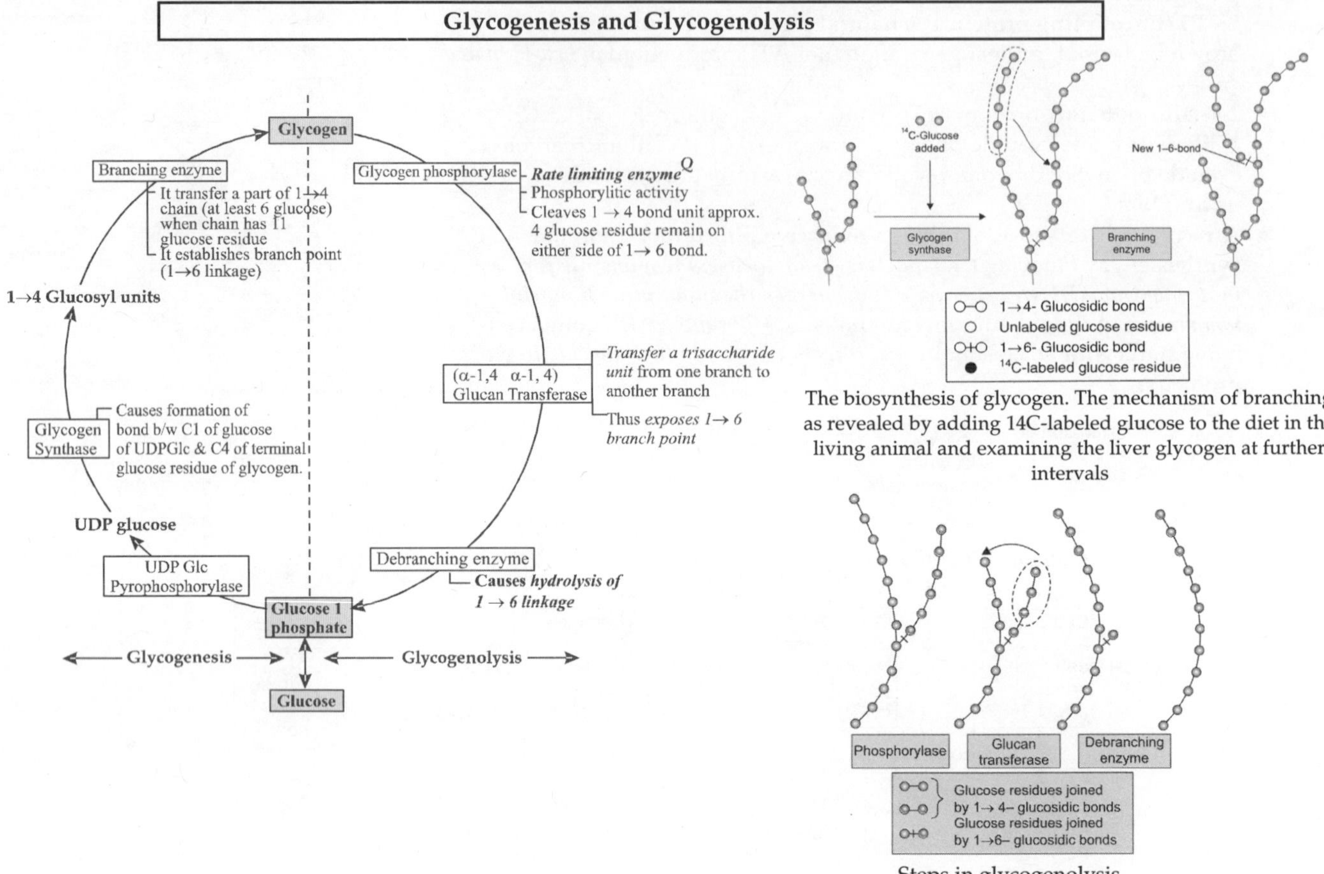

The biosynthesis of glycogen. The mechanism of branching as revealed by adding 14C-labeled glucose to the diet in the living animal and examining the liver glycogen at further intervals

Steps in glycogenolysis

90. B i.e. Glycogen synthase **91. B i.e. Commonly seen in fasting state than in fed state**
92. C i.e. Phosphorylase **93. B i.e. Conversion to Glycogen** **94. D i.e. Storage as glycogen**
95. D i.e. ATP **96. C and E i.e. Oxytocin decreases it and δ subunit is catalytic** **97. D i.e. Insulin**
98. C i.e. Amylo 1, 6 glucosidase **99. A i.e. Phosphorylase, Glucan transferase, Debranching, Phosphorylase**

[Ref: Harper's 28/e p.158-62; Lippincott's 4/e p. 132-33; Chattergea & Shinde 7/e p. 327-30; Lehninger 5th/ed pg 603-04]

- **Main enzyme for glycogen synthesis is glycogen synthase^Q.**
- **Gylcogenolysis** (glycogen metabolism) ***occurs in fasting & starvation***^Q. The main enzyme of glycogenolysis is **glycogen phosphorylase (or phosphorylase),** which is **allosterically inhibited (inactivated) by ATP, glucose $6PO_4$ and free glucose** (1st two in muscle & liver, 3rd only in liver). **Factors activating or maintaining active phosphorylase** include **C-AMP dependent protein kinase** (both in liver & muscle**), 5′ AMP & Ca^{++}** (in muscle only). **Hormones like epinephrine, norepinephrine, glucagon and thyroid hormones** act **indirectly by increasing C-AMP**^Q and so activating C-AMP dependent protein kinase.
- In well fed state (also called *absorptive stage)* ***insulin suppresses glucose –6- phosphatase activity and causes glucose 6 – phosphate to enter glycogenesis***^Q (to form glycogen).
- **Active glycogen phosphorylase** a ***in both tissues (i.e. muscle and liver) is allosterically inhibited and inactivated by ATP and glucose 6- phosphate***^Q. Whereas **in liver, but not in muscle,** ***free glucose is also an inhibitor***^Q**.** Actually when phosphorylase b is activated it is called phosphorylase a.
- Phosphorylase kinase exists in 2 forms – an active phosphorylated 'a' form and inactive dephosphorylated 'b' form. **Active c-AMP dependent protein kinase** phosphorylates inactive b form to active a form. The phosphorylated enzyme can be inactivated by hydrolytic removal of phosphate by **protein phosphatase 1**. This enzyme is activated by ***kinase mediated signal cascade initiated by insulin***^Q.

100. B i.e. Muscle **101. D i.e. Glucose –6 – phosphatase** *[Ref: Harper's 28/e P-146-148, 159; Lippincott 5/e p. 130; Vasudevan 6/e p. 108]*

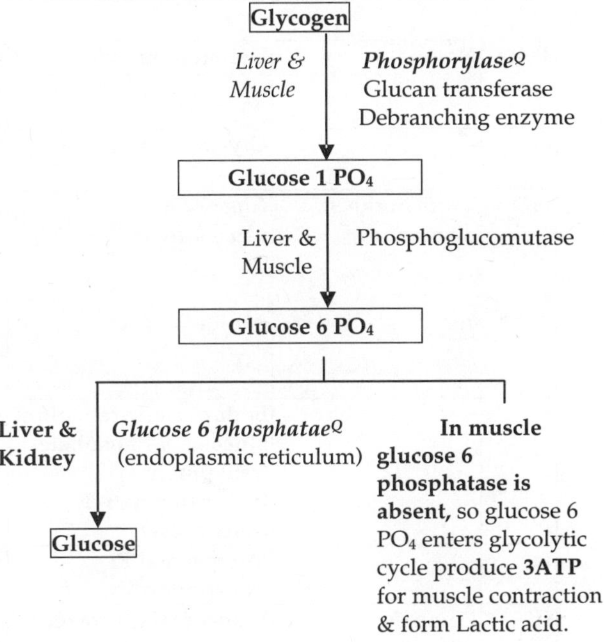

- The *role of glycogen in liver* is to *provide free glucose* for export to maintain the blood glucose level; whereas *in muscles* the role of glycogen is to provide a *source of glucose-6-PO4 for glycolysis* (to supply ATP for muscle contraction).
- This difference of fate of glycogen in liver & muscle is ***d/t absence of glucose -6- phosphatase enzyme in muscle***[Q]. Because of absence of this enzyme, which catalyzes the final step of glycogenolysis, glycogen in muscles can only be converted upto glucose-6- phosphate. Hence ***muscle glycogenolysis does not contribute to blood glucose directly***[Q]. Instead, in muscle, this glucose -6-PO4 can not cross plasma membrane and enters glycolysis producing energy (**3ATP**) needed for muscle contraction. The gain of an extra (1) ATP is d/t bypass of 1st step of glycolysis which requires 1 ATP (If glycolysis starts from glucose only 2 ATPs are produced). Lactic acid produced d/t glycolysis crosses the plasma membrane & reaches liver to form glucose.
- In liver glucose -6. phosphate is transported by glucose- 6- phosphate **translocase** into *endoplasmic reticulum*, where it is converted to glucose by **glucose- 6- phosphatase** (this enzyme is also used in last step of gluconeogenesis). The glucose moves out of ER to cytosol and then released by hepatocytes into blood to maintin blood glucose levels until gluconeogenesis starts.

102. A i.e. Glucose-6-phosphate

Glucose-6-phosphate cannot cross the cell membrane unless it in converted into Glucose by the **enzyme – Glucose-6-phosphatase.**[Q]

Von Gerkes disease in deficiency of Glucose-6-phosphatase leads to accumulation of glucose-6-phosphate (and hence glycogen in the liver). In the absence of this enzyme, glucose-6-phosphate is not converted into glucose and thus cannot enter the blood leading to hypoglycemia.

103. A i.e. I

Type I glycogen storage disease (Von Gierke's) is ***due to deficiency of Glucose – 6- phosphatase***[Q].
As this enzyme is absent in ***muscle, so muscles are not affected in Glycogen storage disease type I.***[Q]. It affects liver, kidney and intestine.

104. A i.e. Von gierke's disease **105. B i.e. Von gierke's disease**
106. C i.e. Fat mobilization is less **107. A i.e More formation of pentose** *[Ref : Chatterjea 7/e P-331; 6/e p. 293]*

Von Gierke's (type Ia glycogen storage) disease d/t deficiency of **glucose 6 phosphatase enzyme**[Q] is autosomal recessive in inheritance. It is characterized by – Cells (of liver, renal tubular epithelium & intestinal mucosa) containing **normal structured metabolically unavailable glycogen, hepato-renomegaly**[Q], doll like face, **hypoglycemia, hyper-lipoemia, hyper cholesterolemia, hyper triglyceridemia (d/t increased fat mobilization)**[Q]**, fatty infiltration of liver, ketosis**[Q], acidemia, ↑ **lactic acid (lactic acidosis)**[Q], ↑ **uric acid and stunted growth**.

108. B i.e. Fabry's disease; D i.e. Fragile syndrome; E i.e. Krabbe's disease
109. B i.e. Debrandhing enzyme **110. A i.e. Glucagon excess** *[Ref: Harper's 28/e P-160, 298; Lippincott 5/e p. 130; Lehninger 5/e p. 599; Chatterjea 7/e p. 330-31; Vasudevan 6/e p. 123, 111; Harrison 17/e p. 2459]*

- **Glucagon l/t hyperglycemia** as it *inhibits glycolysis and stimulates gluconeogenesis*.
- **Glucose 6 phosphatase deficiency (Type Ia/Von Gierke's disease), glycogen synthase deficiency** (Type 0 glycogen storage diseae), liver & muscle debranching enzyme deficiency (limit dextrinosis), liver & muscle phosphorylase deficiency and liver phosphorylase kinase deficiency – cause **fasting hypoglycemia**.
- Hypoglycemia in uremia suggest multiorgan involvement.

Glycogen Storage Diseases (Glycogenosis)

Type	Name	Deficient Enzyme	Organ involved primarily	Clinical Features
O	-	**Glycogen synthase**	Liver	Hypoglycemia (low blood glucose), hyper ketonemia (high ketone bodies), early death.
Ia	**Von Gierke's disease**	*Glucose 6 phosphatase*[Q]	*Liver*[Q]	- Glycogen (**normal structured** but metabolically unavailable) accumulation in liver & renal tubule cells l/t hepatorenomegaly and failure (of both) - **Hypoglycemia, hyper lipemia, hypercholesterolemia, hyper triglyceridemia** ***(d/t increased fat mobilization)***[Q], **hyper ketonemia (ketosis), lactic acidemia (lactic acidosis) and hyper uricemia**
Ib	-	**Endoplasmic reticulum glucose -6-Phosphate transporter (microsomal -6- P translocase)**	*Liver*	- **High susceptibility to recurrent bacterial infections** d/t neutropenia and impaired neutrophil function - Rest as Type Ia
Ic	-	**Microsomal Pi transporter**	*Liver*	As type Ia
II	**Pompe's**	**Lysosomal glucosidase** ($\alpha 1 \rightarrow 4$ & $\alpha 1 \rightarrow 6$) or **Acid maltase**	**Skeletal & Cardiac muscle**	- Fatal accumulation of glycogen in lysosome - **Infantile-juvenile** form: muscle hypotonia & death from **heart failure by age 2**. - **Juvenile-adult form** : myopathy & muscular dystrophy
IIIa	**Forbe's or Cori's, Limit dextrinosis**	**Liver & muscle debranching enzyme**[Q]	**Liver, Skeletal & Cardiac muscle**	- *Hepatomegaly in infants*, myopathy (muscle weakness), fasting hypoglycemia - Accumulation of characteristic branched polysaccharide (**limit dextrin**)
IIIb	**Limit dextrinosis**	**Liver debranching enzyme** (muscle enzyme normal)	**Liver**	As type IIIa but *no muscle involvement (weakness)*
IV	**Andersen's, Amylopectinosis**	**Branching enzyme**	**Liver, Skeletal muscle**	- Hepato-spleenomegaly, myoglobin in urine, death d/t cardiac or liver failure before age 5 - Accumulation of polysachride with few branch points.
V	**Mc Ardle's**	**Muscle (Myo) phosphorylase**	**Skeletal muscle**	- Exercise induced cramps & pain d/t poor exercise tolerance; blood lactate is very low after exercise - Muscle glycogen content is abnormally high (2.5-4%); myoglobin in urine.
VI	**Her's**	**Liver phosphorylase**	**Liver**	Hepatomegaly (d/t accumulation of glycogen), mild hypoglycemia & generally good prognosis.
VII	**Tarui's**	**Muscle & erythrocyte phosphofructo kinase (PFK)-1**	**Muscle, RBC**	As type V with **hemolytic anemia**
VIII		**Liver phosphorylase kinase**	**Liver**	As type VI
IX		**Liver & muscle phosphorylase-kinase**	**Liver, muscle**	As type VI with accumulation of glycogen in muscle.
VIb		**Leukocyte & Liver phosphorylase kinase**	**Leukocytes & Liver**	As type VI
X		C-AMP dependent protein kinase	**Liver**	Hepatomegaly; accumulation of glycogen in liver
XI	**Fanconi-Bickel**	**Glucose transporter (GLUT-2)**	**Liver**	Failure to thrive, hypatomegaly, renal failure and rickets.

★ Fabry's disease and krabbe's disease are sphingolipidoses. **Fragile X- syndrome** is caused by *abnormal expansion of trinucleotide repeats* (CGG/ CCG expansion lead to fragile site on chromosomes)

Disease	Deficiency/Absent Enzyme
Fabry's disease	deficiency of α- ***Galactosidase***Q
Farber's disease	deficiency of ceramidase
Forbe's disease	***Absence of debranching enzyme***Q.

111. A i.e. Glycerol –3-phosphate **112. C i.e. Hexose monophosphate shunt** **113. D i.e. CO_2**
114. A i.e. Glucose 6 phosphate dehydrgenase **115. D i.e. NADPH** **116. C i.e. NADPH**
117. C i.e. Glucose 6 phosphate dehydrogenase **118. C i.e. Transketolase** **119. D i.e. 1 CO_2**
120. C i.e. G-6-P- dehydrogenase **121. A i.e. Liver, C i.e. Lactating mammary gland; D i.e. Gonads**
122. D i.e. HMP – Shunt *[Ref: Lippincott's 5/e p. 145-148; Harper's 28/e p. 174-78; Chattergea & Shinde 7/e p. 332-38;Lehninger 5th/e p. 630]*

*No ATP is directly produced or consumed in HMP shunt. Its major function is to provide NADPH & pentose sugar*Q

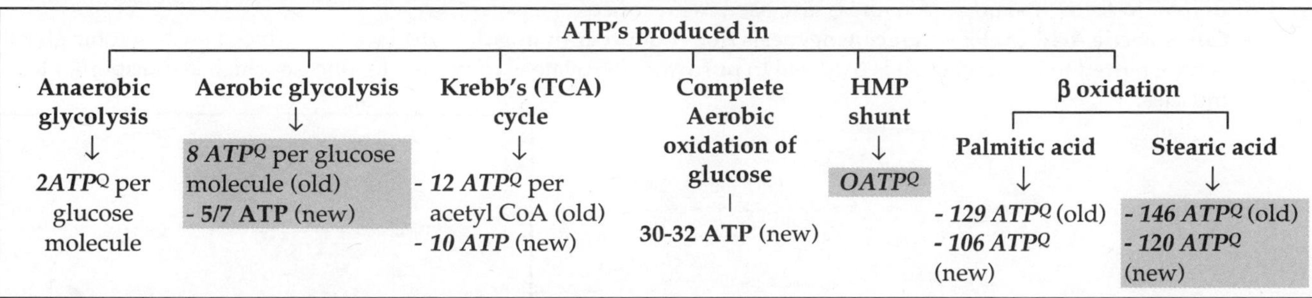

123. A i.e. Glucose-6- PO_4 dehydrogenase *[Ref: Lippincott's 4/e p. 103]*

Glucose 6 phosphate dehydrogenase deficiency is most common and pyruvate kinase deficiency is 2nd most common cause of enzyme deficiency related hemolytic anemiaQ.

124. D i.e. The oxidative phase generates NADPH and non oxidative phase generates pyruvate *[Ref: Lippincott's 4/e p. 147]*
125. D i.e. NADPH *[Ref: Lippincott 5/e p. 152-54; Lehninger 5/e p. 559]*

The **oxidative (irreversible) phase of HMP shunt produce NADPH and ribulose 5 phosphate**Q, whereas **reversible non-oxidative phase** catalyze the interconversion of 3, 4, 5, 6, and 7 carbon sugars, and permit ribulose 5 phosphate to be converted either to **ribose 5 phosphate (needed for nucleotide synthesis) or to intermediates of glycolysis – fructose 6 – PO4 & glyceraldehyde 3- phosphate**Q.

Calvin Cycle, Cori Cycle & Cahill Cycle

126. B, D, C i.e. Sedoheptulose- 1-7- bisphosphatase; Phosphoribulose kinase; Glyceraldehyde 3 PO_4 dehydrogenase
[Ref: Lehninger 5/e p. 774-86]

- **4 Calvin (photosynthetic) cycle enzyme – glyceraldehydes 3- phosphate dehydrogenase, ribulose 5- phosphate kinase, fructose 1, 6- biphosphatase and sedoheptulose, 1, 7- biphosphatase** are activated indirectly by light through thioredoxin- ferredoxin thioredoxin reductase system, which reduce disulfide bonds b/w 2 cysteine residues critical to their catalytic activities.

- Disulfide bonded (oxidized) Cys residue, in dark (night) inactivates these enzymes. In day light, electrons flow from photosystem I to ferredoxin to small, soluble, (oxidized) disulfide containing thiredoxin, reduces it in a reaction catalyzed by *ferredoxin- thioredoxin reductase*. Reduced thioredoxin donates electrons for reduction (activation) of these light activated enzymes.
- **Glucose 6 phosphate dehydrogenase**, the 1st enzyme of oxidative PP pathway is also regulated by light but in opposite sense (i.e. *light induced reduction inactivates it*).

127. **A i.e. Increased release of alanine from muscle**
128. **A i.e. Increased alanine level in muscle**
129. **C i.e. Transaminase enzyme & pyridoxial PO_4 binding is covalent; D i.e. Glutamate is formed**
130. **A, B, C, E i.e. Accepted by α-ketoglutarate; Funneled to L-Glutamate; Prevents oxidative breakdown; SGPT/SGOT...**
131. **C i.e. Inhibited by ADP & activated by GTP** *[Ref: Harper 29/e p 192-93; Lehninger 5/e p 681, 915, 548, 598; Lippincott 5/e p 331-32]*

- During first few days of fasting, there is **rapid breakdown of muscle protein, providing aminoacids (alanine & glutamine mainly) that are used by liver for gluconeognesis**Q.
- In the fasting state, the **output of alanine from skeleton muscle is in far excess of its concentration in the muscle proteins that are being catabolized.** Because it is **also formed by transamination of pyruvate produced by glycolysis of muscle glycogen.** Alanine is exported to the liver, where it is transaminated **back to pyruvate, which serves as a substrate for gluconeogenesis**Q.

132. **C i.e. Transamination of pyruvate to alanine**

- **Cahill's Glucose – Alanine Cycle produces alanine from pyruvate (not lactate) by transamination.** Because **muscles are incapabale of synthesizing urea,** the **α amino groups of aminoacids (i.e. ammonia) is transported from muscles to liver in form of alanine**. Alanine is also used in **gluconeogenesis**.
- **Cori's Lactic Acid Cycle:** As **gluconeogenesis does not occur in muscle**Q, the **lactate** produced by anaerobic glycolysis is **transported to liver,** where it is oxidized to puruvate. Pyruvate is converted to glucose which is transported to muscles.

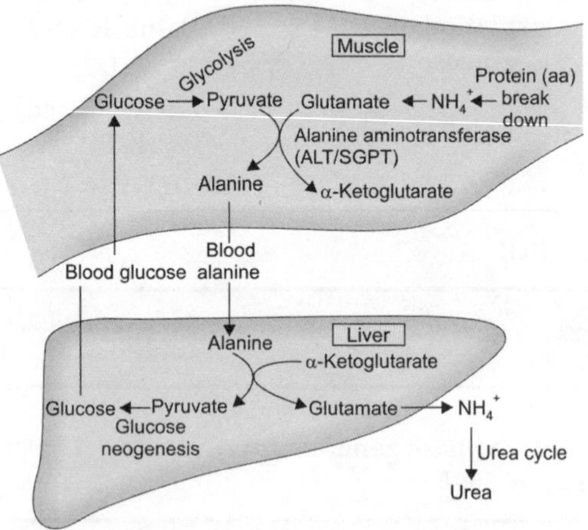

Alanine – Glucose (Cahill) Cycle

Glucose – Alanine cycle: Skeletal muscle transport NH_3 to liver in form of alanine, resulting in reciprocal transfer of glucose to muscle, This cycle is called Glucose – Alanine cycle.

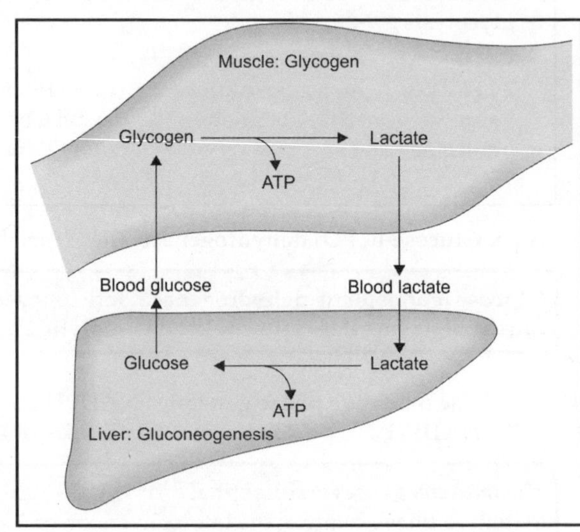

Cori (Lactic Acid) Cycle

133. **A i.e. Fatty acids** *[Ref: Harper 29/e p. 16]*

Organ	Fed	Fasting	Starvation
RBC	Glucose	Glucose	-
Brain	Glucose	Glucose	Ketone bodies
Heart	Fatty acids	Fatty acids	Ketone bodies
Liver	Glucose	Fatty acids	Amino acids
Muscles & Adipose tissue	Glucose	Fatty acids	**Fatty acid (Major source)**Q & **Ketone Bodies** (on prolonged starvation)

Gluconeogenesis

134. **C i.e. Acetoacetate / Fatty acids/Palmitate /GH**
135. **C i.e. Methionine**
136. **D i.e. Lysine**
137. **A i.e. Oleate**

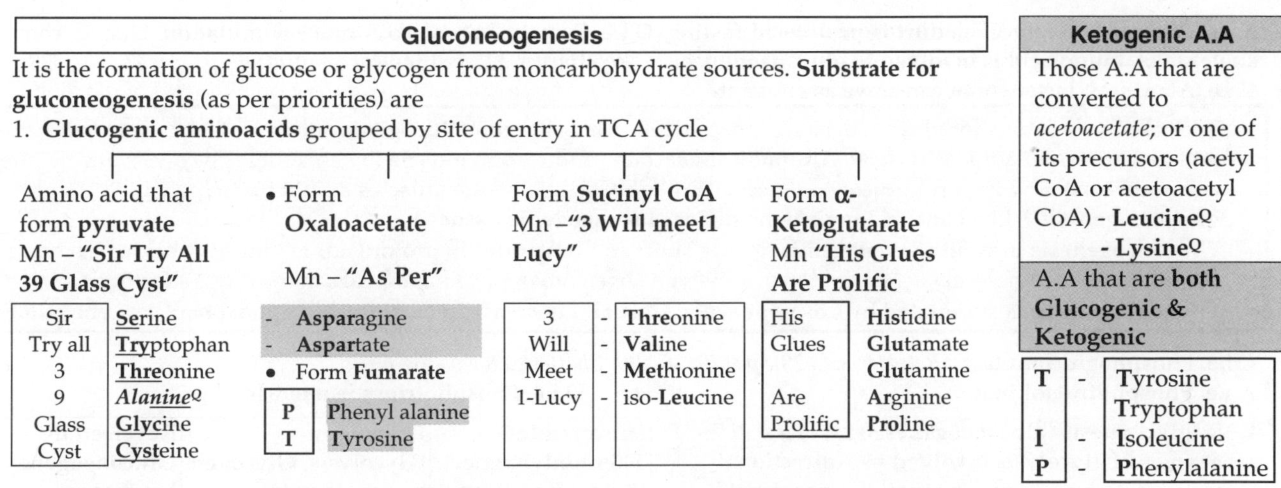

2. *Lactate*[Q] 3. *Pyruvate*[Q] 4. *Glycerol*[Q] (obtained from lipolysis of fat) [Mn "G < P < L"]
5. *Propionic acid*[Q] (important in ruminants)

138. ALL i.e. (Precursor for synthesis of cholesterol.., Form ketone .., Starting material for synthesis .., Arise from glycolysis)

139. B i.e. Malic Enzyme **140. A i.e. Glucose** *[Ref: Harper 29th/e p. 123, 164, 187-189; Chatterjae 8/e p 338, 441; Vasudevan 6/e p. 216, 450, 407; Thomas Miller (2002); Kaplan lecture notes (2007) p-201; Lippincott 4th/ed pg-- 266, 111-12, 220, 96, 119, 192, 195-96 Lehninger 5th/ed pg- 616-17, 695, 557]*

- **Acetyl coenzyme A arises from pyruvate (the end product of aerobic glycolysis) by irreversible oxidative decarboxylation catalyzed by pyruvate dehydrogenase (PDH) complex**[Q]
- **Acetyl CoA is not a substrate for gluconeogenesis and cannot be converted back to glucose**[Q]. This is because **acetyl CoA cannot be converted back to pyruvate**[Q] since its carbon backbone is lost in citric acid cycle as CO2. Hence fatty acids cannot be converted into glucose
- **Substrates for gluconeogenesis** are : **proprionic** acid (in ruminants), **gl**ucogenic amino acids, **gl**ycerol, **py**ruvate and **la**ctate (Mn- **"Proper GPL"**)
- **Acetyl CoA** is used in **oxidative phosphorylation** (in TCA cycle) for energy production; in **acetylation reaction** (coenzyme pantothenic acid) for detoxification & acetyl choline formation. It is also used in **cholesterol synthesis, steroidogenesis** (steroid hormone & vitamin D_3 synthesis), **lipogenesis** (fatty acid synthesis and elongation, synthesis of ether lipids like plasmalogens & PAF) and **ketogenesis** (ketone body formation).
- **Acetyl CoA** is a **precursor or starting material** (& substrate for enzymes) for **synthesis of cholesterol & ketone bodies (= substrate for HMG CoA synthetase) and fatty acid synthesis (=** substrate for **fatty acid synthase, acetyl CoA carboxylase or malonyl CoA synthetase and malonyl transaceylase)**
- **Malic enzyme forms malic acid from pyruvic acid**[Q] in presence of CO_2 & NADPH.

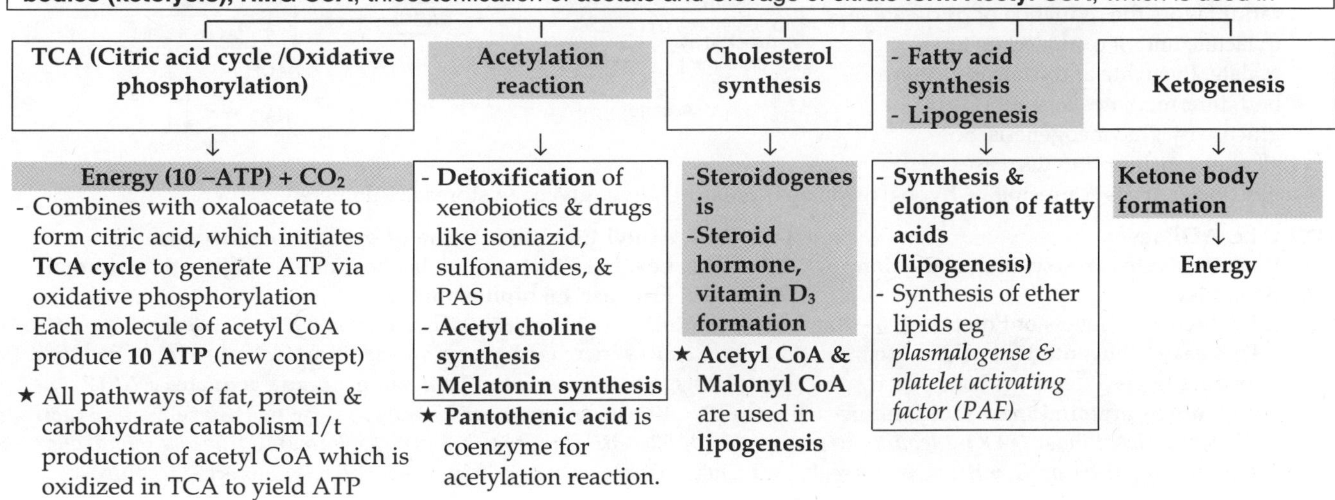

141. A i.e. Prevent hypoglycemia during prolonged fasting; D i.e. Excess of acetyl co A cause stimulation; E i.e. Carbon skeleton of amino acid is involved in gluconeogenesis *[Ref: Harper 29/e p. 187-94; Lippincott 6/e p. 331-32, 326, 329]*

142. C i.e. Alanine & lactate both can serve as substrate

- The **carbon skeletons for gluconeogenesis** are derived primarily from **glucogenic aminoacids & lactate from muscle and glycerol from adipose tissue**[Q]. **Although the lactate produced in muscle** (by anaerobic glycolysis during intense exercise) **is used by liver for gluconeogenesis (through Cori cycle); the muscles do not participate in gluconeogenesis**[Q]. **Liver and kidney are the major gluconeogenic tissues**[Q].
- **Gluconeogenesis prevent hypoglycemia during short and long term (= prolonged) fasting**[Q] i.e. begins 4-6 hours after the last meal becomes fully active as stores of liver glycogen are depleted and peaks at 5-7 days of fasting .
- **Gluconeogenesis is stimulated by excess of acetyl CoA and decrease in fructose 2,6 biphosphate concentration**[Q].

143. C i.e. Phosphoglucomutase *[Ref: Harper's 29/e p. 179, 187-90; Chatterjea 8/e p. 364-69]*

144. A i.e. Phosphofructokinase

- **Neoglucognesis (gluconeogenesis)** involves all **7 enzymes of glycolysis involved in bidirectional reactions** such as (1) ***phosphohexo isomerase***[Q], (2) **aldolase (3) Phosphotriose isomerase (4) glyceraldehyde 3 phosphate dehydrogenase, (5 & 6) *phosphoglycerate kinase/mutase***[Q], and **enolase**. Whereas for thermodynamically irreversible reactions of glycolysis, it uses **pyruvate carboxylase & (7) phosphoenol pyruvate (PEP) carboxykinase**[Q] in place of pyruvate kinase; ***fructose 1, 6 bi phosphatase***[Q] in place of phosphofrctokinase and ***glucose 6 phosphatase***[Q] in place of hexo/glucokinase
- **Phosphoglucomutase** is involved in ***Glycogen metabolism***[Q] ***not gluconeogenesis.***

$$\text{Glucose–6–PO}_4 \xrightarrow{\text{Phosphogluco Mutase}^{Q}} \text{Glucose – 1- PO}_4$$

145. D i.e. Phosphotriose isomerase

Irreversible Thermodynamic Barrier Reactions	Enzyme in Glycolysis, Glycogen metabolism (4th)	Reversed in Gluconeogenesis by key Enzymes
Phosphoenol pyruvate (PEP) → Pyruvate	*Pyruvate Kinase*[Q]	*Pyruvate carboxylase & PEP carboxy kinase*[Q]
Fructose 6 phosphate → Fructose 1, 6 biphosphate	Phospho fructokinase (PFK)1	Fructose 1, 6 biphosphatase
Glucose → Glucose 6 phosphate	*Gluco/Hexo-Kinase*[Q]	*Glucose 6 phosphatase*[Q]
Glycogen → Glucose 1 phosphate	Glycogen phosphorylase, Glucan transferase, Debranching enzyme	UDP Glc phosphorylase, Glycogen synthase, Branching enzyme

146. A i.e. Acetyldehyde *[Ref: Harper's 27/e p. 225-26; Lippioncott's 4/e p. 317-18]*

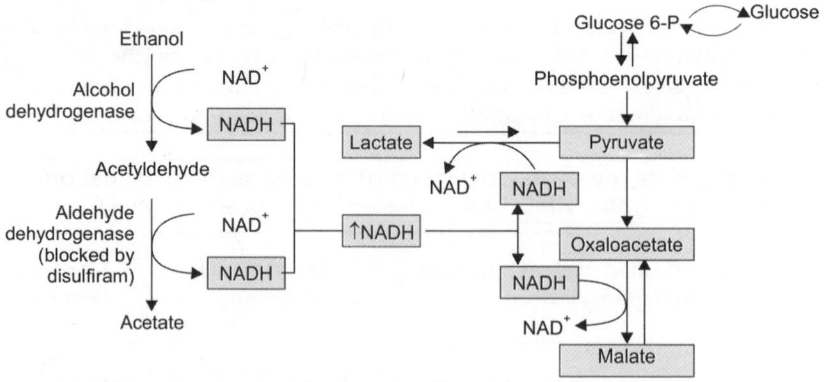

Ethanol is oxidized to acetaldehyde by alcohol dehydrogenase and subsequently to acetate by aldehyde dehydrogenase. Both reactions produce NADH by transferring electrons to NAD+. The **abundance of NADH (increased NADH / NAD+ ratio)** favors the reduction of pyruvate to lactate and of oxaloacetate to malate. Pyruvate and oxaloacetate are both intermediates in synthesis of glucose by gluconeogenesis. So alcohol consumption decreases gluconeogenesis & precipitate hypoglycemia particularly if liver glycogen stores are depleted.

147. C i.e. ADP level

148. B i.e. Acetyl CoA stimulation of pyruvate carboxylase

149. B i.e. Pyruvate carboxylation activation

150. A i.e. Level of Fructose 1, 6- biphosphate is higher than normal

151. B i.e. Liver

152. D i.e. Fructose 1,6 biphosphate

153. C i.e. Increased levels of Fructose 2, 6 – Bisphosphate *[Ref:Harper 29/e p. 187-93; Lippincott 5/e p. 117-122; Lehninger 5/e p. 582-87]*

- **Decreased concentration of glucose** in blood & liver causes **increased glucagon secretion** (&↑ glucagon / insulin ratio) leading to glycogenolysis followed by gluconeogenesis in liver. **Increased levels of glucagon activates c-AMP dependent protein kinase** which inturn **activates F2, 6 BPase (fructose 2, 6 biphosphatase or FBpase 2)** and ***inactivates phosphofructokinase (PFK)-2 leading to conversion of F2, 6 BP (Fructose 2, 6 biphosphatse) to fructose 6 phosphate. So the concentration of F2, 6 BP is decreased***[Q] and fructose 6 phosphate is increased which is converted to glucose.

- **Gluconeogenesis in fasting state is indicated by acetyl CoA induced instantaneous allosteric activation of hepatic pyruvate carboxylase.**[Q]
- **Phosphofructokinase I** takes part in **glycolysis** and **FBPase** 1 in **gluconeogenesis**, by catalyzing the formation & breakdown of fructose 1, 6 biphosphate respectively. Whereas **bifunctional enzyme phosphor fructo kinase 2 (PK-2) also has fructose 2, 6 biphosphatase (FBP ase 2 or F 2, 6 pase) activity** and **plays a unique role in regulation of both glycolysis & gluconeogenesis by determining the levels of fructose 2, 6 bihosphate**[Q].
- **Fructose 2, 6 bihosphate (F2, 6BP) is the most potent allosteric activator of PFK-1** (thereby increase glycolysis) and **inhibitor of fructose 1, 6 biphosphatase /FBP ase 1/ F1, 6 pase** (thereby **decreasing gluconegenesis) in liver**[Q]. The reciprocal action of fructose 2, 6 biPO_4, on glycolysis and gluconeogenesis ensure that both pathways, is not fully active at same time. Therefore, **decreased sensitivity of FBP ase 1 to regulation (inhibition) by fructose 2, 6 biphosphate increases gluconeogenesis; thereby decreasing levels of fructose 1, 6 biphosphate, pyruvate and ATP**[Q]**.**
- **Fructose 1, 6 biphosphate is under negative feed back control of fructose 2, 6 biphosphate**[Q]**.** If fructose 1, 6 biphasphatase becomes less sensitive to the negative feed back of fructose 2, 6 biPO_4, its level of activity will increase. Thus more fructose 1, 6 biPO_4 will be cleaved into fructose 6-PO_4 and levels of fructose 1, 6 biPO_4 will decrease and be lower than normal. The cycle will be shifted more toward gluconeogenesis. **Less ATP would be generated d/t decreased glycolysis**[Q]**.**
- **Glycogenic capability** of cell is **determined by presence (activation) of fructose 1, 6 biphosphatase**[Q]. **The conversion of fructose 1, 6-bisphosphate to fructose6-phosphate, to achieve a reversal of glycolysis, is catalyzed by fructose-1,6-bisphosphatase. Its presence determines whether or not a tissue is capable of synthesizing glycogen not only from pyruvate but also from triosephosphates.** It is present in liver, kidney, and skeletal muscle but is probably absent from heart and smooth muscle.
- **In well fed state gluconeogenesis in liver is inhibited by ADP**[Q]**.**

154. **C i.e. Decreased gluconeogenesis** *[Ref: Lippincott 4th/ed pg-322-23,329; Teitz 6th/ed pg-376,388; Chatterjea 7th/ed pg-363-64]*

Glycolysis increases and gluconeogenesis decreases after feeding[Q].

155. **B i.e. Citrate**

Regulatory & Adaptive Enzymes a/w Carbohydrate Metabolism

Enzyme	Enzyme Activity in		Transcription Regulator		Allosteric Regulation	
	High Energy state (Carbohydrate Feeding)	Low Energy state (Fasting/ Diabetes)	Inducer	Repressor	Activator	Inhibitor
Glycogenolysis, Glycolysis, & Pyruvate oxidation	Increase 1-6 except 2	Decrease 1-6 except 2				
1. Glycogen synthase	↑	↓			Insulin, glucose 6-phosphate	Glucagon
2. Hexokinase	-	-				Glucose 6 phosphate
3. Glucokinase	↑	↓	**Insulin**	Glucagon		
4. Phosphofructo-kinase (PFK)1	↑	↓	**Insulin**	Glucagon	**AMP,** fructose 6-P, fructose 2 , 6 biphosphate, Pi	**Citrate**[Q], ATP, glucagon
5. Pyruvate kinase	↑	↓	**Insulin, fructose**	Glucagon	Fructos 1, 6 biphosphate, insulin	ATP, alanine, glucagon, nor epinephrine
6. Pyruvate dehydrogenase	↑	↓			CoA, NAD+, insulin, ADP, pyruvate	***Acetyl CoA***[Q], NADH, ATP (fatty acid ketone -bodies)
Gluconeogenesis 7. Pyruvate carboxylase 8. PEP carboxykinase 9. Glucose 6-phosphatase			**Glucacortico-steroids, glucagon , epinephrine**	Insulin	**Acetyl CoA**[Q]	**ADP**[Q]
					Glucagon?	-
					-	-

Fructose Metabolism

156. C i.e. Hyperglycemia *[Ref: Harper's 27/e P-183; Harrison 16/e P-2321]*

> **Hereditary fructose intolerance** due to ***deficiency of aldolase B***Q, causes fructose induced ***hypoglycemia***Q despite the presence of high glycogen reserve. The accumulation of fructose 1- PO_4 and fructose 1, 6- PO4 allosterically inhibit liver phosphorylase

157. A i.e. Fructose –1- PO_4 *[Ref: Harper's 27/e P-183-84]*

> **Fructokinase** *convert fructose to fructose –1- PO_4*Q. It is ***deficient in essential fructosuria***

158. A i.e. Glyceraldehyde- 3- phosphate dehydrogenase *[Ref: Harper's 27/e P-183-184; 26/e P-169]*

> ***Glyceraldehyde –3 phosphate dehydrogenase*** **is an enzyme in the pathway *for conversion of fructose to pyruvate*Q.**

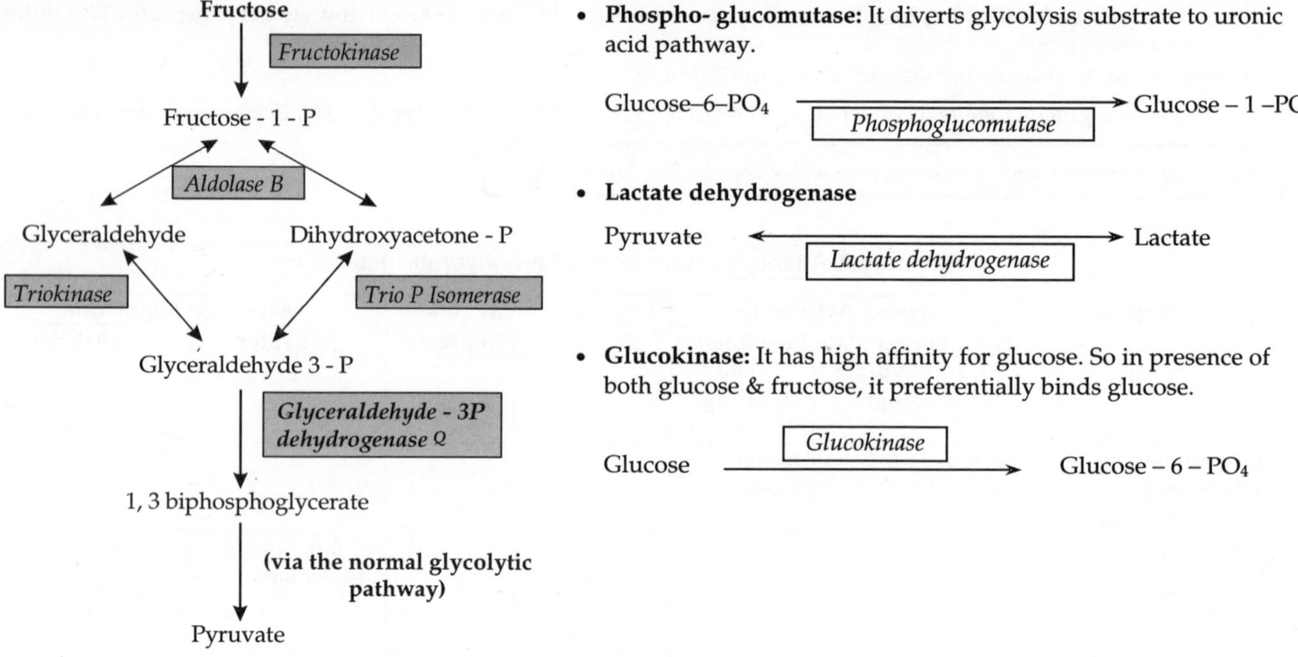

Galactose Metabolism & Intolerance

159. D i.e. All of the above
160. D i.e. Galactose
161. A i.e. Galactose–1–Phosphate uridyl transferase
162. A i.e. Galactose–1–phosphate uridyl transferase
163. A i.e Mental retardation occurs; C i.e Defect in epimerase; D i.e Defect in galactose –1 PO_4 uridyltransferase
164. C i.e. Galactosemia
165. B i.e. Galactosemia
166. D i.e. Galactitol

Glactosemia

An inherited ***Autosomal recessive***Q disorder, in which there is inability to convert galactose to glucose in normal manner. This may occur *due to deficiency* of following enzymes:

Galactose 1-PO_4 Uridyl Transferase (classical & most common)	UDP galactose –4 Epimerase (Rare)	Galactokinase (Minor)
- Manifests with in a few days after birth ***(after ingestion of milk)***[Q] - Failure to thrive - ***Hepto splenomegaly***[Q] - Jaundice, Ascites - ***Hypoglycemia***[Q] - ***Mental retardation***[Q] - ***Cataract***[Q], ***(oil drop cataract)***[Q]	Feature of uridyl trans ferase deficiency + - Nerve deafness - Hypotonia - ↑in cellular UDP Galactose	***Cataract***[Q] Affected infant is other wise asymptomatic.

- Infants are subject to ***bacterial sepsis (especially with E.coli)***[Q] this may be *leading cause of death.*
- **Biochemical & urinary finding**
  - Increase blood galactose level
  - ***Decreased blood glucose***[Q] **(normal oxidase-peroxidase test)**[Q]
  - ***Galactosuria (reducing sugar galactose** in urine gives **positive Benedict's test)***[Q]
  - Albuminuria
  - Amiaciduria: Glycine, Alanine, Serine
- **Treatment: *Galactose free diet***[Q].

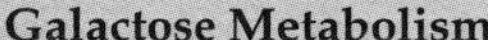

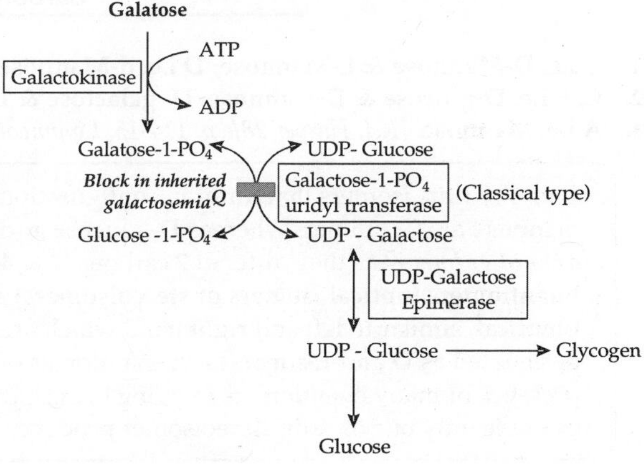

Cataract

In Galactosemia is due to accumulation of galactitol[Q].	In Diabetes is due to accumulation of sorbito[l] in lens.
• The increased galactose conc. in blood and eye is reduced to *Galactitol* by *aldolase reductase,* • Galactitol can not escape from lens cells and accumulates to form cataract.	↑Concentration of glucos[e] in blood & eye is *reduced t[o] sorbitol* by aldolase reductase.

167. **D i.e. Lactase**	168. **D i.e. Sucrase** *[Ref: Harper's 27/e P-184-185; Chatterjea 6/e P- 312-313, 264-65, Nelson 17/e P-1268]*

This patient develops gas and diarrhoea following consumption of dairy products. These are **symptoms of 'Lactose intolerance' due to deficiency of Lactase**[Q]. **Sucrase deficiency presents with similar clinical features as in lactase deficiency**[Q]. As lactase is not given as an option, sucrase is the 2nd best choice.

Lactase deficiency	Sucrase Isomaltase deficiency
• Due to ***deficiency of lactase***[Q]. Lactose —(*Lactase*[Q])→ Galactose + Glucose • Clinical features in response to *ingestion of lactose* (sugar in milk) - ***Bloating (gas)***[Q] - ***Watery diarrhoea***[Q] - Failure to thrive - ***Abdominal cramp***[Q]	• Due to deficiency of sucrose & isomaltase • Clinical features in response to ingestion of sugar (cane sugar and table sugar) - Bloating - Watery diarrhea - Failure to thrive

Enzyme deficiency	Associated disorder
β-galactosidase deficiency	- Galactosidosis - GM1 gangliosidosis - Mucopolysacharidosis IV A: Morquio A
α-glucosidase deficiency	Type II glycogen storage disease (Acid α1, 4 glucosidase deficiency : Pompes disease)

Alcohol Metabolism

169. **B & C i.e. NAD+ & NADPH** *[Ref: Lippincott 4th/ed pg- 317-18; Harper 28th/ed pg- 630-29, 218-20; Lehninger 5th/ed pg-547,664,518]*

In **chronic alcoholism** the **rate limiting** component for alcohol metabolism excluding enzyme are **NAPH** (in MEOS) and **NAD+** (in major pathway).

170. C i.e. D-xylose absorption test

Glycosylated hemoglobin (HbA_{1C}, an index of average glucose level in preceding 12 weeks), **Fasting blood sugar** (FBS ≥ 126 mg/dl), **oral glucose tolerance test (OGTT)** i.e. 2 hour post prandial glucose levels (> 200 mg/dl) and **random blood sugar** (RBS > 200 mg(dl) are used to diagnose diabetes mellitus whereas **D-xylose absorption test** is used to determine absorption of D-xylose in proximal small intestine (duodenum & jejunum) to detect **intestinal malabsorption syndrome**[Q].

Carbohydrate Classification

171. C i.e. D-Mannose & L-Mannose; D i.e. d-Mannose & l-Mannose; E i.e. D-glucose and L glucose
172. C, E i.e. D-glucose & D-mannose, D- galactose & D-glucose
173. A i.e. Mannose *[Ref: Harper 28/e p. 114-15; Lippincott 5/e p. 83-85; Lehninger 5/e p. 236-40]*

- Carbohydrate isomers that differ in configuration around only one carbon atom are called **epimers. D-glucose and D-mannose are** C_2 epimers whereas **D- glucose and D- galactose** differ only at C_4. ***However, D-mannose & D- galactose are not epimers***[Q] as they differ at 2 carbons (2 & 4).
- **Enantiomers (optical isomers or stereoisomers)** are pairs of structures that are **mirror images of each other but not identical**, similar to left and right hand which are the same but opposite. These are non super imposable and are designated as **D and L-sugar**. Each enantiomer often *shows different chemical reactions* with other enantiomers. Because of presence of many enantiomers in living beings, there is usually a marked difference in effects of two stereoisomers. For example only one of drug stereoisomer produces desired effect while the other does not.

174. B i.e. Beta configuration of anomeric C2 *[Ref: Harper 28/e p. 118-19; Lippincott 5/e p. 86-87; Lehninger 5/e p. 246-50; 'Food and Nutrition supplements: Their role in health and disease' (Springer) 1st (2001)/130; 'Colonic Microbiota, Nutrition and Health' by Gibson & Roberfroid 1st (1999)/105]*

Inulin like fructan – prebiotics are non digestible in upper GI tract ***because of their beta (β) configuration of anomeric*** C_2[Q].

Chapter -2 FAT METABOLISM

QUESTIONS

Lipids of Physiological Significance

1. **All are true except** *(PGI 02)*
   A. Linoleic acid is found in soyabean oil ☐
   B. Linolenic & linoleic acids are cis derivatives containing double bonds. ☐
   C. Arachidonic acid contain five double bonds. ☐
   D. Monoenoic acids contain one double bond at 9th position. ☐
2. **Which among the following is a cardioprotective fatty acid?** *(NBE P 13; AI 11)*
   A. Palmitic acid ☐
   B. Stearic acid ☐
   C. Oleic acid ☐
   D. Omega-3 fatty acids ☐
3. **True statement about fatty acid:** *(PGI 11)*
   A. Polyunsaturated FA is essential for membrane structure ☐
   B. Biologically arachidonic acid is essential to life ☐
   C. Hydrogenated vegetable oils contains Trans fatty acid ☐
   D. Most of the naturally occurring unsaturated FA exists as trans-isomer ☐
4. **False about trans fatty acid** *(PGI 10, 09)*
   A. Increase risk of cardiovascular disease ☐
   B. Fried foods have high content of TFA ☐
   C. Hydrogenation increases TFA ☐
   D. Hydrogenation decreases TFA ☐
   E. It ↑ LDL & ↓ HDL ☐
5. **The most essential fatty acid is** *(NBE P 13; AI 05)*
   A. Linoleic acid ☐
   B. Linolenic acid ☐
   C. Arachidonic acid ☐
   D. Palmitic acid ☐
6. **Essential fatty acid is/are:** *(PGI 13)*
   A. Palmitic acid ☐
   B. Linoleic acid ☐
   C. Linolenic acid ☐
   D. Free fatty acid ☐
   E. Oleic acid ☐
7. **Maximum source of linoleic acid is** *(PGI 13; AIIMS 04)*
   A. Coconut oil ☐
   B. Sunflower oil ☐
   C. Palm oil ☐
   D. Vanaspati ☐
8. **Which of these fatty acids is found exclusively in breast milk:** *(NBE P 15; AI 01)*
   A. Linolaete ☐
   B. Linolenic ☐
   C. Palmitic ☐
   D. Docosahexanoic acid ☐
9. **The following fatty acid does not belong to W6 series**
   A. Linoleic acid *(PGI 10; AIIMS 08)* ☐
   B. Arachidonc acid ☐
   C. Gamma linolenic acid ☐
   D. Alpha linolenic acid ☐
10. **Gangliosides consists of:** *(PGI 08)*
    A. Long chain fatty acid (LCFA) ☐
    B. Alcohol- sphingosine ☐
    C. Phosphate ☐
    D. Sailic acid ☐
    E. Glycerol ☐
11. **Which of the following is correct in regards of function of phospholipid:** *(PGI 05)*
    A. Cell-cell interaction ☐
    B. Signal transduction ☐
    C. Surfactant ☐
    D. Acute inflammatory mediator ☐
    E. Activates membrane enzyme ☐
12. **Glycosphingolipidis made up of:** *(PGI 10)*
    A. Glucose ☐
    B. Glycerol ☐
    C. Sphingosine ☐
    D. Fatty acids ☐
    E. Thromboxane A2 ☐
13. **Alcoholic group is found in:** *(PGI 08)*
    A. Ganglioside ☐
    B. Sphingomyelin ☐
    C. Cerebroside ☐
    D. Terpen ☐
14. **Not a predisposing factor for atherosclerotic plaque formation?** *(AI 11)*
    A. Apo E deficiency ☐
    B. Alpha 2 – macroglobulin ☐
    C. Oxidised LDL ☐
    D. Increased homocyctiene ☐
15. **Which of the following phospholipid has antigenic activity-** *(NBE P 14, 15)*
    A. Plasmalogen ☐
    B. Cardiolipin ☐
    C. Phosphatidylcholine ☐
    D. Sphingoyelin ☐

Acylglycerol & Sphingolipid Metabolism

16. **Fatty acids are stored as-** *(NBE P 14, 15)*
    A. Cholesterol ☐
    B. Triglycerides ☐
    C. Sphingomyelin ☐
    D. None ☐
17. **Molecular change in Lysosomal storage disorder is:** *(AIIMS 07)*
    A. Defective fusion of lysosomes and phagosomes ☐

B. Increased synthesis of some substrates ☐
C. Mutation of genes encoding lysosomal hydrolases ☐
D. Membrane defect of lysosomes ☐

18. Which of the following is/are not sphingolipidosis:
A. Tay sach's disease *(PGI 13)* ☐
B. Sandhoff's disease ☐
C. Krabbe's disease ☐
D. Wolman disease ☐
E. Fabry's disease ☐

19. True about gaucher disease: *(PGI 09)*
A. Due to deficiency of enzyme sphingomyelinase ☐
B. Due to deficiency of enzyme Beta-Gluco-cerebrosidase ☐
C. Deposition of glucosylceramide ☐
D. Foam cell depositon ☐
E. PAS staining positive ☐

20. Sphingomyelinase Deficiency is seen in OR Accumulation of sphingomyelin in phagocytic cells is feature of: *(AIIMS 14,12; AI 10)*
A. Niemann-Pick disease *(NBE P 14, 13; PGI 13,15)* ☐
B. Farber's disease ☐
C. Tay Sach's disease ☐
D. Krabbe's disease ☐

21. Gaucher's disease is due to deficiency of enzyme :
A. Sphingomyelinase *(AI 11; PGI 14; NBE P 15,14,13)* ☐
B. β-Glucosidase (Glucocerebrosidase) ☐
C. Hexosaminidase-A ☐
D. β-Galactosidase ☐

22. Splenomegaly seen in A/E: *(PGI 06)*
A. Neimann pick's disease ☐
B. Krabbe's disease ☐
C. GM2 gangliosidosis ☐
D. Gaucher's disease ☐
E. Sialodosis ☐

23. Krabbes disease is due to deficiency of- *(NBE P 15)*
A. SPhingomyelinase ☐
B. Beta galactocerebrosidase ☐
C. Hexosaminidase ☐
D. Arylsulfatase ☐

24. Nieman pick disease is due to deficiency of-
A. Sphingomyelinase *(NBE P 15)* ☐
B. Ceramidase ☐
C. Galactosidase ☐
D. Glucosidase ☐

25. Enzyme deficiency seen in genetic disease like:
A. Tay sach's disease *(PGI 03)* ☐
B. Gaucher's disease ☐
C. Cystic Fibrosis ☐
D. Wilson's disease ☐
E. Familial hypercholesterolemia ☐

26. Enzyme replacement therapy is available for-
A. Gauchers disease *(NBE P 15,13)* ☐
B. Galactosemia ☐
C. Fructosuria ☐
D. None ☐

Lipid Transport

27. Which of the following lipoproteins does not move towards charged end in electrophoresis or Which has least density *(AIIMS 15,13; NBE P 15,14)*
A. VLDL ☐
B. LDL ☐
C. HDL ☐
D. Chylomicrons ☐

28. The human plasma lipoprotein containing the highest percentage of triacylglycerol by weight is OR Triglycerides are maximum in OR Maximum content of triglycerides are found in:
A. VLDL *(NBE P 15,13; AIIMS 14,13; PGI 14,12)* ☐
B. Chylomicrons ☐
C. HDL ☐
D. LDL ☐

29. Dietary triglycerides are transported by
A. Chylomicrons *(AIIMS 15,10)* ☐
B. VLDL ☐
C. LDL ☐
D. HDL ☐

30. Apolipoprotein E is rich in- *(NBE P 15)*
A. Lysine ☐
B. Arginine ☐
C. Histidine ☐
D. Methionine ☐

31. All are true about LDL except- *(NBE P 15)*
A. More dense than chylomicron ☐
B. Smaller than VLDL ☐
C. Transports maximum amount of lipid ☐
D. Contains maximum cholesterol ☐

32. Highest amount of cholesterol is present in OR The most important carrier of cholesterol in plasma is:
A. HDL *(PGI 14,09,02; NBE P 15,14,13)* ☐
B. LDL ☐
C. VLDL ☐
D. IDL ☐
E. Chylomicrons ☐

33. Main transporter of (dietary) cholesterol to peripheral (extrahepatic) tissue is: *(PGI 15,13,11,08; NBE P 14)*
A. HDL ☐
B. LDL ☐
C. IDL ☐
D. VLDL ☐
E. Chylomicron ☐

34. Lipoprotein associated with carrying cholesterol from periphery tissues to liver is- *(NBE P 15)*
A. HDL ☐
B. LDL ☐
C. VLDL ☐
D. IDL ☐

35. In cholesterol transport which is not needed-
A. Liver *(NBE P 15)* ☐
B. Kidney ☐
C. Intestine ☐
D. Fat ☐

36. Lipid with highest mobility is- *(NBE P 15)*
A. HDL ☐
B. LDL ☐
C. VLDL ☐
D. Chylomicrons ☐

37. Apoprotein A is found in : *(AI 09; NBE P 15)*
A. Chylomicrons ☐
B. VLDL ☐
C. HDL ☐
D. LDL ☐

38. Which of the following is maximum in HDL as compared to other lipoproteins? *(AIIMS 16)*
A. Cholesterol ☐
B. Triglycerides ☐
C. Apoproteins ☐
D. Fatty acids ☐

39. Which of the following has highest electrophoretic mobility and least lipid content: *(NBE P 14; PGI 16,14)*
A. Chylomicrons ☐
B. HDL ☐
C. LDL ☐
D. VLDL ☐
E. IDL ☐

40. Good cholesterol found in: *(PGI 12, 07)*
A. HDL ☐
B. LDL ☐
C. VLDL ☐
D. IDL ☐

41. Apo B_{48} and apo B_{100} are expressed as two different apo-proteins because of difference in : *(AI 02)*
A. RNA editing ☐
B. RNA splicing ☐
C. Chromosomal loci ☐
D. Apo-B gene ☐

42. Which helps in the transport of chylomicrons from intestine to liver: *(NBE P 13; AI 10)*
A. Apoprotein B ☐
B. Apoprotein A ☐
C. Apoprotein C ☐
D. Apoprotein E ☐

43. Major apolipoprotein of chylomicrons-
A. B-100 *(NBE P 15)* ☐
B. D ☐
C. B-48 ☐
D. None ☐

44. Endogenous triglycerides in plasma are maximally carried in: *(NBE P 13)*
A. VLDL ☐
B. Chylomicrons ☐
C. LDL ☐
D. HDL ☐

45. VLDL is formed in- *(NBE P 15)*
A. Intestine ☐
B. Liver ☐
C. From chylomicrons ☐
D. Blood ☐

46. Which of the following is an activator of LCAT-
A. Apo B 100 *(DNB 14; JIPMER 02)* ☐
B. Apo B 48 ☐
C. Apo E ☐
D. Apo AI ☐

47. All of the following statements about apoproteins are true Except: *(AI 08)*
A. Apoprotein A-I activates LCAT ☐
B. Apoprotein C-I activates lipoprotein lipase ☐
C. Apoprotein C-II inhibits lipoprotein lipase ☐
D. Apoprotein C- II activates lipoprotein lipase ☐

48. Best marker of dyslipidemia *(AIIMS 09)*
A. TG & cholesterol ☐
B. LDL / HDL ratio ☐
C. Cholesterol ☐
D. APO AI ☐

49. Most important in causing coronary artery disease (CAD) is *(AIIMS 09)*
A. HDL ☐
B. LDL ☐
C. VLDL ☐
D. Triglycerides ☐

50. All of the following statements about LDL are true except: *(AIIMS 04)*
A. It delivers cholesterol to cells ☐
B. It contains only one Apoprotein ☐
C. It is a marker for cardiovascular disease ☐
D. It contains Apo-B_4 ☐

51. All the statements regarding LDL receptors are true except: *(AIIMS 11)*
A. Present only in the extra-hepatic tissues ☐
B. Clathrin-coated pits contain the receptor on cell membrane ☐
C. It is taken into the cells by endocytosis ☐
D. Increased cellular cholesterol down-regulates the synthesis of LDL receptors ☐

52. Cholesterol present in LDL : *(AIIMS 03)*
A. Represents primarily cholesterol that is being removed from peripheral cells. ☐
B. Binds to a receptor and diffuses across the cell membrance. ☐
C. On accumulation in the cell inhibits replenishment of LDL receptors. ☐
D. When enters a cell, suppresses activity of acyl-CoA: cholesterol acytranferase ACAT. ☐

53. All of the following statements are true regarding lipoproteins except:
A. VLDL transports endogenous lipids *(AI 01)* ☐
B. LDL transports lipids to the tissues. ☐
C. Increased blood cholesterol is associated with increased LDL receptors ☐
D. Increased HDL is associated with decreased risk of coronary disease ☐

54. Which receptors are present in liver for uptake of LDL:
A. Apo E *(AIIMS 09)* ☐
B. Apo A and Apo E ☐
C. Apo E and Apo B100 ☐
D. Apo B100 ☐

55. All of the following statements about Lipoprotein Lipase are true, Except *(AI 09)*
A. Found in adipose tissue ☐
B. Found in myocytes ☐
C. Deficiency leads to hypertriacylglycerolemia ☐
D. Does not require CII as cofactor ☐

56. Lipoprotein with scavenging action is OR Concentration of which is inversely related to the risk of coronary heart disease: *(NBE P 15,13; PGI 15, 13, 07)*
A. HDL ☐
B. LDL ☐
C. VLDL ☐
D. None ☐

57. A young male patient presents with LDL 600mg/dl, triglycerides 140 mg/dl. What would be the most likely finding on physical examination *(AIIMS 11)*
A. Tendon xanthoma ☐
B. Planar xanthoma ☐
C. Lipemia retinalis ☐
D. Tuberoeruptive xanthoma ☐

58. A patient was diagnosed with isolated increase in LDL. His father and brother had the same disease with increased cholesterol. The likely diagnosis is:
A. Familial type III hyperlipoproteinemia *(AIIMS 09)*☐
B. Abetaliporoteinemia ☐
C. Familial lipoprotein lipase deficiency (type 1) ☐
D. LDL receptor mutation ☐

59. Which of the following is increased in lipoprotein lipase deficiency: *(AIIMS 02)*
A. VLDL ☐
B. LDL ☐
C. HDL ☐
D. Chylomicrons ☐

60. In Familial hypercholesterolemia there is deficiency of: *(PGI 08; AIIMS 05)*
A. LDL receptor ☐
B. Apo protein A ☐
C. Apo protein C ☐
D. Lipoprotein lipase. ☐

61. Which of the following types of hypertriglyceridemia is associated with an increase in chylomicron and VLDL remnants? *(AI 08)*
A. Type I ☐
B. Type IIa ☐
C. Type III ☐
D. Type IV ☐

62. In Abetaltipoproteinemia result in absence of:
A. Chylomicron *(PGI 02)* ☐
B. LDL ☐
C. VLDL ☐
D. HDL ☐
E. TG ☐

63. A person on a fat free carbohydrate rich diet continues to grow obese. Which of the following lipoproteins is likely to be elevated in his blood?
A. Chylomicrons *(AI 04)* ☐
B. VLDL ☐
C. LDL ☐
D. HDL ☐

64. Endogenous triglycerides in plasma are maximally carried in- *(NBE P 15)*
A. VLDL ☐
B. Chylomicrons ☐
C. LDL ☐
D. HDL ☐

65. Which is an abnormal lipoprotein- *(NBE P 15)*
A. VLDL ☐
B. Chylomicron ☐
C. LP (a) ☐
D. LDL ☐

66. Increased level of lipoprotein(a) predisposes to:
A. Liver cirrhosis *(AIIMS 06)* ☐
B. Atherosclerosis ☐
C. Nephrotic syndrome ☐
D. Pancreatitis ☐

Cholesterol Synthesis & Excretion

67. In cholesterol synthesis, which is rate limiting enzyme:
A. HMG CoA reductase*(NBEP 15,14; AIIMS 15,13,11)* ☐
B. HMG CoA synthetase *(PGI 14,12,06)* ☐
C. 7 alpha hydroxylase ☐
D. Phosphofructokinase ☐

68. Which of the following enzymes is common to the synthesis of cholesterol and ketone bodies: *(AI 12)*
A. HMG –Co-A Reductase ☐
B. HMG-Co-A Lyase ☐
C. HMG-Co-A Synthase ☐
D. Thiokinase ☐

69. Cholesterol structurally belongs to molecule:
A. Steroid *(PGI 03)* ☐
B. Carbohydrate ☐
C. Urea ☐
D. Peptide ☐

70. Fatty acids of cholesterol are mainly: *(PGI 2K)*
A. Oleic acid ☐
B. Linoleic acid ☐
C. Linolenic acid ☐
D. Palmitic acid ☐
E. Stearic acid ☐

71. For reduction of cholesterol, the best management includes: *(PGI 03)*
A. Cholesterol restricted diet ☐
B. High fiber diet ☐
C. Diet with high unsaturated FA and low saturated FA ☐
D. Diet with low unsaturated FA and high saturated FA ☐
E. Cholesterol restricted diet, high fiber and diet with low saturated FA to unsaturated FA ratio ☐

72. Hypolipidemic agents act on: *(PGI 02)*
A. HMG CoA synthetase ☐
B. HMG CoA oxygenase ☐
C. HMG CoA reductase ☐
D. HMG CoA hydratase ☐
E. HMG CoA mutase ☐

73. Bile acids are derived from: *(AIIMIS 07)*
A. Fatty acids ☐
B. Cholesterol ☐
C. Bilirubin ☐
D. Proteins ☐

74. Bile acids synthesized in liver (Primary bile acids):
A. Lithocolic acid *(PGI 2K)* ☐
B. Cholic acid ☐
C. Chenodeoxycholic acid ☐
D. Deoxycholic acid ☐
E. Taurocholic acid ☐

75. Common intermediate in synthesis of steroid hormones is: *(AIIMS 16)*
A. 7 Dihydrocholesterol ☐
B. Cortisone ☐
C. Pregnenolone ☐
D. 7 Hydroxycholesterol ☐

Fatty Acid Synthesis And Metabolism

76. Which biochemical reaction does *not* occur in the mitochondria: *(NBE P 15,14,13; AIIMS 14)*
A. Kreb's cycle/Urea cycle / TCA cycle ☐
B. Fatty acid (β) oxidation ☐
C. Gluconeogenesis/Ketogenesis ☐
D. Fatty acid synthesis/EMP ☐

77. Mitochondria is involved in all of the following, except: *(AIIMS 03)*
A. ATP production ☐
B. Apoptosis ☐
C. Tricarboxylic acid cycle ☐
D. Fatty acid biosynthesis ☐

78. NADPH is required for : *(AI 08)*
A. Gluconeogenesis ☐
B. Glycolysis ☐
C. Fatty acids synthesis ☐
D. Glycogenolysis ☐

79. NADPH is used in: *(AI 05)*
A. Fatty acid synthesis ☐
B. Ketone synthesis ☐
C. Gluconeogenesis ☐
D. Glycolysis ☐

80. In synthesis of fatty acids energy is supplied by:
A. NAD *(AIIMS 02)* ☐
B. FAD ☐
C. GTP ☐
D. NADPH ☐

81. The most important source of reducing equivalents for fatty acid synthesis in the liver is: *(AIIMS 04)*
A. Glycolysis ☐
B. TCA cycle ☐
C. Uronic acid pathway ☐
D. HMP pathway ☐

82. The first step in fatty acid synthesis involves:
A. Acetyl CoA carboxylase *(AI 06)* ☐
B. β-Hydroxyl CoA dehydrogenase ☐
C. Acetyl dehydrogenase ☐
D. Pyruvate kinase ☐

83. Acetyl CoA is necessary for: *(PGI 07)*
A. Aminoacid synthesis ☐
B. Fatty acid synthesis ☐
C. Glucose storage ☐
D. All ☐

84. In fatty acid synthesis CO_2 loss occurs in which step
A. Hydration *(PGI 02)* ☐
B. Dehydration ☐
C. Condensation reaction ☐
D. Reduction ☐

85. Saturated acyl enzyme formation causes:
A. Freeing of PAN-SH site *(PGI 08)* ☐
B. Freeing of Cyst – SH site ☐
C. Both ☐
D. None ☐

86. Carbon atoms added in FA synthesis *(AIIMS 01)*
A. 2 in Ist cycle & 4 in IInd cycle ☐
B. 4 in Ist cycle & 2 in IInd cycle ☐
C. 2 in Ist cycle & 2 in IInd cycle ☐
D. 4 in Ist cycle & 4 in IInd cycle ☐

87. All participate in Fatty acid synthesis except
A. Hydratase *(AIIMS 02)* ☐
B. Reductase ☐
C. Transacylase ☐
D. Dehydrogenase ☐

88. PAN-SH site of fatty acid synthase complex accepts:
A. Acetyl CoA *(PGI 02; AIIMS 04)* ☐
B. Malonyl CoA ☐
C. Propionyl CoA ☐
D. All ☐

89. True about mitochondrial chain elongation of fatty acid is/are *(PGI 09)*
A. Operates under anaerobic conditions ☐
B. Operates aerobically ☐
C. Common pathway ☐
D. Not a common pathway ☐
E. Pyridoxal-Phosphate & NADPH is required ☐

90. In which organelle (s) of hepatocyte, the elongation of long chain fatty acid takes place: *(PGI 08)*
A. Endoplasmic reticulum (ER) ☐
B. Golgi body ☐
C. Mitochondria ☐
D. Lysosomes ☐
E. Ribosome ☐

Triacylglycerol and Phosphoglycerol Synthesis

91. Regarding synthesis of triacyl glycerol in adipose tissue, all of the following are true except: *(AI 07)*
A. Synthesis from Dihydroxyacetone phosphate ☐
B. Enzyme Glycerol kinase plays an important role ☐
C. Enzyme Glycerol 3 phosphate dehydrogenase plays an important role ☐
D. Phosphatidate is hydrolyzed ☐

β - Oxidation Of Fatty Acids

92. The substance essential for transfer of fatty acids across mitochondrial membrane:
A. Ceratine ☐
B. Ceratinine ☐
C. Carnitine ☐
D. Coenyzme A ☐

93. All are true about β-oxidation except: *(AIIMS 13, 11)*
A. Activation of FA is a must ☐
B. Carnitine palmitoyl transferase I is present in outer mitochondrial membrane ☐
C. Carnitine palmitoyl trasferase II is present in mitochondrial matrix ☐
D. FA activation requires 2ATP. ☐

94. β-oxidation of odd-chain fatty acids produces:
A. Succinyl CoA. *(AI 03)* ☐
B. Propionyl CoA ☐
C. Acetyl CoA ☐
D. Malonyl CoA ☐

95. How many ATP's are formed in case of stearic acid by β-oxidation- *(AIIMS 14; NBE P 13)*
A. 7 ☐
B. 18 ☐
C. 56 ☐
D. 147 ☐

96. β-oxidation of palmitic acid yields *(PGI 05)*
A. 3 acetyl CoA ☐
B. 129 ATP net ☐
C. 131 ATP net ☐
D. 16 Acetyl CoA ☐
E. 96 ATP from citric acid cycle ☐

97. Beta-Oxidation is peroxisome is differentiated from that occurring in mitochondria by: *(PGI 03)*
A. Acetyl CoA ☐
B. H_2O_2 formed ☐
C. Different enzymes are found in different sites ☐
D. NADH is required ☐

98. Refsum's disease is due to deficiency of which of the following enzyme? *(AIIMS 08)*
A. Malonate dehydrogease ☐
B. Thiophorase ☐
C. Succinate thiokinase ☐
D. Phytanic alpha oxidase ☐

Eicosanoids

99. Which of the following is a suicide enzyme?
A. Lipoxygenase *(AIIMS 13)* ☐
B. Cyclooxygenase ☐
C. 5′ nucleotidase ☐
D. Thromboxane synthase ☐

Ketogenesis (Ketone Body Formation)

100. All are true about ketone bodies except- *(NBE P 15)*
A. Acetoacetate is primary ketone body ☐
B. Synthesized in mitochondria ☐
C. Synthesized in liver ☐
D. HMG CoA reductase is the rate- limiting enzyme ☐

101. The immediate precursor in the formation of acetoacetate from acetyl Co A in the liver is:
A. Mevalonate *(PGI 09)* ☐
B. HMG CoA ☐
C. Acetoacetyl CoA ☐
D. 3-hydroxy-butyryl ☐

102. Which organ does not utilise ketone bodies:
A. Liver (Hepatocyte) *(NBE P 15,14; AIIMS 08,13)* ☐
B. Brain ☐
C. Skeletal muscles ☐
D. Cardiac muscles ☐

103. Ketone bodies cannot be utilized by: *(AIIMS 13, 15)*
A. Heart ☐
B. Brain ☐
C. Skeletal muscles ☐
D. RBC s ☐

104. In a well fed state, acetyl CoA obtained from diet is least used in the synthesis of: *(AI 02)*
A. Palmity CoA ☐
B. Citrate ☐
C. Acetoacetate ☐
D. Oxalosuccinate ☐

105. In a well fed state, the activity of CPT-I in outer mitochondrial membrane is inhibited by:
A. Glucose *(AIIMS 11)* ☐
B. Pyruvate ☐
C. Acetyl CoA ☐
D. Malonyl CoA ☐

106. All of the following statements are correct about metabolism in brain except: *(AI 03)*
A. Fatty acids are utilised in starvation ☐
B. 60% of total energy is utilized during resting stage ☐
C. Ketone bodies are used in starvation ☐
D. Has no stored energy ☐

107. If starvation exceeds 7 days, the major nutritional supply of the brain comes from *(AI 04)*
A. Fatty acids ☐
B. Ketone bodies ☐
C. Protein breakdown ☐
D. Carbohydrate breakdown ☐

108. Energy source used by brain in later days of Starvation is: *(AI 04)*
A. Glucose ☐
B. Ketone bodies ☐
C. Glycogen ☐
D. Fatty acids ☐

109. In a patient with starvation for 72 hrs which of the following would be seen: *(AIIMS 02)*
A. Increased glycogenolysis ☐
B. Increased ketosis due to break down of fats ☐
C. Degradation of proteins ☐
D. Increased gluconeogenesis ☐

110. All of the following are increased in starvation except:
A. Lipolysis *(PGI 12)* ☐
B. Ketogenesis ☐
C. Gluconeogenesis ☐
D. Glycogenesis ☐
E. Glycogenolysis ☐

111. All of the following metabolic changes occur during prolonged fasting when compared with fasting for 12-24 hours, except: *(AI 12)*

A. Brain use of ketone bodies increases ☐
B. Liver gluoneogenesis increases ☐
C. Muscle protein degradation decreases ☐
D. Brain use of glucose decreases ☐

112. Which of the following metabolic events will not occur following 12-24 hour of fasting *(AI 12)*

A. Increase in free fatty acids ☐
B. Increase in ketone bodies ☐
C. Decrease in Glycogen ☐
D. Decrease in Serum Proteins ☐

113. In starvation, bran utilizes glucose peferentially but not in liver because: *(PGI 2K)*

A. Low km value of hexokinase ☐
B. Low km glucokinase ☐
C. High km glucokinase ☐
D. High blood flow ☐

114. Ketone body formation without glycosuria seen in:

A. DM *(PGI 07)* ☐
B. DI ☐
C. Prolonged starvation ☐
D. Obesity ☐

115. Which substrate is/are used to provide energy for body:

A. Ketone bodies *(PGI 13)* ☐
B. Glucose ☐
C. Free fatty acids ☐
D. Creatine phosphate ☐
E. Collagen ☐

116. In starvation, nitrogen is carried from muscle to liver and kidney by: *(PGI 07)*

A. Alanine ☐
B. Aspartic acid and Serine ☐
C. Glycine ☐
D. Asparagines ☐

117. In a seriously ill patient, addition of amino acids in the diet results in a positive nitrogen balance. The mechanism for this is: *(AIIMS 08)*

A. Increased absorption of amino acids from the intestine ☐
B. Enhanced rates of gluconeogenesis ☐
C. Increased secretion of insulin ☐
D. Increased Growth hormone secretion ☐

118. Starvation and diabetes mellitus can lead on to ketoacidosis which of the following features is in favour of ketoacidosis due to diabetes mellitus.

A. Increase in glucagon/insulin ratio, increased CAMP and increased blood glucose ☐
B. Decreased insulin, increased free fatty acid which is equivalent to blood glucose *(AIIMS 2K)* ☐
C. Decreased insulin, increased free fatty acid which is not equivalent to blood glucose ☐
D. Elevated insulin and free fatty acid, equivalent to blood glucose ☐

119. Rothera's test for detection of: *(AI 10)*

A. Proteins ☐
B. Glucose ☐
C. Fatty acid ☐
D. Ketones ☐

120. A destitute woman is admitted to the hospital with altered sensorium and dehydration; urine analysis shows mild proteinuria and no sugar; what other test would be desirable: *(AI 01)*

A. Fouchet ☐
B. Rothera ☐
C. Hays ☐
D. Benedicts ☐

121. Hay's sulpher test is used to detect which of the following- *(NBE P 15)*

A. Bile salts in urine ☐
B. Reducing sugar in urine ☐
C. Ketone bodies in urine ☐
D. Urobilinogenin urine ☐

ANSWERS & EXPLANATIONS:

Lipids of Physiological Significance

1. **C i.e. Arachidonic acid contain five double bonds** *[Ref: Harpers 28/e P-121-23; Lippincott's 5/e p. 181-82]*

- **Monoenoic acids** (FA with 1 unsaturated double bond) like **palmitoleic, oleic and elaidic** have double bond at **9th position**Q (cis, cis & trans respectively).
- **Linoleic has 2, linolenic** has **3** and **arachidonic acid** has **4 double bonds** (all are **cis**).

2. **D i.e. Omega-3 fatty acids**

Cardioprotective fatty acid is omega (ω) -3 fatty acids (ω-3 PUFA)Q **> monounsaturated fatty acids (like olive oil)**Q

3. **C, B, > A i.e. (Hydrogenated vegetable oils contains Trans fatty acid; Biologically arachidonic acid is essential to life > Polyunsaturated FA is essential for membrane structure)**
4. **D i.e. Hydrogenation decreases TFA** 5. **A i.e. Linoleic acid** 6. **B i.e. Linoleic acid; C i.e. Linolenic acid**
7. **B i.e. Sunflower Oil** 8. **D i.e. Docosahexanoic Acid**

[Ref: Lippincott's 6/e p. 182; Park 16/e p.407; Lehninger 5th/e p. 345, 815-16; Harper 28/e p.122; Vasudevan 6/e p.437]

- **Most of the naturally occurring unsaturated fatty acids are cis-isomers.** Trans-FA do not occur naturally in plants and occurs only in small amounts in animals as **ruminant fat** (eg butter fat) arising from the action of micro organisms in rumen. Cis isomers are less stable than trans FA.
- **Trans fatty acids** formed **during partial hydrogenation or hardening (saturation /deep frying)**Q of vegetable oils – a procedure to improve stability or shelf life. **Trans – FA increase incidence of coronary heart disease by increasing LDL and decreasing HDL**Q.
- **Dietary essential fatty acids in humans are linoleic acid and α- linolenic acid**Q**,** because we lack enzymes needed to synthesize them. Plants provide these EFA. **Linoleic acid is the precursor of ω-6-arachidonic acid** and so prostaglandins. **So the arachidonic acid becomes EFA if linoleic acid is deficient in diet**. α-linolenic acid is precursor of ω-3-fatty acids required for growth and development.
- **Linoelic acid** is the **most important essential fatty acid** because it serves as the basis for production of other EFAs like **arachidonic acid & docosahexanoic acid. Arachidonic acid,** a w-6 PUFA is essential as it is a **precursor of prostaglandins & leukotrienes.**
- **Linoleic acid** is the most important essential fatty acid, maximally found in **Safflower oil**Q**>Corn oil**Q**> Sunflower oil**Q
- **Docosahexanoic Acid (DHA; ω3, 22:6)** which is synthesized from α-linolenic acid or obtained directly from fish oils, is present in high concentrations in retina, cerebral cortex, testis & sperm. DHA is particularly needed for development of brain & retina and is supplied via the **placenta and milk.** Milk is the constant and continuous source of DHA as placenta is not present at all time. Patients with Retinitis pigmentosa are reported to have low levels of DHA.
- Plasma membrane contains both saturated & mono or poly unsaturated FA.

9. **D i.e. Alpha linolenic acid** *[Ref: Harper's 27/e P-123; 26/e P- 113, 191]*

Alpha linolenic acid belongs to **W3 series**Q. Rest others belong to W6 series.
Carbon atoms are numbered from the carboxyl carbon (carbon no. 1). The carbon atoms adjacent to carboxyl carbon are also called. α, β, Y respectively. The terminal methyl carbon is K/as W or n- carbon.

W3 Family	W6 Family	W7 Family	W9
- **Alpha linolenic** Q - Timnodonic - Cervonic	- **Gamma linolenic**Q - **Archidonic**Q - **Linolic**Q	Palmitoleic	- **Oleic**Q - Elaidic

- The first double bond introduced into a saturated fatty acid (to make it unsaturated) is nearly always in Δ9 position. The reaction is catalyzed by Δ9 desaturase in presence of O_2, NADH and cytochrome b5.
- Since animals have Δ9 desaturase, they are able to synthesize W9 (oleic) family.
- Linoleic (W6) or α - linolenic (W3) acids required for the synthesis of other members of W6 or W3 family must be supplied in diet.

10. **A, B, D i.e. Long chain fatty acid (LCFA), Alcohol- sphingosine, Sailic acid**
11. **A i.e. Cell-cell interaction, B i.e. Signal transduction; C i.e. Surfactant; D i.e. Acute inflammatory mediator, E i.e. Activates membrane enzymes** *[Ref: Lehninger 5/e p. 256, 350-55; 829; Chatterjea 7/e p. 45, 58- 61;*
12. **A, C, D i.e. Glucose, Sphingosine, Fatty acids** *Vasudevan 6/e p. 81-82; Lippincott 5/e p. 201-2, 209-10, 217]*

Glycosphingolipid=Ceramide (Sphingosine/amino alcohol+Fatty acid)+Mono/oligo saccharide like glucose, galactose
Ganglioside (acidic glycosphingolipid) = **Ceramide + Oligosaccharide+NANA** (N-acetylneuraminic acid or **sialic acid)**

- **Glyco-sphingolipid** is made up of **ceramide** (which is a long chain fatty acid attached to amino group of sphingosine through an amide linkage i.e. = **sphingosine / amino alcohol + Fatty acid)** attached directly to **mono /oligo saccharide** (polar head) by an O-glycosidic bond. Glycosphingolipids differ from sphingomyelin (phospho-sphingolipid) in that they **do not contain phosphate** (polar group); and differ from **glycerophospholipids** (phosphoglycerides) that they **do not contain glycerol**.
- **Ganglioside** (acidic, negatively charged **glyco-sphingolipid)** contain **sphingosine alcohol (4- sphingenine)** 1 molecule, **long chan fatty acid (1 mol), Oligosaccharide** polar head and 1 or more residues of **N- acetylneurminic acid (Neu 5 Ac), a sialic acid** (often simply called sialic acid) giving it a negative charge, at termini. ***Ganglioside do not contain glycerol and phosphate***[Q].
- **Ceramide** containing **sphingosine amino alcohol** is **present in all sphingolipids (ie. phospho & glyco-sphingolipids)**[Q].

13. **A i.e. Ganglioside, B i.e. Sphingomyelin, C i.e. Cerabrosides***[Ref: Lippincott's 5/e P-211; Harper's 28/e P-208-9]*

Ceramide (i.e. sphingosine amino alcohol + fatty acid) is synthesized in ***endoplasmic reticulum (E R) from amino acid serine***[Q]. It is an important *second messenger* (signaling molecule) in apoptosis (programmed cell death), cell cycle, cell differentiation and senescence. Ceramide is present in **sphingomyelin, gluco/galacto-cerebrosides, globoside and ganglio side**.

14. **B i.e. Alpha 2 – macroglobulin** *[Ref. Harper 28/e p. 216, 232; 575; Vasudevan 6/e p. 292-300, 335]*

- **Atherosclerosis** is a/w **increased LDL (or oxidized LDL), Lp (a) & homocysteine and decreased or defective apo B-100 & E**[Q].
- **Alpha-2 (α-2) macroglobulin**, a large plasma glycoprotein (720 kDa) containing **Zn (zinc)** and a unique internal **cyclic thiol ester bond** (formed between cysteine & glutamine), is a **panproteinase inhibitor** (i.e. neutralize many proteases) and target certain cytokines (like platelet-derived growth factor, transforming growth factor β etc) towards particular tissues or cells. It is **not a predisposing factor for atherosclerosis**[Q].

15. **B i.e. Cardiolipin**

Cardiolipin is only human glycero-phospho lipid which is antigenic[Q]**. It is antigenic and is recognized by antibodies raised against Treponema pallidum (syhillis bacteria)**[Q].

Acylglycerol & Sphingolipid Metabolism

16. **B i.e. Triglycerides**

Triglycerides = Triacyl-glycerol = 3 Fatty Acids + Glycerol

Triglycerides (or TAG, acyl = fatty acid) is main storage form of energy. They are stored in fat cells (adipocytes) of adipose tissue.

17. **C i.e. Mutation of genes encoding lysosomal hydrolases** *[Ref: Harrison 17/e p- 2452-53; Harper's 27/e P-541]*

Lysosomal storage diseases (LSD) are caused by ***mutations in genes encoding lysosomal hydrolases***[Q] responsible for breaking down of macromolecules, which results in accumulation of corresponsing substrate (macromolecule). LSDs are classified on the basis of accumulated substrate into sphingolipidosis, mucolipidosis, mucopolysaccharidoses, glycoproteinoses etc.

18. D i.e. Wolman disease *[Ref: Harper 29/e p. 235, 233; Lippincott's 6/e p. 212, 210; Vasudevan 7/e p. 193, 91-93; Chatterjea 8/e p. 11, 50, 63, 424]*

- Sphingolipidoses include (1) **Neutral glycosphingo lipidoses** (eg **Fabry's, Gaucher's and Niemann Pick disease A and B);** (2) **Generalized GM1 gangliosidoses;** (3) **GM2 gangliosidoses (eg Tay Sachs & Sandhoff's diseases);** (4) **Leukodystrophies** (eg **Krabbe globoid cell leukodystrophy, metachromatic leukodystrophy** and multiple sulfatase deficiency) (5) **Lactosyl ceramidoses** and; (6) **Farber's disease.**
- **Wolman's disease and cholesteryl ester storage diseases are** not sphingolipidoses as these are a/w **accumulation of triglycerides & cholesterol esters (not sphingolipid/ ceramide).**

19. B, C, E i.e. Due to deficiency of enzyme Beta-Gluco-cerebrosidase, Deposition of glucosylceramide, PAS staining positive *[Ref: Harper 28/e p 210; Harrison17/e p- 2452-54; Robbins 7/e p 163-164; Vasudevan 6/e p.168-69; Chatterjea 7/e p 58-59; Lippincott 5/e p 212; Lehninger 5/ 356]*

- **Gaucher's disease** is due to **deficiency of Beta glucocerebrosidase /acid β- glucosidase**Q. This AR (autosomal recessive) disorder results in **accumulation of glucosyl ceramide (gluco cerebroside) usually kerasin** within phagocytic macrophages known as **gaucher cells**. These reticulo endothelial cells are found in liver, spleen, bone-marrow, lymph node, tonsils, thymus, payer patches, and brain.
- **Foam or vacuolated cells** occur in **Niemann Pick disease**Q, Fucosidosis and β-mannosidosis etc. But in contrast to lipid storage diseases **Gaucher cells** are very rarely vacuolated and instead have a **crumpled (or wrinkled) tissue paper appearance of cytoplasm**. The Gaucher cells are **intense PAS (Periodic acid Schiff) staining positive** and show fibrillary crumpled cytoplasm d/t deposition of (glucocerebroside) lipid as bilayered stacks in enlarged & elongated lysosomes. **Shell like inclusion bodies** are seen Tay sachs diselase.
- All sphingolipidoses are AR except Fabry disease which is X-linked; and all can be fatal in early life. Prenatal diagnosis can be made using cultured amniocytes or chorionic villi.

20. A i.e. Niemann-Pick disease **21. B i.e. β-glucosidase** **22. B i.e. Krabbe's disease**
[Ref: Harrison 17/e P 2452-57; Lippincott's 5/e P-208-217; Harper's 28/e P-210, Chatterjea 7/e p. 60, Harrison 16/e p. 2316- 17]

- **Niemann-Pick (A+B) disease** d/t **deficiency of sphingomyelinase**Q **results in defective degradation of phosphosphingolipids (i.e. spingomyelin) and accumulation of sphingomyelin in phagocytic cells**Q.
- Sphingolipidoses occurring d/t defective degradation of glyco-sphingolipid include – **Gaucher disease (deficient β glucosidase**Q**/ glucocerebrosidase); Fabry's disease (α-galactosidase**Q**); Tay-Sach's disease (β- Hexominidase A**Q**); Sandhoff's disease (β-Hexominidase A&B)**Q**; Krabbe's disease (β galactosidase/ galactosyl ceramidase def)**Q**; Farber's disease (acid ceramidase)**Q**; Metachromatic leukodystrophy (aryl sulfatase A**Q**) and GM$_1$, gangliosidase (β galactosidase def**Q**).**
- **Krabbe's disease has no hepatosplenomegaly**Q.

23. B i.e. Beta galactocerebrosidase **24. A i.e. Sphingomyelinase**

25. A i.e. Tay- sach's disease; B i.e. Gaucher's disease *[Ref: Harper's 27/e P-215; Lippincott's 3/e P-210]*

Lysosomal Storage Disease	Deficient Enzyme
Gaucher's disease	β GlucosidaseQ
Niemann- pick ds	SphingomyelinaseeQ
Fabry's ds	α - GalactosidaseQ
Krabbe's ds	β - GlalactosidaseQ
Tay- sach ds	Hexasaminidase AQ
Meta chromatic leucodystrophy	Arylsulfatase AQ

Glycogen Storage Disorder	Deficient Enzyme
Type I (Von Gierke's ds)	G- 6- PhosphataseQ
Type II (Pompe's ds)	Acid maltaseQ
Type III (Forbe's ds)	Debranching enzymeQ
Type IV (Anderson ds)	Branching enzymeQ
Type V (Mc Ardle ds)	Muscle phosphorylaseQ
Type VI (Her's ds)	Liver phosphorylaseQ.

Other Diseases	Defect
Cystic fibrosis	Mutation in CF gene located on chromosome 7
Wilson's ds	Two mutant ATP 7B gene
Familial hyper cholesterolemia	Defective LDL receptor

Lysosomal Storage Disease

Lysosomal storage disorder is accumulation of specific macromolecule within cells that are normally metabolized by cells. This is because of deficiency of one or other lysosomal enzyme.

Mucopolysaccharidoses (MPS)

Type	Syndrome	Enzymatic Defect	Accumulated / Urinary metabolite
I	**Hurler** or **Scheie**	**α- L- Iduronidase**[Q]	- **Dermatan sulfate**[Q] - **Hepran sulfate**[Q]
II	**Hunter**	Iduronate sulfatase	**Heparan sulfate**[Q]
III A	**Sanfilippo A**	Heparan sulfate N- sulfatase (sulfamidase)	
III B	**Sanfilippo B**	α-N- Acetyl glucosaminidase	
III C	**Sanfilippo C**	Acetyl CoA - α-glucosaminidase - N-acetyl transferase	
III D	**Sanfilippo D**	N- Acetylglucosamine 6 sulfatase	
IV A	**Moriquio- A**	N-acetyl Galactosamine –6- sulfatase	- Keratan sulfate - Chondroitin –6 sulfate
IV B	**Morquio -B**	β- Galactosidase	- Keratan sulfate
VI	**Maroteauxlamy**	N- acetyl galactosamine 4-sulfatase (aryl sulfatase β	Dermatan sulfate
VII	**Sly**	β- Glucronidase	- Dermatan sulfate - Heparan sulfate - Chondroitin 4/6- sulfate

Clinical features of MPS: Coarse facies. Valvular heart disease, mental retardation, **hepatosplenomegaly**, skeletal deformity, joint stiffness, corneal clouding, & vacuolated / granulated lymphocytes.

Mucolipidoses (MLS)

	Disorder	Enzyme defect	Accumulated	Clinical features
I	**Sialidosis**	Sialidase (neuraminidase)	Glycoprotein fragments Sialyloligosaccharides	MPS II phenotype – coarse facies, pebbly skin lesions, joint stiffness
II	**I- Cell disease**	UDP- N- acetyl glucosamine: glucoprotein- N- acetylgluco samininylphospho transferase (Acid hydrolases thus lack phosphomannosyl residues)	Glycoprotein fragments Glycolipids	Coarse facies, gingival hypoplasia, absence of mucopolysacchariduria
III	**Phosphotransferase**	As with ML-II but deficiency is incomplete	Glycoprotein fragments Glycolipids	Coarse facies, stiffness of hands & shoulder

Glycoproteinoses

Fucosidosis	α -Fucosidase	Glycopeptides, oligosaccharides
Mannosidosis α, β	Mannosidase α/β	Oligosaccharides
Aspartylglucosaminuria	Aspartylglucosaminidase	Aspartyl glucosamine, glycopeptides
Schindler's disease	α-N- galatosaminidase	

★ Clinical features – Coarse facies, enlarged tongue, angiokeratomas

Neutral glycosphingolipidoses

Disorder	Fabry disease	Gaucher disease	Nieman-Pick disease A&B
Deficient enzyme	**α- Galactosidase A**Q	**Acid-β-glucosidase/glucocerebrosidase**Q	**Sphingomyelinase**Q
Stored material	Globotriacyl ceramide	**Glucosyl ceramide**	**Sphingomyelin**Q
Clinical features	- **Cutaneous angiokeratoma (i.e. reddish purple skin rash)**Q, corneal dystrophy - **Painful acroparesthesis i.e. burning pain in lower extremity)**Q - Hypohydrosis, kidney & heart failure. - X- linked disorder, onset in childhood, - No hepatospleenomegaly, skeletal disease and hematological involvement	- No CNS and opthalmological involvement in type 1 (adult) form - **PAS staining positive Gaucher cells**Q in bone marrow, cytopenia - Lipid as bilayered stacks in elongated distended lysosomes on EM	- Pulmonary infiltrates & lung failure - **Foam cells in bone marrow**Q - Pleomorphic inclusion of lipid in lysosomes concentric parallel lamella (on electron microscopy = EM - Mental retardation, seizures, **hepato spleenomegaly**, macular degeneration - Osteoporosis in type B only

Leukodystrophies

Disorder	Enzyme defect	Accumulated lipid	Clinical Features
Krabbe's disease (globoid cell leukodystrophy)	**Galactosyl ceramidase/ β galactosidase**Q	**Galactosylceramide Galactosyl sphingosine**	- Globoid bodies (glycolipid- laden macrophages) in white matter - Mental & motor retardation - Blindness & deafness
Metachromatic leukodystrophy	**Arylsulfatase A**Q	**Cerebroside sulfate**	- Mental Retardation - Progressive paralysis - Dementia in adult form - Nerve stain yellowish brown with cresyl violet (metachromasia)
Multiple sulfatase deficiency (Active site cysteine to Cα formyl glycine converting enzyme)	**Aryl sulfatases A, B & C and steroid sulfatase**	Sulfogalactosyl ceramide (sulfatide), steroid sulfates, proteoglycans mucopoly saccharides	- Absent activity of all cellular sulfatases - MR, HS omegaly, retinal degeneration, & skeleletal involvement

GM_2 gangliosidoses

Tay Sach's disease	**β- Hexosaminidase A**Q (HAD- A)	**GM_2 gangliosides**	- Mental retardation, seizures, macrocephaly, **hyperacusis and cherry red spot in both**Q. - Hepatosplenomegaly & skeletal involvement only in sandhoff ds.
Sandhoff's disease	β- Hexosaminidase A and B [HAD- A,B]	GM_2 gangliosides	

Disorder of neutral lipids

Wolman disease	Acid lysosomal lipase	Cholesterol esters, triglycerides	Adrenal calcification, hepatospleenomegaly, mild, mental retardation
Cholestery ester storage disease	Acid lysosomal lipase	Cholesteryl ester	Hepatomegaly, cirrhosis
Farber disease	**Acid ceramidase**	Ceramide	Macular degeneration, arthropathy, subcutaneous nodules

26. **A i.e. Gauchers disease**

Enzyme replacement therapy is available for some **lysosomal storage disorders** like (1) **Gaucher's disease**Q **(1st)**, (2) Fabry's ds (3) Glycogen storage ds type II (4) Mucopolysaccharidosis I, II and VI (i.e. **Hurler, Hunter** and VI).

Lipid Transport

27. **D i.e. Chylomicrons** *[Ref: Lippincott 5/e p-227-28; Chatterjea 7/e p 419-18; Harper 28/e p 213]*

Chylomicron does not migrate (or move) towards charged end or anode on electrophoresis and remains at the originQ. The increasing order of mobility on electrophoresis is: ***Chylomicron < LDL (β-regoin) < VLDL (pre β- region) < HDL (α-region)***

28. **B i.e. Chylomicrons** *[Ref: Lippincott's 5/e P-227-28]* 29. **A i.e. Chylomicrons**

Lipoproteins may be differentiated on the basis of their lipid & protein compositions. The lipoproteins containing the largest percentage of triacylglycerol are Chylomicrons (90%). Maximum content of triglycerides (& exogenous TG) is present in chylomicrons which carries exogenous dietary TG's to peripheral tissuesQ.

Triglycerides (TG) are manly found in – ***chylomicrons & VLDL***Q.

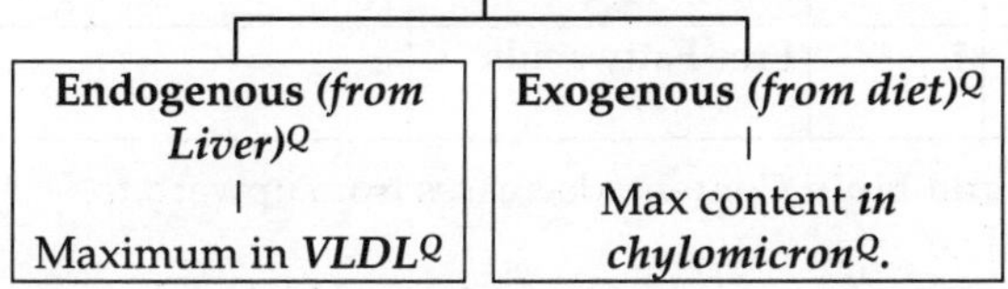

Chylmicrons: are found *in chyle* formed only by the lymphatic system *draining the intestine*. They are responsible for transport of all dietary lipids into circulation.

VLDL: transport *TG from the liver to extrahepatic tissue.*

★ ***The only apolipoprotein, that remains associated with chylomicrons along its entire journey (from intestine to liver) is apo-B48).***Q

30. **B i.e. Arginine**

Arginine rich apo-E (apoprotein-E) is found in VLDLQ.

31. **C i.e. Transports maximum amount of lipid** 32. **B i.e. LDL** 33. **B i.e. LDL** 34. **A i.e. HDL**
35. **B i.e. Kidney** 36. **A i.e. HDL** *[Ref: Harper's 27/e P-218; 26/e P-206, Shinde & Chatterjea: 6/e P- 386]*

Highest amount of cholesterol is present in **LDL** which is the ***most important carrier of cholesterol and provides (transports) choelestrol to extrahepatic peripheral tissue***Q.

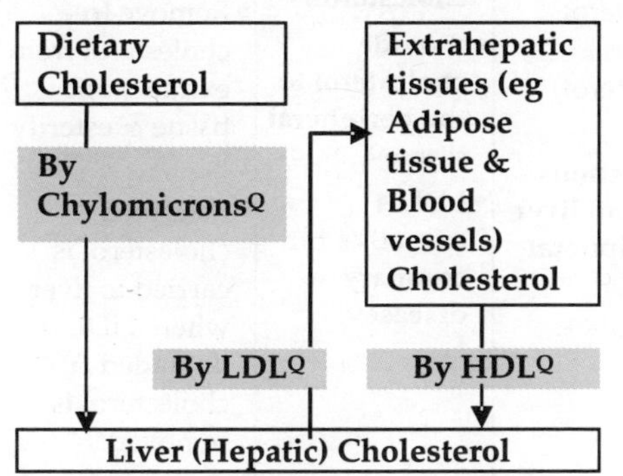

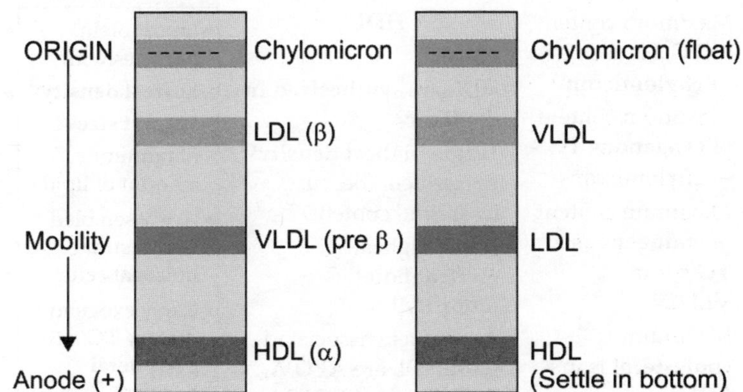

Features of Lipoproteins 

The density of lipoprotein decreases as the proportion of lipid to protein increases.

Lipoprotein	Source	Diameter (nm)	Density (g/mL)	Composition Protein (%)	Composition Lipid (%)	Main Lipid Composition	Apolipoprotiens
Chylomicrons	**Intestine**[Q]	90-1000	<0.95	1-2	98-99	Triacylglycerol	**A-I, A-II, A-IV[1], B-48, C-I, C-II, C-III, E**
Chylomicron remnants	Chylomicrons	45-150	<1.006	6-8	92-94	Triacylglycerol, phospholipids, cholesterol	B-48, E
VLDL	Liver[Q]	30-90	0.95-1.006	7-10	90-93	Triacylglycerol	**B-100, C-I, C-II, C-III**
IDL	VLDL	25-35	1.006-1.019	11	89	Triacylglycerol, cholesterol	B-100, E
LDL	**VLDL**[Q]	20-25	10.19-1.063	21	79	Cholesterol	**B-100**
HDL	Liver, intestine, VLDL, chylomicrons					**Phospholipids**[Q], cholesterol	A-I, A-II, A-IV, C-I, C-II, C-III, D[2], E
HDL$_1$		20-25	1.019-1.063	32	68		
HDL$_2$		10-20	1.063-1.125	33	67		
HDL$_3$		5-10	1.125-1.210	57	43		
Preβ-HDL[3]		<5	>1.210				A-1
Albumin/free fatty acids	Adipose tissue		> 1.281	99	1	Free Fatty acids	

Abbreviations : HDL, high-density lipoproteins; IDL, intermediate-density lipoproteins; LDL, low-density lipoproteins; VLDL, very low density lipoproteins.

1 Secreted with chylomicrons but transfers to HDL
2 Associated with HDL2 and HDL3 subfractions
3 Part of a minor fraction known as very high density lipoproteins (VHDL).

- **Diameter and Lipid Content**: decreases from upward to downward i.e
  - Chylomicron has highest diameter and highest lipid content
  - HDL has lowest diameter & has least lipid content.
- **Density and protein content:** Increases on going downward i.e.
  - HDL has highest density & has max. protein content.
  - **Chylomicron has least density**[Q].

- Maximum content of **TG,s** is seen in → **chylomicron**[Q]
- Maximum content of **exogenous TG's** → chylomicrons
- Maximum content of **endogenous TG's** is in → **VLDL**[Q]
- Maximum **cholesterol** is in → **LDL**[Q].

HDL

- HDL are **synthesized in the liver**[Q].
- This is **highest density**[Q] lipoprotein (because least lipid content)
- **It has highest electrophoretic mobility**[Q]
- Apoprotein associated with HDL are **APO A, APOC II, & APOE**[Q].

Chylomicrons	VLDL	LDL	HLD
• Lipoprotein particles with - **Lowest density**[Q] - **Largest size**[Q] - Maximum amount of lipid • Are assembled **in intestinal mucosal cells**[Q]. • Carry exogenous **dietary TG's to peripheral tissues**[Q].	• Are **produced in the liver**[Q]. • Are composed predominantly of TG (also cholesterol ester & cholesterol) • Carry **endogenous TG from liver to peripheral tissue**[Q].	• **Contain high concentration of cholestrol & cholesterol esters (bad cholesterol)**[Q] • **Provide cholesterol to the peripheral tissue**[Q]. • LDL is **causative for coronary disease**[Q].	• Synthesized in liver & are released into blood by exocytosis. • Remove free cholesterol from extrahepatic tissue & esterify it. • Esterified cholesterol is carried to liver where HDL is degraded & cholesterol is removed. • **Protective in coronary disease (scavenging action)**[Q]

37. **C i.e. HDL** 38. **C i.e. Apoproteins** 39. **B i.e. HDL** 40. **A i.e. HDL**
[Ref: Lippincott's 4/e p 242- 43; Harper 30/e p. 254; Lehninger 5/e p. 836-37]

- HDL contains **good cholesterol**Q. So there is an inverse relation between HDL (HDL_2) concentrations and coronoary heart disease. This is consistent with the **function of HDL in reverse cholesterol transport (i.e. from peripheral tissue to liver)**Q.

- Diseases (eg. diabetes mellitus, lipid nephrosis, hypothyroidism and other considtions of hyperlipedimea) in which prolonged elevations of VLDL, IDL, LCD or chylomicron remnants in blood are often accompanied by premature or severe atherosclerosis. This makes **LDL : HDL cholesterol ratio** a good predective parameter for atherosclerosis & coronary heart disease.

- **HDL** has **highest density**. It has **highest proportion of apoproteins (mainly Apo As) and phospholipids**Q. And HDL **migrates least during electrophoresis.**

41. **A i.e. RNA editing** *[Ref: Harper's 27/e P-218]* 42. **A i.e. Apoprotein B** 43. **C i.e. B-48**

Apo B–48 & apo B-100 *differ due to the RNA editing*Q occurring in the intestinal cells where B-48 is expressed.

Apo B- 48

Apo B- 48: is the **main apolipoprotein of chylomicron**Q.
- It is synthesized in the intestine.
- Apo B – 48 (48% of B- 100) is formed from the same mRNA as apo B –100, after the introduction of stop signal by an RNA editing enzyme.

Apo B–100

Apo B–100 is main apolipoprotein of **LDL**

44. **A i.e. VLDL** 45. **B i.e. Liver**

VLDL is formed in liver from the **triglycerides** mainly. **Endogenous triglycerides** in plasma are maximmaly carried in **VLDL**Q.

46. **D i.e. Apo AI** 47. **C i.e. Apoprotein C II inhibits lipoprotein lipase**
[Ref: Harper's 28/e p. 212-15; Chattergea 7/e p. 419-21; Devlin 5/e p. 712; Lippincott's 100, 177, 189, 227 – 34]

Lipoprotein lipase is activated by phospholipid , apoprotein C I & CII and inhibited by apoprotein AII and apoprotein CIIIQ.

48. **B i.e. LDL / HDL ratio** 49. **B i.e. LDL** 50. **D i.e. It contains Apo-B_4**
Ref: Harper 28th/ed pg-216; Lehninger 5th/ed pg- 843; Journal of American college of nutrition, Vol 27, No-1, 1-5 (2008) Chattarjea 7th/ed pg. – 374-75; Lippincott 4th/ed pg-234-31

LDL has **highest cholesterol and cholesteryl ester content**Q and possesses **only apo B-100 as their major apoprotein**Q. Its **primary function is to provide cholesterol (whether dietary or endogenous) to peripheral (extrhepatic) tissue**Q. So it is **most potent atherogenic lipoprotein, increasing the risk of cardiovascular disease**Q and showing a positive correlation between the incidence and plasma concentration of LDL cholesterol.

51. **A i.e. Present only in the extra-hepatic tissues:** *[Ref: Harper29/e p 242, 255-57; Lehninger 5/e p 837-41; Lippincott 5/e p 233-31]*
52. **C i.e. On accumulation in the cell inhibits replenishment of LDL receptors.**
53. **C i.e. Increased blood cholesterol is associated with increased LDL receptors** 54. **C i.e. Apo E and Apo B100**

- **Liver** and many **extra hepatic tissues** express **LDL (apo- B-100 and E) receptors**Q. LDL receptors are present on **cell membrane pits coated with clathrin (protein) on the cytosolic side**Q; and taken into the **cell by endocytosis**Q (after binding LDL). And **cholesterol present in LDL**, on accumulation in the cell **inhibits replenishment (recruitment i.e. transcription) of LDL receptors via SREBP pathway**Q.
- **Increased cellular cholesterol** coordinately **suppress cholesterol synthesis** (by inhibiting HMG Co A synthase, HMG CoA reductase etc enzymes) **as well as uptake (by down regulating synthesis of LDL receptors)**Q; whereas cholesterol esterification is promoted (by stimulating ACAT activity). Thus the LDL receptor activity on cell surface is regulated by cholesterol requirement for membranes, steroid hormones or bile acid synthesis.

55. **D i.e. Does not require CII as cofactor** *[Ref: Lippincott 4th/e p228-29; Lehninger 5th/e p 837-39; 346, 649; Harper 28th/e p134-35,215-16, 232]*

- In the **capillaries of adipose, heart, skeletal muscle and lactating mammary tissues**Q, **lipoprotein lipase is activated by apo C II aproprotein of chylomicron and VLDL**Q and the enzyme degrades the triacyl glycerol to yield fatty acid and glycerol.
- **Apo CII is essential for activation whereas apo AII and C III inhibits the lipoprotein lipase enzyme**Q. So the patients with a deficient lipoprotein lipase or apo CII (i.e. **Type I hyperlipoproteinemia** or **Familial lipoprotein lipase deficiency**) show a **very high (> 1000 mg/dl) accumulation of chylomicrons containing triacyl glycerol in plasma i.e. hypertriacylglycerolemia even in fasting state**Q.

56. **A i.e. HDL** *[Harper's 27/e P-221-223; 26/e P-209, 210; Chatterjea 6/e P- 386]*

HDL scavanges body cholesterol and blood vessel wall cholesterol by 'reverse cholesterol transport'-[Shinde P- 386]
The transport of cholesterol from the tissue to liver is known as 'reverse cholesterol transport'.

★ **Class B scavenger receptor B1 (SR –B1) and ATP binding cassette transporter A1 (ABCA 1) are involved in reverse cholesterol transport**Q.

★ **Reverse cholesterol** transport involves efflux of cholesterol from peripheral cells to HDL, esterification of cholesterol by PCAT (phosphatidyl choline: cholesterol acyl transferase), binding of cholesterol ester rich HDL (HDL-2) to liver and steroidogenic cells, the selective transfer of the cholesteryl esters into these cells and the release of lipid depleted HDL (HDL-3).

★ The efflux of cholesterol from peripheral cells is mediated by ABCA-1 and the uptake of cholesteryl ester by liver is mediated by SRB1. Hepatic lipase degrade both triacyl glycerol and phospholipid, & participate in conversion of HDL_2 to HDL_3, **(HDL cycle)**. $\mathbf{HDL_2}$ concentrations are inversely related to incidence of coronary atherosclerosis. **HDLc (HDL_1)** is found in diet induced hyper cholesterolemic animals. It is rich in cholesterol & has only apo E apoprotein.

57. **A i.e. Tendon Xanthoma** 58. **D i.e. LDL receptor mutation** 59. **D i.e. Chylomicrons**
60. **A i.e. LDL receptor** 61. **C i.e. III**
[Ref: Harper's 29/e p. 232; Harrison 18/e p. 3148-49; Lippincott's 4/e p. 178, 229- 232, 380; Chattergea 7/e p. 424 – 27]

- **Increased LDL with normal TG levels suggest type II a familial hypercholesterolemia** which may present **with tendon (tuberous) xanthoma**Q.
- **Type I familial hyperlipoproteinemia** is due to **deficiency of lipoprotein lipase**Q & /or **apo- c II. It is characterized by increased chylomicron (↑↑) >> triglycerides (↑)**Q, >> VLDL (pre β lipoprotein) and decreased HDL (α lipoprotein) and LDL (β lipoprotein).
- **Type II familial hyper cholesterolemia (a)** is due to **defective LDL receptor or mutation in ligand region of apo B-100 and is characterized by elevated LDL levels & hyper cholesterolemia in family (autosomal dominant)** Q.
- **Type III familial dysbetalipoproteinemia (broad beta or remnant removal disease) is due to defect in apoprotein E (patient lacs E_3 & E_4 isoforms and have only E_2 which does not react with E receptor)**Q. Since apoprotein E, present on chylomicron & VLDL remnants is required for their removal via hepatic E receptor, **VLDL and chylomicron remnants are not removed adequately and accumulate in the circulation**Q.

62. **A i.e. Chylomicron, B i.e. LDL, C i.e. VLDL, E i.e. TG** *[Ref. Harrison 16/e P-2288; Harper's 27/e P-239]*

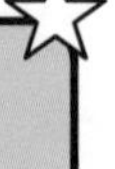

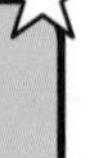

Abetalipoproteinemia: is a rare autosomal recessive disease due to **defective synthesis or secretion of apo B**Q & leads to absent or **low level of chylomicrons, VLDL and LDL**Q. [Apo protein B is major component of chylomicron (B-48), VLDL & LDL (B- 100)]

63. **B i.e. VLDL** *[Ref: Harper's 27/e P-219-220; 26/e P-211-12]*

As **VLDL** is the ***main transporter of endogenous triglycerides***; all the conditions causing increased endogenous triglyceride synthesis will also increase VLDL secretion. And these are-

- Well fed state (not starved)
- High level of circulating free fatty acids
- *Carbohydrate rich diet (especially sucrose & fructose)*Q
- Presence of high level of insulin & low level of glycogen
- Ethanol (alcohol) ingestion

64. **A i.e. VLDL**

VLDL derives Triglycerides from Two sources

- *From hepatic synthesis of F.A* (Liver synthesize TG's from acetyl COA, derived mainly from carbohydrate) → In well fed state, Carbohydrate rich diet
- *From free fatty acids* in circulation → In Fat rich diet, Starvation, Diabetes mellitus

65. C i.e. LP (a) **66. B i.e. Atherosclerosis** *[Ref: Harper 27/e p. 239; Lippincott's 4/e p. 237; Robbins 7/e p. 521]*

Lipoprotein (a) / Lipoprtein little (a) / Lp(a) is associated with **coronary heart disease due to atherosclerosis plus thrombosis d/t inhibition of fibrinolysis**Q.

Lipoprotein (a)

Structure	Circulating levels	Excess cause
- It is identical to LDL. Its distinguishing feature is the presence of an additional apolipoprotein molecule, apo (a), that is covalently linked to apo B – 100. So **Lp (a) = LDL + Apo (a)** - Apo (a) is structurally homologous to plasminogen – the precursor of blood protease whose target is fibrin the main component of blood clot.	- Determined by genetics - Diet rich in trans fatty acid increase Lp (a) - Estrogen decrease both LDL & Lp (a)	- **Coronary heart disease due to atherosclerosis**Q - Thrombosis d/t inhibition of fibrinolysis

Cholesterol Synthesis & Excretion

67. A i.e. HMG COA reductase **68. C i.e. HMG-Co-A Synthase**
69. A i.e. Steroid **70. D i.e. Palmitic acid; E i.e. Stearic acid**
[Ref: Lehninger 5/e p 355-60, 831-35; Vasudevan 6/e p 147-52; Chaterjea 8/e p 431-35; Lippincott 5/e p 196-98; Harper 29/e p 210-13, 251-55]

- **Both cholesterol and ketone bodies are synthesize from (3) beta hydroxyl (3) beta methyl glutary CoA (ie HMG CoA).** So enzymes, **thiolase & HMG CoA synthase involved in conversion of acetyl CoA to HMG CoA are common to synthesis of cholesterol and ketone bodies both**Q. However, **cytoplasmic HMG CoA synthase** is involved in **cholesterol synthesis,** whereas **mitochondrial HMG CoA synthase** is involved **in Ketone body synthesis.**
- **Cholesterol synthesis** is controlled by **regulation of HMG COA reductase, which is a rate limiting enzyme**Q.
- **Cholesterol,** the major **sterol** in animal tissue has **steroid nucleus**Q. Of the cholesterol absorbed, 80-90% is **esterified with long chain fatty acids (mostly saturated) such as palmitic and steric acids**Q. Whereas, substitution of saturated FAs by poly unsaturated FAs in diet has beneficial effects and lowers cholesterol.

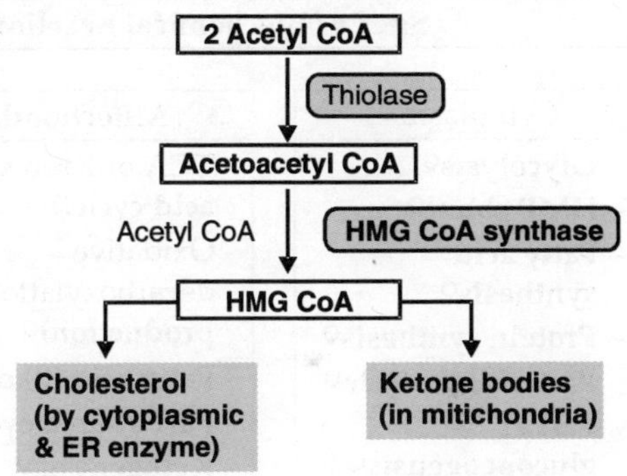

71. E i.e. Cholesterol restricted diet, high fiber diet with low saturated FA... **72. C i.e. HMG COA reductase**
73. B i.e. Cholesterol **74. B i.e Cholic acid; C i.e. Chemodeoxycholic acid. E i.e. Taurocholic acid**
[Ref: Harper's 27/e P-230,236;26/e P-218; Chatterjea 6/e P-374; KDT 5/e P-577]

Choleserol is the **precursor of Bile acids**Q, Corticosteroids, sex hormones and vitamin D.

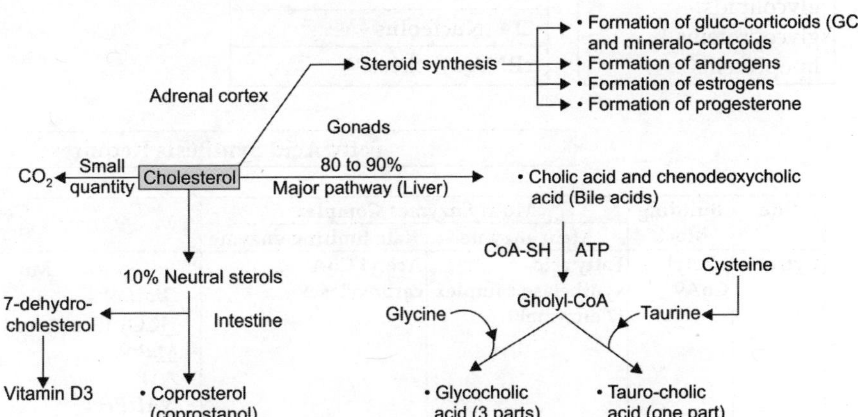

Fate of Cholesterol in the Body

75. **C i.e. Pregnenolone** *[Ref: Harper 30/e p. 503]*

All mammalian **steroid hormones are synthesized from cholesterol** via a **common intermediate pregnenolone**Q through a series of reactions either in mitochondria or ER.

Fatty Acid Synthesis

76. **D i.e. Fatty acid synthesis / EMP** 77. **D i.e. Fatty acid biosynthesis**
78. **C i.e. Fatty acid synthesis** 79. **A i.e. Fatty acid synthesis** 80. **D i.e. NADPH** 81. **D i.e. HMP pathway**
[Ref: Harper's 29/e P-217-24; Lippincott 5/e p. 184-186, 194; Chatterjea 8/e p. 414-419]

- **De novo synthesis of fatty acids (Lipogenesis) occurs in the cytosol**Q.
- **In fatty acid synthesis energy is supplied by NADPH. And the main source of NADPH for lipogenesis is pentose phosphate pathway (or hexose monophosphate/HMP pathway).** NADPH is used as donor of reducing equivalents in both the reduction of 3-keto-acyl and2, 3 – unsaturated acyl derivatives in fatyacid synthesis.

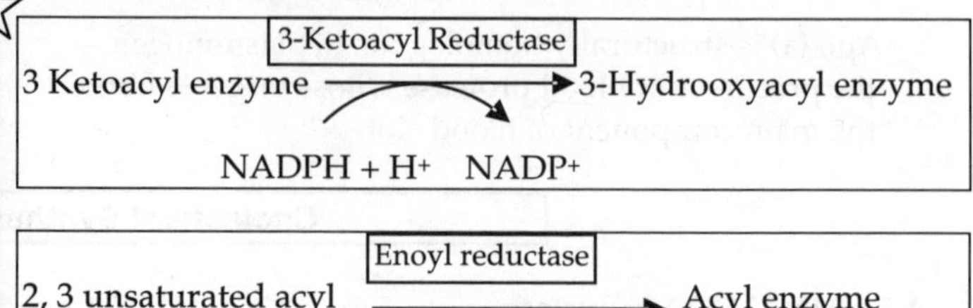

Sites of Biochemical Reaction

❑ Cytoplasm	❑ Mitochondria
- **Glycolysis**Q - **HMP shunt**Q - **Fatty acid synthesis**Q - **Protein synthesis**Q - **Part of urea cycle**Q - **Part of gluconeogensis**Q	- **TCA or Kreb's or Citric acid cycle**Q - Oxidative decarboxylation **(ATP production)**Q - **Fatty acid (β) oxidation**Q - **Part of urea cycle**Q - **Ketogenesis**Q - **Part of gluconeogenesis**Q
❑ **Golgi apparatus**	❑ **Nucleus**
Synthesis & packaging of complexmolecules including glycolipids, glycoproteins & lipoproteins	**DNA & RNA synthesis** ❑ **Lysosomes** Degradation of complex molecule ❑ **Nucleolus** **rRNA synthesis**Q

NADPH: Use & Sources

Uses	Sources
NADPH is used as an electron donor in many reductive syntheses in the body. Examples are: 1. Extra- mitochondrial de-Novo **fatty acid synthesis**Q 2. **Cholesterol synthesis**Q 3. **Steroid synthessis**Q 4. **Sphinigolipid synthesis**Q 5. **Conversion of oxidized glutathione to reduced glutathione**Q 6. Conversion of **Phenylalanine to tyrosine**Q 7. Conversion of **met- Hb to Hb**Q 8. **Uronic acid pathway**Q	- **HMP pathway**Q: Main source of NADPH - **Malic enzyme / Malate dehydrogenase**Q : Malate is oxidatively decarboxylated to pyruvate and NADPH is produced. - **Isocitrate dehydrogenase**Q

Fatty Acid Synthesis Requires

Site	Building Block	Multi Enzymes Complex		Coenzymes & Cofactors
		Main enzyme	Rate limiting enzyme	
CytsolQ	**Acetyl CoA**Q	**Fatty acid synthetase complex (7 enzyme)**Q	**Acetyl CoA carboxylase**Q	Mn- **"Be Human"** - ***Biotin***Q — Be - HCO_3^- (Source of CO_2) — Hu - ***Mn***$^{2+}$Q — M - ATP — A - ***NADPH***Q — N

82. **A i.e. Acetyle CoA Carboxylase;** 83. **B i.e. Fatty acid synthesis** 84. **C i.e. Condensation reaction**
85. **A i.e. Freeing of PAN-SH site** 86. **B i.e. 4 in Ist cycle & 2 in IInd cycle** 87. **D i.e. Dehydrogenase**
88. **B i.e. Malonyl CoA**

- The starting material for the synthesis of fatty acid is **acetyl CoA**Q. Formation of Malonyl-CoA from Acetyl CoA is the **initial and controlling step** in fatty acid synthesis and catalyzed by **acetyl –CoA Carboxylase. (Rate limiting enzyme)**Q. This reaction is also called CO_2- fixation reaction.

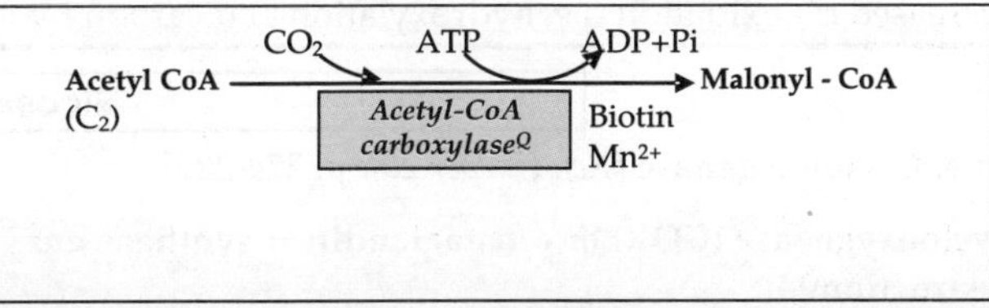

- In **condensation reaction** catabolized by 3 ketoacyl synthase, there is **loss of 1 molecule of CO_2.**
- **Saturated acyl enzyme** formation causes **freeing of PAN-SH site of monomer II which will accept another malonyl group (malonyl CoA)** in each cycle.
- **4 carbon atoms are added in first** and **2 carbon atoms in successive cycles** of FA synthesis.
- **7 enzymes used in FA synthesis** include **acetyl CoA carboxylase, acetyl/malonyl transacylase, 3 ketoacyl synthase (condensation), 3-KA reductase, hydratase (dehydration), enoyl reductase and thioesterase (decyclase)** in this order.

89. **A i.e. Operates under anaerobic conditions; D i.e. Not a common pathway; E i.e. Pyridoxal-Phosphate & NADPH ...**
90. **A & C i.e. ER and Mitochondria** *[Ref: Lippincott 4th/ed pg- 187; Harper 28th/ed pg- 196, 199; Lehninger- 812-15]*

- **Lipogenesis** (i.e. the main pathway for denovo **fatty acid synthesis**) occurs in **cytosol**Q. **Palmitate**, a 16- carbon, fully saturated long chain fatty acid (16: 0) is the principal endproduct of fatty acid synthase system in animal cells. It is the precursor of other long chin fatty acid and may be elongated by addition of 2 carbon unit acetyl groups through the action of **fatty acid elongation system** present in **smooth endo plasmic reticulum (SER) and mitochondria**Q.
- **Mitochondrial FA chain elongation is not a common pathway**Q. It operates under **anaerobic conditions**Q and is favoured by **high NADH / NAD+ ratio and pyridoxal phosphate (coenzyme)**Q.

Triacylglycerol and Phosphoglycerol Synthesis

91. **B i.e. Enzyme glycerol Kinase Plays an important role** *[Ref: Lippincott/s 4/e p. 181-88, 174- 76 , Harper 27/e p. 226, 209-11]*

Triacylglycerol (TAG) is synthesized from acyl- CoA and glycerol 3 phosphate. **Glycerol Kinase** Catalyzes the activation of glycerol to sn- glycerol 3 phosphate. **Because the enzyme glycerol kinase is not expressed in adipose tissue or muscle, glycerol cannot be utilized for provision of glycerol 3 – PO_4, which must be supplied by glucose via glycolysis. So in muscle or adipose tissue, most of glycerol-3 PO_4 is formed from dihydroxy acetone phosphate by glycerol – 3 – phosphate dehydrogenase**Q

β - Oxidation of Fatty Acids

92. **C i.e. Carnitine** *[Ref: Harper's 28/e P-184-86; Lippincott 4/e p. 191]*
93. **C i.e. Carnitine palmitoyl trasferase II is present in mitochondrial matrix**

Long chain activated fatty acid **penetrate the inner mitochondrial membrane only in combination with carnitine**Q. **Carnitine**, a carrier molecule, acts like a ferry boat and transport long chain acyl- CoA across mitochondiral membrane otherwise inner mitochondrial membrane is impermeable to acyl –CoA.

94. **B i.e. Propionyl CoA** *[Ref: Harper's 27/e P-188-89; 26/e P- 182, 181; Shinde & Chatterjea P-348, 347]*

β- oxidation of odd chain fatty acid produces acetyl CoA plus a molecule of **propionyl –CoA**Q. But propionyl CoA is formed only in odd chain fatty acid oxidation (not in even fatty acids)

95. **D i.e. 147** *[Ref: Lehninger 5th/e p. 65-57; Harper 28/e p. 191; 27/e p. 189]*
96. **B i.e. 129 ATP net; E i.e. 96 ATP from citric acid cycle** 97. **B i.e. H_2O_2 formed**

A modified form of β- oxidation is found in peroxisomes and lead to the formation of acetyl CoA and H_2O_2Q

98. **D i.e. Phytanic alpha oxidase** *[Ref: Harper 28th/e p.191, 493; Lippincott 4th/e p.195; Lehninger 5th/e p. 665; Nelson 17/e p.2077]*

Refsum's disease is a rare autosomal recessive disorder caused by **deficiency of phytanic α oxides** (Nelson) / **α-hydroxylase** (Lippincot) / **Phytanoyl CoA hydroxylase** (Lehninger) results in accumulation of phytanic acid due to its decreased α - oxidation (i.e. hydroxylation at α carbon by fatty acid α hydroxylase)

Eicosanoids

99. **B i.e. Cyclooxygenase** *[Ref: Harper 29/e p. 224-226]*

Cyclooxygenase (COX) or prostaglandin H synthase enzyme is a **suicide enzyme responsible for its self catalyzed destruction**Q.

COX has 2 activities, a **cyclooxygenase** (converting arachidonic acid & $2O_2$ to prostaglandin G_2 or PGG_2) and **peroxidase** (converting PGG_2 to PGH_2 an endoperoxide). After this PGH2 can be converted to prostaglandin D & E, prostacyclin (PGI_2) and thromboxane (TXA_2) by isomerase, PC synthase & TX synthase respectively. Switching off of prostaglandin activity is partly achieved by **self catalyzed suicidal destruction property of COX**. However, 15 hydroxy prostaglandin dehydrogenase inactivate prostaglandins rapidly.

Ketogenesis (Ketone Body Formation)

100. **D i.e. HMG CoA reductase is the rate-limiting enzyme** *[Ref: Harper 29/e p 210-14; Lippincott 5/e p 195-97]*
101. **B i.e. HMG CoA** 102. **A i.e. Liver** 103. **D i.e. RBCs** 104. **C i.e. Acetoacetate**

- **HMG CoA** is an intermediate in the pathway of ketogenesis, and this is an **immediate precursor of acetoacetate**Q (Ist ketone body to be formed). Aceto acetyl CoA is the starting material for ketogenesis.It combines with acetyl CoA to form HMG (=3 Hydroxy 3 methylglutaryl) CoA. This **rate limiting step** is catalyzed by **HMG CoA synthase**Q.
- **Liver is the only organ which produces ketone bodies**Q and add to the blood, but it lacks the enzyme responsible for their degradation and utilization. This is the reason why **liver does not utilize ketone bodies**Q. **Liver (>>) and RBCs (d/t lack of mitochondria)** are the **only tissues not able to utilize ketone bodies for energy**Q. **Liver lacks Succinyl CoA-Acetoacetate CoA transferase enzyme** which is required for 1st step i.e. activation of ketone bodies in ketone bodies utilization.
- **Ketosis** is a metabolic adaption to starvation. Thus a ketone body (Acetoacetate) is formed in starvation not in well fed state

Pathways	Rate limiting Enzymes
Glycolysis	**Phospho fructokinase (PFK)-1** Q
Glycogenesis	**Glycogen synthase**Q
Glycogenolysis	**Glycogen phosphorylase**Q
Gluconeogenesis	**Phosphoenol pyruvate (PEP) carboxykinase**Q**; F1, 6 biphosphalase**
Citric acid (TCA) cycle	Alpha- ketoglutarate dehydrogenase
HMP shunt (PPP pathway)	**Glucose 6 phosphate dehydrogenase**Q
Fatty acid synthesis	**Acetyl CoA carboxylase**Q
Cholesterol synthesis	**HMG-CoA reductase**Q
Ketone body formation	**HMG CoA synthesase**Q
Bile acid synthesis	**7-alpha hydroxylase**Q (regulated by **farnesoid x-receptor or FXR)**
Lipolysis of adipose tissue	**Hormone sensitive triacylglycerol lipase**Q
Purine synthesis	PP ribose – P-glutamyl amidotransferase
Uric acid synthesis	**Xanthine oxidase**Q
Urea cycle	**CPS I (mitochondria)**
Pyrimidine synthesis	CPS (carbamoyl phosphate synthetase II)
Purine salvage pathway	**HGPRT ase; APRT ase (adenine phosphoribosyl** transferase)
Heme synthesis	ALA synthase
Catecholamine	DOPA decarboxylase
GTP formation	IMP dehydrogenase
Tetrahydro biopterin formation	GTP cyclohydrolase I

105. D i.e. Malonyl CoA *[Ref: Harper 29/e p 212-14, 247-48; Lippincott 5/e p 330-31, 193-98]*

In well fed state, the activity of CPTI (carnitine palmitoyl transferase I) in outer mitochondrial membrane is inhibited by melonyl CoAQ.

106. A i.e. Usilize fatty acids in Starvation; 107. B i.e. Ketone bodies; 108. B i.e. Ketone bodies

109. D i.e. Increased Gluconeogenesis *[Ref: Ganong 22/e P- 299-301, 342-43, 349- 50; Lehininger 2/e P- 842- 45; Chatterjea 6/e P-362-65, 465; NMS 3/e P-517; Lippincott's 3/e P-294]*

Energy is derived mainly from **glycogenolysis (initial few hours) → gluconeogenesis (upto 72 hours) → Degradation of fast (3 days – 2weeks) → Break down of tissue protein (last 1 weeks)**Q

110. D i.e. Glycogenesis 111. B i.e. Liver gluoneogenesis increases 112. D i.e. Decrease in serum Proteins
[Ref: Lippincott 5/e p 321-33; Mark's (2012) p 35-36; Vasudevan 6/e p 107-108; Chattarjea 8/e p 535-35; Ganong 22/e p 350]

- **Glycogenolysis and liver gluconeogenesis (initially by degradation of glucogenic aminoacids of muscle proteins** followed by glycerol & lactate) are sources of energy in **brief (1st stage) of starvation (ie 12 to 72 hours of fasting). Gluconeogenesis** the main process, **increases during brief fasting but decreases on prolonged fasting. In starvation, glycogenolysis increases and glycogenesis decreases**Q. So in fasting (starvation) there is **increase in glycogenolysis, gluconeogenesis, lipolysis, ketogenesis and proteolysis**Q.
- **During starvation serum proteins are not utilized as a source of energy**Q. Brief fasting is associated with **increased proteolysis (break down) of muscle proteins (not serum proteins) thereby decreasing total muscle proteins, whereas the serum protein levels are unaltered (ie not decreased)**Q. Proteolysis of muscles provide glucogenic aminoacids (alanine & glutamine increasing liver gluconeogenesis
- On **prolonged fasting (starvation), adipose tissue breakdown (beta-oxidation) becomes the main source of energy;** thereby **increasing production of ketone bodies.** However it is important to note that this over produced **ketone bodies are utilized mainly by brain not by muscles** as the utilization of glucose by brain and utilization of ketone bodies by by-muscle **decreases during prolonged starvation.** In the same way, **decreased gluconeogenesis in prolonged starvation** is responsible for **decreased muscle protein degradation and decreased production of urea.**

113. A i.e. Low Km value of hexokinase C i.e. High Km value of glucokinase

Hexokinase has **low Km value i.e. high affinity for glucose**Q and it is present in **all tissue including brain**Q; where as **glucokinase** has **high Km value i.e. low affinity for glucose**Q and it is present in **liver and B- cells**Q. That's why brain can utilize glucose in starvation but the liver can not. The glucokinase functions only when intracellular concentration of glucose in hepatocytes is elevated as in post absorptive state.

114. C i.e. Prolonged Starvation *[Ref: Lippincott's 3/e P-89, 293; Lahninger 2/e P- 840 – 49]*

Diabetes Mellitus	**Differences in Ketosis of**	**Starvation**
- More	**↓ Insulin & ↑Glucagon**	- Less
- More severe	**Ketosis** - Ketonemia (ketone bodies in blood - Ketonuria	- Less severe
- More severe	**Ketoacidosis** (decrease in blood pH or acid buffering capacity of blood buffers)	- Less severe
- PresentQ	**Glycosuria**	**- Absent**Q
- Hyperglycemia	Blood glucose level	- Normal or less

115. A i.e. Ketone bodies; B i.e. Glucose; C i.e. Free fatty acids; D i.e. Creatine phosphate

- **Glucose** (in TCA cycle), **free fatty acid** (in β oxidation), **ketone bodies** (by brain in starvation), **phosphocreatine (creatine phosphate**; in muscles) and **glucogenic aminoacids** are used as **source of energy by body.**
- **Starvation leads to glycogenolysis**(1st stage), **gluconeogenesis** (2nd), **lipolysis** (3rd) and **acidosis (ketoacidosis; 4th stage).**

116. A i.e. Alanine *[Ref: Lippincott 3/e P 294; Lahninger 2/e P 843]*

In starvation, alanine and glutamine are quantitatively the most important gluconeogenic aminoacidsQ. So alanine carries nitrogen from muscle to liver & kidney for further metabolism & energy production during starvation.

117. C i.e. Increased secretion of insulin *[Ref: Ganong 22/e p. 345-46]*

- **Glucose, mannose, aminoacids (such as leucine, arginine, others) and β ketoacids such as acetoacetate (derived from fat catabolism) stimulate insulin secretin and have protein sparing effect**Q.

- **Insulin** has anabolic effect on metabolism. It decreases protein catabolism and fat catabolism for energy production and increases **aminoacid uptake & protein synthesis (positive nitrogen balance)**Q.

118. A i.e. Increase in glucagons / insulin ratio, increased C- AMP & increased blood sugar.
[Ref: Lehnenger 2/e P- 847- 49; Lippincott 2/e P 297; Ganong 22/e P- 350, 336- 49]

Diabetes Mellitus

- In diabetes little glucose is oxidized as fuel, except by the brain. The rest of tissues burn a large amount of fat, particularly the liver where the amount of acetyl COA formed from fatty acids exceeds the capacity of the tricarboxylic acid cycle to oxidize it. The excess acetyl COA is converted to ketone bodies l/t ketonemia, ketonuria & ketoacidosis
- Diabetics not only have a defect in the tissue utilization of glucose but also appears to be metabolically poised to produce maximum amount of glucose from amino acids (gluconeogenesis) and to prevent glucose from being utilized to to form fat. (fat synthesis)
- Insulin is decreased & glucagons is increased l/t ↑**glucagon / insulin ratio**Q. Glucagon acts via elevation **in C- AMP**Q

119. D i.e. Ketones *[Ref. Vasudevan 6/e p. 372, 319, 305, 64, 251-50, 288, 279; Lehninger 5/e p. 241; Satyanarayana 3rd/295; 'Practical Biochemistry for Students' by Malhotra 4th/e 43-47, 'Laboratory Manual of Biochemistry' by Chary & Sharma (2004) / 21]*

Rothera's – nitroprusside – pink/ purple permanganate ring test and **Gerhardt's – ferric chloride – red wine color tests** are used for detection of **ketone bodies** in urine.

120. B i.e. Rotheras *[Ref: Chatterjea 6/e P-652-60]*

- Owing to gradual decline in carbohydrate store & lack of carbohydrates, energy is obtained from burning fat. This leads to an increase in free fatty acids (FFA). As FFA increase, ketogenesis is stimulated and excess of ketone bodies are formed which pass into blood, resulting in ketosis and ketonuria.
- The women is presenting with altered sensorium and dehydration, which may be the presenting features of ketoacidosis. She has already been tested for blood sugar (rules out diabetic ketoacidosis) & protein.
- *The important investigation missed out in this patient is ketone bodies in urine, which is important to reach to the diagnosis of starvation ketosis. Ketone bodies are tested by Rotheras test.*
- There appears no clinical relevance to test for bile salts & bile pigments.

Test	Done for
Fouchet's test	Bile pigments
Hay's sulphur test	Bile salts
Benedicts test	Blood sugar
Rotheras test	*Ketone bodies*Q

121. A i.e. Bile salts in urine

Tests	Used for
Rothera's test (nitroprusside test)	**Ketone bodies in urine**Q**:** acetone and acetoacetate
Gerhard's test (ferric chloride test)	Ketone bodies in urine: acetoacetate
Benedict's test	Reducing sugars in urine
Fehling's test	
Hay's sulphur test	**Bile salts in urine**Q
Fouchet's (borium sulphate test)	Bile pigment: bilirubin
Gmelin's (nitric acid test)	
Vanden Bergh test	
Ehrlich's test	Bilinogens (stercobilinogen, urobilinogen)
Schlesinger's test	Bilins (stercobilin, urobilin)
Ehrlich's aldehyde test	Porphobilinogen and urobilinogen in urine

Chapter -3

STRUCTURE, FUNCTION AND REPLICATION OF INFORMATIONAL MACROMOLECULES

QUESTIONS

Purines and Pyrimidines

1. **Rate limiting step in pyrimidine synthesis-** *(NBE P 15)*
   A. DIhydro-orotase ☐
   B. Ornithine transcarbomolyase ☐
   C. Aspartate transcarbomoylase ☐
   D. Carbamoyl phosphate synthase-1 ☐
2. **Pyrimidine metabolism features a/e** *(PGI 15,10)*
   A. Require CAD polypeptide chain ☐
   B. 6-azauridine l/t oritidinuria ☐
   C. DHOA-dehydrogenase is mitochondrial ☐
   D. Reye syndrome decrease cytosolic carbamoyl phosphate ☐
   E. Urea cycle is linked ☐
3. **What is involved in formation of d-TMP from d-UMP?**
   A. N5, N10-methylene tetra hydrofolate *(PGI 07)* ☐
   B. Form imino folate ☐
   C. N5 formyl folate ☐
   D. Dihydro folate ☐
4. **End product of purine metabolism in non-primate mammals is:** *(NBE P 15,13; AIIMS 14,13,07)*
   A. Uric acid ☐
   B. Ammonia ☐
   C. Urea ☐
   D. Allantoin ☐
5. **In humans, end product of purine metabolism-**
   A. Allantoin *(NBE P 15)* ☐
   B. Uric acid ☐
   C. CO_2 ☐
   D. None ☐
6. **Inositic acid is biological precursor of -**
   A. Uracil and thymine *(Nimhans 07, Jipmer 04)* ☐
   B. Purines and thymine *(UP 05, AMU 06)* ☐
   C. Adenylic acid and guanylic acid ☐
   D. Orotic acid and uridylic acid ☐
7. **False regarding gout is :** *(AI 01)*
   A. Due to increased metabolism of pyrimidines ☐
   B. Due to increased metabolism of purines ☐
   C. Uric acid levels may not be elevated ☐
   D. Has a predilection for the great toe ☐
8. **Gout is a disorder of :** *(AI 06)*
   A. Purine metabolism ☐
   B. Pyrimidine metabolism ☐
   C. Oxalate metabolism ☐
   D. Protein metabolism ☐
9. **What is not true about gout:** *(AIIMS 05)*
   A. Abrupt increase in serum urate levels is more common a cause for acute gout than an abrupt fall in urate levels. ☐
   B. Patient may be asymptomatic with high serum uric acid for years ☐
   C. Development of arthritis correlates with level of serum uric acid ☐
   D. Uric acid crystals are best seen by polarising light microscope ☐
10. **Specific test for gout is:** *(AIIMS 06)*
    A. Raised serum uric acid level ☐
    B. Raised uric acid in synovial fluid of joint ☐
    C. Raised urea level ☐
    D. Raised urease enzyme level ☐
11. **A ten year old child with aggressive behavior and poor concentration is brought with presenting complaints of joint pain and reduced urinary output. Mother gives history of self mutilitative behavior stating that he tends to mutilate his fingers. Which of the following enzymes is likely to be deficient in this child** *(AI 09)*
    A. HGPRTase ☐
    B. Adenosine Deaminase ☐
    C. APRTase ☐
    D. Acid Maltase ☐
12. **Lesch Nyhan syndrome is due to deficiency of:**
    A. Hypoxanthine phosphoribosyl transferase (HGPRTase) *(PGI 08, 12)* ☐
    B. Xanthine oxidase ☐
    C. Purine phosphorylase ☐
    D. Adenosine deaminase ☐
13. **A 12 year old child presents with mental retardation and history of self mutilation. Which of the following tests will help in determining the diagnosis** *(AI 12)*
    A. Serum Lead Levels ☐
    B. Serum Alkaline Phosphatase Levels ☐
    C. Serum Lactate Dehydrogenase Levels ☐
    D. Serum Uric Acid Levels ☐
14. **Which is common metabolic process in human as well as bacteria:** *(PGI 01)*
    A. Purine synthesis ☐
    B. Nitrogen fixation ☐
    C. Mucolipid formation ☐
    D. Nonoxidative photophosphorylation ☐
15. **Apart from occurring in nucleic acids, pyrimidines are also found in:** *(AIIMS 05)*
    A. Theophylline ☐
    B. Theobromine ☐
    C. Flavin mononucleotide ☐
    D. Thiamine ☐
16. **Salvage pathway of purine nucleotide synthesis are used all except-** *(NBE P 15)*
    A. Brain ☐
    B. Liver ☐
    C. RBC ☐
    D. Leukocytes ☐

DNA Structure

17. True statements about DNA structure: *(PGI 06)*
A. All nucleotides are involved in linkage ☐
B. Antiparallel ☐
C. Parallel ☐
D. Bases are perpendicular to DNA ☐
E. Attached by hydroxy bond. ☐

18. mRNA is a complimentary copy of - *(SGPGI 03)* *(Jipmer 02)*
A. TRNA ☐
B. RRNA ☐
C. Ribosomal DNA ☐
D. Both strands of DNA ☐
E. A single strand of DNA ☐

19. Which is not found in DNA: *(NBE P 14,13; AI 04)*
A. Adenine ☐
B. Thymine ☐
C. Guanine ☐
D. Uracil ☐

20. The two strands of DNA are held together by: *(AIIMS 07)*
A. Van-der -Waal bond ☐
B. Hydrogen bond ☐
C. Covalent bond ☐
D. Ionic interaction ☐

21. True about DNA structure: *(PGI 10)*
A. Purines are adenne and guanine & pyrimidines are uracil and cytosine ☐
B. Watson and Crick discovered structure in 1973 ☐
C. Deoxyribose-phosphate backbone with bases stacked inside ☐
D. Mainly consists of left handed helix ☐
E. 5′-3′ phosodiester bonding is present ☐

22. Which form of DNA is predominantly seen: *(NBE P 13)* *(AI 06)*
A. A ☐
B. C ☐
C. B ☐
D. Z ☐

23. Triplex DNA is due to *(NBE P 14; AIIMS 11)*
A. Hoogsteen pairing ☐
B. Palindromic sequences ☐
C. Large no. of guanosine repeats ☐
D. Polypyramidine tracts ☐

24. Chargaff rule state that- *(NBE P 13; UP 08)*
A. A+G = T+C ☐
B. A/T = G/C ☐
C. A = U= T= G= C ☐
D. A + T = G + C ☐

25. A nucleic acid was analyzed and found to contain 32% adenine, 18% guanine, 17% cytosine and 33% thymine. The nucleic acid must be: *(AIIMS 06)*
A. Single-stranded RNA ☐
B. Single-stranded DNA ☐
C. Double-stranded RNA ☐
D. Double stranded DNA ☐

26. In a sample of DNA, if adenine is 23% what will be the amount of guanine present: *(PGI 13, 16)*
A. 23% ☐
B. 25% ☐
C. 46% ☐
D. 27% ☐

27. Triple bonds are found between which base pairs: *(AI 01)*
A. A-T ☐
B. C-G ☐
C. A-G ☐
D. C-T ☐

28. Thermo-stability in DNA is contributed mostly by: *(AI 07; NBE P 13)*
A. A=T ☐
B. G≡C ☐
C. Molecular base ☐
D. Parallel arrangement ☐

29. In Hybrid RNA-DNA, DNA is 5CTTAAG3. The sequence of RNA will be: *(PGI 11, 15)*
A. 5CTTAAG3 ☐
B. 5CUUAAG3 ☐
C. 5GAATTC3 ☐
D. 5GAAUUC3 ☐
E. 5CTTUUG3 ☐

30. Which one of the following is the complementary sequence of 5′ TTAAGCTAC 3′? *(AI 06)*
A. 5′ GTACGCTTAA 3′ ☐
B. 5′ AATTCGCATG 3′ ☐
C. 5′ CATGCGAATT 3′ ☐
D. 5′ TTAAGCGTAC 3′ ☐

31. True about coding strand of DNA: *(PGI 03)*
A. Template strand ☐
B. Minus strand ☐
C. Runs at 5- - 3' direction ☐
D. Runs at 3' – 5' direction ☐
E. Plus strand ☐

32. True a bout coding strand of DNA: *(PGI 03)*
A. DNA acts as template for mRNA ☐
B. Minus strand ☐
C. Plus strand ☐
D. Matches with RNA transcript hat encodes protein ☐

33. 5′ TTACGTAC-3′ after transcription what will be the RNA: *(PGI 08)*
A. 5-TTACGTAC-3′ ☐
B. 3′- TTACGTAC-5′ ☐
C. 5′ CATGCATT-3 ☐
D. 3′- CATGCATT-5 ☐
E. 5′- GUACGUAA-3′ ☐

34. Bromodeoxyuridine is related to DNA in: *(AI 06)*
A. Uracil ☐
B. Adenosine ☐
C. Cytosine ☐
D. Thymidine ☐

35. At the physiological pH the DNA molecules are: *(AIIMS 13, NBE P 14)*
A. Positively charged. ☐
B. Negatively charged. ☐
C. Neutral. ☐
D. Amphipathic ☐

36. True about mitochondrial DNA: *(PGI 14, 11)*
A. Maternal inheritance ☐

B. Same evolutionary origin □
C. Not highly conserved & has high mutation rate □
D. Mitochondrial disease is associated mostly with Mutation & some have deletion □
E. Mostly encodes membrane protein □

37. True about mitochondrial DNA *(NBE P 14; AI 11)*
A. UGA codes for tryptophan □
B. Codes for 13 protein □
C. High content of untranslated sequences □
D. Circular double stranded DNA □
E. Mitochondrial disease occur due to Point Mutations and Large-Scale Rearrangements □

38. Intron is not found in which DNA? *(AIIMS 08)*
A. Nuclear DNA □
B. Mitochondrial DNA □
C. B DNA □
D. ZDNA □

39. NARP syndrome & myopathy is seen in
A. Lysosomal disorder *(AIIMS 15,14,09)* □
B. Glycogen storage disease □
C. Mitochondrial disease □
D. Lipid storage disease □

40. Mitochondrial DNA (gene) true is: *(PGI 14,08,03)*
A. Paternally inherited □
B. Maternally inherited □
C. Horizontal inheritance □
D. Vertical Mendelian inheritance □

41. Mitochondrial DNA is: *(NBE P 15,14; AI 06)*
A. Closed circular □
B. Nicked circular □
C. Linear □
D. Open circular □

42. Circular DNA is found in: *(PGI 11)*
A. Virus □
B. Chloroplast □
C. Bacteria □
D. Mitochondria □
E. Fungus □

43. Total number of genes in a human being is-
A. 800,000 *(DNB 12,08)* □
B. 50,000 □
C. 100,000 □
D. 30,000 □

44. Cellular bearings of herediatary disease seen in:
A. DNA *(DNB 12, 08; PGI 03)* □
B. Ribosome □
C. RNA □
D. Membrane □
E. Proteins □

45. Highly repetitive DNA is seen in: *(PGI 03)*
A. Cloning of DNA □
B. Microsatelite DNA □
C. Telomere □
D. Centromere □

46. True about telomerase or telomere is/are: *(PGI 03)*
A. They are present at the ends of eukaryotic chromosome □
B. Increased telomerase activity favours cancer cells □
C. DNA dependent RNA polymerase □
D. DNA polymerase □

47. Action of 'Telomerase' is *(NBE P 14; UP 04)*
A. DNA repair □
B. Longetivity of cell – Ageing □
C. Breakdown of telomer □
D. None □

48. Ends of chromosomes replicated by: *(PGI 06)*
A. Telomerase □
B. Centromere □
C. Restriction endonuclease □
D. Exonuclease □

49. Which enzymatic mutation is responsible for immortality of cancer cells : *(AIIMS 01)*
A. DNA reverse transciptase □
B. RNA polymerase □
C. Telomerase □
D. DNA polymerase □

50. All of the following cell types contain the enzyme telemerase which protects the length of telomeres at the end of chromosomes, *except*: *(AI 06)*
A. Germinal □
B. Somatic □
C. Hemopoietic □
D. Tumor □

51. True about Histone protein: *(PGI 12, 09)*
A. Ribonucleoprotein □
B. Present inside the nucleus □
C. Acidic □
D. Basic □
E. Glycoprotein □

52. Histone acetylation causes? *(AIIMS 11)*
A. Increased Heterochromatin formation □
B. Increased Euchromatin formation □
C. Methylation of cystine □
D. DNA replication □

53. Components of chromosome are: *(PGI 03)*
A. DNA □
B. tRNA □
C. m RNA □
D. r RNA □
E. Histones □

54. The protein rich in basic amino acids, which functions in the packaging of DNA in chromosomes, is:
A. Histone *(AI 03)* □
B. Collagen □
C. Hyaluronic acid binding protein □
D. Fibrinogen □

55. Histone has post - translational modification by all/except. *(AIIMS 07)*
A. Acylation □
B. Methylation □
C. Phosphorylation □
D. Glycosylation □

56. Euchromatin is the region of DNA that is relatively:
A. Unconcensed *(NBE P 13; AI 06)* ☐
B. Condensed ☐
C. Overcondensed ☐
D. Partially condensed ☐

57. Nucleosome consists of: *(PGI 15, 10)*
A. Histone ☐
B. DNA ☐
C. RNA ☐
D. DNA & RNA both ☐
E. Carbohydrate ☐

58. True about nucleosome: *(PGI 09)*
A. Use only one type of histone protein ☐
B. Each complex is separated from each other by non histone proteins ☐
C. Regular repeating structure of DNA & histone proteins ☐
D. Reflect small nucleus ☐
E. Core of DNA with protein wrapped ☐

59. CG islands in our DNA are important for: *(AIIMS 16)*
A. Acetylation ☐
B. Methylation ☐
C. t-RNA synthesis ☐
D. DNA replication ☐

DNA Synthesis and Replication

60. True about prokaryotic DNA replication: *(PGI 13)*
A. Conservative ☐
B. Semi conservative ☐
C. Unidirectional ☐
D. Bidirectional ☐
E. Semi discontinuous ☐

61. True about DNA supercoiling is all except
A. Underwinding results in negative superhelical density & supercoiling *(PGI 09)* ☐
B. Superhelical density depends on length of DNA ☐
C. Underwinding strain is normally accommodated by strand separation ☐
D. Topoisomerase II change linking number in increments of 2 ☐
E. Most cellular DNA is underwound ☐

62. Okazaki segments are required for OR formed during: *(AIIMS 14; NBE P 15,14,13; AI 10; PGI 14)*
A. DNA synthesis/ replication ☐
B. RNA synthesis ☐
C. Protein synthesis ☐
D. None of the above ☐

63. Okazaki fragments are formed during the synthesis of
A. ds DNA *(AIIMS 15; NBE P 15; AI 08)* ☐
B. ss DNA ☐
C. m RNA ☐
D. t RNA ☐

64. During replication of DNA, which one of the following enzymes polymerizes the Okazaki fragments? *(NBE P 15,14; PGI 14; AI 06)*
A. DNA Polymerase I ☐
B. DNA Polymerase II ☐
C. DNA Polymerase III ☐
D. RNA Polymerase I ☐

65. True-regarding DNA-replication: *(PGI 07)*
A. Occurs in the M-phase of the cell cycle. ☐
B. Sister Chromatids are formed. ☐
C. Follow base pair rule. ☐
D. Semi conservative. ☐
E. Single strand breaknd. ☐

66. Correct sequence of enzymes required for DNA formation is: *(PGI 01)*
A. DNA polymerase → Protein unwinding enzyme → DNA ligase → DNA Isomerase → Polymerase –1 ☐
B. Protein unwinding enzyme → Polymerase 1 → DNA ligase→ DNA Isomerase→ DNA polymerase ☐
C. RNA polymerase → DNA polymerase III → DNA polymerase I → DNA ligase ☐
D. RNA polymerase → DNA polymerase III → dNA ligase → Exonuclease → DNA polymerase I ☐

67. False statements are: *(PGI 11)*
A. In leading strands DNA is synthesized continuously ☐
B. Multiple origins of replication are possible for bacteria ☐
C. DNA replication proceeds in one direction ☐
D. Lagging strand stick by RNA primase ☐
E. DNA polymerase III- processive leading strand synthesis ☐

68. The gaps between segments of DNA on the lagging strand produced by restriction enzymes are rejoined sealed by: *(NBE P 15, 13; AI 09)*
A. DNA Ligases ☐
B. DNA Helicase ☐
C. DNA topoisomerase ☐
D. DNA phosphorylase ☐

69. DNA synthesis requires: *(PGI 16,10)*
A. DNA polymerase ☐
B. DNA ligase ☐
C. DNA topoisomerase ☐
D. Primase ☐
E. RNA polymerase ☐

70. DNA supercoiling is done by :
A. DNA polymerase I *(AIIMS 04, 15)* ☐
B. DNA polymerase II ☐
C. DNA topoisomerase ☐
D. DNA gyrase. ☐

71. Which statements are true about E. coli chromosomal DNA in relation with eukaryotic chromosomal DNA:
A. Circular *(PGI 16,08)* ☐
B. Packed into nucleolus ☐
C. Positively Supercoiled ☐
D. Negatively sepercoiled ☐
E. Nucleoid present ☐

72. Which DNA polymerase is /are involved in repair of mammalian DNA: *(PGI 09)*
A. α ☐
B. β ☐

C. γ ☐
D. ε ☐
E. δ ☐

73. True about DNA polymerase in eukaryotes:
A. Components are α, β, γ, Δ, ε *(PGI 08)* ☐
B. β associated with repair ☐
C. γ associated with repair ☐
D. Δ associated with synthesis of mitochondria DNA ☐
E. Alpha is abundant amount ☐

74. DNA polymerase have: *(PGI 15,10; AIIMS 09)*
A. 3' $\rightarrow$ 5' polymerase activity ☐
B. 5' $\rightarrow$ 3' polymerase activity ☐
C. 3' $\rightarrow$ 5' exonuclease activity ☐
D. 5' $\rightarrow$ 3' exonuclease activity ☐

DNA Damage, Repair and Protooncogene

75. Nucleoside is made up of: *(PGI 13, 10)*
A. Pyrimidine ☐
B. Histone ☐
C. Sugar ☐
D. Purine ☐
E. Phosphate ☐

76. All of the following abbreviations are true except:
A. AMP-Adenosine monophosphate *(PGI 09)* ☐
B. CMP – Cytidine monophosphate ☐
C. GMP – Guanosine monophosphate ☐
D. TMP – Thymine monophosphate ☐
E. UMP – Uracil monophosphate ☐

77. On complete hydrolysis of DNA, we will get all of the following except: *(AI 04)*
A. Adenosine ☐
B. Purine base ☐
C. Phosphoric acid ☐
D. Dexose pentose sugar ☐

78. What will happen to DNA if salt is added to it:
A. Increase Melting point (Tm) *(PGI 08)* ☐
B. Decrease Tm ☐
C. Not affect Tm ☐
D. Melting lead to denaturation of DNA ☐
E. Both increase & decrease in Tm depending on concentration of salt ☐

79. What is meant by melting of double stranded DNA:
A. Splitting of double strands into single strand. ☐
B. Splitting of DNA into fragments. *(AIIMS 08)* ☐
C. Formation of triple helix ☐
D. Separation of bases. ☐

80. Concentration of DNA is measured by:
A. Absorption at 260 nm *(PGI 09)* ☐
B. D-oxyribose estimation ☐
C. Infrared examination ☐
D. Ultrasound examination ☐

81. Incorrect statement are: *(PGI 10)*
A. T4 DNA polymerase has 3'>5' exonuclese activity ☐
B. Klenow fragment of DNA polymerase I function is almost similar to T4 DNA polymerase ☐
C. Restriction endonuclease cut DNA chains at specific location ☐
D. Endonuclease cut DNA at 5' terminus ☐
E. Right handed helix of DNA is more common ☐

82. Photolyase helps in - *(AIIMS 03; DNB 14)*
A. DNA repair ☐
B. DNA replication ☐
C. Protein synthesis ☐
D. None ☐

83. Excessive ultraviolet (uv) radiation is harmful to life. The damage caused to the biological systems by ultraviolet radiation is by OR The primary defect in Xeroderma pigmentosa is: *(AIIMS 10; AI 08)*
A. Formation of thymidine dimmers ☐
B. Poly ADP ribose polymerase is defective ☐
C. Exonuclease is defective ☐
D. Formation of adenine dimers ☐

84. Xeroderma pigmentation is caused due to a group of closely related abnormalities in:
A. Mismatch repair *(NBE P 14; AIIMS 15, 05)* ☐
B. Base excision repair ☐
C. Nucleotide excision repair ☐
D. SOS repair ☐

85. Xeroderma pigmentosum is produced as a result of a defect in: *(AI 04)*
A. DNA polymerase III ☐
B. DNA polymerase I ☐
C. DNA exonuclease ☐
D. DNA ligase ☐

86. A child develops blisters on exposure to sunlight. Irregular dark spots on the skin are also found. He is very likely to have a defect in which of the following mechanisms?
A. Nucleotide excision repair *(AIIMS 12)* ☐
B. Mismatch repair ☐
C. Recombination repair ☐
D. Thymine dimmers ☐

87. 5-methyl cytosine mutation of DNA (DNA methylation) leads to: *(PGI 11)*
A. Deamination to uracil ☐
B. Deamination to thymine ☐
C. Mispair with adenine ☐
D. DNA repair ☐
E. Methylation protects the host DNA from cleavage by its own restriction enzyme ☐

88. DNA repair defect is seen in: *(PGI 11, 08)*
A. Xeroderma pigmentatosa ☐
B. Bloom's syndrome ☐
C. Ataxia telangiectasia ☐
D. Li-Fraumani syndrome ☐
E. Retinoblastoma ☐

89. The normal cellular counterparts of oncogenes are important for the following functions, *except*: *(AI 06)*
A. Promotion of cell cycle progression ☐
B. Inhibition of apoptosis ☐
C. Promotion of DNA repair ☐
D. Promotion of nuclear transcription ☐

90. True about Proto-oncogenes are: *(PGI 07)*
A. Normally involved in cell cycle proliferation ☐
B. Produces tumor ☐
C. Normally involved in suppression of tumour production ☐
D. Proto- oncogens on mutation causes cancer. ☐

91. Anti –carcinogens are: *(PGI 07)*
A. Carotenoids ☐
B. Flavenoids ☐
C. Curcumoids ☐
D. Benzene ☐
E. Lignase ☐

92. Following required for Normal growth: *(PGI 06)*
A. Protooncogenes ☐
B. Tumour suppressor genes ☐
C. Oncogenes ☐
D. DNA repair genes ☐

93. Which is not a tumor suppressor gene? *(AIIMS 08)*
A. WT-1 ☐
B. Rb ☐
C. p53 ☐
D. RAS ☐

94. Maximum damage to DNA is caused by:
A. α-rays *(AIIMS 03)* ☐
B. β-rays ☐
C. γ-rays ☐
D. δ-rays and UV rays ☐

Genetic Code

95. Amino acids not coded by triplet codon: *(PGI 11)*
A. Lysine ☐
B. Hydroxyproline ☐
C. Selenocysteine ☐
D. Pyrrolysine ☐
E. Ornithine ☐

96. True about genetic code except: *(PGI 14, 12, 09)*
A. Degenerate ☐
B. Overlapping ☐
C. Ambigous ☐
D. Universal ☐
E. Commaless ☐

97. Stop codons are A/E:
(NBE P 15,14,13; PGI 16,14, 10; AIIMS 15, 12)
A. UAA ☐
B. UAG ☐
C. UGA ☐
D. UAC ☐

98. True about genetic code: *(PGI 09)*
A. AUA codes for methionine in mitochondria ☐
B. UGA codes for selenocysteine ☐
C. AUG codes for initiator codon in mammalian cell ☐
D. AGA & AGG act as chain terminator in mammalian mitochondria ☐
E. UAA, UAG & UGA are stop codon ☐

99. If there are 4 nucleotides instead of 3 in codon, how many amino acids may be formed? *(AIIMS 11, PGI 07)*
A. 16 ☐
B. 21 ☐
C. 256 ☐
D. 64 ☐
E. 265 ☐

100. A codon consists of - *(AIIMS 03, WB 02)*
A. One molecule of amono acyl-t RNA ☐
B. Two complementary base pairs ☐
C. 3 consecutive nucleotide units ☐
D. 4 individual nucleotides ☐

101. All are true of the genetic code except -
(AIIMS 16,14; DNB 15; NBE P 15,14,13; PGI 15,12)
A. Degenerate ☐
B. Universal ☐
C. Punctuation ☐
D. Non overlapping & Non ambiguous ☐

102. Chain initiation in protein synthesis is by-
A. AUG *(MAHE 04, AIIMS 02, PGI 05)* ☐
B. GLA ☐
C. UGA ☐
D. UAG ☐

103. Nonsense codons bring about- *(AIIMS 13,DNB 15)*
A. Elongation of polypeptide chain ☐
B. Pre-translational modificastion of protein ☐
C. Initiation of protein synthesis ☐
D. Termination of protein synthesis ☐

104. A codon consists of - *(AIIMS 12)*
A. 2 complementary base pairs ☐
B. 3 complementary base pairs ☐
C. 4 complementary base pairs on RNA ☐
D. 4 individual nucleotides ☐

105. A condon consists of - *(DNB 13; Raj 04, UP 05)*
A. Two complementary base pairs ☐
B. Three consecutive nucleotide units ☐
C. An individual ribosome ☐
D. Four individual nucleotides ☐

106. Same aminoacid is coded by multiple codons d/t following: *(AIIMS 12, 11, 06)*
A. Degeneracy ☐
B. Frame-shift mutation ☐
C. Transcription ☐
D. Mutation ☐

107. Wobble hypothesis –regarding the variation true is:
A. 3 - end of anticodon *(PGI 15,14, 06)* ☐
B. 5 – end of anticodon ☐
C. m-RNA ☐
D. t-RNA ☐

Regulation of Gene Expression

108. Steroids act via nuclear receptors which interact with DNA through *(AIIMS 06)*
A. Helix turn helix ☐
B. Zinc finger motif ☐
C. Histidine ☐
D. Leucine zipper ☐

109. Zinc finger is: *(PGI 14, 06)*
- A. Nuclear receptor ☐
- B. Membrane receptor ☐
- C. Receptor associated kinase ☐

110. Steroid receptor regulatory protein: *(PGI 15, 08)*
- A. Zinc finger ☐
- B. Heliz-turn –helix ☐
- C. Leucine zippor ☐
- D. RNA ☐

111. Proteins which is having DNA binding domain in its structure: *(PGI 13, 07)*
- A. Zinc finger ☐
- B. β- sheet ☐
- C. β-band ☐
- D. helix-turn helix ☐
- E. leucine zipper ☐

112. In leucine zipper model, Leucine residue seen after every *(AIIMS 09)*
- A. 3 amino acids ☐
- B. 6 amino acids ☐
- C. 9 amno acids ☐
- D. 12 amino acids ☐
- E. 7 amino acid ☐

113. Binding of proteins to DNA is regulated by: *(AI 07)*
- A. Copper ☐
- B. Zinc ☐
- C. Selenium ☐
- D. Nickle ☐

114. Leucine-Zipper complex is *(AIIMS 06)*
- A. DNA binding protein ☐
- B. Membrane attack complex ☐
- C. B cell epitomes ☐
- D. Receptor ligand protein ☐

115. Which is the smallest fundamental unit coding for DNA synthesis: *(PGI 01)*
- A. Cistron ☐
- B. Operon ☐
- C. Replican ☐
- D. Anticodon ☐

116. True about genes *(AIIMS 08)*
- A. Smallest functional unit of genome ☐
- B. Not capable of independent expression ☐
- C. Promoter & enhancer geens are typical example ☐
- D. Cistron is single functional unit ☐

117. CAP in Lac operon is an example of:
- A. Positive regulator *(AI 09, 07, AIIMS 11)* ☐
- B. Negative regulator ☐
- C. Constitutive expression ☐
- D. Attenuation ☐

118. Which of the following are situated away from the coding region: *(PGI 06)*
- A. Promoter ☐
- B. Enhancer ☐
- C. Operator ☐
- D. Structural gene ☐

119. House keeping genes are *(Jipmer 02, WB 03)*
- A. Inducible ☐
- B. Required only when inducer is present ☐
- C. Mutant ☐
- D. Not regulated ☐

120. True among all is *(BHU 04, UP 04)*
- A. Repressor is dimer and a positive regulator ☐
- B. CRP is gratuitous inducer ☐
- C. Lactose is positive regulator ☐
- D. De-repression is d/t presence of glucose ☐
- E. Catabolite repression is mediated by CRP ☐

121. False statement is *(PGI 04, Jipmer 06, WB 03, KA 04)*
- A. Repressor binds operator gene ☐
- B. Regulator genes produce repressor subunits ☐
- C. IP TG is inducer but not substrate ☐
- D. Regulator gene is inducible ☐

122. Lac operon transcription is induced by
- A. Glucose *(Delhi 03, UP 02, TN 01)* ☐
- B. Glucose with inducer ☐
- C. Inducer without glucose ☐
- D. All ☐

123. All of the following statements about Lambda phage are true, Except: *(AI 09)*
- A. In Lysogenic phase it fuses with host chromosome and remains dormant ☐
- B. In Lytic phase it fuses with host chromosome and replicates ☐
- C. Both Lytic and lysogenic phases occur together ☐
- D. In Lytic it causes cell lysis and releases virus particles ☐

124. In conversion of DNA to RNA, enzyme required:
- A. DNA- Polymerase I *(PGI 08)* ☐
- B. DNA Ligase ☐
- C. DNA-Polymerase III ☐
- D. RNA polymerase ☐
- E. Primase ☐

Transcription

125. The sigma (σ) subunit of prokaryotic RNA polymerase:
- A. Binds the antibiotic rifampicin *(AI 06)* ☐
- B. Is inhibited by α-amanitin ☐
- C. Specifically recognizes the promoter site ☐
- D. Is part of the core enzyme ☐

126. The atachment site of DNA dependent RNA polymerase to a gene is the - (PGI 05; UP 03)
- A. Operator ☐
- B. Promoter ☐
- C. Structural gene ☐
- D. Regulatory gene ☐
- E. Repressor ☐

127. RNA polymerase does not require : *(AI 04)*
- A. Template (ds DNA) ☐
- B. Activated precursors (ATP, GTP, UTP, CTP) ☐
- C. Divalent metal ions (Mn2+, Mg2+) ☐
- D. Primer ☐

128. R-RNA is mainly produced in - *(AIIMS 13, 06)*
- A. Nucleus ☐
- B. Nucleolus ☐
- C. Ribosome ☐
- D. Endoplasmic reticulum ☐

129. Part of eukaryotic DNA contributing to polypetide synthesis: *(PGI 15, 11)*
A. Exon
B. Enhancer
C. Leader sequence
D. tRNA
E. ncRNA

130. Not true about eukaryotic gene: *(PGI 14, 11)*
A. Polycistronic mRNA
B. Noncoding intron
C. Contain nuclear gene & pseudogene
D. Modification of mRNA before transportation from nucleus
E. Noncoding exons

131. The following is a generalized diagram of a typical eukaryotic gene: *(AIIMS 06)*

Promoter Region | Polypeptide Coding Region
INTRON
Direction of transcription

What is the most likely effect of a 2bp insertion in the middle of the intron?
A. Normal transcription, altered translation
B. Defective termination of transcription, normal translation
C. Normal transcription, defective mRNA splicing
D. Normal transcription, normal translation.

132. Part of M-RNA removed during protein synthesis -
A. Interon *(AI 01, MP 05, WB 06)*
B. Codon
C. Exon
D. Suistron

133. Function of endonucleases - *(Kerala 08, TN 07)*
A. Cut DNA at specific DNA sequences
B. To point out the coding regions
C. Enhancers
D. To find out antibiotic resistance

134. Replication and transcription are similar processes in mechanistic terms because both : *(AIIMS 03)*
A. Use RNA primers for initiation.
B. Use deoxyribonucleotides as precursors.
C. Are semi conserved events
D. Involve phosphodiester bond formation with elongation occurring in the 5' - 3' direction.

135. In a DNA the coding region reads 5'-CGT-3'. This would code in the RNA as: *(AIIMS 14, 02)*
A. 5'-CGU-3'
B. 5'GCA-3'
C. 5'-ACG-3'
D. 5'-UGC-3'

136. True about eukaryotic initiation is A/E *(AIIMS 10)*
A. Initiator sequence spans TSS (+1)
B. Distal regulatory element (DRE) is exclusively found in eukaryotes
C. Different σ subunits are responsible for recognition specificity
D. Trans acting factors bind to CAAT/GC box– promoter proximal element.

137. TATA box is seen in- *(NBE P 15, 13)*
A. Promoter region
B. Palindromic region
C. Enhancer region
D. Silencer region

138. A young boy who has difficulty in getting up from sitting position was diagnosed to have Duchene's muscular dystrophy. Which one is true regarding the mutation in the dystrophin gene in promoter region:
A. Initiation of transcription of the dystrophin gene would be affected *(AIIMS 10)*
B. Capping of mRNA of dystrophin gene would be affected
C. Tailing of mRNA of dystrophin gene would be affected
D. Premature termination

139. Non coding RNAs are: *(PGI 15,12, 10)*
A. siRNA
B. miRNA
C. tRNA
D. mRNA
E. rRNA

140. Not product of transcription: *(PGI 14,11)*
A. tRNA
B. mRNA
C. rRNA
D. cDNA
E. New strand of DNA

141. Gene transmitted but not translated: *(AIIMS 04,14)*
A. Glycosyl transferase
B. t-RNA
C. Keratin
D. Histone

142. Which of the following statements regarding mature cytoplsmic messenger RNA is true *(NBE P 14, AI 12)*
A. Transcribed from Nuclear DNA
B. Has Thiamine in place of Uracil
C. Sugar is DeoxyRibose
D. Its molecular weight is more than hn-RNA

143. Nobel prize in 2006 (recently) was given for the discovery of *(AIIMS 09)*
A. Lipoxins
B. RNAI
C. mt DNA
D. β-transcription factor

144. Micro RNA transcribed by: *(PGI 15, 08)*
A. RNA polymerase I
B. RNA polymerase II
C. RNA polymerase III
D. DNA polymerase
E. Drosha

145. Normal role of Micro RNA is: *(AI 09)*
A. Gene Regulation

B. RNA splicing ☐
C. Initiation of Translation ☐
D. DNA conformational change ☐

146. Poly(A) tail translates into (i.e. on translation give rise to): *(AIIMS 11, 08)*
A. Polyproline ☐
B. Polylysine ☐
C. Polyalanine ☐
D. Polyglycine ☐

147. Some mRNA has self splicing activity. The removal of introns is/are done by: *(PGI 11)*
A. Occur in intron that form Ribozyme ☐
B. Spliceosome ☐
C. Self-splicing introns ☐
D. sn RNA ☐
E. Lariats intermediates are formed

148. Introns are exised by *(PGI 05)*
A. RNA splicing ☐
B. RNA editing ☐
C. Restriction endonuclease ☐
D. DNAase ☐
E. Helicase ☐

149. A segment of a eukaryotic gene that is not represented in the mature messenger RNA is known as: *(AI 04)*
A. Intron ☐
B. Exon ☐
C. Plasmid ☐
D. TATA box ☐

150. Splicing Activity is a function of:
A. mRNA *(AI 10, AIIMS 10)* ☐
B. sn RNA ☐
C. r RNA ☐
D. t RNA ☐

151. Which is involve in processing of post-transcriptional modification of mRNA: *(PGI 11)*
A. Lariats formation ☐
B. Splicing ☐
C. Capping at 3'end ☐
D. Poly tail(A) formation at 5'end ☐
E. Methylation ☐

152. Some mRNA has self splicing activity. The removal of introns is/are done by: *(PGI 15,11)*
A. Occur in intron that form Ribozyme ☐
B. Spliceosome ☐
C. Self-splicing introns ☐
D. sn RNA ☐
E. Lariats intermediates are formed ☐

153. Cytoplasmic process during processing is
A. 5' capping *(SGPGI 05, CMC 03)* ☐
B. Poly (A) tailing ☐
C. Methylation of tRNA ☐
D. Attachment of CCA in tRNA. ☐

154. All are processing reactions in t-RNA except *(TN-02)*
A. CCA tailing *(WB-03, Delhi- 04, UP-05)* ☐
B. Methylation of bases ☐
C. Poly (A) tailing ☐
D. Trimming of 5' end ☐

155. Least post translational modification occurs in
A. t-RNA *(CMC 08, Jipmer 09, WB-03)* ☐
B. Prokaryotic r- RNA ☐
C. Eukaryotic r – RNA ☐
D. Prokaryotic mRNA ☐

156. Which of the following is not a post transcriptional modification of RNA?
A. Splicing *(AI 03)* ☐
B. 5'capping ☐
C. 3' polyadenylation ☐
D. Glycosylation ☐

157. In RNA, gene during processing undergoes all, except
A. Chemical hydrolysis *(AIIMS 04)* ☐
B. Terminal addition ☐
C. Nucleoside *modification* ☐
D. Nucleoside cleavage ☐

158. APO B48 & APO B100 is synthesized from the same mRNA; the difference between them is due to:
A. RNA splicing *(AIIMS 11)* ☐
B. Allelic exclusion ☐
C. Deamination of cytidine to uridine ☐
D. Upstream repression ☐

159. Post transcriptional modification includes: *(PGI 13)*
A. All RNA undergo post transcriptional modification ☐
B. Capping of the pre-m RNA Involves the addition of 7-methylguanosine to the 5'end ☐
C. Poly A tailing occur at 3'end ☐
D. Intron excision by spliceosome ☐
E. Primarily occur in cytoplasm ☐

160. True about ribozymes is: *(AIIMS 15, 12)*
A. Cut DNA at specific site ☐
B. GTPase activity ☐
C. Peptidyl transferase activity ☐
D. Participate in DNA synthesis ☐

161. True about ribozymes are A/E *(PGI 12, DNB 11)*
A. Catalytic activity ☐
B. Involved in transesterification ☐
C. Hammerhead metallo enzyme ☐
D. Peptidyl transferase ☐
E. Deamination ☐

162. Acitomycin D interferes with enzyme induction by combining with - *(UPSC 03, AIIMS 04, AI 08)*
A. TRNA ☐
B. DNA ☐
C. R-RNA ☐
D. Repressor protein ☐
E. Negative feedback inhibition system ☐

163. Which of the following blocks DNA replication with getting incorporated in DNA strand: *(PGI 07)*
A. Cytarabine ☐
B. Nalidixic acid ☐
C. Ciprofloxacin ☐
D. Paclitaxel ☐

164. Transcripton is inhibited by: *(PGI 06)*
A. Actinomycin D ☐
B. Amanitin ☐
C. Chloramphenicol ☐
D. Streptomycin ☐
E. Puromycin ☐

165. Inhibitors of DNA synthesis - *(DNB 03, Bihar 08)*
A. Penicillin ☐
B. Polymyxin ☐
C. Chloramphenicol ☐
D. Actinomycin ☐

166. hn RNA seen in : *(AI 07)*
A. Spinal muscular dystrophy ☐
B. Sickle cell disease ☐
C. Hutchinson chorea ☐
D. αThallasemia ☐

167. An enzyme that makes a double stranded DNA copy from a single stranded RNA template molecule is known as:
A. DNA polymerase *(AI 04)* ☐
B. RNA polymerase ☐
C. Reverse transcriptase ☐
D. Phosphokinase ☐

168. True about reverse transcriptase: *(PGI 03)*
A. Forms DNA from RNA ☐
B. Forms RNA from DNA ☐
C. Important for replication of HIV ☐
D. Amplification of DNA ☐
E. DNA dependent RNA polymerase ☐

169. Which of the following require template for it's formation:
A. Carbohydrate *(PGI 01)* ☐
B. Protein ☐
C. Lipid ☐
D. Nucleic acid ☐
E. Phospholipid ☐

170. The anticodon region is an *important* part of the
A. r-RNA *(Kerala 2K, KA 02, AP 03)* ☐
B. m-RNa ☐
C. t-RNa ☐
D. hn-RNa ☐

171. In transcription anticodon is seen in - *(DNB 15,13)*
A. t-RNA ☐
B. m-RNA ☐
C. r-RNA ☐
D. DNA ☐

172. About t-RNA, TRUE is: *(AIIMS 03)*
A. No intrabasal pairing ☐
B. Clover leaf pattern ☐
C. Inverted T appearance ☐
D. Each specific for one m-RNA ☐

173. Which type of RNA has the highest percentage of modified base (modified nucleotides)? OR Which of the following RNA has abnormal purine bases
A. mRNA *(NBE P 15,13; AI 10; AIIMS 14)* ☐
B. tRNA ☐
C. rRNA ☐
D. snRNA ☐

174. Thymidylated RNA present in: *(PGI 11)*
A. mRNA ☐
B. rRNA ☐
C. tRNA ☐
D. 16-s-RNA ☐

Translation (Protein Synthesis)

175. Synthesis of r RNA takes place in- *(NBE P 15,13)*
A. Cytosol *(AIIMS 14)* ☐
B. Nucleus ☐
C. Nucleolus ☐
D. Mitochondria ☐

176. The cellular component for protein synthesis is OR Translation occurs in: *(AI 03, 04)*
A. Ribosomes ☐
B. Mitochondria ☐
C. Nucleus ☐
D. Cytoplasm ☐

177. Aminoacyl t-RNA is not require for- *(NBE P 15)*
A. Proline ☐
B. Lysine ☐
C. Hydroxylysine ☐
D. Methionine ☐

178. True regarding aminoacyl t-RNA synthetase is A/E
A. Isoaccepting t RNA *(SGPGI 06)* ☐
B. Implement genetic code ☐
C. Attachment of amino group to 5′ end ☐
D. Editing function ☐

179. Which enzyme involved in translation is often referred to as 'Fidelity enzyme'; OR Fidelity of protein translation depends on; OR In translation process, proof reading of tRNA is done by: *(NBE P 15,14,13)*
A. DNA polymerase *(AIIMS 15,12, PGI 13)* ☐
B. RNA polymerase ☐
C. Amino acyl-t RNA synthetase ☐
D. Amino acyl-reductase ☐

180. Polypetide chain termination is enhanced by:
A. Stop codon *(PGI 01)* ☐
B. Promoter ☐
C. Ribosomal unit ☐
D. Pepitdyl transferase ☐
E. UAA ☐

181. The hydrolytic step leading to release of polypeptide chain from ribosomes in catalysed by: *(PGI 02)*
A. Stop codons ☐
B. Pepitidyl transferase ☐
C. Release factors ☐
D. AUG codon ☐
E. Dissociation of ribosomes ☐

182. About peptidyl transferase true is *(Jipmer 02)*
A. Used in elongation & cause attachment of peptide chain to A-site of t RNA *(PGI 08)* ☐
B. Used in elongation & cause attachment of peptide chain to P site ☐
C. Used in initiation and cause 43S complex formation ☐
D. Used in initiation & cause 48S complex formation ☐

183. Termination is caused by all except *(AIIMS 06)*
A. RF-1 ☐
B. UAA ☐
C. Peptidyl transferase ☐
D. 48 S complex ☐

184. Ribosome has following enzymatic activity?
A. Peptidyl transferase (AIIMS 08) ☐
B. Peptidase ☐
C. Aminoacyl tRNA synthetase ☐
D. GTPase ☐

185. For 1 peptide bond formation how many high energy phosphate bonds are required: (PGI 07)
A. 0 ☐
B. 1 ☐
C. 2 ☐
D. 3 ☐
E. 4 ☐

186. Which group of amino acid is responsible for peptide bond: (PGI 13)
A. Amino group ☐
B. Carboxyl group ☐
C. Side chain ☐
D. Aldehyde group ☐
E. Amide group ☐

187. Termination process of protein synthesis is performed by: (PGI 10)
A. Releasing factor ☐
B. Stop codon ☐
C. Peptidyl transferase ☐
D. UAA codon ☐
E. AUG codon ☐

188. Which of the following is not required for protein synthesis (in translation) of eukaryotes: (AIIMS 11)
A. RNA polymerase ☐
B. Ribosomes ☐
C. Peptidyl transferase ☐
D. Amino acyl tRNA synthetase ☐

189. Amber codon refers to (AIIMS 01)
A. Mutant codon ☐
B. Stop codon ☐
C. Initiating codon ☐
D. Codon for more than one amino acids ☐

190. Shine-Dalgarno sequence in bacterial mRNA is near:
A. AUG codon (AI 04) ☐
B. UAA codon ☐
C. UAG codon ☐
D. UGA codon ☐

191. tRNA$_f$ met would recognize: (PGI 09)
A. AUG ☐
B. UGC ☐
C. GUG ☐
D. GCU ☐
E. UUG ☐

192. False about eukaryotic protein synthesis is:
A. N formyl Met is the first–RNA to come into action ☐
B. mRNA read from 5′ to 3′ (AIIMS 09) ☐
C. Ef2 shift between GDP to GTP ☐
D. Capping helps in attachment of mRNA to 40 S ribosome ☐

193. Ragarding Cytosolic Eukaryotic gene expression false is: (AI 07)
A. Capping helps in attachment of mRNA to 40 S Ribosome ☐
B. N formyl methionine tRNA will be the first t – RNA to come into action ☐
C. EF2 shifts between GDP & GTP ☐
D. Releasing factor releases the polypeptide chain from the P site. ☐

194. True about translation of protein is (PGI 08)
A. It has 3 steps initiation, elongation & termination ☐
B. IF-2 prevent reassociation of ribosomal subunit ☐
C. IF-3 and 1A cause binding of initiating codon ☐
D. IF 2 has α and β units ☐

195. 43S preinitiation complex include all except:
A. IF3 (AIIMS 03) ☐
B. IF1A ☐
C. IF2β ☐
D. IF-4F ☐

196. IF4F include all except (PGI 05, JIPMER 09)
A. 4A ☐
B. 4G ☐
C. 4E ☐
D. 4S ☐

197. Which of the following does not undergo phosphorylation by protein kinases in Eukaryotes:
A. Threonine (AI 12) ☐
B. Tyrosine ☐
C. Serine ☐
D. Asparagine ☐

198. Component of 50s subunit is/are: (PGI 11)
A. 23s ☐
B. 28s ☐
C. 5s ☐
D. 5.8s ☐
E. 16s ☐

199. Components of 60 S subunit of ribosome are:
A. 5.8 S (PGI 09) ☐
B. 23 S ☐
C. 16 S ☐
D. 18 S ☐
E. 28 S ☐

200. True about ribosomes: (PGI 09)
A. Conserved in nature ☐
B. Role is to bring t-RNA and m-RNA together ☐
C. DNA forms RNA and rotein are formed from RNA ☐
D. They are always free ☐
E. Have two subunits ☐

201. Regarding ribosome all is true except
A. 16 S ribosome identifies shine- dalgarno sequence ☐
B. Cytosolic ribosomes synthesize proteins of peroxisome (Jipmer-04, CMC-05) ☐
C. Large subunit catalyzes peptide bond formation ☐
D. Binding of aminoacyl tRNA uses 2ATP ☐

202. Vitamin required for post translational modification of coagulants is : (AI 07)
A. Vitamin A ☐
B. Vitamin C ☐
C. Vitamin B6 ☐
D. Vitamin K ☐

Immunoglobin

203. Correct pair of Ig subclass with their heavy chain: *(PGI 10)*
A. IgM - α (alpha) ☐
B. IgG -γ (gamma) ☐
C. IgM - δ (delta) ☐
D. IgE- γ- (gamma) ☐
E. IgA -γ (gamma) ☐

204. Correct order of switching of Ig: *(PGI 10)*
A. IgM to IgG ☐
B. IgA to IgG ☐
C. IgM to IgA ☐
D. IgM to IgD ☐
E. IgE to IgG ☐

205. True about IgM *(PGI 10)*
A. Fix complement ☐
B. Increased in primary response ☐
C. Fab region is composed of variable region ☐
D. Fc is antibody –binding portion ☐

206. True about Ig gene rearrangement & Ig diversity: *(PGI 10)*
A. Somatic mutations theory ☐
B. One loop and two loop joining theory ☐
C. DNA rearrangement ☐
D. Appropriate class switching ☐

207. True about location of Ig chromosome: *(PGI 10)*
A. κ- 2 ☐
B. κ - 6 ☐
C. κ - 14 ☐
D. λ – 22 ☐
E. λ- 10 ☐

208. What factor is responsible for deciding whether an antibody will remain membrane bound or get secreted? OR Synthesis of an immunoglobulin in membrane bound or secretory form is determined by: *(AIIMS 14, 08; AI 11)*
A. RNA splicing ☐
B. Class switching ☐
C. Differential RNA regulation (processing) ☐
D. Allelic exclusion ☐

Intracellular traffic & Sorting

209. Secretory proteins are synthesized in: *(AIIMS 05)*
A. Cytoplasm ☐
B. Endoplasmic reticulum ☐
C. First in cytoplasm and then in Endoplasmic Reticulum ☐
D. First in Endoplasmic Reticulum and then in cytoplasm ☐

210. Signal peptides are synthesized in *(Jipmer 06, TN 05)*
A. ER ☐
B. Free ribosomes ☐
C. Membrane bound ribosomes ☐
D. Golgi body ☐

211. Elongation arrest occurs due to *(AP 05, KA 05, WB-06)*
A. SRP- R ☐
B. SRP ☐
C. Signal peptide ☐
D. Docking protein ☐

212. Sequence which is responsible for retaining proteins in membrane *(UP 05, AMU 06, Delhi 03)*
A. Translocon ☐
B. Sec 61 complex ☐
C. Docking protein ☐
D. Halt signal ☐

213. Not true among the following is *(PGI 05, TN 06)*
A. Sec 61 translocon complex form passage way ☐
B. SRP-R is docking protein ☐
C. SRP blocks elongation ☐
D. SRP-R releases elongation block ☐
E. SRP-R is ATP bound ☐

214. Which of the following groups of proteins assist in the folding of other proteins? *(NBE P 14; AI 08, 04)*
A. Proteases ☐
B. Proteosomes ☐
C. Templates ☐
D. Chaperones ☐

215. The primary role of chaperones is to help in: *(NBE P 13; AI 03)*
A. Protein synthesis ☐
B. Protein degradation ☐
C. Protein denaturation ☐
D. Protein folding ☐

216. Folding protein are: *(PGI 09)*
A. GLUT-1 ☐
B. Calnexin ☐
C. Cytochrome 450 ☐
D. Insulin receptor ☐
E. Protein disulfide isomerase ☐

217. All are true about chaperones except- *(NBE P 15)*
A. Cause folding of proteins ☐
B. Are lipid in nature ☐
C. May have ATPase activity ☐
D. Include heat shock proteins ☐

218. True statement about chaperones: *(PGI 15, 12)*
A. Belong to heat shock proteins ☐
B. Wide range of expression ☐
C. Present from bacteria to human ☐
D. Ubiquitin is the most important chaperones ☐
E. Also k/a stress proteins ☐

219. Proteins targeted for destruction in eukaryotes are covalently linked to: *(AI 04)*
A. Clathrin ☐
B. Pepsin ☐
C. Laminin ☐
D. Ubiquitin ☐

220. Proteins are sorted by : *(AI 08)*
A. Golgi Bodies ☐
B. Mitochondria ☐
C. Ribosomes ☐
D. Nuclear Membrane ☐

221. Not a disorder of protein misfoldig? *(AI 11)*
A. Alzheimer's disease ☐
B. Tuberculosis ☐
C. Cystic fibrosis ☐
D. CJD (Creutzfeld-Jakob disease) ☐

222. The secondary structure of prion particles is: (AIIMS 08)
A. Alfa helix
B. Beta bends
C. Beta sheets
D. Beta turns

223. Defect in folding of the protein result in which of the following clinical disease: (AIIMS 02)
A. Kuru
B. Migraine
C. Hypothyroidism
D. Myopia

224. If cellular proteins do not fold into a specific conformation, their function are affected. Certain disorders arise, if specific proteins are misfolded. Which of the following disorders arises due to conformational isomerization: (AIIMS 05)
A. Familial fatal insomnia
B. Hepatitis delta
C. Pernicious anemia
D. Lesch-Nyhan syndrome

Gene Duplication

225. Gene duplication plays an important role in the evolution of (AIIMS 11)
A. mRna
B. rRna
C. tRna
D. hn Rna

Mutation

226. Small scale mutations include all except: (AIIMS 12)
A. Substitution
B. Deletion
C. Paracentric inversion
D. Insertion

227. Base substitution of GAC (Asp) to GAG (Glu) is an example of: (PGI 11)
A. Point mutation
B. Silent mutation
C. Non-sense mutation
D. Conserved mutation
E. Non-conserved mutation

228. Which of these is a conservative mutator: (AIIMS 08)
A. Glutamic acid- glutamine
B. Histidine-glycine
C. Alanine- leucine
D. Arginine-aspartic acid

229. In sickle cell anaemia, the defect can be explained as having arisen from - (PGI 04, UP 02)
A. A base insertion in DNA
B. A base deletion in DNA
C. A base substitution in DNA
D. None of the above

230. Hbs has defect in aminoacid position- (DNB 14, 12)
A. 4
B. 6
C. 11
D. 12

231. One of the following mutation is potentially lethal - a) (Delhi 10)
A. Substitution of adenine for cytosine
B. Substitution of methylcytosine for cytosine
C. Substitution of guanine for cytocine
D. Insertion of one base

232. Sickle cell ancmia is the clinical manifestation of homozygous genes for an abnormal haemoglobin molecule. The event responsible for the mutation in the B chain is - (DNB 10)
A. Insertion
B. Deletion
C. Nondisjunction
D. Point mutation

233. Null mutation is : (AI 04)
A. Mutation occuring in Non Coding region.
B. Mutation that does not change the amino acid or end product
C. Mutation that codes for a change in progeny without any chromosomal change
D. Mutation that leads to no functional gene product

234. A mutation in the codon which causes a change in the coded amino acid, is known as: (AIIMS 02)
A. Mitogenesis
B. Somatic mutation
C. Missense mutation
D. Recombination

235. Somatic mutations involve: (PGI 02)
A. Deletion
B. Plasmid mediated
C. Frame-shift alteration in coding nucleotides
D. Trinucleotide repeat mutations
E. Non-sense alteration of DNA

236. Frame shift mutation does not effect complete amino acid sequence if it occurs in multiple of- (NBE P 15)
A. 1
B. 2
C. 3
D. None

237. Base substitution mutations can have be following molecular consequence except: (AI 06)
A. Changes one codon for an amino acid into another codon for that same amino acid
B. Codon for one amino acid is changed into a codon of another amino acid
C. Reading frame changes downstream to the mutant site
D. Codon for one amino acid is changed into a translation termination codon

238. Transition mutation of GATCCT is: (PGI 06)
A. GGTCCT
B. GTTCCT
C. GABCCT
D. GrUGGT
E. GTTUCT

239. Trinucleotie repeats are found in: *(PGI 09, 15)*
A. Huntington's disease ☐
B. Spinocerebellar ataxia ☐
C. Amyotropic latera sclerosis ☐

240. Which of the following is an example of trinucleotide repeat mutation- *(NBE P 15)*
A. Huntington's chorea ☐
B. Fragile-x-syndroem ☐
C. Friedreich ataxia ☐
D. All fo the above ☐

241. In a mutation if valine is replaced by which of the following would not result in any change in the function of protein:
A. Proline *(AIIMS 02)* ☐
B. Leucine ☐
C. Glycine ☐
D. Aspartic acid ☐

242. Which of the following can be a homologous substitution for valine in hemoglobin? *(AI 04)*
A. Isoleucine ☐
B. Glutamic acid ☐
C. Phenylalanine ☐
D. Lysine ☐

243. True about silent mutation in gene:
A. No change in mRNA *(PGI 09)* ☐
B. No change in Amino acid sequence in protein ☐
C. No expression of protein ☐
D. No change in expression of protein ☐
E. Termination of protein synthesis ☐

244. True about Sickle cell disease are all, Except:
A. Single nucleotide change results in change of Glutamine to Valine *(AIIMS 10)* ☐
B. Deoxygenated Hb l/t exposure of sticky end d/t replacement of nonpolar residue by polar residue ☐
C. HbS confers resistance against malaria in heterozygotes ☐
D. RFLP results from a single base change ☐

245. In sickle cell anemia replacement is: *(PGI 08)*
A. Valbglu in b6 ☐
B. Glu by val in b6 ☐
C. Hist val b8 ☐
D. 6A ☐

246. Sickling in 'HbS' disease is primarily caused by
A. Decreased Solubility *(AI 09)* ☐
B. Decreased Stability ☐
C. Altered function ☐
D. Altered O_2 binding capacity ☐

247. All of the following are true about Sickle cell disease, Except *(AI 09, AIIMS 11, 10)*
A. Single nucleotide change results in change of Glutamine to Valine ☐
B. RFLP results from a single base change ☐
C. 'Sticky patch' is generated as a result of replacement of a non polar residue with a polar residue ☐
D. HbS confers resistance against malaria in heterozygotes ☐

248. Technique (s) used to detect Gene Mutation is/are
A. RT-PCR *(PGI 12)* ☐
B. Denaturing gradient gel electrophoresis ☐
C. DNA sequencing ☐
D. Restriction fragment polymorphism (RFLP) ☐
E. Single-strand conformational polymorphism ☐

249. All the following can be used to detect mutation, except: *(AI 02)*
A. Single strand conformational polymorphism ☐
B. Ligase chain reaction ☐
C. Polymerase chain reaction ☐
D. DNA Sequencing ☐

ANSWERS & EXPLANATIONS:

Purines and Pyrimidines

1. **C i.e. Aspartate transcarbomoylase**

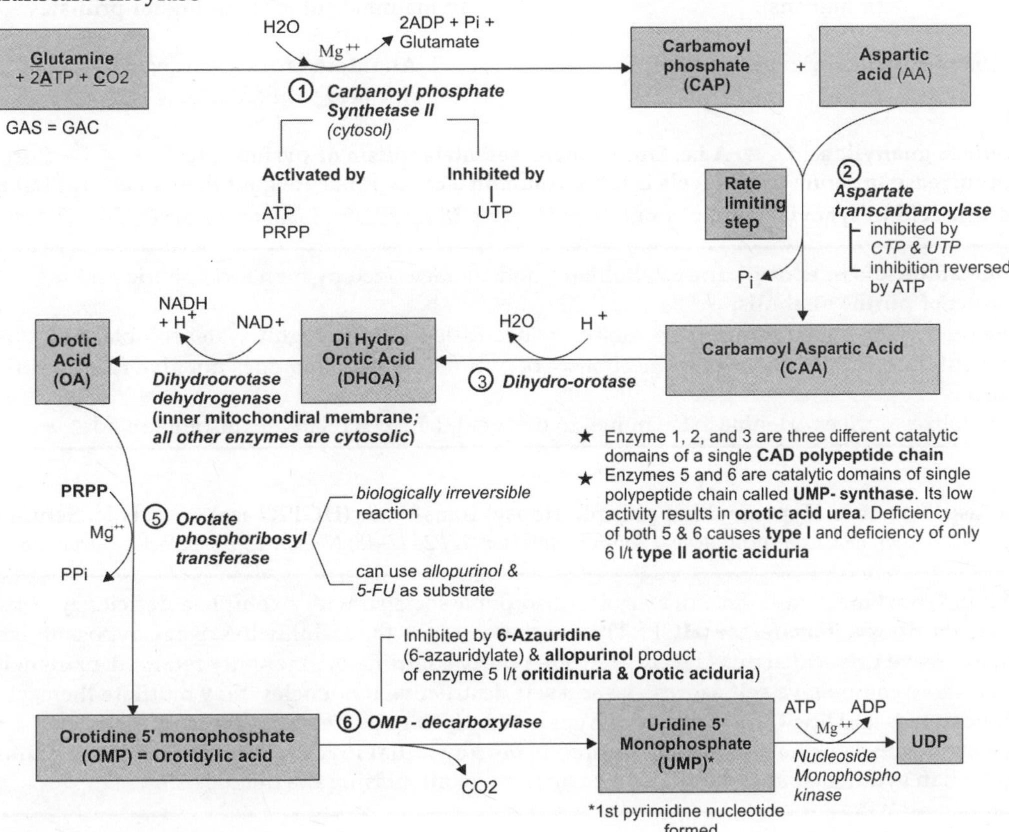

2. **D i.e. Reye syndrome decrease cytosolic carbamoyl phosphate**
3. **A i.e. N5 – N10 methylene tetrahydrofolate**

[Ref: Harper's 28/e P- 298; Chattergea 7/e p. 214-17; Lippincott 5/e p. 302-5; Lehninger 5/e p. 892-94]

- d-UMP (deoxy-uridine monophosphate) is converted to d-TMP (deoxy-thymidine monophosphate) **which uses N5, N10 – methylene tetra hydrofolate as a source of methyl group (1 carbon & 2 hydrogen)Q.)**. This is an unusual reaction in that THF (tetrahydrofolate) contributes not only 1 carbon unit but also 2 hydrogen atoms from pteridine ring, which causes oxidation of THF to DHF. Disorders of **folate & vitamin** B_{12} metabolism cause deficiency of TMP.
- Thymine analog, antitumor drug **5-flurouracil (5Fu)** is converted to 5-F dUMP, which becomes **permanently bound to the inactive thymidylate synthaseQ**. So 5FU is a **suicide inhibitor. Methotrexate (Mtx) and antibacterial trimethoprim inhibits dihydrofolate reductase, an enzyme which reduces DHF to THFQ.**

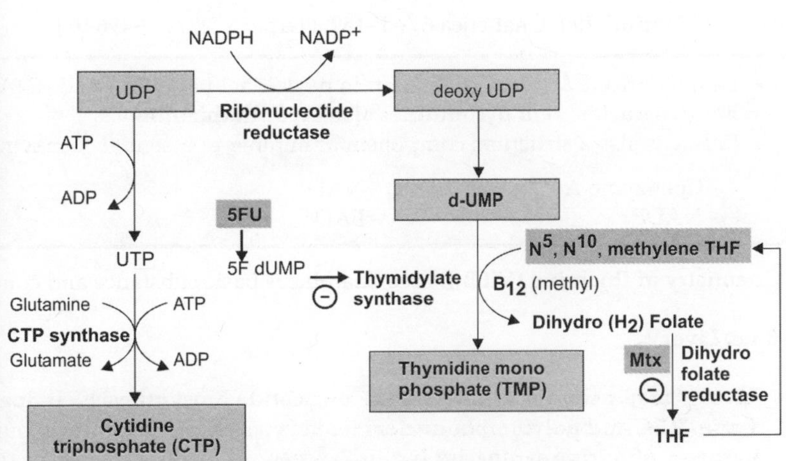

4. **D i.e. Allantoin** 5. **B i.e. Uric acid**

End product of catabolism of purine (adenosine & guanosine) nucleotides

- **In humans**
  - **Uric acid**Q (lack uricase enzyme)
- **In mammals other than higher primates**
  - **Allantoin**Q (uricase converts uric acid to allantoin)

6. **C i.e., Adenylic & guanylic acid** 7. **A i.e. Due to increased metabolism of pyrimidines** 8. **A i.e. Purine metabolism**
9. **A i.e. Abrupt increase in serum urate levels is more common a cause for acute gout than an abrupt fall in urate levels**
10. **B i.e. Raised uric acid in synovial fluid of joint** *[Ref: Harper's 28/e p.292-99; Lippincott's 5/e P-294-302; Harrison 16/e P 2046]*

- **Gout** is a **metabolic disorder of purine catabolism**Q, and characterized by high level of uric acid in the blood . **Uric acid is end product of purine catabolism**Q
- **Pyrimidine nucleotide** unlike purine rings can be opened & degraded to highly water soluble structure like, β- alanine, β- amino isobutyrate, NH_3 & CO_2. Excess meabolism of pyrimidine therefore **does not give rise to clinical manifestation**Q
- Human catabolizes purine (Adenine & Guamine) to uric acid, which is relatively insoluble acid.

11. **A i.e. HGPRTase** 12. **A ie. Hypoxanthine phosphoribosyl transferase (HGPRTase)** 13. **D ie. Serum Uric Acid Levels** *[Ref: Lehninger 5/e p. 893, 882; Lippincott 4th/e p 296-97; Harrison 17/ 2447-48; Nelson 18/e p-629-30; Harper 28th/ed pg- 298-99]*

Lesch – Nyhan syndrome is an X- linked, recessive disorder associated with a **complete deficiency of hypoxanthine guanine phosphoribosyl transferase (HGPRT)**Q and therefore has the inability to salvage hypoxanthine or guanine, from which excessive uric acid are produced. They are **poorly coordinated, mentally retarded, extremely hostile male children** who show **compulsive self aggressive and self destructive tendencies; they mutilate themselves by biting off their fingers, toes and lips**Q. The features of **hyper ureamia & gout** are also presented.
Uric acid (urate) levels in urine and plasma (serum) is the key initial investigation in purine metabolism disorder (like Lesch Nyhan syndrome) and should be measured to avoid missing the diagnosisQ.

14. **A i.e.Purine synthesis** [Ref: Harper's 27/e P-301]

All forms of life (except protozoa) synthesize purine and pyrimidine nucleotides

15. **D i.e. Thiamine** [Ref: Chatterjea 6/e P-159; Harper's 27/e P-496-97]

- Usually purine & pyrimidine occur in nucleic acid i.e. DNA and RNA
- **Besides nucleic acid pyrimidines also occur in thiamine**Q
- Purine is also a structural component of number of essential coenzyme:

- Coenzyme A	- NAD^+
- $NADP^+$	- FAD^+

Chemistry of thiamine (Vit B_1): Free thiamine is basic substance and contains: a) **Pyrimidine**Q; b) Thiazole ring; c) Sulphur

16. **B i.e. Liver**

- **Liver is major site for denovo purine nucleotide biosynthesis**Q**. It does not use salvage pathway**Q.
- **Brain, RBC and polymorphonuclear leukocytes** can not synthesize purine by denovo pathway. So they **use salvage pathway of purine synthesis**Q (i.e. use exogenous purines formed by degradation of purines synthesized in liver).

DNA Structure

17. **A i.e. All nucleotides are involved in linkage; B i.e. Antiparallel; D i.e. Bases perpendicular to DNA**
18. **E i.e. A single strand of DNA** 19. **D i.e. Uracil** 20. **B i.e. Hydrogen bond**
21. **C i.e. Deoxyribose-phosphate backbone with bases stacked inside** 22. **C i.e. B**
[Ref: Harper 28/ed 289-90, 302-304; Chattarjae 7/e 225-27; Lippincott 5/e 396-98; Lehninger 5/e 277-82]

The most common form of DNA is B- DNA[Q]. Within the cells most of DNA is B –DNA, although regions rich in guanine and cytosine base pairs may assume Z- conformation.

23. **A i.e. Hoogsteen pairing** *[Ref: Harrison 17th /1764; Harrison's 18th/2312]*

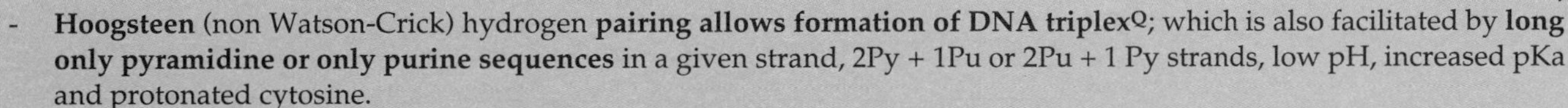

- **Hoogsteen** (non Watson-Crick) hydrogen **pairing allows formation of DNA triplex**[Q]; which is also facilitated by **long only pyramidine or only purine sequences** in a given strand, 2Py + 1Pu or 2Pu + 1 Py strands, low pH, increased pKa and protonated cytosine.
- **DNA helix bends** whenever **≥4 adenosine (A) residues** appear sequentially in row in one strand (6 A produce 18° bend). **Hairpins or cruciform (cross shaped) structures** are formed when **self complementary palindromic sequence (of DNA or RNA) form intrastrand base pairing** in single or both strands respectively. **Four stranded DNA (tetraplex or quadruplex)** occurs only for DNA sequences with **very high proportion of guanosine residue** (or very stable **guanosine /G tetraplex**).

24. **A i.e. A+G = T+C** 25. **D i.e. Double stranded DNA**
26. **D i.e. 27%** *[Ref: Lehninger 5/e p. 278; Lippincott 6/e p. 291, 397; Satyanarayan 3/ e p. 73]*

Chargaff's Rules for Double stranded (ds) DNA

- In all cellular DNAs, regardless of species-
  - number of **adenosine residues is equal to number of thyrmidine residues** (i.e. **A=T**)
  - number of **guanosine residues is equal to the number of cytidine residues (G ≡ C)**
- From these relationships it follows that sum of **purine residues equals the sum of pyrimidine residues;**
  - $A + G = T + C$
  - Ratio of purine to pyrimidine is always around 1
  - $\frac{A+G}{T+C} = \sim 1$

- The base composition of DNA generally varies from one species to another
- DNA specimens isolated from different tissues of same species have the same base composition
- The base composition of DNA in a given species does not change with an organism's age, nutritional state or changing environment.

Because in DNA, A=T and G=C; and A is 23%. So thymine (T) will also be = 23%. This makes 46% (23+23). The remaining 54% of DNA will be guanine (G) and cytosine (C). But because the amount of G is equal to C each G & C will be 54/2 =27%.

27. **B i.e. C- G** 28. **B i.e. G ≡ C** *[Ref: Harper's 27/e P-311]*

Thermostability in DNA is contributed mostly by C ≡ G[Q] because there are **3 Hydrogen bonds between C & G**[Q]. G ≡ C bonds are much more resistant to denaturation or melting than A= T rich region (2 Hydrogen bonds)

29. **B i.e. 5CUUAAG3** 30. **A i.e. 5'GTACG CTTAA'3'** *[Ref: Harper 29/e p-343-46; Lippincott 5/e p 396-98]*

- **Complementary DNA sequence of 5' TTAAGCTAC3' is 3'AATTCGCATG5' or 5'GTACGCTTAA3'.**
- **Complementry RNA sequence of 5CTTAAG3** template strand of DNA is **3GAAUUC5 or 5CUUAAG3**

Base Pairing Rule And Complementary Sequence

- **Cytosine (C) is always paired with guanine (G)** in both DNA & RNA.
- **Adenine (A) is always paired with Thiamine (T) in DNA and Uracil (U) in RNA** (ie DNA-RNA hybrid)

C ≡ G
A = T (in DNA) / **U** (in RNA-DNA hybrid)

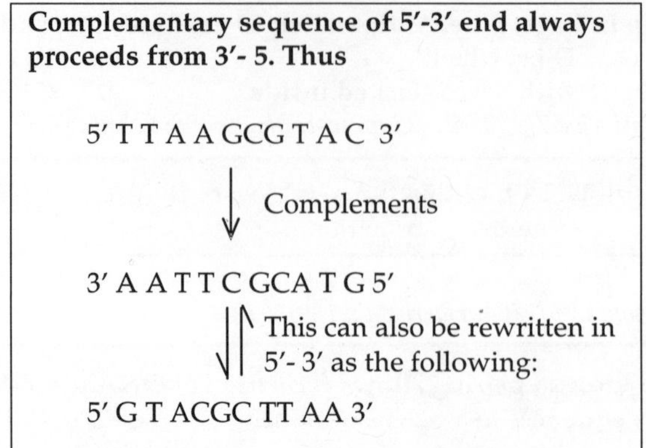

5′CTTAAG3′
↓ Complements
3′GAATTC5′ (in DNA) or
3′ GAAUUC 5′ (in RNA)
↓ Can be rewritten as
5′CTTAAG (in DNA)
5′CUUAAG (in RNA hybrid)

31. **C i.e. Runs at 5′- 3′ direction** *[Ref: Harper's 27/e P-348-350]*
32. **D i.e. Matches with RNA transcript that encodes protein.**

In double stranded DNA the 2 strands are

Template strand
- The strand that is copied into RNA molecule
- The information of this strand is **read in 3′ → 5′ direction**Q.
- The template strand for each gene will not necessarily be the same strand of DNA double helix.

Coding strand
- The other strand (other than Template) is coding strand because it **matches the RNA transcript that encodes protein**Q
- The **information is read in 5′ → 3′ direction**Q

Minus strandQ:
- Is synthesized from RNA
- Acts as a template for synthesis of *plus strand*
- Most retroviral recombination occur during minus strand synthesis.

Thus plus & Minus strands are met with replication of retrovirus.

33. **E i.e. 5′- GUACGUAA**-3′ *[Ref: Lippincott 4th/ed p. 419, 430]*

- The **template strand** (5′-TTACGTAC-3′) is **read in 3′-5′** direction and **RNA product** after transcription has sequence that is complementary to the sequence of template strand but **Thymine (T) is replaced by Uracil (U)** in RNA.
- The **coding strand** of DNA is complementry to its template strand. So it matches the RNA transcript except that *T is replaced by U*. The information is read in 5′→3′ direction. So

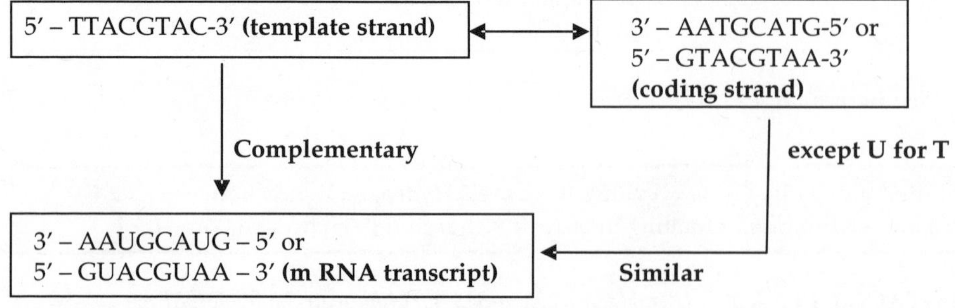

34. **D i.e. Thymidine** *[Ref: NMS 3/e P-222; Harper's 27/e P-298-99]*

Bromodeoxyuridine is a thymidine analogueQ
As in DNA thymine is present instead of uracil, bromodeoxy uridine (5 halogenated derivative of uracil) is analogus to Thymidine of DNA.

35. **B i.e. Negatively Charged** *[Ref: Ronald Hofman hematology 2/e P-2202]*

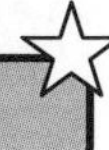

DNA molecules are ***negatively charged***[Q], this is evident as it is stained by *a cationic dye (Methylene blue).*

36. **A i.e. Maternal inheritance; C i.e. Not highly conserved & has high mutation rate; D i.e. Mitochondrial disease is ..**
37. **A, B, D, E i.e. UGA codes for tryptophan, Codes for 13 protein, Circular double stranded DNA, Mitrochondrial disease occur due to Point Mutations and Large-Scale Rearrangements**
38. **B i.e. Mitochondrial DNA** 39. **C i.e. Mitochondrial disease** 40. **B i.e. Maternally inherited**
41. **A i.e. Closed Circular** *[Ref: Lehninger 5th/ed pg-738-42; Harper 28th/ed pg-319-20; Robbin's 7/e p. 185; Teitz 6th/ed pg-269; Eberhard: Colour atlas of genetics 3/ed pg-134; Acta Neuropathol (2006) 111: pg-610-16]*

- **Mitochondrial DNA (mt DNA)** is a ***closed circular double stranded***[Q] molecule that is ***transmitted by maternal inheritance***[Q] and ***contains no or very few interons (untranslated sequences)***[Q]. It is ***not highly conserved has high mutation rate (d/t point mutation, large scale rearrangements & some deletions) and leads to mitochondrial myopathies, MELAS, Leber's hereditary optic atrophy, Leigh syndrome and NARP syndrome***[Q].
- Mt DNA has **37 genes** encoding. 2mt rRNAs, 22 mt tRNAs and **13 proteins**; with a slightly different genetic code i.e. **UGA** is **tryptophan** (not stop codon), **AUA** is **methionine** (not isoleucine) and **AGA/AGG** are **stop codons** (not arginine).

42. **A i.e. Virus; B i.e. Chloroplast; C i.e. Bacteria; D i.e. Mitochondria** *[Ref: Greewood 16/e p 10-11; Ananthanarayana 8/e p 10-13; Jawetz 25/e p 2-4- 97- 100]*

- **Circular DNA** is found in **viruses** (eg polyoma virus has double stranded & porcine virus has single stranded circular genome), **prokaryotes (most bacterial DNA is circular), blue green** algae as well as in eukaryotic cells like **mitochondrial DNA or plasmid DNA and in chloroplast.**

- A distinguishing characteristic of prokaryotes is their capacity to exchange small packets of genetic information carried on **plasmids**. Plasmid are **small, specialized genetic element** that are capable of replication within at least one cell line or exhibit broad hoast range and may carry sets of specialized genetic information (eg drug resistance) through a population. Plasmids were identified as small genetic elements carrying genes and *capable of independent replication in prokaryotes (bacteria & yeast)*. Unlike viruses, plasmids are naked DNA and donot carry genes necessary to encase genetic material for transfer to new host. Sometimes plasmids may be found in eukaryotes like saccharomyces cerevisiae). In genetic engineering, plasmid is a small genetic (DNA) element that is *separate from and can replicate independently of the chromosoml DNA. So introduction of DNA restriction fragment into a plasmid allows the fragment to be amplified many times.*

43. **D i.e. 30,000** 44. **A i.e. DNA** *[Ref: Harper's 28/e P-316-18; Lehninger 5/e p. 950]*

Hereditary information is preserved in DNA. ***Thus all genetic diseases are due to change in DNA***[Q].

45. **C i.e. Telomere; D i.e. Centromere; B ie. Microsatelite DNA** *[Ref: Harper 28/e 315-19; Lipincott 5/e 475; Lehninger 952-53]*

Highly repetitive sequences also called **simple sequence DNA** or **simple sequence repeats (SSR)** or **satellite DNA** is mostly clustered in ***centromeres and telomeres***[Q].

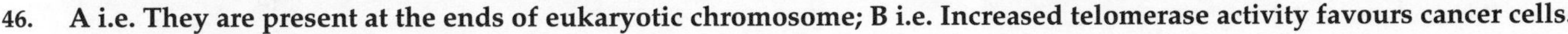

46. **A i.e. They are present at the ends of eukaryotic chromosome; B i.e. Increased telomerase activity favours cancer cells.**
47. **B i.e. Longetivity of cell- aging**
48. **A i.e. Telomerase** 49. **C i.e. Telomerase** 50. **B i.e. Somatic**
[Ref: Lehninger 5/e 1053-55, 953; Harper 28/e 315-19; Robbins 7/e p 308-9; Lippincott 5/e 408-7; Ganong 22/e p 20]

Telomerase is a multisubunit RNA containing complex related to **viral RNA- dependent DNA polymerase (reverse transcriptase)**, the enzyme which is **responsible for telomere synthesis & thus for maintaining the length of telomere**[Q]. **Telomerase, a RNA dependent DNA polymerase (reverse transcriptase)**, is the **enzyme responsible for telomere synthesis and thus for maintaining the length of telomere**[Q]. **Germinal (germ line), cancer and hemopoetic stem cells**[Q] with telomerase activity do not under go **cellular aging and apoptosis (death).** Whereas, **somatic cells** without telomerase activity undergo cellular aging and death after 40-60 replication cycles d/t critical shortening of telomere.

51. **B i.e. Present inside the nucleus; D i.e. Basic** 52. **B i.e. Increased Euchromatin formation**
53. **A i.e. DNA; E i.e. Histones** 54. **A i.e. Histone** 55. **D i.e. Glycosylation**
56. **A i.e. Uncondensed** 57. **A, B i.e. Histone, DNA** 58. **C i.e. Regular repeating structure of DNA & histone..**
[Ref: Chatterjea 8/ p 83, 240; Harper 28/ed 312-13; Lehninger 5/e 963-66; Lippincott 5/e 409-11, 422; Satyanarayan 3/e p 79; Vasudevan 6/e 471-72]

- **Histones** are small ***basic proteins rich in basic aminoacid arginine & histidine with alkaline isoelectric pH. It is a simple protein***[Q] ie its complete hydrolysis only yields amino acids. They are soluble in water, salt solution & dilute acids but not in ammonia and do not easily coagulate on heating. Histones are ***synthesized in cytoplasm and migrate to nucleus to form conjugated nucleoprotein (chromatin) with nucleic acid (DNA)***[Q]. Histones act as repressor of template activity of DNA in RNA synthesis. Histones also conjugate with porphyrins. Globin, the protein part of hemoglobin is an atypical histone and it has *predominance of histidine & lysine instead of arginine.*
- **Nucleosome**, the *fundamental organizational units of chromatin (chromosome)*, consists of regular repeating **"beads on a string"** arrangement in which **histone octamer** i.e. $(H_3-H_4)_2-(H_2A-H_2B)_2$ forms the **core (bead)** around which *146 base pair double stranded DNA is wrapped* and **30 bp/54 bp linker DNA and H_1 histone protein** forms **string**.
- **Histone acetylation (by histone acetyl transferase = HAT)** causes ***increased (trancriptionally active) relatively uncondensed euchromatin formation***[Q]. Acetylation or phosphorylation of lysine residue at aminoterminal **decreases positive (+) charge of basic histone protein**, there by decreasing their association with negatively (-) charged DNA, thus releasing nucleosomes and allowing access to DNA. **Histone deacetylation (by histone deacetylase = HDAC)** removes acetyl group, restores positive charge and causes **increased formation of transcriptionally inactive hetero chromatin (relatively condensed).**
- Histone is post translationally modified by **ribosylation, ubiquitin binding, phosphorylation, acetylation and methylation (RUPAM).**

59. **B i.e. Methylation** *[Ref: Harper 30/e p. 735; Lippincott 6/e p. 409,460; MTx]*

- **Microsatellite Repeat Sequences (MiRS)** of 2-6 base pairs eg AC, **CG**, CA & AT produce **heritable polymorphism** and are used in **constructing genetic linkage map.** (See Tx of Highly repetitive sequences).

Epigenetic Modifications

Are **non mutational changes** to histone proteins & DNA that **influence gene expression.** These include

1. **Post- translational modifications of histone such as acetylation, methylation, phosporylation & ubiquitylation.**
2. **Methylation/demethylation of cytosine residue (nest to guanine) in CG islands of DNA**[Q].

- **One X chromosome in females is condensed and inactivated to prevent overexpression of X linked genes. This X inactivation occurs by hypermethylation of cytosine in CG islands and deacetylation of histone proteins.**
- **Methylation/ demethylation of cytosine (in CG island)** and **acetylation of histone H3 & H4** have been found in **cancer cells. Methylation of C (by methyl transferase) turns off gene**[Q].
- Many epigenetic changes are **reversible. 5′ Azadeoxycytidine** is an **inhibitor of methyl transferase** and **SAHA (Suberoyl anilide hydroxamic acid/Vorinostat) deacytylate histones.** So both agents are used in leukemias & lymphomas.

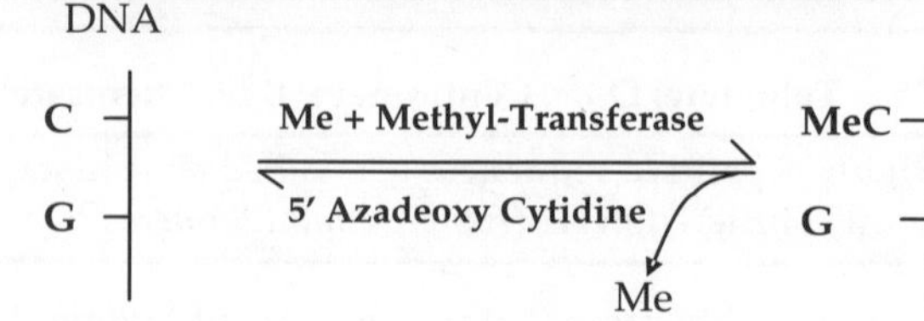

DNA Synthesis and Replication

60. **B i.e. Semi conservative; D i.e. Bidirectional; E i.e. Semi discontinuous**
61. **B, C i.e. Superhelical density depends on length of DNA, Underwinding strain is normally accommodated by strand...**
62. **A i.e. DNA synthesis / replication** 63. **A i.e. ds DNA** 64. **C i.e. DNA Polymerase III**
65. **B i.e. Sister chromatids are formed C i.e. Follows base pair rule D i.e. Semi conservative E i.e. Single strand breakend.**
66. **C i.e. RNA polymerase → DNA polymerase III → DNA Polymerase I → DNA ligase.**

67. **B i.e. Multiple origins of replication are possible..; D i.e. Lagging strand stick by RNA..; C i.e. DNA replication ...**
68. **A i.e. DNA Ligases** 69. **A,B,C,D,E i.e. DNA polymerase,DNA ligase,DNA topoisomerase, Primase, RNA polymerase**
70. **D i.e. DNA gyrase** *[Ref: Lippincott 5/e p 399-405; Lehninger 5/e p 954-58, 977-92; Harper 29/e p 365-72; John Baynes 3/e p 418]*

- **DNA replication is semiconservative** (since half of the original DNA is conserved in each of the daughter DNA), **semi-discontinuous** (i.e. continuous in leading & discontinuous in lagging strands) and **bidirectional** (d/t replication bubble/ fork) in both pro and eukaryotes. **Although prokaryotes have single and eukaryotes have multiple origins.**
- **Okazaki fragments** are **short (small) discontinuous segments of DNA synthesized on the lagging strand in 5′ → 3′ direction, during the process of double stranded (ds) DNA replication (synthesis)**[Q]. On lagging strand, first an RNA primer is synthesized by **primase** and then **DNA polymerase III** binds to this RNA primer and **synthesizes Okazaki fragments** by adding deoxyribonucleotides **(=polymerization)** along the single stranded template. After this **DNA polymerase I removes the RNA primer and fills the created gap by DNA (nick translation). DNA ligase seals the nick** created by removal of DNAPI in lagging strand (**Nick sealing or sticking**)

DNA Replication (Elongation)

Leading strand
RNA primer (made by primase)
DNA chain made by DNA polymerase III (addition of deoxyribonucleotides or polymerization)

Lagging strand
RNA primer (made by Primase)
DNA made by DNA polymerase III
(in short Okazaki fragment, in an antiparallel fashion)
Excision of RNA primer by **DNA polymerase I**
DNA gap filled by **DNA polymerase I**
Remaining nuclei sealed by **DNA ligase.**

- **DNA replication** occurs in **S phase** of cell cycle, is **semi conservative** process that **follows base pair rule** and yields two pairs of **sister chromatids** from each chromosome. ***For replication DNA is breakened (unwound) into single strands***[Q].
- **Replication loops** always initiate at a *unique point in DNA* termed *origin* (indicated by *denaturation mapping of Ross inman*). Both (or one) ends of replication loop are dynamic points, termed **replication forks**, where parent DNA is unwound and separated strands quickly replicated – l/t **bidirectional** (or **unidirectional**) DNA replication.
- DNA synthesis always proceeds in a **5′ → 3′ direction and is semidiscontinuous**. The **nascent DNA** is always ***synthesized in the 5′→3′ direction because DNA polymerase can add a nucleotide only to the 3′ end of a DNA strand***[Q]. This also means that the template is read from its 3′ end towards its 5′ end.
- **Leading or Forward (5′ →3′) strand** is synthesized **continuously** and in the **same direction as replication fork moves. Lagging (retrogade) (3′→5′) strand** is synthesized **discontinuously** in short pieces (**Okazaki fragments**) in a direction **opposite** to that in which replication fork moves. Genetic information found in DNA is copied & transmitted to daughter cells through DNA replication.
- **Nick translation** (i.e. filling the gap produced by removal of DNA or RNA strand such as RNA primer paired to DNA templet) ***is done by 5′- 3′ exonuclease activity of DNA polymerase I***[Q] whereas **nick sealing** (i.e. filling the gap produced by removal of DNA polymerase I on lagging strand) is done by ***DNA ligase***[Q].
- **DNA gyrase,** a **type II topoisomerase** found in bacteria & plants ***introduce negative supercoils***[Q] in relaxed circular DNA using ATP (energy). This facilitates the future replication of DNA because the negative supercoils neutralize the positive supercoils introduced during opening of double helix.
- Process of **eukaryotic DNA replication** closely follows that of prokaryotic DNA synthesis except that **it has multiple origins of replication (Ori)** and RNA primers are removal by **RNase H and FEN1** (rather than by DNA polymerase) in eukaryotic cells. **Prokaryotes have single Ori.**

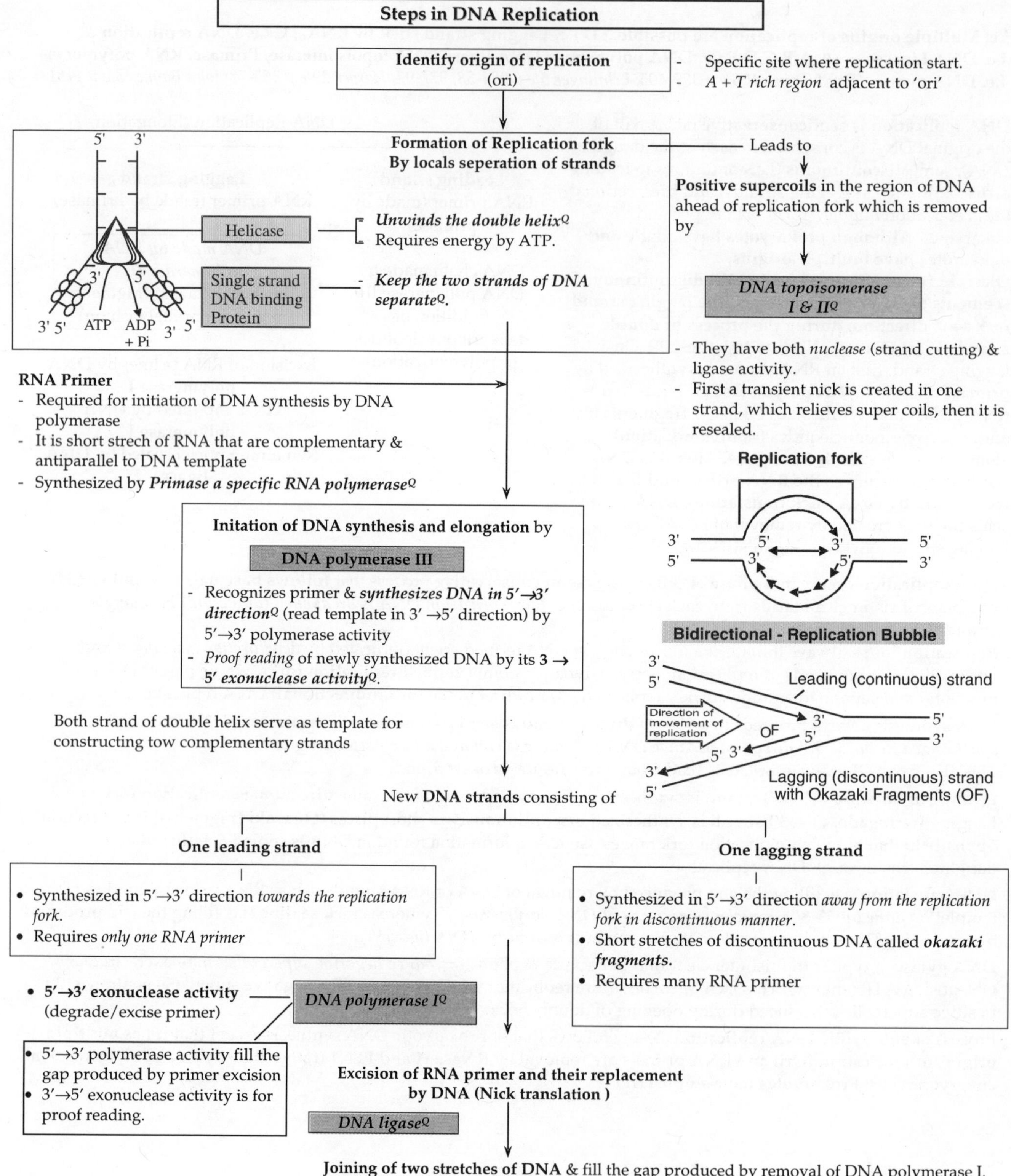
Steps in DNA Replication
Identify origin of replication (ori)
- Specific site where replication start.
- A + T rich region adjacent to 'ori'
Formation of Replication fork
By locals seperation of strands
5' 3'
Helicase
- Unwinds the double helixQ
- Requires energy by ATP.
Single strand DNA binding Protein
- Keep the two strands of DNA separateQ.
3' 5' ATP ADP + Pi 3' 5'
Leads to
Positive supercoils in the region of DNA ahead of replication fork which is removed by
DNA topoisomerase I & IIQ
- They have both nuclease (strand cutting) & ligase activity.
- First a transient nick is created in one strand, which relieves super coils, then it is resealed.
RNA Primer
- Required for initiation of DNA synthesis by DNA polymerase
- It is short strech of RNA that are complementary & antiparallel to DNA template
- Synthesized by Primase a specific RNA polymeraseQ
Replication fork
Bidirectional - Replication Bubble
Initation of DNA synthesis and elongation by
DNA polymerase III
- Recognizes primer & synthesizes DNA in 5'→3' directionQ (read template in 3' →5' direction) by 5'→3' polymerase activity
- Proof reading of newly synthesized DNA by its 3 → 5' exonuclease activityQ.
Leading (continuous) strand
Direction of movement of replication
OF
Lagging (discontinuous) strand with Okazaki Fragments (OF)
Both strand of double helix serve as template for constructing tow complementary strands
New DNA strands consisting of
One leading strand
• Synthesized in 5'→3' direction towards the replication fork.
• Requires only one RNA primer
One lagging strand
• Synthesized in 5'→3' direction away from the replication fork in discontinuous manner.
• Short stretches of discontinuous DNA called okazaki fragments.
• Requires many RNA primer
• 5'→3' exonuclease activity (degrade/excise primer)
DNA polymerase IQ
• 5'→3' polymerase activity fill the gap produced by primer excision
• 3'→5' exonuclease activity is for proof reading.
Excision of RNA primer and their replacement by DNA (Nick translation)
DNA ligaseQ
Joining of two stretches of DNA & fill the gap produced by removal of DNA polymerase I. So it seals the nick on lagging strand (Nick sealing)

DNA Polymerase Complex

Prokaryotic DNA Polymerase

- **DNA polymerases III (pol III) catalyzes the highest rate of chain elongation (polymeriztion)** and is the **most processive** (polymerizing 0.5 Mb DNA in one cycle on leading strand).
- Pol III is > 1MDa (large), multi (13) subunit protein complex. Its association with 2 identical **beta subunits of DNA sliding clamp** markedly increases the **stability, rate of chain elongation** (20-50 nt/s) **and processivity** (100 to > 50 thousand nucleotides) of DNA polymerase III enzyme.
- **DNA polymerase I & II (pol I & II)** are mostly involved in **proof reading and DNA repair.**

Feature	DNA Polymerase		
	I	II	III
5′→ 3′ Polymerase activity[Q]	+	+	+
3′→ 5′ Exonuclease activity (Proof reading)[Q]	+	+	+
5′→ 3′ Exonuclease activity[Q] **(Excision – repair/nick translation)**	+[Q]	-	-
Repair	+	+	-
Polymerization rate (nucleotide/s)	16-20	40	250-1000
Processivity (nucleotides added before polymerase dissociates)	3-200	1500	≥5 lacs
Subunits	1	7	≥10
Structural genes	pol A	pol B	**pol C (dnaE)**

Endonucleases are enzymes that **cleaves internal bonds in DNA & RNA**[Q].

Eukaryotic DNA Polymerase (Lippincott)

- At least of 5 type & are designated by Greek letter rather than roman numbers (i.e. α, β, γ, δ, ε)
- **α is a multi subunit enzyme.**
  - One subunit has **primase activity**, which initiates strand synthesis on leading strand & at beginning of each Okazaki fragment on lagging strand.
  - Primase subunit synthesizes a short RNA primer that is extended by **α5′ → 3′ polymerase** activity, which adds a short piece of DNA
  - **Pol δ** is then recruited to complete DNA synthesis of leading strand & elongate each Okazaki fragment, using 3′→5′ exonuclease activity to proofread the newly synthesized DNA
  - DNA polymerase δ associates with proliferating cell nuclear antigen protein, which serves as a **sliding DNA clamp** (similar to β subunit of DNA polymerase III ensuring high processivity).

DNA polymerase	Function	Proof Reading
Pol α	Contains **primase Initiates DNA synthesis**	-
Pol β	**Repair**	-
Pol ε	**Repair**	+
Pol γ	**Replicates** mitochondrial DNA	+
Pol δ	**Elongates** leading strands & okazaki fragment	+

Comparison (Harper)

All DNAP complex share 3 features

1. **Chain Elongation**: accounts for nucleotide per second rate (nt/s) at which **polymerization** occurs
2. **Processivity**: is number of nucleotides added to nascent chain before the DNA polymerase disengages from the template.
3. **Proof reading**: is identification of copying errors and correcting them.

E.coli	Eukaryotic	Function
I		**Gap filling (synthesis) of lagging strand** following DNA replication, repair & recombination
II		DNA proof reading & repair
	β	**DNA repair**[Q]
	γ	**Mitochondrial DNA synthesis**[Q]
III	ε	Procssive, leading strand synthesis
DNA G	α	Primase
	δ	Processive, lagging strand synthesis.

71. **A, D, & E i.e. Circular, Negatively sepercoiled & Nucleoid present** *Ref: Lehninger 5th/ed pg- 949-50; Greenwood 16/ed pg- 10-12*

> E. coli (bacteria) has **single, closed, circular, double stranded (ds) negatively supercoiled DNA chromosome of about 1.7 mm (46, 39, 675 bp) long in their nucleioid**[Q]. Bacteria have no nucleus and nuclear membrane.

72. **B, D i.e. β; ε** *[Ref: Lippincott 4th/ed pg- 407; Harper 29/367; Lehninger 5th/ed pg. 989]*
73. **A, B, & C i.e. Components are α, β, γ, Δ, ε, β associated with repair, & γ associated with repair**
74. **B i.e. 5′→ 3′ Polymerase activity; C i.e. 3′→ 5′ exonuclease activity; D i.e. 5′→ 3′ exonuclease activity**

DNA Damage, Repair and Protooncogene

75. **A, C, D i.e. Pyrimidine, Sugar, Purine** *[Ref: Lehninger 5/e 271-75; Chatterjae 7/e 206-8; Vasudevan 6/e 457-59-296;*
76. **D, E i.e. TMP – Thymine monophosphate, UMP – Uracil monophosphate** *Lippincott 5/e 291-93; Harper 28/e 285-87]*

- **Nucleosides** are N-glycosides formed by addition of **pentose sugar (D-ribose or 2 deoxy D-ribose)** to a **purine (adenine, guanine) or pyrimidine (cytosine, thymine & uracil) bases**. Nucleosides with purine bases (A, G) have – **'sine'** suffix viz – **adenosine, guanosine**[Q], whereas pyrimidine nucleosides have '**dine**' suppix viz – **cytidine, thymidine and uridine**[Q].
- **Nucleotides** are phosphorylated nucleosides. Suffix – **sine /-nylate /-nylic acid for purine & - dine /-dylate /-dylic acid for pyrimidine** are used. So UMP is uridylate or uridine now phosphate and TMP is thymidylate or thymidine mono phosphate

77. **A i.e. Adenosine**

- Nitrogen base + sugar = **Nucleoside**
- Nucleoside + phosphate = **Nucleotide**
- Nucleotides linked together by. 3′ 5′ phosphodiester bond = **Nucleic acid.**

Adenosine is a *nucleoside composed* of -
- Adenine (Nitrogen base)
- Ribose (Pentose sugar)

On complete hydrolysis, Adenosine should yield the above two component individually.

The complete hydrolysis of Nucleic acid yields the basic component, which include:

Nitrogen bases	Pentose sugar	Phosphate sugar
- Purine: Adenine & Guanine - Pyrimidine: Thymine & Cytosine (uracil in RNA)	- Deoxyribose (in DNA) - Ribose (in RNA)	

78. **A & D i.e. Decrease Tm & Melting lead to denaturation of DNA**
79. **A i.e. Splitting of double strands into single strand.** *[Ref: Lippincott's 4/397-98,Harper's 28/303-4;Chatterjea 7/228-229;Lodish 6/e p117]*

Seperation of double stranded (ds) DNA into single stranded DNA[Q] is known as **denaturation or melting of DNA**. It is **promoted by increasing temperature or decreasing salt concentration. So increased salt (monovalent cation) concentration increases Tm**[Q].

80. **A i.e. Absorption at 260 nm** *[Ref: Harper 28/e 288; Lehninger 5/e 276]*

Concentration (and quality) **of nucleotides and ncleic acid (DNA /RNA)** is measured in terms of "**absorbance at 260 nm**[Q]" with a **Ultraviolet (UV) spectrophotometer**.

81. **D i.e. Endonuclease cut DNA at 5′ terminus** *[Ref: Lehninger 5/e 979-82; Harper 28/e 311-404; Vasudevan 6/e 475]*

- **B-DNA** with **right handed helix is most common**[Q]. Nucleic acid (i.e. DNA & RNA both) is degraded by **nuclease** and specifically RNA by **ribonucleases (RNases)** and DNA by **deoxy ribonucleases (DNases)**. **Exonucleases** degrade nucleic acid **from one end** of molecule **in only 5′→3′ or 3′→5′** direction, **removing nucleotides only from 5′ or 3′ end (terminal)**[Q] respectively of one strand of a double stranded or a single stranded DNA.
- **Endonucleases** are capable of cleaving **internal phosphodiester bonds** to produce either 3′ – OH and 5′ – PO4 terminals or 5′ – hydroxyl and 3′ – phosphoryl terminals. Hence endonucleases cut (degrade) in the internal site of nucleic acid to produce nicks, reducing it to smaller & smaller fragments. **Restriction endonucleases cleave DNA only at specific nucleotide sequences**[Q].
- **DNA polymerase I (Korenberg's enzyme)** has **5′ → 3′ polymerase activity** (responsible for polymerization), **3′ →5′ exonuclease** activity (responsible for **proof reading**) and specific (or exclusive) **5′ →3′ exonuclease** activity (responsible for **nick translation** and excision repair). Due to 5′→3′ exonuclease activity, DNA polymerase I can replace a segment of DNA or RNA paired to template strand, in a process k/a nick translation. Most other DNA polymerases lack 5′→3′ exonuclease activity and when this is removed the remaining **large fragment** of DNA polymerase I is k/a **Klenow fragment**, which retains the polymerization & proof reading activities.
- **DNA polymerase of T4 bacteriophage of E.Coli and Klenow fragment (of DNA polymerase I) have almost similar functions**[Q] but the 3′→5′ exonuclease activity of T4 DNA polymerase is 200 times higher than that of klenow fragment making it preferable for blunting DNAs with 3′ over hangs. While klenow fragments are preferred for oligonucleotide mutagenesis reactions as it displaces oligonucleotides downstream as it polymerizes.

82. **A i.e. DNA repair** *[Ref: Chattergea 7/e p. 239-40]*

Photoreactivation (light induced repair), recombinational repair, mismatch repair (or sister strand exchange), and excisional repair[Q] are various **DNA repair mechanisms.**

83. **A i.e. Formation of thymidine dimmers**
84. **C i.e. Nucleotide excision repair**

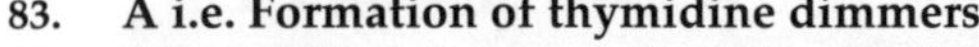

85. **B i.e. DNA Polymerase I > D i.e. DNA ligase** *[Ref: Harper's 27/e P-345-46,343; Lehninger 5/e p. 1003]*
86. **A i.e. Nucleotide excision repair**

- The damage produced by UV rays is caused **due to formation of pyrimidine (mainly thymine) dimers**Q. The thymine dimmer **prevent DNA polymerase from replicating**Q the DNA strand beyond the dimmer, thus inhibiting the repair of defective DNA.
- In Xeroderma Pigmentosa mechanism for repair **('nucleotide excision repair')**Q of damaged DNA is defective d/t formation of **Thymidine dimers**Q.

Xeroderma Pigmentosa

- An *autosomal recessive condition* in which cells can not repair the damged DNA
- The clinical syndrome include ***marked sensitivity to sun light***Q resulting in
  - ***Skin cancers***Q
  - ***Premature death***Q
- Arises because of ***defect in 'nucleotide excision' pathway*** of repair due to defect in either of three:
  - ***UV specific endonuclease (most common defect)***Q
  - ***DNA polymerase 1***Q
  - ***DNA ligase***Q

Repair of thymine (pyrimidine) dimmer by Excision repair

UV rays

↓

Damage of DNA by formation of thymine dimerQ

↓ *UV specific endonuclease.*

Damaged sequence is recognized and cleaved

↓ *DNA polymerase I*
- Synthesize new DNA strand in 5'- 3' direction using sister strand as template
- 5'- 3' *exonuclease* activity removes the damaged sequence

Removal of damaged DNA & formation of new DNA strand

↓ DNA ligase

Joining of new DNA strand with the main chain

87. **B i.e. Deamination to thiamine; D i.e. DNA repair > E i.e. Methylation protects the host DNA from cleavage by its own restriction enzyme** *[Ref: Vasudeven 6/e p477; Harper 29/e p370-74; Lippincot 5/e p 398, 460-62, 422; Lehninger 5/e p 289-92, 302, 993-95]*

Deamination of cytosine forms uracil and deamination of 5 methyl cytosine forms thymine. TDG & MBD4 DNA uracil glycosylase remove either U or T residues paired with G, generated by deamination.
DNA methylation of adenine at 5' GATC repair mismatched base pairs. And methylated parental (template) strand is protected from cleavage / digestion by its own restriction enzyme.

88. **A, B & C i.e. Xeroderma pigmentatosa, Bloom's syndrome & Ataxia telangiectasia**
[Ref: Harper-28th/ed pg- 330-33; Chatterjea 7th/ed pg-239-41; Lehninger 5th/ed pg- 1003-992; Harrison 17/ed pg-396]

Ataxia telangiectasia, Bloom's syndrome, Fanconi's anemia, Xeroderma pigmentosa, hereditary non polyposis colon cancerQ and few breast cancers are due to **DNA repair defects**.

89. **B i.e. Inhibition of apoptosis** *[Ref: Robbins 7th/293,295; ww.lungcancerbooksandnewsletter.com/what_is_cancer.htm]*

Oncogenes may function by inactivation of DNA repair genes, but not by promotion of DNA repair. Promotion of DNA repair is protective from oncogenesis and is hence the answer of exclusion.

- **Oncogenesis and DNA repair:** (Inactivation of DNA repair genes leads to oncogenesis)
  - Cancer generally involves multiple incidents of DNA damage.
  - Inactivation of DNA repair genes allow build up of genetic mistakes with each succeeding round of cell division.
  - This 'genetic instability' may lead to oncogenesis.
- **Apoptosis**: (Inhibition of apoptosis leads to oncogenesis)
  - Apoptosis or programmed cell death is an inherent method of protection against development of cancer
  - Inhibition of apoptosis by oncogenes promotes cancers.
- **Cell cycle progression:** (Enhanced cell cycle progression leads to oncogenesis)
  - Cell cycle is a highly ordered sequence of events that lead to cell growth and division
  - In normal cells 'Cell Cycle Control genes' control the progression of cells through cell division cycles.
  - Deregulation of signals controlling the progression of cell through cell division cycles leads to oncogenesis.
- **Nuclear transcription** (Factors causing enhanced nuclear transcription cause oncogenesis.
  Transcriptional factors enter the nucleus bind the DNA and cause proliferation and oncogenesis.

90. A i.e. Normally involved in cell cycle proliferation; D i.e. Proto- onchogenes on mutation cause cancer
91. A i.e. Carotenoids *[Ref: Casciato: Onchology 5/e p-22, 25; Harrison 16/e p- 1072, Robbins 7/e p. 100, 288, 292- 95]*

- **Protooncogenes** are ***normal cell genes that participate in cellular functions related to growth and proliferation***[Q]. Proteins encoded by protooncogenes may function as ***growth factor, ligands and receptors, signal transducers, transcription factors and cell cycle regulators***[Q].
- ***Protooncogenes on activation become oncogenes that induce cancer***[Q]. The process of activation include gene amplification, **point mutation**, insertion mutation, retroviral transduction (integration), chromosomal translocation and protein- protein interaction.
- Onchoproteins encoded by oncogenes have similar functions as their normal counterparts but they are constitutively expressed and endow the cell with self sufficiency in growth. ***Carotinoids are anticarcinogens***[Q].

92. A ie. Proto-oncogenes; B ie. Tumor suppressorgene; D ie. DNA repair genes **93. D i.e. RAS** *[Ref: Robbins 7/e p 289-309]*

- Genes that promote autonomous cell growth in cancer cells are called **oncogenes** and their ***normal cellular counterparts***[Q] ***are called proto-oncogenes***[Q]. ***RAS is an oncogene***[Q].

Growth factor		**Growth factor receptors**		**Proteins involved in signal transduction**		**Nuclear regulatory proteins**	
Protooncogene	Encode	Protooncogene	Encode	Protooncogene	Related to	Protooncogene	Related to
HST-1, 1NT-2	Fibroblast growth factor	ERB-B2 & ERB-B1 (ECRF)	EGF-receptor family	RAS-K/H/N	GTP binding	**MYC-C/N/L**	***Transcriptional activator***[Q]
TGF α	Transforming growth factor-α	FMS	Colony stimulating factor (CSF)-1	ABL	Nonreceptor tyrosine kinase	**Cell cycle regulators**	
HGF	Hapatocyte growth factor	RET	Receptor for neuro-trophic factors	BRAF	RAS signal transduction	**Cyclin D/E**	Cyclins
SIS	Platelett growth factor β-chain	KIT	Receptor for stem cell (steel)factor	β-catenin	WNT-signal transduction	CDK-4	Cyclin dependent kinase

- **MYC – protooncogene** is expressed in almost all eukaryotic cell. MYC – protein is translocated to nucleus (sometimes as hetrodimer with MAX protein) and is *a potent transcription activator*. MYC activation causes *cell proliferation*, induces histone acetylation, protein synthesis and cell motality & decreases cell adhesion & proteinase activity. ***Cells in culture undergo apoptosis if MYC activation occurs in absence of growth factors***[Q], but it is not clear whether MYC induced apoptosis occurs in vivo.
- *Retinoblastoma susceptibility protein (RB)*, in *hypophosphorylated* state, prevents cell from replicating by forming *complex with transcription factor E2F* (E2F/D P1/RB – complex). Phosphorylation of RB dissociates the complex, release E2F, eliminates main barrier to cell cycle progression & promotes cell replication. **Cyclin D**, which is *the first cyclin* to increase in cell cycle, (appears in *G_1 phase* but becomes detectable in *S phase*) activates CDK4 and form cyclin D- CDK4 complex that phosphorylates RB. During M phase RB is again hypophosphorylated.

Normal growth requires – protooncogenes not oncogenes , tumor suppressor genes, genes involved in apoptosis and DNA reapir[Q]**.**

94. A i.e. α-rays *[Ref: Grainger 4/e P-139; Park 17/e P-521]*

Maximum damage to DNA is caused by α- Rays[Q].

Radiation	Content	Penetrating Power	Ionizing Power	Damaging Power
α-particle	Helium nuclei (i.e. 2 protons & 2 neutrons)	**Poorest**[Q] **(1)**	**Maximum**[Q]	**Most damaging**
β-particle	Either high energy electron or antimatter counter part positron	Greater than α-particle (100)	Lesser than α-particle	< α-particle
X-Ray	**Low energy photons**[Q]	More than β-particles	Lesser than β-particle	< β-particle
γ-Radiation	**Very high energy photons**[Q]	More than X Rays (10000) i.e. **Most Penetrating**[Q]	**Minimum Ionizing**[Q]	**Least damaging**

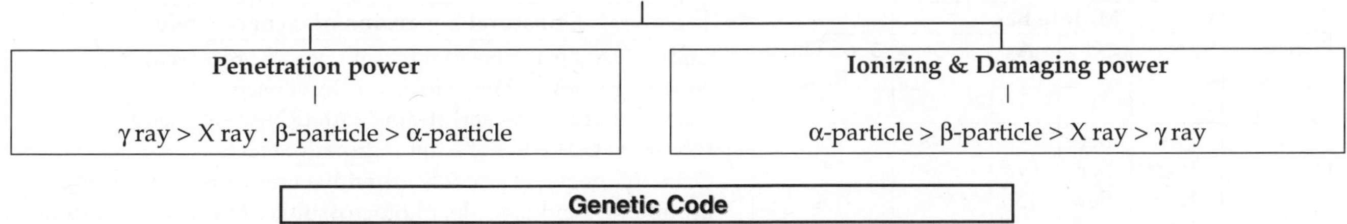

Genetic Code

95. B i.e. Hydroxyproline; E i.e. Ornithine **96. B, C i.e. Overlapping, Ambigous** **97. D i.e. UAC**

98. A, C, D, E i.e. AUA codes for methionine in mitochondria, AUG codes for initiator codon in mammalian cell, AGA & AGG act as chain terminator in mammalian mitochondria, UAA, UAG & UGA are stop codon

99. C i.e. 256 **100. C i.e. 3 consecutive nucleotide units** **101. C i.e. Punctuation**

102. A i.e. AUG **103. D i.e. Termination of protein synthesis** **104. B i.e. 3 complementary base pairs**

105. B i.e. 3 consecutive nucleotide unit **106. A i.e. Degeneracy** **107. B i.e., 5-end *of* anticodon**

[Ref: Lippincott 5/e p 432; Harper's 29/e P- 270; Lehninger 5/e p 1085

Genetic Code and Codons ☆

Genetic code is a dictionary that identifies a corrospondence b/w a sequence of nucleotide bases and a sequence of amino acids. And **codon** is each individual *genetic word* of this dictionary that is ***composed of 3 nucleotide bases***Q.

- Condons are present in m- RNA in language of **A** (adenosine), **G** (guanine), **C** (cytsine), and **U** (uracil) nucleotides.
- There nucleotide sequences are always written *from 5′ to 3′* end. Each codon consist of a ***sequence of 3 nucleotides***Q i.e. it is a **triplet code.**
- Since there are only **4 different nucleotides** (A, G, U,C) in m- RNA and codon consists of sequence of 3 nucleotides; each codon must consist of *>1 purine or pyrimidine* nucleotide and there are ***64 (4^3) different combinations of codon***Q.
- 61 of 64 genetic codons code for 20 common amino acids **– phenylalanine (Phe), leucine (Leu), isoleucine (Ile), methionine (Met), Valine (Val), serine (Ser), proline (Pro), threonine (Thr), alanine (Ala), tyrosine (Tyr), histidine (His), glutamine (Gln), asparagine (Asn), lysine (Lys), aspartic acid (Asp), glutamic acid (Glu), Cysteine (Cys), tryptophan (Trp), arginine (Arg), and glycine (Gly).** ***AUG designating methionine is initiating codon***Q.
- 3 codones – **UAA, UAG, UGA** do not code for any amino acid and are known as **stop (termination or nonsense) codon**. When one of these appear in m-RNA sequence, it **indicates that synthrhesis of protein coded by that mRNA is completed**Q.

If codon consisted of	Number of codons
2 nucleotide sequence eg. AU	$(4)^2$ = ***16***Q
3 nucleotide sequence eg AUG	$(4)^3$= ***64***Q
4 nucleotide sequence eg AUG	$(4)^4$= ***256*** Q

Characteristics of Genetic Code

- **Specificity (Unambiguous):** which means *a particular codon always codes for the same amino acid.*
- **Universal:** which means the specificity of genetic code is conserved from very early stages of evolution to mammals (between species) and among different tissues in a species. The exceptions are
- *Mitochondrial* translational machinery reads *four codons differently* from t-RNA molecules in cytoplasm of even same cell. So mitochondria requires only *22 t- RNA* molecules to read their genetic code, where as cytoplamic translation system has a full complement of *3′ tRNA.*

Codon	Cytoplasm	Mitochondria
AUA	Ile	Met (**Methionine**)
UGA	Termination codon	Trp (**Tryptophan**)
AGA AGG	Arginine	**Stop** or **chain termination codon**

- **Degeneracy (Redudancy):** which means ***some aminoacids are coded by multiple codons***Q. For example six diffrent codons specify serine as well as arginine
- **Non overlapping, non punctuated and commaless:** which means the code is read from a fixed starting point as a continuous sequence of bases taken 3 at a time *without any overlapping or comma (punctuation)* between the codons. For example ABCDEFGHI is ABC/DEF/GHI.

5′ or First Base	Middle Bas				3′ or Third Base
	U	C	A	G	
U	Phe	Ser	Tyr	Cys	U
	Phe	Ser	Tyr	Cys	C
	Leu	Ser	Stop	Stop	A
	Leu	Ser	Stop	Trp	G
C	Leu	Pro	His	Arg	U
	Leu	Pro	His	Arg	C
	Leu	Pro	Gln	Arg	A
	Leu	Pro	Gln	Arg	G
A	lle	Thr	Asn	Ser	U
	lle	Thr	Asn	Ser	C
	lle	Thr	Lys	Arg	A
	Met	Thr	Lys	Arg	G
G	Val	Ala	Asp	Gly	U
	Val	Ala	Asp	Gly	C
	Val	Ala	Glu	Gly	A
	Val	Ala	Glu	Gly	G

Natural Expansion (Evolution) of Genetic Code

- There are **actually 22 rather than 20 amino acids specified by known genetic code. The 21st amino acid selenocysteine** (Sec) **is coded by UGA and 22nd amino acid pyrrolysine (Pyl) is encoded by UAG**. So in effect, UGA and UAG doubles as a codon for both termination and (very occasionally) selenocysteine (in bacteria with *formate dehydrogenase* or in mammals with *glutathione peroxidase* protein) and **pyrrolysine (in methanogens** or methane producing anaerobic archaea).
- ***Unlike hydroxyl lysine or hydroxyproline, selenocysteine arises cotranslationally*** during its incorporation into peptides. Unlike selenocysteine – pyrrolysine was attached directly to a dedicated tRNA by a cognate *pyrrolysyl tRNA synthetase*.

Unnatural Expansion of Genetic Code

- **Codon UAG** is the best target (of scientific research) for encoding a new aminoacid as it is least used of the three termination codons and strains with tRNAs selected to recognize UAG do not exhibit growth defects.
- Over 30 unnatural aminoacids with a unique reactive chemical group like ketone, azide, photocrosslinker (a functional group designed to form a covalent bond with a nearby group when activated by light), a highly florescent amino acid, aminoacid with a heavy atom (Br) for use in crystallography and aminoacid with long chain cysteine analog that can form extended disulfide bonds have been added to genetic code.

Induced Variation in Genetic Code: Nonsense Suppression

- **Nonsense mutation** produce a termination codon in interior of gene, prematurely halting translation, producing inactive incomplete polypeptide. The gene can be restored to normal function if a 2nd **restorative mutation (k/a nonsense suppressors)** either suppresses the effects of termination codon or converts the misplaced termination codon to a codon specifying an aminoacid.
- Mostly nonsense suppressors involve mutations in t-RNA genes to produce **altered (supprssor) t RNA** (mostly *with a single base substitution in their anti codon) that can recognize the termination codon and insert an aminoacid at that position.*
- A cell usually has several copies of each tRNA. Nonsense suppression does not completely disrupt normal information transfer in cell because these suppressor mutations usually involve minor (weakly expressed) t RNA, leaving the normal tRNA to read its codon normally. However nonsense suppression can produce enough full length active protein from a gene with nonsense mutation to allow the cell to survive.
- Nonsense suppression *does not always lead to abnormally long proteins or creation of suppression t-RNA with mutation in anticodon.* Eg suppression of UGA nonsense codon generally involves tRNA trp that normally recognize UGG and inserts Trp at that position. Alteration of G to A at 24 position in arm of tRNA allows it to read both UGA and UGG (& insert Trp).

Regulation of Gene Expression

108. B i.e. Zinc finger motif **109. A i.e. Nuclear receptor** **110. A i.e. Zinc finger**
111. A i.e., Zinc finger D i.e., Helix turn helix E i.e., Leucine zipper *[Ref: Harper's 28/e p. 381-84; Lippincott's 5/e p. 423, 450, 18]*
112. E i.e. 7 Amino acid **113. B i.e. Zinc** **114. A i.e. DNA binding protein**

> **Binding of transcription regulatory proteins to DNA is regulated by several motifs**Q – the **helix turn helix, the leucine zipper** and the **zinc finger**. However, the **binding motif for steroid receptor family and thyroid (nuclear) receptor family is zinc finger**Q.

115. A i.e. Cistron *[Ref: Chatterjae 7/e 253; Vasudevan 6/e 473-561-60; Harrison 17/e p-385; Harper 28/e 370-71; Lehninger 271-477-948]*
116. A, C, D i.e. Smallest functional unit of genome, Promoter & enhancer geens are typical example, Cistron is single ...
117. A i.e. Positive regulator

> *CAP – cAMP regulator is a positive regulator for Lac operon*Q because its presence is required for gene expression.

Operon is the segment of DNA strand, consisting of *cluster of several genes involved in metabolic pathway.*

Operon = **structural genes** coding for enzymes of metabolic pathway + **regulatory genes** that determine their transcription

Structural genes for Lac operon	Coded protein
Lac Z	β galactosidase
Lac y	Permease
Lac A	Acetylase

Regulator genes/ proteins & inducers	
Positive regulator	*CRP = CAP + CAMP*[Q]
Negative regulator	*Lac I gene*[Q] Repressor protein
Inducer	*Lactose*[Q] IPTG (gratuitous inducer)

118. **A i.e. Promoter; B i.e. Enhancer; C i.e. Operator** *[Ref: Harper's 28/e p. 370-373; Lippincott's 5/e p. 449-53; Chattergea 7/e p. 253-58]*
119. **D i.e., Not regulated**
120. **E i.e., Catabolite repression is mediated by CRP**
121. **D i.e., Regulator gene is inducible**
122. **C i.e. Inducer without glucose**
123. **C i.e. Both Lytic and lysogenic phases occur together**

Depending upon the nutritional state of host cell (E. coli), the temperate virus bacteriophage lambda (λ) DNA will **either** integrate into the host genome and remain dormant **(lysogenic pathway)** until activated, or it will commence replicating until it has made about 100 copies of complete, protein packed virus, leading to lysis and killing of bacterial host **(lytic pathway)**.

124. **D i.e. RNA polymerase**

DNA dependent RNA polymerase is ***key enzyme in transcription (i.e. DNA to RNA conversion)***[Q]. Whereas, ***DNA polymerase, DNA ligase and primase are used in DNA replication***[Q].

Transcription

125. **C i.e. Specifically recognizes the promoter site**
126. **B i.e. Promoter**
127. **D i.e. Primer**
128. **B i.e., Nucleolus**

[Ref: Lippincott's 5/e p. 419, 422, 424; Harper's 28/e p. 337, 345; Lehninger 5/e p. 1024-32; Chatterjea 7/e p. 242-43]

- **The sigma (σ) subunit (factor)** ***enables RNA polymerase to recognize promoter regions on DNA***[Q].
- Like DNA polymerase, RNA polymerase uses *nucleoside triphosphate* as substrates & releases pyrophosphate each time a nucleoside monophosphate is added to growing chain. And as with replcation, transcription is always in 5′ → 3′direction. However, ***incontrast to DNA polymerase, RNA polymerase (both in eukaryotes and prokaryotes) does not require primer and has no known proofreading activity***[Q].

129. **A i.e. Exon > B i.e. Enhancer**
130. **A i.e. Polycistronic mRNA; E i.e. Non coding exon**
131. **D i.e. Normal transcription, normal translation** *[Ref: Harper 29/e p 360-64]*
132. **A i.e. Interon**
133. **A i.e. Cut DNA at specific DNA seq.**

- **Interons** are *non coding region of gene* which are *processed out of primary transcript*. Hence any change (insertion or removal of base pairs) in intron ***will not effect transcription or translation***[Q].
- **Exons (coding regions)** ***of gene are expressed as m-RNA and contribute to polypeptide synthesis***[Q]. **Enhancer** and **repressor (silencer)** are **cis acting** (ie located on same chromosone, whose transcription affect) distal regulatory elements that regulate (increase & decrease respectively) the rate of initiation of transcription by pol II in eukaryotes.
- **Leader sequence at 5′ end of mRNA, 3′ flanking sequence and non coding (nc) or non protein coding (npc) or non messenger (nm) or small (s) or functional (f) RNA like rRNA, t-RNA, sn RNA, sno RNA**, sca RNA, st RNA, mi RNA, si RNA, etc **do not translate into protein.**
- **Endonucleases** cut DNA at specific sequence *with in the molecule* (as opposed to **exonuclease** which digest *from the ends* of DNA) are key tools in recombination DNA research. These enzymes were called **restriction enzymes** because their presence in a bacteria restricted the growth of certain bacterial viruses called bacteriophage.

- In eukaryotic cells, small mobile **DNA elements** k/a **jumping DNA** or **jumping genes**, that clearly are not viruses are capable of transpoising themselves out and in of the host genome in way that affect the junctioning of neighbouring DNA sequences. These mobile jumping genes can carry flanking regions of DNA and therefore profoundly affect evolution. **Alu family** of moderately repeated DNA sequences has structural similarity to termini of retrovirus, allowing the latter to move in and out of mammalian genome. **Processed genes** (eg for alpha globin molecules) provide direct evidence for transposition in human genome. **Processed genes consist of DNA sequences identical or nearly identical to those of m-RNA for appropriate gene product** (ie the 5′ non translated region, the coding exon region without intron representation, and 3′ poly A tail are all present contiguously). This processed DNA sequence arrangement must have resulted from the *reverse transcription of an appropriately processed m-RNA* from which introns had been removed and poly (A) tail added. And the only known mechanism this reverse transcriptase could have used to integrate into human genome is a transposition event. That's why processed genes have short terminal repeats at each end like transposed sequences in lower organisms.
- In absence of transcription & genetic selection for function, many processed genes are randomly altered through evolution so that they now contain nonsense codons that preclude their ability to encode a functional intact protein. These are k/a **pseudogenes**
- Thus a **eukaryotic gene contains neuclear & mitochondrial genes, pseudo genes and processed genes; coding exons and non coding introns.**
- **Monocistronic mRNA** encodes only single polypeptide (protein) chain (like in **most eukaryotes**), whereas **polycistronic mRNA** encodes >1 or many proteins eg prokaryotes (bacteria), lac operon.
- Exons are spliced together to form mRNA and introns are spliced out of precursor RNA. However, **eukaryotic- heterogenous nuclear (hn) RNA or pre-m RNA or primary transcript must undergo several post transcriptional** modifications like capping , splicing & addition of poly (A) tail before it is exported from nucleus to cytoplasm for protein synthesis.

Eukaryotic gene

Coding Regions = Exons	**Non coding regions (Interons)**
* Double helical DNA is packaged into a more compact structure d/t basic protein *histone* * *Enhancers* are the DNA sequences in gene that increase the rate of transcription & *silencers* repress transcription	Interpose between exons and are always removed from precursor RNA before transport into cytoplasm occurs.. The process by which interons are removed and exons are ligated together is called **RNA splicing**

134. **D i.e. Involve phosphodiester bond formation with elongation occurring in the 5′- 3′ direction.**
[Ref: Harper's 27/e P-348; Chatterjea 6/e P-232]

> **In both DNA and RNA synthesis**, the general steps of **initiation, elongation and termination occur in 5′- 3′ direction with the formation of phosphodiester bonds**Q.

135. **A i.e. 5′ – CGU – 3′** *[Ref: Harper's 28/e p. 336-46; Lippincott 5/e p. 418-22]*

> - In **transcription**, the **template strand** of DNA serves as a template for RNA synthesis and is always read in **3'→5' direction**. So the primary transcript **(m-RNA) is complementary to template stand**Q.
> - The **opposite non template DNA strand** (which is complementary to template strand) is also called **coding strand** because it is **identical in base (nucleotide) sequence to mRNA** transcribed from that DNA (gene), **with U in mRNA in place of T in coding strand of DNA. So 5'GCT3' coding strand means 5'CGU3' mRNA transcript.**

136. **C i.e. Different σ subunits are responsible for recognition specificity**
137. **A i.e. Promoter region**
138. **A i.e. Initiation of transcription of the dystrophin gene would be affected**
[Ref: Lippincott 5/e 430-423; Harper 28/e 553-54; Harrison 17/e 2682-83; Chattarjae 7/e 243; Robbins 7/e p-1337]

Let me rephrase this question to make it straight forward, and then it would be – what is the consequence of **alteration (i.e. mutation) in promoter region**?

> - **Promoter region of transcription unit is** the portion of DNA having **specific consensus sequences** (like **TATA box /CAAT box /GC box** etc) which is identified by the **RNA polymerase enzyme** for binding and formation of **preinitiation complex (PIC)** in prokaryotes or **RNA polymerase II/pol II-transcription complex** in eukaryotes – a process ultimately resulting in **initiation of transcription**.

- So this becomes very obvious, that any **alteration /mutation / damage in** promoter would typically **prevent formation of PIC or pol II transcription complex**, resulting in a **decrease in the initiation of m-RNA synthesis (transcription)** l/t decreased protein synthesis. And similarly **promoter induction** would *increase the transcription rate*Q.
- **Capping, tailing, termination and splicing** are **not associated with promoter** and so are not a consequence of promoter mutations. However, capping & tailing defects can result in m RNA with decreased stability and splicing defects in mRNA in which to few or too many introns have been removed.

139. A, B, C, E i.e. siRNA, miRNA, tRNA, rRNA *[Ref: Harper 28/e 307-10; Lehninger 5/e 1146-1060-33-1076]*

- **Noncoding (nc) RNAs** are *all RNAs that do not encode protein*. They are also called *non protein coding (npc) RNA, non-messenger (nm) RNA, small (s) RNA, and functional (f) RNA*. The gene (DNA sequence) from which a nc-RNA is transcribed as end product is called **non coding RNA gene** or **RNA gene**.
- **Non coding (nc) RNAs** include **ribosomal (r) RNA, transfer (t) RNA, small nuclear (sn) RNA, small nucleolar (sno) RNA, sca RNA, small temporal (st) RNA, micro (mi) RNA, small interfering (si) RNA**Q, pi RNA, rasi RNA, linc RNA, antisense RNA, and long nc RNAs like Xist & HOTAIR.
- **Messenger (m) RNA** is a **coding RNA.**

140. D i.e. C-DNA; E i.e. New strand of DNA

Genetic information stored in genes (chromosome) transmitted to daughter cells through DNA replication, is expressed through transcription to RNA and in cases of mRNA, subsequent translation into proteins. ***tRNA and rRNA are not translated***Q.

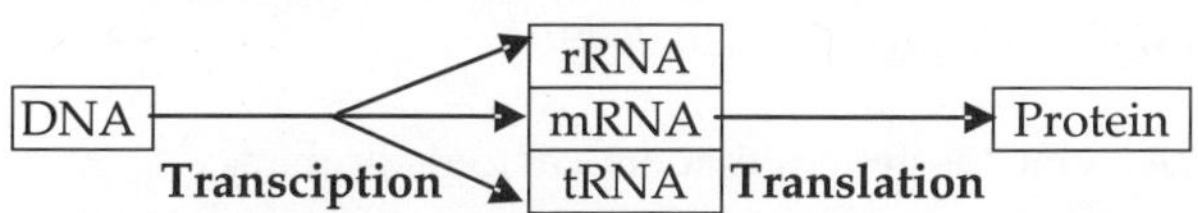

141. B i.e. t RNA

All RNA molecules (eg **r RNA, tRNA, mRNA** etc) are ***produced from transcription of DNA***Q. Whereas, as a **new strand of DNA** is formed by **DNA polymerase III** enzyme in process of **DNA synthesis / replication**. And **complementary (c) DNA** is prepared ***by using mRNA as a template by enzyme reverse transcriptase (= RNA dependent DNA polymrase)***Q in process of reverse transcription.

142. A i.e. Transcribed from Nuclear DNA

- **m-RNA is transcribed from one strand of ds nuclear DNA**Q. In eukaryotes, the primary transcript (immediate product of transcription) in nucleus is **heterogenous nuclear (hn) RNA** not mature mRNA. This hn RNA is very heterogenous, can be **>10-50 times longer (with higher molecular weight)** containing both exons & introns, and is very unstable. By post transcriptional modification (processing) eg splicing hn RNA is converted to **smaller molecular weight final transcript (ie mature mRNA).**

Component	DNA	RNA
Sugar	**2-deoxy D-ribose**	**D-ribose**
Nucleotides	Adenine (A), Cytosine (C), Guanine (G), and **Thymine (T)**	Adenine (A), Cytosine (C), Guanine (G) and **Uracil (U)**

- **DNA** contains **deoxy ribose sugar** and **thymine (T) nucleotide**, whereas **RNA (including mRNA)** contains **ribose sugar** and **uracil (U) nucleotide**.

143. B i.e. RNAI **144. B & E i.e. RNA polymerase II & Drosha** **145. A i.e. Gene Regulation**

Ref: Harper 28th/e p. 348-50, 306-10,366; Lehninger 5th/ed pg- 1030-33, 1145, 1045-46,1146; Lippincott 4th/ed pg- 422-24; Lodish-Molecular Biology 6/ed pg-348

- **Micro-RNA (mi-RNA) is transcribed by RNA polymerase II**Q as primary mi-RNA (pri-mi-RNA). It is processed by 2 endoribonucleases of RNase III family:

1. **Drosha** (with DGCR8, in nucleus to precursor mi-RNA or pre-mi-RNA) and
2. **Dicer** (with TRBP in cytoplasm to nearly mature mi-RNA or **small interfering RNAs = si –RNAs or small temporal RNAs = st RNAs** paired with a short RNA complement)

- **RNA helicase** removes the complement and mature mi- RNA is incorporated into protein complexes to form **RNA induce silencing complex (RISC).**
- By this process of **gene silencing** by **RNA interference (Nobel prize** 2006 given to Andrew Fire & Craig mello) **mi-RNA, st- RNA and si – RNA play a important role in gene regulation by inhibition of gene expression (& so translational process)**Q

146. B i.e. Polylysine *[Ref: Harper's 27/e p. 366; Lippincott's 4/e p. 432, 424-27 ; Genes & development 21 : 519- 524, 2007]*

Codon	**AAA**	**GGG**	**CCC**	**TTT / UUU**
Translation product	**Lysin**Q	Glycine	Proline	Phenylalanine

Poly A tail translates into polylysineQ

147. A i.e. Occur in intron that form Ribozyme; C i.e. Self-splicing introns; E i.e. Lariats intermediates are formed
148. A i.e. RNA splicing **149. A i.e. Intron** **150. B i.e. snRNA**
[Ref: Harper 28th/ed pg- 307, 346-48; Lippincott 5th/ed pg- 426-27; Lehninger 5th/ed pg- 1146, 1043-44]

- **Self splicing introns function as ribozyme and do not require external protein enzymes or high energy cofactors (eg ATP). Intron forms lariat in group II** but not in group I self splicing introns.
- **Splicing is process of removing introns (i.e. the segment of gene that is not represented in mature m-RNA) from primary transcript and joining (or ligating together) exons (RNA sequences that code protein)**Q**. It is mediated by sn RNP or snrups formed from sn RNA**Q.
- **Small nuclear RNAs (sn RNAs)** are involved in **RNA splicing**Q; **small nucleolar RNAs (sno RNAs)** are involved in r **RNA modifications**Q; **micro RNAs (mi RNAs) & small temporal RNAs (st RNAs)** are involved in **inhibition (regulation) of gene expression (gene silencing)**Q; **small interfering RNAs (si RNAs)** are involved in **RNA interference (RNAi)**Q; and **B2 RNA** binds to pol II and block transcription of many genes during heat shock
- Mammalian genomes seem to encode more non coding RNAs (nc RNAs) than coding m RNAs. nC RNAs are RNAS that do not encode proteins including r RNAS, t RNAs, mi RNAs, si RNAs, st RNAs and sn RNAs.

151. A i.e. Lariats formation; B i.e. Splicing; E i.e. Methylation
152. A i.e. Occurs in introns that form ribozyme; C i.e. Self splicing introns; E i.e. Lariat intermediates are formed
153. D i.e. Attachment of CCA in tRNA. **154. C i.e. Poly (A) tailing** **155. D i.e. Prokaryotic mRNA**
156. D i.e. Glycosylation **157. A i.e. Chemical hydrolysis** **158. C i.e. Deamination of cytidine to uridine**
[Ref: Vasudevan 6/e p 485-86; Harper 29/e p 389-94; Lippincott 5/e p 427, 457-58; Lehninger 5/e p 1036-49]

- **Least post translational modification** occurs in **prokaryotic mRNA**, which is generally identical to its primary transcript.
- Post translational modification of t-RNA includes **removal of introns from anticodon loop, trimming of 5' & 3' ends, methylation** / reduction / deamination / alkylation / rearranging glycolsidic bond to **produced modified bases like methylated bases, dihydrouracil (D) & pseudo uracil (Ψ) bases** in **nucleus, whereas cleavage** and attachment of **CCA tailing occur in cytoplasm**Q.
- In RNA, gene during processing undergoes **nucleoside modifications, nucleoside cleavage and terminal addition but not chemical hydrolysis**Q.
- **Post translational modification of mRNA** involves **5' capping , 3' polyadenylation (addition of poly 'A' tail at 3' end), splicing** (removal of non coding intervening or intron sequences and ligation / joining of coding exons) **by Sn RNA / Sn RNPs / Snurps** or **self splicing d/t ribozyme activity of self splicing introns** with formation of **lariat intermediates, RNA editing and secondary methylation**Q.
- Apo B-48 and Apo B-100 are synthesized from same Apo B gene and same ApoB- m-RNA. **Apo B 100 is a 100 kDa protein synthesized in liver by full length translation** of corresponding mRNA of Apo B gene. Apo – B-100 forms part of LDL, IDL and VLDL. **Apo B-48** is a 48 KDa protein (48% shorter form of Apo B-100) **synthesized in intestine by partial translation of same mRNA of Apo B gene**. Apo B 48 forms part of **chylomicron & chylomicron remnant**. This difference between the sizes of Apo B100 and Apo B48 occurs because **post transcriptional processing (editing)** of Apo B mRNA , **deaminates the cytidine (C) to uracil (U) in intestine** at 2153 position. After **cytidine deamination** the **CAA codon** (which codes **glutamine in liver**) becomes **UAA (nonsense or stop codon)** in intestine. This results in shorter apo B-48 protein being made in intestine (and incorporated into chylomicron) than is made in the liver full length Apo B-100, incorporated in to VLDL.

159. A i.e. All RNA undergo post transcriptional modification; B i.e. Capping of the pre-m RNA Involves the addition of 7-methylguanosine to the 5'end; C i.e. Poly A tailing occur at 3'end; D i.e. Intron excision by spliceosome

- **Nearly all eukaryotic & prokaryotic RNA (except prokaryotic m-RNA) are extensively processed primariy with in the nucleus (for eukaryotes) before they become functional**Q.
- Post transcriptional modification of mRNA includes **capping (i.e. 7 methyl guanosine addition to 5' end), poly A tail addition at 3' end, removal of introns & joining of exons by spliceosome**Q.

160. C i.e. Peptidyl transferase activity **161. E i.e. Deamination** *[Ref: Harper 29/e p. 68, 348]*

Ribozyme is RNA with catalytic activityQ. Examples include **peptidyl transferase, selfsplicing group I introns, RNase P, & hammerhead metallo enzyme**Q of virusoids (requiring Mg^{2+}). These are involved in **transesterification, phosphodiester bond hydrolysis (cleavage)**, RNA metabolism (splicing & endoribonuclease), **peptide bond formation (peptidyl transferases) and site specific RNA cleavage**Q.

162. B i.e. DNA **163. A i.e. Cytarabine** **164. A i.e. Actinomycin D - B i.e. Amanitin** **165. D i.e. Actinomycin**
[Ref: Chatterjea 7/e p. 245, 252; Lippincott's 4/e p. 424, 397; Harrison 16/e p. 479, 794, 635, Harper 27/e p. 351, 378]

166. A i.e.Spinal muscular dystrophy *[Ref: Lippincott 5/e 425-26; Harper 28/e 317-348-49-308; Lehninger 5/e 1035-40; Vasudevan 6/e p. 484-85]*

β-thalassemia and **spinal muscular atrophy** occur due to defective splicing of **hetrogenous nuclear (hn) RNA**.

167. C i.e. Reverse transcriptase *[Ref: Harper's 27/e P-316, 410; Lippincott's 3/e P- 405]*
168. A i.e. Forms DNA from RNA; C i.e. Important for replication of HIV

Reverse transcriptase (RT) is an **RNA dependent DNA polymerase that produces double stranded DNA copies of RNA template**Q. In retrovirus (eg HIV), reverse transcriptase uses RNA as its template (Genome of retrovirus is single stranded RNA) **for synthesis of viral DNA**Q.
RT moves along the template in 3'→5' direction, synthesizing DNA in 5' →3' direction.

DNA polymerase	Synthesize ***DNA from DNA***Q
RNA polymerase	Synthesize ***RNA from DNA***Q
Phosphokinase	***Adds a phosphate moiety***Q

★ ***Amplification of DNA*** is done ***by Polymerase Chain reaction (PCR)***Q.

169. B i.e. Protein; D i.e. Nucleic acid *[Ref: Harper's 27/e P-314, 316]*

Template is required for protein and nucleic acid synthesisQ.
- Nucleic acid synthesis require DNA as a template
- Protein synthesis require mRNA as a template

170. C i.e. t – RNA **171. A i.e. t – RNA** **172. B i.e. Clover leaf pattern** **173. B i.e. t-RNA**

The t-RNA's contain many modifications of the standard bases A,U,G, and C, including methylation, reduction, deamination and rearranged Glycosidic bonds.

174. C i.e. t RNA

The Tψ C arm of **tRNA** has sequence of **thymidine**Q, Pseudouridine, and cytosine.
The T ψ C arm of tRNA is involved in binding of amino acyl – tRNA to the ribosomal surface at the site of protein synthesis.

hn RNA is heterogenous nuclear RNA, they are processed to generate the mRNA, which then enter the cytoplasm to serve as template for protein synthesis.

Translation (Protein Synthesis)

175. C i.e. Nucleolus **176. A i.e. Ribosome** **177. C i.e. Hydroxylysine**
178. C i.e. Attachment of amino group to 5' end **179. C i.e. Amino acyl t- RNA synthetase**
180. A i.e. Stop Codon; E i.e. UAA; D i.e. Peptidyl **181. B i.e. Peptidyl transferase; C i.e. Release factors**
182. A i.e. Used in elongation & cause attachment of peptide chain to A-site of t RNA
183. D i.e. 48 S complex **184. A i.e. Peptidyl transferase** **185. E i.e. 4** **186. A i.e. Amino group; B i.e. Carboxyl ..**
187. A, B, D i.e. Releasing factor, Stop codon, UAA codon **188. D i.e. Amino acyl tRNA synthetase**
[Ref: Harper 29/e p 400-408; Lippincott 5/e p 438-45; Lehninger 5/e p 1075-95]

- **Translation** is the **process by which 'Ribosomes' convert the information carried by mRNA to the synthesis of protein**Q. Thus Ribosome is a cellular component on which all interaction take place to **synthesize protein**Q.
- Initial step of protein synthesis is activation of **aminoacid by t-RNA** to **form aminoacyl t-RNA**. This reaction is ctalyzed by **amino aceyl t RNA synthase**. Because **hydroxyproline & hydroxylysine** are not represented in genetic code (as they **are synthesised post translationally) so they do not have t-RNA capable of acccepting them**Q.
- **Aminoacyl tRNA synthetase** is **responsible for proof reading, editing & high fidelity of translation (protein synthesis)**Q as it **attaches aminoacids to their corresponding (isoaccepting) tRNAs**- an interaction that is also called **second genetic code**. It attaches aminoacyl groupto **3' position** of terminal residue.
- **Peptidy transferase (a ribozyme)** catalyze **peptide bond formation**Q and causes attachment of growing peptide chain to tRNA of A site. The **formation of peptide bonds** (for protein chain elongation) is catalyzed by **peptidyltransferase**, an activity **intrinsic to 23 S r RNA found in 50 S ribosomal subunit**Q (Lippincott) /**28S rRNA of 60S ribosomal subunit**Q (Harper). Because the peptidyl transferase activity **resides in rRNA component of ribosome, it is a ribozyme and indicates – direct role of r-RNA in protein synthesis. Energy required for formation of 1 peptide bond is 4 high energy phosphate bonds (2ATP + 2GTP)**Q.
- **Peptide bond is formed between amino group** (of amino acyl tRNA at A site) and **carboxyl group carbon** (of peptidyl t RNA in P site).
- **Termination of protein synthesis** occurs when a stop codon (UAA, UAG, UGA) appears in 'A' site. These codons are recognized by release factors (RF-1, RF-3). **RF with GTP & peptidyl transferase promotes hydrolysis of bond between the peptide & t RNA occupying the 'P' site**Q.
- **RNA polymerase** is **required for transcription (mRNA synthesis) not for translation (protein synthesis)**Q

Functions of

Nucleolus

Site of r-RNA synthesisQ

Ribosomes

- Exists free in cytoplasm
- Contains 65% r- RNA & 35% protein
- *Synthesize protein (i.e. translate m-RNA) that remain within cells*Q.

Rough Endoplasmic Reticulum

- Coated with Ribosomes
- Responsible for protein synthesis (only integral membrane protein & protein that are to be exported)
- Initial folding of polypeptide chains with formation of disulfide bond.
  [Thus this is Ribosome which is responsible for protein synthesis in RER]

Smooth Endoplasmic reticulum

- *Steroid synthesis*Q
- Detoxification process
- Plays important role in cardiac & skeletal muscle contraction.

★ Central **Dogma**: The *flow of information from DNA to RNA to protein*Q.

189. B i.e Stop Codon **190. A i.e. AUG Codon** **191. A i.e. AUG** **192. A i.e. N formyl Met is the first – RNA ...**
193. B i.e. N formyl methionine t RNA will be first t RNA to come into action.
194. A i.e. It has 3 steps initiation, elongation & termination; D i.e. IF-2 has α &β units **195. D ie. IF-4F** **196. D i.e. 4S**

- Three codons are called as Stop codons or nonsense codons. These are **UAA (Ochre), UAG (Amber), UGA (Opal)**Q
- **Shine Dalgarno sequence** is a **sequence of nucleotide bases (5' – UAGGAGG-3') located 6- 10 base upstream of AUG codon on mRNA molecule**Q. It helps ribosomes in recognizing the nucleotide sequence that is essential for initiation of translation.
- Although amino acid **methionine (Met)** has only one codon **AUG**, all organism have 2 types of t RNA for methionine tRNA ^{fMet} incorporating **N-formyl methionine (f-met)** in response to **initiation codon** AUG and **tRNA**^{Met} incorporating **methionine (Met)** in response to AUG codon in **internal position**.
- **Methionine** having anticodon **UAC** is the first amino acid required in binding to the initiation codon AUG on mRNA. In **bacteria (prokaryotes)** & **mitochondria** the **initiator t-RNA carries an N – formylated methionine aminoacid**Q, whereas in **eukaryotes**, the **initiator tRNA carries a methionine that is not formylated**Q.
- Translation has 3 steps initiation elongation & termination. IF2 has α – β subunits. IF4F has 4A, 4G, & 4E (ie AGE) components. 40/43 s preinitiation complex has 1A, 2β and 3 initiation factors (IF).

197. **D i.e. Asparagine:** *[Ref: Lehninger 5/e p 1096-97, 224-26; Smith 8/e p 96-221]*

- **Serine, threonine and tyrosine undergo phosphorylation by protein kinase (in eukryotes) during post translational modifications**
- Extra **carboxyl** group is added to **glutamate** residue of blood clotting protein prothrombin (**carboxylation**). **Lysine undergo methylation** in some muscle proteins (mono & dimethyllysine), and **calmodulin** (trimethyl lysine); **carboxy group of glutamate** undergo methylation removing their negative charge.

198. **A i.e. 23s; C i.e. 5s**

199. **A, E i.e. 5.8 S, 28 S**

200. **A, B, C, E i.e. Conserved in nature, Role is to bring t-RNA and m-RNA together, DNA forms RNA and rotein are formed from RNA, Have two subunits** *[Ref: Lehninger 5/e 3, 1076-79; Harper 28/e 308-10; Lippincott 5/e 436; Vasudeven 6/e 493-487]*

201. **D i.e. Binding of aminoacyl tRNA uses 2ATP**

- **Component of 50s subunit** are **23s & 5s**; and components of **60s subunit are 28s, 5.8s and 5s.**
- **Ribosome** is a **highly conserved natural machine for protein synthesis that brings m-RNA & t-RNA together**Q. It has 2 subunits the **large subunit** catalzes **peptide bond formation** whereas **small subunit** is responsibl for **accuracy**. 16s rRNA component of 30s subunit **identifies & binds shine Dalgarno sequence**. Binding of aminoacyl tRNA to A site uses **1 GTP**. Free cytosolic ribosomes synthesize proteins required in cytosol, nucleus, mitochondria & peroxisomes. Whereas RER bound ribosome form proteins for various plasma membranes.

202. **D i.e. Vitamin K**

Generation of biologically active clotting factors involves the post translational modification of Glutamate residues of the precursor proteins to γ carboxyglutamate residue by a specific carboxylase enzyme that is dependent on 'vitamin K'. **Vitamin C is also involved in post translational modification, but not of coagulants.**Q

Immunoglobin

203. **B i.e. IgG -γ (gamma)**

204. **A, C i.e. IgM to IgG, IgM to IgA**

205. **A, B, C i.e. Fix complement, Increased in primary response, Fab region is composed of variable region**

206. **A, C, D i.e. Somatic mutations theory, DNA rearrangement, Appropriate class switching**

207. **A, D i.e. κ- 2, λ – 22** *[Ref: Lehninger 5/e 1014-16, 1040-41, 170-73; Harper 28/e 349, 361, 322, 576-80; Lippincott 5/e 461-62-426; Vasudevan 6/e 561-62, 554-58; Anantnarayan 7/e p 96; Harrison 17/e p 2036; Chattarjae 7/e 256]*

- In humans, genes for **light chains-Kappa (κ)** is in **chromosome 2**; for **light chain lambda (λ)** is in **chromosome 22** and genes for **heavy chains** are in ***chromosome 14***Q.
- Each of the 5 classes of immunoglobulin has a characterstic type of heavy chain – **alpha (α)** in IgA, **gamma (γ)** in IgG, **delta (δ)** in IgD, **mu (μ)** in IgM and **epsilon (ε)** in IgE.
- **Immunoglobin** has **2 identical light (L) & 2 identical heavy (H) chains**, each containing **variable (V) & constant (C) regions. Variable regions of light- & heavy chains (i.e. VL & VH)** bind to specifc antigen and form **a part of Fab (antigen binding fragment).**
- **IgM** is **natural antibody** produced in **primary response** to antigen. **It does not cross placenta**, therefore, the fetus even though it carries an incompatible antigen, is protected from natural antibodies of mother. It ***fixes complement***Q (like IgG) and agglutinates bacteria (like IgA & G). It has **antigen receptors on B cells**, surface (IgD is found on surface of B cells where it acts as a receptor for antigen).
- **Newly** mature **B cells** produce both IgM and IgD, which can switch to other class of immunoglobulin (i.e. IgG, IgA or IgE) in a process k/a **isotype/class switching**.

208. **C i.e. Differential RNA regulation** *Ref: Lehninger 5th/ed pg- 1014-16; Tasuku: Immunoglobulin genes 2/e pg-237*

Synthesis and diversity immunoglobin in membrane bound or secretory form is ***determined by differential /alternative RNA processing*** of heavy, Kappa and lambda light chains and *immunoglobin gene rearrangements.*

Intracellular traffic, sorting and folding, Chaperons

209. **B i.e. Endoplasmic reticulum** *[Ref: Vasudevan 6/e p. 493; Harper 28/e p. 487-91]*

The secretory proteins and transport proteins are synthesized in ribosomes attached to the endoplasmic reticulumQ. Where as proteins which have to be delivered in cytosol are synthesized in free polyribosomes.

210. **C i.e. Membrane bound ribosomes**
211. **B i.e. SRP**
212. **D i.e. Halt signal**
213. **E i.e. SRP-R is ATP bound**
214. **D i.e. Chaperones**
215. **D i.e Protein folding**
216. **B, E i.e. Calnexin, Protein disulfide isomerase**
217. **B i.e. Are lipid in nature**
218. **A, B, C, E i.e. Belong to heat shock proteins; Wide range of expression; Present from bacteria to human; Also k/a stress proteins** *[Ref: Harper 28/e p- 39, 496-97; Devlin Biochemistry 5/e p- 255; Ganong 22/e p.25, 297-96, Chatterjea 8/e p 269-270]*

- **Chaperones (heat shock or stress proteins) are present in wide range of species from bacteria to humans**Q**. Most exhibit ATPase activity.**Q
- **Chaperones** are **proteins that play a role in the assembly or proper folding of other proteins without themselves being component of the later**. They prevent faulty folding and unproductive interactions of other proteins by stabilizing partially folded or unfolded intermediates, allowing them time to fold properly.
- **Chaperones are folding** proteins which prevent faulty folding and unproductive interactions. These include **chaperonins like mt Gro EL** (from complex barrel like structures in which unfolded protein is retained for proper folding); **BiP (immunoglobulin heavy chain binding protein), GRP-94** (glucose related protein), **calnexin and calreticulin**Q and enzymes such as **PDI** (protein disulfide isomerase) & **PPI** (petidyl prolyl cis-trans-isomerase). All these are located in rough endoplasmic reticulum (RER).

219. **D i.e. Ubiquitin** *[Ref: Lippincott's 3/e P-244; NMS 4/e P-375; Harper 28/e p. 497-987; Ganong 22/e p. 296-98, 25]*

- **Ubiquitine is a small, highly conserved protein (76 amino acid polypeptide),** that plays a key role in **marking** (targeting) & **escorting many intracellular protein mainly abnormal newly produced protein and aged normal protein for degradation**Q (ticket of degradation) in multisubunit proteolytic particles the 26 S proteasome. It is also involved in activation of NF_kB, cell cycle regulation (degradation of cycles), DNA repair, viral infections etc.

- **Clathrin** is a peripheral membrane protein, that helps in endocytosis. **Pepsin** is proteolytic enzyme secreted by chief cells of stomach and is used for digestion. **Laminin** is found in extracellular matrix a most abundant glycoprotein present in basement membrane

220. **A i.e. Golgi bodies**

Trans – golgi is involved in sorting of proteinsQ.

Role of golgi apparatus in membrane synthesis

- **Processing of oliosaccharide chains** of membrane and N- linked glycoprotein and
- Contains enzymes involved in **O-glycosylation**
  - **By all parts of golgi apparatus**Q

Sorting & seggregation of various proteins prior to their delivery to their appropriate intracellular destination
- **Trans- port of golgi apparatus is particularly involved**Q.

221. **B i.e. Tuberculosis** *[Ref: Harper 28/e p 497-98, 493; Vassudevan 6/e 590, 495]*

Alizheimers, cystic fibrosis and prions diseases (eg Creutzfeld Jakob's disease, Kuru, fatal familia insomnia etc)Q occur due to **protien misfolding.**

222. **C i.e. Betasheets** *[Ref: Harper's 28/e p. 39; Lippincott's 4/e p. 22; Harrison 17/e p. 2646]*

There is no difference in amino acid & gene sequence, primary structure & post translational modifications between normal cellular isoform of non infectious (host) prion protein (PrP^c) and infectious (pathological) prion proteins (PrP^{sc}). **The key to becoming infectious lies in 3 dimensional conformation i.e. a number of α-helices present in non infectious PrP^c are replaced by β sheets in infectious (PrP^{sc}) form**Q.

223. A i.e. Kuru *[Ref: Harper's 28/e P-39, 496-97; Lippincott's 3/e P- 21- 22]* **224. A i.e Familial fatal insomnia**

Kuru, familial fatal insomnia & Creutzfeldt Jacob's disease are d/t protein misfolding.

Gene Duplication

225. A i.e. mRna *[Ref: Lehninger 5/e p. 1060-61, 325, 34, 30]*

Gene duplication and mutation is a path to **generate new enzymatic activities by evolution of superfluous (extra) gene producing new mRNA & new enzyme** with new substrate specificity.

Mutation

226. C i.e. Paracentric inversion

- **Chromosomal (or large scale) mutations** involve large part of chromosome eg entire gene, many nucleotides etc. Examples include **inversions (paracentric & pericentric), translocations** (reciprocal, Robertsonian/ centric fusion, intrachromosomal, inter chromosomal), **duplications** and deletions (**terminal deletion & interstitial deletions).**
- **Small scale (base pair or gene) mutations** occur in individual base pair (nucleotide) or a small group of base pairs (gene). Examples include **base pair substitution or point mutation (transition,** transversion, silent/ missense/ nonsense mutation) and **frame shift mutation (d/t deletion or insertion).**

227. A i.e. Point mutation; D i.e. Conserved mutation **228. C i.e. Alanine – leucine**
229. C i.e. A base substitution in DNA **230. B i.e. 6** **231. D i.e. Insertion of one base**
232. D i.e. point mutation **233. D i.e. Mutation that leads to no functional gene product** **234. C i.e. Missense mutation**
235. C i.e. Frame shift alteration in coding nucleotide; D i.e. Trinucleotide repeat mutation; E i.e. Nonsense alteration of DNA
236. C i.e. 3 **237. C i.e. Reading frame changes down stream to the mutant site** **238. A i.e. G G T C C T**
239. A i.e. Hutingtoris disease B i.e. Spinocerebellar ataxia **240. D i.e. All fo the above** **241. D i.e. Aspartic acid**
242. B i.e. Glutamic acid **243. B, D i.e. No change in amino acid sequence, No change in expression of protein**
[Ref: Harper 28/e 355-58; Lippincott 5/e 433-34, 460, 427; Chattarjae 7/e 258-60; Lehninger 5/e 29-289,947,993; Vasudevan 6/e 501-503-262; Harrison 16/e p 370]

- **Conserved mutation** is a type of **acceptable missense mutation** that is caused by **single base substriction (or point mutation)** and **results in translation of aminoacid that has same properties as of original aminoacid eg glutamic acid (Glu) to aspartic acid (Asp)**[Q].
- Genetic code **GAA & GAG** encode **Glutamic acid (Glu)**; and **GAC and GAU encode Aspartic acid.**

Mutation

Mutation is defined as any *alteration in primary nucleotide sequence of DNA regardless of functional consequences*. It can involve (i) **Germ cells** to get transmitted to progeny or, (ii) **somatic cells**, which is *non hereditary* and may result in cancers etc. Types include.

I. Base Substitution (or Point) Mutation

- It involves **substitution (replacement or change) of one nucleotide base with another base**[Q] and can be of 2 types

Transition	Transversion
Purine base is replaced by another purine base or pyrimidine is replaced by another pytimidine base[Q]. **Purine (A) ↔ purine (G)** **Pyrimidine(T)↔Pyrimidine (C)**	It changes **purine to either of two pyrimidines or pyrimidines to either of 2 purines.** **Purine** A/G ↔ **Pyrimidine** T/C

II. Mutations **altering the amount or structure of protein** produced by translation.

1. Frame Shift Mutation

Insertion type **Deletion type**

- Insertion or deletion of **one or two** or **non multiples of 3 nucleotides** into the coding gene results in an m-RNA in which the **reading frame is distorted** upon translation. This **reading frame change**

- It may result in **disappearance** of already present restriction site **or creation** of a new **restriction site** by a particular restriction endonuclease (RE) l/t *generation of larger or smaller fragmens resectively* on digestion with that RE. In otherwords, **point mutation may l/t RFLP**Q (restriction fragment length polymorphism).

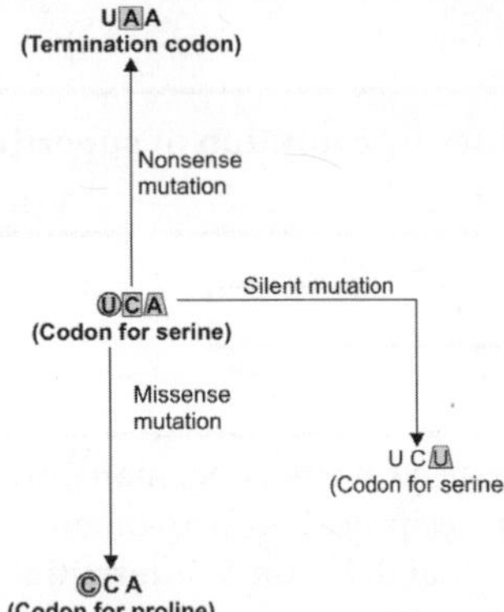

Possible effect of changing a single nucleotide base in the coding region of an mRNA chain

- The resulting **m-RNA will show a change only at a point complementary to a base change** at the corresponding locus. Point mutation or changing a single nucleotide base on mRNA chain may l/t any of these 3 effects. Effects of point mutation may be

Silent Mutation

- If mutation affects **non-essential DNA** or if it has a **negligible effect** on function of a gene, it is k/a silent mutation.
- The codon containing the changed base may **code for same amino acid.** This occurs **d/t redundancy /degeneracy** of genetic code.
- **No apparently detectable** effect usually occurs d/t **change in 3rd nucleotide of** genetic code. And because of **wobble phenomenon** translation of a gene is least sensitive to a change at 3rd position.
- **For example CUU, CUA, CUG, and CUC all code** leucine **and both UCU & UCA code serine**
- Example: **Homologous substitution** of **valine** at 67th position of **β-chain-**

Missense Mutation

- Codon containing the changed base may **code for a different aminoacid.** The substitution of a **mistaken/ missense/** or **incorrect** amino acid is called a missense mutation.
- The incorporation of mistaken different aminoacid, depending upon its location in

Nonsense Mutation

- The codon containing the changed base may ***become a stop/termination codon***Q. This creation of stop codon at inappropriate site is called a non sense mutation.
- It would result in **premature termination** of peptide chain and **only a fragment of intended protein molecule** will be produced.
- There is high probability that *prematurely terminated partially produced peptide or protein fragment will not*

/alteration/distortion in an mRNA, all the way down to the mutant site is a **feature of frame shift mutation & is not seen in point mutations.**

- The machinery translating the mRNA can not recognize that a base is missing (deleted) or added (inserted), *since there is no punctuation in reading of codons* – is the reason of altered reading frame.
- This can result in production of **garbled protein** (i.e. protein with completely/radically different amino acid sequence) or **truncated/short /prematurely terminated** – proteins (d/t premature creation of termination codon) or perhaps reading through the normal termination codon until another nonsense codon is encountered. (d/t deletion/insertion just prior to or within non sense codon)
- Following an insertion in a gene, a deletion (or vice versa) can restore the proper reading frame. And the corresponding mRNA on translation would contain a garbeled amino acid sequence b/w insertion & deletion and a correct sequence after that.
- If **3 or multiples of 3 nucleotides** are deleted/inserted in a coding region, the **corresponding number of aminoacids is missing/added in the protein**Q. Loss of 3 bases *maintains the reading frame* but can result in serious pathology like *cystic fibrosis* **(CF).**
- In CF, deletion of one codon (i.e. 3 bases) result in loss of 1 aminoacid **phenyl-alanine at 508th position (ΔF508) in CFTR (cystic fibrosis trans membrane conductance regulator) protein.** CFTR protein normally is a **chloride channel** in epithelia cells & its loss l/t production of thick, sticky secretion in lungs & pancreas causing damage to both.

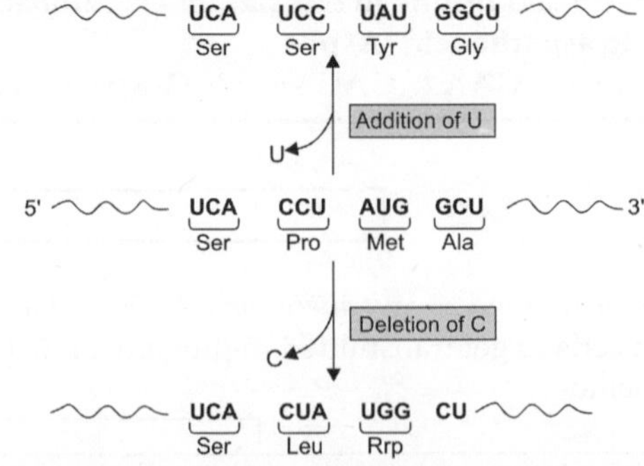

Frame Shift mutation d/t insertion & deletion of 1 base l/t production of garbled protein

2. Trinucleotide Repeat Expansion/Dynamic Mutation

- A sequence of 3 nucleotide bases that is repeated in tandem becomes amplified in number, so that too many copies of triplet occur.
- If this occurs in **coding region**, the protein will **contain many extra copies of one aminoacid** Eg CAG amplification in Hutington disease l/t insertion of many extra glutamine aa in Hutington protein making

HbA with another aminoacid has **no apparent effect** and result **in functionally normal hemoglobin** types.

Hemoglobin type	Homologous substituted aminoacid at 67th position on β-chain of Hb-A
Normal Hb A	Valine
Hb-Milwaukee	*Glutamic acid*Q/*glutamate*
Hb-Bristol	*Aspartic acid*Q/aspartate
Hb-Sydney	*Alanine*Q

specific protein – might be *acceptable (mostly), partially acceptable or unacceptable*

function in its assigned role. Eg. β-thalassemia

- If a *stop codon is changed into a coding codon*, this l/t elongation of protein to produce **run on polypeptide.** Eg Hb constant spring (α-thalassemia).

	Acceptable Mutations	**Partially Acceptable**	**Unacceptable mutations**
	- Change in aa has no functional consequence i.e. it **does not alter the normal function of protein** - **Conserved mutation** means altered aa has the same properties of original aa eg **glutamic acid to aspartic acid**. Most point mutation would result in replacement of one aa by another with rather similar functional groups –a natural mechanism to avoid drastic changes. The resulting protein may not be distinguishable from the normal one.	- It will result in a protein molecule with **partial but abnormal function** - **HbS** *hinders normal function* since it l/t sickle cell anemia when mutant gene is present in homozygous state and is considered *partially acceptable* because HbS does not bind & release O_2 abnormally.	- It results in **totally non functional protein,** that may be incompatible with normal life. - For example **HbM** mutation generate molecules that oxidize Fe^{2+} of heme to Fe^{3+}, producing **methemoglobin,** which cannot transport oxygen
Protein	**Hb-Hikari (β-chain)**	**Hb-S/Sickle Cell (β-chain)**	**Hb-M (Boston), α-Chain**

it unstable that accumulates causing neurodegenerative disorder.

- If amplification occurs in **non coding regions,** the result may be decrease in amount of protein produced, eg, **fragile X syndrome** & **myotonic dystrophy**. In fragile X syndrome the amplification results in gene silencing through **DNA hyper methylation** (as we know transcriptionally active **DNA is hypomethylated** whereas hypermethylation silences gene expression).

Disease	Repeat	Gene product
Hutington disease	CAG	Hutington
Spinocrebellar ataxia 1, 2, 3 (Machado Joseph disease), 6, 7, 12	CAG	Ataxin 1, Ataxin 2, SC3 (MJD1), Alpha 1A voltage dependent Ca++ channel, Ataxin 7, Protein phosphatas 2A
Dentorubral pallidoluysiane atrophy (DRPLA)	CAG	Atrophin
X-chromosome spinobulbar muscular atrophy (DRPLA)	CAG	Androgen receptor
Friedreich ataxia	GAA	Frataxin
Fragile –X-syndrome	CGG /GCC	FMR ½ protein
Dystrophia myotonica	CTG / CUG	Myotonin protein kinase

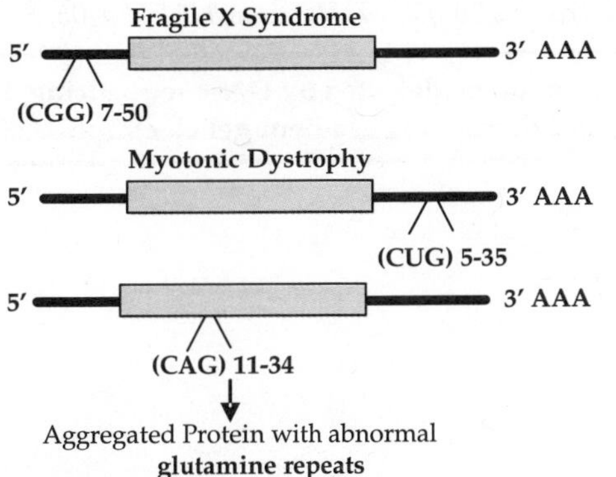

3. Splice Site Mutation

- Improper splicing can alter the way in which introns are removed from pre mRNA l/t production of aberrant proteins.
- Eg incorrect splicing of β-globin mRNA l/t **β-thalassemia** and in **myotonic dystrophy** gene silencing occurs d/t splicing alterations.

Suppressor Mutations

- Suppressor mutations can suppress/counteract some effects of missense, nonsense & frame shift mutations

Aminoacid change	In HbA-**β-chain-61 position**, lysine is replaced by **asparagine** **61 Lysine →Asparagine**	In HbA-**(β-chain)-6th position glutamate** is replaced by **valine** **6,Glutamic acid→valine**	In HbA-**α-chain- 58th position**, histidine is replace by **tyrosine** **58Histidine →Tyrosine**
Codon change	**Transversion** AAA or AAG ↓ ✕ ↓ AAU or AAC	**Transversion** **GAA or GAG** ↓ ↓ **GUA GUG**	CAU or CAC ↓ ↓ UAU UAC

★ **Null mutation** l/t no functional gain

by producing abnormally functioning, mutated, **suppressor t-RNA molecules** with alterations in anticodon region. These are capable of binding to & decoding altered mutated codones, thereby suppressing the effects of mutations in distinct mutated mRNA encoding structure genes.

- Suppressor t RNA usually result in *decreased viability* as these are incapable of distinguishing b/w a normal & a mutated codon. Eg **nonsense S-tRNA** can suppress normal termination signals to allow a read through when it is not desirable and a **frameshift S-tRNA** may read a normal codon plus a component of a juxtaposed codon to provide a frame shift when it is not desirable.
- Since reading through of translation has on occasion been observed, S-tRNA may exist in mammalian cells.

244. B i.e. Deoxygenated Hb l/t exposure of sticky end d/t replacement of nonpolar residue by polar residue
245. B i.e. Glu by val in b6 **246. A i.e. Decreased Solubility**
247. C i.e. 'Sticky patch' is generated as a result of replacement of a non polar residue with a polar residue
[Ref: Harper 28th/ed pg-49, 357, 397-98; Lippincott 5/e p. 475-77; Robbins 7th/ed pg- 402, 628; Eichler medical Biochemistry (2006) p-44; Gribben-Molecular hematology (2009) pg-9; John Baynes & Marek Dominiczak medical Biochemistry 3/rd pg-53-55,438,475; Lehninger 5th/ed pg 168-69]

- **In sickle cell anemia- Glutamic acid is replaced by valine at sixth position in β - globin chainQ.**
- **Sticky patch** is generated as a result of **replacement of polar residue (negatively charged glutamate amino acid) with a nonpolar hydrophobic residue (valine)Q**. This change makes HbS (sickle cell hemoglobin) **less soluble, when deoxygenated and cause sicklingQ.**
- **HbS confers resistance against malaria in heterozygotesQ.**

248. ALL i.e. (RT-PCR, Denaturing gradient gel electrophoresis, DNA sequencing, Restriction fragment polymorphism (RFLP), Single-strand conformational polymorphism
249. B i.e. Ligase chain reaction
[Ref: Harrison's 18th/508-7; Harrison 17th/e/d p406; Eming's Elemens of Medical Genetics by Muller & Young P-63].

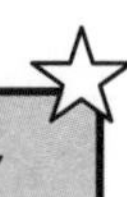

Mutations can be detected by DNA sequencing, PCR, RT PCR, single strand conformational polymorphism (SSCP), RFLP, and denaturing gradient gel electrophoresisQ.

Chapter -4 CYTOGENETICS AND MOLECULAR GENETICS, RECOMBINANT DNA & GENOMIC TECHNOLOGY

QUESTIONS

Cytogenetics

1. **The long and short arms of chromosomes are designated respectively as:** *(NBE P 13; AI 06)*
   A. p and q arms ☐
   B. m and q arms ☐
   C. q and p arms ☐
   D. 1 and s arms ☐
2. **Karyotyping under light microscopy is**
   A. L Banding *(AIIMS 14, 09)* ☐
   B. G banding ☐
   C. C Banding ☐
   D. FUdR banding ☐
3. **Rapid method of chromosome identification in intersex is:**
   A. FISH *(AIIMS 07)* ☐
   B. PCR ☐
   C. SSCP ☐
   D. Karyotyping ☐
4. **Which of the following technique can be used for exact localization of a genetic locus?** *(AIIMS 13)*
   A. Chromosome painting ☐
   B. Western blot ☐
   C. Comparative genomic hybridization ☐
   D. FISH ☐
5. **Subtelomeric rearrangement of genes is frequently associated wih mental retardation. All of the following techniques can be used to diagnose them except:**
   A. FISH *(AIIMS 15, 11)* ☐
   B. MAPH ☐
   C. cGH array ☐
   D. MALDI ☐
6. **Which of the following is used to detect the chromosomal differences between neoplastic cells and their normal counterparts?** *(NBE P 13, AIIMS 12)*
   A. PCR ☐
   B. Comparative genomic hybridization ☐
   C. Spectral karyotyping ☐
   D. Western blotting ☐
7. **Nanotechnology has found tremendous application in the diagnosis of cancers because of all of following advantages, except:** *(AIIMS 12)*
   A. Nanocrystals exibit bright, photostable fluorescence ☐
   B. Nanocrystals have a narrow spectrum wavelength ☐
   C. Peak spectrum wavelength is tunable ☐
   D. Nanocrystals exhibit a narrow difference between their excitation and emission peak spectra ☐
8. **Transfer of genetic material in 1 meiotic division between 2 non-homologous chromosomes:**
   A. Translocation *(PGI 12, 10)* ☐
   B. Non- disjunction ☐
   C. Inversion ☐
   D. Isochromose ☐
   E. Deletion ☐
9. **Aneuploidy is due to:** *(AI 04)*
   A. Non-disjunction at meiosis ☐
   B. Mosaicism ☐
   C. Deletion ☐
   D. Translocation ☐
10. **Differential expression of same gene depending on parent of origin is referred to as:** *(AI 08)*
    A. Genomic imprinting ☐
    B. Mosaicism ☐
    C. Anticipation ☐
    D. Nonpenetrance ☐
11. **Normal parent with 2 siblings having osteogenesis imperfecta. Pattern of inheritance is**
    A. Mutation *(AIIMS 10)* ☐
    B. Anticipation ☐
    C. Genomic imprinting ☐
    D. Germline mosacism ☐
12. **Prenatal diagnosis at 16 weeks of pregnancy can be performed using all of the following, except:**
    A. Amniotic fluid *(AI 06)* ☐
    B. Maternal blood ☐
    C. Chrionic villi ☐
    D. Fetal blood ☐
13. **Rich source of IgG is:** *(AIIMS 04)*
    A. Stomach ☐
    B. Visceral peritoneum ☐
    C. Small intestine ☐
    D. Large intestine ☐
14. **Rh factor is** *(AI 08)*
    A. IgM antibody ☐
    B. Mucppolysaccharide ☐
    C. IgG antibody ☐
    D. Fatty acid ☐
    E. Glycoprotein ☐
15. **Barr body is found in the following phase of the cell cycle:**
    A. Interphase *(AI 05)* ☐
    B. Metaphase ☐
    C. GI phase ☐
    D. Telophase ☐
16. **Movement of protein from nucleus to cytoplasm can be seen by** *(AIIMS 11)*
    A. FISH ☐
    B. FRAP ☐
    C. Confocal microscopy ☐
    D. Electron microscopy ☐

Luminescence

17. Fluorescence means *(AIIMS 11)*
- A. Spontaneous illumination in dark ☐
- B. Release of longer wavelength light on absorbing light of shorter wavelength ☐
- C. Release of shorter wavelength light on absorbing light of longer wavelength ☐
- D. Release of equal wavelength light at constant rate ☐

18. Which statement is incorrect? *(AIIMS 09)*
- A. Chemiluminescence: excited electron in higher orbit comes to lower orbit by emitting energy in form of photon ☐
- B. Bioluminescence: is a form of chemiluminescence ☐
- C. Photoluminiscence: absorbed radiation emitted as light ☐
- D. Electrophotochemiluminescence: Light-emitting reaction which take place by the use of electrical current ☐

19. Firefilies produce light due to: *(NBE P 13; AIIMS 08)*
- A. NADH ☐
- B. GTP ☐
- C. ATP ☐
- D. Phosphocreatinine ☐

20. Nephelometry is based on the principle of
- A. Light attenuated in intensity by scattering ☐
- B. Refraction of light *(AIIMS 07)* ☐
- C. Reduced transmission of light ☐
- D. Filtration of solutes by kidney ☐

21. DNA estimation can be done by *(AIIMS 12)*
- A. Spirometer ☐
- B. Spectrophotometer ☐
- C. pH meter ☐
- D. Sphygmometer ☐

22. Immunoflorescent probes are used in: *(PGI 15, 13)*
- A. FRET ☐
- B. Microarray ☐
- C. RIA ☐
- D. Recombinant DNA ☐
- E. ELISA ☐

Restriction Endonuclease

23. RFLP, True are: *(PGI 08)*
- A. Endonuclease cuts DNA at nucleotide level: ☐
- B. It acts at specific site ☐
- C. Only cohesive ends are produced ☐
- D. Only blunt ends are produced. ☐

24. Restrinction Endonucleas function → true about:
- A. Cut both the strands of ds DNA *(PGI 06)* ☐
- B. The cut ends produced are sticky ☐
- C. The cut ends produced are blunt. ☐
- D. Cuts single strand of DNA ☐

25. Restriction endonuclease is : *(NBE P 15, 13, AI 07)*
- A. Break single stranded DNA ☐
- B. Break double stranded DNA ☐
- C. Break peptide chain ☐
- D. Break RNA ☐

26. Correct statements regarding restriction endonuclease is/are: *(PGI 03)*
- A. Restriction endouclease recognizes specific sites of DNA sequence ☐
- B. Restriction endonuclease recognizes short sequence of DNA ☐
- C. It acts at 5' – 3' direction ☐
- D. It acts at 3' – 5' direction ☐

27. DNA fragments formed by the action of Restriction Endonucleases, are separated by: *(NBE P 14, AI 08)*
- A. Gel electrophoresis ☐
- B. Agarose gel eletrophoresis ☐
- C. Paper Chromatography ☐
- D. High pressure liquid chromatography ☐

28. DNA restriction is done by the following method:
- A. Paper chromatography *(AI 06)* ☐
- B. Electrophoresis agargel method ☐
- C. Spectrophotometer ☐
- D. Spectrometry ☐

29. After digestion by restriction endonucleases DNA strands can be joined again by *(AIIMS 11, 10)*
- A. DNA polymerase ☐
- B. DNA ligase ☐
- C. DNA topoisomerase ☐
- D. DNA gyrase ☐

30. True about Restriction enzymes: *(PGI 15, 09)*
- A. Palindromic ☐
- B. Produce DNA sticky end ☐
- C. Restrict replication of DNA ☐
- D. Restriction sites are not specific ☐
- E. Breaks at sugar-phosphate bond ☐

31. True statement about Restriction endonuclease:
- A. Palindromic sequences observed *(PGI 12)* ☐
- B. Protects bacteria from infection by virus ☐
- C. Present only in eukaryotes ☐
- D. Restrict replication of DNA ☐

32. Which of the following represents the most charachteristic function of Type II Restriction Enzyme
- A. Prevent folding of proteins *(NBE P 14, AI 12)* ☐
- B. Remove formed DNA ☐
- C. Prevent supercoiling ☐
- D. Cut DNA at palindromic sites ☐

33. True about DNA methylation: *(PGI 10)*
- A. Alters gene expression ☐
- B. Genetic code remains intact ☐
- C. Role in carcinogenesis ☐
- D. Protective mechanism against cleavage by restriction endonuclease ☐

34. Bacteria aquires restriction endonuclease by horizontal transfer. The result would be
- A. Bacteria can undergo mutation *(AIIMS 10)* ☐
- B. Bacteria causes death of host DNA ☐
- C. Bacteria cannot survive because it lacks DNA methylase that protects the host DNA ☐
- D. It helps in DNA proof reading in bacteria ☐

Polymorphism and RFLP

35. True about polymorphism is: *(PGI 14, 08)*
A. Single locus → multiple normal alleles ☐
B. Single locus → multiple abnormal alleles ☐
C. Single phenotype:Single locus → multiple normal alleles ☐
D. Single phenotype: Single locus → multiple abnormal alleles ☐

36. Correct statement about Restriction fragment gene
A. Detected by Southern blot *(PGI 15,11)* ☐
B. Detected by Northern blot ☐
C. Used for identification of gene for genomic mapping ☐
D. RFLP is a DNA variation sequence ☐

37. Restriction fragment length polymorphism is used for:
A. Analysis of chromosome structures *(AI 03)* ☐
B. DNA estimation ☐
C. Synthesis of nucleic acid ☐
D. Detecting proteins in a cell ☐

38. For measurement of long DNA molecules (50-100 KB) following is used *(NBE P 13, AIIMS 08)*
A. Chromosome walking ☐
B. Nitch ☐
C. RFLP ☐
D. SSLP ☐

39. RFLP, true is /are: *(PGI 06)*
A. Detects mutation ☐
B. Recognizes triuncleotide repeates ☐
C. Detects deletion ☐
D. Blunt ends are produced ☐
E. Always short ends are produced ☐

40. Microsatellite sequence is: *(NBE P 15, AI 06)*
A. Small satellite ☐
B. Extra chromosomal DNA ☐
C. Short sequence (2-5) repeat DNA ☐
D. Looped-DNA ☐

DNA Fingerprinting

41. DNA fingerprinting is based on possessing in DNA of:
A. Constant Tandem Repeat *(PGI 14, 08)* ☐
B. Variable Number Tandem Repeats (VNTR) ☐
C. Non- repeatative sequence ☐
D. Exon ☐
E. Intron in eukaryotes ☐

42. DNA fingerprinting was founded by: *(PGI 06)*
A. Watson ☐
B. Galton ☐
C. Jeffrey ☐

43. DNA finger printing is done by: *(PGI 07)*
A. Splitting DNA ☐
B. DNA of WBC ☐
C. DNA from nucleated cells ☐
D. All of the above ☐

PCR

44. True about polymerase chain reaction (PCR):
A. Carried out by thermostable DNA polymerase ☐
B. Exponential *(PGI 15, 09)* ☐
C. Additive ☐
D. Specific ☐
E. Single-stranded DNA is required ☐

45. In PCR: *(PGI 14, 08)*
A. Thermostable enzyme is needed ☐
B. 211 copies formed after 'n' numbers of multiple ☐
C. Non specific ☐
D. Thermolabile enzyme ☐
E. Primer is needed. ☐

46. True about polymerase chain reaction is:
A. Enzymatic DNA amplification *(NBE P 13, AI 09)* ☐
B. Recombinent DNA amplification ☐
C. Seperation of protein fragments is serum ☐
D. None ☐

47. Which of the following is not true about PCR:
A. Thermostable enzyme is used *(AI 04, PGI 05)* ☐
B. Annealing is done after DNA denaturation ☐
C. Specific primers re required ☐
D. Required atleast 1 week time for synthesis ☐
E. DNA polymerase has to be added on each cycle ☐

48. The enzyme used in polymerase chain reaction (PCR) is: *(AIIMS 09,13)*
A. Thermostable enzyme ☐
B. Enzyme stabiliser ☐
C. Inorganic ion ☐
D. Inorganic metal ☐

49. True statements about PCR: *(PGI 08)*
A. Protein amplification ☐
B. DNA amplification ☐
C. Same as western blot test ☐
D. Detection of infecting organisms ☐

50. True about PCR: *(PGI 13,10)*
A. Primers required ☐
B. DNA dependent RNA polymerase ☐
C. DNA polymerase ☐
D. RNA dependent DNA polymerase ☐

51. Enzyme(s) used in polymerase chain reaction is/are:
A. Restriction endonuclease *(PGI 11)* ☐
B. DNA polymerase ☐
C. Alkaline phosphate ☐
D. RNA polymerase ☐
E. Reverse transcriptase ☐

52. Which of the following is/are features of polymerase used in recombinant synthesis: *(PGI 2K)*
A. Thermostable ☐
B. Doesn't require primer ☐
C. Unusually active ☐
D. Replicates double stranded DNA ☐

53. In PCR Acquaticus thermophilus is preferred over E.coli. because: *(PGI 07)*
A. Thermostable at temperature at which DNA liquefies. ☐

B. Proof reading done. ☐
C. Done in more precisely. ☐
D. Does not require primer. ☐
E. Better DNA replication. ☐

54. True about DNA polymerase used in PCR: *(PGI 13)*
A. Obtained from virus ☐
B. Obtained from bacteria ☐
C. Used for joining the two strands ☐
D. It is heat stable ☐
E. Add nucleotide ☐

55. Which of the following is used in PCR? *(AIIMS 07)*
A. Ca++ *(NBE P 15)* ☐
B. Mg++ ☐
C. Li+ ☐
D. Na+ ☐

56. For PCR which of the following is not required:
A. Taq polymerase *(AIIMS 14)* ☐
B. d-NTP *(PGI 15; NBE P 14,13)* ☐
C. Primer ☐
D. Radiolabelled DNA probe ☐

57. For PCR which of the following is not required:
A. Taq polymerase *(NBE P 13, AIIMS 11)* ☐
B. d-NTP ☐
C. Dideoxynucleotides ☐
D. Magneswium ☐

58. SYBR Green Dye is used for: *(AIIMS 07)*
A. HPLC ☐
B. Immunofluorescence ☐
C. PCR ☐
D. ELISA ☐

59. Real time PCR is used for: *(AIIMS 13)*
A. Multiplication of RNA ☐
B. Multiplication of proteins ☐
C. Multiplication of specific segments of DNA ☐
D. To know how much amplification of DNA has occurred ☐

60. Prenatal diagnosis of Hemophilia is best done by:
A. PCR *(AI 10)* ☐
B. Linkage analysis ☐
C. Cytometry ☐
D. Microarray ☐

Ligase Chain Reaction

61. DNA Amplification is done in: *(PGI 06)*
A. PCR ☐
B. NASBA (Nucleic acid sequential based amplification) ☐
C. Ligase chain reactions ☐
D. DNA sequencing ☐

Cloning

62. In molecular cloning, Blue-white screening is used for:
A. To screen for recombinant vectors *(AIIMS 08)* ☐
B. To detect gene mutations ☐
C. To identify desired chromosomal DNA insert in plasmid vectors ☐
D. To detect host DNA in situ ☐

63. True about Monoclonal antibody: *(PGI 11, 08)*
A. Produced by hybridoma technology ☐
B. Non-specific ☐
C. Requires in small quantity ☐
D. Used for blood grouping ☐

64. True about Hybridoma: *(PGI 08)*
A. Immortalise myeloma cell ☐
B. Hybridoma cell produced by fusion of T-cell & myeloma ☐
C. Cell is of human origin ☐
D. Prior immunization is done ☐
E. Produce monospecific & monoclonal Ab ☐

65. Methods of producing fusion of cells are A/E
A. Attaching inactive viral particles on cell membrane ☐
B. Adding polyethylene glycol *(AIIMS 10)* ☐
C. Applying a small electric current *(AI 11)* ☐
D. Reducing surface tension ☐

66. In gene cloning, largest fragment can be incorporated in:
A. Plasmid *(AIIMS 05)* ☐
B. Bacteriophage ☐
C. Cosmid ☐
D. Retrovirus ☐

67. In DNA transfer the vectors used from smallest to largest is:
A. Cosmids, Plasmids, Bacteriophage *(PGI 07)* ☐
B. Plasmids, Bacteriophage, Cosmids ☐
C. Bacteriophage, Cosmides, Plasmids ☐
D. Cosmids, Bacteriophage, Plasmids ☐
E. Plasmids, Cosmids, Bacteriophage ☐

68. Which is true about phage DNA *(PGI 07)*
A. Antibiotic susceptibility ☐
B. Restriction enzyme sites ☐
C. Hexagonal DNA ☐
D. Carries short segment of DNA ☐

Site Directed Mutagenesis

69. Which test uses oligomer with single base pair substitution as primer *(AIIMS 09)*
A. PCR ☐
B. RFLP ☐
C. Error coded mutation analysis with PCR ☐
D. Site directed mutagenesis ☐

Site Specific Recombination

70. Site specific recombination is *(AIIMS 09)*
A. Palindromic ☐
B. Ser-form Holliday intermediate ☐
C. RE + ligase ☐
D. Inversion in same orientation / Non precise ☐

Linkage Analysis

71. Which of the following statement is true about Linkage analysis? *(AIIMS 07)*
A. Detection of Characteristic DNA polymorphism in a family is associated with disorders ☐
B. Useful to make pedigree chart to show affected and non-affected family members ☐
C. Used to make a pedigree chart to show non-paternity ☐
D. Non-Gene maping method of genetic study ☐

Analyzing Technique

72. True about western blot: *(PGI 11, 09)*
A. Separation of proteins are based on mass ☐
B. SDS-PAGE electrophesis is used for separation ☐
C. Enzyme linked antibodies are used ☐
D. Confirmatory in AIDS ☐

73. Antigen antibody reaction is detected by: *(PGI 09)*
A. ELISA ☐
B. Southern blot ☐
C. Northern blot ☐
D. Western blot ☐
E. Eastern blot ☐

74. Southern blot is used to visualize- *(NBE P 15,14)*
A. RNA ☐
B. DNA ☐
C. Protein ☐
D. Antibody ☐

75. Western blot technique is done for *(AIIMS 14, 09)*
A. Mitochondrial RNA ☐
B. Double strand DNA ☐
C. r- RNA ☐
D. Protein ☐

76. Nothern blot is used for the separation of: *(AI 07, NBE P 13)*
A. mRNA ☐
B. DNA ☐
C. Protein ☐
D. Protein DNA interaction ☐

77. Northern blot test is used for: *(NBE P 14, AIIMS 15, 08)*
A. DNA analysis ☐
B. RNA analysis ☐
C. Analysis of proteins ☐
D. Enzyme analysis ☐

78. Probe used in western blot: *(PGI 14, 08)*
A. Antibody ☐
B. M-RNA ☐
C. DNA ☐
D. t-RNA ☐
E. PCR ☐

79. The following methods can be used to detect the point mutation in the beta (β)-globin gene that causes sickle cell anemia, *except:* *(AI 06)*
A. Polymerase chain reaction with allele-specific oligonucleotide hybridization ☐
B. Southern blot analysis ☐
C. DNA sequencing ☐
D. Northern blot analysis ☐

80. Which of following techniques is used for detection of variations in DNA sequence and Gene expression: *(AI 11)*
A. Northern Blot ☐
B. Southern Blot ☐
C. Western Blot ☐
D. Microarray ☐

81. Which of the following tests is not used for detection of specific aneuploidy: *(AI 10)*
A. FISH ☐
B. RT-PCR ☐
C. QF-PCR ☐
D. Microarray ☐

82. Gene expression can be detected by all except: *(PGI 14,12,11)*
A. RT-PCR ☐
B. cDNA microarray ☐
C. Southern blot ☐
D. Northern blot ☐
E. Immunohistochemistry ☐

Gene Library

83. True about gene library: *(PGI 14,12,11)*
A. Also known as chromosome ☐
B. Library that contains books on gene ☐
C. Computer base with all gene knowledge ☐
D. DNA Nucleotide or fragment ☐
E. Complete collection of gene copies of one organism ☐

Recombinant DNA Technology or Genetic Engineering

84. Biotechnology is/are used for *(PGI 09)*
A. Viral vaccine production ☐
B. To cure genetic disorder ☐
C. Genetic crop ☐
D. Gene production ☐
E. Production of genetic products ☐

85. Starting material for production of insulin from bacteria is: *(AIIMS 11)*
A. Genomic DNA from beta pancreatic cells of human ☐
B. Genomic DNA from lymphocytes of human ☐
C. mRNA from beta pancreatic cells of human ☐
D. mRNA from lymphocytes of human ☐

86. Reverse transcriptase is: *(PGI 11)*
A. DNA dependent RNA polymerase ☐
B. RNA dependent DNA polymerase ☐
C. DNA dependent DNA polymerase ☐
D. RNA dependent RNA polymerase ☐
E. RNA polymerase ☐

87. True about DNA reconstruction technology: *(PGI 08)*
A. Restriction endonucleases involved ☐
B. DNA ligase is used ☐
C. Acid phosphatase is used ☐
D. Reverse transcriptase needed ☐

88. Enzymes used in DNA research programme are except: *(PGI 07)*
A. Polymerase ☐
B. Exonuclease ☐
C. Nuclease ☐

D. Alkaline phosphatase ☐
E. None ☐

89. Which of the following is a strategy used to increase the yield of protein produced in recombinant protein synthesis?
A. Promoter induction *(AI 11)* ☐
B. Genes for protease inhibitors ☐
C. Translation initiation ☐
D. Translation and transcription termination ☐

90. Study of structure and products of gene is:
A. Genomics *(PGI 05)* ☐
B. Protenomics ☐
C. Bioinformatics ☐
D. Cytogenetics ☐
E. Pharmacogenomics ☐

91. Study of multiplication of proteins in disease process is called: *(AI 07)*
A. Proteomics ☐
B. Genomics ☐
C. Glycomics ☐
D. Nucleomics ☐

92. Techniques used for protein expression proteomics study include(s): *(PGI 12)*
A. Gene Array Chips ☐
B. Mass Spectroscopy ☐
C. PolyAcrylamide Gel Electrophoresis (PAGE) ☐
D. RT-PCR ☐
E. Two-Dimensional Electrophoresis ☐

Transgenic Organism

93. Mutation that completely disrupt the function of the gene used in which of the following technique:
A. Knock-out *(PGI 09)* ☐
B. Non-sense mutation ☐
C. Restrictin fragment length polymorphism ☐
D. Targeted gene disruption ☐
E. Knock –in ☐

94. True statement about transgenic mice: *(PGI 10)*
A. Developed from DNA insertion into fertilized egg ☐
B. Have same genome as parents except one or more genes ☐
C. Identical genome to parent mice ☐
D. Produced by breeding over several generations ☐
E. Homozygous are selected ☐

95. Which of the following methods is most suited to assess function of a gene: *(AI 12)*
A. Southern blot ☐
B. Northern blot ☐
C. Gene knockout animals ☐
D. Transgenic animals ☐

96. Nude mouse is used in genetics because of the following properties: *(PGI 11)*
A. Absence of thymus ☐
B. Xenograft can be sustained for weeks ☐
C. Severe combined immunodeficiency mice is same as nude mice ☐

97. Two transgenic plants are grown. One plant has a gene encoding a fluorescent pigment incorporated in its genome. The other plant has a fire fly luciferase gene incorporated in its genome. Which of the two plants will glow in the dark?
A. Both plants will glow *(AI 11)* ☐
B. Neither will glow ☐
C. First one will glow ☐
D. Second one will glow ☐

Gene Therapy

98. Purpose of Gene therapy: *(PGI 03)*
A. Replacement of abnormal gene by normal gene ☐
B. Replacement of normal gene by abnormal gene ☐
C. Knock out of abnormal gene ☐
D. Introduction of viral gene ☐

99. Gene therapy methods are: *(PGI 03)*
A. Electroporation ☐
B. Intranuclear injection ☐
C. Site directed mutagenesis ☐
D. Retrovirus ☐

100. The first gene therapy (somatic enzyme) was successfully done in: *(PGI 07)*
A. SCID ☐
B. Phenylketonuria ☐
C. Thalassemia ☐
D. Cystic fibrosis ☐
E. Alkaptonuria ☐

Genetic Disorder

101. True abut 'X' Chromosome inactivation:
A. X gene *(PGI 06)* ☐
B. RNA interference ☐
C. Seen in Male ☐
D. Seen in Female ☐

102. Which of the following are X- linked recessive disorders:
A. Marfan Syndrome *(PGI 08)* ☐
B. Phenylketonuria ☐
C. Neurofibromatosis ☐
D. Duchenne muscular dystrophy ☐
E. G-6-P dehydrogenase deficiency ☐

103. Father to son inheritance is never seen in case of:
A. Autosomal dominant inheritance *(AIIMS 03)* ☐
B. Autosomal recessive inheritance ☐
C. X- linked recessive inheritance ☐
D. Multifactorial inheritance

104. An affected male infant born to normal parents could be an example of all of the following, *except:* *(AI 06)*
A. An Autosomal dominant disorder ☐
B. An Autosomal recessive disorder ☐
C. A polygenic disorder ☐
D. A vertically transmitted disorder ☐

105. Autosomal recessive disease are: *(PGI 08)*
A. Tuberous sclerosis ☐

B. Duchenne muscular dystrophy ☐
C. Cystic fibrosis ☐
D. Ataxia telangiectasia ☐
E. Factor VIII deficiency ☐

106. A child with a small head, minor anomalies of the face including a thin upper lip, growth delay, and developmental disability can have all of the following, *except*: *(AI 06)*
A. A chromosomal syndrome ☐
B. A teratogenic syndrome ☐
C. A mendelian syndrome ☐
D. A polygenic syndrome ☐

107. In a family, the father has widely spaced eyes, increased facial hair and deafness. One of the three children has deafness with similar facial features. The mother is normal. Which one of the following is most likely pattern of inheritance in this case? *(AI 06)*
A. Autosomal dominant ☐
B. Autosomal recessive ☐
C. X-linked dominant ☐
D. X-linked recessive ☐

108. Gene for major histocompatibility complex and HLA gene is located on: *(AIIMS 08, 09)*
A. Long arm of chromosome 8. ☐
B. Short arm of chromosome 8 ☐
C. Long arm of chromosome 6 ☐
D. Short arm of chromosome 6 ☐

109. True about MHC: *(PGI 03)*
A. Transplantation reaction ☐
B. Autoimmune disease ☐
C. Immunosupression ☐
D. Involved in T-cell function ☐
E. Situated at long arm of chromosome ☐

110. MHC class II antigens are located on which of the following cells: *(PGI 2K)*
A. Platelets ☐
B. Dendritic cell ☐
C. RBC ☐
D. T-cell ☐
E. G-cell ☐
F. B-cell ☐

111. MHC II is/are presented by: *(PGI 12)*
A. Macrophage ☐
B. Dendritic cells ☐
C. Lymphocyte ☐
D. Epithelial cells ☐
E. Platelets ☐

112. Which of the follwoing molecular phenomenon in I_g genes is responsible for affinity maturation of antibody response
A. Chain shuffling *(AI 08)* ☐
B. Junctional diverity ☐
C. Somatic hypermutation ☐
D. Altered RAA splicing ☐

ANSWERS & EXPLANATIONS:

Cytogenetics

1. **C i.e. q and p arms** *[Ref: Robbins 7th/170-73; http://www.ring-chromosome-20.org/what_are_chromosomes.aspx]*

The short arm of chromosome is desingated as 'p' (for petit) and the long arm is refered to as 'q' (the next letter of alphabet).

2. **B i.e. G banding** *[Ref: Nagesh Rao: Human genetics (1988) 78. 21-26]*
3. **A i.e. FISH** *[Ref: Robbin's 7/e p. 171- 73; http://members.aol.com/chrominfo/fishinfo.htm]*

FISH, chromosome painting and spectral karyotyping (SKY) are rapid methods of chromosome identification[Q].

4. **D i.e. FISH** *[Ref: Harper 29/e p. 442]*

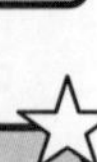

- **Gene maping** localizes specific gene to distinct chromosomes and thus define a **map of human genome.** This **exact localization of genetic locus can be done by FISH** (very sensitive technique which utilizes fluorescence rather than radioactively labeled porbes), **somatic cell hybridization** and **in situ hybridization** (simpler, more direct procedure adding **radioactive probe to metaphase spread chromosome**).
- **Chromosomal painting** hybridizes multiple (coloured) fluorescent labeled DNA probes to chromosomal DNA. This produces a **multicolored or painted effect** with a unique color at each site of hybridization in metaphase or inter phase cells. So CP identifies both **numerical & structural choromosomal aberrations** with high sensitivity and specificity.

5. **D i.e. MALDI** *[Ref: Teitz 6/e p 1225-28; Harrison 18/e p 510-12 665; Harper 29/e p-442]*

Subtelomeric rearrangements of gene eg chromosomal duplications or deletions too small to be detected by conventional cytogentic analysis are detected by **c-GH (comparative genomic hybridization), multiprobe FISH (fluorescence in situ hybridization), MAPH** (multiplex amplifable probe hybridization) and **MLPA** (multiplex ligation-dependent probe amplification). Subtelomeric rearrangements are significant cause of idiopathic & familial mental retardation.

6. **B i.e. Comparative genomic hybridization**

Comparative genomic hybridization (FISH-CGH) can be **used to detect chromosomal differences between neoplastic cells and their counterparts[Q].**

7. **B i.e. Nanocrystals have a narrow spectrum wavelength**

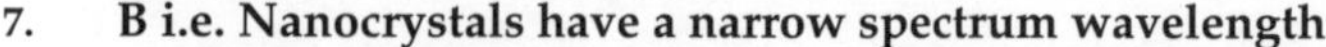

Nanocrystals (or Quantum dots) are inorganic, semiconductor crystals which exhibits ***very bright (strong) photostable fluorescence emissions***[Q]. It can be used as fluorescent probes in biological staining and diagnosis. Compared with conventional fluophores; the nanocrystals are **photochemically & optically stable (i.e. very durable)** and their ***electronic & optical properties (i.e. absorption band and emission spectra wave length) can be adjusted (or tuned) by changing their size***[Q] or by growing it smaller or larger. So nanocrystal size controls a **widely tunable absorption band resulting in widely tunable emission spectra**. So ***nanocrystals have tunable broad & continuous excitation spectrum (i.e. broad spectrum wave length)***[Q] because of greater chemical (size) flexibility. **But they have a narrow, tunable (adjustable), symmetric emission (peak) spectra** (in comparison to conventional fluorophores).

8. **A i.e. Translocation** *[Ref: Robbins 7/e p-173 –75; Harrison 16/e p. 384- 85]*
9. **A i.e. Non disjunction at meiosis**

- **Aneuploidy** is a condition in which a cell contains other than haploid number of chromosomes or an exact multiple of it. It produced by ***non- disjunction of chromosomes at meiosis***[Q] and is *common in cancer cells.*
- Term *'Ploidy'* is used to refer number of chromosomes in cells. *Euploid*: Normal resting diploid cell. *Tetraploid*: Cells just before division.

Cytogenetic Disorders (Chromosomal Mutations)

I. Due to abnormal number of chromosomes

- **Euploid** means any exact multiple of haploid number (23) and **aneuploidy** means chromosomes *not in exact multiple of 23.*
- The usual cause of aneuploidy are

Non disjunction

Occurs when a ***homologous pair of chromosome fails to disjoin at 1st meiotic division***[Q], or two chromatids fail to seperate either at 2nd meiotic division or in somatic cell divisions resulting in 2 aneuploid cells. If this occurs in gametogenesis, gametes formed have either *an extra (n+1) or one less (n-1) chromosome*. Fertilization of such gametes by normal gametes result in – **trisomic (2n+1)** or **monosomic (2n-1)** zygotes

Anaphase lag

- ***One homologous chromosome in meiosis or one chromatid in mitosis lags behind***[Q] & is left out of cell nucleus. The result is one normal cell and one with monosomy
- All autosomal monosomies are fatal d/t loss of too much genetic information
- Monosomies & trisomies of sex chromosomes & trisomy of 21 autosomal chromosome are compatabile with life.

Deletion

II. D/t alteration in structure of chromosomes

- **Deletion** means *loss of portion of chromosome* & may be of 2 types
  - **Terminal deletion** at ends
  - **Interstitial deletion** refers to 2 breaks within chromosome arms f/b loss of material b/w the breaks & fusion of broken ends (most common type)
- **Ring chromosome** is special form of deletion, produced when break occurs at both ends of chromosomes with fusion of damaged ends.
- **Inversion** refers to rearrangement that involves two breaks within single chromosome with *inverted reincorporation of segment.*
  - **Paracentric** inversion involves only one arm of chromosome
  - **Pericentric inversion** has breaks on opposite side of centromere
- **Isochromosome** results when one arm of chromosome is lost and the other is duplicated resulting in a chromosome containing *2 short arms or 2 long arms only*. Most common isochromosome (in live birth) involves long arm of X [i (x) (q 10)]. & is associated with monosomy for genes on short arm of X and trisomy for genes on long arm of X
- **Translocation** l/t ***transfer of a segment of chromosome to another nonhomologous chromosome***[Q]
  - **Reciprocal translocation** is ***mutual swapping of ends between any two non homologous chromosomes***[Q]. It may be balanced or unbalanced (eg during meiosis).
  - **Robertsonian translocation (or centric fusion)** is *tanslocation b/w two acrocentric chromosomes (13, 14, 15, 21, & 22).* The *break occurs close to centromere* of each chromosome and transfer of segments l/t one very long & one extremely small chromosome. 14-21 fusion may cause Down syndrome.

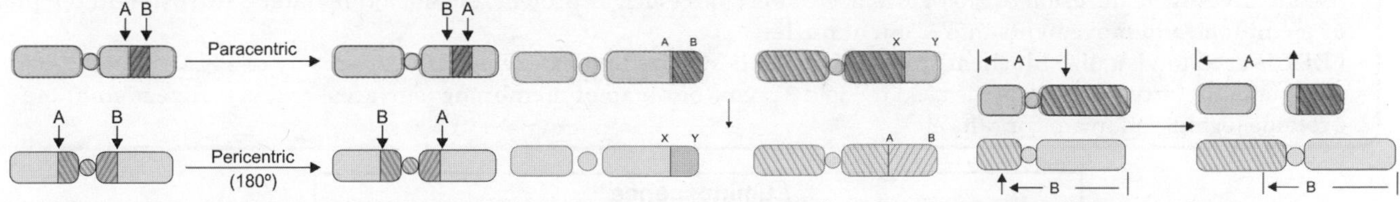

10. A i.e. Genomic Imprinting *[Ref: Robbins 7/e p 186; Harrison 16/e p. 375]* **11. D i.e. Germline mosacism**

- **Differential expression of same gene depending on parent of origin is referred to as genomic imprinting.**
- **Germline (Gonadal) mosaicism** results from a mutation **only affecting cells destined to form gonads – postzygotically during early embryonic development. So the individual (parent) is phenotypically normal but can transmit the disease to offsprings through mutant gametes**[Q]. And because the progenitor cells of gametes carry mutation, there is a high possibility that more than 1 child of such parent would be affected.

Genomic Imprinting

It is selective *inactivation of a gene or set of genes on either the maternal or paternal chromosome*Q. It occurs in ovum or sperm before fertilization & then is stabily transmitted to all somatic cells through mitosis and so can be of two types

Maternal genomic imprinting

- It is **inactivation of maternal allele (genes or chromosome)** Q
- Paternal allele are functional
- Example is **Angleman syndrome**Q

Paternal genomic impringint

- It is inactivation of paternal allele (gene or chromosome)
- Functional allele are provided by only maternal chromosomes
- Example is **Prader Willi Syndrome**Q

12. **D i.e. Fetal blood** *[Ref: Dutta 6th/108; www.americanpregnancy.org/prenatal testing]*

'Cordocentesis is performed under local anaesthetic usually after 18 weeks of gestation'-Dutta 6th/108
Cordocentesis is a procedure that takes a blood sample from one of the blood vessels in the baby's umbilical cord, to directly test the baby's blood. **Cordocentesis can only be done later in the pregnancy, from about 18-24 weeks, when the umbilical cord has adequately developed.**

Prenatal diagnosis

Chorionic villus sampling (choronic villi)	Amniocentesis (Amniotic fluid)	MSAFP (Maternal blood)	Cordocentesis (Fetal blood)
10-12 weeks 10weeks to term (transabdominal)	14-16 weeks	15-18 weeks	18-20 weeks.

Prenatal diagnosis at 16weeks can therefore be performed using all of the above except fetal blood.

13. **C i.e. Small intestine** (Most probably) Most abundant immunoglobin in blood → IgG.
14. **A i.e. IgM antibody >> E i.e. Glycoprotein** *[Ref: Harrison 17/e p. 2155; Chakraborty Microbiology 1/e p. 141; Davidson 20/e p. 1074]*

- **Rheumatoid (Rh) factor** in rheumatoid arthritis is an ***autoantibody of IgM class directed against Fc fragment of IgG***Q.

- Antibodies (immunoglobins) are *glycoproteins*. And Rh factors is an autoantibody of any immunoglobin class directed against Fc fragment of IgG immunoglobin (Davidson).

15. **A i.e. Interphase** *[Ref: Tortora Principles of Anatomy & Physiology 10/e P-1098; Robbins 7/e P-178; Chandrasoma Taylor 3/e P- 227]*

The inactive X can be seen in the interphase nucleus as a darkly staining small mass in contact with the nuclear membrane known as the Barr body or X chromatin. Barr body is the inactivated X chromosome. In non dividing interphase cells it remains tightly coiled and can be seen as a dark staining body within the nucleus.

16. **B i.e. FRAP** *[Ref: Lehninger 5/e p 383, 434-36, 760]*

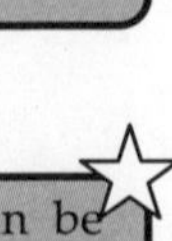

- **FRAP (fluorescence recovery after photobleaching)** primarily measures **rate of lateral diffusion** of lipids and it can be used to investigate diffusion of biological macromolecules (such as proteins etc) including **lateral diffusion in the plane of membrane and movements into & out of nucleus.**
- **FRET** is used to **visualize biochemistry of living cells such as to measure cAMP and activity of PKA.**
- **AFM (atomic force microscopy)** is used to yield **3D contour map of membrane (surfaces) and visualize membrane proteins** (eg microdomains or rafts etc)

Luminescence

17. **B i.e. Release of longer wavelength light on absorbing light of shorter wavelength**
18. **None** *[Ref: Lehninger 5th/e p. 435, 509; Teitz 6th/ed pg- 63, 79-80, 167-68, 179]*

Fluorescence means release of longer wavelength (lower energy) light on absorbing light of shorter wave length (higher energy)Q

19. **C i.e. ATP** *[Ref: Lehninger 5th/ed pg- 509, 332; Teitz 6th/ed pg -79]*

In **firefly, ATP** is used in a set of reactions that **convert chemical energy into light energy**[Q]. So fire fly flashes are glowing reports of ATP **(i.e. flashes in firefly indicate presence of ATP & SOLIFE)**[Q]

20. **A i.e. Light attenuated in intensity by scattering** *[Ref: Tietz 6/e p. 80-179]*

Nephelometry determines turbidity by measuring intensity of scattered light[Q].

When light passes through a medium with dispersed particles of different refractive index, it is attenuated in intensity by scattering. The intensity of scattered light depends on *its wave length & particle size*. However scattering is *directly proportional to the concentration of particulate matter*. This principal is used to measure turbidity by;

Turbidimetry	Nephelometry
Intensity of unscattered transmitted light is measured[Q]	***Intensity of scattered light***[Q] usually but not necessarily at right angle to the incident beam is measured.

21. **B i.e. Spectrophotometer** *[Ref: Lehninger 5/e p. 78; Teitz 5/e p 152]*

Quantitative estimation of DNA (or RNA) can be done by **UV spectrophotometer at about 260** (-280nm) and **densitometry** (after gel electrophoresis).

22. **A i.e. FRET; B i.e. Microarray; C i.e. RIA; E i.e. ELISA** *[Ref: Chatterjea 8/e p. 834; Lippincott 6/e p. 472]*

Immunoflorescent probes are used in **radioimmunoassay** (RIA), immunoradiometric assay (IRMA), **ELISA**, FIA (fluorescence IA), chemiluminescence (C)IA, **FRET (fluorescence resonance energy transfer)** and **microarray.**

Restriction Endonuclease

23. **B i.e. It acts at specific site**
24. **A i.e. Cut both strands of ds DNA; B i.e. Cut ends produced are sticky; C i.e. Cut end produced ..**
25. **B i.e. Break double stranded DNA**
26. **A i.e. Restriction endonuclease recognizes specific sites of DNA; B i.e. Restriction endonuclease reconises short sequence of DNA**
27. **B i.e. Agarose gel electrophoresis**
28. **B i.e. Electrophoresis agar gel method**
29. **B i.e. DNA ligase**
30. **A, B, C, E i.e. Palindromic, Produce DNA sticky end, Restrict replication of DNA, Breaks at sugar-phosphate..**
31. **A, B, D i.e. Palindromic sequences observed; Protects bacteria from infection by virus; Restrict replication ...**
32. **D i.e. Cut DNA at palindromic sites** *[Ref: Harper 29/e p 434-36; Chatterjea 7/e 261-63; Lippincott 5/e 465-66; Lehninger 5/304-7,1052-55]*

- **Restriction endonuclease (restriction enzyme)** makes 2 incisions through **sugar phosphate backbone (phospho diester bond) of each strand of ds DNA**[Q] at specific sequence k/a **recognition sequences or restriction site.** So **RE restricts viral (bacteriophage - DNA) replication**[Q] **and protects bacteria (prokaryote) from infection by virus**[Q].
- RE cuts both strands of double stranded (ds) DNA at specific restriction sites with **palindromic (inverse repeat)** arrangement; thus producing smaller, manageable fragments with short sequenes and **sticky / blunt ends**[Q]. These restriction fragments can be **isolated by agarose gel /polyacrylamide – electrophoresis**[Q] or HPLC.
- **After digestion by restriction endonucleases the DNA ends can be ligated (joined / annealed) by ' DNA-ligase**[Q]

Features	Type I RE	Type III RE	Type II RE
Structure, components & activities	**Single large, multisubunit, multifunctional** enzyme containing both **endonuclease (nuclease) & methylase activities in one enzyme**	**Single large, multisubunit, multifunctional** enzyme containing both **endonuclease (nuclease) & methylase activities in one enzyme**	Simple **homodimers** (2 identical proteins linked together) with **separate nuclease & methylase** activities (ie both not in one enzyme).
Nuclease subunit structure & Requirements for cleavage	- **Hetero – trimer** - **Require ATP** for cleavage - Cofactors **ATP, Mg^{++}, SAM** - **2** recognizition sites in **any orientation**	- **Hetero-dimer** - **ATP not required** for cleavage - Cofactors **Mg^{++}, SAM** - **2** recognizition sites in **head to head orientation**	- **Homodimer** - ATP not required for cleavage - Cofactors **Mg^{++}** - **Single** recognizition site

Site of DNA cleavage and methylation	- Cleaves at **random sites that can be > 1000 base pairs** (bp) away from recognition sequence (RS) - Methylates at RS	- Cleaves DNA, 25 bp (24-26) from recognition site (towards 3′ end) - Methylates at RS	- Cleaves DNA within recognized sequence itself (ie at or near RS) - Methylates at RS
DNA translocation	- Present - **Require ATP for moving along DNA**	- Absent - Require ATP for moving along DNA	- Absent - **Require no ATP**
Restriction modification	By single multifunctional enzyme	By separate enzymes sharing a common subunit	Separate restriction (nuclease) & modification (methylase)
Enzyme turnover	Absent	Absent	Present

Type II RE is first isolated by Hamilton Smith (Beta Hind 1) and Daniel Nathans first used them to cut DNA for mapping & analyzing genes & genome.

33. **A i.e. Alters gene expression; B i.e. Genetic code remains intact; C i.e. Role in carcinogenesis; D i.e. Protective mechanism against cleavage by restriction endonuclease** *[Ref: Lehninger 5/e 994-96, 292, 223, 233; Wikipedia]*

- **DNA methylation alters the gene expression** pattern in cells-for example it may cause ***X-chromosome inactivation, tumor suppressor gene silencing (in cancer cells)***[Q], suppression of expression of repetitive clements / deleterious elements / viral genes that have been incorporated into genome of host over time
- E. coli has 2 prominent **DNA methylation system**, both using *S-adenosyl methionine (SAM) as a methyl group donor.*
- Adenine or cytosine methylation in **restriction – modification system**, serves as ***a part of defence mechanism against cleavage by restriction endonuclease***[Q]. It helps the cell to distinguish its DNA from foreign DNA by marking its own DNA with methyl group and destroying (foreign) DNA without the methyl group.
- **Mismatch repair** mediated by Dam methylase improves the overall fidelity of DNA replication by fctor of $10^2 – 10^3$. **Dam** (**D**NA **a**denine **M**ethylation) methylase, methylates adenosine residue to N^6- methyl adenosine within the palindromic (5^1) GATC (3) sequence. This can serve to distinguish parent/template strand (which is methylated) from unmethylated (transient state) newly synthesized strand. So replication mismatch in vicinity of hemi-methylated GATC sequence are then repaired a/t the information the methyated parent strand.
- In eukaryotic cells ~ *5% of cytidine* in DNA are methylated to 5 methyl cytidine. Methylation is most common it **CpG islands** (a *C G rich region,* upstream of promoter region and P signifies *phosphodiester bond between them*) producing methyl –CpG symmetrically on both strands of DNA.

34. **C i.e. Bacteria cannot survive because it lacks DNA methylase that protects the host DNA**

- Any bacteria is protected against its own restriction endonuclease (RE) by a companion enzyme **site specific DNA *methylase which methylates the restriction sites recognized by that particular RE***[Q]. In other wors, every bacteria has its own pair of RE & site specific DNA methylase
- So if any **bacteria aquires new / different RE by horizontal transfer (i.e. from other bacteria)** this restriction enzyme will ***cleave (lyse) the bacterial DNA and kill bacteria***[Q] because the restriction sites for this RE are not methylated & protected.

Polymorphism and RFLP

35. **C i.e., Single phenotype, single locus, multiple normal allelle**
[Ref: Harper's 27/e p. 413-16; Lippincott's 4/e p. 473-79; Robbins 7/e p. 189-91, 146, 150]

Polymorphism is presence of **single normal phenotype with multiple normal allele (DNA sequence varioations) in single locus (site)**[Q] in >1% population.

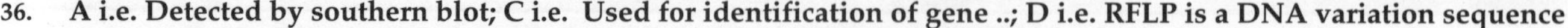

36. **A i.e. Detected by southern blot; C i.e. Used for identification of gene ..; D i.e. RFLP is a DNA variation sequence**
37. **A i.e. Analysis of Chromosal structure** 38. **C i.e. RFLP**
39. **A i.e. Detects Mutation B i.e., Recognizes trinucleotide repeats C i.e., Detects deletion D i.e., Blunt end produced**
[Ref: Lehninger 5/e p 319; Lippincot 5/e p 474-76]

- **RFLP** is a ***DNA sequence variation observed by cleaving the DNA into fragments by restriction endonuclease (RE) enzyme***[Q]. These restriction fragments are separated by **agarose gel electrophoresis on the basis of size** and detected by ***southern blot***[Q].
- **RFLP results from single nucleotide polymorphism (SNPs), single base changes (mutation), deletions, insertions (copy number variations = CNVs), length polymorphism / variable number of tandem repeats (VNTR),** like mini satellite repeats and microsatellite or **short tandem repeats (STR)**. All of these *result in gain / loss of a restriction site; thereby producing an extra / fewer fragments.*

- RE cuts both strands of double stranded (ds) DNA at specific restriction sites with **palindromic (inverse repeat)** arrangement; thus producing smaller, manageable fragments with short sequenes and ***sticky (cohesive, overlapping, staggered)/ blunt ends***Q. These restriction fragments can be ***isolated by agarose gel /polyacrylamide – electrophoresis***Q or HPLC.
- RFLP is used for ***identification of gene for genomic maping***Q, **establishing linkage (thus analyzing chromosomal structure** and measurement / identification of DNA fragments or molecules of different size), which by process of **chromosomal walking** will eventually **define disease locus and isolate any gene in unknown location** of large DNA.

40. **C i.e. Short sequence (2-5) repeat DNA** *[Ref: Robbins 7th/307; Harrisons 16th/449; http://oneweb.utc.edu/~Margaret-Kovach/microsat.html]*

'Microsatellites are tandem repeats of one to six nucleotides scattered throughout the genome'

DNA Fingerprinting

41. **B i.e. Variable Number Tandem Repeats (VNTR)**

Variable number of tandem (one after another) repeats (VNTR), is unique for any individual & therefore serves as **molecular DNA finger print.** VNTR may be short tandem (microsatellite) or large tandem (minisatellite) repeats.

42. **C i.e. Jeffrey** 43. **D i.e. All of the above** *[Ref: Lehninger 5/e p. 319-21; Lippincott's 5/e p. 83, 475; Harper 28/e p. 404]*

PCR

44. **A, B, D i.e. Carried out by thermostable DNA polymerase; Exponential; Specific**
45. **A & E i.e. Thermostable enzyme is needed & Primer is needed.** 46. **A i.e. Enzymatic DNA amplification**
47. **D i.e. Required atleast 1 week time for synthesis; E i.e. DNA polymerase has to ....** 48. **A i.e. Thermostable enzyme**
49. **B i.e. DNA amplification; D i.e. Detection of infecting organism** 50. **A i.e. Primers required, C i.e. DNA polymerase**
51. **B i.e. DNA Polymerase** 52. **A i.e. Thermostable, D i.e. Replicates double stranded DNA**
53. **A i.e. Thermostable at temperature..** 54. **B i.e. Obtained from bacteria; D i.e. It is heat stable; E i.e. Add nucleotide**
55. **B i.e. Mg^{++}** 56. **D i.e. Radiolabelled DNA probe** 57. **C i.e. Dideoxynucleotides** 58. **C i.e. PCR**

[Ref: Vassudevan 6th/e p. 616-18; Lehninger 5th/e p. 317-18; Chattarjea 7th/e p. 267-72; Harper 28th/e p. 395, 319; Lippincott 5th/e p. 479-82; Harrison 17th /1764; Harrison's 18th/2312]

- **Polymerase chain reaction (PCR)** is a **sensitive, selective (specific), and exponentially rapid (2^{cycle}) in-vitro** (test tube) **enzymatic method** of **amplifying (xeroxing) a desired (selected or target) DNA sequence**Q of 50 base pairs to 10 kb.
- **Each cycle** of heat **denaturation (separation /melting) → priming (annealing) → polymerization, doubles the amount of double stranded DNA**Q. PCR uses a **pair of primers** (synthetic oligonucleotide of 20-35 bp; one for each strand), **all 4 dXTPs or dNTPs (deoxy neucleoside triphosphate of A,G,C,T) in excess, heat stable DNA polymerase such as thermostable Taq polymerase** derived from Thermus aquaticus bacteria that lives at 90°C and **magnesium (Mg++) ion.** The advantage of thermostability is that the **enzyme itself is not denatured & therefore does not have to be added at each successive cycle**Q.
- **DNA polymerase used in PCR** is **obtained from bacteria (not virus), is heat stable and adds nucleotide to 3' OH end of primer**Q (not joins strands).
- **Probes are required in blot (southern, western, northern) tests but not in PCR**Q**. PCR uses Taq Man, molecular becon & syber Green dyes**Q**.**

59. **D i.e. To know how much amplification of DNA has occurred**

PCR is a method of amplifying DNA. And **real time (RT)-PCR** as well as **realtime quantitative (RQ) PCR** are **used to know how much amplification of DNA has occurred** because the increase in fluorescence signal is directly proportional to the amount of PCR product.

60. **A i.e. PCR** *[Ref: Hall – Advances in genetics (1995) vol 32 p-121; Chen. Atlas of genetic diagnosis & counciling (2006) p-478]*

- **Prenatal diagnosis of hemophilia (and diseases in which mutation nucleotide sequence is known like sickle cell anemia, cystic fibrosis, β-thallasemia etc)** is **best** done by **direct mutation analysis using PCR**Q, in chorionic villus sample (at 11-13 weeks) because it specifically identifies mutation or base pair change responsible for disease with out analyzing multiple family members.
- However **indirect, linkage analysis** can also be used for prenatal diagnosis but its uses has been restricted to genetic disorder if mutant gene is not known. Because it is less specific and requires analysis of multiple family members.

Ligase Chain Reaction

61. **A i.e. PCR > B i.e. NASBA; C i.e. Ligase chain reaction** *[Ref: Lippincott]s 4/e p. 479-83; Chatterjea 7/e p. 267- 71; Robbins 7/e p- 361]*

DNA amplification techniques include – **polymerase chain reaction (PCR), real time PCR, nucleic acid sequence based amplification (NASBA), ligase chain reaction (LCR) and Gap LCR**Q. These are also k/a nucleic acid amplification tests (NAAT's).

Cloning

62. **C i.e. To identify desired chromosomal DNA insert in plasmid vectors.**
63. **A i.e. Produced by hybridoma technology; C i.e Requires in small quantity; D i.e. Used for blood grouping**
64. **A, D, & E i.e. Immortalise myeloma cell, Prior immunization is done & myeloma & Produce monospecific & monoclonal Ab** *[Ref: Harper 29/e p 647-48; Vasudevan 6/e p 617]*

- **Hybridoma** is an **immortal (permanent) cell**Q produced by **cell fusion of B cells (previously immunized or injected with antigen) and myeloma cells of mouse**Q (or suitable animal). It produces **monospecific monoclonal antibodies**Q which can be **humanized** (used in humans) by attaching the complementarity – determined regions [CDRs], (the site that binds antigens) onto appropriate sites in human immunoglobulin molecule. Attempts to produce human monoclonal antibodies are underway.
- **Monoclonal antibodies** are produced by **hybridoma technology (in vitro)** or by one clone secreting specific type of antibody in **multiple myeloma (in vivo)**. It is **required in minute (only microliter) quantities and can be used for blood grouping**Q.

65. **D i.e. Reducing surface tension** *[Ref: Harper 28/e 580]*

Cell fusion (eg. as used in hybridoma technique to produce monoclonal antibodies) can be brought about by

- **Exposure to polyethylene glycol gel**Q
- **Electric field induced (i.e. applying small electric current) cell fusion**Q
- Laser induced cell fusion
- **Attaching inactive viral particles**Q like inactivated rota virus and Sendai virus.

66. **C i.e. Cosmid** *[Ref: Harper's 27/e P-406-08]*

Larger fragment of DNA can be **cloned in cosmide**Q as it combine the best features of plasmide & phage.

67. **B i.e. Plasmid, bacteriophage, cosmid** *[Ref: Chattergea 7/e p. 262]*

★ **Plasmid is smallest & most commonly used vectors**
★ 1Kb = 1000 nucleotide long base

Vector / Vehicle-DNA	DNA insert size (i.e. can accept DNA fragment of)
Plasmid (PBR 322)	0.01 – 10 kb ***(smallest)***Q
Bacteriophage (Lambda charon 4A)	10 –20 kb
Cosmids	35 – 50 kb ***(largest)***Q

68. **B i.e. Restriction enzyme sites** *[Ref: Harper's 27/e P- 407; Anantha Narayan 6/e p. 426- 28]*

Bacteriophage (or **phages**) are viruses that *infect bacteria* and play an important role in gene transfer between bacteria by mechanism of transduction that ***confer antibiotic resistance***Q. They usually have ***linear DNA molecule***Q into which ***foreign DNA can be inserted at several restriction enzyme sites***Q. ***It can carry 10- 20 kb long DNA segment***Q.

Site Directed Mutagenesis, Site Specific Recombination, Linkage Analysis & Analyzing (Hybridization) Techniques

69. **D i.e. Site directed mutagenesis** *[Ref: Lehninger 5/e p. 312-13]*

Site directed mutagenesis and **oligonucleotide directed mutagenesis uses oligomer with single base pair substitution as primer**Q to create a specific DNA sequence change (in gene), thus producing modified proteins with changes in primary structure of protein. This helps researchers to examine the effect of these changes on 3-D structure, folding & activity of protein.

70. **C i.e. RE+ligase** 71. **A i.e. Detection of characteristic DNA polymorphism in a family is associated with disorder**
72. **A i.e. Separation of proteins..; B i.e. SDS-PAGE electrophesis..; C i.e. Enzyme linked antibodies..; D i.e. Confirmatory..**
73. **A, D i.e. ELISA, Western blot** 74. **B i.e. DNA** 75. **D i.e. Protein**
76. **A i.e. m- RNA** 77. **B i.e. RNA analysis** *[Ref: Harper 29/e p 439-40; Vasudevan 6/e p 612-14; Lippincott's 5/e p. 485; Lehninger 5/e p. 174, 1010-1012; Robbins 7/e p-189-91; Human genetics 2000, 8:738-43]*

- **Blotting techniques separate fragments on the basis of their mass (size) by agarose or SDS- polyacrylamide gel electrophoresis (SDS-PAGE) and then transfer the pattern to nitrocellulose /nylon paper** (blotting or adsorption). Then **enzyme/radioactive/or fluorescence labeled probe is added** complementing, hybridizing & detecting the desired fragment. **Southern** blotting, **Northern** blotting and **Western blotting techniques** (Mn – **"See No West"**) are used respectively to analyze **DNA, mRNA and proteins sample**Q (sequence of protein synthesis). And the probes used in these techniques are **c-DNA, cDNA and antibody respectively.**
- **Antigen-antibody reaction** is detected by **ELISA** (enzyme linked immune sorbent assay) and **Western (immuno) blot. ELISA is sensitive and Western blot is confirmatory in AIDS diagnosis**Q

Analysis of Gene (DNA) and Products of Gene Expression (mRNA and Proteins)

Technique	Sample analyzed	Gel used	Probe	Purpose
Southern blot	*DNA*Q	Yes	Radioactive DNA probes	Detects DNA changes & mutation
Allele specific oligonucleotide (ASO)	DNA	No	Allele specific oligo nucleotide probe	Detects DNA mutation
Microarray	M-RNA or C-DNA	No	DNA probe	- ***Genotyping*** **(i.e., gene variation or mutation) by using DNA sample.** - ***Gene expression analysis*** (i.e., patterns of m-RNA production) by using m-RNA & converting it to c-DNA by reverse transcriptase. - Analyze thousands of gene & mRNA at same time - **Tumor fingerprint or transcriptional profile** used to determine the differing (global) pattern of gene expression in two different cells types eg normal & cancer cells (in order to develop most appropriate form of chemotherapy).
Northern blot	*RNA*Q	Yes	**DNA probe**	Measures ***mRNA***Q amounts & sizes
Western (immuno) blot	***Protein*** Q	Yes	**Labeled antibody**Q	Measure protein amounts
South Western blot	**Protein,** DNA (?)	Yes	**Labelled nucleic acid (DNA) probe**	Examines **protein – DNA (protein-nucleic acid) interactions**
ELISA	Protein or antibodies	No	***Antibody***Q (specific for protein to be measured)	Detects proteins (antigens) or antibodies
Proteomics	***Protein***Q	Yes	-	Measures abundance, distribution, post translational modifications, function & interactions of cellular proteins

The base sequence of DNA that have been cloned & purified can be determined in the laboratory by – **Sanger dideoxy enzymatic (manual) method** and **Maxam & Gilbert chemical (manual) method**.

78. **A i.e. Antibody** *[Ref: Lippincott's 4/e p. 470- 74, 483-84; Harper's 27/e p. 409-12, 313-14]*

Western blot (immuno blot) ***analyses protein by antibody labeled probe***Q. **Northern blot** analyses *m-RNA* by a *radioactive probe* and **southern blot** analysis *DNA* by *radioactive probe.*

79. **D i.e. Northern blot analysis** *[Ref: Harrisons 16th/365, 378, 595]*

Definitive diagnosis of a point mutation in the beta globin gene requires DNA analysis. Northern blot test is a technique used to study the RNA, rather than DNA and hence is the answer of exclusion.

Polymerase chain reaction, DNA Sequencing and southern blot testing are rapid methods for DNA analysis, and can all be used to detect the point mutation in the globin gens.

'The advent of polymerase chain reaction (PCR), allele specific oligonucleotide hybridization and automated DNA sequencing has made it possible to identify globin gene mutations in a few days'. **'The southern blot technique is a fast way of analyzing a small number of DNA fragments, for instance the sickle cell mutation. Before PCR and cheap fast sequencing became available, the southern blot was the universal workhorse.**

The northern blot is a technique to analyze RNA rather than DNA. This is thus the answer of exclusion.

80. **D i.e. Microarray** *[Ref: Lippincott 5/e 483-85; Vassudeven 6/e 614; Lehninger 5/e p. 325-28]*

DNA Microarrays (DNA-Chips) is used for ***detection or screening of variations in DNA sequences and gene expression***Q analysizing thousands of gene at a same time.

81. **D i.e. Microarray** *[Ref: Harrison 17/e p 406, 390; Robbin's 7/e p 171-73]*

- **FISH (Fluorescent in situ hybridisation)** and **PCR (polymerase chain reaction)** like *RT-PCR and QF PCR tests can* ***detect specific anemploidy***Q**.**
- Whereas, **microarray based CGH (comparative genomic hybridization) test** can be used as high resolution whole genome scan for the detection or screening of unknown (non specific) abnormalities, mutation or genomic imbalance including deletions, duplication and aneuploidies. Microarray based CGH cannot detect balanced translocations or inversions.

- So **FISH** and **PCR** can **detect specific (known) chromosomal abnormalities** whereas **microarray based CGH** is better suited for **screening unknown (non specific)** chromosomal abnormalities.

82. **E i.e. Immuno histochemistry >> C i.e. Southern Blot** *[Ref: Harrison 18/e p 508; Lippincott 5/e p 465-85]*

Immunohisto chemistry detects antigens (eg proteins) in abnormal (eg cancerous) or normal cells of a tissue by antibodies binding specifically to that antigen (so immune means antigen-antibody binding and histo means in tissue). It is used to find distribution & localization of biological marker in various tissues.

Gene Library

83. **D, E i.e. DNA Nucleotide or fragment, Complete collection of gene copies of one organism** *[Ref: Lehninger 5/e 315; Lippincott 5/e 469-70; Chatterjea 7/e p-265; Vassudeven 6/e p 516; Satyanarayan 3/e p 596-97]*

Genomic DNA (gene) library contain a **copy of every DNA nucleotide sequence in genome**Q, whereas. **c-DNA (gene) libraries** contain those DNA sequences that transcribe as m RNA.

Recombination DNA Technology or Genetic Engineering

84. **A, B, C, D, E i.e. Viral vaccine production; To cure genetic disorder; Genetic crop; Gene production, Production of genetic products** *[Ref: Lehninger 5/e 337; Vasudevan 6/e 512-14; Chattarjea 7/e-275, 279]*
85. **C i.e. mRNA from beta pancreatic cells of human:** *[Ref: Harper 28/e p388; Lehninger 5/e p 334-37, 316]*

Starting material for production of insulin from bacterial cells (E.coli) using recombination DNA technology is ***mRNA from beta pancreatic cells of human***Q.

86. **B i.e. RNA dependent DNA polymerase** *[Ref: Harper's 29/436; Cjhatterjea 7th/e p. 261-63; Lehninger 5/e p. 305]*
87. **A, B & D i.e. Restriction endonucleases involved, DNA ligase is used, Reverse transcriptase..** 88. **E i.e. None**

Enzymes used in recombination DNA technology are nuclease (BAL-31, S1), exonuclease (III, λ), endonuclease (restriction), DNase I, DNA polymerase I, DNA ligase, reverse transcriptase (RNA dependent DNA polymerase) Q, **polynucleotide kinase, terminal transferase and alkaline phosphatase (not acid phosphatase)**Q

89. **B i.e. Genes for protease inhibitors** *[Ref: Herper 28/e 392]*

- **Expression vector** is a vector which synthesize/produce/express the protein coded by a gene introduced via DNA recombination technology. So it is used to produce protein by genetic engineering and detect specific c-DNA molecules in library.
- Expression vectors are specially constructed so that they contain **very active inducible promoters, proper in phase translation initiation codons,** ***both transcription & translation termination signals***Q (to increase transcription & translation) and appropriate protein processing signals, if needed (to produce processed function protein).

- **To enhance the final yield of protein product, some expression vectors even contain genes that code for protease inhibitors**Q.

90. **A i.e. Genomics**   91. **A i.e. Protenonomics**

92. **A, E > B, C i.e. (Gene Array Chips, Two-Dimensional Electrophoresis >Mass Spectroscopy; PolyAcrylamide Gel Electrophoresis (PAGE)** *[Ref: Lippincott's 4/e p. 484-85; Harper 29/e p 28-33; Stedman's dictionary 27/e p-739]*

- Study of structure & products of gene is **genomics.** Genomics enables protein to be identified from small amount of sequence data.
- Study of multiplication of proteins in disease process is called **proteomics**. The goal of proteomics is **to identify the entire complement of proteins elaborated by a cell under diverse conditions**Q.
- **Two dimensional electrophoresis, gene arrays (DNA chips), multidimensional protein identification technology (Mud PIT)** employing successive rounds of **chromatography** are used to survey **protein expression in proteomics.** After 2D electrophoresis, individual polypeptides are extracted & analyzed by **Edman sequencing** or **mass spectroscopy**.
- **Protein purity** is most widely assessed by **polyacrylamide gel electrophoresis (PAGE) – SDS** (sodium dodecyl sulfate). **Isoelectric focusing (IEF) is used in conjunction with SDS-PAGE** for 2D (two dimensional) electrophoresis, which seperates polypeptides based on pI on one dimension and molecular mass (Mr) in second. 2D electrophoresis is particularly used for separating the components of complex mixtures of proteins.

Transgenic Organism

93. **A, D i.e. Knock-out, Targeted gene disruption**

94. **A i.e. Developed from DNA insertion into fertilized egg; B i.e. Have same genome as parents except one or more genes; E i.e. Homozygous are selected:**

95. **D i.e. Transgenic animals** *[Ref: Harrison 18/e p 490-94; Harper 29/e p 447; Lippincott 5/e p 486; Leheninger 5/e p 334; Vasudevan 6/e p 621]*

- Mutations that **completely disrupt the function of a gene**Q are called **knock out mutation**. And the techniques for disrupting or knocking out of a specific gene in a specific cell, tissue or organ is called **conditional /directed knock outs** or **targeted gene disruption (ablation).**
- **Transgenic animals** can be produced **by micro injecting one or few cloned genes into the nuclei of fertilized egg (ovum)**Q. If the new gene becomes successfully integrated into a chromosome, it will be present in the germline of few animals. By careful breeding **homozygous transgenic line** can be established.
- Although Southern /Northern blot tests can assess changes in DNA /RNA and suggest a function of gene but it is necessary to conduct a specific genetic analysis in genetically modified animals to correctly define gene function. **Many of gene knock outs do not have an apperent phenotype, either because of redundant functions of other genes or because the phenotype is subtle**Q. Whereas **homozygous transgenic animals** (homozygous for new gene or genes) cause many features of disorder.

96. **A i.e. Absence of thymus; B i.e. Xenograft can be sustained for weeks**
[Ref: Harrison 18/e p 2699-2701, 490-93; Harper 29/e p 447; www.genetic-nude mouse-1768]

- **Nude (hair less) mouse** is a transgenic mouse with **absent thymus and T cell function resulting in lack/slow xeno and allograft rejection**Q
- **SCID (Severe combined immune deficieny) mouse** has thymus (±), spleen follicles and lymphoids and is **virtually devoid of lymphocytes (T cells, B cells and NK lymphocytes)**

97. **A i.e. Both plants will glow** *[Ref: Lehninger 5/e 316, 434, 332]*

- Both the plants expressing genes for **firefly luciferase** and **(green /yellow /blue /cyan) fluorescent protein of jelly fish** (Aequorea victoria) will ***glow in dark***Q.

- Fluorescent probes are derived from green fluorescent protein (GFP) of jelly fish. It is an 11-stranded β-barrel and light absorbing /emitting center (chromatophore) of protein comprises a modified (oxidized) form of tripeptide – Ser^{65} - Tyr^{66} – Gly^{68} located within the barrel. Oxidation of tripeptide is catalyzed by GFP itself, with **no other protein or cofactor required other than oxygen**Q. So it can be cloned into virtually any cell, where it can serve as a fluorescent marker for itself or for any protein to which it is fused. When exited by absorption of photon of light GFP emits fluorescent, photon in green region. A related protein (**m RFP1**) fluoresces red light.
- Actually **luciferase containing transgenic plants** emit quite weak light and a prolonged exposure (~ 24 hour) pictures show them glowing in dark.

Gene Therapy

98. **A i.e. Replacement of abnormal gene by normal gene.**
99. **A i.e. Electroporation, B i.e. Intranuclear infection, C i.e. Site directed mutagenesis, D i.e. Retrovirus**
100. **A i.e. SCID** *[Ref: Harper's 28/e P-380, 400, 504, 625; Lippincott's 5/e P- 485-56; Lehninger 5/e p. 331-35, 312, 1004; Chatterjea 7th/e p. 278-87]*

- The goal of gene therapy is **replacement of abnormal mutant gene by normal gene**Q.
- **Technique to transfer genes** (foreign material) into cells include – **transfection, microinjection, electroporation, site directed recombination, transduction using adenovirus or retrovirus and plasmid liposome complex**Q etc.
- **SCID (Severe combined imuunodeficiency disease)** or **bubble baby syndrome** is the **first disease treated successfully by gene therapy.**

Genetic Disorder

101. **A i.e. X-gene; D i.e. Seen in females** *[Ref: Kumar & Clark 6/e p. 172-73; Harrison 16/e p. 375]*

Although females have 2X chromosomes (XX), but due to inactivation (lyonization) genes on one X chromosome becomes transcriptionally inactive. Thus **X inactivation prevents expression of most genes on one of the X- chromosome in every cell of female**Q.

102. **D & E i.e. Duchenne muscular dystrophy & G-6-P dehydrogenase deficiency**
103. **C i.e. X– linked recessive inheritance** *[Ref.: Chandrasoma Taylor 3rd/e P-234, 235, 236; Robbins 6th/e P-146]*

Single X-chromosome of son is achieved from his mother, not father; so x-linked diseases never transmit from father to sonQ.

104. **A i.e. Autosomal dominant disorder** *[Ref: Harrison 16/e P- 374]*

Autosomal dominant disease cannot occur in offspring of an unaffected individualsQ. Because the allele is dominant it will always express phenotypically (clinically) and hence both parents can't be normal in autosomal dominant disorders even if they have a single abnormal gene.

105. **C & D i.e. Cystic fibrosis & Ataxia telangiectasia** *[Ref: Harrison 17/ed pg- 398-401, 494; Robbins 7th/ed pg- 151-52]*

Ataxia telangiectasia & cystic fibrosis are autosomal recessive disordersQ. **Tuberous sclerosis is AD**Q **and Duchene / Becker muscular dystrophy and hemophilia A (factor – 8 deficiency)**Q are **X-linked recessive disorders.**

106. **D i.e. A polygenic syndrome** *[Ref: www.som.tulane.edu/departments/peds_respcare/genetic.htm]*

A syndrome with facial anomalies including a thin upper lip, growth delay and developmental disabilities is likely to result from either a teratogenic congenital malformation, a single gene defect (Mendelian) or a chromosomal disorder. A trait is called polygenic if multiple genes are thought to contribute to the phenotype and includes conditions like diabetes and hypertension. A polygenic disorder is the least likely diagnosis amongst the options provided and the single best answer of exclusion.

- **Mendelian Syndrome presenting with above features is the Cornelia de Lange syndrome. (Amsterdam Dwarf Syndrome).** This is a mendelian syndrome with either autosomal recessive or autosomal dominant inheritance, and is characteristically associated with a thin upper lip, small head size (microcephaly) and other developmental disabilities.

- **Teratogenic syndrome presenting with features in question is the fetal alcohol syndrome.** Fetal alcohol syndrome results from the teratogenic effects of alcohol on the fetus during pregnancy and characteristic features include a thin upper lip, small head size (microcephaly) and other developmental abnormalities.
- **An example of a chromosomal disorders presenting with features in question is the Miller Dicker Syndrome. (MDS).** Miller Dicker Syndrome is a chromosomal syndrome with a mendelian pattern of inheritance. Chromosomal anomalies include deletion of short arm of chromosome 17 (17 p 13.3) and characteristic features include a thin lip, microcephaly and other developmental disorders.

107. **A i.e. Autosomal dominant (most likely)** *[Ref: http://www.babyhearing.org/HearingAamplification/ Causes/BasicGenetics.pdf; http://www.emedicine.com/ped/topic2422.htm]*

Waardenburg's Syndrome (WS) is a rare **autosomal dominant syndrome** characterized by pigmentary disturbances (skin, **hair**, iris), **sensorineural hearing loss**, and other developmental anomalies such as **dystopia canthorum (widely spaced eyes)** and blepharophimosis.

The syndrome that closest matches the features provided in the question is Waardeburg syndrome type-I. This is inherited as an autosomal dominant fashion and hence is the answer of exclusion.

As the question does not provide us with details as to the sex of the three children, a sex linked inheritance pattern cannot be worked out. Also the combined presentation of an affected father, unaffected mother and one affected child among three children is possible with both an autosomal dominant and an autosomal recessive inheritance pattern. **In absence of any more details, the answer to this question cannot be deduced through the exploration of various permutations and combinations.** How both autosomal dominant and autosomal recessive inheritance can be responsible for the above combination:

Autosomal Dominant	Autosomal recessive
(A-affected allele and a normal allele) If the disease is transmitted in an Autosomal Dominant then : Father (affected) will be either 'AA' or 'Aa' Mother (unaffected) will be 'aa' **If father is AA and mother aa, the offsprings will be** 1. aA – 100% affected **If father is Aa and mother aa, the offsprings will** 1. Aa – 50% affected 2. aa - 50% not affected ***The scenario in the above question therefore is possible autosomal dominant inheritance if father is Aa and mother is aa***	*('A'-affected allele and 'a' normal allele)* If the disease is transmitted in an Autosomal recessive form : Father (affected) will be 'AA' Mother (unaffected) may be 'aa' or 'Aa' **If father is AA and mother aa, the offsprings will be** 1. aA – 100% not affected, (but carriers) **If father is AA and mother Aa, the offsprings will be** 1. Aa – 50% not affected, carrier 2. AA - 50% affected ***The scenario in the above question therefore is possible with autosomal recessive inheritance if father is aa and mother is Aa***

108. **D i.e. Short arm of chromosome 6** *[Ref: Harrison 18/e p.497, 2680, 2685-94; Ganong 22/e P- 526; Robbins 7/e P 203]*
109. **A i.e. Transplantation reaction; B i.e. Autommune disease; D i.e. Involved in T –Cell function**
110. **B i.e. Dendritic cells; F i.e. B-cell**
111. **A, B i.e. Macrophage; Dendritic cells; C i.e. Lymphocytes**

- Genes encoding **major histocompatibility complex (MHC) or human leucocyte antigen (HLA) complex** (named so because MHC encoded antigens were initially detected on leucocytes) are clustered on **small (4 megabase) region on short arm of chromosome 6**Q. It is involved in transplantation reaction & autoimmune diseases.
- **MHC II** are expressed (presented) by antigen presenting cells eg **dendritic cells, macrophages, Langerhans cells, B cells and activated T cells**Q.

112. **C i.e. Somatic Hypermutation** *[Ref: Principles of Cellular & Molecular Immunology by Austin and Wood 1993/408, 449, 450]*

Affinity Maturation refers to the increased affinity of antibodies for their specific antigen as the antibody response continues. This phenomenon is not seen in IgM responses.

Those B-cells expressing receptors with a higher affinity for the antigen are selctively expanded, even as the levels of antigen fall. Thus B-cells with higher affinity are generated during the 1° & 2° immune respones in large part **due to Somatic hypermutations that occur in V_H genes**Q.

(V_H=Variable region of Heavy chain).

Chapter -5 STRUCTURE & FUNCTIONS OF PROTEINS AND ENZYMES

QUESTIONS

Structure of Protein

1. **The primary structure of a protein refers to:** *(AIIMS 04)*
   A. Linear structure and order of the amino acids present ☐
   B. Regular confirmational forms of a protein ☐
   C. Complete three-dimensional structure of the polypeptide units of a given protein ☐
   D. Subunit structure of the protein ☐
2. **Alpha helix and Beta pleated sheet are examples of:**
   A. Primary structure *(NBE P 13; AI 04)* ☐
   B. Secondary structure ☐
   C. Tertiary structure ☐
   D. Quaternary structure ☐
3. **Which one of the following is not true for an α-helix:**
   A. It is one of the most important secondary structure ☐
   B. It has a net dipole moment *(AIIMS 04)* ☐
   C. All hydrogen bonds are aligned in the same direction ☐
   D. Long stretches of left handed α-helices occur in proteins ☐
4. **An amino acid which does not participate by αhelix formation is:** *(AI 06)*
   A. Leucine ☐
   B. Glycine ☐
   C. Proline ☐
   D. Lysine ☐
5. **An alfa helix of a protein is most likely to be disrupted if a missense mutation introdues the following amino acid with in the alpha helical structure:** *(AIIMS 02)*
   A. Alanine ☐
   B. Aspartic acid ☐
   C. Tyrosine ☐
   D. Glycine ☐
6. **Folding of protein chain is due to :** *(AIIMS 97)*
   A. Amide bond ☐
   B. Hydrogen bonds ☐
   C. Phosphodiesterase bonds ☐
   D. Disulphide bond ☐
7. **The 3 dimensional shape of a protein is maintained mainly by:** *(AIIMS 03)*
   A. Strong covalent interactions ☐
   B. Interactions with other proteins ☐
   C. Multiple weak interactions ☐
   D. Interactions with prosthetic groups ☐
8. **Proteins are linear polymers of amino acids. They fold into compact structures. Sometimes, these folded structures associate to form homo-or hetero-dimers. Which one of the following refers to this associated form?** *(AI 06)*
   A. Denatured state ☐
   B. Molecular aggregation ☐
   C. Precipitation ☐
   D. Quaternary structure ☐
9. **An Immunoglobulin molecule represents the following level of organized protein structure:** *(AI 12)*
   A. Primary structure ☐
   B. Secondary structure ☐
   C. Tertiary structure ☐
   D. Quartenary structure ☐
10. **True about Isopeptide bond:** *(PGI 11)*
   A. It makes protein resistant ☐
   B. Bond is formed b/w carboxyl terminus of one protein and the amino group of a lysine residue on another ☐
   C. Involves in post-transcriptional modification of protein ☐
   D. Enzyme acts as catalyst for the bond formation ☐
11. **Stability of the toxoid in snake's venom is due to:**
   A. Disulfide bonds *(NBE P 14; AIIMS 09)* ☐
   B. Hydrogen bonds ☐
   C. Ionic bonds ☐
   D. Van Der Wall's bond. ☐
12. **Keratin in skin is softer than keratin in nail because keratin in skin has:** *(AI 12)*
   A. Less number of disulphide bonds ☐
   B. Less number of salt bridges ☐
   C. High sodium content ☐
   D. Different affinity for water ☐
13. **Keatin contains-** *(NBE P 15)*
   A. Arginine ☐
   B. Histidine ☐
   C. Lysine ☐
   D. All ☐
14. **Biomineralization is seen in:** *(AIIMS 13)*
   A. Pinna ☐
   B. Molluscs shell ☐
   C. Hooves of cattle ☐
   D. Nails ☐
15. **Different sequence of amino acids having similar structure of proteins is an example of**
   A. Divergence *(AIMS 07)* ☐
   B. Convergence ☐
   C. Opportunistic ☐
   D. Incidental ☐
16. **There are more than 300 variants of human hemoglobin gene. Among these only a few are fatal. Hence, the most important factor to be conserved in a protein for its function is the:**
   A. Amino acid sequence *(AI 06)* ☐
   B. Ligand binding residues ☐
   C. Structure ☐
   D. Environment ☐

17. Which of the following is not true in relation to glycoproteins: *(PGI 05)*
A. Are proteins to which oligosaccharide are covalently attached ☐
B. The carbohydrate units of glycoprotein have several repeats ☐
C. Carbohydrate content is same but proteins are different ☐
D. Carbohydrate chain is often linear ☐

18. Which of the following is a component of polysaccharide- *(PGI 04)*
A. Synovium ☐
B. Glucosamine ☐
C. Glucoronic acid ☐
D. Ascorbic acid ☐

19. Regarding proteoglycans, false is: *(AI 07)*
A. Chondroitin sulfate is a Proteoglycan ☐
B. They hold less amount of water ☐
C. They are made up of sugar and aminoacids ☐
D. They carry charge ☐

20. Compounds with large amount of carbohydrate & small amount of protein *(Jipmer 06, SGPGI 07)*
A. Glycoprotein ☐
B. Glycosaminoglycan ☐
C. Proteoglycan ☐
D. Glycocalyx ☐

21. Which of the following aminoacids in a protein commonly acts as a potential O-Glycosylation site for attachment of an oligosaccharide unit: *(AI 12)*
A. Glutamine ☐
B. Cysteine ☐
C. Serine ☐
D. Asparginine ☐

22. All steps of N- glycosylation occur in ER except
A. Dolichol synthesis *(Jipmer 04, TN 05)* ☐
B. Glycosyl transferase ☐
C. Protein- oligosacharide transferase ☐
D. Final trimming ☐

23. Glycosyl transferase of O-glycosylation is found in
A. RER *(WB 03, Assam 04)* ☐
B. SER ☐
C. Golgi ☐
D. Lysosome ☐

24. Difference between High mannose & complex glycoprotein *(AMU 03, UP 02)*
A. Core pentasacharide ☐
B. Protein chain ☐
C. Asparagine ☐
D. Presence of GlC – NAc – Gal – NANA in complex glycoprotein ☐

25. Following organelles are involved in the formation of N- glycosylated product: *(PGI 07)*
A. Golgi apparatus ☐
B. Nucleolus ☐
C. SER ☐
D. RER ☐
E. Peroxisomes ☐

26. Characteristics of glycoprotein: *(PGI 07)*
A. Protein linked with glycosidic bond ☐
B. Core protein ☐
C. Sugar residues are long in carbohydrate portion of glycoprotein. ☐
D. Participate in cell surface recognition. ☐

27. All are true about denatured proteins except:
A. Amino acid sequence remains intact ☐
B. The biological function remains intact ☐
C. The isoelectric pH changes *(AIIMS 08)* ☐
D. Recovery after denaturation is not possible ☐

28. True about denaturation of proteins is all except:
A. Unfolding occurs *(AIIMS 08)* ☐
B. Disruption of secondary structure occurs ☐
C. Sequence of amino acids remain the same ☐
D. Biological activity is retained ☐

29. Random arrangement of molecule results in
A. Crystallization *(AIIMS 08)* ☐
B. Precipitation ☐
C. Denaturation ☐
D. High Solubility ☐

30. Protein that precipitates on heating to 45° C and redissolves on boiling is: *(AI 12, 07)*
A. Bence Jones Protein ☐
B. Gamma globulin ☐
C. Albumin ☐
D. Myosin ☐

31. Optical transmission through a solution depends on:
A. Time *(PGI 03)* ☐
B. Concentration ☐
C. Scale ☐
D. Path length ☐
E. Spectrophotometer

32. Cytochrome C of the bacteria has 50% identity of amino acid sequence with that of human. Which of the following is the most conserved parameter in these two proteins?
A. Quarternary structure *(AI 04)* ☐
B. Tertiary structure ☐
C. Amino acid sequence ☐
D. Loop and turn segments ☐

33. Which of the following is a denaturing substance?
A. Guanosine *(AIIMS 05; AI 06)* ☐
B. Guanidine ☐
C. Glutamate ☐
D. Glycine ☐

34. The structural proteins are involved in maintaining the shape of a cell or in the formation of matrices in the body. The shape of these proteins is: *(AI 06)*
A. Globular ☐
B. Fibrous ☐
C. Stretch of beads ☐
D. Planar ☐

35. Structural proteins OR Keratin is OR In a centrifugal distribution, protein that is precipitated first:
A. Fibrous *(AIIMS 08) (NBE P 14)* ☐
B. Globular ☐

C. Branched ☐
D. Compound ☐

36. True about Collagen: *(PGI 11)*
A. Triple helix ☐
B. Beta- pleated structure ☐
C. Vit C is necessary for post-translational modification ☐
D. Glycine residue at every third position ☐

37. Which of the following are intracellular events occurring in fibroblast during synthesis of collagen:
A. Hydrolysis of procollagen to collagen *(PGI 08)* ☐
B. Glycosylation of proline ☐
C. Formation of triple helix ☐
D. Formation of covalent cross link b/w fibrils ☐
E. Self assembly of tropocollagen molecules into fibrils ☐

38. The 40 nm gap in between the tropocollagen molecule in collagen which serve as the site of bone formation is occupied by which of the following- *(AIIMS 11, 06)*
A. Carbohydrate ☐
B. Ligand moiety ☐
C. Ca^{++} ☐
D. Fe^{+++} ☐

39. Albumin and globulin are classified as: *(PGI 07)*
A. Conjugated proteins ☐
B. Simple globular proteins ☐
C. Unconjugated proteins ☐
D. Derived proteins ☐

40. Which is /are not transport protein (s): *(PGI 12)*
A. Transferrin ☐
B. Collagen ☐
C. Ceruloplasmin ☐
D. Hemoglobin ☐
E. Albumin ☐

41. Which of the following is/are storage protein :
A. Myoglobin *(PGI 11)* ☐
B. Ovalbumin ☐
C. Ricin/Hepcidin ☐
D. Ferritin ☐
E. Glutelin ☐

42. A Protein estimation test is confused with: *(AI 06)*
A. Phosphates ☐
B. Nitrates ☐
C. Sulphates ☐
D. Bile salts ☐

43. Intact peptide bond is necessary for which test:
A. UV diffraction *(PGI 08)* ☐
B. Ninhydrin ☐
C. Diazo reaction ☐
D. All ☐

44. All of the following assays are used for estimation of total serum protein, except *(AI 12)*
A. Biuret ☐
B. Bradford ☐
C. Lowry's ☐
D. Bromocresol green ☐

45. Which of the following estimates blood creatinine level most accurately *(AIIMS 06)*
A. Jaffe method ☐
B. Kinetic jaffe method ☐
C. Technicon method ☐
D. Enzyme assay ☐

46. False positive test of protein in dipstick test seen in:
A. Chlorpropamide *(PGI 07)* ☐
B. IV contrast agent ☐
C. Viral infection ☐
D. IV administration of drugs ☐

Methods of Protein Separation (Purification)

47. Protein separation based on mass / molecular weight (size) is /are done in all except: *(PGI 12)*
A. Ultrafiltration ☐
B. Native gel electrophoresis ☐
C. 2D gel electrophoresis ☐
D. Gel Filtration chromatography ☐
E. Ultracentrifugation ☐

48. Protein fragments separation is /are done by:
A. Western blot *(PGI 10)* ☐
B. Chromatography ☐
C. Centrifugation ☐
D. Ultrafiltration ☐
E. Electrophoresis ☐

49. In SDS-PAGE (Sodium Dodecyl Sulfate-Polyacrylamide Gel Electrophoresis) proteins are separated on basis of: *(PGI 09)*
A. Mass ☐
B. Charge ☐
C. Density ☐
D. Molecular weight ☐
E. Solubility ☐

50. Proteins are separated on the basis of size by:
A. SDS-PAGE *(PGI 03)* ☐
B. HPLC ☐
C. Affinity Chromatography ☐
D. Ion-exchange Chromatography ☐

51. Separation of proteins based on size is done by:
A. Affinity chromatography depending on charge ☐
B. SDS-Polyacrylamide gel electrophoresis *(PGI 01)* ☐
C. Ion exchange chromatography ☐
D. High performance liquid chromatography ☐
E. Electrophoresis ☐

52. Protein purification and separation can be done by all except:
A. Chromatography *(AI 07)* ☐
B. Centrifugation ☐
C. Electrophoresis ☐
D. Densitometry ☐

Ammonium Sulfate Fractionation

53. Protein is purified using ammonium sulfate by: (AIIMS 14, 09)
A. Salting out ☐
B. Ion exchange chromatography ☐
C. Mass chromatography ☐
D. Molecular size exclusion ☐

Chromatography

54. The following separation technique depends on the molecular size of the protein: *(AI 03)*
A. Chromatography on a carboxymethyl (CM) cellulose column ☐
B. Iso-electric focussing ☐
C. Gel filtration chromatography ☐
D. Chromatography on a diethylaminoethyl (DEAE) cellulose column ☐

55. Molecular separation of two proteins with same charge can be done by: *(PGI 07)*
A. Ion exchange chromatography ☐
B. Dialysis ☐
C. Gel diffusion chromatography ☐
D. Electrophoresis ☐

56. The best method to differentiate proteins is by: *(PGI 09)*
A. Gel chromatography ☐
B. Affinity chromatography ☐
C. Ion exchange electrophoresis ☐
D. None of the above ☐

57. In chromatography mass movements of the substances is due to: *(AIIMS 01)*
A. Diffusion ☐
B. Electrophoresis ☐
C. Paper chromatography ☐
D. Osmosis ☐

58. In which type of chromatography, the proteins are bound to another substance: *(AIIMS 01)*
A. Hydrophobic chromatography ☐
B. Affinity chromatography ☐
C. Paper chromatography ☐
D. Gel chromatography ☐

59. Method of chromatography in which molecules that are negatively charged are selectively released from stationary phase into the positively charged molecules in mobile phase is termed as: *(AI 10)*
A. Affinity chromatography ☐
B. Ion-Exchange chromatography ☐
C. Adsorbtion chromatography ☐
D. Size-Exclusion chromatography ☐

60. Fastest moving amino acid in methanol- chloroform electrophoresis is OR Which amino acid migrates fastest on chromatography on carboxy methylcellulose medium? *(AIIMS 14, 09, 08)*
A. Glycine ☐
B. Aspartic Acid ☐
C. Valine ☐
D. Leucine ☐

Electrophoresis

61. True regarding electrophoresis are all except *(PGI 09)*
A. Isoelectric focusing use ampholytes & pI ☐
B. Adversely affect structure & function ☐
C. Depends on size not on shape ☐
D. Commonest method of purifying protein ☐
E. Use electric field & quickly estimate no. of proteins ☐

62. Supercoiled DNA is separated by relaxed DNA by: *(AIIMS 14, 12)*
A. ELISA ☐
B. Gel electrophoresis ☐
C. DNA footprinting ☐
D. DNA fingerprinting ☐
E. Microarray assay ☐

63. Which process separates the fragments of DNA : *(AIIMS 07)*
A. Gel centrifugation ☐
B. Paper chromatography ☐
C. High speed centrifugation ☐
D. Thin layer chromatography ☐

64. The two fragments of DNA are separated by: *(AIIMS 06)*
A. High speed centrifugation ☐
B. Thin layer chromatography ☐
C. Paper chromatography ☐
D. Gel chromatography ☐

65. The molecular weight of a protein can be determined by - *(AIIMS 04)*
A. Native Poly Acrylamide Gel Electrophoresis (PAGE) ☐
B. Sodium Dodecyl Sulphate PAGE ☐
C. Isoelectric focussing ☐
D. Ion Exchange Chromatography ☐

66. A protein with molecular weight of 100 kD is subjected to SDS PAGE electrophoresis. The SDS PAGE electrophoresis pattern show two widely separated bands of 20kD and 30kD after addition of Mercaptoethanol. The true statement regarding this will be. *(AI 09)*
A. The protein has undergone complete lysis ☐
B. The protein is a monomer of 20 kD and 30kD protein ☐
C. The protein is a dimmer of two 20kD and 30kD proteins ☐
D. The protein is a tetramer of 20kd and 30kD proteins ☐

67. Hemoglobin electrophoresis is based on *(AIIMS 07)*
A. Molecular weight ☐
B. Charge ☐
C. Solubility ☐
D. Calorimetric properties ☐

Detection of Protein Structure & Amino acids

68. Method (s) to determine protein structure is /are: *(PGI 09, 10)*
A. X-RAY Crystallography ☐
B. NMR Spectroscopy ☐
C. Electrophoresis ☐
D. Infra red spectroscopy ☐

69. **All of the following can determine the protein structure, Except:** *(AIIMS 08)*
A. High performance liquid chromatography ☐
B. Mass spectrometry ☐
C. X- ray crystallography ☐
D. NMR spectrometry ☐

70. **Sequence in a long chain of protein is identified by-**
A. Restriction fragment length polymorphism (RFLP) ☐
B. Chromosome walking *(AIIMS 08)* ☐
C. Leucine Zipper ☐
D. SSOP ☐

71. **The tertiary structure of protein is detected by:**
A. X- ray diffraction /crystallographs. *(AIIMS 09)* ☐
B. Spectrophotometry ☐
C. Electrophoresis. ☐
D. Chromatography. ☐

72. **Trypsin cleaves :** *(PGI 10)*
A. Arginine ☐
B. Glutamate ☐
C. Lysine ☐
D. Proline ☐

73. **All is true about fragment cleavage in 1° structure determination Except** *(PGI 09)*
A. Trypsin cleaves lysine residue (C) ☐
B. Trypsin cleaves arginine next to proline ☐
C. Trypsin & lysyl endoproteinase cleave C terminal of lysine ☐
D. Cysteine reduced by 2 mercapto ethanol ☐
E. Performic acid break disulfide bond

74. **Chymotrypsin cleaves carbonyl terminal of:** *(PGI 11)*
A. Phenylalanine ☐
B. Arginine ☐
C. Lysine ☐
D. Tryptophan ☐
E. Tyrosine ☐

75. **Molecular size is assesed by :** *(PGI 04)*
A. Sedimentation ☐
B. Absorption mass spectroscopy ☐
C. Liophilization ☐
D. Salting out ☐

76. **The substance present in the gall bladder stones or the kidney stones can be best identified by the following techniques:**
A. Fluorescence spectroscopy *(AI 03)* ☐
B. Electron microscopy ☐
C. Nuclear magnetic resonance ☐
D. X-ray diffraction ☐

77. **Ninhydrin test is used for-** *(NBE P 15)*
A. Bile salts ☐
B. Amino acids ☐
C. Nucleic acid ☐
D. Lipids ☐

Enzyme: Kinetics

78. **Substance which binds to substrate other than catalytic enzyme is-** *(NBE P 15)*
A. Competitive inhibitor ☐
B. Non-competitive inhibitor ☐
C. Reversible inhibitor ☐
D. None of the above ☐

79. **In competitive inhibition-** *(PGI 12, 05)*
A. Vmax unchanged ☐
B. Apparent Km unchanged ☐
C. Apparent Km decreased ☐
D. Vmax decreased ☐
E. Rate independent of substrate concentration ☐

80. **Disopropyl phosphofluoridate (DFP) reacts with serine proteases irreversibly and therefore is:** *(PGI 06, 04)*
A. Allosteric inhibitor ☐
B. Competitive inhibitor ☐
C. Non competitive inhibitor ☐
D. A repressor ☐

81. **The type of enzyme inhibition (in which succinate dehydrogenase reaction is inhibited by malonate) is an example of:** *(AIIMS 06)*
A. Non competitive ☐
B. Uncompetitive ☐
C. Competitive ☐
D. Allosteric ☐

82. **True about reversible non-competetive inhibitors:**
A. Lower Vmax *(PGI 13,10,09)* ☐
B. Lower Km ☐
C. Not affect Km ☐
D. Not affect Vmax ☐
E. Affect both V max & Km ☐

83. **True about competitive inhibition of enzyme:**
A. ↑ Km *(PGI 13,10)* ☐
B. ↓ Km ☐
C. ↑ Vmax ☐
D. No change in Km and Vmax ☐
E. V max remain same ☐

84. **In noncompetitive antagonism the true statement is:** *(NBE P 14,13; PGI 16,14,12)*
A. Km value decrease; V max normal ☐
B. Km value decreased; V max decreased ☐
C. Km value normal; V max decreased ☐
D. Km value decreased; V max increased ☐

85. **Km increased but Vmax same enzyme is:** *(PGI 14,09,08)*
A. Competitive *(NBE P 15,14)* ☐
B. Non competitive ☐
C. Irreversible ☐
D. Uncompetitive ☐

86. **Km value is defined as:** *(PGI 04)*
A. Substrate concentration at Vmax/2 ☐
B. Substrate concentration of twice Vmax ☐
C. Substrate concentration of thrice Vmax ☐
D. Substrate concentration of one third Vmax ☐

87. **Enzyme specificity is given by-** *(NBE P 14)*
A. K_M ☐
B. V_{max} ☐
C. Both ☐
D. None ☐

88. True about Km *(PGI 09)*
A. Half the substrate concentration at which velocity is maximum ☐
B. Substrate concentration at which reaction rate is half the maximum ☐
C. Michaelis constant ☐
D. Dissociation constant of enzyme-substrate complex ☐
E. Dissication constant of enzyme-product complex ☐

89. Hormone substrate concentration affects the velocity of enzymatic action, this is known as - *(UP 01)*
A. Zimmerman reaction *(DNB 2K, AIIMS 04)* ☐
B. Salkowski reaction ☐
C. Michales Menton reaction ☐
D. Lieberman-Burchard reaction ☐

90. Michaelis-Menten hypothesis states that -
A. Rate of enzymatic reaction is independent of substrate concentration *(DNB 01, MP 02, Jhar 04)* ☐
B. Rate of non enzymatic reaction is proportinal to substrate concentrate ☐
C. Km is the enzyme-substrate complex association constant ☐
D. Enzyme-substrate complex formation is essential in enzymatic reaction ☐

91. Which of the following enzymes are activated in dephosphorylated state: *(PGI 09)*
A. HMG Co A reductase ☐
B. Glycogen phosphorylase ☐
C. Glycogen phosphorylase kinase ☐
D. Citrate lyase ☐
E. Glycogen synthase ☐

92. Enzyme regulated by phosphorylation: *(PGI 08)*
A. Glucokinase ☐
B. Glycogen synthetase ☐
C. Pyruvate dehydrogenase ☐
D. Isocitrate ☐
E. Citrate lyase ☐

93. All of the following enzymes are regulated by calcium or calmodulin, except: *(AI 06)*
A. Adenylate cyclase ☐
B. Glycogen synthase ☐
C. Guanylyl cyclase ☐
D. Hexokinase ☐

94. "All enzymes are not proteins." This statement is justified by: *(AI 02)*
A. All enzymes do not follow the Michaelis Menton hypothesis ☐
B. RNAs act as ribozymes ☐
C. Antibodies take part in the catalysis of many reactions ☐
D. Metals are involved in attachment to enzymes and catalysts. ☐

95. Definition of Ribozyme: *(PGI 06)*
A. RNA molecular that acts catalytically to change it self or another RNA molecule ☐
B. t-RNA ☐
C. m–RNA ☐
D. Ribosome ☐
E. Ribonucleoprotein ☐

96. One of the following enzyme is not a protein:
A. DNAase *(AIIMS 02)* ☐
B. Abzyme ☐
C. Eco RI ☐
D. Ribozyme ☐

97. Ribozymes is/are : *(PGI 02)*
A. Splicing of heterogenous RNA (hnRNA) to form mRNA ☐
B. Splicing of polypeptide chain and mRNA ☐
C. Transcription of mRNA ☐
D. Recognition of codons in introns ☐
E. RNA polymerase ☐

98. Enzyme activity is expressed as: *(PGI 06)*
A. Millimoles /lit? ☐
B. Milli gm/lit? ☐
C. Mg/dl ☐
D. Micromoles/min ☐

99. True about enzyme specificity: *(PGI 01)*
A. Amount of enzyme required per second, per mole or product formation ☐
B. Number of sites per substrate ☐
C. Amount of enzyme binding with various substrates ☐
D. Number of enzyme units per milligram of enzyme protein ☐
E. Amount of enzyme causing transformation of 1 μmol of substrate per minute under standard conditions ☐

100. Enzymes Ea,Eb and Ec are under allosteric control of S2 and P1 and P2 respectively. If Ec is defective what would occur -
A. Accumulation of S1 *(AIIMS 01)* ☐
B. Accumulation of P1 ☐
C. Accumulation of S2 ☐
D. Decrease of S2 ☐

101. Non- functional enzymes are all except:
A. Alkaline phosphatase *(AIIMS 08)* ☐
B. Acid phosphatase ☐
C. Lipoprotein lipase ☐
D. Gamma glutamyl transpeptidase ☐

102. True about isoenzymes is: *(AIIMS 11)*
A. Same quaternary structure ☐
B. Same distribution in different organs ☐
C. Same enzyme classification with same umbers ☐
D. Catalyze the same reaction ☐

103. True about isoenzymes is/are: *(PGI 01)*
A. Different km value ☐
B. Act on different substrate ☐
C. Consist of multimeric complex ☐
D. Same electrophoretic mobility ☐
E. Have different physical properties ☐

104. The predominant isozyme of LDH in cardiac muscle is:
A. LD-1. *(AI 05)* ☐
B. LD-2. ☐
C. LD-3. ☐
D. LD-5. ☐

105. In which of the following conditions the level of creatinine kinase-1 increases? *(AI 04)*
A. Myocardial Ischemia ☐
B. Brain Ischemia ☐
C. Kidney damage ☐
D. Electrical cardioversion ☐

106. Force not acting in an enzyme substrate complex :
A. Electrostatic *(AI 01)* ☐
B. Covalent ☐
C. Van der waals ☐
D. Hydrogen ☐

107. The serine proteases do not include *(AIIMS 03)*
A. Pepsin ☐
B. Trypsin ☐
C. Elastase ☐
D. Chymotrypsin ☐

108. Active sites of serine protease contain: *(PGI 03)*
A. Histidine ☐
B. Lysine or threonine ☐
C. Arginine ☐
D. Serine ☐

109. If chymotrypsin molecule undergoes a ser-195-ala mutation then : *(AI 08)*
A. Chymotrypsin will not bind the substrate ☐
B. Chymotrypsin will bind the substrate as well as cause cleavage ☐
C. Chymotrypsin will bind the substrate but will not cause cleavage ☐
D. No affect will be observed ☐

110. Tyrosinase is - *(AIIMS 06, UP 12)*
A. Oxidase ☐
B. Transferase ☐
C. Lyase ☐
D. Isomerase ☐

111. Hexokinase is a: *(AIIMS 13, NBE P 15)*
A. Transferase ☐
B. Reductase ☐
C. Oxidoreductase ☐
D. Oxidase ☐

112. Fumarase / Decarboxylase is: *(PGI 14, NBE P 15,13)*
A. Oxidoreductase ☐
B. Transferase ☐
C. Oxidase ☐
D. Lyases ☐

113. Enzymes mediating transfer of one molecule to another are OR Enzymes that move a molecular group from one molecule to another are known as: *(AI 08,05)*
A. Transferases ☐
B. Oxidases ☐
C. Lysases ☐
D. Peptidases ☐

114. Addition of water in C-C bond is by the enzyme:
A. Hydroxylase *(PGI 04)* ☐
B. Dehydrogenase ☐
C. Hydrolase ☐
D. Hydratase ☐

115. Which of the following enzymes does not participate in oxidation-reduction reactions? *(AIIMS 13)*
A. Oxygenases ☐
B. Peroxidases ☐
C. Hydroperoxidases ☐
D. Dehydrogenases ☐

116. All of the following enzymes are involved in oxidation – reduction reactions, Except *(AI 09)*
A. Dehydrogenases ☐
B. Hydrolases ☐
C. Oxygenases ☐
D. Peroxidases ☐

117. Detoxification of drugs is controlled by: *(AP 10)*
A. Cytochrome ☐
B. Cytochrome P450 ☐
C. Cytochrome C ☐
D. Cytochrome A ☐

118. All of the following are true regarding oxygenases except :
A. Incorporate 2 atoms of oxygen *(AIIMS 11, AI 07)* ☐
B. Incorporate 1 atom of oxygen ☐
C. Required for hydroxylation of steroids ☐
D. Required for carboxylation of drugs. ☐

119. Which of the following is not a rate limiting enzyme:
A. HMG CoA Reductase *(AIIMS 13,11,08)* ☐
B. Phosphofructokinase ☐
C. Acetyl CoA carboxylase ☐
D. Malanoate dehydrogenase ☐

120. In which of the following reactions is Magnesium required:
A. ATPase *(AI 02)* ☐
B. Dismutase ☐
C. Phosphatase ☐
D. Aldolase ☐

121. Coenzymes are ....organic compounds :- *(PGI 04)*
A. Lipoprotein ☐
B. Proteinaceous ☐
C. Non-protein ☐
D. Any of the above ☐

122. The combination of main supporting enzyme is called:
A. Apoenzyme *(PGI 03, AIIMS 01)* ☐
B. Coenzyme ☐
C. Holoenzyme ☐
D. Constitutive enzyme ☐

123. Which of the following acts as co-enzymes and not as co-factors: *(PGI 06)*
A. Pyridoxine ☐
B. Biotin ☐
C. Thiamine ☐
D. Folic acid ☐
E. Co-balamin ☐

124. Coenzyme, in an enzymatic reaction usually functions to :
A. Activate the substrate *(AIIMS 06)* ☐
B. Increase the active sites of apoenzyme ☐
C. Enhance the specificity of aponzyme ☐
D. Accept one of the cleavage products ☐

125. Thiamine deficiency decreases cellular metabolism because:
A. Thiamine is a coenzyme for pyruvate dehydrogenase and alfa-ketoglutarate dehydrogenases *(AIIMS 08)* ☐
B. Activity of transketolase is inhibited ☐
C. It is required for the process of transamination ☐
D. It is a cofactor in oxidative reduction ☐

126. Vitamin K is required for: *(AIIMS 14, 07)*
A. Carboxylation ☐
B. Hydroxylation ☐
C. Oxidation ☐
D. Reduaction ☐

127. Which coenzyme is responsible for carboxylation reaction? OR Treatment of Multiple Carboxylase Deficiency is: *(NBE P 14, 13; AIIMS 08, AI 10)*
A. Biotin ☐
B. FAD ☐
C. NADH ☐
D. Thiamine pyrophosphate ☐

128. Which of the following acts as cofactor after it's modification: *(PGI 01)*
A. Vit-C ☐
B. Pantothenic acid ☐
C. Biotin ☐
D. Zinc ☐
E. Copper ☐

129. Zinc is cofactor for: *(AIIMS 09)*
A. Alcohol dehydrogenase ☐
B. Pyruvate Carboxylase ☐
C. Pyrvate Carboxylase ☐
D. Alpha- KG dehydrogenase ☐

130. Zinc acts as co-factor in A/E: *(PGI 14,12,08)*
A. Lactate dehydrogenase ☐
B. Carbonic anhydrase ☐
C. Glutathione peroxidase ☐
D. Alkaline phosphatase ☐
E. Superoxide dismutase ☐

131. Carboxypeptidase contains which mineral-
A. Copper *(NBE P 15)* ☐
B. Zinc ☐
C. Iron ☐
D. None ☐

132. Selenium deficiency causes: *(PGI 13, 12)*
A. Dermatitis ☐
B. Cardiomyopathy ☐
C. Diarrhoea ☐
D. Alopecia ☐
E. Gonadal atrophy ☐

133. Selenium is co-factor for : *(NBE P 15,14,13; AI 08)*
A. Glutathione peroxidase *(PGI 14)* ☐
B. Glutathione reductase ☐
C. Glutathione synthetase ☐
D. Glutathione dehydrogenase ☐

134. Abzyme is a/an *(AIIMS 08)*
A. Isoenzyme ☐
B. Allosteric enzyme ☐
C. Abnormal enzyme ☐
D. Antibody with a catalytic activity ☐

135. Ceruloplasmin contains- *(NBE P 15)*
A. Zn ☐
B. Cu ☐
C. Se ☐
D. Fe ☐

136. Copper containing enzymes is/are All except: *(NBE P 15,14; AIIMS 14; PGI 15,14,12)*
A. Superoxide dismutase ☐
B. Cytochrome oxidase ☐
C. Myeloperoxidase ☐
D. Tyrosinase & Amine oxidase ☐

137. Biological role of metallothioneins is to sequester harmful metal ions. These bind *(AIIMS 04)*
A. Cd^{++}, Cu^{++} & Zn^{++} ☐
B. Al^{+++}, Hg^{++} & NH_4^+ ☐
C. Pt^{++}, As^{+++} & PO_4^- ☐
D. Fe^{+++}, Na^+ & K^+ ☐

138. Increased copper excretion in urine is seen in all except
A. Primary sclerosing cholangitis *(AIIMS 07)* ☐
B. Wilson's disease ☐
C. Primary biliary cirrhosis ☐
D. Hepatocellular carcinoma ☐

ANSWERS & EXPLANATIONS:

Structure & Functions of Proteins

1. **A i.e. Linear structure and order of amino acids present**
2. **B i.e. Secondary structure**
3. **D i.e. Long stretches of left handed α- helices occur in proteins**
4. **C i.e. Proline**
5. **B i.e. Aspartic acid**
6. **B i.e. Hydrogen bond**
7. **C i.e. Multiple weak interaction**
8. **D i.e. Quaternary structure**
9. **D i.e. Quartenary structure**

[Ref: Lehninger 5/e p 140-117, 92; Lippincott 5/e p 16-17; Vasudevan 6/e p 32-33; Harper 29/e p 36-40; Chattarje 8/e p 89-91]

- Discription of **all covalent bonds (mainly peptide and disulfide bonds) linking aminoacid residues in a linear structure refers to primary structure of protein.**
- **Secondary structure of protein** refers to **description of steric relationship (spatial arrangement) between aminoacids located relatively near each other in a selected segment of main polypeptide chain,** without regard to the conformation of its side chains or its relationship to other segments. Examples of secondary structures include **α-helix, β pleated sheet and β turns** etc.
- Naturally occurring L-aminoacids can (theoretically) form either right or left handed α-helices, ***but extended left handed α-helices are theoretically less stable and have not been observed in proteins***[Q].
- **Proline** and **glycine** have the ***least tendency (proclivity) to form α-helices***[Q].
- Large number of ***charged aminoacids like aspartate (aspartic acid)***[Q], glutamate (glutamic acid), arginine, lysine or histidine can also disrupt α-helix by forming ionic bonds or electrostatically repelling each other.
- **Secondary structure** is *stabilized by hydrogen bonds & disulfide bonds; Cooperative hydrogen bonding* in repeating secondary structures have an ***important role in guiding the protein folding process***[Q]. However , **location of bends (including β turns)** in polypeptide chain and the direction and angle of these turns are determined by the numer & location of ***specific bend producing aminoacid residues, such as Pro, Thr, Ser, and Gly. Interacting segments of polypeptide chains are held in their characteristic tertiary (3-dimensional) positions by several kinds of weak interactions***[Q] (mainly hydrophobic bonds, vanderwall forces, ionic interactions) and sometimes by covalent bonds (such as disulfide cross links) between the segments.
- Some proteins contain ≥2 **polypeptide chains or subunits which may be identical (homo) or different (hetero). Quarternary structure** of protein refers to three dimensional arrangement of these protein subunits. Therefore, ***homo-or hetero-dimers formed between 2 polypeptide chains is an example of quaternary structure***[Q]. Similarly an *immunoglobin molecule represents hetero-tetrameric quarternary structure between 4 polypeptide (2 heavy + 2 light) chains.*

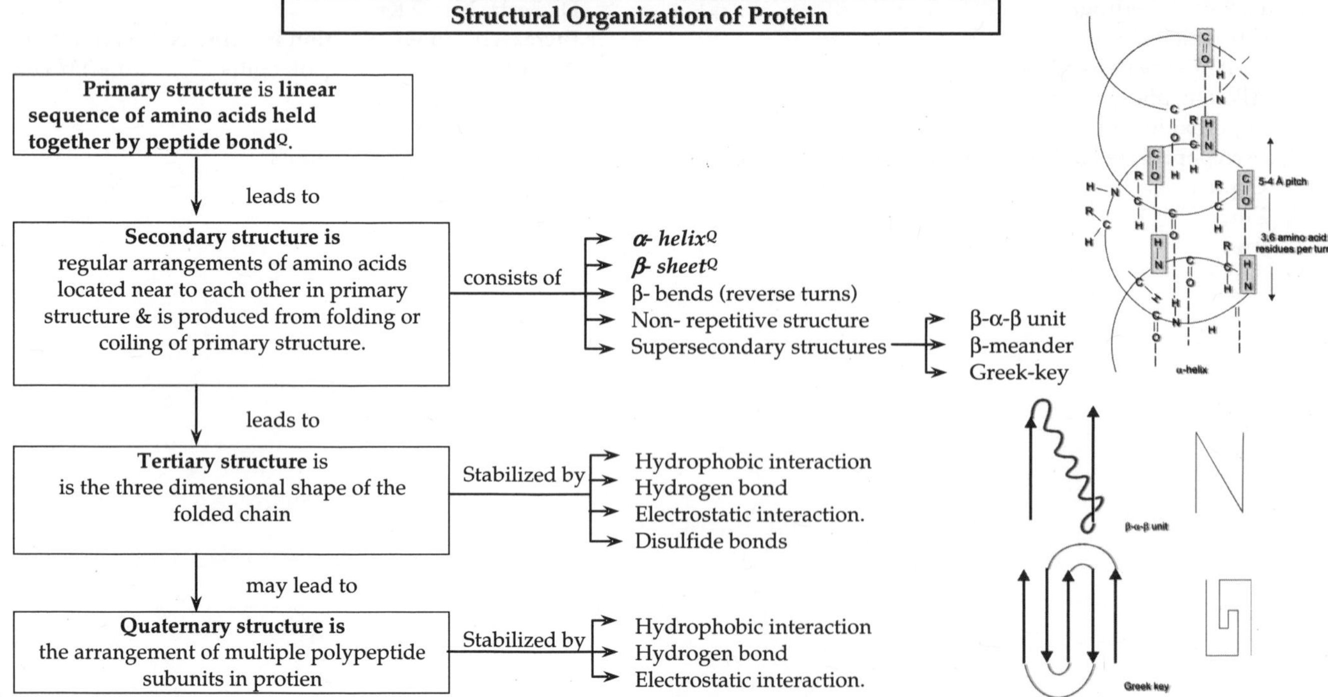

★ **Secondary and tertiary structure** of protein maintain the 3- dimensional shape of protein and the main bonds involved are weak non covalent bonds. (Thus **3-D shape is maintained by multiple weak interaction)**[Q].

10. **All i.e. (It makes protein resistant, Bond is formed b/w carboxyl terminus of one protein and the amino group of a lysine residue on another, Involves in post-transcriptional modification of protein, Enzyme acts as catalyst for the bond formation)**

> **Isopeptide bond** is an amide bond formed **between the side (not main) chain carboxy terminal of one protein** (with either glutamate or aspartate) and **amino group of lysine** residue on side chain of another target protein. Bond formation is either **spontaneous or enzyme (transglutminase) catalyzed, involves post translational modification and makes protein resistant.**

11. **A i.e. Disulfide bond** *[Ref: Lippincott's 3/e P-19; Harper's 27/e P-33-35]*

A disulfide linkage contribute to stability of three dimensional shape of protein molecule.
Many *disulfide bonds are found in proteins that are secreted by cell,* to stabilize the structure and *prevent them from becoming denaturated in the extracellular environment.*
Since ***snake's venom is a protein secretion it is most probably stabilized by disulfide bond***Q.

12. **A i.e. Less number of disulphide bonds** 13. **D i.e. All**
[Ref: Vasudevan 6/e p 584; Harper 29/e p 626-27, 43-44; Lehninger 5/e p 71, 123]

> ***Keratin in skin is softer than keratin in nail, horn & hooves because skin keratin has less number of disulfide bonds***Q between Cys residues of **adjacent polypeptide chains. Keratin contains Histidine, Arginine & Lysine (Mn: HAL**Q **in 1:12:4).**

14. **B i.e. Molluscus shell** *[Ref: Internet]*

> - **Biomineralization** (ie mineralization caused by cell mediated phenomenon in living organisms to harden or stiffen existing tissues) is seen in **molluscus shell, sea shells** (i.e. calcium carbonate in invertebrates), **bone & teeth in mammals and birds** (i.e. $CaCO_3$ & $CaPO_4$ in vertebrates), **silicates in algae & diatoms**, and copper, iron, gold in bacteria.
> - **Hoof and nails are thickened keratin.**

15. **B i.e. Convergence** *[Ref: Convergent evolution among immunoglobins F : M Frick;]*

Convergence is an evolutionary process by which distinctly unrelated organisms (protein) aquire morphologically similar traits, (function), where as **divergence** produces different traits (functions) in related same ancestor organisms (proteins).
Convergence may be

Sequence convergence	Structural convergence	Mechanical convergence	Functional convergence
≥1 aminoacids or aminoacid sequence of two different proteins come to resemble	**Proteins of different aminoacid sequences assume similar motif structures**Q	**Proteins with different aminoacid sequences & strucure come to act by similar mechanism**Q	Proteins with different amino acid sequences, structure and mechanisms come to serve same function.

16. **B i.e. Ligand binding residues** *[Ref: Lehninger 4th/160; Harper's 27/e P-369]*

Function in biochemistry revolves around a reversible protein ligand interaction.
A molecule bound reversibly by a protein is called a 'Ligand'. A ligand binds at a site on the protein called the 'binding site', which is complementary to ligand in size, charge and hydrophobic or hydrophillic character. As long as the ligand binding residues are preserved to allow interaction between the ligand and the binding sites the function will essentially be preserved.

- Amino acid sequence alterations are compatible will functionally normal haemoglobin: (Acceptable missense mutations) eg. Haemoglobin Hikari has been found in at least two families of Japanese people. This haemoglobin has asparginine substituted for lysine at position 61 in IL β chain. (change in AA sequence). This replacement of specific lysine with arginine apparently does not alter the normal function of the β chain in these individuals.
- As long as the domains/Ligand receptors are preserved, a variation in **structure** is still compatible with normal function.
- Environmental changes do not explain why only a few out of 300 variants of human globin gene are incompatible will function.

17. **C i.e. Carbohydrate content is same but proteins are different D i.e. Carbohydrate chain is often linear**
18. **B i.e. Glucosaminoglycan** 19. **B i.e. They hold less amount of water** 20. **C i.e. Proteoglycan**
21. **C i.e. Serine** 22. **D i.e. Final trimming** 23. **C i.e. Golgi**
24. **D i.e. Presence of GlC – NAc – Gal – NANA in complex glycoprotein** 25. **D i.e. RER > A i.e. Golgi apparatus**
[Ref: Lippincott 5/e p 444; 166-70; Vasudevan 6/e p 124]

- **O-glycosylation** involves addition of a specific oligosaccharide unit (sugar chain) to the terminal (OH) group of **serine or threonine aminoacids** (commonly) and **tyrosine, hydroxylysine or hydroxyproline** (rarely). **Glycosyl transferase responsible for O-glycosylation** is found in **golgi complex**Q.
- **Dolichol synthesis, glycosyl transferase and protein oligosaccharide transferase** steps of **N-glycosylation** occurs in **endoplasmic reticulum (ER)**. Whereas final trimming & completion occurs in golgi complex
- **N linked complex oligosaccharide (glycoproteins) contain Glc NAC, NANA & Fuc**, whereas high mannose contain pramiraly Man (mannose).

26. **A i.e. Protein linked with glycosidic bond; D i.e. Participate in cell surface recognition**
27. **B i.e. Biological function remains..** 28. **D i.e. Biological activity is retained** 29. **C, B ie. Denaturation, Precipitation**
30. **A i.e. Bence Jones proteins** *[Ref: Harper's 27/e P-45-46; Leninger 2/e P- 141, 160, 63, 66- 61; Lippincott's 4/e p. 20, 171; Ananthanarayan 7/e p. 90; Harrison 16/e p. 251]*

- **Bence Jones protein** in urine can be identified by its characteristic property of **coagulation (precipitation or clumping due to denaturation) when heated to 50 – 60° C. But the clumps begin to desappear (d/t renaturation) when the sample is further heated to boiling point (70 – 100°C)**Q Again on cooling clumps reappear **(Heat test)**.
- **Cryoglobulins** (immunoglobulin proteins) precipitate when cooled and dissolve on heating to higher temperatures
- **Pyroglobulins** (associated with multiple myeloma, macroglobulinemia & other neoplastic disorders) resembles Bence Jones proteins in that both precipitate on heating to about 50°C but do not dissolve when cooled.

31. **B i.e. Concentration; D i.e. Path Length** *[Ref: Lehninger 3/e P- 121; 2/e 314, 207]*

Measurement of light absorption is an important tool for analysis of nucleotides and nucleic acids. The fraction of the incident light absorbed by a solution at a given wave length is related to the ***thickness of absorbing layer (i.e. path length) and the concentration of absorbing spaces***Q. The two relations hips are combined into the **Lambert Beer law** given in integrated form as-

$$\text{Log}\ \frac{I_o}{I} = \varepsilon c l$$

Where,
I_0 = Intensity of incident light
I = Intensity of transmitted light
ε = Molar absorption coefficient (in liters /mole- centimeter)
C = Concentration of absorbing species in moles /liters
l = thickness of light absorbing sample in centimeters
log I_0/I = Absorbance, and low assumes that the incident light is parallel and monochromatic (of single wave length) and solvent and solutes are randomly oriented.

32. **B i.e. Tertiary structure** *[Ref: Homology of pseudomonas cytochrome C-551 with eukaryotic Ctyochrome C by northwest university school of medicine]*

- Tertiary structure of cytochrome C in bacteria and humans are highly conserved. Pseudomonas (bacterial)cytochrome C differs from eukaryotic (human) cytochrome in
  - total no. of amino acids
  - amino acid sequence.
- Comparison of primary protein structure with the tertiary structure revealed that functionally crucial a.a residues fold closely together in tertiary structure while they were distant to each other in primary structure.

33. **B i.e. Guanidine** *[Ref: Lippincott's 3/e P-21, 23, Lehninger 3/e P 192]*

Guanidine is a **denaturating substance**Q, results in loss of secondary & tertiary structure of proteins

Denaturation of Protein

Results in the unfolding and disorganization of the protein's secondary and tertiary structures (3-D structure), sufficient to cause loss of function. The **primary structure is intact**Q. Some denaturant are

- **Heat**Q	- **Urea**Q	- **Guanidine hydrochloride**Q
- **Extremes of pH**Q	- **Detergents**Q	- Organic solvents eg. alcohol & acetone

↓

Loss of secondary and tertiary structureQ leading to Loss of function

34. **B i.e. Fibrous proteins** 35. **A i.e. Fibrous** *[Ref: Harper's 27/e P-38; 26/e P-30; Chatterjea 6/e P-78; Lehninger 5/e p. 125]*

- **Proteins responsible for maintaining the structural strength of cells (i.e. cytoskeleton) and tissues include collagens, keratin and myosin etc. These proteins are classified as fibrous proteins. 'Structural proteins' are usually fibrous protein**Q, and include proteins of skin, cartilage, nail (such as collagen and proteoglycan). **Fibrous protein centrifuge more rapidly**Q because of their rod like shape.
- Collagen is the most abundant of the fibrous proteins. Other prominent fibrous proteins include keratin and myosin. These proteins represent a primary source of structural strength for cells (the cytoskeleton) and tissues.

Fibrous protein	Globular protein
- When the axial ratio of length: width of a protein molecule is more than 10, it is called fibrous protein. Polypeptide chains **are arranged in long strands or sheets.** - Usually consists largely of single type of secondary structure - Structures that provide support, shape and external protection to vertebrates are fibrous protein. Thus **structural proteins are usually fibrous proteins**Q. - Examples: **Collagen, α- keratin of hair etc, (i.e. structural protein)**Q	- When the axial ratio of length: width of a protein is less than 10, it is called globular protein. Polypeptide chain is folded into spherical or globular shape - Often contain **several types of secondary structures** - Most enzymes & regulatory proteins are globular protein - Examples: Myoglobin, Hemoglobin (i.e. storage proteins or transport proteins)

36. **A i.e. Triple helix** 37. **C i.e. Formation of triple helix** *[Ref: Harper 28th/ed pg-528-30; Lippincott 4th/ed pg- 43-49]*

- Collagen is a **triple helical structure**Q in which **3 α chains are wound into right handed superhelix with occurance of glycine residue at every 3rd position**Q of triple helix of α-chain. **Vitamin C (ascorbic acid) is necessary (as cofactor) for hydroxylation of proline & lysine while procollagen is converted into collagen during post translational modification**Q.
- Removal of **leader or signal sequence** (to form pro α- chains), **hydroxylation** (not hydrolysis) of proline & lysine residues, **glycosylation** of some hydroxylysine not proline residues with glucose or glucosyl galctose, **interchain and intrachain disulfide bond** formation at carboxy terminal propeptide extension (while amino terminal extension propeptide forms only intrachain disulfide bonds) and **triple helix formation**Q are **intracellular events of collagen formation.**
- **Cleavage of amino & carboxy terminal propeptide extensions** (by N & C procollagen peptidases) releasing triple helical tropocollagen; **spontaneous self assembly of tropocollagen** molecules **to form collagen fibrils**; assembly of collagen fibrils in orderd, **quarter overlapping, parallel, staggered alignment; oxidative deamination** of E aminogroups of lysyl and hydroxyl lysyl residues to aldehydes; and formation of intra and inter chain covalent cross links via Schiff bases and aldehyde condensation products l/t mature collagen formation are **extracellular events of collagen formation.**

38. **C i.e. Calcium**

40 nm gap between the typrocollagen molecues serve as nucleation site for deposition of hydroxyapatite [$Ca_5(PO_4)_3(OH)$] with some phosphate] crystals in boneQ.

39. **B i.e. Simple globular protein** *[Ref: Chatterjea 7/e p. 81-82; Lehninger 5/e p. 85]*

Plasma proteins like **albumin and globulin are simple globular protein**Q.

40. **B i.e. Collagen:** *[Ref: Harper's 29/e p 48, 632; Chattarjae 8/e p 105-06]*

Albumin, ceruloplasmin, transferrinn and **hemoglobin are transport proteins** whereas **collagen is a structural protein.**

41. **B, D, E > A i.e. Ovalbumin, Ferritin, Glutelin > Myoglobin** *[Ref: Chatterjaea 8/e p 617, 83-85; Satyanarayan 3/e163; Harper 29/e 635]*

- **Ricin** is a **phytotoxin**. Whereas **, ovalbumin, ferritin and glutelin are storage proteins.**
- **Hepcidin** is the ***chief regulator protein known to play a central role in systemic iron hemostasis***[Q]. It bind to cellular iron exporter ferroportin and triggers its internalization and degradation. When plasma iron levels are high, hepatic synthesis of hepcidin increases, thus reducing iron absorption in intestine (mucosal block); preventing recycling of iron from macrophages and reducing placental iron transfer. This leads to reduction in circulating iron levels (hypoferremia). The opposite occurs when plasma iron levels are low.

42. **A i.e. Phosphates** *[Ref: Chatterjea 6/e P- 657]*

A protein estimation test is confused with phosphates[Q]- as presence of phosphate give false positive test

43. **B i.e. Ninhydrin** *[Ref: Lippincott's 3/e P- 14- 15]*

Amino acids can be detected and quantified by reaction with ninhydrin after seperation of amino acid from mixtures. The test ***requires intact peptide bonds***[Q].

44. **D i.e. Bromocresol green** *[Ref: Teitz 6/e p 687, 80-179]*

Bromocresol purple (BCP) and bromcresol green (BCG) dye binding assay (ie Alb_{BCP} & Alb_{BCG}) is a method for **estimation of total serum albumin (not total protein).**

45. **D i.e. Enzyme assay** *[Ref: Reliability of plasma creatinine method in infants & children marie Jose clermont – Clinical pediatrics, vol. 25, No 11, 569- 572 (1986); Recommendations for improving serum creatinine methods- Gary L. Myers, Clinical chemistry 52 : 5 – 18 – 2006; Measurement of serum creatinine – Micheal whiting].*

Gas chromatography – isotope dilution mass spectrometry (GC- IDMS) is considered the method of choice for establishing the true concentration of creatinine in serum because of its excellent specificity > ***HPLC > Enzyme assay > Alkaline picrate methods***[Q].

46. **B i.e. IV Contrast agent; A i.e. Chlorpropamide** *[Ref: Schnier: Manual of nephrolgy 6/e p- 116- 17]*

Protein – dipstick test

False positive		False negative
- Concentrated urine - Gross hematuria - Presence of mucus, semen or leukocytes	- Highly alkaline urine (> 7ph) - **Iodinated IV contrast agent**[Q] - Contaminated with chlorhexidine, benzoalkonium, penicilline, aspirins, oral hypoglycemic agents	- Non albumin proteins - Albumin in small amount

Methods of Protein Separation (Purification)

47. **B, C i.e. Native gel electrophoresis; 2D gel electrophoresis**
48. **B, C, D, E i.e. Chromatography, Centrifugation, Ultrafiltration, Electrophoresis** 49. **A, D i.e. Mass; Molecular wt**
50. **A i.e. SDS- PAGE** 51. **B i.e. SDS- Polyacrylamide gel electrophoresis** 52. **D i.e. Densitometry**
[Ref: Chatterjea 6/e P-749- 50, NMS 4/e P 19- 23; Harper's 27/e p. 21-24]

SDS polyacrylamide gel electrophoresis is method of protein seperation & purification ***on the basis of molecular size***[Q]. Whereas electrophoretic mobility of protein in **native (non-denaturating) gel electrophoresis and 2-D gel electrophoresis** depends on both **charge (PI)** and its **mass (hydrodynamic size). Densitometry** is a method to ***quantitate protein in tissue***[Q].

Method of Separation & Purification of Protein

(based on)

Molecular size

Technique	Property used
Denaturing gel/ SDS-PAGE (polyarcylamide gel) electrophoresis[Q]	**Molecular weight (mass)**
Gel filtration (size exclusion) chromato-graphy[Q]	Molecular weight (size)
Dialysis/Ultra filtration	Size
Ultracentrifugation	Mass/density

★ **pI** is **pH** at which the net charge of molecule is zero. And electrophoresis in general is for separation of **charged molecules.**

Charge & or Iso electric point (pI, pH) and combined

Chromatography	Property used
High performance liquid chromatography (HPLC)	Charge, size, affinity
Ion exchange chromatography	Charge
Chromato focusing chromatograpgy	pI
Electrophoresis	**Property used**
Isoelectric focusing (IEF) electrophoresis	pI
Native gel electrophoresis	Mass/Charge
2D gels electrophoresis	Molecular weight & pI

Solubility

- **Ammonium sulfate precipitation (bulk method) i.e.**
  - **Salting in**
  - **Salting out**
- **Partition chromatography**

Hydrophobicity

- **Reversed phase** chromatography
- **Hydrophobic interaction** chromatography

Biological activity or affinity binding

- Affinity (absorption) chromatography
- Precipitation by antibodies

★ Ammonium sulphate, precipitation, centrifugation, and filtration are **bulk methods**

Ammonium Sulfate Fractionation

53. **A i.e. Salting out** *[Ref: Lehninger 5th/ed pg-85-92; John Baynes Mechanical Biochemistry 3rd/ed pg- 14-15; Harper 28th/ed pg-21]*

The **solubility of proteins** is generally lowered at high salt concentration. So **addition of salts (eg ammonium sulfate)** in right amount can **selectively precipitate some proteins, an effect called salting out**[Q]. It is used to purify protein.

Ammonium Sulfate / $(NH_4)_2SO_4$ = (Salt) Fractionation

Early purification (fractionation) utilize differences in **protein solubility** which depends on *pH, temperature, salt concentration etc.*

Salts of **divalent ion** such as ammonium sulfate / $(NH_4)_2SO_4$ and magnesium chloride ($MgCl_2$) are far more effective than salts of monovalent ions eg NaCl, KCl, and NH_4Cl. ***Ammonium sulfate is particularly effective and is often used to salt out protein***[Q].

Salting In

In **low concentrations,** salt increase the solubility of many proteins, a phenomenon known as **salting in**

Salting out

- The solubility of proteins is lowered at **high salt concentration**, an effect called salting out
- **Increasing the ionic strength (or salt concentration) gradually decrease the solubility of proteins.** So addition of certain salts eg ammonium sulfate can selectively precipitate some proteins, while others remain in solution
- At 33-40% saturated $(NH_4)_2SO_4$, human immunoglobins are precipitated (salted out) while albumin remains soluble. Most proteins will precipitate from an 80% saturated $(NH_4)_2SO_4$. Saturated ammonium sulfate is about 4.1 mmol/L

Chromatography

54. C i.e. Gel filtration Chromatography **55. C i.e. Gel diffusion Chomatography** **56. A i.e. Gel Chromotography**
57. A i.e. Diffusion **58. B i.e. Affinity chromatography**
[Ref: Chatterjea: 7/e p. 769-72; Harper's 28/e p. 21-23; Vasudevan 6/e p. 601-4]

- **Gel filtration chromatography** separates protein according to their molecular sized **(molecular weight).**Q
- **Proteins whose charges are same, can be separated by Gel diffusion chromatography.**Q
- **Affinity Chromatography** separates proteins by their binding specificities. The **proteins retained on the column are those that bind specifically to a ligand**Q (substance) that has an inherent ability to bind with the target molecule to be purified.

59. B i.e. Ion-Exchange chromatography **60. B i.e. Aspartic acid**
[Ref:Lehninger 5th/e p. 85-88, 173, 364-65; John Baynes Mechanical Biochemistry 3rd/e p. 16; Harper 28th/e p.22; Vasudevan 6/e p. 601-4]

In **cation exchange chromatography** solid stationary matrix has negatively charged groups (**i.e. –ve charged carboxy methyl cellulose**, O – CH2 – COO⁻ is used as cation exchanger). So in the mobile phase, **proteins with a net positive charge (i.e. cations) move slowly than those with net negative charge (anion)**Q. Hence **aspartate (aspartic acid)** being a negatively charged amino acid will **move fastest in carboxymethyl cellulose** or methanol chloroform (cation exchanger) ion exchange chromatography.

Electrophoresis

61. C & D i.e. Depends on size not on shape & Commonest method of purifying protein
62. B i.e. Gel electrophoresis **63. A i.e. Gel centrifugation** **64. D i.e. Gel chromatography**
[Ref: Lehninger 5th/ed pg- 958-56; Teitz 6th/ed pg- 278; Micklos: DNA science 2/ed pg-438-39; Pierce: Genetics 2/e p-515; John Baynes Mechanical Biochemistry 3rd/ed pg- 467-66]

The fragments of DNA produced by endonuclease can be **isolated by electrophoresis on agrose or polyacrlamide gels**Q. **Relaxed DNA is separated from supercoiled & linear DNA by gel (agarose / polyacrylamide) electrophoresis**Q

65. B i.e. Sodium Dodecyl Sulphate PAGE **66. C i.e. The protein is a dimmer of two 20kD and 30kD proteins**
[Ref: Lehninger 5th/ed pg- 88-91; Harper 28th/ed pg-23-24; John Baynes Mechanical Biochemistry 3rd/ed pg-16-17]

Most widely used **method for determination of purity and molecular weight** of proteins is **SDS- PAGE** i.e. polyacrylamide gel electrophoresis **in the presence of anionic detergent sodium dodecyl sulfate**Q

SDS PAGE gel electrophoresis separates proteins on the basis of their relative *molecular weight alone*. Since the results of SDS PAGE electrophoresis show two bands only, *the protein that underwent SDS-PAGE is composed of polypeptides with two different molecular weights (One of 20 KD and the other of 30kD)*. If the protein in question was a monomer its molecular weight should have been 50kD. Since the protein has a molecular weight of 100kD, the protein is likely to be a dimmer of two 20 kD proteins (Which form one band) and two 30 kD proteins (Which form the other band).

67. B i.e. Charge *[Ref Cahill, Mathew. Handbook of Diagnostic Tests. Springhouse, 1995. ;Jacobs, David S., et al. Laboratory Test Handbook. 4th ed.; Pagana, Kathleen Deska. Mosby's Manual of Diagnostic and Laboratory Tests. St. Louis1998]*

Hemoglobin electrophoresis is based on chargeQ

Hemoglobin electrophoresis is a test that measures the different types of hemoglobin in the blood. Hemoglobin (Hgb) is comprised of many different types, the most common being A_1, A_2, F, S, and C. Hgb A_1 is found in normal red blood cell, Hgb A_2 is a minor component of normal hemoglobin, Hgb F in the fetus, Hgb S in **sickle cell disease,** Hgb C in **hemolytic anemia.** ***Each of the major hemoglobin types has an electrical charge of a different degree, so the most useful method for separating and measuring normal and abnormal hemoglobins is electrophoresis.***
This process involves *subjecting hemoglobin components from dissolved red blood cells to an electric field*. The components then *move away from each other at different rates*, and when separated *form a series of distinctly pigmented bands*. The bands are then *compared with those of a normal sample*. Each band can be further *assessed as a percentage of the total hemoglobin, thus indicating the severity of any abnormality*.

Detection of Protein Structure

68. **A, B, E i.e. X-RAY Crystallography, NMR Spectroscopy, Electrophoresis** *[Ref: Vasudeven 6/e 34; Harper 28/e 23-27-37-39; Lehninger 5/e 75-90; Lippincott 5/e 21; John Baynes 3/e p 15-17, 55*
69. **A i.e. High performance liquid chromatography**
70. **B i.e. Chromosome walking**
71. **A i.e. X-ray diffraction / Crystallography**

- **High performance (pressure) liquid chromatography (HPLC)** is a modern refinement of column chromatography and is **used for protein separation, purification**Q and identification. **It can not determine protein structure**Q.
- **Electrophoresis** separates (& purifies) proteins based on migration of charged proteins in an electric field. **It can not determine protein structure**Q.
- **Higher level (2°, 3° & 4°) of protein structure is studied by X-ray crystallography, NMR sepectroscopy, infrared and ultraviolet spectroscopy**Q.

72. **A i.e. Arginine; C i.e. Lysine**
73. **B i.e. Trypsin cleaves arginine next to praline**
74. **A,D,E i.e. Phenylalanine; Tryptophan; Tyrosine**

[Ref: Harrison 17th /1764; Harrison's 18th/2312Lehninger 5th/ed pg-95-96; Vasudevan 6/e p. 33; Harper 28/e p. 462; John Baynes Mechanical Biochemistry 3rd/ed pg- 18-19]

Reagent & Cleavage Point

- **Trypsin cleaves peptide bonds on C- terminal side of arginine and lysine residues, provided the next residue is not proline**Q. **Chymotrypsin** cleaves peptide bond on **carbonyl (C) terminal of phenylalanine, tryptophan and tyrosine**Q
- **Lysyl endopeptidase cleaves c- terminal side of lysine**Q and cyanogens bromide cleaves C- terminal side of methionine.
- Disulfide bonds interfere with sequencing procedure. So before cleavage **proteins with cysteine** and **cystine** residue are either **oxidized by performic acid**Q to **cysteic acid or reduced by dithiothreitol (or β mercaptoethanol)**Q and idoacetate (to carboxymethylated cysteine) to **irreversibly break disulfide bonds**. This avoids spontaneous formation of inter or intra molecular disulfides during analysis.
- For **determination of structure of protein:** Purified protein (by process of salting out →dialysis → ion exchang & gel filtration chromatography →SDS PAGE) is cleaved by **protelytic degradation**. The cleaved peptides fragments are again purified by reverse phase HPLC and then sequenced on automated protein sequencer, using **Edman's degradation technique**, Now **Mass spectrometry, MALDI – TOF, ESI –MS** and indirect hybrid techniques are also used to determine 1° protein structure.

Reagent (Biological source)	**Cleavage point**
Trypsin (bovine pancrease)	- **Lysine, Arginine (C) provided next residue is not proline**Q - Elastase esters of small neutral aliphatic aminoacids, chymotrypsin esters of aromatic aminoacids.
Lysyl endoproteinase C (bacterium Lysobacter enzymogenes)	Lysine (C) carboxy terminal
Submaxillarus protease (mouse submaxillary gland)	Arginine (C) terminal
Cyanogen bromide chemical	Methionine (C)
V8 protease (staphylococcus aureus)	Aspartate, Glutamate (C)
Asp – N- protease (Pseudomonas fragi)	Aspartate, Glutamate (N terminal)
Chymotrypsin (bovine pancreas)	Phenylalanine, Tryptophan, Tyrosine (C) or Leucine
Pepsin (Porcine stomach)	Leucine, phenyalanine (Phe), Tryptophan (Trp), Tyrosine (Tyr) – **N** amino side

75. **B i.e. Absorption mass spectroscopy**
76. **D i.e. X-ray diffraction** *[Ref: Harper's 28/e P-26-27; Campbells Urology 8/e P- 3274]*

Polarizing microscopy, X-ray diffraction and infrared spectroscopy are techniques for analysing renal and gall bladder stones.

77. **B i.e. Amino acids** *[Ref: Chatterjee 5/e p. 88]*

Sanger's & Edman's Reaction

Used to determine Aminoacid sequence in polypeptide chain by tagging (N) amino terminal with **Sanger's reagent (1 fluro-24-Dinitrobenzene)** or **Edman's reagent (Pheny-isothio-cyanate).** Tagged aminoacid is hydrolysed and identified.

Test/Reaction	Used to Identify Aminoacids (group or specific)
Ninhydrin	**All α aminoacids**
Xanthophoretic	**Aromatic aminoacids**[Q]
Aldehyde test & Hopkins-Cole-Reaction	Tryptophan (Indole ring)
Sulphur/Nitroprusside Test	Cysteine (Sulphydryl group)
Millan (Nasse) Test	Tyrosine (Phenol group)
Pauli's Diazo Test	Histidine (Imidozole gp) or Tyrosine
Sakagauch's Test	Arginine (Guanidinium gp)
Biurate Reaction	**Peptide Bond**[Q]

Enzymes

78. **B i.e. Non-competitive inhibitor**

In non competitive inhibition, there is **no competition between substrate & inhibitor** because inhibitor is **structurally different and it binds to enzyme at a site other than substrate binding (catalytic) site**[Q]**.**

Enzyme Inhibition 

Any substance that can *decrease the velocity of an enzyme catalyzed* reaction is k/a **inhibitor (I)**. The inhibition can be **reversible** or irreversible. **Reversible inhibitors** bind to enzymes through *non covalent bonds and can be dissociated (removed)* from its binding site (by dilution) without loosing its enzyme activity. Whereas, **irreversible inhibitors** bind to enzyme through *covalent bonds* and can be removed from its site of binding only at the loss of enzymatic activity (i.e. **irreversible inhibitors poison enzymes**). Two most common types of reversible inhibiton are competitive & non competitive. However the non- competitive can also be irreversible.

	Competitive Inhibition	Non-Competitive – Inhibition
Direction	***Reversible***[Q]	***Reversible or irreversible***[Q]
Structure of inhibitor (I)	Resemble substrate (structure) and so are termed **substrate analogs.**	Bear **no** (or little) structure **resemblance** to substrate
Binding site	Inhibitor binds to **substrate binding portion of active site** (i.e. both inhibitor & substrate bind to **same site** and so inhibitor competes with the substrate (S) for that site) thereby blocking access by the substrate	Inhibitors bind enzymes at sites **distinct from substrate binding site** (i.e. substrate (S) and inhibitor (=I) bind enzyme (=E) at **different sites**) and so there is *no competition* between inhibitor & substrate for enzyme.
EIS complex	- Inhibitor can not bind to enzyme – substrate (ES) complex - Either EI or ES complex is formed and EIS is not possible	- Inhibitor can bind to ES complex - Both EI and **EIS complexes** can form; however EIS generates product at negligible rate.
Raising substrate concentration (i.e. dilution)	**Overcomes inhibiton** (i.e. at sufficiently high substrate concentration, **Vmax will be same** as observed in absence of inhibitor)	**Can not be overcome** (i.e. inhibitor **decreases Vmax**)
Substrate affinity to enzyme	- **Decreased** (i.e. once inhibitor binds to enzyme, the enzyme cannot bind to substrate) - So more substrate is needed to achieve ½ Vmax (i.e. **Km↑**)	- **Does not change** (i.e. non competitive inhibitors donot interfere with binding of substrate to enzyme) - Same amount of substrate is needed to achieve ½ Vmax (i.e. **Km is unaffected)**
V max **Km**	**Same**[Q] **Increased (↑)**[Q]	**Lowered (↓)**[Q] **Same**[Q]

Michaelis – Menten equation	$V = \frac{V_{max}[S]}{Km\frac{1+(I)}{Ki}+S}$	$V = \frac{V_{max}[S]}{Km\left[\frac{1+(I)}{Ki}\right][Km]+[S]}$
Lineweaver – Burk plot	$\frac{1}{V}=\frac{Km}{V_{max}}[1+\frac{(I)}{Ki}]\times\frac{1}{[S]}+\frac{1}{V_{max}}$ For Non-Competitive – Inhibition $\frac{1}{V}=\frac{Km}{V_{max}}\left[1+\frac{(I)}{Ki}\right]\times\frac{1}{[S]}+\frac{1}{V_{max}}+\left[1+\frac{(I)}{Ki}\right]$	$\left[\frac{1}{V}\right]$ Non-competitive Competitive No inhibitor Vmax decreased Vmax same ⊖ Km same, Km increase, O ⊕ $\left[\frac{1}{S}\right]$ **Line-Weaver Burk (Double reciprocal) plot**
Eadic – Hofstee plot	No change in Y intercept (Vmax) but possesses steeper slope and smaller x intercept.	No change in slope (-Km) but Y intercept is lowered and x intercept declines in value

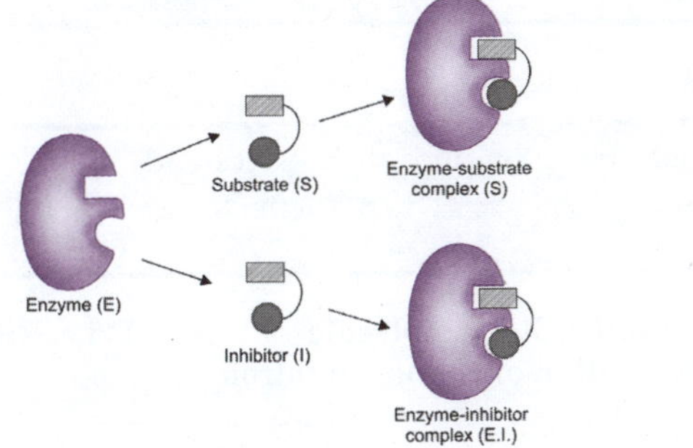

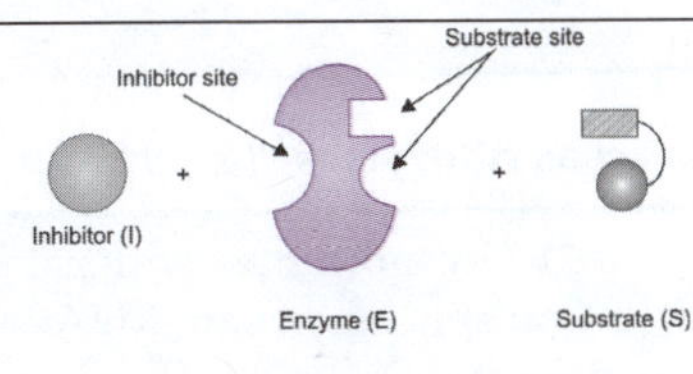

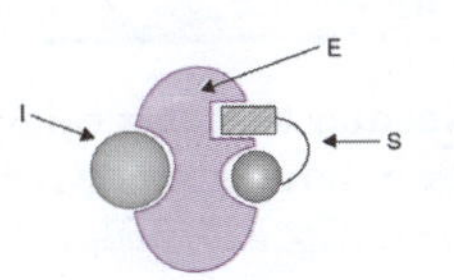

79. **A i.e. V_{max} unchanged** 80. **C i.e. Non competitive inhibitor** 81. **C i.e. Competitive**
82. **A, C i.e. Lower Vmax, Not affect Km** 83. **A, E i.e. ↑ Km, V max remain same**
84. **C i.e. Km value normal; V_{max} decreased** 85. **A i.e. Competitive** 86. **A i.e. Substrate concentration at $V_{max}/2$**
87. **A i.e. K_M** *[Ref: Chattarjea 7/e p 121-24; Harper 28/e 70-74-77-79; Lippincott 5/e 62-64; KDT 6/e p 40]*

In non competitive inhibition, there is **no competition between substrate & inhibitor** because inhibitor is **structurally different and it binds to enzyme at a site** other than **substrate binding (catalytic) site**Q.

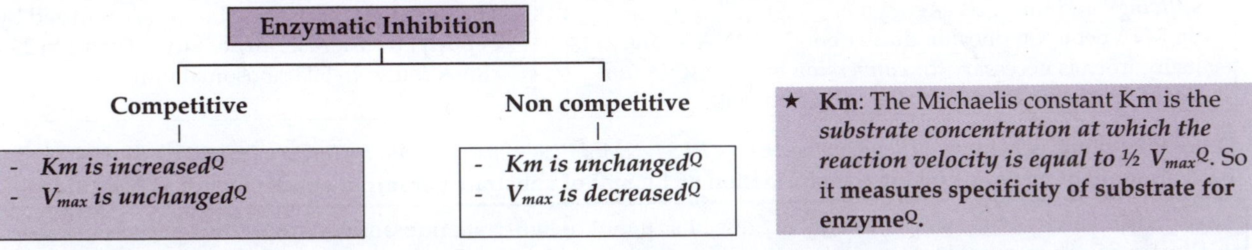

88. **B, C i.e. Substrate concentration at which reaction rate is half the maximum; Michaelis constant**
89. **C i.e. Michales–Menton reaction** 90. **D i.e. Enzymes substrate complex formation is essential in enzymatic reaction**
91. **A, E i.e. HMG CoA; Glycogen synthase** 92. **B,C,E ie. Glycogen synthetase, Pyruvate dehydrogenase & Citrate lyase**
Ref: Lippincott 4th/e p.63, 110; Lehninger 5th/e p. 220-27, 571-77; Harper 28th/e p.81; Chattarjea & Shinde 7/e p. 118- 19]

Phosphorylation is the most important type of regulatory modification

- It involves addition or removal of phosphate group from *serine, threonine, tyrosine or histadine residue of enzyme*
- *ATP* is used as PO_4 donor
- **Protein kinase** enzyme catalyzes phosphorylation (i.e addition of PO_4) and **phosphoprotein phosphatase** catalyzes dephosphorylation (i.e. removal of PO_4 group).

- Some enzymes are regulated by reversible covalent modification
- Common modifying group include: phosphoryl, acetyl, adenylyl, uridyl, methyl, amide, carboxyl , myristoyl, palmitoyl, prenyl, hydroxyl, sulfate and adenosine di phosphate ribosyl groups

Enzyme P = Phosphorylated D = Dephosphorylated	Activity state	
	Low (Inactive)	High (Active)
Acetyl – CoA carboxylase	P	D
Glycogen synthase	P	D
Pyruvate dehydrogenase	P	D
HMG – CoA – reductase	P	D
Glycogen phosphorylase	D	P
Citrate lyase	D	P
Phosphorylase b kinase	D	P
HMG-CoA reductase kinase	D	P

- Even entire proteins eg *ubiquitin & sumo* are used as specialized modifying groups **Ubiquitin** is added to protein as a tag that pre destines them for ***proteolytic degradation***Q. Sumo is attached to eukaryotic nuclear proteins with role in regulation of transcription, chromatin structure & DNA repair.
- ADP ribosylation (derived from NAD) occurs in bacterial enzyme *dinitrogenase reductase* (l/t regulation of biological N_2 fixation), diphtheria toxin & cholera toxin

93. **D i.e. Hexokinase** *[Ref: Harper's 28/e p. 450; Vasudevan 6/e p. 412, 587; Lehninger 5/e p. 436-37]*

Adenyl cyclase, guanylate cyclase and glycogen synthase enzymes (but not hexokinase)Q are activated by **calcium and calmodulin**.

94. **B i.e. RNAs act as ribozymes** *[Ref: Harper's 27/e P-315, 318, 364]*

Ribozymes are **RNA molecules with catalytic activities**Q, which acts upon phosphodiester bonds in RNA & cause its hydrolysis [intron splicing event]. RNAs are not protein, but meet all the classic criteria of enzymes therefore all enzymes are not protein.

95. **A i.e., RNA molecular that acts catalytically to change itself or another RNA molecule**
96. **D i.e. Ribozyme**
97. **A i.e. Splicing of heterogenous RNA to form mRNA; D i.e. Recognition of codons in intron** *[Ref: Harper's 27/e P-315, 318, 364; 26/e P-308, 356; Lippincott's 3/e P-436]*

Ribozymes are RNA molecules with intrinsic catalytic activity. These are generally involved in transesterification reactions, & most are concerned with RNA metabolism (splicing and endoribonuclease). Example: Sn RNAs, rRNA

Ribozymes

Sn RNA	rRNA
- **Small nuclear RNAs (Sn RNA)** in assosiation with small nuclear ribonucleoprotein particles (Sn RNPs) ***facilitate splicing***Q and thus acts as enzyme. - Sn RNA act upon phosphodiester bond of RNA & causes its hydrolysis necessary for ***conversion of pre mRNA (hn RNA) to mature RNA***Q. [Intron splicing event]	- **rRNA** is involved in elongation of polypeptide chain during eukaryotic protein synthesis - The formation of peptide bonds is catalyzed by peptidyl transferase, an activity intrinsic to 23S rRNA found in 508 ribosomal unit.

98. **D i.e. Micromoles / Minute** *[Ref: Lippincott's 3/e P- 54, NMS. Biochemistry 4/e P-59-60; Vasudevan 4/e p- 44]*
99. **E i.e. Amount of enzyme causing transformation of 1 μ mol of substrate per minute under standard condition**

The specific activity of enzyme is usually **expressed as μ mol of substrate transformed to product per minute per milligram of enzymes under optimal condition of measurement**Q.

1 international unit (IU) = *1 micromole / minute*Q
Modern unit of enzyme activity, ***1 katals (kat) = 1 mole / second*** *(i.e. conservation of 1 moles of substrate per second)*
Enzymes are highly specific, interacting with one or few specific substrates & catalyzing only one type of chemical reaction Rate of metabolic processes may thus be regulated by changes in the catalytic efficiency of specific enzymes.

100. **C i.e. Accumulation of S_2** *[Ref: Harper's 27/e P-75-77; 26/e P- 74]*

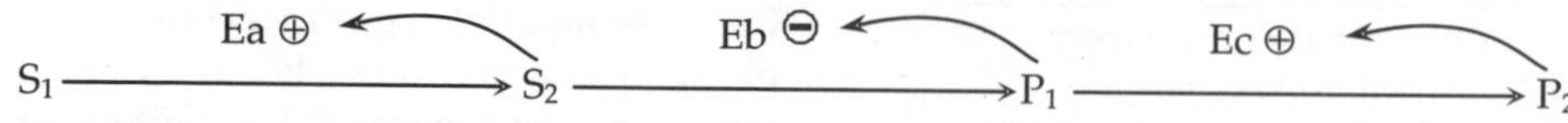

- Defective Ec would block the conversion of P_1 to P_2 & thus P_1 start accumulating.
- This increased P_1 exerts a *negative feedback effects* on Eb and decreases the conversion of S_2 to P_1 & thus S_2 accumulates.
- Increased S_2 exerts a *positive feedback* on Ea & increases the conversion of S_1 to S_2. The more S_2 accumulates the more enzyme Ea is activated to convert S_1 to S_2 & thus S_2 goes on accumulating.

101. C i.e. Lipoprotein lipase *[Ref: Harper 28th/e p. 59]*

Lipoprtein lipase is a **functional enzyme (i.e. has physiological role) that hydrolyze lipids in lipoproteins (chylomicrons & VLDL) into free fatty acids and glycerol molecule**Q.

102. D i.e. Catalyze the same reaction
103. A i.e. Different Km value; C i.e. Consist of multimeric complex; E i.e. Have different physical properties
104. A i.e. LD-1 **105. B i.e. Brain Ischemia**
[Ref: Chatterjea 8/e p 123, 644-647, 522; Lippincott 5/e p 65-66; Das 8/e p 94; Harper's 29/e P-63-65; Harsh Mohan 4/e 296; Debajyoti Das 8/e P 94]

- **Isozymes (iso enzymes) catalyze the same reaction but at different rates**Q. **They differ from each other structurally (d/t difference in quarternary structure), electrophoretically (d/t different number of charged acidic or basic amino acids), physically ie in physical properties such as heat resistance (d/t genetically determined differences in aminoacid sequence).** They **differ in pH optima, Km and V_{max}** values as well as in **enzymatic classification numbers.** Isoenzymes have **different tissue distribution** and may **contain various combinations of different subunits of multimeric complex**Q.
- **Isoenzyme LDH-1** with four 'H' subunit **predominates in cardiac tissue**Q, since heart expresses the H subunit almost exclusively. **CPK-1 is found in brain ischemia**Q

106. C i.e. Vander Waals *[Ref: Textbook of Biochemistry Thomas M.Devlin 4/e P 156]*

'Vander Walls' forces are too weak, to actively participate in formation of enzyme- substrate complex.

Various models have been proposed to explain the substrate specificity of enzymes e.g. 'Lock & Key' method

- Substrate fits in the binding site of enzyme just as key fits into proper lock (strong interaction). Forces contribute in binding are:- **Hydrogen bonding**Q
  - Ionic (electrostatic) bondingQ
  - Hydrophobic interaction
- Enzymes function to decrease the activation energy so that reactions can occur at normal body temperature. The substrate form a ***covalent bond***Q with the enzymes active site, & accelerates the reaction.

107. A i.e. Pepsin **108. D i.e. Serine** *[Ref: Harper's 27/e P-53-55]*
109. C i.e. Chymotrypsin will bind the substrate but will not cause cleavage

Serine- 195 is a highly reactive residue of chymotrypsin molecule. It endows chymotrypsin with its 'Reactivity' and not its ability to bind to substrate. **In absence of Ser- 195 residue, chymotrypsin is inactivated i.e., it will not cleave, however, it still has the ability to bind (by virtue of other remaining residues).**

110. A i.e. Oxidase **111. A i.e. Transferase** **112. D i.e. Lyases**
113. A i.e. Transferase **114. C i.e. Hydrolase** **115. None >>> B i.e. Peroxidase**
116. B i.e. Hydrolases **117. B i.e. Cytochrome P 450** **118. D i.e. Required for carboxylation of drugs**
[Ref: Chattergea & Shinde 7/e p. 469, 116; Harper's 28/e p. 52; Lippincott's 5/e p. 53-54; Lehninger 5th/ed pg- 816, 518-20]

- Transferase – **enzymes catalyze** transfer of a particular group (containing C-, N- or P-) from one substrate to anotherQ. **Whereas,** hydrolase **bring about** hydrolysis by addition of waterQ.
- Fumarase **is a** lyaseQ, glutamine synthetase is ligaseQ, tyrosinase **is** oxidaseQ **and** hexokinase **is a** transferaseQ.
- **Enzymes involved in oxidation (removal of e-) and reduction (gain of electrons) are called** oxido – reductase **and are classified into 4 groups:** oxidase, oxygenase, dehydrogenase, hydroperoxidase (peroxidase and catalase)Q.
- **Hydrolase is another class of enzyme that catalyzes hydrolysis i.e. cleavage of bonds by addition of water.**
- **Carboxylase enzyme, which belongs to ligase class is required for carboxylation**Q
- **Oxigenase (which belongs to oxido-reductase class) cause incorporation of 2 atoms of O_2 (dioxygenase) or 1 atom of O_2 (monoxygenase or hydroxylase)**

6 – Classes of enzymes (International Union of Biochemistry = IUB) Mn – "TO HILL"

Class	Feature	Example
Transferase	**Catalyze transfer of C – N-, or P-containing group from one substrate to another**Q, such as Serine ⇌ Glycine (SHT)	- Aspartate & alanine transminase (AST/ALT) - **Hexokinase**Q, Hexose 1- phosphate uridyl transferase - Phosphoglucomutase - Ornithine carbamoyl transferase - Serine hydroxy methyl transferase (SHT)
Oxidoreductase	Catalyze oxidation reduction reactions, such as Lactate ⇌ Pyruvate (*Lactate dehydrogenase*)	- Alcohol dehydrogenase, lactate dehydrogenase, glucose – 6 – phosphate dehydrogenase - Glutathione reductase - Xanthine oxidase, **Tyrosinase**Q
Hydrolases	**Catalyze hydrolysis i.e., cleavage of bonds by addition of water**Q, such as $Urea + H_2O \xrightarrow[Urease]{} CO_2 + 2NH_3$	- Pepsin, trypsin, esterases - Glucose 6 phosphatase, glycoside hydrolases - **Urease**Q
Isomerases	Involved in isomerization of substrate i.e., catalyze racemization of optical or geometric isomers, such as Methyl Malonyl CoA ⇌ Succinyl CoA (MMCoAM)	- Triose phosphate isomerase, retinal isomerase - UDP- glucose epimerase, racemase - Methyl malonyl CoA mutase (MMCM)
Lysases	Catalyze cleavage of C – C, C – S, & certain C – N bonds and facilitate removal of small molecules from a large substrate $Pyruvate \xrightarrow[decarboxylase]{Pyruvate} Acetaldehyde$	- **Fumarase**Q, Argino- succinase - Histidine **decarboxylase**Q - Pyruvate **decarboxylase**Q
Ligases	Catalyze formation of bonds between carbon and O, S, N coupled to hydrolysis of high energy phosphates and involved in joining together two substrates. $Pyruvate + CO_2 \xrightarrow{PC} Oxalo\ acetate$ (ATP → ADP)	- DNA ligase, Pyruvate carboxylase (PC) - Alanyl t-RNA synthetase - **Glutamine synthetase**Q

119. **D i.e. Malonate dehydrogenase**

Reactions	Rate Limiting Enzymes
Glycolysis	**Phosphofructokinase**Q
Glycogen synthesis	**Glycogen synthetase**Q
Glycogenolysis	**Glycogen phosphorylase**Q
TCA Cyle	**Isocitrate dehydrogenase**Q
Fatty acid synthesis	**Acetyl COA Carboxylase**Q
Cholesterol synthesis	**HMG COA reductase**Q
Ketone body synthesis	**HM COA synthetase**Q
Bile acid synthesis	**7- α- hydroxylase**Q
Catecholamine synthesis	**Tyrosine hydroxylase**Q
Urea synthesis	**Carbamoyl transferase**Q

120. **C i.e. Phosphatase** *[Ref: Harper's 27/e P-78-79; Chatterjea 6/e P-559]*

Magnesium is required as co-factor in:
[Mnemonic: **"C T PARK"**]
C - Carboxylase
T - Transketolase
P - PhosphataseQ
 - Peptidase
A- **A**denyl cyclase
R- **R**ibonuclease
K- Kinase

Magnesium is required in covalent modification of enzymes by phosphorylation, dephosphorylation of seryl residues.

ATP → ADP (Mg^{2+}, Kinase)
Enz – Ser -OH ⇌ Enz – Ser $-O-PO_3^{2-}$
Phosphatase (Mg^{2+})
Pi ← H_2O

121. C i.e. Non protein **122. C i.e. Holoenzyme**

123. A i.e. Pyridoxine; B i.e. Biotin; C i.e. Thiamine; D i.e. Folic acid **124. D i.e. Accept one of the cleavage products**

125. A i.e. Thiamine is a coenzyme for pyruvate dehydrogenase & α ketoglutarate ... **126. A i.e. Carboxylation**

[Ref: Lippincott's 4/e p. 54- 55, 101, 110, Harper's 27/e p. 50-51,490; Chattergea & Shinde 7/e p. 114- 16 ; Vasudevan 4/e p. 37- 39]

Except for **ribozyme,** ***which is RNA***[Q], all the enzymes are protein in nature with large molecular weight. Some enzymes require, molecules other than proteins for enzymic activity. **Holoenzyme** is active enzyme with its nonprotein component, whereas the enzyme without its nonprotein moiety is termed an apoenzyme and is inactive. So the *protein part of enzyme* is called **apoenzyme,** non-protein part – **coenzyme, cofactor or prosthetic group,** and the complete structure **holoenzyme.**

127. A i.e. Biotin *[Ref: Nelson 17/e p. 412]*

Multiple carboxylase deficiency is a group of disorder resulting from defective utilization of biotin. Since **biotin is a coenzyme for carboxylase enzymes (carboxylation),** it results in malfunction of all carboxylases and organic acedimia. It is *treated by biotin*[Q].

128. B i.e. Pantothenic acid *[Ref: Harper's 27/e P-503]*

The active form of pantothenic acid is CO- enzyme A (COA) & the Acyl carrier protein (ACP). **Pantothenic acid acts as a cofactor after its modification**[Q]

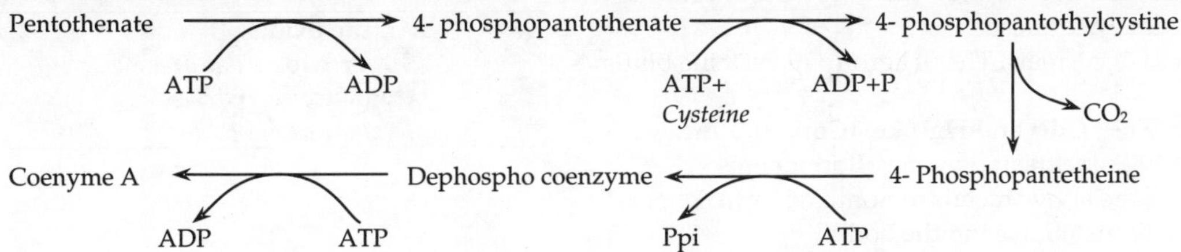

129. A i.e. Alcohol dehydrogenase **130. C i.e. Glutathione peroxidase** **131. B i.e. Zinc**

Functions of Zinc

Role in Enzyme action		Other functions
Zinc forms an integral part of several enzymes (metallo enzymes) in the body: • ***Superoxide dismutase***[Q] in cytosol: Cu-Zn protein complex with two Zn^{++} per molecule of the enzyme. • ***Carbonic anhydrase***[Q] present in RBC, parietal cells and renal tubular epithelial cells, one Zn^{++} per molecule • **Leucine- Amino- peptidase** of intestinal juice • **Carboxyl peptidase A** – of *pancreatic* juice	• **Others:** - ***Alcohol dehydrogenase, lactate dehydrogenase***[Q], glutamate dehydrogense, malate dehydrogenase, Carbon monoxide dehydrogenase, D-2 hydroxy acid dehydrogenase, galactitol 1 PO4 5 dehydrogenase - ***Alkaline phosphatase***[Q], δ ALA dehydratase - Retinine reductase, DNA & RNA polymerase, histone deacetylase - β lactamase, lactoylglutathione lyase, insulin degrading enzyme. - Glutamae carbboxypeptidase II, glutamyl aminopeptidase - ADAM (a disintegrin & metalloprotease domain) of proteinases (eg TACE i.e. TNF α converting enzyme)	• **Role in Vit A metabolism** - Stimulate release of Vit A from liver - Participate in the regeneration of Rhodopsin in eye during dark adaptation (as present in *Retinine reductase*) • Role in *insulin secretion* • Role in *growth & Reproduction* • Role in *wound healing*

132. B i.e. Cardiomyopathy **133. A i.e. Glutathione Peroxidase**

[Ref: Harper 29/e p 118, 201, 270, 541; Harrison 18/e p 604; Chattrjea 8/e p 211, 630-31, 560, 801; Indian Journal of Medial Science 1190; 44(7): p. 173-7]

- **Selenium** in form of **selenocysteine** is a component (as a prosthetic group) of **glutathione peroxidase, thioredoxin**, and **deiodinase** that converts thyroxine to triodothyronine.
- **Selenium deficiency** causes **Keshan disease (endemic cardiomyopathy) and Kaschinbeck disease (endemic degenerative osteoarthritis or osteopathy** particularly affecting children). Low selenium levels also increase the risk of **thrombotic episode, cancer** (specially GI , more so oesophegeal & orolaryngeal cancers). Concomitant deficiency of Se & iodine may *worsen clinical manifestations of cretinism.*

134. D i.e. Antibody with catalytic activity *[Ref: NMS Biochemistry 4/e P- 109]*

Abenzymes are catalytic antibodies (antibody + enzyme)Q

135. B i.e. Cu **136. C i.e. Myeloperoxidase** **137. A i.e. Cd^{++}, Cu^{++} & Zn^{++}** *[Ref: Harper 29/e p 640]*

- **Metallothioneins** regulate tissue levels of **copper (Cu^{2+}), zinc (Zn^{2+}), cadmium (Cd^{2+}), and mercury (Hg^{2+})**
- **Copper containing enzymes include ferroxidase (ceruloplasmin), lysyl oxidase, ascorbic acid oxidase**Q**, amine oxidae, cytochrome oxidase, superoxide dismutase and tyrosinase**Q

Metallothioneins

- Are group of small proteins (6.5 KDa), found in cytosol of cells, particularly of liver, kidney & intestine
- They have high content of cysteine. The SH group of cysteine binds the metal
- **Tissue levels of Cu^{2+}, Zn^{2+}, Cd^{2+} and Hg^{2+} i.e. (Copper, Zinc, Cadmium & mercury)**Q are regulated by metallothioneins
- It may function to store the above metals in nontoxic form & are involved in their over all metabolism in the body.
- The concentration of metallothionines in tissue is increased by acute intake of metals or administration of certain hormones or cytokines.

Enzymes that contain Copper

- **Amine oxidase**Q
- **Superoxide dismutase**Q
- **Cytochrome oxidase**Q
- **Tyrosinase**Q

138. D i.e. Hepatocellular carcinoma *[Ref: Robbins 7/e p. 910; Harper's 27/e p. 595-97; Chattergea 7/e p. 584-86]*

- Copper is excreted in the bile into GI tract from which it is not reabsorbed. So normally urine contains only traces of copper. Since ***copper homeostasis is maintained almost exclusively by biliary excretion***Q, any disease which hampers its biliary excretion will lead to accumulation of Cu in liver → increased blood levels & increased urinary excrition. ***So cholestatic hepatitis, primary biliary cirrhosis and primary sclerosing cholangitis show increased copper excretion in urine***Q.
- **Wilson disease** has defect in *copper binding P type ATPase (ATP 7B protein)* which cause defective excretion of copper into bile & reduction in incorporation of copper into apoceruloplasmin l/t accumulation of Cu in liver, brain, kidney & RBC.

Chapter -6 METABOLISM OF PROTEIN & AMINO ACIDS

QUESTIONS

Fate of Amino Group

1. **Transfer of an amino group from an amino acid to an alpha keto acid is done by?** *(AI 11)*
   A. Transaminases ☐
   B. Aminases ☐
   C. Transketolase ☐
   D. Decarboxylase ☐
2. **Transmination of pyruvate with glutamate produces** *(AI 03)*
   A. Oxaloacetate & aspartate ☐
   B. Alanine & asparate ☐
   C. Oxaloacetate & α-ketoglutarate ☐
   D. Alanine & α-ketoglutarate ☐
3. **Trans-amination of pyruvate and glutamic acid leads to the formation of** *(AI 06)*
   A. Oxaloacetate ☐
   B. α-ketoglutarate ☐
   C. Aspartate ☐
   D. Malate ☐
4. **All are involved in non toxic transport of ammonia except**
   A. Glutamine synthetase *(WB 10, UP 09)* ☐
   B. Glutaminase ☐
   C. Alanine cycle ☐
   D. SGPT ☐
5. **The amino acid which serves as a carrier of ammonia from skeletal muscle to liver is:** *(NBE P 15,14; AI 06)*
   A. Alanine ☐
   B. Methionine ☐
   C. Arginine ☐
   D. Glutamine ☐
6. **Glutamine in blood acts as:** *(PGI 08)*
   A. NH_3 transporter ☐
   B. Toxic element ☐
   C. Stored energy ☐
   D. Abnormal metabolite ☐
7. **Which end product of citric acid cycle is used in detoxification of ammonia in brain** *(AIIMS 01)*
   A. Oxaloacetate ☐
   B. Alphaketoglutarate ☐
   C. Succinate ☐
   D. Citrate ☐
8. **In Metabolic alkalosis, which is true about excretion in urine:** *(PGI 03)*
   A. More of NH_3 ☐
   B. Less of aceto acetic acid ☐
   C. Betahydroxy butyric acid ☐
   D. Less ammonia ☐
9. **Ammonia is detoxified (removed as) in brain to:**
   A. Urea *(NBE P 15,13; AIIMS 16,15; AI 09)* ☐
   B. Glutamine ☐
   C. GABA ☐
   D. Uric acid ☐
10. **Glutamine synthetase is a -** *(AIIMS 03, Delhi 05)*
    A. Isomerase ☐
    B. Ligase ☐
    C. Lyase ☐
    D. Transferase ☐
11. **Source of ammonia in urine** *(Jipmer 02)*
    A. Glutaminase ☐
    B. Urease ☐
    C. Glutamate dehydrogenase ☐
    D. Arginase ☐
12. **The amino acid producing (major source of) ammonia in kidney is:** *(AIIMS 07,13)*
    A. Glutamine ☐
    B. Alanine, Aspartate ☐
    C. Methionine ☐
    D. Glycine ☐
    E. Glutamate
13. **Oxidative deamination is catalyzed by-**
    A. Glutaminase *(NBE P 15)* ☐
    B. Glutamine synthase ☐
    C. Glutamate dehydrogenase ☐
    D. None of the above ☐

Urea Cycle

14. **In urea cycle, hydrolysis of arginine forms-** *(NBE P 15)*
    A. Citrulline ☐
    B. Ornithine ☐
    C. Carbomoyl phosphate ☐
    D. Arginosuccinase ☐
15. **Which of the following enzyme (s) is/are not involved in urea cycle:** *(PGI 12)*
    A. Glutamate dehydrogenase ☐
    B. Argininosucinate synthetase ☐
    C. α-KG dehydrogenase ☐
    D. Isocitrate dehydrogenase ☐
    E. Fumarase ☐
16. **Urea cycle occurs in :** *(NBE P 14; AI 11)*
    A. Liver ☐
    B. G.I.T. ☐
    C. Spleen ☐
    D. Kidney ☐
17. **Urea cycle enzymes are:** *(PGI 14, 09)*
    A. Glutaminase ☐
    B. Asparginase ☐
    C. Arginosuccinate synthetase ☐
    D. Ornithine transcaroxylase ☐
    E. Glutamate dehydrogenase ☐
18. **Urea is produced by the enzyme-** *(NBE P 13; PGI 12)*
    A. Urease ☐
    B. Uricase ☐
    C. Arginase ☐
    D. Glutaminase ☐

19. Urea is mainly formed in liver and to small extent in-
A. Spleen *(DNB 15; AMU 03)* ☐
B. Heart ☐
C. Muscle ☐
D. Brain ☐

20. Which of the following is true in relation of urea cycle:
A. First 2 steps in cytoplasm *(PGI 05)* ☐
B. First 2 steps in mitochondria ☐
C. Defect of enzyme of any step can cause deficiency disease ☐
D. Urea is formed by NH_3, glutamic acid and CO_2 ☐
E. Citruline is formed by combination of carbomoyl phosphate and L. Ornithine ☐

21. Sources of the nitrogen in urea cycle are: *(AI 01)*
A. Aspartate and ammonia ☐
B. Glutamate and ammonia ☐
C. Arginine and ammonia ☐
D. Uric acid ☐

22. Urea cycle, true is all except *(AMU 10, UP 09)*
A. Aspartate converted to fumarate ☐
B. Ornithine-citrulline transporter aminoacids ☐
C. N-acetyl glutamate is allosteric inhibitor ☐
D. Aspartate-arginino succinate shunt ☐

23. A child presents with metabolic lactic acidosis along with hyperammonemia and convulsion is due to
A. Reye's syndrome *(AIIMS 2K)* ☐
B. Mitochondrial enzyme disorders (MELAS) ☐
C. Urea cycle defect ☐
D. Phenylketonuria ☐

24. Hyperammonaemia inhibit TCA cycle by depleting:
A. Oxaloacetate *(PGI 09)* ☐
B. α-ketoglutarate ☐
C. Citrate ☐
D. Succinyl Co-A ☐
E. Fumarate ☐

Amino Acids

25. Cystine s formed by- *(NBE P 15)*
A. Hydroxylation of cysteine molecule ☐
B. Carboxylation of cysteine molecule ☐
C. Peptide bond between two cysteine molecule ☐
D. Disulfide bond between cysteine molecule ☐

26. Initial amino acid in prokaryotic protein synthesis-
A. Arginine *(NBE P 15)* ☐
B. Methionine ☐
C. Formyl-methionine ☐
D. Alanine ☐

27. Tryptophan is glucogenic & ketogenic by producing-
A. Acetyl coA & alanine *(NBE P 15)* ☐
B. Acetoacetate & fumarate ☐
C. Acetoacetate & arginine ☐
D. Arginine & alanine ☐

28. A common feature of all serine proteases is: *(AI 06)*
A. Autocatalytic activation of zymogen precursor ☐
B. Tight binding of pancreatic trypsin inhibitor ☐
C. Cleavage of protein on the carboxyl site of serine residues ☐
D. Presence of Ser-His-Asp catalytic triad at the active site ☐

29. Guanido acitic acid is formed in....from....-
A. Kidney; Arginine+Glycine *(AI 11, DNB 15)* ☐
B. Liver; Methionine + Glycine ☐
C. Liver; Cysteine + Arginine ☐
D. Muscle; Citrulline + Aspartate ☐

30. Creatinine is synthesised from - *(DNB 10; NBE P 14,13)*
A. Glycine, arginine and methionine ☐
B. Glycine and methionine ☐
C. Ornithine and glycine ☐
D. Thymine and ornithine ☐

31. Creatine is made up of all, except- *(NBE P 15)*
A. Glycine ☐
B. Alanine ☐
C. Methionine ☐
D. Arginine ☐

32. All of the following amino acids are converted to succinyl-CoA, *except*: *(AI 06)*
A. Methionine ☐
B. Isoleucine ☐
C. Valine ☐
D. Histidine ☐

33. Which one of the following can be a homologous substitution for isoleucine in a protein sequence?
A. Methionine *(AI 06)* ☐
B. Aspartic acid ☐
C. Valine ☐
D. Arginine ☐

34. At physiological pH, the carboxy-terminal of a peptide is: *(AIIMS 05)*
A. Positively charged ☐
B. Negatively charged ☐
C. Neural ☐
D. Infinitely charged ☐

35. Iso electric pH is: *(AIIMS 05)*
A. Point at which all amino acids are in zwitter ion form ☐
B. Point at which pH of ions are same. ☐
C. Point at which pH of ions does not alter. ☐
D. Point at which positive and negative charges on the amino acid are equal. ☐

36. At isoelectric pH protein: *(PGI 03)*
A. Have Net charge 'O' ☐
B. Are positively charged ☐
C. Are negatively charged ☐
D. Don't migrate ☐

37. The amino acid residue having an iminoside chain is:
A. Lysine *(AI 05)* ☐
B. Histidine ☐
C. Tyrosine ☐
D. Proline ☐

38. Sulphur containing amino acid is/are: *(PGI 15,12,06)*
A. Aspartic acid ☐
B. Glutamine ☐
C. Methionine & Cysteine ☐
D. Glycine ☐
E. Serine ☐

39. **Replacing alanine by which amino acid will increase UV absorbance of protein at 280 nm wavelength:**
A. Leucine *(AIIMS 08)* □
B. Proline □
C. Arginine □
D. Tryptophan □

40. **Property of photochromosity is seen amongst the following amino acids OR The property of proteins to absorb ultraviolet rays of light is due to:** *(AI 11, 09)*
A. Unsaturated aminoacid □
B. Aromatic aminoacid □
C. Monocarboxylic acid □
D. Dicarboxylic acid □

41. **Aromatic amino acids are A/E OR Aromatic ring is present in all except-** *(NBE P 15, 14,13; AIIMS 15,13)*
A. Tryptophan □
B. Tyrosine □
C. Lysine □
D. Phenylalanine □

42. **Hydrophobic aminoacids are:** *(PGI 10)*
A. Methione □
B. Isoleucine □
C. Tyrosine □
D. Alanine □
E. Asparagine □

43. **Polar amino acid (s) is/are:** *(PGI 15, 12)*
A. Serine □
B. Tryptophan □
C. Tyrosine □
D. Valine □
E. Lysine □

44. **Non Polar Amino Acids are:** *(PGI 10)*
A. Alanine □
B. Tryptophan □
C. Isoleucine □
D. Lysine □
E. Tyrosine □

45. **Which of the following side chains is least polar**
A. Methyl *(AI 09)* □
B. Carboxyl □
C. Amino □
D. Phosphate □

46. **Leucine is a aminoacid with a:** *(AI 08)*
A. Nonpolar side chain □
B. Polar side chain □
C. Negatively charged side chain □
D. Positively charged side chain □

47. **Polar amino acid are all except-** *(NBE P 15)*
A. Glutamic acid □
B. Histidine □
C. Glutamine □
D. Methionine □

48. **Most non polar Amino Acid is :** *(AI 11)*
A. Leucine □
B. Glycine □
C. Arginine □
D. Lysine □

49. **Neutral amino acid is-** *(NBE P 15)*
A. Aspartate □
B. Arginine □
C. Glycine □
D. Histidine □

50. **Acidic amino acids are-** *(PGI 10,03)*
A. Asparagine □
B. Arginine □
C. Glutamine □
D. Lysine □

51. **Basic amino acids are:** *(AI 01; AMU 04)*
A. Aspartate and glutamate □
B. Serine and glycine □
C. Lysine and arginine □
D. None of the above □

52. **Most basic amino acid out of the following is:**
A. Alanine *(NBE P 13)* □
B. Arginine □
C. Histidine □
D. Lysine □

53. **Basic amino acid (s) is /are A/E OR At physiological pH, which of these amino acids has a positive charge?:**
A. Arginine *(PGI 16,15,09; AIIMS 16,15)* □
B. Proline □
C. Lysine □
D. Histidine □

54. **Which of these amino acids will migrate slowest to the anode end at the physiological pH-** *(AIIMS 02)*
A. Aspartic acid □
B. Glycine □
C. Lysine □
D. Valine □

55. **Non-Essential amino acid is -** *(AI 08, DNB 09)*
A. Tyrosine *(AIIMS 15,13)* □
B. Phenylalanine □
C. Lysine □
D. Threonine □

56. **An essential amino acid in man is -**
A. L-methionine *(AIIMS 14, 12)* □
B. L-tyrosine □
C. L-serine □
D. L-proline □

57. **Aminoacid that enters the TCA cycle for gluconeogenesis & Ketogenin in nature-** *(PGI 06)*
A. Pheylalanine □
B. Alanine □
C. Glycine □
D. Serine □

58. **Essential amino acid is-** *(NBE P 15,14,13)*
A. Alanine □
B. Serine □
C. Arginine □
D. Proline □

59. **All ar essential amino acid except-**
A. Phenylalanine *(AIIMS 14; AI 08; NBE P 15,14,13)* □
B. Lysine □
C. Leucine □
D. Glycine □

60. Essential amino acid amongst the following-
A. Arginine *(NBE P 15,14,13)* □
B. Lysine □
C. Threonine □
D. All □

61. Semiessential amino acids are- *(PGI 15,13)*
A. Arginine □
B. Histidine □
C. Glycine □
D. Phenylalanine □

62. Negative nitrogen balance is produced in humans by elimination from the diet of all of the following amino acids except - *(DNB 13; Delhi 10)*
A. Leucine □
B. Methionine □
C. Lysine & Threonine □
D. Serine □

63. All of the following are essential aminoacids except:
A. Methionine *(AIIMS 15, 07)* □
B. Lysine □
C. Alanine □
D. Leucine □

64. Substitution of which one of the following amino acids in place of alanine would increase the absorbance of proteins at 280 mm: *(AIIMS 05)*
A. Leucine □
B. Arginine □
C. Tryptophan □
D. Protein □

65. Which one of the following amino acids is most likely to be found in the transmembrane region of a protein
A. Lysine *(AIIMS 04)* □
B. Arginine □
C. Leucine □
D. Aspartate □

66. All biologically active proteins are *(AIIMS 03)*
A. L-forms □
B. D-forms □
C. Mostly D form □
D. D and L form □

67. The conversion of an optically pure isomer (enantiomer) into a mixture of equal amounts of both dextro and levo forms is called as: *(AI 03)*
A. Polymerization □
B. Stereoisomerization □
C. Racemization □
D. Fractionation □

68. Amino acid with double chiral is- *(NBE P 15)*
A. Phenyalanine □
B. Threonine □
C. Tryptophane □
D. Tyrosine □

69. Amino acid which lacks chirality is: *(NBE P 14; AI 10)*
A. Lysine □
B. Leucine □
C. Histidine □
D. Glycine □

70. Which of these amino acids does not have anomeric carbon atom OR Optically inactive Amino Acid is OR Flexibility of protein depends on:
A. Valine *(NBE P 13; AIIMS 14,02; PGI 10)*□
B. Alanine □
C. Tyrosine □
D. Glycine □

71. Major from of folic acid to transfer one carbon is-
A. Methylene THF *(NBE P 15)* □
B. Formyl THF □
C. Methyl THF □
D. ALL □

72. Vitamin involved in 1 carbon metabolism OR Which vitamin is required for transfer of 1- carbon unit:
A. Folic acid *(NBE P 15,13; PGI 15,14; AIIMS 14)* □
B. Thiamine □
C. Pyridoxine □
D. Vitamin A □

73. Which vitamin is related to a co-factor in glycine Metabolism is- *(AIIMS 03)*
A. V, E □
B. Folic acid □
C. Thiamine □
D. Pantothenic acid □

74. Conversion of glycine to serine requires: *(PGI 02)*
A. Folic acid □
B. Thiamine □
B. Vit. C. □
C. Fe^{2+} □
D. Pyridoxal phosphate □

75. Amino acid with dissociation constant closest to physiological pH is OR Most stable amino acid at the physiological pH is OR Maximum influence of local milieu on ionization is on OR Which of the following amino acid is active at neutral pH OR Which amino acid can protonate & deprotonate at neutral pH OR At physiological pH buffering action in blood is caused by: *(NBE P 15, 14,13; AIIMS 13,10; PGI 14, 09)*
A. Serine □
B. Histidine □
C. Threonine □
D. Proline □

76. Which of the following is true about glutathione
A. Contain sulfhydral group *(PGI 14,13)* □
B. Forms met Hb from Hb □
C. It does not detoxity superoxide radicals □
D. Transport aminoacid across cell membrane □
E. Part of enzymes □

77. In glutathione which amino acid is reducing agent-
A. Glutamic acid *(AIIMS 07)* □
B. Glycine □
C. Cysteine □
D. Alanine □

78. Regarding glutathione which of the following is/are true:
A. It helps in absorption of certain amino acids □
B. It inactivates some enzymes *(PGI 02)* □
C. It helps in membrane transport □
D. It helps in conjugation reactions □

79. Amino acids secreted in cystinuria are all except:
A. Ornithine *(AIIMS 01)* □
B. Histidine □
C. Arginine □
D. Lysine □

80. Cystinuria is associated with excretion of which A.A in urine: *(PGI 09)*
A. Cystine, lysine, Tyrosine and alanine □
B. Cystine, lysine, ornithine and alanine □
C. Cystine, ornithine, lysine and arginine □
D. Cystine, ornithine, leucine and arginine □

81. Aminoacid containing indole ring is -
A. Arginine *(DNB 12, PGI 10)* □
B. Tryptophan □
C. Tyrosine □
D. Histidine □

82. The following is false about Tryptophan *(NBE P 14,13)*
A. Non essential amino acid *(DNB 08; AI 06)* □
B. Involved in serotonin synthsis □
C. Involved in niacin synthesis □
D. Involved in melatonin synthesis □

83. The amino acid that can be converted into a vitamin
A. Glycine *(NBE P 13)* □
B. Tryptophan □
C. Phenylalanine □
D. Lysine □

84. Which of the following amino acids is involved in the synthesis of thyroxine - *(NBE P 13,11)*
A. Glycine □
B. Methionine □
C. Threonine □
D. Tyrosine □

85. An amino acid not involved in urea synthesis is -
A. Ornithine *(DNB 07, 13)* □
B. Citrulline □
C. Arginine □
D. Aspartic acid □

86. Melatonin is synthesised from-
A. Tryprophan *(PGI 14,12; AIIMS 15; NBE P 15,13)* □
B. Serotonin □
C. Phenylalanine □
D. Histidine □

87. Which of the following is precursor of adrenalin and thyroxine synthesis - *(AIIMS 14,12; UP 08)*
A. Phenyl alanine □
B. Tyrosine □
C. Tryptophan □
D. None of the above □

88. Which of the following is not synthesised from tyrosine - *(AIIMS 14, 12, 08)*
A. Norepinephrine □
B. Melatonin □
C. Thyroxine □
D. Dopamine □

89. The substance from which ammonia is produce by the kidney is- *(AIIMS 06, CMC 08, Jipmer 09)*
A. Glycine □
B. Alanine □
C. Glutamine □
D. Methionine □

90. Ammonia is detoxified in brain by-
A. Uric acid *(JIPMER 01, AMU 08, J&K 03)* □
B. Glutamine □
C. Creatinine □
D. Urea □

91. The urea in the brain is derived from- *(AI 01, MP 06)*
A. Glutamine □
B. Glutamine acid □
C. Lactate □
D. Uric acid □

92. Phenylalanine is the precursor of all the following, except:
A. Tyrosine *(AI 02)* □
B. Epinephrine □
C. Thyroxine □
D. Melatonin □

93. Increased risk of Myocardial infarction is associated with which amino acid *(AIIMS 04)*
A. Methionine □
B. Homocystine □
C. Ornithine □
D. Valine □

94. All will predispose to atherosclerosis except:
A. Homocystinemia *(PGI 05)* □
B. Fibrinogen □
C. Calcium □
D. Lipoprotein A □

95. In phenylketonuria the main aim for first line therapy is: *(AI 11)*
A. Limiting the substrate for deficient enzyme □
B. Giving the missing amino acids by diet □
C. Replacement of enzyme □
D. To replace deficient product □

96. PKU is a congenital amino acid metabolic disorder. In one of the following rare variants of PKU Dihydro Biopterin synthesis is affected. The enzyme deficient is: *(PGI 08)*
A. Histidine decarboxylase □
B. Phenylalanine hydroxylase □
C. Dihydropterin reductase □
D. Tyrosine deficiency □

97. What results due to incomplete oxidation of phenylpyruvic acid: *(AIIMS 03)*
A. Albinism □
B. Alkaptonuria □
C. Phenylketonuria □
D. Tyrosinemia □

98. Ferric chloride test in PKU gives: *(PGI 06, 08)*
A. Red □
B. Green □
C. Blue □
D. Yellow □

99. Mousy odour urine is seen in: *(PGI 11, 07)*
A. Maple syrup urine □
B. Phenylketonuria □
C. Isovalericaciduria □
D. Cystinuria □

100. Tyrosinemics are more susceptible to develop:
A. Adenocarcinoma colon (*AIIMS 07*) ☐
B. Melanoma ☐
C. Retinoblastoma ☐
D. Hepatic carcinoma ☐

101. A 40 yr old woman presents with progressive palmoplantar pigmentation. X-ray spine shows calcification of intervertebral discs. On adding Benedict's reagent to urine, it gives greenish brown precipitate and blue-black supernatant fluid. What is the diagnosis? (*AIIMS 10*)
A. Phenylketonuria ☐
B. Alkaptonuria ☐
C. Tyrosinemia type-2 ☐
D. Argininosuccinic aciduria ☐

102. If urine sample darkens on standing: the most likely condition is : (*AI 01*)
A. Phenylketonuria ☐
B. Alkaptonuria ☐
C. Maple syrup disease ☐
D. Tyrosinemia ☐

103. Metabolites of tryptophan can give rise to: (*PGI 02*)
A. Diarrhoea ☐
B. Vasoconstriction ☐
C. Flushing ☐
D. Can predispose to albinism ☐
E. Phenylketonuria ☐

104. In maple syrup urine disease the amino acids. excreted in the urine are-(*PGI 15,13,10; NBE P 14,13; AIIMS 14,09*)
A. Leucine ☐
B. Isoleucine ☐
C. Valine ☐
D. a, b & c ☐

105. Which of the following aminoacid is excreted in urine in maple syrup urine disease : (*AI 09*)
A. Tryptophan ☐
B. Phenylalanine ☐
C. Leucine ☐
D. Arginine ☐

106. Branched chain ketoacid decarboxylation is defective in (*NBE P 13; AI 11*)
A. Maple Syrup urine disease ☐
B. Hartnup disease ☐
C. Alkaptonuria ☐
D. GMI Gangliosidosis ☐

107. Disease of branched chain amino acid includes:
A. Phenylketonuria (*PGI 15,13*) ☐
B. Maple syrup disease ☐
C. Taysach's disease ☐
D. Isovaleric acidemia ☐
E. Niemann-pick disease ☐

108. Orotic aciduria is due to deficiency of- (*NBE P 15*)
A. Decarboxylase ☐
B. Tyrosinase ☐
C. Isomerase ☐
D. Homogentisate oxidase ☐

109. Sweaty feet odor in body fluids occur d/t deficiency of
A. Biotin (*KA 09, AI 06*) ☐
B. FAD linked dehydrogenase ☐
C. Thiamin linked decarboxylase ☐
D. Leucine transaminse ☐

110. Correct combination of urine odour in various metabolic disorders: (*PGI 13*)
A. Phenylketonuria-Mousy odour ☐
B. Tyrosinemia-Rotten cabbage ☐
C. Hawkinsuria-Potato smell ☐
D. Maple syrup disease-Rotten tomato ☐
E. Alkaptonuria-Rotten egg ☐

111. Phosphorylation of amino acid by: (*PGI 08*)
A. Serine ☐
B. Tyrosine ☐
C. Leucine ☐
D. Tryptophan ☐

112. Succinyl Co-A is formed by: (*PGI 08*)
A. Histidine ☐
B. Leucine ☐
C. Valine ☐
D. Lysine ☐

113. A baby presents with refusal to feed, skin lesions, seizures, ketosis organic acids in urine with normal ammonia; likely diagnosis is: (*AI 01*)
A. Proprionic aciduria ☐
B. Multiple carboxylase deficiency ☐
C. Maple syrup urine disease ☐
D. Urea cycle enzyme deficiency ☐

114. The comparison of the amino acid sequence of Cytochrome C from different species shows many variations. Most of these variations are found:
A. Randomly (*AI 06*) ☐
B. Only in helical regions ☐
C. Only in strand regions ☐
D. Mainly in loop regions ☐

Hemoglobin, Bile Pigment & Porphyrin

115. Hemoproteins are: (*PGI 14,09*)
A. Cytochrome C (Oxidase) ☐
B. Cytochrome 450 ☐
C. Myoglobin ☐
D. Hemoglobin ☐
E. Catalase ☐

116. Haemoglobin is a buffer because of OR In hemoglobin, iron is bound to - (*NBE P 15,13*)
A. Histidine residue (*AIIMS 14,12*) ☐
B. Glycoprotein nature ☐
C. Weak acidic nature ☐
D. Iron molecule ☐

117. False statement about hemoglobin structure?
A. Hb has 2 polypeptide (*AIIMS 12,10*) ☐
B. Iron is present in ferrous state ☐
C. Hb structurally similar to myoglobin ☐
D. Ferrous ions are in porphyrin rings ☐

118. In hemoglobin the innate affinity of heme for carbon monoxide is diminished by the presence of:
A. His F8 (*AIIMS 15,10,02*) ☐
B. His E7 ☐
C. Gly B6 ☐
D. Thr C4 ☐

119. True statement about hemoglobin is- (*NBE P 15*)

A. Each hemoglobin molecule is made of 4 polypeptides of each subunit ☐
B. Two alpha and two beta subunits having a O_2 attached to each subunit ☐
C. Each hemoglobin molecule binds to only one O_2= molecule ☐
D. Each hemoglobin has one heme molecule ☐

120. Heme is which porphyrin- *(NBE P 15)*
A. Type 1 ☐
B. Type II ☐
C. Type III ☐
D. Type IV ☐

121. Haemoglobin unlike myoglobin shows: *(PGI 12, 08)*
A. Parabolic curve of oxygen association ☐
B. Co-operative effect of combine O_2 ☐
C. Cooperative index of 81 ☐
D. Hill's coefficient of 1 ☐

122. Which of the following statement characterize both Hemoglobin and Myoblogin: *(PGI 03)*
A. Non-helical ☐
B. Subunits which are held together by hydrogen bonds. ☐
C. Binds with 2 Heme ☐
D. Heme at hydrophobic pockets ☐
E. Bind with 1 molecule of O_2 ☐

123. Which is an allosteric protein: *(AIIMS 05)*
A. Transferrin ☐
B. Ceruloplasmin ☐
C. Phosphofructokinase ☐
D. Haemoglobin ☐

124. True regarding conversion of deoxyhemoglobin to oxyhemoglobin is : *(AIIMS 02)*
A. Binding of O_2 causes release of H^+ ☐
B. One mole of deoxyhemoglobin binds two moles of 2,3 DPG ☐
C. pH of blood has no affect on the binding of O_2 ☐
D. Binding of O_2 causes increased binding of 2,3,DPG ☐

125. Decreased glycolytic activity impairs oxygen transport by hemoglobin due to: *(AI 03)*
A. Reduced energy production ☐
B. Decreased production of 2,3-bisphosphoglycerate ☐
C. Reduced synthesis of hemoglobin ☐
D. Low levels of oxygen ☐

126. Bilirubin is absent in urine because it is:
A. Distributed in the body fat *(AIIMS 09)* ☐
B. Conjugated with glucoronide ☐
C. Not filterable ☐
D. Lipophilic. ☐

127. Pigment providing colour to stool is: *(PGI 07)*
A. Stercobilinogen ☐
B. Urobilinogen ☐
C. Mevobilirubin ☐
D. Bilirubin ☐

128. The conjugation of bilirubin to glucuronic acid in the liver; *(AIIMS 03)*
A. Converts a hydrophilic compound to a hydrophobic one ☐
B. Converts a hydrophobic compound to a hydrophilic one ☐
C. Enables the bilirubin molecule to cross the cell membrane ☐
D. Is increased during neonatal jaundice ☐

129. Bilirubin in conjugation with glucoronic acid conjugation has properties: *(PGI 07)*
A. Able to cross cell membrane ☐
B. Hydrophillic to hydrophobic ☐
C. Hydrophobic to hydrophilic ☐
D. Lipid soluble ☐

130. Detergent action of bile salts is due to: *(AIIMS 07)*
A. Hydropathic ☐
B. Acts as a zwitter ion ☐
C. Amphipathic ☐
D. All ☐

131. All are true except- *(NBE P 15)*
A. Porphyrinogens are coloured ☐
B. Porphyrins emit flurorescence by UV light ☐
C. Pyrrole rings of porphyrins are joind by methenyl bridges ☐
D. Pyrrole rings of porphyrinogens are joind by methylene bridge ☐

132. Which of the following is luminous (coloured): *(AI 11)*
A. Porphyrin *(NBE P 13)* ☐
B. Zymogen ☐
C. Chromatin ☐
D. Albumin ☐

133. Prophobilinogen in urine produces pink colour with:
A. Fouchet's reagent *(AI 03)* ☐
B. Benedict's reagent ☐
C. Sodium nitropruside ☐
D. Ehrlich's aldehyde reagent ☐

134. All of the following types of porphyrias are autosomal dominant except: *(AI 12)*
A. Acute intermittent porphyria ☐
B. Porphyria cutanea tarda ☐
C. CEP (Congenital Erythropoietic Porphyria) ☐
D. Hereditary coproporphyria ☐

135. The enzyme deficient in erythropoietic porphyria is:
A. PBG deaminase *(PGI 04)* ☐
B. Uroporphyrin II cosynthetase ☐
C. Coprophyrin ☐
D. Ferrochelatase ☐

136. Hepatomegaly is an essential feature of A/E
A. Von Gierke's disease *(AIIMS 10)* ☐
B. Nieman Pick disease ☐
C. Hurler syndrome ☐
D. Hepatic porphyria ☐

137. Heme synthesis requires *(PGI 02)*
A. Ferrous iron ☐
B. Glycine ☐
C. Alanine ☐
D. Succhyl CoA ☐
E. Lead ☐

ANSWERS & EXPLANATIONS:

Fate of Amino Group

1. **A i.e. Transaminases** *[Ref: Lehninger 5/e p 677-83; Lippincott 5/e p 250-53; Harper 29/e p 274-78; Chatterjea 7/e p 443-50; Vasudevan 6/e p 174-76]*

Transaminase (Amino-transferases) transfer an α-amino (NH_3^+) group from L amino acid to an alpha keto acid[Q].

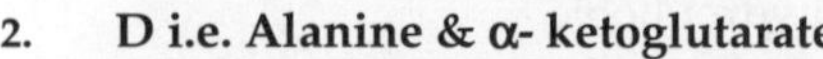

2. **D i.e. Alanine & α- ketoglutarate** 3. **B i.e. α- ketoglutarate**

Transamination of pyruvate and glutamic acid (or glutamate) l/t formation of **alanine and α-keto (oxo) glutarate[Q].**

4. **B i.e. Glutaminase** 5. **A i.e. Alanine**

The amino acid used primarily by muscle, for transport of ammonia to liver is alanine. Most other tissues however use glutamine

6. **A i.e. NH_3 transporter** 7. **B i.e. Alphaketoglutarate** 8. **D i.e. Less of NH_3** 9. **B i.e. Glutamine**
[Ref: Lippincott's 3/e P-254, 255; Harper's 27/e P-247-250]

Glutamine is the **sole form of transport of ammonia in brain[Q]**.
Glutamine is an amide of glutamic acid which is **formed from alpha – ketoglutarate. (Product of TCA cycle)[Q].**
In metabolic alkalosis, there is decreased ammonia excretion[Q] in urine.

Transport of Ammonia to Liver

Ammonia is transported to Liver from peripheral tissue for its ultimate conversion to urea. Two mechanisms are available in humans for this transport

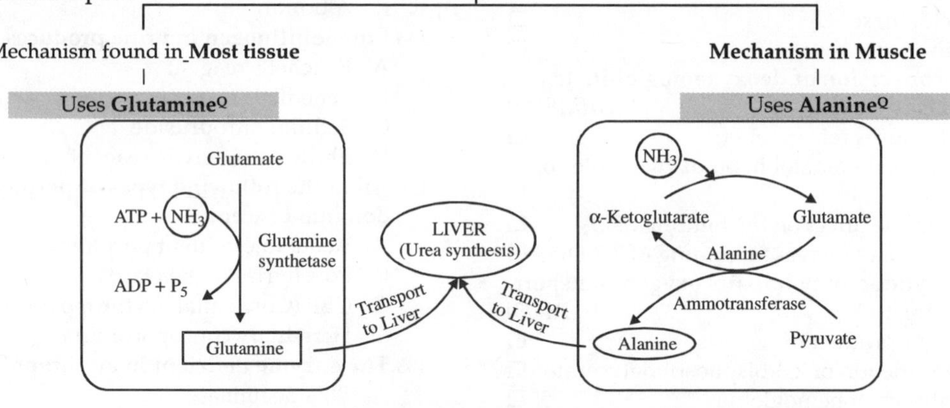

Ammonia Transport

Enters Urea Cycle	As Glutamine[Q]
- **Most important rout of disposal** - Formation of urea in liver & then excreted in urine from kidney - A portion of urea diffuses from blood into intestine & is cleaved to NH_3 & CO_2 by bacterial urease	- Provide a **nontoxic storage & transport form of NH_3[Q]** - **Major mechanism for removal of NH_3 in brain[Q].** - Formation of glutamine from glutamate & NH3 occurs primarily in muscle & Liver - Glutamine is an amide of glutamic acid (glutamate) which is **formed from α- Ketoglutarate[Q].**

Ammonia production (NH_4^+ ion) from renal amino acid (eg glutamine) **increase in metabolic acidosis and decrease in metabolic alkalosis[Q].** [To maintain acid- base balance]

Metabolism of Ammonia

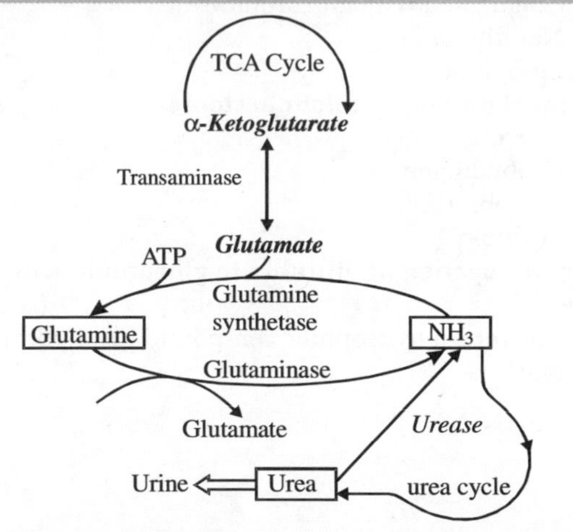

10. B i.e. Ligase **11. A i.e. Glutaminase** **12. A i.e. Glutamine**

[Ref: Harper's 28/e p. 242-46; Lippincott's 4/e p. 250-53; Ganong 22/e p. 721; Chatterjea 7/e p. 116]

- **Glutamine synthase is a mitochondrial enzyme of ligase^Q class.** Ligase enzymes are involved in joining together two substrates.
- **In renal tubular cells (kidney), ammonia (NH_3) is produced by hydrolysis of glutmine (by enzyme glutaminase)^Q.** Secretion of NH_4^+ in urine maintains acid base balance and conserve cation.

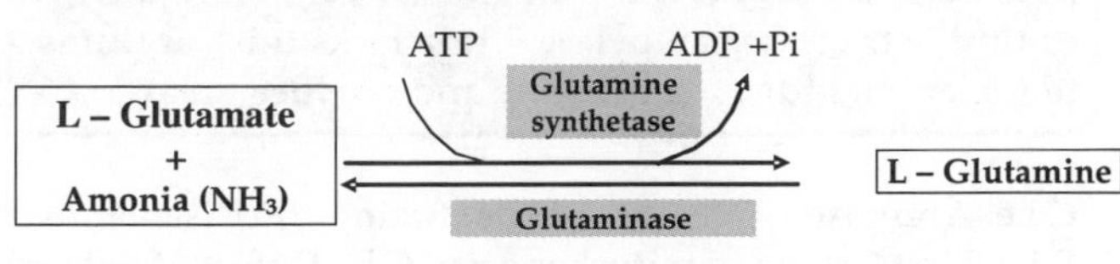

13. C i.e. Glutamate dehydrogenase

- **Oxidative deamination is catalyzed by D & L-aminoacid oxidase.**
- **But oxidative deamination of L-Glutamate is done by L-Glutamate dehydrogenase (GDH)^Q.**

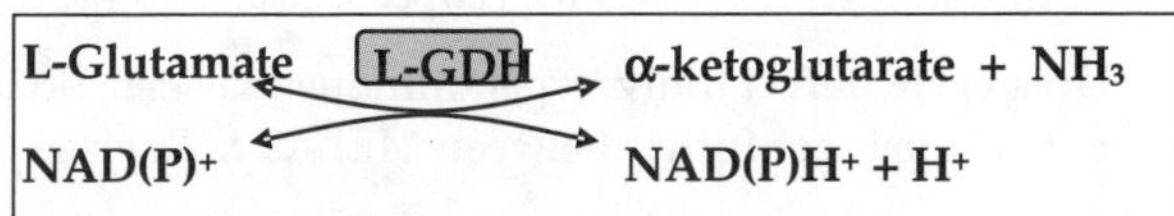

Urea Cycle

14. B i.e. Ornithine *[Ref: Harper's 29/e p 267, 274-78; Chattargea 8/e p 476-77]*

15. A, C, D, E i.e. Glutamate dehydrogenase; alpha-KG dehydrogenase; Isocitrate dehydrogemase; Fumarase

- α-KG dehydrogenase, isocitrate dehydrogenase and fumarase are enzymes of citric acid (TCA) cycle.
- **L- glutamate dehydrogenase**, deaminates L-glutamic acid (glutamate) to α-ketoglutaric acid (α-keto glutarate) and NH_3.
- **Enzymes of urea cycle** include **carbamoyl phosphate synthase I (rate limiting = pacemaker enzyme)^Q, L-ornithine transcarbamoylase, arginosuccinate synthase (defect l/t citrullinemia type 1), arginosuccinate lyase (defect l/t arginosuccinic acidemia), arginase , N-acetylglutamate synthase**, mitochondrial membrane ornithine permease (encoded by **ORNT1 gene** is mitochondrial ornithine carrier and deficiency results in **HHH syndrome** ie hyperornithinemia, hyperammonemia, and homocitrulinuria syndrome) and mitochondrial **aspartate / glutamate carrier enzyme CTLN2** (defect l/t citrullinemia type 2).

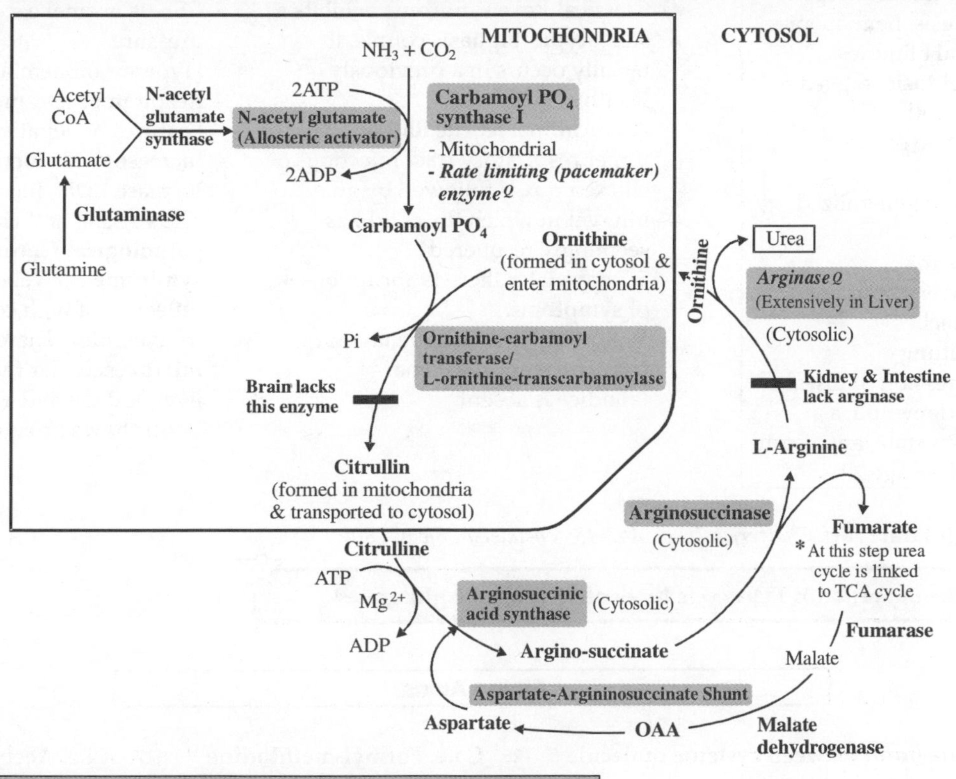

Sources of Carbon & Nitrogen in Urea (NH_2CONH_2)

Mn: **"OCC-ASA"** i.e.

Ornithine + Carbamoyl → Citrullin → Argino-Succinate → Arginine

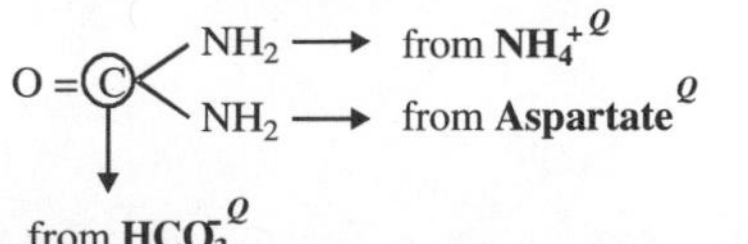

16. **A i.e. Liver** 17. **C, D i.e. Arginosuccinate synthetase , Ornithine transcaroxylase**

Urea cycle occurs in liverQ and involve **carbamoyl PO_4 synthetase 1 (rate limiting /pace maker mitochondrial enzyme), ornithine trans carbamoylase (brain lacks this), argininosuccinate synthetase, argininosuccinase and arginase enzymes (deficient in kidney & intestine and produce urea)**Q.

18. **C i.e. Arginase** 19. **D i.e. Brain** *[Ref. Nelson 16/e P-1214, 1246; Harper's 27/e P-100-101]*
20. **B i.e. First 2 steps in mitochondria; C i.e Defect of enzyme of any step can cause deficiency disease; E i.e. Citruline is formed by combination of carbomoyl phosphate and L. Ornithine**
21. **A i.e. Aspartate and ammonia** 22. **C i.e. N-acetyl glutamate is allosteric inhibitor** 23. **A i.e Reye's syndrome**
[Ref: Lehninger 5/e p. 683-85; Harper 28/e p. 243-46; Lippincott 5/e p. 253-57; Vasudevan 6/e p. 177-79; Chatterjea 7/e p. 448-50]

Urea cycle defect (only hyperammonemia seen, no lactic acidosis, no convulsions) & **Phenylketonuria can be easily ruled out.** There is confusion between MELAS & Reye's syndrome.

MELAS (Mitochondrial Encephalopathy, Lactic Acidosis & Stroke like episodes)

Children with MELAS may be normal for the first several years, but they gradually display delayed motor and cognitive development and short stature. **The clinical syndrome is characterized by-**

- Recurrent **stroke like episodes** manifesting as hemiparesis, hemianopia or cortical blindness.
- **Lactic acidosis**, ragged red fibres or both
- At least two of the following:
  - focal or generalized seizures
  - dementia
  - recurrent migraine headaches
  - vomitting
- Full expression of disease leads to dementia, a bedridden state, and death often before age 20.

Reye's Syndrome
(Syndrome of acute encephalopathy and fatty degeneration of liver)

- No known etilogical factor has been proved. **Aspirin or salicylates used for certain viral respiratory infections** might precipitate Reye's syndrome.
- The **major site of injury is the mitochondria**. The activities of hepatic intramitochondrial enzymes, involving Ornithine transcarbamylase(OTC), Carbamoylphosphate synthatase(CPS) and pyruvate dehydrogenase are reduced, often to less than half of their normal values. **Hyperammonemia**Q may result from decreased activities of OTC and CPS. **Lactic acidosis**Q results from decreased activity of pyruvate dehydrogenase.

- **Clinical features :**
  - Classical Reye syndrome exhibits a stereotypic, biphasic course. It usually occurs in a previously healthy child.
  - A prodromal febrile illness, an upper respiratory tract infections or chicken pox is followed by an interval in which the child has seemingly recovered.
  - 5-7 days later there is abrupt onset of symptoms.
  - Vomitting, irrational behaviour, seizures, stupor & coma.
  - Jaundice is absent

- **Laboratory features :**
  - CSF- is normal except for elevated pressure
  - Hyperammonemia
  - Respiratory and metabolic acidosis
  - Features of hepatic failure
  - Increase AST, Increase ALT, Increase LDH, Increase PT
  - The striking and **characteristic gross pathological feature of Reye syndrome** is a yellow to white liver, reflective of high content of triglycerides. There is **microvescicular fatty steatosis***of liver, kidney and brain.
  - Brain shows gross cerebral edema.

24. **B i.e. α-ketoglutarate** *[Ref: Chatterjea 7/e p. 447-48; Vasudevan 6/e p. 180]*

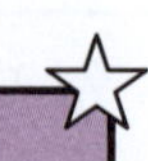

Hyper ammonaemia inhibit TCA cycle by depleting α-keto glutarateQ

Amino Acids

25. **D i.e. Disulfide bond between cysteine molecule** 26. **C i.e. Formyl-methionine** 27. **A i.e. Acetyl coA & alanine**

Amino Acids: Summary

Glycine	Histidine	Glutamine
- **Simplest**[Q] a.a - **Optically inactive**[Q] - **Lacks chirality**[Q] - **Synthesize Creatine**[Q] (with arginine & methionine) - Used **in heme synthesis**[Q].	- **Most stable a.a at physiological pH**[Q] - Acts as buffer **at pH 7**[Q] - **Protonate & deprotonate at neutral pH**[Q] - **Precursor of histamine**[Q].	- **Storage and transport form of ammonia**[Q]. - Major pathway for removal of NH_3 in brain - Precursor of purines and pyrimidines

Phenylalanine / Tyrosine	Cysteine	Methionine
• Phenylalanine is precursor of tyrosine • Tyrosine is a precursor of: - **Catecholamines**[Q] - **Thyroxine**[Q] - **melanin**[Q]	- Sulphur containing amino acid - **Two cysteine join by disulphide bond to form cystine**[Q] - Can be synthesize in body from methionine. - **Responsible for reducing action of glulathione**[Q]	- Sulphur containing a.a - Methionine form **S-adenosylmethionine (SAM),** major **methyl group donor in body**[Q] - **Precursor of homocysteine**[Q]- metabolite **associated with atherosclerotic vascular disease**[Q]. - In **eukaryotes, initial aminoacid in protein synthesis (or aa carried by initiator tRNA) is methionine.** Whereas, in **prokaryotes** & in **mitochondria** it is **N-formyl methionine (i.e. methionine modified by transformylase or Formyl transferase.)**

Tryptophan	Arginine	Alanine
- Precursor of **niacin and serotonin**[Q] - Serotonin form melatonin - **60mg tryptophan give rise to 1mg Niacin**[Q]. - **Also kla α - amino β -3 indole propionic acid**[Q] - **Precursor of Vitamin niacin and serotonin** - Tryptophan is **both glucogenic (by producing alanine) & ketogenic (by producing acetyl CoA)**[Q]	- Member of urea cycle - ***Precursor of nitric oxide***[Q]	- ***Most basic amino acid***[Q] - *Transport form of ammonia from muscle.*

28. **D i.e. Presence of Ser-His-Asp catalytic triad at the active site:**
29. **A i.e. Kidney; Arginine + Glycine**
30. **A i.e. Glycine, arginine and methionine**

[Ref: Harper's 27/e P- 274 – 77; Lippincott's 4/e p. 287- 88]

- **A common feature of all serine proteases is presence of Ser-His-Asp catalytic triad at the active site.**
- **Glycine, arginine and methionine all participate in creatine biosynthesis**[Q]**. Mn- "GAM"**

Serine Protease

- These are *protein digesting enzymes.* They contain ***serine residue at the active center***[Q]
- They form *charge relay network* with histidine and asparate. This charge relay network functions as *proton shuttle.* This proton shuttle *donate a proton* to serine & activate it. The activated serine *breaks down peptide.* Serine proteases include **- *Trypsin***[Q]**, *Elastase***[Q]**, Thrombin, *Chymotrypsin***[Q]

31. **B i.e. Alanine**
32. **D i.e. Histidine** *[Ref: Lippincott's 3/e P-261]*

Methionine, Valine, Isoleucine and Threonine are the four aminoacids that form succinyl- CoA. Histidine forms α ketoglutarate and not Succinyl CoA.

33. **C i.e. Valine** *[Ref: Harper's 27/e P-15]*

Isoleucine is an aminoacid with an aliphatic side chain.
Amongst the options provided valine is the only other amino acid with an aliphatic side chain and is the answer of choice here. Substitution of isoleucine with valine in a protein sequence is an example of a homologous or conservative substitution.

34. **B i.e. Negatively Charged**
35. **D i.e. Point at which positive and negative charges on the amino acids are equal.**
36. **A i.e. Have net charge 'O'** *[Ref: Lippincott's 3/e P- 1]*

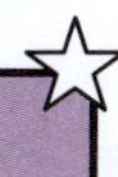

At physiological pH (7.4), all amino acids have both a **negatively charged carboxyl ion (COO^-)**[Q] and a positively charged ammonium ion ($-NH_3^+$). The amino acids are therefore dipolar ion **(Zwitter ions**[Q]**)**

Zwitter Ion
Molecules that contain an equal number of ionizable groups of opposite charge and therefore bear no net charge. Carboxyl and aminogroup of amino acid can protonate & deprotonate depending on the pH of surrounding medium. Thus the net charge depends on surrounding pH

Isoelectric Point
The **pH at which an amino acid bears no net charge**Q i.e. where the **sum of the positive charges equals the sum of negative charges**Q.

37. **D i.e. Proline** 38. **C i.e. Methionine & Cysteine** 39. **D i.e. Tryptophan**
40. **B i.e. Aromatic amino acid** 41. **C i.e. Lysine** 42. **A, B, C, D i.e. Methione, Isoleucine, Tyrosine, Alanine**
43. **A, C, E i.e. Serine, Tyrosine, Lysine** 44. **A, B, C > E i.e. Alanine, Tryptophan, Isoleucine > Tyrosine**
45. **A i.e. Methyl** 46. **A i.e. Nonpolar side chain** 47. **D i.e. Methionine** 48. **A i.e. Leucine**

Ref: Lehninger 5th/e p.73-76; Lippincott 5th/e p. 2-9; Harper 30th/e p.15-21; Vasudevan 6/e p. 20-23; Chatterjea 7/e p. 74-76]

- **Proline is a unique amino acid and has an immino group**Q **(=NH) instead of an amino (NH_2) group found in other amino acid.**
- **Methionine & Cysteine are sulfur containing aminoacids**Q. **Methionine is nonpolar (hydrophobic) aa**Q.
- **The property of photochromicity (i.e. absorbance of ultraviolet light at 250-290nm esp 280nm) is seen with aromatic amino acid (tryptophan > tyrosine > phenylalanine).**
- **Hydrophobic (non polar) aminoacids** have no charge on their R group or side chain. **Aliphatic (eg methyl, methylene, thioether & imino) side chains** and aromatic side chains are nonpolar. So **methyl (CH_3) side chain of alanine**; propyl (C_3H_7) side chain of **valine**; butyl (C_4H_9) side chain of **leuicine & isoleucine**; thioether side chain of methionine; and **imino group / pyrrolidine containing side chain of proline**Q are nonpolar.
- **Methyl (CH_3) side chain of alanine is nonpolar**Q. **Serine, threonine, tyrosine containing hydroxyl group and cysteine containing sulfhydryl group, are polar aminoacids with neutral/uncharged/nonionic side chain. Positively charged basic amino** (NH_3^+) group side chain of histidine, arginine and lysine ; and negatively **acidic carboxyl (COO^-)** side chain of aspartic acid and glutamic acid is **polar.**

49. **C i.e. Glycine** 50. **A i.e. Asparagine; C i.e. Glutamine**

(L-α)- Amino acid Classification (Based on Side Chain)

Polarity and Solubility

Hydrophobic (Nonpolar) Neutral aa *(Lehninger)*

T	Tryptophan*
	Tyrosine**
M	Methionine
L	Leucine
V	Valine
I	Isoleucine
A	Alanine
P	Phenylalanine
	Proline
G	Glycine*

Mn – **"Try To Meet Lucy in Valley Is All Phen's problem– G" or "TAMIL VAP-G"**

However in aromatic side chain aa tyrosine > tryptophan are more polar than phenylalanine. ★ = Relative

Hydrophillic (Polar) aa

- **Uncharged (Neutral)**
  - **Serine**Q
  - Threonine
  - **Tyrosine**Q
  - Aspargine
  - Cysteine
  - Glutamine
- **Acidic (Negatively charged – Proton donors)**
  Mn: "**Acidic as Glue**"
  - Aspartic acid
  - Glutamic acid
  - Asparagine★
  - Glutamine★
- **Basic (Positively charged – Proton acceptor)**
  Mn: **"His basics are loose"**
  - **His**tidine (weakly basic or neutral) ★
  - Hydroxy lysine
  - Arginine (most basic)Q
  - **Lysine**Q

Side Chain Content

Aliphatic

- Glycine
- Alanine
- Valine
- Leucine
- Isoleucine
- Proline
- Methionine

Mn: **'GAVLI-PM'**

Aromatic

- Tyrosine
- Tryptophan
- Phenylalanine
- Histidine

Mn: **"Try To Pen His Arrow"**

Hydroxyl (OH) group

- Tyrosine
- Threonine
- Serine

Mn: **"OH! Try Three sari"**

Sulfur atoms

- Cysteine
- Methionine

Mn: **"Meet Sulphuric Cyst"**

Immino acid/ (Secondary amino group)

ProineQ

Basic group

- **Arginine**Q
- **Lysine**Q
- **Histidine**Q

Acidic Group

- **Aspartic acid (aspartate)**Q
- **Glutamic acid (glutamate)**Q

Amides of acidic group

- Asparagine
- Glutamine

51. **C i.e. Lysine and arginine** 52. **B i.e. Arginine**
53. **B i.e. Proline** 54. **C i.e. Lysine**

- At physiological pH *basic aminoacid (positive charged a.a) will move slowest towards anode*[Q] (positively charged electrode). **Basic amino acids are:** *Arginine*[Q] (Most basic), *Lysine*[Q] and *Histidine*[Q] (Weekly basic).
- **Acidic amino acids include aspartic acid (aspartate) & glutamic acid (glutamate)[Q]. Others are neutral aa.**

55. **A i.e. Tyrosine**
56. **A i.e. L- methionine**
57. **A i.e. Phenyalanine**
58. **C i.e. Arginine**
59. **D i.e. Glycine**
60. **D i.e. All**
61. **A i.e. Arginine B i.e. Histidine**
62. **D i.e. Serine**
63. **C i.e. Alanine**

[Ref: John Baynes 3/e p. 248; Lehinger 5/e p. 686]

Threonine, Lysine, Phenylalanine, Methionine, Isolcucine & Leucine, Tryptophan, Valine > Histidine >> Arginine are **nutritionally essential amino acids**. Among these last two (histidine & arginine) are semi- essential, and arginine is more essential than histidine.

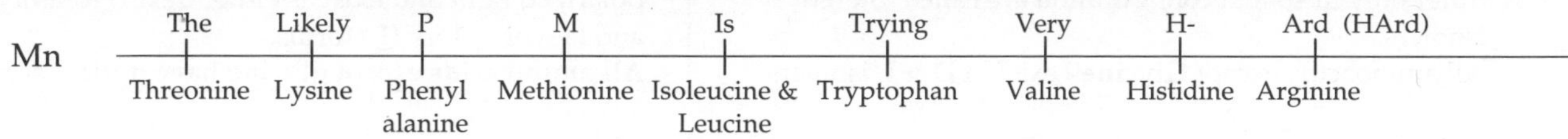

Classification of Amino Acids on the Basis of Metabolism

Essential Amino Acid

Lu-	Leucine	Vali-	Valine
Ly-	Lysine	Iso-	Isoleucine
Thi -	Threonine	Phenyl-	Phenylalanine
Her-	Histidine } *Semi-*	Metho-	Methionine
Argi -	Arginine } ***essential***[Q]	Trypto-	Tryptophan

[Mn: **'LuLi Thi His Argi Vali Iso Phenyl Metho Trypto'**] or **"Please Visit To TIM HALL"**

Conditionally Essential

Required to some degree in young growing animals & during illness
- Arginine – Glutamine – Proline
- Cysteine – Glycine – Tyrosine

Non essential Amino Acids

- Alanine – Aspartate - Serine
- Asparagine - Glutamine

Ketogenic A . A	Glucogenic A. A.		Both Glucogenic & Ketogenic A.A.
Leucine	**V**	- Valine	Isoleucine
Lysine	**C / see**	- Cysteine, Serine	Tyrosine
	All	- Alanine	Tryptophan
	His	- Histidine	**Phenylalanine**
	Three	- Threonine	
	Asses	- Aspartate	
	Are	- Arginine	
	Grass	- Glycine, Glutamate	
	Prone	- Proline / **Hydroxy proline**	

★ In Lehninger, **Histidine** is essential and **Arginine** is conditionally essential.

	Ketogenic	Glucogenic & Ketogenic	Glucogenic
Essential	**Leucine Lysine**	**Isoleucine Phenyl alanine Tryptophan**	**Methionine Threonine Valine** Histidine*
Semi Essential	-	-	Histidine Arginine
Non - Essential	Hydroxy -lysine	**Tyrosine**	**Arginine* Alanine Asparagine Aspartate Cysteine Glutamate Glutamine Glycine Proline,** hydroxyproline **Serine**

64. **C i.e. Tryptophan**

Most amino acid do not absorb visible light & are thus colourless. The only amino acids that may absorb light are Aromatic amino acids i.e. **Tryptophan, Tyrosine, Phenylalanine & Histidine[Q].** Mn: **"Try To Pen His Arrow". Aromatic aminoacids absorb ultraviolet light**[Q] (250- 290 nm). Tryptophan makes 'major contribution to ability of most proteins to absorb light in the region of 280 nm.

65. **C i.e. Leucine** *[Ref: Lippincott's 3/e P-3- 4]*

Hydrophobic or Non polar aminoacid are present in transmembrane region[Q]. Hydrophillic or polar amino acids are present on outer surface of membrane. **Leucine is a hydrophobic a.a so it lies in transmembrane region[Q]**

Cell membrane

- Cell membrane is a complex structure composed of lipid, proteins and carbohydrate. Membrane lipids form bilayer. The unique characteristic of this layer is that it has its hydrophobic ends in the centre of membrane while its hydrophilic ends lie on the outer surface of membrane.
- Membrane proteins are associated with lipid bilayer. So
- The **hydrophilic amino acids** of the protein should **protrude at the inside & outside faces of membrane.**
- While **hydrophobic a.a should lie in the centre (transmembrane region)[Q].**

66. **A i.e. L- forms** *[Ref: Harper's 28/e P-14; Chatterjea 6/e P-25]*

67. **C i.e. Racemization**

Natural protein of animals and plants **generally contain L- amino acids**Q. D- amino acid occur in bacteria.
Racemic or DL mixture: When equal amount of D & L isomers are presentQ, the resulting mixture has no optical activity and called Racemic mixture.

Asymmetric Carbon: A carbon atom to which 4 different atoms or group of atoms are attached. **Glycine lacks asymmetrical carbon atom so does not exhibit isomerism**Q.

Isomerism

Two types of isomerism are shown by a.a, because of the presence of asymmetrical carbon atom.

Stereoisomerism	Optical isomerism
- Compound which are identical in composition and differ only in spatial configuration are called 'Stereo isomers' - All aminoacids except **Glycine**Q exist in D & L isomers	- Optical isomers or 'enantiomorphs' rotate the plane polarized light and exist as either dextro rotatory (d) and laevorotatory (L) forms. - **All amino acids except glycine have optical activity**Q

68. **B i.e. Threonine** 69. **D i.e. Glycine** 70. **D i.e. Glycine**

All aminoacids have one chiral (or asymmetric) α carbonQ which has 4 different groups attached to it except

Glycine	Aminoacid which **lacks chirality or does not have anomeric (asymmetric/chiral) carbon** and so is **optically inactive**.
Threonine & Isoleucine	Aminoacid with **2 chiral centers (with double chirality)**Q.

Glycine

- **Glycine** does **not posses asymmetric carbon atom and is therefore optically inactive i.e. lacks chirality (handedness)**Q.
- The α- Carbon of each a.a is attached to four different chemical groups & is therefore chiral or optically active. Glycine is an exception because its α- carbon has two Hydrogen atoms & therefore is optically inactive.

- **Smallest**Q and **simplest**Q amino acid
- Amino acid **responsible for flexibility of proteins**Q.
- Is **optically inactive**Q, does not exist in isomeric form.
- It **lacks chirality**Q.
- Glycine with **a**rginine & **m**ethionine (GAM) **synthesize creatine**Q.
- Glycine (with succinyl COA) is used for **Heme synthesis**Q.

71. **A i.e. Methylene THF** 72. **A i.e. Folic Acid** 73. **B i.e. Folic Acid**

Tetrahydrofolic acid and S- adenosyl methionine act as a carrier compound for single carbon unitsQ. **Methylene THF is major form of folic acid to transfer one carbon**Q.

One Carbon Units

- One carbon units can exist in form of ***methane, methanol, formaldehyde, formic acid and carbonic acid***, all of which except methane can be incorporated in various synthetic pathways.
- Sources of one carbon unit are ***serine, glycine, choline, histidine, and formate***Q
- ***Tetrahydrofolate and S-adenosyl methionine are carrier of one carbon units***Q. The **active form of folic acid, tetra hydrofolic acid (THE) can carry carbon unit bound to nitrogen N_5 or N^{10} or to both N_5 and N^{10} in form of formyl, formimino, or methyl** (attached to N_5), **methylene, methenyl group** (bridging N_5 & N^{10}) and **formyl** (attached to N^{10}).

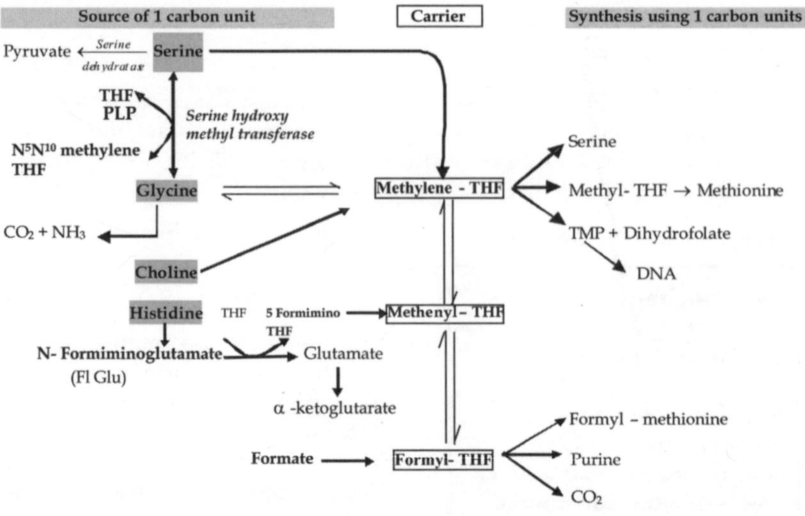

★ Biotin functions as coenzyme to transfer CO_2 in carboxylation reactions (enzyme carboxylase). But **CO_2 is not considered as member of 1 carbon pool**.

74. A i.e. Folic acid

Glycine is converted to serine by addition of methylene group from N^5, N^{10} – methylenetetra hydrofolic acid[Q] and requires **pyridoxal phosphate as coenzyme for serine hydroxymethyl tranaferase**[Q].

75. B i.e. Histidine

Histidine	
- **Most stable amino acid at physiological pH**[Q] - **Can serve as best buffer at pH 7**[Q] - Can **protonate & deprotonate at neutral PH**[Q]	**Histidine** is unique, since pKa of its imidazole group permits it at pH7 (physiological) to function either as a base or as an acid catalyst i.e. it **has capacity to protonate or deprotonate at neutral pH**[Q]. **Minor change in pH, changes the ionization charge on histidine to buffur pH change**[Q]. Therefore it **can serve as a buffer & is most stable amino acid at physiological pH**[Q].

76. A i.e. Contain sulfhydral group ; D i.e. Transport aminoacid across cell membrane; E i.e. Part of enzymes
77. C i.e. Cysteine *[Ref: Harper's 27/e P-636; Lippincott's 3/e P-4, 5, 146; Harper's 27/e P-17-18; Lippincott's 3/e P- 4, 5]*
78. C i.e. It helps in membrane transport, D i.e. It helps in conjugation reaction

Glutathione acts as a reducing agent in body and its cysteine residue is responsible for its reducing property[Q].
Glutathione (GSH) is a **tripeptide**[Q] of three amino acids: [Mn:**GGC**]: Glycine, Cysteine (Provides SH group), Glutamate

79. B i.e. Histidine **80. D i.e. Cystine, Ornithine, Lysine, Arginin** **81. B i.e. Tryptophan** **82. A i.e. Non essential A.A.**
83. B i.e. Tryptophan **84. D i.e. Tyrosine** **85. C i.e. None** **86. A i.e. Tryptophan**
87. B i.e. Tyrosine **88. B i.e. Melatonin** **89. C i.e. Glutamine** **90. B i.e. Glutamine**
91. A i.e. Glutamine **92. D i.e. Melatonin** *[Ref: Harper's 27/e P-259-62; 26/e P- 257; Lippincott's 5/e p. 250; Chatterjea 7/e p. 477]*

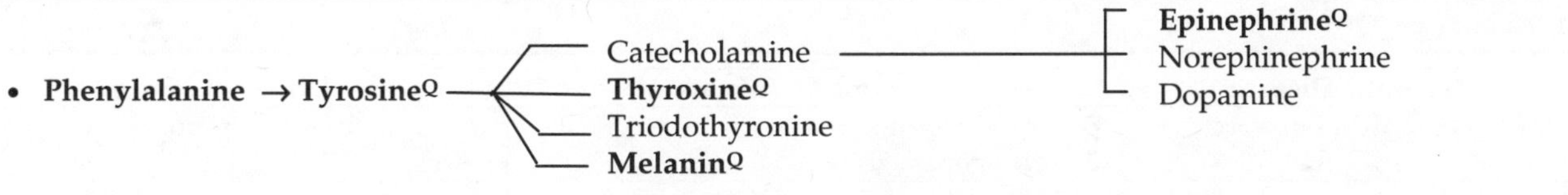

- **Melatonin** is formed **from tryptophan**[Q].

Tryptophan → **serotonin**[Q] → **melatonin**[Q]
↓
Niacin[Q]

93. B i.e. Homocytine **94. C i.e. Calcium** *[Ref: Harrison 16/e P. 1430, 1432]*

- There is a **strong Co- relation between hyperhomocytinemia and coronary events (MI)**[Q].
- Fortification of food with folic acid to reduce NTD has lowered homocystine level in population.

95. A i.e. Limiting the substrate for deficient enzyme **96. C i.e. Dihydropterin reductase**
97. C i.e. Phenylketonuria **98. B i.e. Green** **99. B i.e. Phenylketonuria**
[Ref: Lippincott's 5/e P- 270-71;Lehninger 5/e p. 696-99; Chatterjea 7/e p. 469-70; Harper's 28/e P-254-55, 237; Harrison 17/e p. 2471-70; Nelson 18/e p. 530]

Phenylketonuria is caused by **deficiency of phenylalanine hydroxylase & /or dihydrobiopterin (BH_2) reductase, which regenerates BH4 from BH_2**[Q]. It presents with **mousy (musty)** odour in urine and **emerald green colour in $FeCl_3$ test**[Q]. The **aim of first line therapy** is **to limit the substrate (i.e. phenylalanine) for deficient enzyme**[Q]

100. D i.e. Hepatic carcinoma *[Ref: Lehninger 5/e p.696-97; Chatterjea: 7/e P- 471; Harper's 28/e P-254; Lippincott 5/e p. 269; Vasudevan 6/e p. 209-10]*

In **Tyrosinemia type I**, ***hepatocellular carcinoma***[Q] occurs in children who survive beyond 2 yrs.

101. B i.e. Alkaptonuria **102. B i.e. Alkaptonuria**
[Ref: Lehninger 5/e 694-698; Vasudeven 6/e 208-10; Chatterjae 7/e 470-71; Harper 28/e 254; Lippincott 5/e 269, 274; Harrison 17/e 2470-73; Nelson 18/e p 534; Weedon skin pathology 2/e p 440]

Alkaptonuria a condition d/t **defective homogentisate 1, 2- dioxygenase**Q (l/t defective tyrosine degradation) **usually presents after age of 40**Q with characteristic triad of **Homogentisic aciduria (which blacken/darkens on exposure to air /standing and is strongly Benedict's positive), Ochronosis (i.e black pigmentation of cartilage & collagenous connective tissue), and Arthritis of large joints**Q, (Mn – "**Alkaptonuria – Black-HOA** = हुआ")

103. **A i.e. Diarrhoea; B i.e. Vasoconstriction; C i.e. Flushing** *[Ref: Chatterjea: 6/e P- 451; Harper's 27/e P-262]*

- **Trytophan** is an essential amino acid and is precursor of Serotonin, Melatonin & Niacin.
- **Clinical effects of Serotonin or 5Htase:** Symptoms occur due to effect on smooth muscle.
  - Cutaneous vasomotor episodes of **flushing**Q.
  - Potent **vasoconstriction**Q.
  - **Chronic diarrhoea**Q
  - Respiratory distress & bronchospasm.
- Albinism accompanies defective melanine, product of tyrosine biosynthesis

104. **D i.e. a, b & c**
105. **C i.e. Leucine**
106. **A i.e. Maple Syrup urine disease**
107. **B i.e. Maple syrup disease; D i.e. Isovaleric acidemia** *[Ref: Harper 29/e p. 284, 293-95; Lippincott 6/e p. 266; Vasudevan 7/e p.230; Chatterjea 7/e p. 493; Satyanarayan 3/e p. 376; Lehninger 5/e p. 694-701]*

Diseases of branched chain aminoacids include (1) **maple syrup (burnt sugar) urine disease** or **branched chain ketonuria (BCKU)** and **intermittent BCKU** (less severe) both due to **defect of branched chain α ketoacid dehydrogenase**Q **resulting in defective oxidative decarboxylation of leucine, isoleucine & valine**Q; (2) **Isovaleric acidemia** d/t defective **isovaleryl CoA dehydrogenase**Q and; (3) **Hypervalinemia** d/t defective **valine transaminase**.

108. **A i.e. Decarboxylase**
109. **B i.e. FAD linked dehydrogenase**
110. **A i.e. Phenylketonuria-Mousy odour; B i.e. Tyrosinemia-Rotten cabbage**

Sweaty feet odor in body fluids a/w neurological problems occur in **deficiency of FAD linked dehydrogenase specific for isovaleryl COA**Q.

Metabolic Disease	Enzyme Deficient	Urinary Feature
Maple syrup urine disease	**Branched chain ketoacid dehydrogenase**Q	**Sweat maple syrup (burnt sugar) odour**Q
Methyl-melonic aciduria	Methyl-malonyl CoA mutase (isomerase)	
Isovaleric academia	**Isovaleryl-CoA dehydrogenase**	**Sweaty feet (cheesy) odor in body fluids & breath**
Tyrosinemia (Tyrosinosis) I	Fumarylacetoacetate hydroxylase	**Boiled or rotten cabbage/mushroom like odour**
Tyrosinemia II	Tyrosine transaminase (Tyrosine aminotransferase)	
Neonatal tyrosinemia	Hydroxyphenyl pyruvate hydroxylase	
Albinism	Tyrosinase	
Alkaptonuria	**Homogentisate oxidase**Q	**Urine turns black** on air exposure or standing
Phenylketonuria	**Phenylalanine hydroxylase**Q	**Mousy (musty) urine odour**Q
Orotic aciduria	OMP decarboxylase	
Homocystinuria	Cystathionine synthatase	
Lesh-Nyhan Syndrome	Complete deficiency of enzyme HGPRT	
Cystinosis	Cystine reductase	
Hawkinsinuria		**Swimming pool odour**Q

BCAA Disease	Defective Enzyme
MSUD (BC Ketonuria)	BCKA Dehydrogenase
Intermittent branched chain ketonuria	BCKAD (less severe)
Isovaleric acidemia	Isovaleryl CoA dehydrogenase
Hypervalinemia	Valine transaminase

111. **A i.e. Serine, B i.e. Tyrosine** *[Ref: Chatterjea 6/e P-446; Harper's 27/e P-78-79]*

Selective phosphorylation, specific for ***serine & tyrosine***Q residue or threonine and subsequent dephosphorylation is catalyzed by protein kinase & phosphatase.
In human, activity of many enzymes are regulated by covalent modification such as ATP dependent phosphorylation & subsequent dephosphorylation.

112. C i.e. Valine

Succinyl COA is formed by ***Valine***Q, Isoleucine, Methionine. [Mn: "**Succesful V I M**"]

113. B i.e. Multiple carboxylase deficiency *[Ref: Nelson 16/e P-356]*

In the *degradation of valine, leucine, isoleucine* (essential, branched chain aminoacids), the intermediate metabolites are all *'organic acids'*, and deficiency of any of the degradative enzymes (except for transaminases) causes *acidosis due to accumulation of organic acids* before the enzymatic block. The patient in question has ketosis as well as skin manifestation and thefore the answer is Multiple carboxylase deficiency. Normal levels of ammonia rule out urea cycle enzyme deficiency.

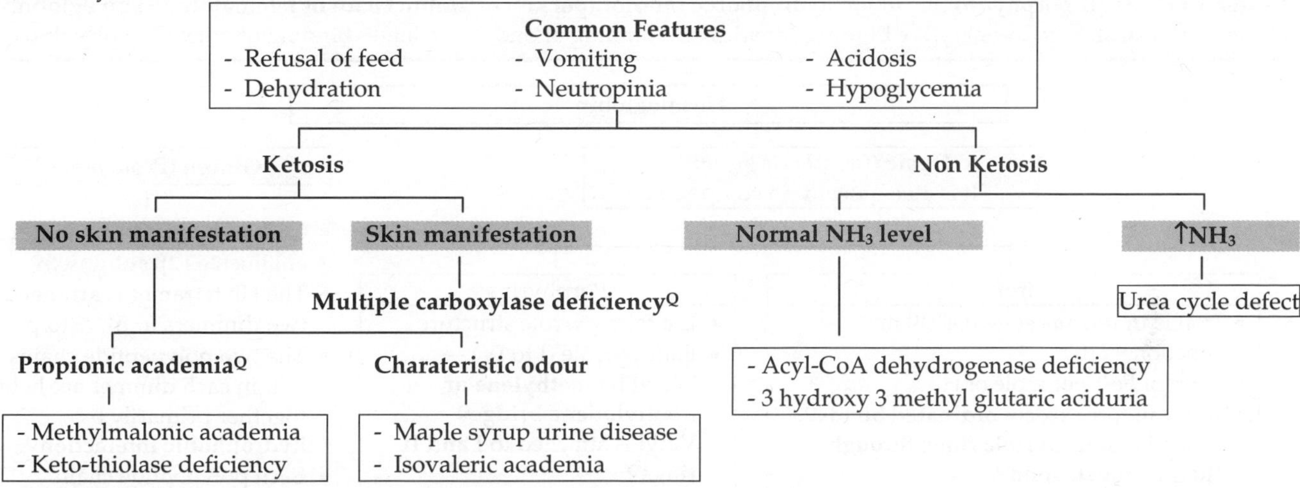

114. A i.e. Randomly (Most probable answer of exclusion)

Most variations in aminoacid sequence of cytochrome c affect primary structure in a way not to affect the secondary and tertiary structures which are more important for function. The amino acids that cannot be replaced without a major modification of the enzymic properties of the cytochrome c are not altered. Thus the amino acids at locations that determine the secondary structure of protein (loops, helix or strands) are preserved while aminoacids that do not contribute to the determination of secondary and tertiary structure are preferentially altered. **These alterations are likely to be distributed randomly** as they result from point mutations on the responsible gene and this is the single best answer of exclusion here.

Also note that it is the tertiary structure which is most important for function and hence it is the most conserved parameter. Some changes in the secondary structure (helix, loop or strands) may be seen as a result of random changes in the polypeptide sequence of amino acids. **These changes may affect the 'helical regions' or the 'loops' or the 'strands' randomly and should not be confined to only the helical regions, the loops or the strands.**

Hemoprotein, Hemoglobin, Porphyrins & Bile Pigment

115. A, B, C, D, E i.e. Cytochrome C; Cytochrome 450; Myoglobin; Hemoglobin; Catalase *[Ref: Harper 28/e 271-72; Chattarjae 7/e 82; Lippincott 5/e 25, 34; Lehninger 84-85]*

Hemoproteins are a group of chromo proteins that contain *heme* as a tightly bound prosthetic group. And heme is a complex of *protoporphyrin IX and ferrous (Fe2+) ion*. The iron is held in center by bonds to *4 nitrogens of porphyrin ring*. The heme iron can form two additional bonds. In hemoglobin & myoglobin one of these is with histidine residue of globin and other is available to bind O_2.

Hemoproteins	Function
Hemoglobin **Myoglobin**	Transport O_2 in blood Storage of O_2 in muscle
Cytochrome C (oxidase) **Cytochrome P – 450**	Electron transport chain Hydroxylation of xenobiotics
Catalase	Degradation of H_2O_2
Tryptophan pyrrolase	Oxidation of tryptophan
Per-oxidase	Oxidative enzyme

116. A i.e. Histidine residue

117. A i.e. Hb has 2 polypeptide chain

[Ref: Harper's 27/e P- 41-45; 26/e P- 40; Chatterjea 6/e P-133-34]

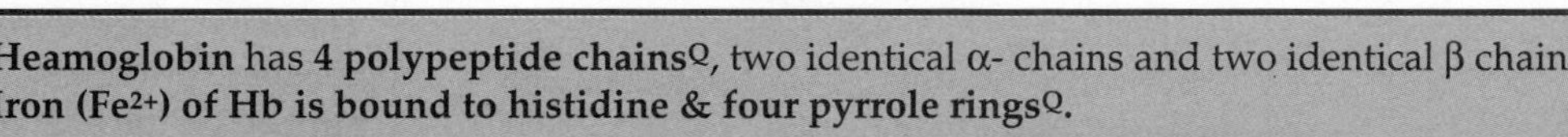

Heamoglobin has **4 polypeptide chains**Q, two identical α- chains and two identical β chains.
Iron (Fe^{2+}) of Hb is bound to histidine & four pyrrole ringsQ.

118. B i.e. His E 7 *[Ref: Harper's 27/e P-44; 26/e P- 40]*

> The heme has high affinity for carbon monoxide (about 25000 more than for O_2). **But when heme molecule is associated with Histidine E 7 (as occurs in myoglobin), its affinity for CO is drastically reduced**Q because His E 7 creates a hindered environment for CO by disturbing the orientation of atoms in heme molecules.

119. A i.e. Each hemoglobin molecule is made of 4 polypeptides of each subunit

120. C i.e. Type III

121. B i.e. Co-operative effect of combine O_2

122. D i.e. Heme at hydrophobic pockets

[Ref: Harper's 27/e P- 42-44; Chatterjea 6/e P-134, Lippincott's 3/e P-26]

> - **Heme (a type III porphyrin) lies in the hydrophobic interior (pocket) of globin chain of hemoglobin & myoglobin**Q.
> - **Hemoglobin shows Co-operative binding kinetics**Q i.e. binding of one O_2 facilitates binding of other O_2 molecules.

Heamoglobin

Heme *(Prosthetic group)*Q
It is a Fe- porphyrin compound

Iron	Porphyrins
• Iron is **in ferrous state (Fe^{2+})**Q in functional Hb • 4 gm of Fe^{2+} per mole of Hb • Iron can form six co- **ordinated bonds**Q - Linked to four **pyrrole rings through their nitrogen atom**Q. - **5th linkage to nitrogen of imidazole ring of histidine of polypetide**Q. - On other side co-ordinated position of Fe2+ is available to bind to O_2	• Is a tetra pyrrole structure • Four pyrrole (I to IV) → joined by **methylene or Methylodene bridge**Q • Vinyl is attached to **I and II rings**Q. • Propionic acid at 6th & 7th position of heme of III & IV Pyrroles

- Within the pH range of 7.0 to 7.8, most of the **physiological buffering action of Hb is due to imidazole group of amino acid histidine**Q.
- Imidazole H+ group can give up H+ (Proton) and accept H+ depending on pH of medium.
- Other dissociable buffering group responsible for buffering capacity of Hb
  - a) Acidic-COOH group
  - b) Basic-NH2 group
  - c) Guanidino group

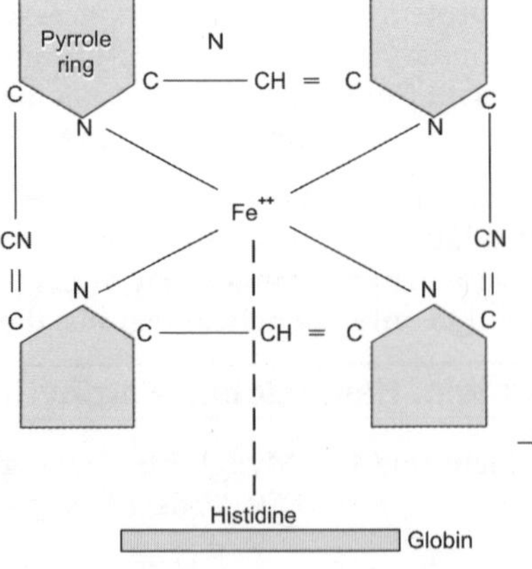

Globin (Protein part)

- Composed of **4 polypeptide chains (2α+2β subunits)**Q
- The Hb tetramer is arranged a two dimmers $(\alpha\beta)_1$ & $(\alpha\beta)_2$
- The two polypeptide chains within each dimmer are held together primarily by **hydrophobic interaction**Q.
- Each polypeptide chain **contains a 'heme' in heme Pocket**Q. Thus 1 Hb contains 4 heme units
- Hb contains mostly hydrophobic amino acids internally **(forming 'heme pockets')**Q & hydrophilic a.a on their surfaces.
- **The 'Heme pocket' of α-subunit are adequate for entry of O_2 while β- subunits heme pockets blocks entry O_2 by valine residue**Q.

123. D i.e. Hemoglobin *[Ref: Lehninger 3/e P-214, 278]*

Hemoglobin is allosteric proteinQ **and Phosphofructokinase is allosteric enzyme**Q.

Allosteric property of hemoglobin

- Results from its **quaternary structure**Q.
- There are four subunits in Hb & each subunit can bind an O_2 molecule. The binding of O_2 to one subunit increases the affinity of other subunits for O_2
- Hb binds O_2 with a **sigmoid binding curve**Q because of its allosteric property. (Myoglobin binds O_2 with a hyperbolic binding curve)

Allosteric Protein	Allosteric Enzymes
- Is one in which binding of a ligand to one site affects the binding properties of another site on the same protein - Allosteric proteins are those having 'other shapes' or conformation induced by binding of ligands referred to as modulators. - The conformational changes induced by modulator inter convert more active & less active forms of protein. Modulator may be either inhibitor or activator	- Is one in which binding of a modulator to the enzyme induces a conformational change in the enzyme making it more active or less active. - The same concept of allosteric protein is applied on the enzymes.

124. A i.e. Binding of O_2 causes of H^+ *[Ref: Harper's 27/e P- 42-45]*

Binding of O_2 to deoxyhemoglobin in lungs causes release of proton (H+)Q. This is responsible for **Bohr effect.**

125. B i.e. Decreased production of 2, 3- biphosphoglycerate

2, 3- DPG is produced by an alternative pathway in glycolysis. It is **formed form 3-phosphoglyceraldehyde, which is a product of glycolysis via Embden- Meyerh of pathway**Q. It is very plentiful in red cells. If the glycolytic activity is decreased, the level of 2, 3- DPG in RBCs will decrease. **Decreased level of 2, 3 DPG concentration:**

- Shifts the **O_2-Hb curve to left**Q
- **Increases the O_2 affinity of Hb**Q (impairs O_2 transport).

2, 3 – Biphosphoglycerate Pathway in Erythrocytes

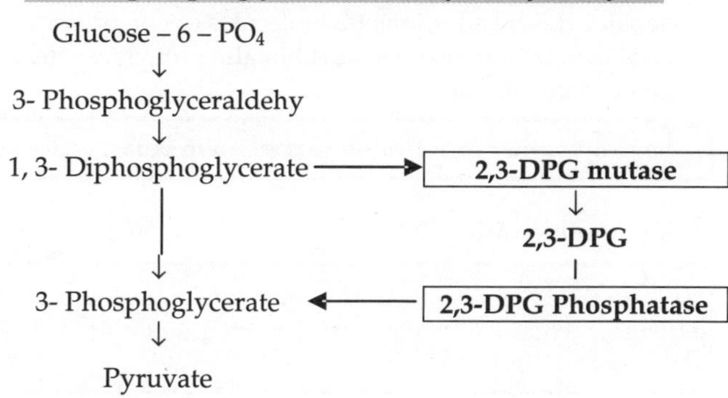

126. D i.e. Lipophilic **127. A i.e. Stercobilinogen** *[Ref: Lippincott's 3/e p 287, 281; Chatterjea 6/e p. 476, 478; Harper's 27/e 155]*

- **Unconjugated bilirubin is absent in urine because it is highly lipid soluble (lipophilic)**Q but conjugated bilirubin can be present in it. I think that the question is about unconjugated bilirubin as 90% bilirubin in serum is unconjugated.
- **Brown color of stool is due to stercobilin**Q.

• RBC (old, senescent 80%)
• Ineffective erythropoiesis
• Other sources

Hb – Heme – Biliverdin – Bilirubin **Spleen, liver**

In blood

Bilirubin + albumin (unconjugated bilirubin)

Liver Bilirubin – Bilirubinglucoronid (conjugated)

Intestine
Bilirubin - glucoronide
Glucoronide is removed by gut bacteria
Bilirubin
Urobilinogen
Oxidised by bacteria
Stercobilinogen (brown pigment of feces)

Uro-bilinogen – Urobilin

In urine (giving its yellow color)

128. B i.e Converts a hydrophobic compound to a hydrophilic one *[Ref: Lippincott's 3/e P-281; Chatterjea 6/e P-478]*

Liver uptakes unconjugated bilirubin (hydrophobic) & conjugates it with glucoronic acid generating **bilirubin glucoronide which is water soluble**Q.

Bilirubin is produced in reticuloendothelial cells of spleen and liver.

Unconjugated bilirubin :
- *Lipophilic*Q
- *Not soluble in water*
- Bound to albumin for its transfer in plasma

- Liver uptakes unconjugated bilirubin & Conjugation with glucuronic acid

↓

Conjugated bilirubin: - ***Water soluble***Q
(Bilirubin glucuronide)

129. A i.e. Able to cross cell membrane; C i.e. Hydrophobic to hydrophilic *[Ref: Lippincott 4/e p. 282; Harper's 27/e p. 289]*

- Bilirubin is only sparingly (slightly) soluble in water, but its solubility in plasma is increased by non covalent binding to albumin. Each albumin molecule has one high & one low affinity site for bilirubin. Only 25 mg of bilirubin can be tightly boud to albumin at its high affinity site in 100 ml plasma. The excess amount bound loosely & can be easily detached.
- Bilirubin enters hepatocytes via facilitated transport system and binds to cytosolic proteins (ligandin, protein Y), which to keep it solubilized & prevent its efflux back into blood stream before conjugation.
- **Bilirubin is nonpolar & would persist in cells if not rendered water soluble**Q. Solubility of bilirubin is increased in hepatocytes by addition of 2 molecules of glucuronic acid to convent it to a polar form. This process k/a **conjugation** is catalyzed by microsomal bilirubin glucuronyl transferase and use uridine diphosphate – (UDP) – glucuronic acid as glucuronate donor.

- So **conjugation of bilirubin makes them polar, water soluble, hydrophilic and able to cross cell membrane**Q

130. C i.e. Amphipathic *[Ref: Ganong 21/e P 477, 505]*

Fats are finely emulsified in the small intestine by the detergent action of bile salts, lecithin and monoglycerides. *Detergent action of bile salts* are due to their ***amphipathic***Q nature i.e., they have both hydrophilic and hydrophobic domains.

- Bile salts tend to form cylindrical disks called micelles with hydrophilic surface facing out & hydrophobic surfaces in.
- These micelles take up lipids, solubilzes them & provide a mechanism for their transport to the enterocytes.

131. A i.e. Porphyrinogens are coloured **132. A i.e. Porphyrins** *[Ref: Harper's 27/e P-282; 26/e P- 273]*

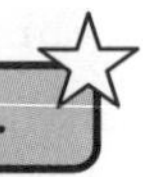

Porphyrins are **colored (luminous) and fluorescence**Q wherase **porphyrinogens are colorless (non-luminous)**Q.

- When porphyrins dissolved in strong mineral acids or in organic solvents are ***illuminated by ultraviolet light, they emit a strong red fluorescence***Q.
- The *double bonds joining the pyrrole rings* in porphyrin are responsible for characteristic absorption & fluorosence.
- **Soret band:** - The sharp *absorption band near 400nm.* shown by porphyrin solution (in 5% HCl)
  - Is *characteristic of all porphyrins* regardless of the side chain present.

Feature	Porphyrinogen	Porphyrins
Color, Fluorescence and Luminosity	**Colorless & Do not emit fluorescence (nonluminous)**Q	**Colored** compounds and **emit red fluorescence** on UV illumination (i.e. are **luminous)**Q
Pyrolle ring join by	**Methylene (-CH_2-) bridge** Q	**Methenyl (-HC =) bridge)**
At 400nm	No absorbance	Characteristic absorbance

Porphyrinogens are reduced porphyrins as they contain extra 6 hydrogens. They can be autooxidized (by light) to their respective porphyrins.

133. D i.e. Ehrlich's aldehyde regent *[Ref: Practical boochemistry, C Raj Gopal and B D Toora 1/e P 47]*

Reagent	Substance
Ehrlich's aldehyde	**Porphobilinogen & Urobilimogen**Q
Fouchet's reagent	Bile Pigment
Benedict's reagent	**Glucose**Q
Sodium nitroprusside	**Ketones**Q

Ehrlich's aldehyde reagent test for porphobilinogen & urobilinogen

Take 5ml of urine +5 ml of Ehrlich's reagent
(Mix and allow to stand for 10 minutes)
↓
Add 5ml of saturated sodium acetate & mix Next add 5ml chloroform & shake for few seconds
(allow layer to separate)

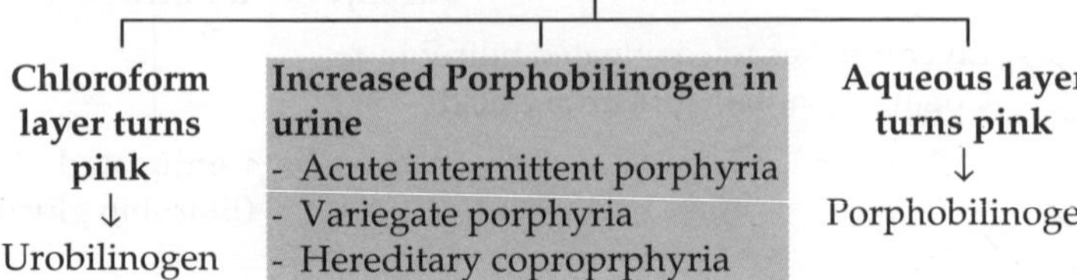

134. C i.e. CEP **135. D i.e. Ferrochelatase**

[Ref: Harper's 27/e P-283-286; Vasudevan 6/e p. 245-50; Chatterjea 6/e P-472- 73, Lippincott's 3/e P-279]

- **Erythropoietic protoporphyria** is due to **deficiency of enzyme ferrochelatase**Q.
- **All porphyrias are autosomal dominant (AD) except congenital erythropoietic porphyria** (autosomal recessive, AR), **ALA dehydratase (porphobilinogen) deficiency (AR)** and **X-linked protoporphyria (X-linked).**

136. D i.e. Hepatic porphyria

Hepatomegaly is an essential feature of **von Gierek's disease** (all glycogen storage diseases except type 2, 5, 7), **Hurler (Scheic) syndrome** (& all mucopolysaccharidosis) and **Nieman-Pick disease. But the hepatic involvement of hepatic porphyria is variable**Q. Patients with chronic hepatic porphyria (porphyria cutanea tarda), however may show liver enlargement d/t fatty infiltration but frank sings of hepatomegaly and iron overload are rare.

137. A i.e. Ferrous ion; B i.e. Glycine; D i.e. Succinyl CoA *[Ref: Harper 26/e Pg 271-275]*

Heme Synthesis

- First step is – Formation of ALA from **succinyl-COA & Glycine.**Q
- ALA is synthetised in mitochondria then enters the cytosol to form porphobilinogen.
- Porphobilinogen is converted to uroporphyrinogen in presence of uroporphyrinogen synthatase. (Intermediate product is hydroxy methyl bilane)

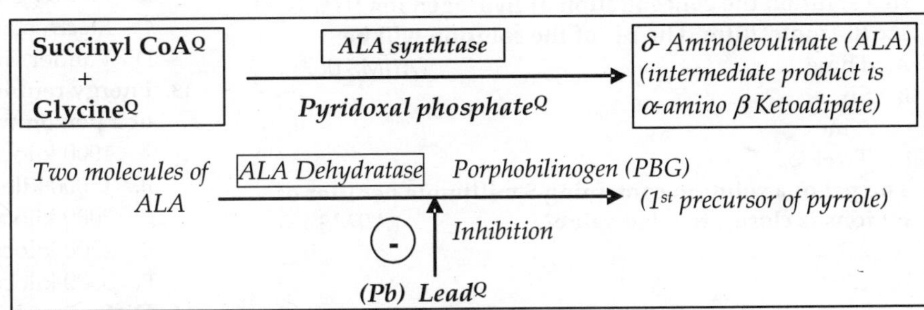

- Uroporphyrinogen is converted to coproporphyrinogen by uroporphyrinogen decarboxylase.
- Coproporphyrinogen enters the mitochondria where it form protoporphrinogen and then converted to protoporphyrin.
- Protoporphyrin with ferrous ion form heme in the presence of Ferrochelatase (Heme synthtase).

Chapter -7 GENERAL BIOCHEMISTRY

QUESTIONS

Water, pH, Buffers & Bioenergetics

1. **Metabolic water is-** (NBE P 15)
   A. Ingested water ☐
   B. Water infused iv ☐
   C. Water produced by metabolism ☐
   D. None ☐
2. **Monoprotic acid are** (PGI 09)
   A. Formic acid ☐
   B. Carbonic acid ☐
   C. Acetic acid ☐
   D. Citric acid ☐
   E. Nitric acid ☐
3. **In a solution the concentration of hydrogen ion [H^+] is 1 x 10^{-6} moles/litre. The pH of the solution will be:**
   A. Three (AIIMS 06) ☐
   B. Six ☐
   C. Nine ☐
   D. Twelve ☐
4. **The pH of a solution containing 5 millimole per liter of H^+ ions is closest to what value?** (AIIMS 16)
   A. 2.3 ☐
   B. 1.7 ☐
   C. 3.5 ☐
   D. 4.2 ☐
5. **The buffering capacity of a buffer is maximum at pH equal to** (AI 03)
   A. 0.5 pKa ☐
   B. pKa ☐
   C. pKa+1 ☐
   D. 2pKa ☐
6. **A buffer that is most effective at a pH of about 4.5 is;**
   A. Acetate buffer. (AIIMS 14, 03) ☐
   B. Bicarbonate buffer ☐
   C. Phosphate buffer ☐
   D. Tris buffer ☐
7. **HCO_3/H_2CO_3 is the best buffer because it is?**(AIIMS 16)
   A. pKa near physiological pH ☐
   B. Its components can be increased or decreased in the body as needed ☐
   C. Good acceptor and donor of H+ ions ☐
   D. Combination of a weak acid and weak base ☐
8. **The presence of 2 extra pairs of electrons on the oxygen in water molecule results in :** (AIIMS 02)
   A. Makes water a non-polar solvent ☐
   B. Forms covalent bonds in the ice. ☐
   C. Electro negative charge on water molecule ☐
   D. Electro positive charge on water molecule ☐
9. **Strongest bond out of the following is :** (AI 08)
   A. Electrostatic ☐
   B. Hydrogen ☐
   C. Hydrophobic ☐
   D. Vanderwall's ☐
10. **True statement regarding covalent bonds is :** (AI 07)
    A. Electrons have same spin ☐
    B. Electrons have opposite spin ☐
    C. They are weak bonds ☐
    D. None of the above ☐
11. **Strongest bond amongst the following is** (AI 06)
    A. Hydrophobic ☐
    B. Electrostatic ☐
    C. Hydrogen bond ☐
    D. Wander wall's ☐
12. **Weakest bond is :** (AIIMS 07)
    A. Covalent ☐
    B. Hydrogen ☐
    C. Electrostatic ☐
    D. Vander wall ☐
13. **Energy required for maintenance of bodily functions of a person weighing 40 kgs is:** (PGI 01)
    A. 1000 kilocalories ☐
    B. 15000 kilocalories ☐
    C. 2000 kilocalories ☐
    D. 2500 kilocalories ☐
    E. 3500 kilocalories ☐
14. **Difference between reversible and irreversible reaction is** (AIIMS 03)
    A. Entropy ☐
    B. Temperature ☐
    C. Work done ☐
    D. Amount of heat production ☐
15. **Regarding a crystal, the true statement is :** (AI 02)
    A. Molecules are arranged in same orientation with different confirmation ☐
    B. Molecules are arranged in different oreintation with different confirmation ☐
    C. Molecules are arranged in same orientation and same confirmation ☐
    D. Molecules are arranged in different oreintation but with same confirmation ☐

Xenobiotics

16. **All are true about glutathione except:** (AIIMS 10,08)
    A. It is a tripeptide ☐
    B. It converts hemoglobin to methemoglobin ☐
    C. It conjugates xenobiotics and it is co-factor of various enzymes ☐
    D. It scavenges free radicals and superoxide ions ☐
17. **True about Glutathione except-** (NBE P 15)
    A. TRIpeptide ☐
    B. Formed form glutamic acid, glycine, cysteine ☐
    C. Act as antioxidant in reduced state ☐
    D. All of the above ☐

18. Which of the following elements is known to influence the body's ability to handle oxidative stress?
A. Calcium *(AI 04)* ☐
B. Iron ☐
C. Potassium ☐
D. Selenium ☐

19. Which of the following enzyme are associated with break down of H_2O_2. *(PGI 11)*
A. Catalase ☐
B. Perioxidase ☐
C. Oxidase ☐
D. Oxygenase ☐
E. Hydrolase ☐

20. H_2O_2 is breaked or formed by which of the following enzyme: *(PGI 03)*
A. Oxidase ☐
B. Oxygenase ☐
C. Hydrolase ☐
D. Peroxidase ☐
E. Catalase ☐

21. Which of the following is not a phase I Reaction:
A. Oxidation *(AI 12)* ☐
B. Reduction ☐
C. Hydrolysis ☐
D. Conjugation ☐

22. The main enzyme responsible for activation of xenobiotics is
A. Cytochrome P-450 *(AI 03)* ☐
B. Glutathione S-transferase ☐
C. NADPH cytochrome P-450-reductase ☐
D. Glucuronyl transferase ☐

23. The conjugation of bilirubin to glucuronic acid in the liver; *(AIIMS 03)*
A. Converts a hydrophilic compound to a hydrophobic one ☐
B. Converts a hydrophobic compound to a hydrophilic one ☐
C. Enables the bilirubin molecule to cross the cell membrane ☐
D. Is increased during neonatal jaundice ☐

24. What is metabolised like xenobiotics *(AIIMS 05)*
A. Myoglobin ☐
B. Bilirubin ☐
C. Biliverdin ☐
D. Haemoglobin ☐

25. Bile salts undergo xenobiotics: *(PGI 07)*
A. After conjugation with taurine and glycine ☐
B. After conjugation with lysine ☐
C. After conjugation with betaglucuronic acid ☐
D. After conjugation with derived proteins ☐

Free Radicals

26. Which of the following reduces oxidative stress except:
A. Superoxide dismutase *(PGI 11)* ☐
B. Catalase ☐
C. Glutathione peroxidase ☐
D. Xanthine oxidase ☐
E. Ceruloplasmin ☐

27. All of the following act as antioxidants except:
A. Vit. D *(PGI 15,13,09; AIIMS 16,08; NBE P 15,14,13)* ☐
B. Vit. C & E ☐
C. Selenium ☐
D. Glutathione peroxidase ☐

28. The mineral having action like vitamin E-
A. Calcium *(NBE P 15,13)* ☐
B. Iron ☐
C. Selenium ☐
D. Magnesium ☐

29. The main function of vitamin C in the body is-
A. Coenzyme for energy metabolism *(NBE P 15,14)* ☐
B. Regulation of lipid synthesis ☐
C. Involvement as antioxidant ☐
D. Inhibition of cell growth ☐

30. Major function of vitamin E in the body- *(NBE P 15)*
A. Regulation of energy metabolism ☐
B. Carboxylation reaction ☐
C. Blood clotting ☐
D. Protection of biological membrane from free radical damage ☐

31. Reperfusion injury is caused by: *(PGI 06)*
A. Vitamin E ☐
B. Superoxide ion ☐
C. Calcium ion ☐
D. Magnesium ion ☐

32. Which of these have antioxidant properties: *(PGI 12)*
A. Tocopherol ☐
B. Reduced Glutathione (GSH) ☐
C. Citrulline ☐
D. Lycopene ☐

33. True about Glutathione reductase: *(PGI 01)*
A. Sulphur containing enzyme ☐
B. Important in methemoglobinemia ☐
C. Free radical scavenger ☐
D. All ☐

34. Enzyme responsible for respiratory burst reaction
A. Dehydrogenase *(AIIMS 08)* ☐
B. Peroxidase ☐
C. Hydroxylase ☐
D. NADPH – oxidase ☐

35. Reactive oxygen intermediates are released by:
A. Catalase *(AI 08)* ☐
B. NADPH oxidase ☐
C. Glutathione peroxidase ☐
D. Superoxide dismutase ☐

Minerals

36. Which is non essential mineral: *(AIIMS 10)*
A. Sodium ☐
B. Manganese ☐
C. Iron ☐
D. Lead ☐

Vitamins

37. **Which of the following is a Water Soluble Vitamin?** (AI 08)
    A. Folic Acid ☐
    B. Vitamin A ☐
    C. Vitamin K ☐
    D. Linolenic Acid ☐
38. **NAD acts as a cofactor for** (PGI 09)
    A. Citrate Synthetase ☐
    B. Isocitrate dehydrogenase ☐
    C. α-ketoglutarate dehydrogenase ☐
    D. Malate dehydrogenase ☐
    E. Succinyl thiokinase ☐
39. **ALL are involved in energy metabolism except-** (NBE P 15)
    A. Vitamin B_1 ☐
    B. Vitamin B_3 ☐
    C. Vitamin B_7 ☐
    D. Vitamin B_{12} ☐
40. **Gene for folic acid absorption is present on** (AIIMS 08)
    A. Chromosome X ☐
    B. Chromosome XXI ☐
    C. Chromosome V ☐
    D. Chromosome Xi ☐
41. **The gene for folic acid transporter is located on which chromosome:** (AIIMS 08)
    A. 5 ☐
    B. 15 ☐
    C. 21 ☐
    D. X ☐
42. **Which of the following statement about thiamin is true?** (AIIMS 08)
    A. It is a co-enzyme of lactate deydrogenase ☐
    B. Its deficiency is associated with scurvy ☐
    C. Its co enzyme function is done by thiamine monophosphate ☐
    D. Its co-enzyme for pyruvate dehydrogenase and α-ketoglutarate dehydrogenase ☐
43. **Thiamine requirement increases in excessive intake of:** (AIIMS 09)
    A. Carbohydrate ☐
    B. Amino acid ☐
    C. Fat ☐
    D. Lecithine ☐
44. **Thiamine level is best monitored by:** (AI 12; NBE P 15,14,13; AIIMS 15,13)
    A. Transketolase level in blood (RBC) ☐
    B. Thiamine level in blood ☐
    C. G6PD activity ☐
    D. Reticulocytosis ☐
45. **Enzyme activity measured in beri beri is**: (PGI 15,13,05)
    A. RBC Transketolase ☐
    B. Transaminase ☐
    C. Decarboxylase ☐
    D. Deaminases ☐
46. **Thiamine acts as a cofactor in:** (AI 04)
    A. Conversion of pyruvate to acetyl-CoA ☐
    B. Transamination reactions ☐
    C. Oxidation in respiratory chain ☐
    D. Conversion of pyridoxal to pyridoxal phosphate ☐
47. **Thiamine is essential for** (AI 05)
    A. Isocitrate dehydrogenase ☐
    B. Succinate dehydrogenase ☐
    C. Pyruvate dehydrogenase ☐
    D. Acetyl CoA synthetase ☐
48. **Thiamine is not used in which of the following reactions** (AIIMS 01)
    A. Lactate to pyruvate ☐
    B. Alphaketoglutarate to succinyl CoA ☐
    C. Glucose to pentose ☐
    D. Oxidative decarboxylation of α-keto amino acids ☐
49. **Which of the vitamin deficiency lead to lactic acidosis** (AIIMS 10)
    A. Riboflavin ☐
    B. Thiamine ☐
    C. Niacin ☐
    D. Pantothenic acid ☐
50. **Riboflavin deficiency is assessed by-** (NBE P 15)
    A. Transketolase ☐
    B. Glutathione reductase ☐
    C. PDH ☐
    D. None ☐
51. **Which vitamin deficiency causes glossitis and cheilosis-** (NBE P 15)
    A. Thiamin ☐
    B. Riboflavin ☐
    C. Folic acid ☐
    D. Vitamin A ☐
52. **The activity of the following enzyme is affected by biotin deficiency**: (AIIMS 03, AI 06)
    A. Transketolase, ☐
    B. Dehydrogenase. ☐
    C. Oxidase. ☐
    D. Carboxylase. ☐
53. **Active moiety of CoA is** (WB 10, TN 09)
    A. Acetyl group ☐
    B. Pantoic acid ☐
    C. Thiol of β-alanine ☐
    D. Thiol of pantetheine ☐
54. **Which vitamin is necessary for coenzyme A synthesis** (AI 05)
    A. Pantothenic acid ☐
    B. Ascorbic acid ☐
    C. Biotin ☐
    D. Pyridoxine ☐
55. **Panthothenic acid is coenzyme of which of the following reaction (s):** (PGI 08)
    A. Dehydrogenation ☐
    B. Oxidation ☐
    C. Decarboxylation ☐
    D. Reduction ☐
    E. Acetylation ☐
56. **Patient presenting with pellagra, parkinsonism, convulsions, anemia and kidney stones has deficiency of** (AI 05)
    A. Coenzyme A ☐
    B. FADH ☐
    C. Niacin ☐
    D. Pyridoxal phosphate ☐

57. Which is not pyridoxine dependant: *(AIIMS 08)*
A. Homocystinuria ☐
B. Maple syrup urine disease ☐
C. Oxaluria ☐
D. Xanthinuria. ☐

58. Cause(s) of homocystinuria: *(PGI 12)*
A. Deficiency of vit B6 ☐
B. Deficiency of vit B 12 ☐
C. Deficiency of folic acid ☐
D. Deficiency of pantothenic acid ☐

59. Co-enzyme used in transamination *(AIIMS 03)*
A. NAD ☐
B. Biotin ☐
C. Pyridoxal phosphate ☐
D. Riboflavin ☐

60. Intrinsic factor of Castle is secreted by
A. Chief cells *(AIIMS 10)* ☐
B. Parietal cells ☐
C. Mucous cells ☐
D. β cells ☐

61. Vitamin B_{12} deficiency has A/E *(PGI 10, WB 10)*
A. Folate trap ☐
B. Decreased methyl malonyl CoA ☐
C. SACD ☐
D. Megaloblastic anemia ☐

62. Vitamin B_{12} is absorbed in the *(NBE P 14; AI 06)*
A. Stomach ☐
B. Duodenum ☐
C. Ileum ☐
D. Colon ☐

63. Cobalt forms a component of which vitamin
A. Biotin *(AI 05)* ☐
B. Vitamin B12 ☐
C. Vitamin A ☐
D. Tocopherol ☐

64. Not a dietary source of vit. B12- *(AIIMS 08)*
A. Fish ☐
B. Meat ☐
C. Soyabean ☐
D. Liver ☐

65. Vitamin B_{12} and folic acid supplementation in megaloblastic anemia leads to the improvement of anemia due to: *(AI 02)*
A. Increased DNA synthesis in bone marrow ☐
B. Increased Hemoglobin production ☐
C. Erythroid hyperplasia ☐
D. Increased iron absorption ☐

66. Vitamin B_{12} acts as co-enzyme to which one of the following enzymes? *(AIIMS 14,12; PGI 13; AI 10)*
A. Isocitrate dehydrogenase ☐
B. Homocysteine methyl transferase ☐
C. Glycogen synthase ☐
D. G-6-P dehydrogenase ☐

67. All are true about vitamin B_{12}, except- *(NBE P 15)*
A. Active form is methylcobalamine ☐
B. Requires for conversion of homocysteine to methionine ☐
C. Requires in metabolism of methylmalonyl CoA ☐
D. Requires for conversion of pyruvate to lactate ☐

68. Vitamin which is excreted in urine is : *(AIIMS 07)*
A. Vitamin A ☐
B. Vitamin C ☐
C. Vitamin D ☐
D. Vitamin K ☐

69. All of the following are required for hydroxylation of proline in collagen synthesis except : *(NBE P 13)*
A. O_2 ☐
B. Vitamin C ☐
C. Dioxygenases ☐
D. Pyridoxal phosphate ☐

70. Vitamin required for hydroxyproline to proline conversion: *(NBE P 14; PGI 07)*
A. Vitamin C ☐
B. Vitamin E ☐
C. Pyrodoxal PO_4 ☐
D. Biotin ☐

71. During the formation of hydroxyproline and hydroxylsine, the essential factors required is/are:
A. Pyridoxal phosphate *(PGI 03)* ☐
B. Ascorbic acid ☐
C. Thiamine pyrophosphate ☐
D. Methylcobalamine ☐
E. Biotin ☐

72. Aminoacyl t-RNA is required for all except : *(AI 02)*
A. Hydroxyproline ☐
B. Methionine ☐
C. Cystine ☐
D. Lysine ☐

73. Gamma carboxylation of glutamic acid in clotting factor II, VII and protein C is dependent on
A. Vitamin K *(NBE P 14, 13; AI 08)* ☐
B. Vitamin C ☐
C. Vitamin A ☐
D. Vitamin E ☐

74. The Similarity between Vit C & Vit K is: *(AI 09, 05)*
A. Both help in conversion of proline to hydroxyproline ☐
B. Both help in post-translational modification ☐
C. Both have anti infective activity ☐
D. Both are involved in coagulation cascade ☐

75. In vitamin C deficiency, post translational modification of which amino acid is defective:
A. Lysine *(AIIMS 07)* ☐
B. Alanine ☐
C. Glycine ☐
D. Arginine ☐

76. Vitamin K is ivolved in the posttranslational modification? *(AI 11)*
A. Glutamate ☐
B. Aspartate ☐
C. Leucine ☐
D. Lysine ☐

77. Carboxylation of clotting factors by vitamin K is required to be biologically active. Which of the following amino acid is carboxylated? *(AIIMS 15,13,08)*
A. Histidine ☐
B. Histamine ☐
C. Glutamate ☐
D. Aspartate ☐

78. HDN is seen due to deficiency of vitamin: *(PGI 09)*
A. A ☐
B. C ☐
C. K ☐
D. E ☐

79. Vitamin required for post translational modification of coagulants is : *(AI 07)*
A. Vitamin A ☐
B. Vitamin C ☐
C. Vitamin B6 ☐
D. Vitamin K ☐

80. Vit K is needed for which of these post transational modification processes- *(AIIMS 01)*
A. Methylation ☐
B. Carboxylation ☐
C. Hydroxylation ☐
D. Transketolation ☐

81. The vitamin used for post-translational modification of glutamic acid to γ-Carboxy-glutamate is *(AI 04)*
A. Vitamin D ☐
B. Vitamin E ☐
C. Vitamin A ☐
D. Vitamin K ☐

82. Vitamin K dependent coagulation factors include:
A. II and III *(AI 10)* ☐
B. IX and X ☐
C. III and V ☐
D. VIII and XII ☐

83. Vitamin K dependent clotting factor is:
A. Factor VII *(AIIMS 10)* ☐
B. Factor I ☐
C. Factor XI ☐
D. Factor XII ☐

84. Which of the following is a component of the visual pigment rhodopsin: *(AIIMS 05)*
A. β-Carotene ☐
B. Retinal ☐
C. Retinol ☐
D. Retinoic acid ☐

85. Vitamin A is stored mainly as retinol esters in:
A. Kidney *(AIIMS 05)* ☐
B. Muscle ☐
C. Liver ☐
D. Retina ☐

86. Which of the following combinations of biologically active molecules does vitamin A consists of
A. Retinol, retinal and retinoic acid *(AIIMS 04)* ☐
B. Retinol, retinal and tetrahydrofolate ☐
C. Retinal, conjugase and retinoic acid ☐
D. PABA, retinal and retinaldehyde ☐

87. Vitamin A intoxication causes injury to
A. Lysosomes *(AIIMS 07)* ☐
B. Mitochondria ☐
C. Endoplasmic reticulum ☐
D. Microtubules ☐

88. Metabolic bone disease is caused by excess intake of which vitamin: *(PGI 02)*
A. A ☐
B. B ☐
C. C ☐
D. D ☐
E. E ☐

89. Which of the following does not contain keratin
A. Potato *(AIIMS 04)* ☐
B. Tomato ☐
C. Carrot ☐
D. Spinach ☐

ANSWERS & EXPLANATIONS:

Water, pH, Buffers & Bioenergenetics

1. **C i.e. Water produced by metabolism** *[Ref: Naik 1/e p. 271]*

Metabolic water is water produced during metabolism of food. It is ~ **150-350 ml/day.**

2. **A, C, E i.e. Formic acid, Acetic acid, Nitric acid**

Monoprotic acids (donating 1 proton) are ***hydrochloric acid (HCl), nitric acid (HNO_3), formic acid (HCOOH), acetic acid (CH_3COOH) and benzoic acid***Q. **Biprotic acids** are sulfuric acid (H_2SO_4) and ***carbonic acid (H_2CO_3)***Q and **triprotic acids** are phosphoric acid (H_3PO_4) and ***citric acid***Q

3. **B i.e. Six** *[Ref: Harper's 30/e P-10-13]*

pH = -log [H+] i.e. pH is the *negative log of hydrogen ion concentration.*

In this case pH = - log [10^{-6}]
= - (-6) = + *6.0*

In case if H^+ conc. is 3.2 x 10^{-6}

pH = - log [3.2 x 10^{-6}]
= - log [3.2] – log [10^{-6}]
= - [0.5] – [-6]
= - 0.5 + 6 = 5.5

So you can see that as ***H^+ conc. increases pH decreases***

I would like to tell this much about dissociation constant 1 gm of water contains 3.46 x 10^{22} molecules. To state that the probability that a hydrogen exists as an ion is 0.01 i.e. that a hydrogen atom has 1 chance in 100 of being an ion and 99 chances out of 100 of being part of water molecule. The actual probability of hydrogen atom in pure water existing as a hydrogen ion is ~*1.8x10*$^{-9}$ and as molecule is *1*. Stated another way ***for every hydrogen ion and hydroxyl ion in pure water there are 1.8 billion or 1.8x 10^9 water molecules.***

Dissociation constant of $H_2O \rightarrow K = \frac{[H^+][OH^-]}{[H_2O]}$

Ion product for water Kw= (K) [H_2O] = [H^+] [OH^-]

Bracket represents molar concentration (strictly speaking molar activities). Since one mole (mol) of water weighs 18g, one liter (L) (1000g) of water contains 1000/18 = 55.56 mol Since the probability that a hydrogen ion in pure water will exist as a hydrogen ion is 1.8x10^{-9} the molar conc. of H^+ (or OH^-) in pure water is 1.8x 10^{-9} times of molar conc. of pure water (55.56) = ~ *10^{-7}*

Dissociation constant, $K = \frac{[10^{-7}][10^{-7}]}{55.56} = \boldsymbol{1.8 \times 10^{-16}\ mol/L}$

Ion product Kw = (1.8x10^{-16} mol / L) (55.56 mol / L) = **10^{-14} mol^2 / L^2**

Kw equals 10^{-14} (mol /L)^2 for all aqueous solutions, even solutions of acids or bases. We shall use Kw to calculate pH of acidic & basic solutions.

4. **A i.e. 2.3**

pH = - log [H^+] = -log [5 × 10^{-3}] = -log (5) – log [10^{-3}]
= -log(5) – (-3) = -log (10/2) + 3 = -1 + log 2 +3
= 3 – 1 + log 2 = 2+ log 2 = 2+0.3 = **2.3**Q

★ [log 10 = 1 & log 2 = 0.3010]

5. **B i.e. pKa** *[Ref: Harper's 30/e P-11-13; Guyton 11/e p. 385]*

6. **A i.e. Acetate Buffer**

"At values close to pKa, the buffer solution resists changes in pH most effectively", i.e. a buffer system is most effective when the pH of the system is near its pka valueQ.

Buffers

- Buffering is the tendency of a solution to resist a change in pH more effectively after addition of a **strong acid or base** than does an equal volume of water.
- Solutions of weak acids & their conjugate bases (& vice versa) exhibit buffering. Strong acid/bases do not have buffering quality as great as the weak acid/bases. **pKa** refers to the ***pH at which the concentration of the acid equals that of the base***Q.

	Buffer Systems (BS)
ICF	**Phosphate** BS
Both in ICF & ECF	**Protein** BS (i.e. **Hb, plasma protein & amino acid** BS)
ECF	**Carbonic acid–Bicarbonate**

At pH = pKa	At pH < pK	At pH > pK
the solution would contain acid and base in equal amounts, and therefore would resist a change most effectively in either direction.	i.e. more acidic environment much of the acid buffering capacity of the solution has already been neutralized so adding even minute quantities of acid would decrease the pH, i.e. it no more has buffering capacity to acids, but it would still have buffering capacity towards bases.	i.e. more alkaline environment, much of the alkaline buffering capacity has been neutralized after all that's the reason why the pH rose above pK in the first place so adding even minute quantities of alkali would increase the pH.

Buffer	Pka
Phosphate	6.8
Bicarbonate	**6.1**[Q]
Acetate	4.76
Tris [hydroxymethyl aminomethane]	8.3

Note: The **effective range of a buffer is one pH unit higher or lower than pKa**[Q].

7. **B i.e. Its components can be increased or decreased in the body as needed**

- **Bicarbonate – carbonic acid buffer system has low element concentration and has pK of 6.1 (physiological pH is 7.4)** which means the buffer operates where the slope is low or buffering power is poor (as the pH & pK difference is > 1).
- **Despite these facts, the bicarbonate buffer system is the most powerful (best) extracellular buffer in the body.** This **apparent paradox** is mainly due to the fact that the two components of this buffer system i.e. **HCO_3^- & CO_2 (bicarbonate & carbon dioxide) are regulated by kidney and lungs respectively in the body as needed**[Q].

8. **C ie Electronegative charge on water molecule** 9. **A i.e. Electrostatic** 10. **B i.e. Electrons have opposite Spin**
11. **B i.e. Electrostatic** 12. **D i.e. Vander wall** *[Ref: Harper's 27/e P- 5-7; Lehninger 2/e P- 39- 45; Chatterjea 6/e P- 84]*

In **decreasing order of strength** various bons are **covalent bond (strongest)**[Q] > **disulphide bond> electrostatic (salt bridges)**[Q] > hydrogen bond > **vander wall forces (weakest)**[Q]

★ **Disulphide bond** is strong high energy covalent bond between two cysteine residues.

13. **A i.e. 1000 Kcal** *[Ref: CMDT 1263; Park's SPM 424]*

Energy required for basal metaboism = 1 K.cal/hr/kg of body weight[Q]

So in 24 hours for a 40kg individual, it is 40x24 = 960 K cal.

Basal energy Expenditure is 10% less than resting energy Expenditure

14. **C i.e. Work done** *[Ref: Lehninger 2/e P 390-92; Bahl 24/e P-270-74; 200]*
15. **C i.e. Same conformation & molecules are arranged in same orientation** *[Ref: Chemistry by Mishra, Bhushan, Sharma/105]*

A crystal lattice is a three dimensional, highly ordered and regular arrangement of atoms, molecules or ions. A crystal is formed from small units, (that have the same orientation and same conformation[Q]**), such that when these units are repeated in all possible directions, the structure of the crystal is still maintained.**

Xenobiotics

16. **B i.e. It converts hemoglobin to methemoglobin** 17. **D i.e. All of the above** 18. **D i.e. Selenium**
[Ref: Lippincott's 4/e p. 148; Harper's 27/e p. 620, 636-37, 180- 81, 96; Chattergea 7/e p. 478-79]

- **Selenium in the form of 'selenocysteine' is a component of enzyme glutathione peroxidase**[Q]. 'Glutathione peroxidase serve to protect proteins, cell membranes, lipid and nucleic acids from oxidant molecules'. **Glutathione prevents oxidation of hemoglobin to methemoglobin**[Q]**. It acts as antioxidant in reduced state**[Q]**.**
- Reduced glutathione is **tripeptide thiol (γ- gluatamyl cystein glycine) consisting of 3 amino acids – glutamic acid, cysteine and glycine**[Q]. The glutamate is linked to cysteine through γ – carboxyl linkage. And **sulfhydryl (SH) or thiol group of cysteine, which accounts for its strong electron donating (nucleophilic) character of glutathione**[Q], is the business part of molecule.

19. **A i.e. Catalase; B i.e. Perioxidase** 20. **A i.e. Oxidase; D i.e. Peroxidase; E i.e. Catalase** *[Ref: Harper's 27/e P-96, 204]*

Oxidase & superoxide dismutase generate H_2O_2, where as catalase and peroxidase are associated with breakdown of H_2O_2[Q].

21. **D i.e. Conjugation** *[Ref: Harper 29/e p 6767-682; Vasudevan 6/e p 447-50]*
22. **A i.e. Cytochrome P-450** 23. **B i.e. Converts a hydrophobic compound to a hydrophilic one**
24. **B i.e. Bilirubin** 25. **C i.e. Conjugation with β glucoronic acid**

- **Phase I biotransformation reactions** include **Hydrolysis, Hydroxylation, Reduction, Oxidation, Oxidative Deamination, Dealkaylation and Epioxidation. Mn "High RODE".** Whereas **phase II reactions** include **Glucronidation, Sulfation, Conjugation (with glucronic acid, glutathione, sulfate or aminoacids), Acetylation and Methylation.** Mn **"5G-SCAM".**
- **Cytochrome p450** ***monoxygenase is the main enzyme responsible for activation of xenobiotics (phase I hydroxylation reaction)***[Q].
- **Bilirubin** is metabolized like xenobiotics; it is conjugated with beta glucronic acid in hepatocytes to ***convert a nonpolar hydrophobic bilirubin to a polar hydrophilic one which is readily excreted in bile***[Q].

Free Radicals

26. **D i.e. Xanthine oxidase** 27. **B, C, D i.e. Vit.C & E, Selenium, Glutathione peroxidase** 28. **C i.e. Selenium**
29. **C i.e. Involvement as antioxidant** 30. **D i.e. Protection of biological membrane from free radical damage**
31. **B i.e. Superoxide ion** *[Ref: Harper 28/e 482-85; Chattarjae 7/e 198; Lippincott 5/e 148; Vassudevan 6/e 241-388-409-429]*

- **Xanthine oxidase increases oxidative stress by generating superoxide free radicles**[Q]
- **Ischemic reperfusion injury** is caused by **reactive oxygen species (ROS)/free radical or pro oxidant like superoxide ion**[Q]
- **Antioxidants** blocking free radical formation include **vitamin A (Beta carotene), C and E; superoxide dismutase, catalase and selenium containing glutathione peroxidase enzymes**; ceruloplasmin, transferrin, ferritin, and lactoferrin transport proteins etc.
- **Main function of vitamin E is antioxidation**[Q]. **It prevents oxidation of other antioxidants (eg vitamin A, C & carotenes). It protects biological membrane from free radical damage**[Q] formed by peroxidation of PUFA. So it **prevents rancidity of fats.**

32. **A i.e. Tocopherol; B i.e. Reduced Glutathione(GSH); D i.e. Lycopene**
33. **C i.e. Free radical scavanger** *[Ref: Harper 29/e p. 200-201]*

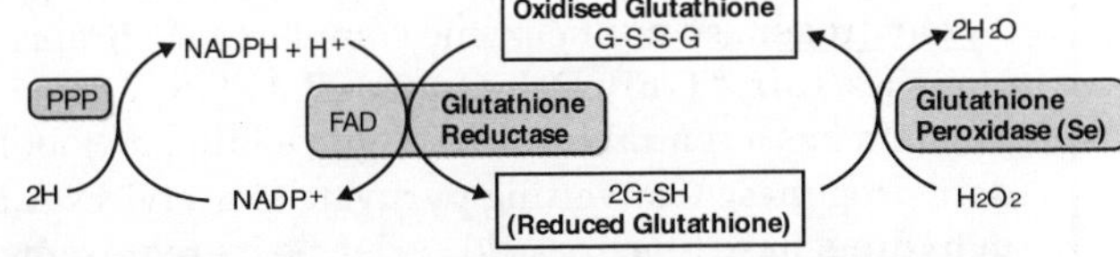

- **Tocopherol (vitamin E), lycopene** (in red tomatoes) and **reduced glutathione (GSH) have antioxidant properties.**
- In RBC, the **pentose phosphate pathway** is the only source of NADPH for reduction of oxidized glutathione by enzyme glutathione reductase. **Glutathione reductase**, a flavo protein enzyme containing FAD ***catalyzes oxidised glutathione to reduced glutathione***[Q]. **Reduced glutathione (GSH) removes H_2O_2** in a reaction catabolized by **glutathione peroxidase (a selenocysteine** i.e. contains **selenium analog of cysteine). Since** H_2O_2 accumulation in RBC causes oxidative damage to cell membrane l/t hemolysis & decreased life span. **The PPP, glutathione peroxidase and reduced glutathione (GSH) protect erythrocyte against oxidative damage** (i.e. have antioxidant properties).

★ **Glutathione = Glycine + Cysteine + Glutamate**

★ *Methhemoglobin reductase* is important for conversion of methhemoglobin back to hemoglobin.

34. **D i.e. NADPH – oxidase** 35. **B i.e. NADPH oxidase**

[Ref: Harper 28/e p. 482-85; Robbins 7/e p. 16-17, 60-61; Guyton 11/e p.16; Ganong 22/e p. 518]

Minerals

36. **D i.e. Lead** *[Ref: Vasudevan 6/e p 411; Styanarayan 3/e p 403; Chatterjea 7/e p 707-570]*

Aluminium, cadmium, mercury and lead minerals are toxic and should be avoided[Q].

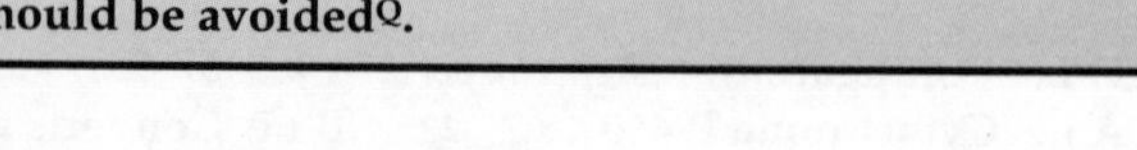

Vitamin

37. **A i.e. Folic Acid** *[Ref:; Lippincott's 4/e p- 373; Ganong 22/e p. 313- 16; Devlin 5/e p- 1154, Harper's 28/e P- 468]*

Vitamin B complex and C are water soluble, whereas vitamin A, D, E and K are fat soluble[Q].

38. **B, C, D i.e. Isocitrate dehydrogenase, α-ketoglutarate dehydrogenase, Malate dehydrogenase** *[Ref:Chatterjea 7/e p 171;Lehninger 5/e p 518]*

Niacin (Vitamin B_3) in biologically active form of **NAD^+** (nicotinamide adenine dinucleotide) and **NADP+** (nicotinamide adenine dinucleotide phosphate). **NAD^+ act as cofactor for various enzymes such as malate**/alcohol/lactate/glyceraldehyde 3-P/ α-glycero-P/**α-ketoglutarate & pyruvate dehydrogenase.** $NADP^+$ is cofactor for G6PD & glutathione reductase. **$NADP^+$ or NAD^+** act as cofactor for **glutamate & isocirate dehydrogenase**[Q].

39. **D i.e. Vitamin B_{12}**

5 Vitamins of B group involved in **energy metabolism are (1) B1 (Thiamin)**[Q], **(2) B2 (Riboflavin)**[Q], **(3) B3 (Niacin)**[Q], **(4) B5 (Pentothenic acid)**[Q] and **(5) B7 (Biotin/Vitamin H)**[Q].

40. **B i.e. Chromosome XXI** 41. **C i.e. 21**

Folic acid transporter gene (SLC 19 AI solute carrier family 19) is located on ***long arm of chromosome 21* (21q)** [Q] at band 22.3. Transport of folate occurs by potocytosis which functionally couples folate receptor, folate transporter and V- type h+ pump.

42. **D i.e. Its co-enzyme for pyruvate dehydrogenase and α-ketoglutarate dehydrogenase** 43. **A i.e. Carbohydrate**
44. **A i.e. Transketolase level in blood** 45. **A i.e. Transketolase** 46. **A i.e. Conversion of Pyruvate to acetyl COA**
47. **C i.e. Pyruvate dehydrogenase** 48. **A i.e. Lactate to Pyruvate** 49. **B i.e. Thiamine**
[Ref: Harper 28/e p. 154, 273-74; Lippincott 5/e p 111, 266, 145-46, 378-79; Vasudevan 6/e p 391-92; Lehninger 5/e p 549-51; Chatterjea 7/e p. 166-67]

- **Vitamin B_1 (Thiamine)** in form of **thiamin diphosphate (TDP)** or **TPP** act as a coenzyme for **tr**ansketolase (in PPP) and 3 **dehydrogen**ase multienzyme complexes i.e. **B**ranched chain, **A**lpha ketoglutarate and **P**yruvate – dehydrogenase enzymes. (**Mn "Truly Dehydrated- B AP"**)
- Thiamin has a central role in energy yielding metabolism (especially of carbohydrates) as it is required for **pyruvate dehydrogenase (converting pyruvate to acetyl CoA in carbohydrate metabolism)**[Q] and **α-ketoglutarate dehydrogenase** (in citric acid cycle). So **its requirement increases on excess intake of carbohydrate**[Q]. And for the same reasons **thiamine deficiency causes decreased energy production**[Q].
- Because of role of TDP in pyruvate dehydrogenase; thiamin deficiency in subjects on high carbohydrate diet results in increased plasma pyruvate and lactate eventually l/t potentially life threatening **lactic and pyruvic acidosis**[Q].
- Thiamin deficiency l/t – **beriberi, Wernicke- korsakoff syndrome**[Q], **polyneuritis and lactic acidosis**[Q]. Thiamin nutritional status is **best assessed** by **erythrocyte transketolase activation**[Q].

50. **B i.e. Glutathione reductase** 51. **B i.e. Riboflavin**
52. **D i.e. Carboxylase** *[Ref: Lippincott 5/e p. 381, 266; Harper 28/e p. 479; Vasudevan 6/e p. 400; Chatterjea 7/e p. 179-80]*

- **Riboflavin deficiency is assesses by glutathione reductase**[Q].
- **Biotin** is a **coenzyme of carboxylase enzymes**[Q], that catalyze CO_2 transfer reactions (CO_2 fixation reaction).

Vitamin	Vit B_2 (Riboflavin)	Vit B_3 (Niacin)	Folic acid
Coenzyme	FMN & FAD	NAD & NADP	**Tetrahydro folate** (TH_4F)
Function	• FMN and FAD are 2 coenzymes of this vit, and are **electron carriers**Q in oxidoreduction reaction • Consituent of: - **Cytochrome C- reductase** - **Warburg yellow enzyme** - Fumarate dehydrogenase	• NAD and NADP are its active forms which operate as hydrogen & electron transfer agent • **Deficiency seen in:** - **Maize eater**Q - **Carcinoid syndrome**Q - **Heartnup disease**Q	Its active form, Tetrahydrofolate is a **carrier of one carbon unit**; synthesis of methionine, thymine and purine
Deficiency	- Seborrhic dermatitis - **Angular stomatitis, Glossitis**Q - **Cheilosis**Q	**Pellagra**Q c/b "3Ds" - Diarrhoea - Dermatitis - Dementia	- **Megaloblastic anemia**Q - **Neural tube defect**Q.
Features	- Heat & acid resistant - Destroyed by light & alkali - Used as food additive because of its yellow color - **Deficiency detected by measurement of RBC glutathione reductase**Q	- In body **synthesized from tryptophan**Q - 60mg tryptophan= 1mg niacin - High doses used to **treat hyperlipidemia**Q - In overdose causes cholestatic jaundice	- **Folic acid reduces risk of Neural tube defect &** - **Hyperhomocystinemia**Q

53. **D i.e. Thiol of pantetheine** 54. **A i.e. Pantothenic acid**
55. **E i.e. Acetylation** *[Ref: Harper 28/e p. 479; Chatterjea 7th/ed pg 177-76; Lippincott 5th/ed pg-381; Vasudevan 6/e p. 398-99]*

Pantothenic acid is necessary for **synthesis of coenzyme A (CoA)**Q, **which functions as a coenzyme for acetylation reactions**Q

56. **D i.e. Pyridoxal phosphate** 57. **B i.e. Maple syrup urine disease**
58. **A i.e. Deficiency of vit B_6; B i.e. Deficiency of vit B_{12}; C i.e. Deficiency of folic acid** 59. **C i.e. Pyridoxal phosphate**
[Ref: Harper 28/e p. 252-58, 475-76; Lippincott 5/e p. 378; Vasudevan 6/e p. 396-97; Chatterjea 7/e p. 172-73; Lehninger 5/e p. 864-65, 878-83]

- **Pyridoxal phosphate (active B_6) dependent conditions** (in which it is used in treatment) are **Homo**cystinuria, **O**xaluria, **Cystathion**inuria and **Xan**thurenic acid uriaQ, Mn – **"HOCX or Homo Ox Siton Zen"**
- **Homocystinuria is vitamin B6, B12 and folate. dependent**Q
- **Maple syrup urine disease** is d/t defective **branched chain α-ketoacid dehydrogenase enzyme**; and it may be a/w **thiamin (vitamin B_1) deficiency**Q
- **Methylmalonyl aciduria is seen in vitamin B_{12} deficiency**Q.
- **Figlu (N- formimimino-glutamate) uria** following a dose of histidine occurs in **folate (folic acid) deficiency (Histidine load test). AICAR** (amino imidazole carboxamide ribosyl 5'-P) **uria** also occurs in **folate deficiency**.

60. **B i.e. Parietal cells** 61. **B i.e. Decreased methylmalonyl CoA**
62. **C i.e. Ileum** 63. **B i.e. Vitamin B_{12}** 64. **C i.e. Soyabean** 65. **A i.e. Increased DNA synthesis in bone marrow**
[Ref: Harper's 28/e P-500-02, 476-77; Lippincott 5/e p. 374-76; Vasudevan 6/e p. 403-5; Chatterjea 5/e p. 185-89]

Cobalt containing Vitamin B_{12} is found **only in food of animal origin and is absorbed from distal ileum**Q. B_{12} & folic acid supplements **treat pernicious (megaloblastic) anemia by increasing DNA synthesis in bone marrow**Q.

66. **B i.e. Homoeystine Methyl transferase** *[Ref: Lippincott 3rd/373; Chetterjea Shinde 6th/181]*

Vitamin B_{12} is required as a coenzyme to homocystine methyl transferase involved in the synthesis of methionine from homocystine.

Metabolic role of Vitamin B_{12}

Biologically active forms of vitamin B_{12} are called as 'cobamide coenzymes' and act as coenzymes with several enzymes for various metabolic reactions. These include

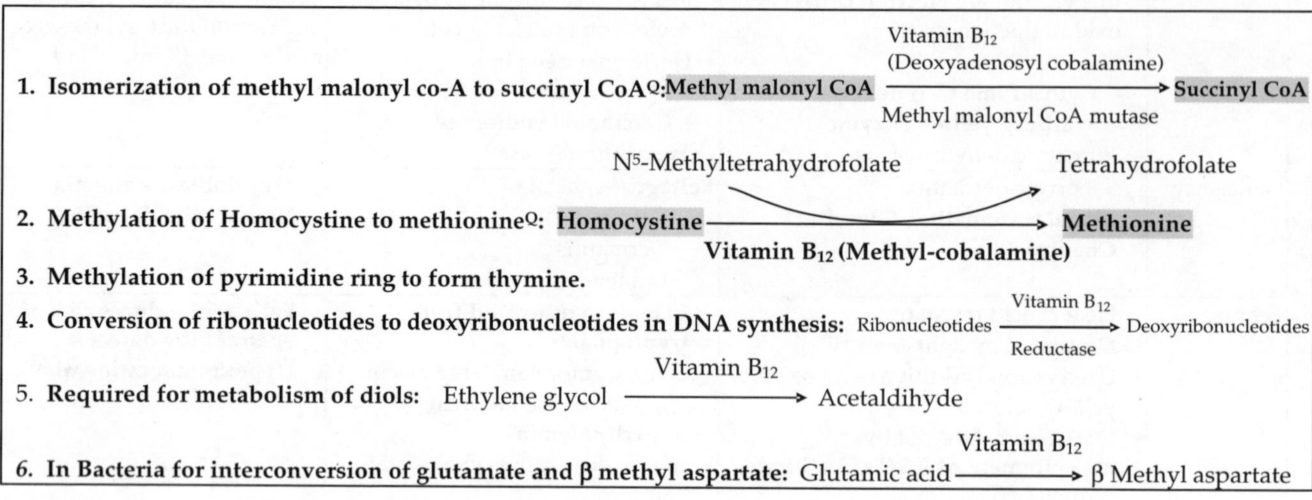

67. **D i.e. Requires for conversion of pyruvate to lactate**

Deficiency of Vitamin B12

- 3 enzymes **methyl malonyl CoA mutase (or isomerase), leucine amino mutase, and methionine synthase** are B_{12} dependent

Methyl malonic acid uria

- Methyl malonyl CoA is formed as an intermediate in catabolism of valine, threonine, isoleucine & methenine aminoacids and (by carboxylation of propionyl CoA arising in catabolism of) cholesterol side chains, isoleucine & fatty acids with odd numbers of carbon atoms or directly from proprionate

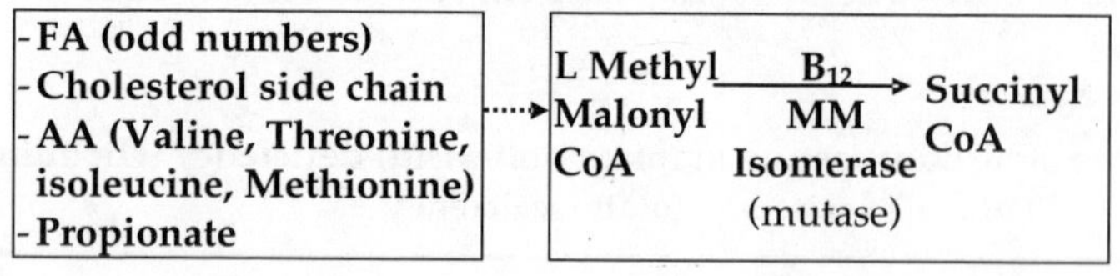

- In B_{12} deficiency methyl malonyl accumulates and its *urinary excretion provides a means of assessing B_{12} nutritional status.*
- Accumulation of unusual fatty acids and their incorporation in cell membrane of nervous system may account for neurological manifestations.
- ***Hyper homocysteinemia, homo cystinuria l/t cardiovascular diseases, like atherosclerosis, thrombosis, hypertension and MI[Q]***

Folate Trap and Pernicious Anemia

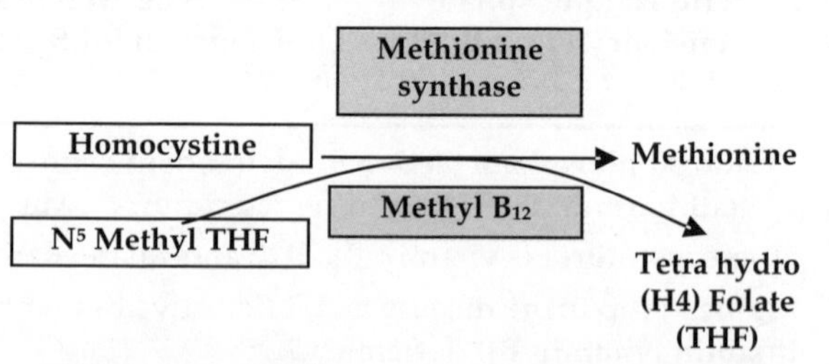

- Effect of B_{12} def. is most pronounced in rapidly dividing cells of *bone marrow erythropoietic tissue & intestinal mucosa* as these need both the N_5 N_{10} methylene & N_{10} formyl forms of THF for ***synthesis of nucleotides required for DNA replication[Q]***
- In B_{12} deficiency, d/t dysfunction of methionine synthase methylation of homocysteine by N_5 methyl THF is hampered l/t accumulation of both.
- Because methylated form cannot be directly converted to other forms of tetrahydro folate (THF), the **folate is trapped in N_5 methyl form**, which accumulates. The level of other form decreases l/t **functional folate deficiency** (*needed for purine & TMP synthesis*). Decreased DNA synthesis disturbs erythropoiesis, causing immature precursor of RBC to be released in circulation l/t **megaloblastic / pernicious anemia.**

- **Subacute combined degeneration (SACD) & Demyelination**
  - D/t methionine deficiency in CNS, there is irreversible degeneration of spinal cord, as a result of failure of methylation of one arginine residue on myelin basic protein. Therefore inadequate methylation of phosphotidyl ethanolamine to phosphatidyl choline l/t deficient formation of myelin sheath of nerves and demyelination.

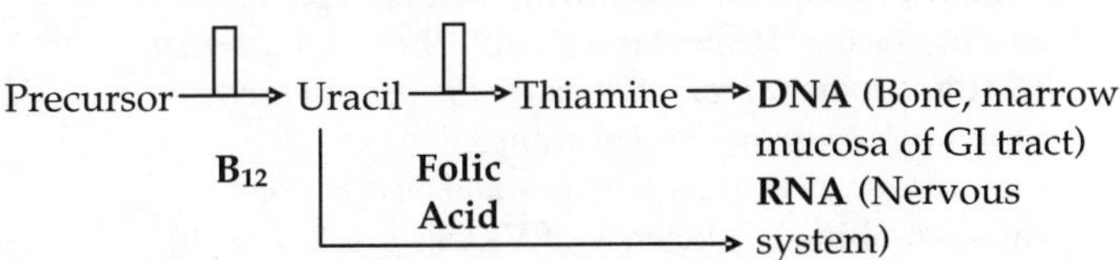

  - **Nieweg's hypothesis** explain why only B_{12} def. is a/w neurological lesions whereas, both B12 and folic acid deficiency cause megaloblastic anemia. This occurs because folate is only concerned with DNA synthesis, whereas B_{12} is required for both DNA & RNA synthesis.
- ***Both B_{12} & folate correct megaloblastic anemia by increasing DNA synthesis***Q. Only folate supplements may put some people at risk as this would rectify (correct) megaloblastic anemia but may hasten development of irreversible nerve damage.
- Schilling **(radioactive lebelled Cobalt-60) test is done to assess B12 deficiency.**

68. **B i.e. Vitamin C** *[Ref: Harrison 16/e p- 406-07, 2469]*

- **Vitamin C** is a *water soluble vitamin*, which is ***mainly excreted in urine***Q. Its intake above *100 mg/day* results in saturation of its metabolic capacity and excretion into urine. So large doses (1 gm TDS/81p) are used to acidify urine in preventing and treating UTI as some drugs act better in acidic urine.
- **Vitamin A, D, E, K** are fat soluble and so excreted mainly in bile and very minimally in urine.

69. **D i.e. Pyridoxal phosphate** 70. **A i.e. Vitamin C** 71. **B i.e. Ascorbic acid** 72. **A i.e. Hydroxyproline**

- **Collagen** most abundant protein of mammalian tissue, contains- *Glycine & Proline*
- Hydroxyproline: is formed by the post translational hydroxylation of proline by *prolyl hydroxylase.*
- There is ***no t-RNA capable of accepting hydroxyproline or hydroxylysine***Q and inserting them into an elongating polypeptide chain. Thus preformed hydroxyproline & hydroxylysine of ingested food proteins are not incorporated into collagen

Hydroxylation of Proline Require

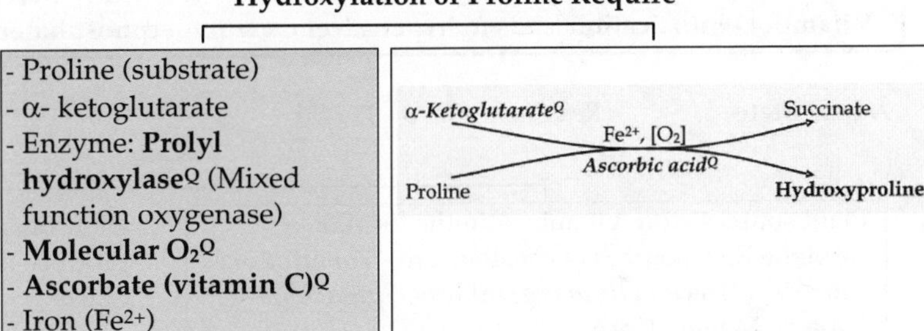

73. **A i.e. Vitamin K** 74. **B i.e. Both help in post translational modification** 75. **A i.e. Lysine**
[Ref: Harper's 28/e P-472-473, 479-80; Lippincott's 5/e p. 377-78, 389-90; Vasudevan 6/e p. 407-10; Devlin 5/e p. 1146]

- **Both vitamin C and vitamin K are required for post translational modification**Q.
- **Vitamin C** is required for **post translational modification of proline & lysine in collagen synthesis**Q.
- **Vit K** is required for **post translational modification of glutamate residue for generation of clotting factors**Q.

76. **A i.e. Glutamate** 77. **C i.e. Glutamate** 78. **C i.e. K** 79. **D i.e. Vitamin K**
80. **B i.e. Carboxylation** 81. **D i.e. Vitamin K**

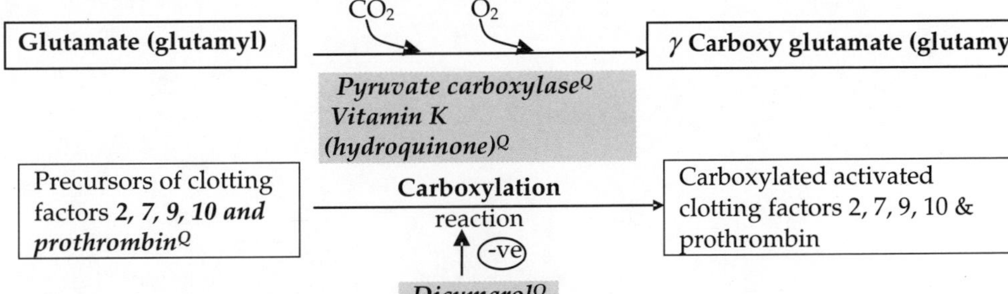

Vit K function as a *coenzyme for carboxylase*Q enzyme responsible **for post translational modification of blood clotting factors** II, VII, IX, X and prothrombin. These proteins are initially synthesized as inactive precursors containing glutamyl residues. ***Vit K activates these clotting factors by carboxylation of their glutamic acid residues***Q. Carboxylated glutamyl residues on activated clotting factors confer them the capacity to bind Ca^{++} and phospholipid surface.

82. B i.e. IX and X *[Ref: Ganong 23/e 535]*

- **Vitamin K dependent clotting factors (VKCF)** are clotting factors **II *(prothrombin)*, VII *(Proconvertin)*, IX *(Christmas factor)*, X *(Stuart Prover Factor)*, protein C, protein S and protein Z**^Q^.
- *Liver diseases, Warfarin over dose and mlabsorption* cause combined deficiency of VKCFs (i.e. 2, 7, 9, 10, C, S & Z) and leads to bleeding.
- Two types of autosomal recessive (AR) disorder i.e. VKCF deficiency 1 (VKCFD1) is a/w point mutation in *gamma-glutamyl carboxylase gene* (GGCX) and VKCF deficiency 2 (VKCFD-2) is a/w point mutation in *vitamin K epoxide reductase gene* (VKOR).

83. A i.e. Factor VII

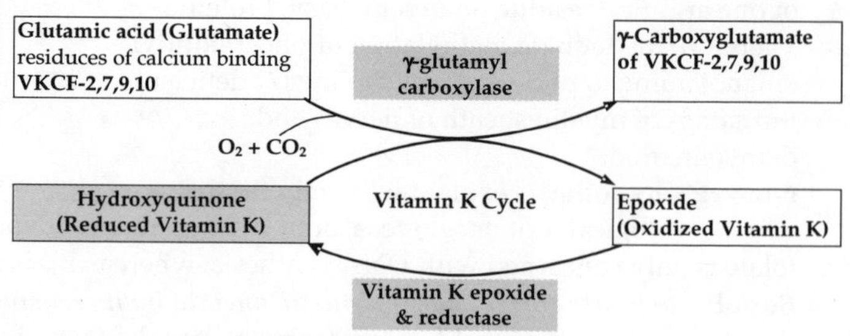

84. B i.e. Retinal

85. C i.e. Liver

86. A i.e. Retinol, Retinal, and Retinoic acid

87. A i.e. Lysosome *[Ref: O.P. Ghai 6/e p. 121; Harrison 16/e p. 408]*

Vitamin D intoxication leads to rupture of lysosomal membrane^Q^.

88. A i.e. A; D i.e. D *[Ref: Harper's 27/e P-492-94]*

Vitamin –A intoxication leads to **demineralization of bone, hypercalcemia, hyperostosis**^Q^.
Vitamin D intoxication leads to **hypercalcemia & hyperphosphatemia**^Q^

89. A i.e. Potato *[Ref: Chatterjea 6/e P-145]*

Diet

Plant sources store vitamin A in the form of carotene Rich sources of carotene are - ***Tomatoes***^Q^, ***Carrots***^Q^, ***Green yellow vegetables***^Q^, ***Spinach***^Q^, Papaya, Mango, Corn	Diet consisting of following will produce deficiency of vitamin A - Maize, Wheat, Rice, ***Tubers (Potatoes)***^Q^

BIOCHEMISTRY

Review Notes with High Yield Text

Chapter 1. CARBOHYDRATE METABOLISM: REVIEW NOTES

Energy Production per Molecule of Glucose

Common in both aerobic & anaerobic conditions

- **Steps at which energy is utilized** (ATP consumption)

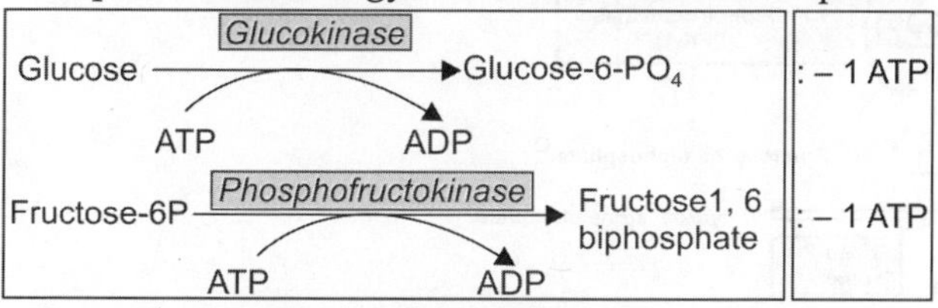

- **Steps where energy (ATP) is produced**

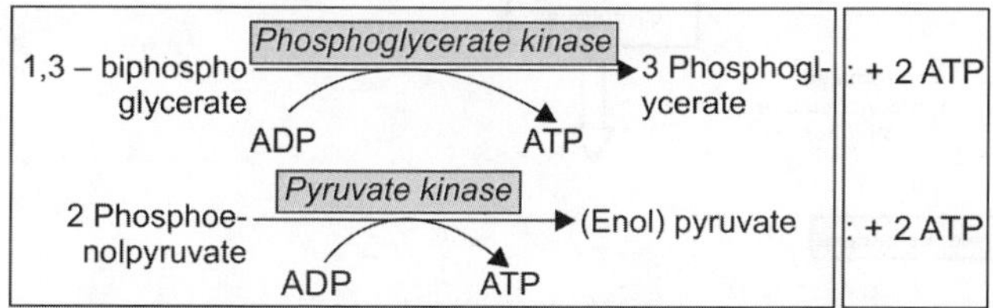

Net ATP produced in anaerobic condition=4-2=*2ATP*[Q]

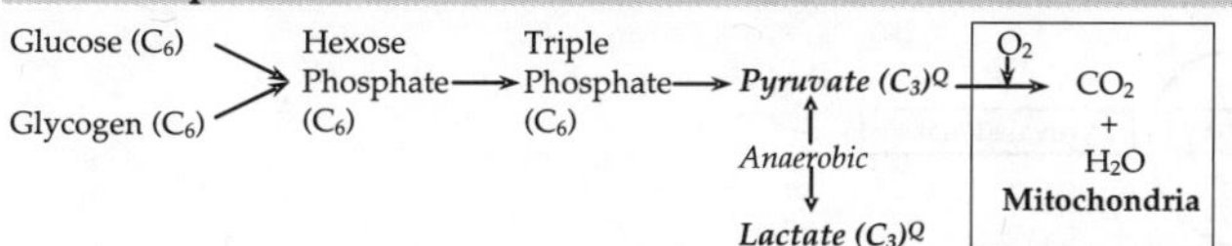

Reaction occurring in aerobic conditions only

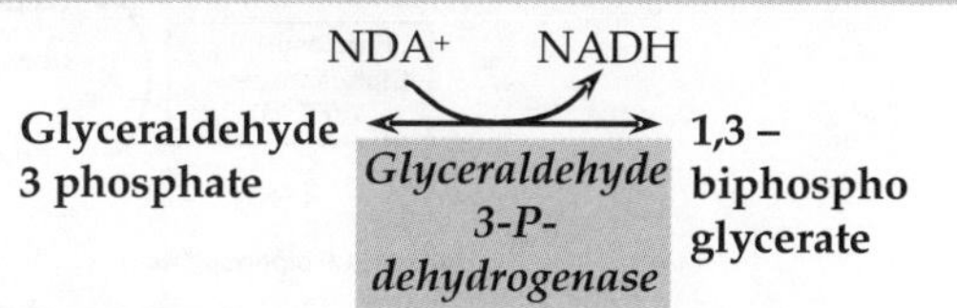

- In absence of oxygen, reoxidation of NADH at glyceraldehyde –3P – dehydrogenase stage cannot take place in electron transport chain.
- ATP gained from 1NADH according to old concept is 3ATP but according to new concept it is **1.5** or **2.5** depending on shuttle. So for 2NADH, 5 ATP will be produced (or 6 a/t old concept)
- Because **1 glucose molecule** yields **2 molecules of glyceraldehydes 3-phosphate**, the overall production of NADH per molecule of glucose is 2
- So for **2 NADH; 5ATP** will be produced (or 6 a/t old concept)
- Hence the net ATP gain in glycolysis in **Aerobic conditions** is 5 (from NADH) + 4 -2 = **7 ATP** (a/t new concept) / 6 (from NADH) + 4-2 = **8 ATP** (a/t old concept)

Embden-Meyerhof Pathway of Glycolysis ☆

Glycolysis is the cytosolic pathway of all mammalion cells for the ***metabolism of glucose (or glycogen) to pyruvate and lactate***[Q].

- In glycolysis glucose (C_6) is ***converted into 3C units substances; pyruvate (C_3) and lactate (C_3)***[Q].
- All the enzymes of glycolysis are present in ***cytosol***[Q].

Aerobic Condition	Anaerobic Condition
Under aerobic condition final product is ***pyruvate***[Q]	- ***Lactate***[Q] is a final product - Erythrocytes, which lacks mitochondria (O_2 supply) completely reliant on glucose as their metabolic fuel.

- This is ***not a complete breakdown***[Q] of glucose as *pyruvate further enters mitochondria* to completely degraded into CO_2 and H_2O.
- It is unique in the sense that it can function either aerobically or anaerobically.

- **Fructose – 2, 6 Biphosphate** is *not a part of glycolytic* pathways *but is formed during glycolysis.*
- When the body has abundant supply of glucose:
  Fructose 2,6 biphosphate is formed *from fructose –6 PO_4 by* the action of *phosphofructokinase –2 (PFK-2).*
- If Glucose supply is not adequate:
  Fructose 2, 6 biphosphate is converted back to Fructose – 6- PO_4 by PFK –2 which now acts as fructose – 2, 6 biphosphotase
- Phosphofructokinase –2 is a bifunctional enzyme.
- Fructose 2, 6 biphosphate has a ***unique role to play in the regulation of Glycolysis and Gluconeogenesis***[Q].
- ***Positive allosteric effector of phosphofructokinase –1***[Q] (rate limiting enzyme of glycolysis)
- ***Inhibitor of Fructose 1, 6 Biphosphatase***[Q] (enzyme of Gluconeogenesis)
- At each of 3 points where glycolytic reactions are bypassed by alternative gluconegenic reactions, simultaneous operation of both pathways would consume ATP without accomplishing any chemical or biological work, ie ATP is hydrolysed and large amount of chemical energy is dissipated as heat without any useful metabolic work being done. Therefore these uneconomical bypass processes are called **futile cycle**. However, **substrate cycle** is a better name because these provide *advantages for controlling pathways*.

That means

↑ed Fructose 2, 6 – Biphosphate → **↑ Glycolysis, ↓ Gluconeogenesis**

↓ed Fructose 2, 6- Biphosphate → **↓ Glycolysis, ↑Gluconeogenesis**

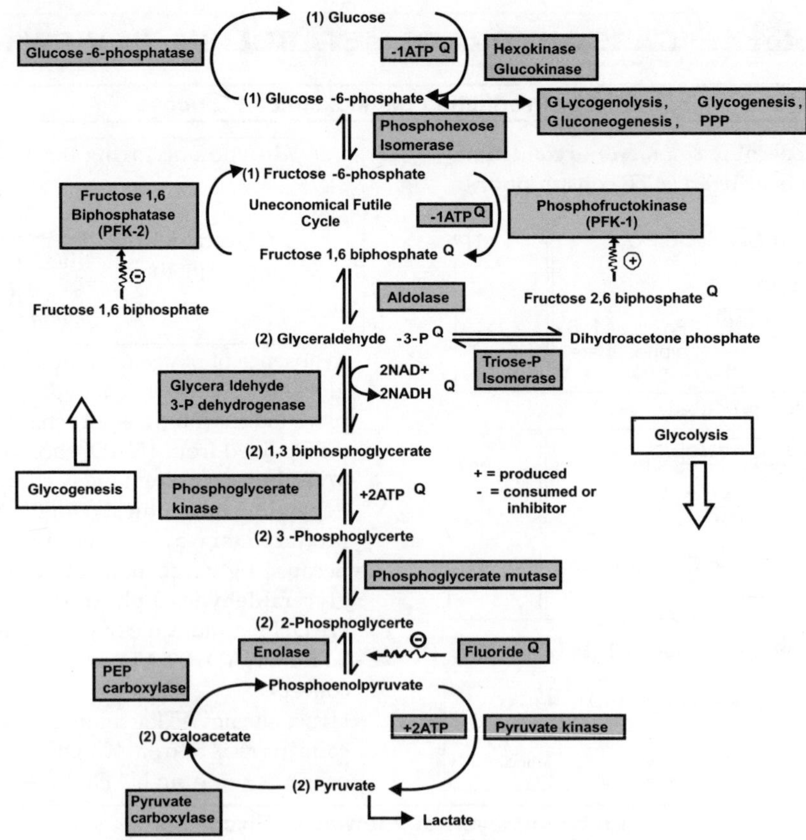

Opposing pathways of Glycolysis & Gluconeogenesis

Oxidase – Peroxidase Test Strips

It is new highly specific method for estimating glucose in blood & urine. **Glucose oxidase** enzyme produce hydrogen **peroxide** & gluconic acid from glucose. And peroxidase catalyzes the reaction of H_2O_2 with colourlesspotassium iodide to brown iodide. This produces a colour change, the intensity of which may indicate glucose concentration in some tests (such as Boehringer, Diastix). **Horseradish peroxidase** (HRP) are used for histochemistry & ELISA because of their excellent stability, low molecular weight and its ability to produce chromogenic products (such as peroxidase labelled antibodies).

$$\textbf{Glucose} + H_2O + O_2 \xrightarrow{\textbf{Oxidase}^Q} \mathbf{H_2O_2} + \text{Gluconic acid } (\delta\text{-gluconolactone})$$

*Peroxidase*Q ↓ ← KI

Brown Iodide

Inhibitors of Metabolic Pathway

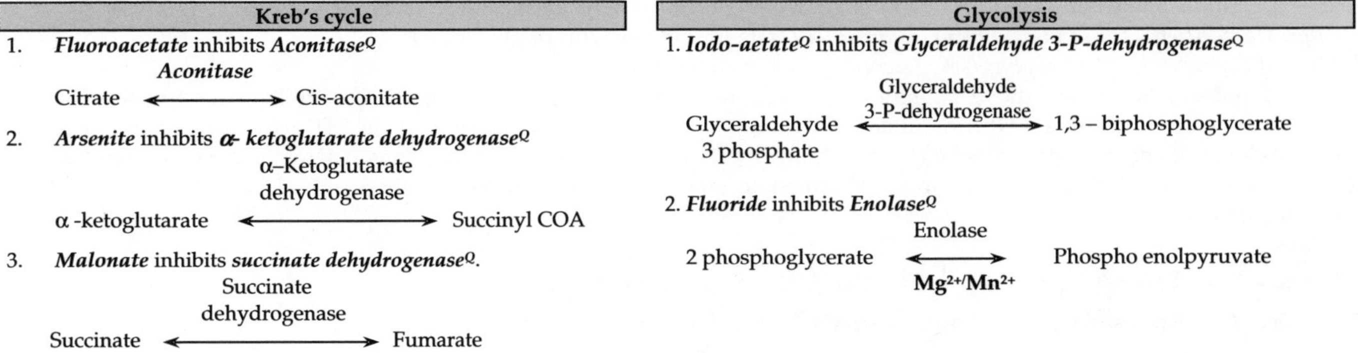

Kreb's cycle

1. *Fluoroacetate* inhibits *Aconitase*Q

   Citrate ←*Aconitase*→ Cis-aconitate

2. *Arsenite* inhibits ***α- ketoglutarate dehydrogenase***Q

   α -ketoglutarate ←α–Ketoglutarate dehydrogenase→ Succinyl COA

3. *Malonate* inhibits ***succinate dehydrogenase***Q.

   Succinate ←Succinate dehydrogenase→ Fumarate

Glycolysis

1. *Iodo-aetate*Q inhibits ***Glyceraldehyde 3-P-dehydrogenase***Q

   Glyceraldehyde 3 phosphate ←Glyceraldehyde 3-P-dehydrogenase→ 1,3 – biphosphoglycerate

2. *Fluoride* inhibits ***Enolase***Q

   2 phosphoglycerate ←Enolase / **Mg^{2+}/Mn^{2+}**→ Phospho enolpyruvate

Enzyme (Genes) and Pathways regulated by Insulin

Increased Expression

In Glycolysis
- ***Hexokinase II***[Q]
- ***Hexokinase IV (i.e. glucokinase)***[Q]
- Phosphofructokinase (PFK-1)
- Pyruvate kinase

In regulation of glycolysis/ gluconeogenesis
- PFK-2 / FBP ase-2

In Pentose phosphate pathway (NADPH)
- Glucose-6-phosphate deydrogenase
- 6- phosphogluconate dehydrogenase

In Fatty acid desaturation
- Stearoyl CoA deydrogenase

In Triacyl glycerol synthesis
- Acyl-CoA- glycerol transferase

In Fatty acid synthesis
- Pyruvate dehydrogenase
- Acetyl CoA carboxylase
- Malic enzyme (NADPH)
- ATP citrate lyase (provides acetyl CoA)
- Fatty acid synthase complex

Decreased Expression

PEP carboxykinase	Gluconeogenesis
Glucose-6-phosphatase	Glucose release to blood

Hexokinase and Glucokinase

- **Hexokinase**, which *catalyzes the entery of glucose into glycolytic* pathway (by converting glucose to glucose 6 PO_4), is a *regulatory enzyme*. Humans have 4 isoenzymes (I to IV)
- Predominant isoenzyme type of **myocyte (muscle)** is **hexokinase II > I**. It has low Km and high affinity fo glucose. It normaly acts at or near its maximal rates (because Km=0.1 is much lower than blood glucose conc. 4-5 mM) and is allosterically inhibited by their product glucose 6 – phosphate
- Predominant hexokinase isoenzyme of **liver** is **hexokinase IV (glucokinase)** which differs from hexokinase I-III of muscle in 3 respects

1. **Km** or **glucose concentration at which glucokinase is half saturated (10 mM) is higher** than usual concentration of glucose in blood. Because an efficient glucose trasporter **(GLUT-2)** rapidly equilibrates glucose concentration in cytoplasm (of liver cell) & blood, the high km of glucokinase allows its direct regulation by blood glucose level.

High blood glucose level
(After carbohydrate rich meal)

Excess glucose transported into hepatocytes & converted to glucose – 6 PO_4 by glucokinase. Because it is only half saturated at 10 mM glucose, its activity continues to rise as glucose concentration rises to >10 mM
So its ***main function is to clear glucose from blood at levels > 100 mg/dl***[Q].

Low blood glucose level
(after fasting)

Glucose concentration in hepatocyte is low due to its *low affinity* (high km) and the glucose generated by gluconeogenesis leaves the cell before being trapped by phosphorylation.
So it ***makes glucose available to tissue at lower blood glucose levels***[Q].

Features	Hexokinase (I-III)	Glucokinase (Hexokinase IV)
Found in	*All tissues including fetal & adult liver*	***Adult liver only***[Q]
Km **Affinity** (for glucose)	***Low (0.1 mm)***[Q] **High**	***High (10 mM)***[Q] **Low**
Stability	More	Less (labile)
phosphorylate	Any hexose (non specific)	Glucose (specific)
Allosteric inhibition	***Glucose – 6-*** PO_4[Q]	***Fructose-6-phasphate***[Q]
Glucose feeding	No change	Increased
Fasting /DM	Not much change	Decreased
GH, Glucocortico-steroids	Inhibit	Inhibit
Insulin	Induce	Induce
Function	Make glucose available to tissues for oxidation at lower blood glucose level	Clear glucose from blood after meals (leves > 100 mg/dl)

2. ***Glucokinase is not inhibited by glucose-6 –*** PO_4[Q] and it can therefore continue to operate when the accumulation of glucose – 6- PO_4 completely inhibits hexokinase I- III.
3. Glucokinase is inhibited by reversible binding of **regulatory protein** specific to liver (and more tightly in presence of **allosteric effector fructose -6- phosphate)**. Glucose competes with fructose 6-PO_4 for binding & cause dissociation of regulatory protein from hexokinase (in nucleus), relieving the inhibition. Whereas during fast, (glucose <5 mM), fructose 6-PO_4 triggers inhibition of glucokinase by regulatory protein, so liver does not complete with other organs for scarce glucose

★ Glucose enter into cells by *GLUT – 2* in the liver *under control of insulin*. GLUT –2 has higher km value for glucose hence transport glucose only when blood sugar is high.

★ **GLUT-4** Work *in muscle* cells and *adipocytes*.

Shuttle System

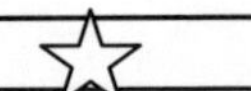

Mitochondrial (inner) membrane is impermeable to NADH. The NADH generated in **glycolysis** are transported from cytoplasm to mitochondria for oxidation by shuttles (mainly matale)

Malate shuttle

- This is more common and universal shuttle used mainly in liver, kidney & heart
- *Oxidation of reduced* ***NADH + H+*** in mitochondria *yields* ***3 ATPQ (old)/ 2.5 ATP (new)***
- When body utilized malate shuttle, net ATP production by glycolysis – TCA cycle per glucose molecule oxidized will be ***38 ATPQ*****/32 ATP** (new).
- The complexity of this system is d/t impermeability of mitochondrial membrane to O.AA, which must react with glutamate & transaminate to aspartate and α - ketoglutarate before transport through mitochondrial membrane & reconstitution to O.A.A in cytosol.

Glycerophosphate shuttle

- This is present in some tissue (*e.g. brain, white skeletal muscle*) and absent in others (e.g. Heart muscle)
- ***FADQ*** dependent so *only* ***2 ATPQ*** *(old)*/**1.5 ATP** (new) are produced.
- When body utilizes this system, net ATP production is ***36 ATPQ*** (old)/**30 ATP** (new.)

Malate shuttle
Mitochondrial membrane
Cytosol
Mitochondrion
NAD⁺
Malate
Malate
NAD⁺
Malate dehydrogenses
Malate dehydrogenses
NADH + H⁺
O.A.A.
O.A.A.
NADH + H⁺
Glutamate
Glutamate
Transaminase
Transaminase
α-Keto glutarate
Aspartate
Aspartate
α-Keto glutarate
Respiratory chain

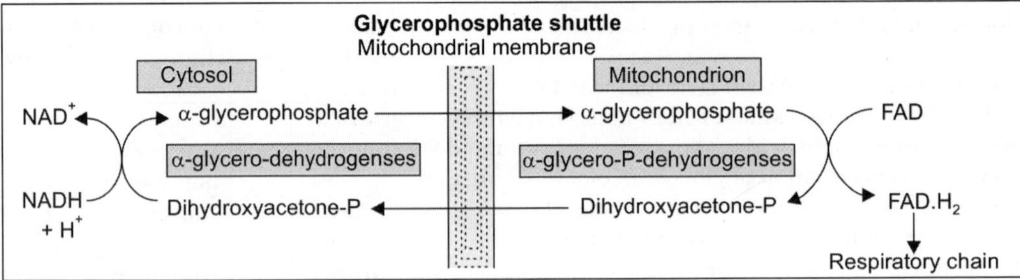

Fate of Pyruvate

- *7 reversible reactions* of glycolysis are used in synthesis of glucose from lactate to pyruvate (i.e. gluconeogenesis). But the *3 irreversible reactions* must be circumvented by 4 alternate reactions that enegetically favour the synthesis of glucose. And these reactions are unique to gluconeogenesis. **The first road block in synthesis of glucose from pyruvate (gluconeogenesis)** ***is irreversible conversion of PEP to pyruvate by pyruvate kinase in glycolysisQ***. In gluconeogenesis, pyruvate is first carboxylated by pyruvate carboxylase to OAA, which is then converted to PEP by PEP – carboxykinase.
- Conversion of phosphoenol pyruvate(PEP) to pyruvate is one of the three irreversible step (barrier) in simple reversible glycolysis. So this conversion is achieved by 2 enzymes.

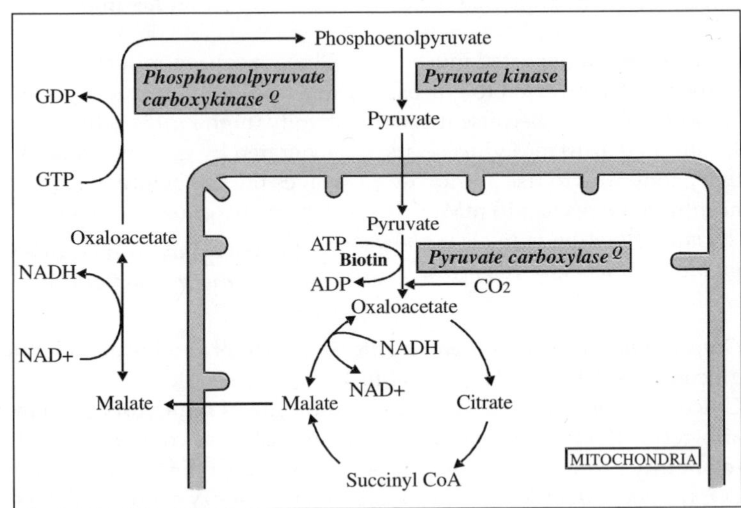

- **Pyruvate carboxylase:** Pyruvate has to be first converted to oxaloacetate in mitochondria.
- **Phosphoenol pyruvate carboxykinase:** OAA is then converted to phosphoenolpyruvate in cytosol

Fate of Pyruvate (End product of glycolysis)

Oxidative decarboxylation by *pyruvate dehydrogenase complex*, in tissues with *high oxidative capacity* such as cardiac muscle, irreversibly converts pyruvate to **acetyl CoA** (a **major fuel of TCA cycle and a building block** *for fatty acid synthesis*)

Carboxylation by *biotin dependent pyruvate carboxylase* converts pyruvate to ***oxaloacetate*** **(OAA)**. This replenishes the citric acid cycle intermediates and provides substrate for gluconeogenesis.

Anaerobic glycolysis occurs in tissue which are poorly vascularized/or lack mitochondria such as *exercising muscle, cornea & lens of eye, kidney medulla, testes, leucocytes & RBC.* **Lactate** formed by action of *lactate dehydrogenase* is the final product.

Transamination by *alanine amino transferase (ALT/SGPT)* converts pyruvate to ***alanine***[Q]

Arsenic (As) poisoning

Arsenite (trivalent As) inhibits (dehydrogenases) enzymes **that require lipoic acid co-enzyme** (primary mechanism)

- **E_2 of pyruvate dehydrogenase (PDH) complex**[Q]
- **α-ketoglutarate dehydrogenase**[Q]
- **Branched chain α- ketoacid dehydrogenase**[Q]

Arsenate (Pentavalent As) *competing with inorganic phosphate as a substrate* (also occurs)

- Arsenate competing as a substrate for **glyceraldehydes -3- phosphate dehydrogenase**, forms a complex that spontaneously hydrolyzes to form 3-phosphoglycerate. By bypassing the synthesis of 1, 3-BPG and phosphate transfer from it, the cell is usually deprived of energy usually obtained from glycolysis. So it inhibits net ATP & NADH production without inhibiting the pathway itself.
- As also replaces phosphate on F1 domain of ATP synthase resulting in formation of ADP- arsenate that is rapidly hydrolyzed.

Citric Acid Cycle/Krebb's Cycle 

Citric acid cycle is a series of reaction in ***mitochondria***[Q] that *oxidize acetyl CO-A* and reduce coenzyme that upon reoxidation are linked to the formation of ATP.

Mn = "C, Cis, I, O, α, S², F, M, O"

- ❖ In bracket carbon content of each compound is written
- ❖ Release of CO_2 l/t decrease in one carbon atom
- ❖ Two irreversible steps of TCA are
  - *Oxaloacetate → citrate*
  - *α-ketoglutarate → succinyl CoA*
- ❖ ⊖—— indicates inhibitors of TCA

★ New concept
1NADH = 2.5 ATP
1 $FADH_2$ = 1.5 ATP

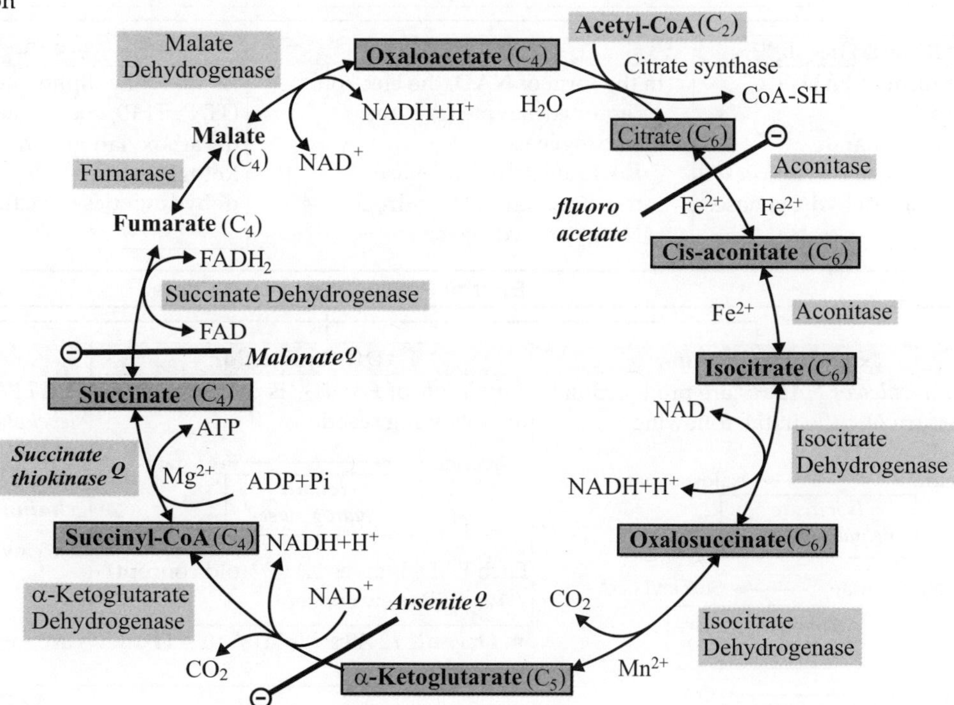

Inhibitors of TCA (Citric Acid /Kreb's) Cycle

- **Aconitase** which isomerizes citrate to isocitrate, is *non competitively inhibited* by a ***rat poison fluoroacetate***[Q]. **Fluoroacetate (with acetyl CoA)** is converted to **fluoroacetyl CoA**, which ***condenses with oxaloacetate to form***[Q] **fluoro-citrate** – a potent *non competitive inhibitor of aconitase* – resulting in **citrate accumulation.**
- **Alpha ketoglutarate dehydrogenase** enzyme (which converts *α-ketoglutarate to succinyl CoA by oxidative decarboxylation) is non-competitively inhibited* by **arsenite (trivalent arsenic)** causing the substrate alpha ketoglutarate to accumulate. Arsenite forms a stable complex *with thiol group of lipoic acid* making it unavailable to serve as a coenzyme.
- *Oxidation of succinate to fumarate* by **succinate dehydrogenase** is competitively inhibited by **malonate**. Succinate dehydrogenase is the only enzyme of TCA cycle that is embedded in inner mitochondrial membrane and so also functions as **complex II of electron transport chain.**
- **Hyperammonemia** (↑NH_3) usually due to urea cycle defect inhibits TCA cycle by ***depleting α-ketoglutarate***[Q].

Inhibitor of TCA cycle	Enzyme	Inhibition Type
Fluoroacetate (Rat poison)	*Aconitase*[Q]	**Non-competitive**
Arsenite (Trivalent Arsenic)	**Alpha-ketoglutarate dehydrogenase**	Non-competitive
Malonate	*Succinate dehydrogenase*[Q]	Competitive
Ammonia Intoxication	***By depleting Alpha-ketoglutarate***[Q]	

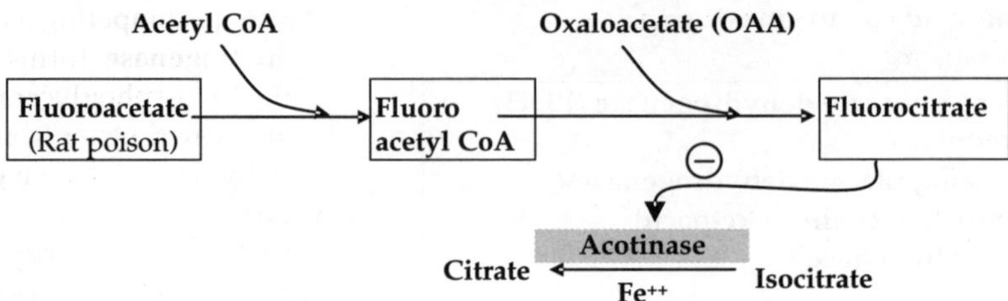

4-B Complex Vitamins are Essential in the TCA (Citric Acid) Cycle

Riboflavin[Q] **(B_2)**
In the form of **FAD**, a cofactor in
- α- ketoglutarate dehydrogenase complex
- succinate dehydrogenase.

Niacin
In the form of **NAD**, the electron acceptor coenzyme for three dehydrogenase
- Isocitrate dehydrogenase
- α- ketoglutarate dehydrogenase
- Malate dehydrogenase

Thiamine[Q] **(B_1)**
As thiamine diphosphate (TDP/TPP), coenzyme for decarboxylation in **α-ketoglutarate dehydrogenase** reaction.

Pentothenic acid
As part of **coenzyme A**, the cofactor attached to active carboxylic acid residue such as acetyl CoA & succinyl CoA.

Energy Production in TCA Cycle ☆

NADH Production

- ***3 molecules of NADH***[Q] are produced in one turn of cycle in the following reaction
  - Isocitrate ⟷ Oxalosuccinate (*Isocitrate dehydrogenase*[Q])
  - α- ketoglutarate ⟶ Succinyl CoA (***α- ketoglutarate dehydrogenase***[Q])
  - Malate ⟷ OAA (*Malate Dehydrogenase*[Q])
- Each NADH gives **3 ATP** (old concept) / **2.5 ATP** (new concept). So NADH oxidation in one TCA cycle provides ***9ATP***[Q] (old) / **7.5 ATP** (new).

$FADH_2$ Production

1 molecule of FADH$_2$[Q] is produced in the following reaction
- Succinate ⟷ Fumarate (*succinate dehydrogenase*[Q])

Each $FADH_2$ gives *2ATP*[Q] (old concept) / **1.5 ATP** (new concept)

ATP / GTP synthesis

1 GTP/ATP[Q] is produced by *substrate level phosphorylation* [It is production of ATP 'at the substrate level' without ***the participation of electron transport chain.]***[Q]

Succinyl CoA ⟷ Succinate (*Succinate thiokinase*[Q])

★ ***Over all 12 ATP***[Q] (old) / **10 ATP** (new) are formed **per turn of the citric acid cycle.**

Substrate	ATP Production	
	New value	Old value
NADH	2.5	3
FADH	1.5	2
Glucose	32	38
Acetyl CoA	10	12
Palmitate	106	129

Regulation of Citric Acid Cycle by

Availability of ADP[Q]	Supply of NAD+[Q]	Regulation of selective enzyme activity
- ↑ADP → Stimulates TCA cycle - ↑ATP/ ↓ADP→ cycle depressed	- ↑NAD^+ → Stimulates cycle - ↑NADH →Inhibits cycle	- Citrate synthase - ***Isocitrate dehydrogenase***[Q] - α- ketoglutarate dehydrogenase complex

- In addition to above

Succinate dehydrogenase is inhibited by OAA, and availabiy of OAA depends on *malate dehydrogenase* which is controlled by NADH / NAD^+ ratio.

Involvement of the Citric Acid Cycle in Transamination and Gluconeogensis

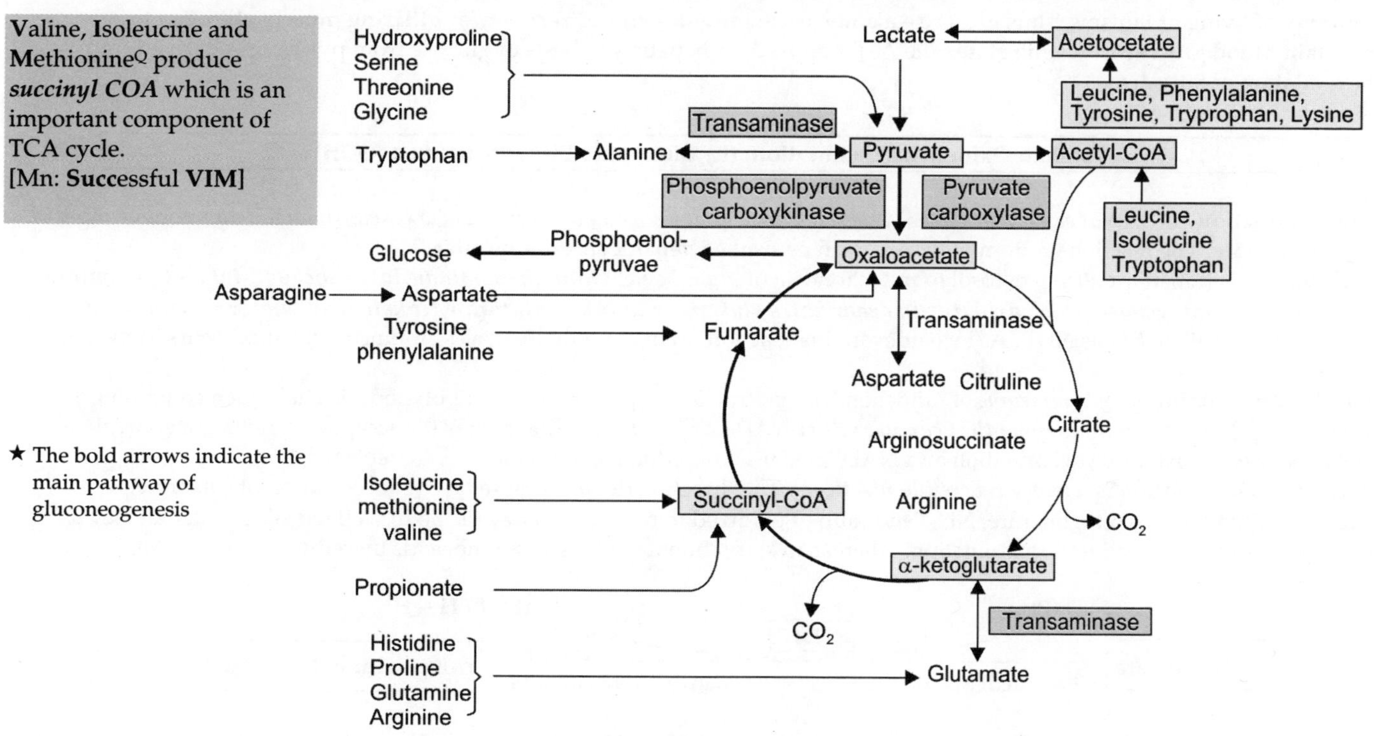

Glucose – Alanine Cycle

- **Alanine transportes toxic ammonia (amino group) from skeleton muscles to liver** via a pathway called glucose – alanine cycle.
- It is important to remember that **resting muscles use fatty acids** as its major fuel source. Whereas **exercising muscles initially use glycogen stores** (by anaerobic glycolysis & convert it to lactate / pyruvate) **and then use free fatty acids** provided by mobilization of TAG from adipose tissue (when glycogen reserves are depleted) so these aminoacids are not directly utilized as fuel source by muscles.
- During first few days of fasting, there is ***rapid breakdown of muscle protein, providing aminoacids (alanine & glutamine mainly) that are used by liver for gluconeognesis***[Q]. *Because muscles do not have glucagon receptors, muscle proteolysis is initiated by fall in insulin and is sustained by the rise in glucocorticoids.* Alanine & glutamine are produced by catabolism of branched chain aminoacids. By ***several weeks of fasting, rate of muscle proteolysis decreases paralleling a decline in the need for glucose as a fuel for the brain which has started using ketone bodies as a source of energy***[Q].
- In tissues that degrade aminoacid for fuel (mainly skeletal muscle), amino group is collected in form of L-glutamate (d/t transamination)

- This **glutamate** (containing toxic α-amino group) can be transported to liver by converting it to glutamine or it can transfer its α-amino group to **pyruvate**, a easily available product of muscle glycolysis by the action of **alanine aminotransferase (ALT/SGPT)**. The **alanine** so formed passes into blood to liver.
- In liver cell cytosol **alanine aminotransferase (ALT/SGPT)** transfers amino group from alanine to α-ketoglutarate forming pyruvate (which enters gluconeogenesis) and glutamate (under go oxidative deamination)
- Vigrously contracting muscles operate anerobically producing pyruvate & lactate (from glycolysis) and NH_3 (from aa break down). **Alanine-glucose cycle** in concert with Cori cycle send these products to liver where pyruvate & lactate are incorporated into glucose (by gluconeogenesis and returned back to muscle) and NH_3 is converted to urea for excretion. So the **energetic burden of gluconeogenesis is imposed on liver and all available ATP in muscle is devoted to muscle contraction.**
- In the fasting state, the **output of alanine from skeleton muscle is in far excess of its concentration in the muscle proteins that are being catabolized**. Because it is **also formed by transamination of pyruvate produced by glycolysis of muscle glycogen**. Alanine is exported to the liver, where it is transaminated ***back to pyruvate, which serves as a substrate for gluconeogenesis***[Q]. **The use of alanine to transport ammonia from skeleton muscles to liver is an example of intrinsic economy** of living organisms. Thus glucose – alanine cycle **provides an indirect way of utilizing muscle glycogen to maintain blood glucose in fasting state**. The ATP required for hepatic synthesis of glucose from pyruvate is derived from the oxidation of fatty acids.

Reversible Oxidative Deamination: (L) Glutamate Dehydrogenase (GDH)

- **Transamination** (1st step in catabolism of aa) *transfers amino group of many α-amino acids to α-keto glutarate*, thus converting it to **L-glutamate**. The reaction predominatly occurs in **cytosol of hepatocytes (liver cells)**.
- L glutamate is transported from cytosol to mitochondria of hepatocyte. ***Only (predominantly) mitochondrial matrix contain glutamate dehydrogenase which oxidatively deaminates glutamate to α-ketoglutarate (α-keto acid) and free amonia***[Q] (α-amino group is liberated as NH_3). A/t vasudevan this reaction occurs in only liver; a/t Lippincott 252 this occurs in liver & kidney.
- GDH, a **Zn containing** *metalloenzyme* of mitochondrial matrix, is a tetramer (i.e. has 4 polypeptide chain each containing 1 Zn molecule). It is the ***only enzyme that can use either NAD+ or NADP+ as coenzyme***[Q] (or acceptor of reducing equivalent). NAD^+ is used in oxidative deamination and NADPH is used in reductive amination (i.e. reverse reaction).
- ***Oxidative deamination is a freely reversible reaction***[Q]. The direction depends on relative concentration of substrate, product (glutamate, α-ketoglutarate, NH_3) and ratio of oxidized to reduced coenzyme. So in well fed state glutamate levels are high resulting in oxidative deamination, whereas in starvation it synthesize amino acids by reductive amination.

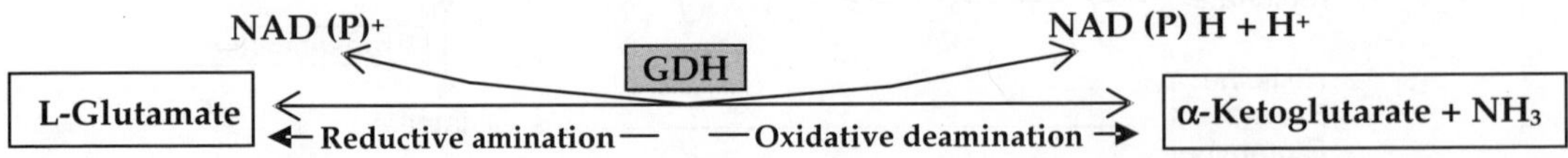

- **Liver GDH** is ***allosterically activated by ADP and inhbited by ATP, GTP and NADH***[Q]. Thus when energy levels are low in cell, amino acids are catabolized by GDH for energy production. Mutations that alter GTP binding site cause permanent activation of GDH, & result in hyper insulinism-hyper-ammonia syndrome characterized by ↑NH3 and ↓glucose in blood.
- **Trans deamination** is sequential action of *transamination f/b oxidative deamination*, and provide a pathway where by the amino groups of most amino acids can be released as NH3. *Transamination takes place in cytoplasm of all cells of body (mainly liver, kidney, muscle, heart etc)* and form glutamate. Toxic glutamate is transported to liver as non-toxic glutamine (most tissue) and alanine (from muscles), and finally oxidatively deaminated in mitochondria of liver (mainly).
- Minor pathways of deamination are L/D/Mono-amino oxidase; dehydrase, desulfhydrase and histidase (non oxidative) etc.

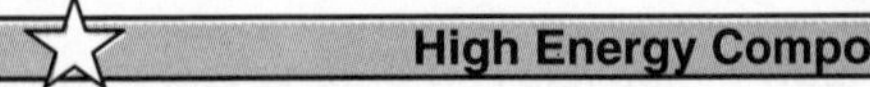

These compounds release **at least 7 Kcal /mol (i.e. > 7 K cal/mol or > 25 KJ/mol)** on hydrolysis; they have large Δ G° (free energy of hydrolysis) from *7-15 Kcal/mol*. The high energy bond is indicated by a *squiggle bond (~)*. These include

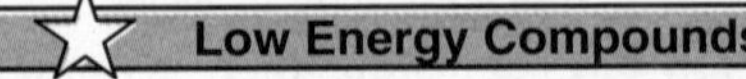

These liberate **< 7 Kcal/mol** on hydrolysis at pH7 (i.e. lower than energy liberated by hydrolysis of ATP to ADP + Pi)

High Energy Compounds	Δ G° (Kcal/ mol)	Energy release (KJ/mol)
• **Phosphate Compounds**		
1. Pyrophosphates: Nucleotides like **ATP, GTP, UTP, UDP-glucose**		
- ATP → ADP + Pi	7.3	30.5
- ATP → AMP + PPi	10.7	45.6
2. Phosphagens: like **Creatine phosphate (CP) or phosphocreatine**	10.5º	43.1
3. Acyl phosphates: like **1, 3-Biphosphoglycerate (BPG)**	10.1	49.4
4. Enol phosphates like **phosphoenol pyruvate (PEP)**	14.8	61.9
5. **Carbamoyl phosphate**	12.3	51.4
6. **Amino acyl adenylate (amino acyl AMP/cycline AMP)**	12.0	50.0
7. **Acetyl phosphate**	10.3	
8. **Arginine phosphate**	10.0	
9. **Inorganic pyrophosphate**	8.0	
• **Sulfur Compounds**		
10. Sulfonium compounds like **S- adenosyl methionine (SAM)**	8.0	
11. Thioester **CoA derivatives like Acetyl CoA, Succinyl CoA, Fatty acyl CoA, HMG CoA**	7.7	
12. **Adenosine phosphosulfate** (active sulfate)		

These include

Low Energy Compounds	Δ G° (Kcal/mol)
1. **ADP** – AMP + Pi	6.5
2. **Glucose 1 phosphate**	5.0
3. **Fructose 6 phosphate**	4.0
4. **Glucose 6 phosphate**	3.5
5. **Glycerol 3 phosphate**	2.2

★ All valuses of Δ G° and energy released are negative (-)

Redox Potential (Eo) & Electron Transport Chain (ETC)

- Mitociondrial ETC consists of a series of sequentially acting electron carriers, accepting & donating either 1 or 2 electrons. Free energy is released as electrons are transferred from an **electron donor (reducing agent / reductant)** to an **electron acceptor (oxidizing agent / oxidant)**. 3 types of electron transfer occur and term reducing equivalent is used to designate a *single electron equivalent* in any form.
  - Direct transfer of **electrons (e-) to cytochromes** for reduction of **Fe3+ to Fe^{2+}**
  - Transfer as a **hydrogen atom, ($H^+ + e^- = \bullet H$)** to **FMN, FAD** and **coenzyme Q (Ubiquinone)**
  - Transfer as **hydride ion (:H^-)** bearing 2 electrons to **NAD^+**
- Oxidation (loss of e^-) of one substance is always accompanied by reduction (gain of e^-) of another substance. For example oxidation of NADH to NAD^+ is accompanied by (a/b) reduction of FMN to $FMNH_2$. So oxidation – reduction reactions are sum of 2 separate half reactions one an oxidation & other a reduction reaction. Thus NAD^+ /$NADH_2$ form a **redox pair** and FMN /$FMNH_2$ forms other.
- **Standard recuction potential / Redox potential (E°)** in *volts*, is a *quantitative measurement of the tendency of a redox pair (couple) to donate or accept electron under standard potential*. The pairs are ordered from most negative to most positive E° i.e. is in increasing order of E°. **More negative** the E°, the greater is the tendency of reductant member of that pair to **lose electron. More positive** the greater is the tendency of oxidant member of that pair to **accept electron**. *So electron flow spontaneously from lower to higher (i.e. more negative to more positive) redox potential.*
- The change in free energy (Δ G°) is directly related to Δ E° (i.e. E° of electron accepting pair – E° of electron donating pair). The standard free energy required for phosphorylation of ADP to ATP is + **7.3 Kcal/mol.**

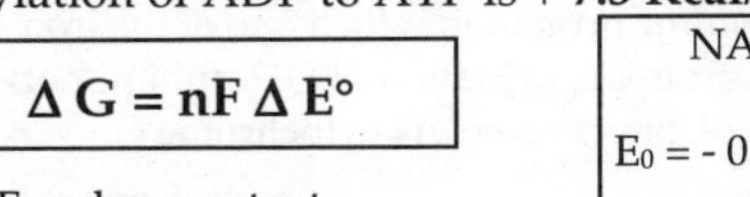

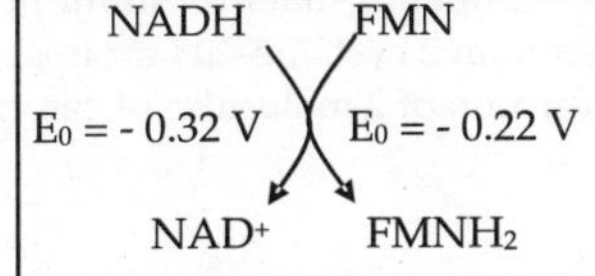

F = Faraday constant (23.1 K Cal/Volt-mol)
n = Numbers of e- transferred (1 for cytochrome, 2 for NADH, $FADH_2$ and CoenzymeQ)

Redox Pair		Redox potential (E° volts)
Ferredoxin (Fe^{+3} /Fe^{+2})		- 0.432
$2H^+/H_2$ (at pH7)		- 0.414
α-Ketoglutarate /Isocitrate		- 0.38
Acetoacetate /β Hydroxy butyrate		- 0.35
NADP+ / NADPH		- 0.324
NAD+ / NADH		- 0.320
Lipoate (ox /red)		- 0.29
Glutathione (ox /red)		- 0.23
FAD / $FADH_2$		- 0.22
Pyruvate / Lactate		- 0.19
Oxaloacetate / Malate		- 0.17
$2H^+$ / H_2 (at PH0)		0
Fumarate / Succinate		+ 0.03
Ubiquinone / Ubiquinol		+ 0.045
Fe^{3+} / Fe^{2+} in Cytochromes	b	+ 0.077
	C_1	+ 0.22
	C	+ 0.254
	a	+ 0.29
	a_3	+ 0.35
Fe^{+3} / Fe^+		+ 0.771
O_2 / H_2O		1+ 0.82

Transport of a pair of e- from NADH (complex I) to O_2 via ETC produces 52.58 Kcal and so produce 3 ATPs from 3 ADP & 3 Pi (3 x 7.3 = 21.9 K Cal/mol) per O atom reduced. Hence **P:O ratio** is **3:1** for NADH (and 2:1 for $FADH_2$ because complex I is bypassed). The remaining energy is used in anciliary reactions or released as heat. But now recent studies have shown that 2.5 ATP is produced per **0.5** mol (1/2 O_2) = per atom of O from NADH (P:O ratio = **2.5:1**). And $FADH_2$ generate 1.5 ATP (P:O ratio = 1.5:1)

Electron Transport Chain (ETC)/Respiratory Chain

- Energy rich molecules like glucose are ultimately metabolized to CO_2 and water. The metabolic intermediates of these oxidation reactions donate electrons to NAD /FAD to form energy rich coenzymes **NADH/FADH₂.**
- These energy rich reduced coenzymes, in turn, donate electrons to *a specialized series of electron carriers / donors arranged a/t redox potential (E°)* – collectively called ETC.
- ETC is present in **inner mitochondrial membrane** & is the final common pathway in aerobic cells by which electrons obtained from different fuels of body flow to oxygen. This requirement of O_2 makes the ETC the **respiratory chain**, which accounts for the greatest portion of body's use for oxygen.
- Electrons flow through the ETC through a redox span of **1.1 volts** from NAD^+ / NADH to O_2 /H_2O
- The components of respiratory chain contain 4 large protein complexes (initial 2 are flavoproteins & last 2 are cytochromes) and 2 mobile electron carriers – coenzyme Q & cytochrome C.
- The chain reaction of e- transport starts with formation of NADH (by various **substrate dehydrogenases** removing hydrogen atom as in TCA cycle – isocitrate / α-ketoglutarate / malate - dehydrogenase). Transfer of hydride ion (:H^-, bearing 2 electrons) and a free proton (H^+) to NAD^+ l/t formation of NADH (having 2 e^-) plus a free proton (H^+). ETC consists of

Component of ETC	**Prosthetic Group/Electron flow**	**Features**
Complex I: NADH dehydrogenase/ NADH-Ubiquinone (CoQ) oxidoreductase / NADH-CoQ reductase	**FMN**, non heme iron sulfur proteins **(FeS)** NADH→FMN ↓ Fes ↓ CoQ	- It is a large L shaped 42 subunit protein which accepts $2e^-$ & 1 H^+ from NADH and transfer it to CoQ - **12 Kcal/mol** of released energy is utilized to pump **4 protons (H^+)**Q out of mitochondria into inter membranous space.
Complex II: Succinate dehydrogenase /Succinate –Q-Reductase	**FAD, FeS** Succinate→FAD ↓ Fes ↓ CoQ	- It is a small 4 subunit protein which accepts e- from succinate & transfer it to CoQ. - It is **not a proton pump** as energy liberated is not enough to pump protons. - It also contain **heme b** that is not in direct path of e^- transfer but serve to **reduce** the frequency with which **e^- leak out of system**, moving from succinate to molecular O_2 to produce reactive oxygen species
Coenzyme Q (CoQ)/Ubiquinone/Q		- This **only nonprotein** member of ETC is a *lipid soluble benzoquinone with long hydrophobic isoprenoid tail (side chain).* - It is called ubiquinone as it is *ubiquitous (present everywhere) quinone derivative. Menaquinone (of bacteria) & plastoquinine (of chloroplast)* have analogous roles - It can accept 1 or 2 electrons to become semiquinone or ubiquinol respectively. So it can act at the junction of 2e- donor & 1e- acceptor (Q cycle). - Because it is small & hydrophobic, Q is a **mobile carrier** freely diffusible within the lipid bilayer of inner mitochondrial membrane and can shuttle b/w other less mobile e- carriers. - It has a central role in coupling e- flow to proton (H+) movment as it carries both e- & H+. - **For transferring to complex III it accepts hydrogen atom (e- & H+) from.** 1. $FMNH_2$ produced in **complex I** (from FMN) 2. $FADH_2$ produced in **complex II** 3. $FADH_2$ produced in β-oxidation by **acyl CoA dehydrogenase** (through **ETF-ubiquinone- oxidoreductase**) and by **glycerol 3 phosphate dehydrogenase**. These bypass complex II & I.
Complex III: Cytochrome bC₁ complex /Ubiquinone cytochrome C oxido-reductase / Cytochrome reductase	Fe-S, **Heme** group (a porphyrin ring & iron, which is reversibly converted from Fe^{3+} to Fe^{2+} form) Q →Cyt **b** ↓ Cyt **C₁** ↓ CytC	- It transfers electron from CoQ to cytochrome C. – 10 Kcal/mol of released energy is utilized to **pump 4 protons**Q out of mitochondria into inter membranous space. - **Q cycle** couples e- & H+ transport in complex III & involves **cytochrome b_1, b_H (b562, b566), cytochrome C_1 and Rieske Fe – S** (an unusual iron sulfur protein in which one of the iron atom is linked to 2 histidine –SH rather than 2 cysteine- SH groups) , oxidation of QH_2 (ubiquinol) to Q (ubiquinone) is coupled to reduction of 2 molecules of cytochrome via cytochrome C

Cytochrome c	- Soluble carrier protein of intermembrane space - After its single heme group accepts an electron from complex III, cytochrome c moves to complex IV to donate electron to a binuclear copper centre	
Comple IV Cytochrome c oxidase / cytochrome oxidase	2 Heme groups (of cyt a, a_3), **2 copper ions** of Cu_A, Cu_B **Cyt C→ CuA ↓ Cyta ↓ Cyt a3 ↓ CuB ↓ O_2**	- It transfer electrons from cytochrome C to the final acceptor O_2 converting (reducing) it to water (H_2O). - O_2 remains tightly bound to complex IV (a_3) until it is fully reduced to H_2O, this minimizes the release of ROS. - It pumps **2 proton (H+)** out into inter membrane space for every pair of electron passing down the chain by complex IV

Oxidative Phosphorylation

- As electrons (e^-) are transported down the ETC, they *lose* much of *their free energy*. Some part of this energy is **captured & stored as ATP** (from ADP + Pi) in a process called **oxidative phosphorylation.** The remainder (not trapped as ATP) energy is used for ancilliary reactions like *Ca^{+2} transport into mitochondria & to generate heat.*
- Electron transfer down the ETC is energetically favoured because NADH is a strong electron (e^-) donor and O_2 an avid acceptor.
- **Mitchelle- chemiosmotic hypothesis** of proton pump & ATP synthase
- It states that ETC is responsible for ATP production b/o electro-pH gradient produced d/t associated proton pumping (i.e. proton pump is a link b/w ETC and oxidative phosphorylation).
- As we know, electron transport through **complex I, III and IV** also transports (pumps) **4, 4 and 2 protons (H+)** respectively across inner mitochondrial membrane from matrix to inter membrane space.
- This associated proton transport creates **an electrical gradient** (*outside is positive* relative to inside) of 0.15-0.20V; and a **pH gradient** (*outside pH is lower* than inside d/t more H+ ion concentration) of 0.75 -1.4. This generates a proton motive force (PMF) of 0.224V corresponding to a free energy change of 5.2 Kcal/mol of protons.
- The energy generated by proton gradient is enough to synthesize ATP by **ATP synthase (complex V).** So the proton gradient is a link that couples oxidation (ETC) to phosphorylation (ATP synthesis)
- **Complex V: ATP synthase** (also k/a **F_1/F_0 ATPase** because it can also catalyze hydrolysis of ATP to ADP + Pi) has F_0 and F_1 subunits. **F_o unit** spans inner mitochondrial membrane and serves as **proton channel,** whereas **F1 unit phosphorylates ADP to ATP.**
- Protons that have been pumped out to inter membrane space, creating electrical and pH gradient, they **reenter** the **mitochondrial matrix by passing through a proton channel in F_o domain of ATP synthase (complex V).**
- This re-entery of protons *rotates F_0 unit thus producing conformational changes in extra membranous F_1 domain,* and at the same time, dissipating the pH and electrical gradients. The conformational changes of F_1 unit allow phosphorylation of ADP + Pi to ATP, and release ATP.
- **Paul Boyer's Binding Change mechanism** of **rotational catalysis**
- It states that ATP synthesis by proton gradient is comparable to a *'water driven hammer minting coin'*. F_0 is wheel, flow of proton is water fall, and structural changes in F_1 l/t ATP coin being minted for each turn of wheel.
- 3 Beta (catalytic sites) sub units of F1 has 3 conformational states

1. **L state** binds to substrate & product with with loose affinity
2. **T state** binds substrate tightly & catalyzes ATP synthesis
3. **O state** is open and does not bind to substrate or product; i.e. release product (ATP)

- For complete rotation of F_1 unit through 3 states **10 protons** are translocated. As the ATP is released, the original conformation of enzyme (F_1) is assumed
- So the energy is actually required for producing conformational change (not for ATP synthesis). And the energy surplus produced by proton gradient is stored as chemical energy ATP.

Mitchell's Chemi-Osmotic Theory

Mitchell's chemiosmotic theoryQ postulates that energy from oxidation of respiratory chain components is coupled to the translocation of hydrogen ions (proton, H^+) from the inside to outside of inner mitochondria membrane Respiratory chain ***complexes I, III & IV***Q acts as a **proton pump**. Inner mitochondrial membrane is impermeable to ions in general but particularly to protons which accumulates outside the membrane creating **a electro- chemical potential difference** ($\Delta\mu H^+$)
The $\Delta\mu H^+$ is used to drive a membrane located **ATP synthase** which functions as a *rotary motor to form ATP.*

F_0 Subunit complex	F_1 Subunit complex
- A *membrane protein* complex which forms ***proton channel***Q - It is a *disk of "C" protein* subunit - Attached to it is ***"bent axle"*** formed by ***Y-subunit & ε- subunit***Q - Protons passing through the disk of "C" units cause it & attached Y- unit to rotate - Uncoupling agent dinitrophenol allow leakage of H^+ across the membrane, thus collapsing the electrochemical proton gradient. *Oligomycin specifically blocks conduction of H^+ through F_0 subunit*	- Composed of 9 polypeptide chains (3α, 3β, 1γ, 1 σ & 1ε) project into *matrix* and contain *phosphorylation mechanism* - ***3 α & 3- β subunits, which are fixed to the membrane and do not rotate***Q - The Y- subunit fits inside F_1 sub complex - *ADP & Pi are taken up sequentially by the β subunits to form ATP,* which is expelled as the rotating Y subunite squeeze each β subunit in turn. Thus ***3 ATP molecules are generated per rotation***Q.

★ **Ionophores** are lipophilic molecules that complex specific cations & facilitate their transport eg *valinomycin (K^+), dinitrophenol.*

★ **Familial infantile mitochondrial myopathy & renal dysfunctions** involves severe diminution or absence of most oxido reductases of the respiratory chain. **MELAS** (**m**itochondiral **e**ncephalopathy **l**actic **a**cidosis & **s**troke) is caused by mutation in mitochondrial DNA & is d/t NADH: ubiquinone oxidoreductase (complex I) or cytochrome oxidase deficiency. It may be involved in *Alzheimer is disease & diabetes mellitus.*

Transporter System in Inner Mitochondrial Membrane

Although the outer membrane is freely permeable to most ion & small molecules, the inner mitochondrial membrane is **impermeable to most small ions** like H^+, Na^+, K^+; and **small molecules** such as ADP, ATP, Pyruvate and other metabolites important to mitochondrial function. The relative impermeability of inner mitochondrial membrane necessitates exchange transporters

Inner mitochondrial membrane is freely permeable to unchanged small molecules such as,

- O_2 - H_2O
- CO_2 - NH_3
- Monocarboxylic acids such as 3-OH-butyric acid, acetoacetic & acetic

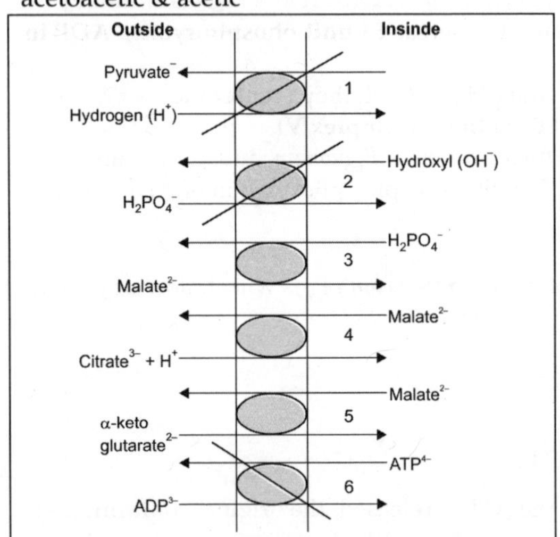

★ **N- ethyl- Maleimide, hydroxycinnamate** and **atractyloside** inhibit *pyruvate symport, phosphate transporter and adenine nucleotide transporter*

★ Transporters are named on the name of product they take inside mitochondria

Transporters	Exchange / Transport
1. **Pyruvate symport**	Transport pyruvate & hydrogen ions in same direction (inwards)
2. **Phosphate transporter**	Exchange phosphate for hydroxyl ions
3. **Dicarboxylate transporter**	Exchange dicarboxylate (malate 2-) ions for phosphate
4. **Tricarboxylate transporter**	Exchange tricarboxylate (citrate) for malate
5. **α-ketoglutarate transporter**	Exchange alpha ketoglutrate for malate
6. **Adenine Nucleotide transporter**	Exchange ADP for ATP
7. **Glutamate-Aspartate transporter**	Glutamate is converted to aspartate and aspartate is exchanged for H^+ ion

Transporters are required for

- *Long chain fatty acids* require carnitine system
- *Pyruvate*
- Dicarboxylate & tricarboxylate anions and aminoacids
- ***ADP enter & ATP exit***Q
- *NADH* is transported by **malate and glycerophosphate shuttle**
- ***NADPH***Q
- Mitochondria accumulate cations such as K^+, Na^+, Ca^{2+} and Mg^{2+} & *Pi*
- **Creatine phosphate shuttle** bring outside the ATP generated in mitochondria
- Alpha-ketoglutarate transporter and glutamate/aspartate transporter are used in **malate shuttle** for transfer of reducing equivalents from cytosol into mitochondria.
- Transporter for glutamine, ornithine, neutral amino acids and carnitite (**carnitine acyl carnitine translocase**).

Poisons Inhibiting the Respiratory Chain 

1. Inhibitors of Electron Transport Chain (ETC)

- ETC inhibitors, **prevent the passage (transport) of electrons** by binding to a specific component of chain, thus blocking the **oxidation-reduction reaction**. So all electron carriers located before the block are fully reduced, whereas those located *after the block are oxidized*.
- Inhibition of ETC *blocks ATP synthesis* as both processes are tightly coupled. And *reactive oxygen species (ROS)* like superoxide (O_2^{-}•), hydroxyl radicals (OH•) and hydrogen peroxide (H_2O_2) are produced d/t incomplete reduction of O_2 to H_2O. ROS can damage DNA, proteins & cause lipid peroxidation.

Site of action	Inhibitor (Poison)	Mechanism
Complex I: NADH-CoQ reductase (or NADH dehydrogenase complex)	- **Amobarbital** (amytal) & **seco barbitals** = Barbiturates - **Rotenone** (fish poison & insecticide) - Myxothiozole	Blocks e- transfer through complex I (i.e. from Fe S to CoQ / *ubi quinone*)
	- **Piericidin A** (antibiotic)	Blocks e- transfer by ***competing with CoQ***
	- Chlorpromazine (tranquilizer) - Guanethidine (a hypotensive alkyl guanide)	
Complex II: Succinate –CoQ Reductase (Succinate dehydrogenase)	- ***Malonate***[Q]	Competitive inhibitor of complex II inhibiting e- transfer from succinate to FAD
	- Carboxin - TTFA	Inhibit e- transfer from Fe S to CoQ (through complex II)
Complex III: CoQ – Cyt C reductase (Cytochrome reductase)	- **Antimycin A** - **BAL** (British anti lewisite or **Dimercaprol**), antidote of war gas - Napthoquinone - Phenformin (hypoglycemic drug)	Inhibits transfer of e- from cyt b to C_1.
Complex IV: Cytochrome oxidase (Cyt c oxidase)	- **Carbon monoxide (CO)**[Q]	Capture O_2 binding site
	- **Cyanide (CN-)** - **Hydrogen sulfide (H_2S)** - **Azide (N_3^-)**	**Inhibit terminal e⁻ transfer from a_3 to molecular O_2 (arrest respiration)**[Q]

★DCMU (Dichlorophenyl dimethyl urea) competes with Q B for binding site in PS II

2. Inhibitors of Oxidative Phosphorylation (ATP synthesis)

- **Oligomycin** (antibiotic) - **Venturicidin**	- **Atractyloside** (glycoside) - **Bongregate** (pseudomonads toxin)	**Ionophores**
- **Binds to Fo domain of ATP synthase, closing the proton (H+) channel, blocking reentry of protons** through ATP synthase into mitochondrial matrix - This l/t *accumulation of H+ at higher concentration in inter membrane space.* Because the pH & electrical gradient cannot be dissipated, e- transport stops b/o difficulty of pumping any more protons against steep proton gradient. - Inhibition of phosphorylation inhibits e- transport - So Oligomycin completely blocks oxidation & phosphoryla-tion by blocking the flow of protons through ATP synthase and prevents stimulation of O_2 uptake by ADP & phosphorylation of ADP to ATP	- **Blocks adenine nucleotide transporter (translocases)** responsible for ***movement of ADP into & ATP out of the mitocho-ndria***[Q] ***across the inner mitochondrial membrane***[Q] - It ***Inhibits ATP-ADP exchange***[Q]. - Adequate supply of ADP is blocked thus preventing phosphorylation and ATP formation.	- Ionophores are lipid soluble compounds that increase the permeability if lipid bilayer to certain ions. - These are of 2 types 1. **Valinomycin** (mobile ion carrier) 2. **Gramicidin** (channel formers) - Valinomycin allow K+ to permeate mitochondria and dissipate proton (H⁺) gradient.

Oligomycin & venturicidin inhibits F_o & CF_o ; **DCCD** (dicyclohexyl carbodimide) blocks proton flow through F_o & CF_o; and **aurovertin** inhibits F1 domain of **ATP synthase (complex V)**

3. Uncouplers of Oxidative Phosphorylation

- Uncouplers *uncouple oxidation (electron transport chain) from phosphorylation*. This dissociation of oxidation from phosphorylation will allow oxidation to proceed, but the energy instead of being trapped into ATP by phosphorylation is dissipaled as heat.
- Uncouplers create a **proton leak removing proton gradient** i.e. allowing protons to re-enter mitochondrial matrix without capturing any energy as ATP. The energy is released as heat and the process is called **non-shivering thermogenesis.**
- Uncouplers are (mostly) *toxic in vivo*, causing respiration to become uncontrolled, since the *rate is no longer limited by concentration of ADP or Pi*. These allow mitochondria to use O_2 regardless of whether or not there is any ADP or Pi available.
- Uncouplers (eg DNP) are amphipathic & *increase permeability of lipoid inner mitochondrial membrane to protons, thus reducing electro- chemical potential & short circuiting ATP- synthase.* In this way oxidation can proceed without phosphorylation (i.e., without ATP synthesis). So energy is lost as heat (**chemiosmotic theory**). So these are toxic in vivo. Examples are

Natural/Physiological Uncouplers	Synthetic Uncouplers
- **Uncoupling proteins (UCP)** occur in *inner mitochondrial membrane (of mammals* including humans) *adipocytes*. **Thermogenin (UCP-1)** is responsible for non shivering thermogenesis (heat production) in **brown fat** to maintain body heat, in response to cold in *neonates* and during arousal in *hibernating animals*. UCP-1 is activated by *fatty acids* and brown fat (unlike white fat) uses almost 90% of its respiratory enrgy for thermogenesis. UCP-2 and 3 are also found in humans but their importance remains unclear. - **Long chain fatty acids (FA)** in brown fat - Essential fatty acid (EFA) deficiency - Excess of **thyroxine hormone** - Unconjugated *hyperbilirubinaemia*	- **2, 4 Dinitrophenol★** (2,4-DNP) - **2, 4 Dinitrocresol★** (2,4-DNC) - **CCCP★** (Chloro carbonyl cyanide phenyl hydrazone; the most active uncoupler) - **FCCP★** (tri fluora carbonyl cyanide phenyl hydrazone) - **Dicoumarol** (vitamin K analogue, anti coagulant) - **Aspirin** & other salicylates in high doses; this is the reason of fever d/t toxic overdose - ***Valinomycin*** (produced by streptomyces; **a K^+ ionophore**, transport K^+ from cytosol to matrix & H^+ viceversa thus decreasing proton gradient) - **Calcium** (Ca^{++} transport into mitochondria is coupled with uptakes of Pi and oxidative phosphorylation. But the energy produced is spent to pump the Ca^{++} into mitochondria. So e^- transport proceeds but no energy is stored as ATP) ★ Are hydrophobic proton carriers

Mechanism of Apoptosis

Extrinsic (death- receptor- initiated) pathway

- **Death receptors** are members of **TNF** (tumor necrosis factor esp *TNF1*) family that contain a **cytoplasmic death domain** involved in protein-protein interaction. The pathway is initiated by engagement of cell surface death receptor.
- When **Fas** binds to its ligand FasL (a death receptor) their cytoplasmic death domain binds with **FADD (Fas associated death domain)**, which in turn binds an inactive form of ***caspase – 8 (& in humans caspase- 10)***.
- Multiple procaspase 8 molecules cleave one another to generate active caspase –8. This pathway can be inhibited by **FLIP**.

Intrinsic (mitochondrial) pathway

- Growth factors & survival signals stimulate antiapoptotic. **Bcl – 2 protein** (named after B cell lymphoma & is homologous to C. elegans protein C ed 9)
- **Antiapoptotic Bcl- 2 & Bcl- x** proteins normally reside in mitochondria & cytoplasm
- When cells are deprived of survival signals or subjected to stress Bcl – 2 / Bcl-x are lost from mitochondrial membranes & replaced by **pro-apoptotic Bak, Bax**, and **Bim**. So the permeability of mitochondrial membrane increases and **cytochrome C** & **AIF** leaks out.
- Cytochrome C binds to **Apaf-1 (apoptosis activating factor 1**, homologous to Ced 4 of c. elegans) and complex activates **caspase – 9**
- **Apoptosis inducing factor (AIF)** enter cytosol & bind to various inhibitors of apoptosis.

Glycogen Phosphorylase and Glycogenolysis

- Mobilization of stored glycogen is caused **by glycogen phosphorylase**, which degrades *glycogen to glucose 1 phosphate*. It is often referred to simply as **phosphorylase** – so honoured because it was the first phosphorylase to be discovered. It was the first enzyme shown to be allosterically regulated & controlled by reversible phosphorylation and for which detailed 3 dimensional structures of active & inactive forms were revealed by x-ray crystallography.
- Phosphorylase exists in 2 inter convertible forms: **phosphorylase a** which is catalytically active, and **phosphorylase b** which is less active (or inactive). This conversion from inactive to active phosphorylase is done by active phosphorylase kinase b or **phosphorylase kinase a**, an enzyme responsible for transferring a phosphoryl group to ser residues in each of the 2 identical subunits of glycogen phosphorylase.
- **Epinephrine & nor epinephrine (in muscle** during activity) or **glucagon** (in **liver** when blood glucose level is too low) *increase concentration* of **C-AMP**, which inturn activates **C- AMP dependent protein kinase (protein kinase A, or PKA).** PKA then **phosphorylates & activates phosphorylase b kinase (to phosphorylase kinase a)**, which catalyzes phosphorylation and activation of serine residues of **glycogen phosphorylae** , and thus stimulating glycogen breakdown. In muscle this provides fuel for glycolysis to sustain muscle contraction whereas in liver it counters the low blood glucose levels.
- Both phosphorylase and phosphorylase kinase (a) are dephosphorylated and inactivated by **phosphorylase α phosphatase or phosphoprotein phosphatase 1** (PP1). In resting muscles. Protein **inhibitor 1**, when activated after phosphorylation by cAMP dependent protein kinase,inhibit PP1. In liver insulin increases activity of **phosphodiesterase** (which hydrolyze C-AMP) and indirectly stimulate PP1 resulting in decreased glycogenolysis.
- In liver, cAMP independent glycogenolysis occurs in response to α_1 adrenergic stimulation by epinephrine or norepinephrine. This involves stimulation of **Ca^{++} / calmodulin sensitive phosphorylase kinase** by Ca++. It is also activated by **vasopressin, oxytocin, & angiotensin II**Q acting either through Ca^{++} or PIP2
- **Ca^{++} ion is responsible for intiation & synchronization of both muscle contraction and glycogenolysis (or activation of phosphorylase)**Q. Muscle phosphorylase kinase (c activates phosphorylase) is a tetramer of α, β, γ, and δ subunits.
  - **α**, and **β**, subunits contain serine residue that are activated by cAMP dependent protein kinase.
  - **δ** subunit is identical to Ca++ binding protein calmodulin & binds 4 Ca^{++}
  - **γ catalytic subunit** is activated (by δ- calcium binding) even while the enzyme is in dephosphorylated state b; the fully activated & phsphorylated a form occurs in high concentrations of calcium.

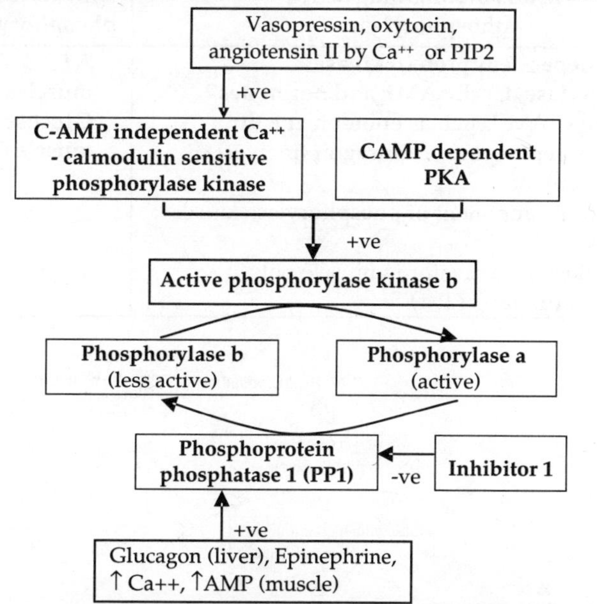

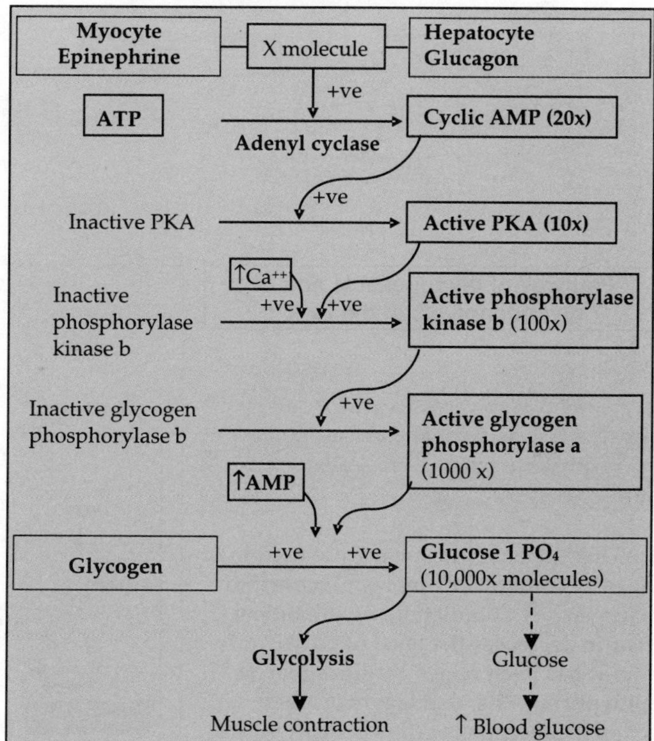

- **Allosteric control** of phosphorylase occurs through

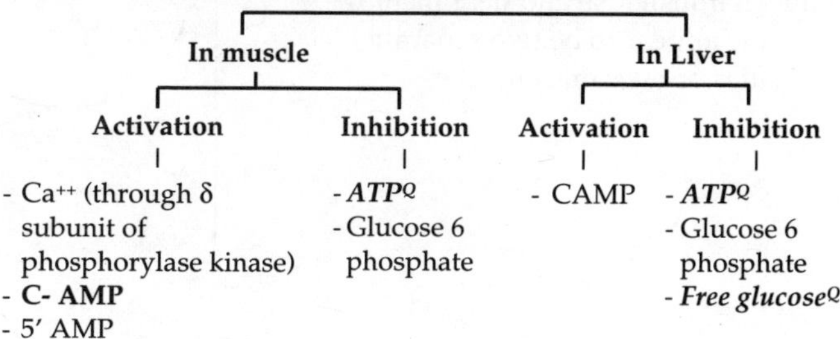

Factors maintaining active phosphorylase	Allosteric Inhibitors of glycogen phosphorylase (inactivating it)	Factors maintaining inactive phosphorylase
- **C- AMP dependent protein kinase**Q - **Adenyl cyclase, Cyclic AMP and hormones**Q increasing C-AMP.such as **epinephrine (in muscle)**, norepinephrine, **glucagon** (in liver) & thyroid hormone - Calmodulin component of phosphorylase kinase - **Calcium**Q - **5AMP** (allosteric activator in muscle only) - **Inhibitor-1** (inhibits PP-1)	- **ATP & Glucose 6 phosphate (in muscles & liver both)**Q - **Glucose (in liver but not in muscles)** Q	- **Protein phosphatase 1**Q (PP-1) - **Glucose 6 phosphate**Q - **Insulin**Q - Phosphodiesterase (hydrolyze cAMP)

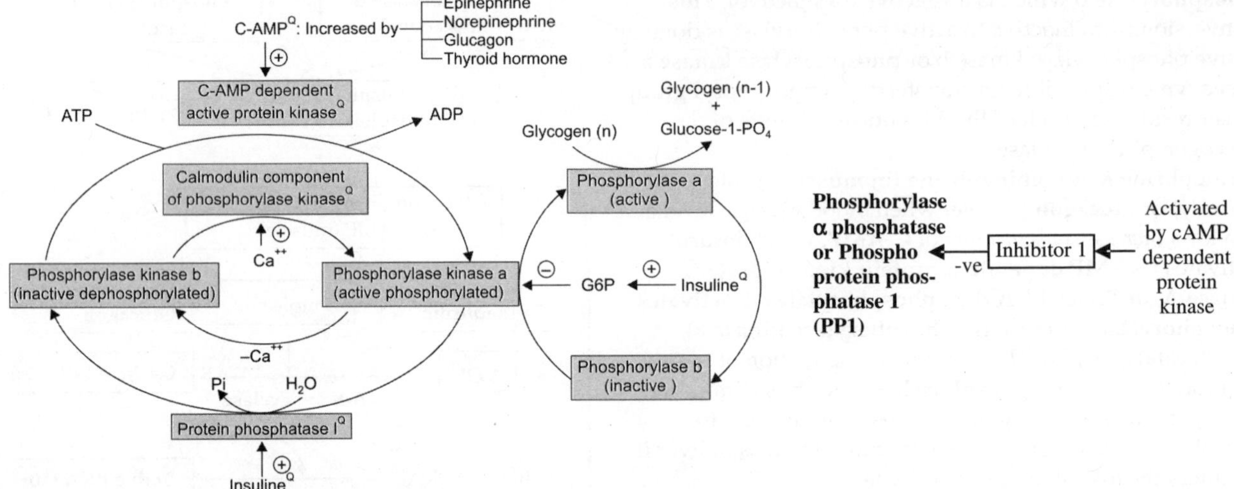

Pathway of glycogenesis and of glycogenolysis in the liver

In well fed state (also called absorptive stage) **insulin suppresses glucose –6-phosphatase activity and causes glucose 6 – phosphate to enter glycogenesis**Q (to form glycogen).

Two high-energy phosphates are used in the incorporation of 1 mol of glucose into glycogen. (+), stimulation; (-), inhibition. **Insulin decreases the level of cAMP only after it has been raised by glucagons or epinephrine – i.e. it antagonizes their action**Q. Glucagon is active in heart muscle but not in skeletal muscle. At asterisk: Glucan transferase and debranching enzyme appear to be two separate activities of the same enzyme.

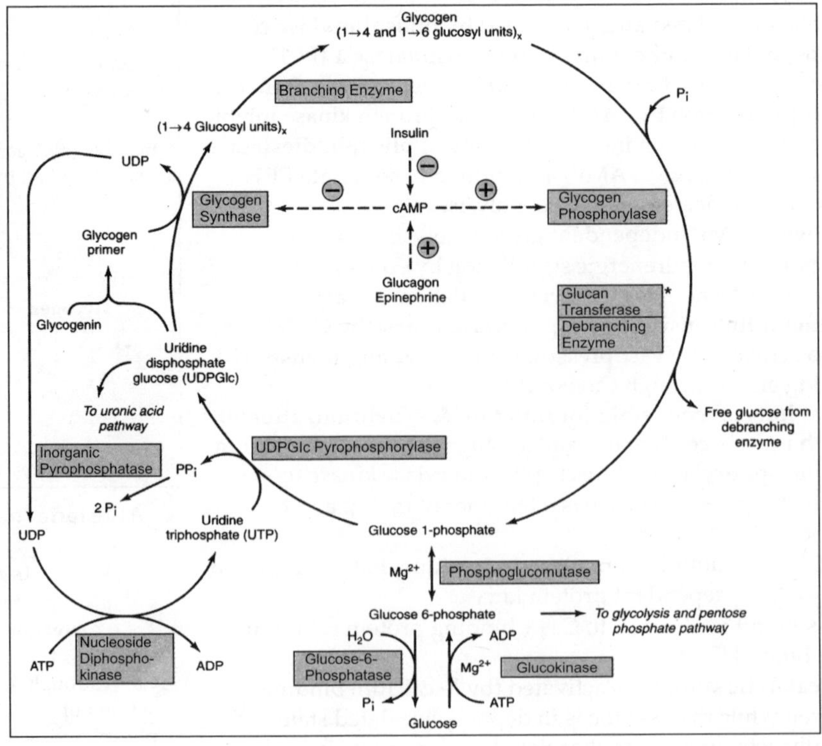

Von Gierke's Disease (Type Ia Glycogen storage Disease)

Inheritance **Chromosome**	**AR**Q 17
Enzyme defect	*Glucose 6 phosphatase*Q
Organs affected	**Liver** (primary), kidney, intestinal mucosa
Glycogen Stored	***Normal in structure but metabolically not available***Q
Appearance	*Doll like face* with fatty cheeks, thin extremities and protuberant abdomen (d/t **hepato-reno megaly)**

Glucose 6 phosphatase (present in liver but not in muscle) *converts glucose 6-PO4 (obtained from glycogenolysis) to glucose*. So deficiency l/t **hypoglycemia**.

Metabolic Abnormalities & Clinical Presentation

- **Fasting hypoglycemia** d/t unavailability of glycogen
- **Hyper lipemia (hyper lipidemia), acidaemia & ketosis** occurs as a result of utilizing fat as energy source (i.e. **increased fat mobilization**).
- Excess acetyl CoA obtained from β- oxidation is diverted for **increased cholesterol, fatty acid** and **ketone body synthesis** resulting in xanthomas, fatty infiltration of liver, hepatorenomegaly (protuberant abdomen) & doll like face with fatty cheeks
- Persistent hypoglycemia has 2 effects
  - *Inhibits insulin secretion* which *inturn inhibits protein synthesis* l/t *stunted growth (dwarfism) and thin extremities*
  - *Stimulates secretion of catecholamines* which cause muscle glycogen to break down producing *lactic acidosis*
- Hyperuricemia an gout (d/t more pentose ***formation and decreased excretion)***Q. It has 2 reasons

1. Increased production:
   - ***Accumulated G-6- Phosphate enters the HMP shunt and l/t increased production of pentoses***Q
   - Pentose acts as substrate for *PRPP synthetase* (Phospho Ribosyl pyro phosphate synthetase) and result in *increased production of purines*
   - Purines are catebolized to uric acid.
2. Decreased renal excretion of uric acid is caused by *increased lactic acid level which competes with uric acid for excretion.*

Glucose-6-PO_4 Dehydrogenase (G6PD) Deficiency

- It is a ***X-linked recessive disorder***Q that causes episodic hemolytic anemia because of ***decreased ability of RBCs to deal with oxidative stresses, due to impaired generation of NADPH***Q.
- ***G6PD is the first and rate limiting enzyme of the HMP shunt which is responsible for the production of NADPH in the cells***Q.

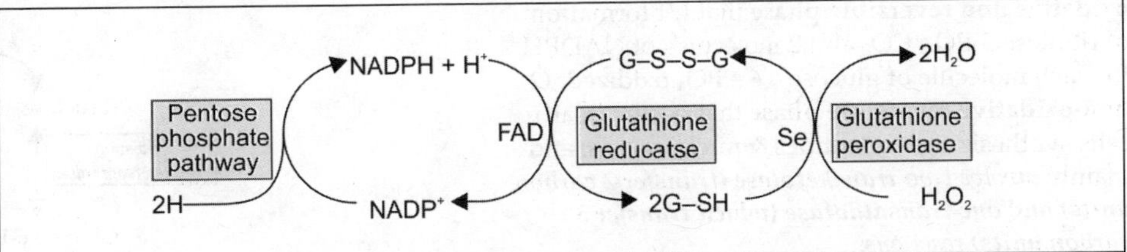

Role of the pentose phosphate pathway in the glutathione peroxidase reaction of erythrocytes. (G-S-S-G, oxidized glutathione; G-SH, reduced glutathione; Se, selenium cofactor)

- NADPH acts as a ***cofactor for glutathione reductase***Q that generates reduced form of glutathione.
- Reduced glutathione is a potent antioxidant and removes H_2O_2 by enzyme ***glutathione peroxidase***
- In the absence of reduced glutathione, H_2O_2 accumulates and decrease the life span of RBC by causing oxidative damage to cell membrane leading to hemolysis.
- **Favism** by eating **Fava beans** (eg as an ingredient of falafel- a Mediterranean food) *l/t hemolytic anemia, jaundice, even kidney failure & death may occur in peoples with G6PD deficiency.*

6- Phosphogluconate Pathway / Hexose Mono Phosphate (HMP) Shunt / Pentose Phosphate Pathway (PPP)/Warburg-Dickens-Lipman-Pathway

- It is an *alternate pathway for complete oxidation of glucose,* which is not ***meant for production of energy (ATP)***Q. Like glycolysis, enzymes of PPP are ***cytosolic***Q. But unlike glycolysis
- the **irreversible oxidative portion of PPP** occurs in specialize tissue like ***liver, lactating mammary glands & adipose tissue***Q which are active in fatty acid synthesis, in ***adrenal cortex***Q which is active in NADPH dependent synthesis of steroids and in ***erythrocytes***Q which require NADPH to require glutathione reduced. It also occurs in ***lens, cornea, testes and ovary but not in non lactating mammary gland and unimportant in skeletal muscle***Q. Whereas glycolysis occurs in all tissues.
- It is *multicyclic process,* 3 molecules of glucose 6 phosphate gives rise to 3 molecules of CO2 and 3 molecules of 5 carbon sugar, which rearranges to give 2 molecules of glucose 6- phosphate and 1 molecule of glyceraldehyde 3- phosphate. ***CO_2 is produced in HMP shunt which is never produced in E.M. pathway***Q.

6 Carbon Glucose –6 P (3 molecules)	→	5 Carbon Sugar (3 molecules) +3CO_2
		↓ Rearrange
		6 carbon Glucose– 6–P (2 molecules) + 3 carbon Glyceraldehyde–3-P (1 molecule)

- ***Oxidation is achieved by dehydrogenation using $NADP^+$ not NAD^+ as hydrogen acceptor***Q.
- HMP shunt can be divided into 2 phases: (1) **oxidative non reversible phase** that l/t formation of ribulose 5-PO_4, CO_2 and 2 molecules of NADPH for each molecule of glucose – 6 – PO_4 oxidized. (2) **non-oxidative reversible phase** that occurs in all cells synthesizing nucleotides & nucleic acids; and mainly *involve* ***two transketolase (transfer 2 carbon units) and one transaldolase (which transfer 3 carbon units)*** *reactions.*
- ***Glucose 6 PO_4 dehydrogenase is the rate limiting enzyme and uses $NADP^+$ as a coenzyme***Q. **Transketolase** ***requires thiamine pyrophosphate (TPP)***Q. Other enzymes requiring TPP are ***pyruvate de carboxylase***Q of pyruvate dehydrogenase complex, ***α – ketoglutarate dehydrogenase***Q of TCA cycle, & ***branched chain α -keto acid deydrogenase***Q of branched chain aminoacid metabolism.
- ***No ATP is directly produced or consumed in HMP shunt***Q. Its ***major function is to provide NADPH***Q (required for fatty acid & steroid synthesis) ***and pentose sugar***Q (for nucleic acid & nucleotide synthesis). Summary of PPP is

3 glucose – 6- PO_4 + $NADP^+$	→	2 glucose – 6- PO_4 + 1 glyceraldehyde–3- PO_4 + 3CO_2 + 6NADPH + 6H^+

★ **Insulin** & **thyroid hormone** enhance the activity of HMP shunt

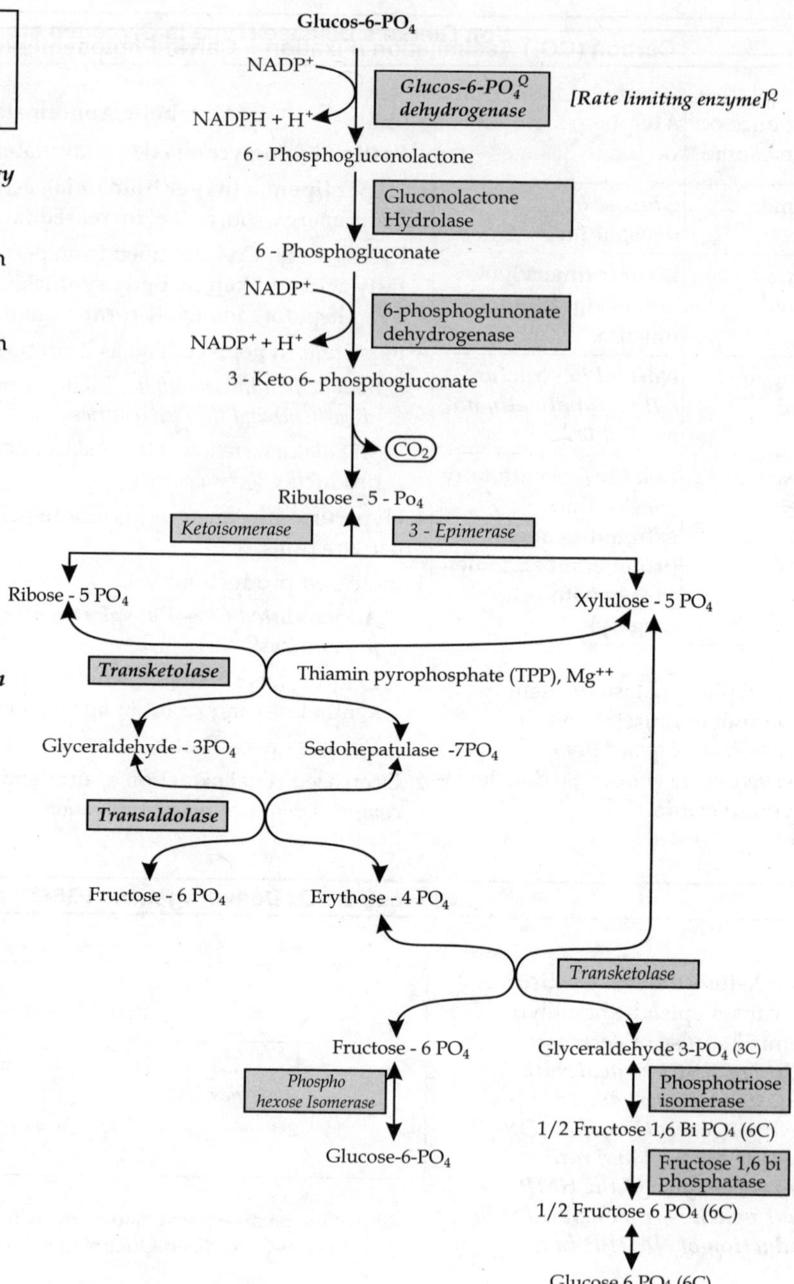

**** It is multicyclic process, 3 molecules of glucose-6PO_4 enter the cycle, producing 3 mols of CO_2 and 3 mols***

Carbon (CO_2) Assimilation /Fixation = Calvin Photosynthetic Carbon Reduction Cycle

- Plants synthesize carbohydrate from CO_2 and water by process of photo synthesis in plastids (chloroplast). It occurs in 3 stages – fixation of CO_2 into 3 phosphoglycerate, conversion of 3 phosphoglycerate to glyceraldehydes 3 phosphate and regeneration of ribulose 1, 5 biphosphate from triose (glyceraldehydes 3) phosphate.
- Overall 3 molecules of ribulose 1, 5 biphosphate fixes 3 molecules of CO_2 to form 6 molecules of glyceraldehyde 3 phosphate (18 carbons) in equilibrium with dihydroxy acetone phosphate. The formation of glyceraldehyde from 3 phosphoglycerate *is reversal of corresponding glycolysis steps, with one exception that cofactor is* NADPH rather than NADH.
- In 3rd stage 5 of 6 molecules of triose (glyceraldehyde 3) PO_4 (=15C) are used to regenerate 3 molecules of starting material ribulose 1, 5 biphosphate (15 carbons) involving many of the same reactions used in oxidative **pentose phosphate pathway** (but in reverse direction). This **reductive pentose phosphate pathway** also uses few extra enzymes like sedoheptulose, 1, 7 biphosphatase etc that make the reductive cycle irreversible.
- **Fructose 6 phosphate** is a key intermediate in stage 3 and can lead either to regeneration of ribulose 1, 5 biphosphate or to synthesis of starch.
- **6 NADPH and 9 ATPs** are required for synthesis of each triose phosphate (glyceraldehyde 3 PO_4) from CO_2 & H_2O. so summary of calvin cycle is

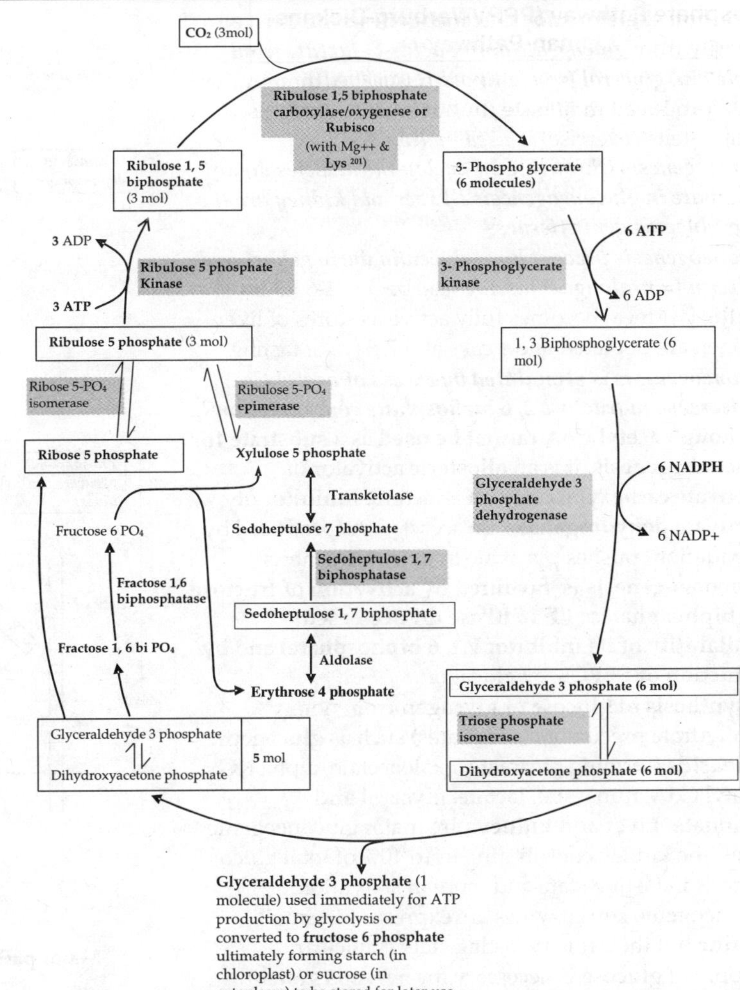

$$3CO_2 + 5H_2O + 6NADPH + 9\ ATP \rightarrow \text{Glyceraldehyde 3 phosphate (G3P)} + 6NADP^+ + 9\ ADP + 2H^+ + 8Pi$$

Fate of

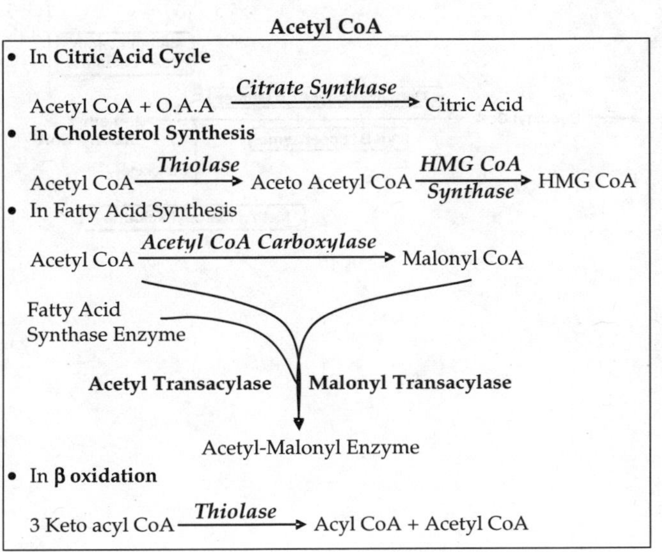

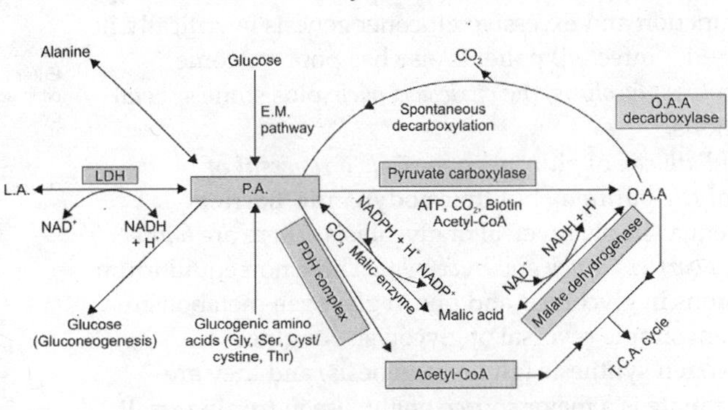

★ **Acetyl CoA carboxylase is also known as Malonyl CoA Synthetase**

Gluconeogenesis

- The **carbon skeletons for gluconeogenesis** are derived primarily from ***glucogenic aminoacids & lactate from muscle and glycerol from adipose tissue***[Q]. **Although the lactate produced in muscle** (by anaerobic glycolysis during intense exercise) ***is used by liver for gluconeogenesis (through Cori cycle); the muscles do not participate in gluconeogenesis***[Q]. ***Liver and kidney are the major gluconeogenic tissues***[Q].
- ***Gluconeogenesis prevent hypoglycemia during short and long term (= prolonged) fasting***[Q] i.e. begins 4-6 hours after the last meal becomes fully active as stores of liver glycogen are depleted and peaks at 5-7 days of fasting .
- ***Gluconeogenesis is stimulated by excess of acetyl CoA and decrease in fructose 2, 6 biphosphate concentration***[Q].
  1. **Although acetyl CoA cannot be used as a substrate for gluconeogenesis,** it is an **allosteric activator** of pyruvate **carboxylase** and an **allosteric inhibitor of pyruvate dehydrogenase.** So acetyl CoA (produced by β oxidation) pushes pyruvate to gluconeogenesis
  2. **Gluconeogenesis is favoured by activation of fructose 1,6 biphosphatase (F 16 BPase d/t decreased availability of its inhibitor F,1, 6 biphosphate)** and by **induction of PEPCK** by glucagon.
- It is **synthesis of glucose or glycogen from** non carbohydrate precursors (substrates) such as **glucogenic aminoacids** (forming **pyruvate**, oxaloacetate, alpha KG, succinyl CoA, fumarate), **lactate, glycerol and propionate. Liver and kidneys** are major gluconeogenic tissues; the kidney contributing upto 40% of total glucose synthesis in fasting state and more in starvation. Gluconeogenic key enzymes are expressed in **small intestine** but their role in fasting state is unclear.
- A supply of **glucose** is necessary for **nervous system (brain) & erythrocytes (RBC)**. Glucose is important in *maintaining the level of intermediates of citric acid cycle* even when fatty acids are the main source of acetyl CoA. Gluconeogenesis also *clears lactate produced by muscles & erythrocytes, and glycerol produced by adipose tissue.* Failure of gluconeogenesis is fatal b/o hypoglycemic brain dysfunction and excessive gluconeogenesis in critically ill (injured / infected) patients also has poor outcome.
- It *involves glycolysis*, the *citric acid cycle* plus some special reactions.
- *Main Pathway* of gluconeogenesis *is* ***a reversal of glycolytic pathway*** but **thermodynamic 'barriers'** prevent a simple reversal of glycolysis. There are *four such energy barriers which are irreversible.* Three non equilibrium reactions in glycolysis and one in glycogen metabolism prevent simple reversal of glycolysis for glucose /glycogen synthesis (gluconeogenesis) and they are
- **Propionate** is a major source of glucose in **ruminants**. It **non ruminant** (eg **humans**) propionate arises from ***beta-oxidation of odd chain fatty acids (eg ruminant lipids), oxidation of isoleucine & side chain of cholesterol***[Q], and is a minor substrate for gluconeogenesis.

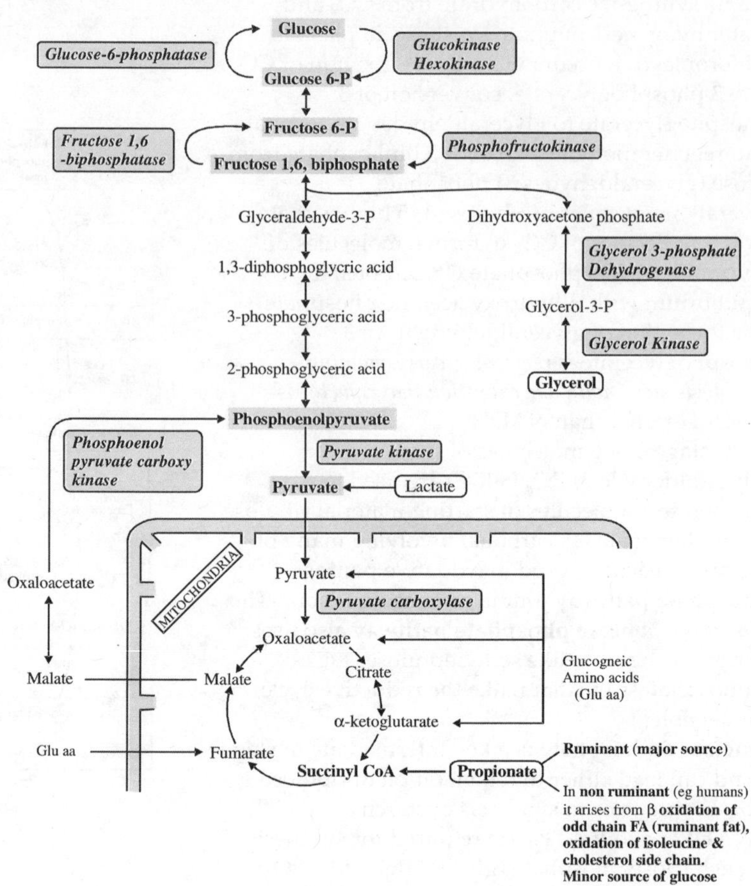

Major pathways of gluconeogenesis and glycolysis in liver

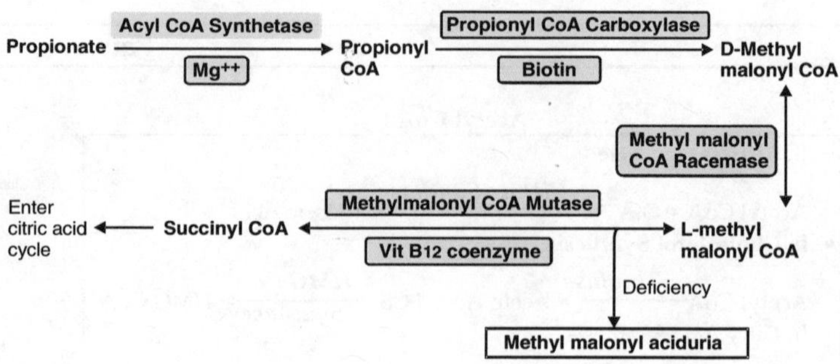

Regulation of Gluconeogenesis & Glycolysis

- Since glycolysis and gluconeogenesis share the same pathwy but in opposite directions, they must be regulated reciprocally. **Availability of glucogenic precursors (substrates)** is the most important factor, along with **circulating level of glucagon**, in movement to movement **regulation of gluconeogenesis.**
- In carbohydrate metabolism enzyme activity is **regulated by 3 mechanisms**

Slow Adaptive changes in enzyme activity (Induction & Repression) from alteration in rate of Enzyme Synthesis or Degradation or both.

- Induction & repression of key enzymes (*catalyzing physiologically irreversible non equilibrium reactions*) is **slow & requires several hours.**
- Activity of enzymes catalyzing reactions in opposite direction varies **reciprocally** so the effects are reinforced.
- For example **insulin** secreted in response to excess of blood glucose enhance synthesis of *key enzymes of glycolysis and antagonize* the effect of epinephrine, glucocorticoids and glucagon stimulated cAMP thereby suppressing synthesis of *key enzymes of gluconeogenesis.*

Excess of glucose (Carbohydrate Feeding)

- **Increased Insulin** → **Increased activity of enzymes involved in glucose utilization (glycolysis &** lipogenesis)
- **Decreased Glucocorticoid, Glucagon, Epinephrine** → **Decreased** activity (synthesis) of key enzymes of **gluconeogenesis**

Covalent Modification by Reversible Phosphorylation

- It is **rapid**
- In response to **fasting** (decrease in blood glucose), **glucagon & epinephrine,** inhibit glycolysis and stimulate gluconeogenesis in liver by **increasing cAMP concentration. c-AMP dependent protein kinase activity** leads to phosphorylation & inactivation of **pyruvate kinase**

Fasting / Diabetes

- **Decreased insulin & glycolysis enzymes**
- **Increased glucocorticoids, glucagon (cAMP), epinephrine** and enzymes of **gluconeogenesis**

Allosteric Modification

It is **instantaneous** and examples of allosteric regulation include

A. Allosteric activation of hepatic pyruvate carboxylase by acetyl CoA increases gluconeogenesis and **reciprocal inhibition of pyruvate dehydrogenase** by acetyl CoA sparing pyruvate from oxidation (in TCA).

- **Gluconeogenesis in fasting state** is ***indicated by increased activity (activation) of pyruvate carboxylase by Acetyl CoA***Q. As a result of increased lipolysis (in fasting state & diabetes), the liver is flooded with fatty acids. The rate of formation of acetyl CoA by beta- oxidation of these fatty acids exceeds the capacity of liver to oxidize it to CO_2 & H_2O. As a result, **acetyl CoA accumulates and cause allosteric activation of hepatic pyruvate carboxylase.** At the same time acetyl CoA **inhibits pyruvate dehydrogenase** (by activating PDH kinase). Thus acetyl CoA can divert pyruvate towards gluconeogenesis and away from TCA.

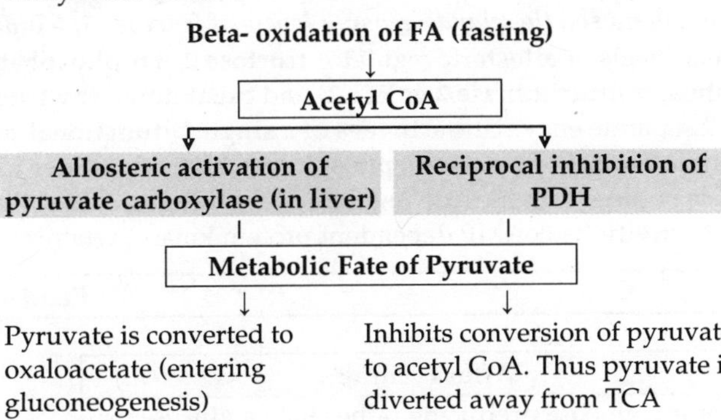

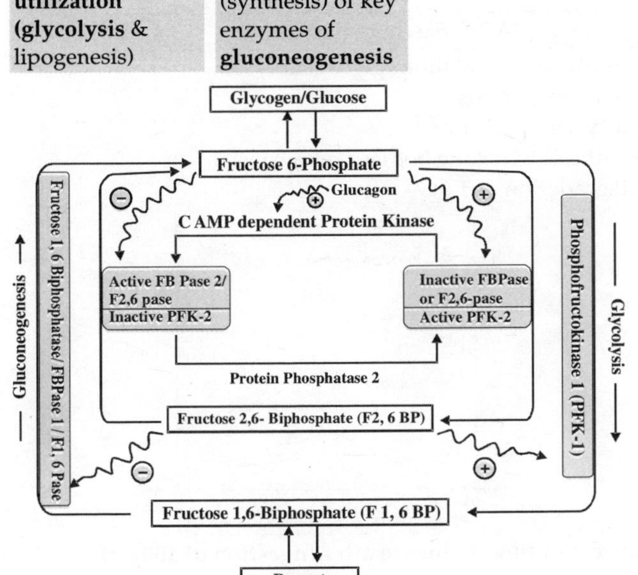

B. Allosteric regulation by Energy levels within cells

- **5′AMP acts as an indicator of energy status of cells.** A small decrease in ATP (d/t its use in energy requiring proesses) causes a several fold increase in AMP so that AMP acts as a **metabolic amplifier (sensitive signal) of change in energy status of cell.**
- Energy rich state of cell (ie high ATP & low AMP levels) stimulate gluconeogenesis (an energy requiring pathway). Whereas energy poor state (elevated levels of AMP) increase glycolysis (for energy / ATP formation)

PFK-1 and Fructose 1, 6 Biphosphatase are reciprocally regulated (allosterically) by AMP

- **Fructose 1, 6 biphosphatase is allosterically inhibited by AMP** (decreasing gluconeogenesis) and simultaneously AMP **activates phosphofructokinase (phosphofructokinase 1)** increasing glycolysis & **phosphorylase** increasing glycogenolysis.

- **PFK1 occupies a key position in regulating glycolysis** in response to energy status of cell. It is activated by 5′ AMP and is inhibited by citrate & normal ATP concentrations. As a consequence of inhibition of PFK-1, glucose 6 phosphate accumulates, which in turn inhibits uptake of glucose in extrahepatic tissue by inhibition of hexokinase.

C. PFK-1 & FBP ase1are reciprocally regulated (allosterically) by Fructose 2, 6 Biphosphate

- **Fructose 2, 6 Biphosphate** is most potent positive allosteric **activator of phosphor fructokinase 1** (increasing glycolysis) and **inhibitor of fructose 1, 6 biphosphatase /FBPase 1 /or F 1, 6 pase** (decreasing gluconeogenesis). Thus it ***(F2, 6 BP) plays a unique role in regulation of glycolysis & gluconeogenesis in liver***[Q].
- **PFK1 is virtually inactive in the absence of F2, 6 biphosphate (d/t inhibition caused by ATP, citrate glucagon).** F2, 6 biphoshate increases PFK1's affinity for its substrate fructose 6 phosphate and reduces its affinity for allosteric inhibitors ATP & citrate; thereby increasing glycolysis. F2, 6 BP has opposite effect on FBPase1 : it inhibits FBpase 1 (or fructose 1, 6 biphosphatase) by reducing its affinity or increasing km for its substrate fructose 1, 6 biphosphate

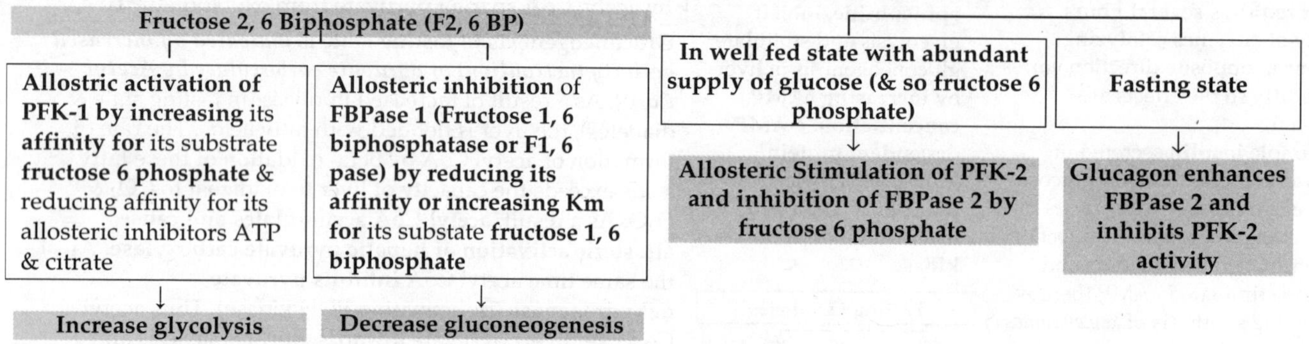

- Therefore **decreased sensitivity of FBpase 1 to regulation (inhibition) by fructose 2, 6 biphosphate increases gluconeogenesis;** ***thereby decreasing levels of fructose 1, 6 biphosphate, pyruvate and ATP***[Q].
- Cellular **levels of allosteric regulator fructose 2, 6 biphosphate (F2, 6BP) depends on the relative rates of its formation (by phosphofructokinase 2 or PFK2) and breakdown (by fructose 2, 6 biphosphatase or FBPase 2).** PFK-2 and FBPase 2 are 2 separate enzymatic activities of a **single bifunctional protein (enzyme)**. This bifunctional enzyme is **under allosteric control of fructose 6 phosphate which stimulates kinase (PFK-2) and inhibits phosphatase** (FBpase 2). The balance of these activities are **regulated by glucagon & insulin; as glucagon enhances FBPase 2 activity & inhibits PFK-2 activity** (via cAMP dependent protein kinase) whereas insulin has opposite effect.

Feed – Fast Cycle

After Feeding

- Liver is a glucose producing rather than a glucose using tissue. However after a meal containing carbohydrate, the liver becomes a net consumer of glucose, retaining ~ *60 of every 100 gm of glucose* presented by portal system.
- Hepatic metabolism of glucose is increased by

- ↑phosphorylation of glucose - ↑ glycogen synthesis - ↑ activity of HMP - ↑ glycolysis - ↓ gluconeogenesis

- Fat metabolism: ↑ Fatty acid & TAG synthesis
- Aminoacid metabolism: ↑protein synthesis and ↑ amino acid degradation
  But the liver has limited capacity to degrade branched chain aminoacids leucine, isoleucine and valine; they pass through the liver essentially unchanged and are preferentially metabolized in muscle.

After Fasting (starvation)

- ↑ glycogen degradation (glycogenolysis)
- ↑ gluconeogenesis
- ↑ fatty acid oxidation
- ↑synthesis of ketone bodies (ketogenesis)
- ↑ degradation of TAG

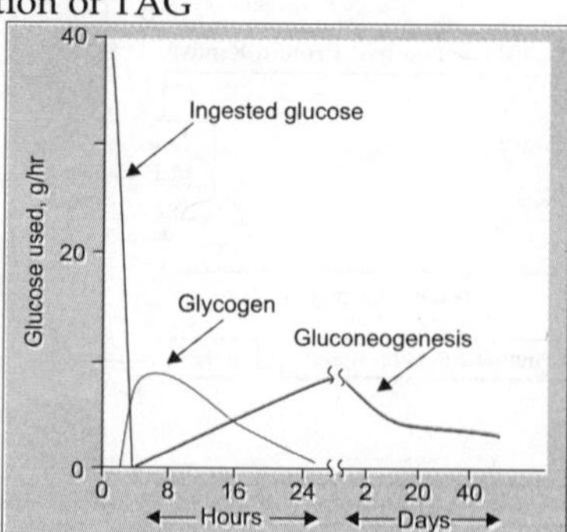

Sources of blood glucose after ingestion of 100g of glucose

Fructose Metabolism

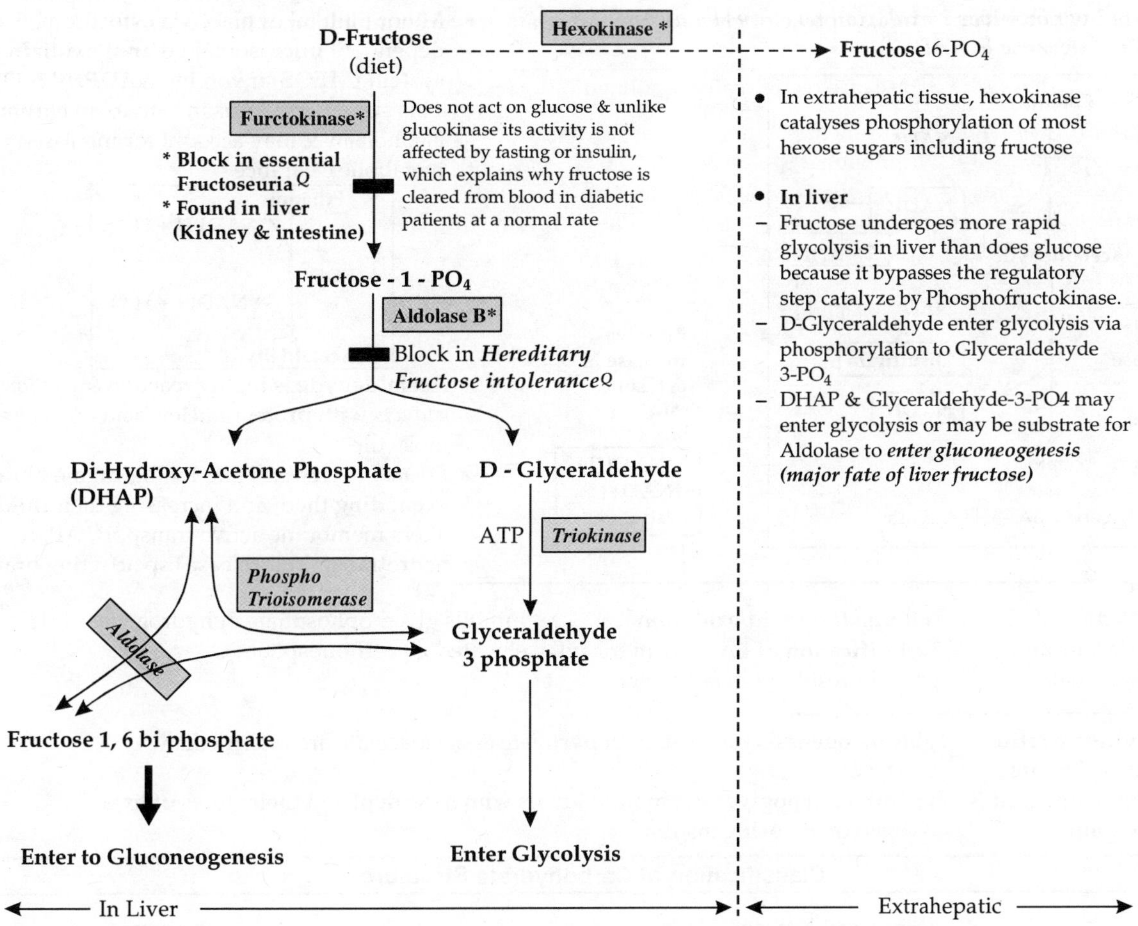

Hereditary Fructose Intolerance

Hereditary fructose intolerance is due to ***deficiency of fructose 1, 6- biphosphate aldolase B in the liver, kidney and intestine***Q.

Mechanism	Clinical Presentation
• Aldolase B catalyzes fructose 1-PO_4 to DHAP and D- glyceraldehyde. • Its deficiency causes *excessive rise of **fructose –1- PO_4 and fructose in blood***Q ↓ *Hypoglycemia*Q	• This is severe disease of infants that appears with the ingestion of fructose containing food • Administration of fructose or sucrose leads to ***Hypoglycemia***Q accompanied by nausea, vomiting, convulsion & profuse sweating. • Continued intake leads to - ***Hepatomegaly***Q - ***Jaundice***Q - ***Proximal renal tubular dysfunction***Q - ***Intellectual impairment***Q

Treatment: Complete elimination of all sources of sucrose, fructose and sorbitol from the diet.

Ethanol (Alcohol) Metabolism

Major path in liver involves 2 oxidation reactions by alcohol & aldehyde dehydrogenase & NAD+[Q]

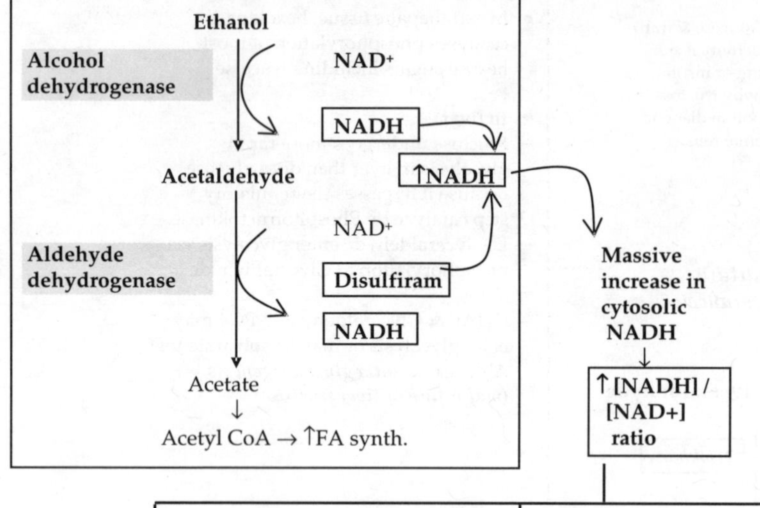

- Minor path takes place via cytochrome P450 dependent **microsomal ethanol oxidizing system (MEOS)** involving *NADPH*[Q] & O_2
- This system increases in activity in chronic alcoholism & may account for increased metabolic clearance

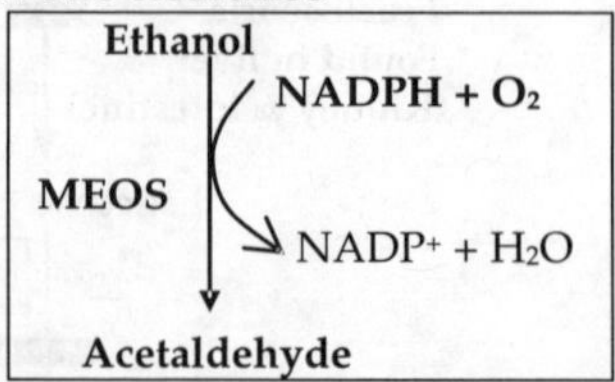

★ **Acetaldehyde** is highly reactive & can *form adducts* with protein nucleic acids & other molecules

★ *Ethanol interpolates* into biological membranes, expanding them and increasing their fluidity. It alters membrane active transport, AP, & neurotransmitter release esp affecting brain.

Favours reduction of pyruvate to lactate and oxaloacetate to malate

- ↑**lactate / pyruvate ratio**
  - **Hyperlacticacidemia**
  - ↓ excretion of uric acid
  - Aggravate **gout**
- ↓**gluconeogenesis** (because both pyruvate & oxaloacetate are intermediates)
  ↓
  Precipitate hypoglycemia in individuals who have depleted their stores of liver glycogen or are using insulin.

- **Inhibits fatty acid oxidation**
- ↑**esterification of FA** to form triacyl glycerol resulting in fatty liver

Inhibits glycerophosphate dehydrogenase l/t elevated glycerophosphate

Classification of Carbohydrate Structure

Aldose and Ketose

- Monosacchrides are classified a/t the number of carbon atoms they contain eg triose for 3C, tetrose for 4C etc. Most oxidized functional group of **aldoses** is aldehyde and **ketoses** is ketone. In other words, if the carbonyl group is at an end (C_1) of carbon chain (in an aldehyde group) the monosacchride is aldose and if the carbonyl group is at any other position (eg C_2 in a ketone group) the monosaccharide is a ketose. Most aldoses have –ose (except few like glyceraldehyde) and ketoses have – ulose (except few like fructose) suffix.

Epimers

- Carbohydrate isomers that differ in configuration around only one carbon atom (with the exception of carbonyl carbon) are called **epimers**. For example

- **Erythrose and threose** are C_2 epimers
- **Ribose** is epimer of **arabinose** (at C_2) and **xylose** (at C_3) but arabinose and xylose are not epimers as they differ in C_2 & C_3 positions.
- **Lyxose** is epimer of **Xylose** (at C_2) and **arabinose** (at C_3) but arabinose and Xylose are not epimers as they differ in C_2 & C_3 positions.
- **Glucose** is epimer of **mannose** (at C_2) and **galactose** (at C_4) but mannose & galactose are not epimers.
- **Allose** is epimer of **altrose** (C_2), **glucose** (C_3) and **gulose** (C_4) but altrose, glucose & gulose are not epimers
- **Talose** is epimer of **galactose** (C_2), **idose** (C_3) and **mannose** (C_4) but galactose, idose & mannose are not epimers.

Isomers

Isomers are compounds that *have same chemical formula but have different structures*. For example glucose, fructose, galactose, mannose, idose, talose, gulose, allose, and altrose all are isomers with same chemical formula $C_6H_{12}O_6$.

Carbon	Generic	Aldoses	Ketoses
3	**Trioses** ($C_3H_6O_3$)	**Glycerose** (glyceraldehyde)	**Dihydroxy-acetone**
4	**Tetroses** ($C_4H_8O_4$)	**Erythrose, Threose**	**Erythrulose**
5	**Pentoses** ($C_5H_{10}O_5$)	**Ribose, Xylose** Arabinose, Lyxose	**Ribulose Xylulose**
6	**Hexoses** ($C_6H_{12}O_6$)	**Glucose, Gulose, Galactose, Mannose,** Allose, Altrose, Idose, Talose	**Fructose,** Psicose, Sorbose, Tagatose
7	**Heptoses** ($C_7H_{14}O_7$)	-	**Sedoheptulose**
9	**Nonoses** ($C_9H_{18}O_9$)	**Neuraminic Acid**	

¹CHO	CHO	CHO	CHO	CHO	CHO	CHO	CHO
H – ²C - OH	OH – C – H	H – C – OH	HO – C – H	H – C – OH	HO – C – H	H – C – OH	HO – C – H
H – ³C – OH	H – C – OH	HO– C - H	HO – C -H	H – C – OH	H – C - OH	HO– C - H	HO– C - H
H – ⁴C – OH	H – C – OH	H – C – OH	H – C – OH	HO– C – H	HO– C – H	HO – C – H	HO – C – H
H – ⁵C – OH	H – C – OH	H – C – OH	H – C – OH	H – C – OH	H – C – OH	H – C – OH	H – C – OH
⁶CH₂OH	CH₂OH	CH₂OH	CH₂OH	CH₂OH	CH₂OH	CH₂OH	CH₂OH
D-Allose	D-Altrose	D-Glucose	D-Mannose	D-Gulose	D-I dose	D-Galactose	D-Talose

Enantiomers (Optical/Stereo-Isomers)

- **Enantiomers (optical isomers or stereoisomers)** are pairs of structures that are **mirror images of each other but not identical**, similar to left and right hand which are the same but opposite. These are non super imposable and are designated as **D and L-sugar**. Each enantiomer often *shows different chemical reactions* with other enantiomers. Because of presence of many enantiomers in living beings, there is usually a marked difference in effects of two stereoisomers. For example only one of drug stereoisomer produces desired effect while the other does not.
- Isomers that are mirror images of each other are called **enantiomers (optical isomers)** and the 2 membes are designated as 'D' or 'L' sugars. In **L** form the OH group on the **asymmetric (chiral) carbon** *(i.e. a carbon linked to 4 different atoms or groups)* farthest from carbonyl carbon is on **left**, whereas in **D isoform** it is on the **right**. **Racemase** enzymes inter convert D & L enantiomers. In general, a molecule with n chiral centers have **2^n stereoisomers** (enantiomers). Glyceraldehyde (triose) has 1 chiral carbon so $2^1 = 2$ stereoisomers, whereas hexoses have 4 chiral carbons so $2^4 = 16$ stereoisomers.
- The *presence of asymmetric carbon atoms provides optical activity to compound.* A beam of polarized light, when passed through a solution of optical isomer, is rotated either to **right, dextro rotatory (+)** or to **left, (levorotatory (-)**. *Stereochemistry (D/L forms) is independent of the direction of rotation of polarized light*, so D (+), D (-), L (+) or L (-) forms exist. Glucose being dextrorotatory is also called dextrose and naturally occurring fructose is D (-).

Fischer Projection Formula; Diastereomers (Anomers)

- **In Fischer projection formula** to represent 3 dimensional sugar structure on paper, horizontal bonds project out of plane of paper *towards* the reader, whereas vertical bonds project behind the plane of paper, away from reader.
- $\geq$ 99% of sugars with 5 or more carbons exist in **cyclic (ring) form** (i.e. $\leq$ 1% is in **open chain** or **acyclic form**) in which the aldehyde group (of aldose) or Keto group (of ketose) has reacted with the alcohol (OH) group on the same sugar to form **hemiacetals** or **hemiketals**. This cyclization makes the carbonyl carbon (C_1 of aldose & C_2 of ketose) asymmetric (now called **anomeric carbon**) generating **alpha and beta anomers**. Because these are not mirror images of each other they are also called **diastereomers**, and can be spontaneously inter converted by **mutarotation process**. The **alpha anomer** has **same side** and **beta anomer** has **opposite side orientation of hydroxyl (OH) group at anomeric & farthest chiral centers**, in Fischer projection. Biological enzymes use alpha or Beta forms preferentially like glycogen is synthesized from alpha where as cellulose from Beta – D glucopyranonose.

Pyran/Furan; Haworth Projection; Chair Conformation

- The ring structure of monosaccharides are either similar to **pyran** (a *6 membered ring consisting of 5 carbon & 1 oxygen*) or **furan** (a 5 membered ring consisting of 4 carbon & 1 oxygen) and are called **pyranose** or **furanose**.
- Cyclic structures are drawn in **Haworth projection** in which *bonds nearest to the viewer* (viewing from side & above the plane of ring) *are bold and thickened* and OH groups are above or below the plane of ring. However, the 6 membered pyranose ring is *actually in form of (two) chair conformation* and is not planar as Haworth perspective suggested. Two **conformations** (like chair) are **interconvertible *without the breakage of covalent bond whereas 2 configurations (like Alpha & Beta) can be inter converted only by breaking a covalent bond.***
- If the hydroxyl group of anomeric carbon of ring sugar is not linked to other compound by a glycosidic bond, the ring can open and the sugar is called **reducing sugar**. Because it acts as a reducing agent with **chromogenic Benedict's** or **Fehling's solutions**. So the reagent gets reduced and sugar becomes oxidized. Only state of oxygen in aldehyde group decide if sugar is reducing or non reducing.

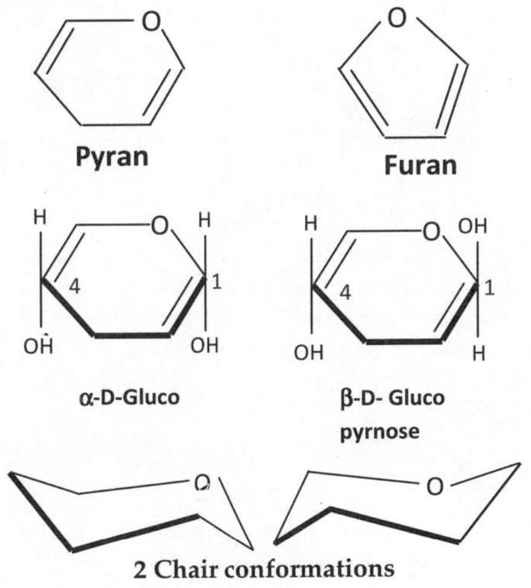

2 Chair conformations

Inulin like Fructan Prebiotics (ILF)

- **Prebiotics** are *nondigestible food ingredients* that should *pass harmlessly through upper gastrointestinal tract* to be a *substrate for advantageous probiotic agents (colonic bacteria) in the large bowel.* These beneficially affect the host by *selectively stimulating the growth or activity of health promoting colonic bacteria like lactobacilli & bifidobacteria.*
- Inulin is a polysaccharide of fructose (& so a **fructosan**) found in roots & tubers of dandelions, dahlias and artichokes. It is easily soluble in water and is used to **determine GFR**. But it is not hydrolyzed by intestinal enzymes and acid. So **non digestible oligosaccharide (NDO)- inulin like fructans** are most widely used & studies prebiotics.
- Inulin like fructans are **non digestible** in upper digestive tract b/o their **β-configuration of anomeric C_2Q**. Their **Beta glycosidic bonds (linkages)** resist the hydrolysis by enzymes & acid. As human digestive enzymes **α–amylase (in saliva)** and **disaccharidases** (like isomaltase, maltase, sucrase, lactase synthesized by small intestinal mainly jejunal mucosal cells) can break **α (1 → 4) and α (1 → 6) glycosidic bonds** respectively; trehalase breaks α (1 → 1) bond.
- Humans lack β- (1 → 4) endoglucosidase and therefore are unable to digest cellulose containing *β(1 → 4) glycosidic bonds between glucose residue* and chitin (exoskeleton of arthropods) containing *β(1 → 4) glycosidic linkage b/w N-acetyl glucosamine residue.*
- ILF pass through small bowel without degradation and with out inhibiting (even actually promoting) the absorption of nutrients & minerals like Fe^{+2}, Ca^{+2} and Mg^{+2} (i.e. harmless passage through upper digestive tract).
- ILF reach colon in intact form and become substrates for *beneficial health promoting probiotic bacteria like bifidobacteria and lactobacilli.*

Chapter 2. FAT METABOLISM: REVIEW NOTES

Fatty Acids

F.A. are aliphatic carboxylic acids. The chain may be saturated (containing *no double bonds* & end in –'**Anoic**') or unsaturated (containing one or more double bond & end in – '**Enoic**'). Carbon atoms are numbered from carboxyl carbon (carbon No 1). The carbon atoms adjacent to carboxyl carbon (Nos. 2, 3 & 4) are also k/a α, β & γ respectively, and the *terminal methyl carbon* is K/a *ω or n- carbon.* Δ indicates number & position of double bonds eg Δ^9 = a double bond between carbons 9 & 10; ω9 = a double bond on the 9th carbon counting from ω carbon. So

$$\underbrace{\overset{1}{C}-\overset{2}{\underset{\alpha}{C}}-\overset{3}{\underset{\beta}{C}}-\overset{4}{\underset{\gamma}{C}}-C-C-C-C-\overset{9}{C}}_{\Delta 9}=\underbrace{\overset{10}{C}-C-C-C-C-C-\overset{16}{\underset{\omega}{C}}}_{\omega 7}$$

this is 16 carbon atom monoenoic acid (unsaturated fatty acid with one double bond) that is Δ^9 *and ω7*

Saturated Fatty Acids (SFA)

- Saturated fatty acids (having no double bond) are major component of meat product (beef fat) making it white, greasy & *solid at room temperature*. Other main sources are *dairy product* and some vegetable oils such as coconut & palm oils (used in latin American & Asian food).
- Consumption of saturated fat is a/w **increased incidence of coronary heart disease (by increasing total plasma cholesterol & LDL cholesterol), and increased risk of prostate & colon cancer**. So limiting intake of saturated fats is strongly advised.
- SFA with 14 (Myristic) & 16 (palmitic) carbon chain lengths are most potent in increasing serum cholesterol. Whereas, stearic acid (18 carbon) found in chocolate etc has little effect on blood cholesterol.

Name	Number of (Atoms)
Acetic	2
Propionic	3
Butyric	4
Valeric	5
Caproic	6
Capric	10
Lauric	12
Myristic	14
Palmitic	**16**
Stearic	**18**
Lignoceric	**24**

Unsaturated Fatty Acids (UFA)

- Contain one (**monounsaturated**) or more double bond (**polyunsaturated**). Are named *monoenoic, dienoic trienoic, tetra enoic, pentaenoic & hexaenoic* according to numbers of double bond 1,2 3, 4, 5, & 6 respectively
- **Monounsaturated fatty acids (MUFA)** like **olive oil rich in oleic acid** (when substituted for saturated FA in diet) **lower both total plasma cholesterol & LDL cholesterol, but maintain or increase HDL cholesterol; thus decreasing incidence of coronary heart disease.**
- Effect of polyunsaturated fatty acid (PUFA) on cardiovascular disease is influenced by location of double bond (ω_3 = at 3rd bond position / ω_6 = at 6th bond position starting from methyl end).
- Consumption of ω_6 or n-6 PUFA (mainly **linoleic acid**, 18:2 (9, 12)) when substituted for SFA, **lower plasma cholesterol & LDL cholesterol**, but **HDL** which protects against coronary heart disease is **also lowered**. So the powerful benefits of lowering LDL are only partially offset because of decreased HDL. *Nuts, avocados, olives, soyabean* and various vegetable oils including *sesame, cottonseed, corn oil, sunflower oil, canola oil, safflower oil* etc are common sources of ω_6 PUFA.
- Dietary **ω_3 PUFA** *suppress cardiac arrhythmias, reduce serum triacyl glycerols, decrease tendency of thrombosis, lower BP and substantially reduce risk of cardiovascular mortality* (i.e. are **cardioprotective**) but they have *little effect on LDL or HDL cholesterol level*. The ω_3 PUFA mainly Alpha-linolenic acid, 18:3 (9, 12, 15) are found in plants (its acceptable range is 0.6 – 1.2% of total calories). Flax seed oil, canola oil, soyabean oil are rich in ω-3 PUFA. **Fish oil (salmon fat)** containing long chain ω-3- **DHA** (docosahexaenoic acid) and **EPA** (eicosapentaenoic acid) are ω-3 PUFAs. Two fatty fish meals per week are recommended.
- **Mediterraneen diet rich in MUFA (olive oil) and ω-3 fatty acids (from fish oils & some nuts)** but low in saturated fats is a/w ↓ LDL & total cholesterol but little change in HDL: hence decreased risk of coronary heart disease. Plasma triacyl glycerols are unchanged.
- Arachidonic acid a precursor of prostaglandins & leukotrienes is ω-6 PUFA.

No. of Carbon atoms	No. of double bonds	Position of double bonds	Family	Common Name	Systemic Name	Occurrence
16	1	Δ^9	ω^7	**Palmitoleic**	Cis- 9- Hexadece- noic	In nearly all fats
18	1	Δ^9	ω^9	**Oleic**	Cis- 9- octadecenoic	Possibly the most common fatty acid in natural fats (olive oil)
18	1	Δ^9	ω^9	**Elaidic**	Trans-9- actadecenoic	Hydrogenated and ruminant fats
18	2	9, 12	ω^6	**Linoleic**	all –cis- 9,12- octadeca dienoic	Corn, peanut, cottonseed, soyabean, and many plant oils
18	3	9, 12, 6	ω^6	**γ - Linolenic**	all – cis- 6, 9, 12- octadeca trienoic	Some plants, eg. oil of evening primrose, borage oil; minot fatty acid in animals
18	3	9, 12, 15	ω^3	**α - Linolenic**	all –cis- 9,12, 15 octa-decatrienoic	Frequently found with linoleic acid but particularly in **linseed** oil
20	4	5, 8, 11, 14	ω^6	**Arachidonic**	all –cis-5,8, 11, 14- Eicosatetraenoic	Found in animals fats and in peanut oil; important component of phospholipids in animals
20	5	5, 8, 11, 14, 17	ω^3	**Timnodonic**	all –cis- 5, 8, 11, 14, 17- Ecosapentaenoic	Important component of fish oils eg. **cod liver, mackerel, menhaden, salmon oils.**
22	6	4, 7, 10, 13, 16, 19	ω^3	**Cervonic**	all –cis- 4, 7, 10, 13, 16, 19- Docosahexaenoic	Fish oils, phospholipids in brain.
24	1	15		**Neurvonic acid**		

Fatty acid type	Metabolic Effect		Clinical Effect
	LDL	HDL	
Trans fatty acid	↑	↓	**Increased** incidence of **coronary heart disease**
Saturated fatty acid	↑	Little effect	**Increased** incidence of **coronary heart disease** Increased risk of **prostate & colon cancer**
Monounsaturated fatty acid (MUFA)	↓	↓	**Decreased** incidence of coronary heart disease
ω-6 polyunsaturated fatty acid (PUFA)	↓	↓	**Decreased** incidence of coronary heart disease
ω-3 Polyunsaturated fatty acid (PUFA)	Little effect	Little effect	**Decreased** incidence of **coronary heart disease** Decreased risk of **sudden cardiac death** **Decreased** tendency for **thrombosis**, reduce **BP** & serum **triacylglycerols** and suppress **cardiac arrhythmias**

Trans Fatty Acids (TFA)

Procedure & Purpose

- Lipid rich food, when exposed too long to oxygen (air), may *spoil and become rancid d/t oxidative cleavage of double bond in unsaturated fatty acids*, which produces aldehyde and carboxylic acids of shorter chain length & therefore *higher volatility*.
- To improve/increase the shelf life and volatility (stability at high temperature in deep frying), commercial vegetable oils are subjected to **partial hydrogenation / hardening**.
- Hardening *converts many cis double bonds in FA to single bonds*

Biological Significance

- Trans fatty acids do not occur naturally in plants, but occur in small amount in animals (**ruminant fat** arising from action of microorganisms in the rumen)
- Many fast foods are **deep fried in partially hydrogenated vegetable oils** & therefore contain high levels of trans fatty acids. So TFA is a major component of many commercial baked goods, like cookies, cakes and most deep

and increase the melting temperature of oils, so that they are more nearly *solid at room temperature.* **Margarine** is produced from liquid vegetable oils by partial hydrogenation.

- But the undesirable effect of partial hydrogenation procedure is production of trans fatty acids i.e ***some cis double bonds are converted to trans double bonds***Q. So trans fatty acids are chemically unsaturated fatty acids but behave like saturated fatty acid (i.e. they are atherogenic).
- Soft margarine, low in trans fatty acid (or containing not at all) is produced by refined technology

Trans	Cis
H—C=C—H (trans)	—H, —H (cis)

Fatty Acid

fried foods. A clue to presence of TFA is "**partially hydrogenated**" word used in the list of ingredients.

- Dietary intake of trans fats **raise the level of triacyl glycerol & LDL (bad) cholesterol,** increase the body's inflammatory response (another risk factor for heart disease) and **decrease the level of HDL (good) cholesterol** and so a/w higher incidence of cardiovascular disease, and avoiding these fats in diet substantially reduces the risk of coronary heart disease.
- Consumption of trans fatty acid is a/w ***increased risk of cardiovascular disease, diabetes mellitus***Q (d/t increased insulin resistance) and adversely affect endothelial function.

Essential Fatty Acid

- ***Dietary essential fatty acids in humans are linoleic acid and α-linolenic acid***Q, because we lack enzymes needed to synthesize them. Plants provide these EFA. **Linoleic acid is the precursor of ω-6-arachidonic acid** and so prostaglandins. **So the arachidonic acid becomes EFA if linoleic acid is deficient in diet**. α-linolenic acid is precursor of ω-3-fatty acids required for growth and development.
- Those fatty acids that ***cannot be synthesized by human bodies***Q and must be provided in diet. The most important essential fatty acid is → ***Linoleic acid***Q (because it serves as a basis for the production of other EFA)

EFA	Dietary Source
Linoleic acidQ	Safflower oil
Linolenic acidQ	*Soyabean oil*Q
Arachidonic acid	*Meat, egg, milk*Q
Eicosapentaenoic acid	*Fish oil*Q
*Docosahexanoic Acid*Q	*Breast milk*

Dietary sources of linoleic acid	
*Safflower oil*Q	*73%*Q *(max)*Q
*Corn oil*Q	57%
*Sunflower oil*Q	56%
*Soyabean oil*Q	51%

- Humans require but do not have the enzymatic capacity to synthesize omega-3 PUFA α linolenic acid (ALA; 18:3 ($\Delta^{9, 12, 15}$), and must therefore obtain it in diet. However from ALA; humans can synthesize 2 other omega PUFAs: eicosapentaenoic acid (EPA; 20 : 5 ($\Delta^{5, 8, 11, 14, 17}$) and docosahexaenoic acid (DHA; 22:6 ($\Delta^{4, 7, 10, 13, 16, 19}$). An imbalance between dietary ratio of omega 6 & omega 3 (optimal is between 1:1 and 4: 1) PUFAs is associated with increased risk of cardiovascular disease.
- Mammalian hepatocytes can introduce ***double bonds at Δ^9 position of FA but not between C-10 and methyl terminal end. So mammas can not synthesize linoleate, 18:2 ($\Delta^{9,12}$) or α- linolenate 18:3 ($\Delta^{9, 12, 15}$)***Q.

  However, plants can synthesize both; the desaturases that introduce double bonds at Δ^{12} and Δ^{15} positions are located in ER and chloroplast. So these are **essential fatty acids** for mammals; they must be obtained from dietary plant material. ***Once ingested linoleate may be converted to other PUFAs, particularly γ-linolenate***Q, eicosatrienoate and eicosatetraenoate (arachidonate), all of which can be **made only from linoleate**

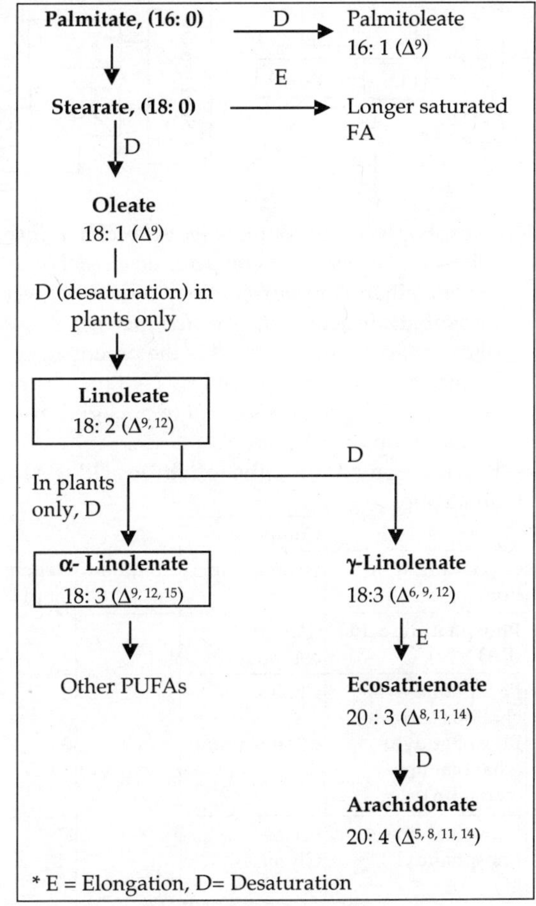

(Polar) Membrane Lipids

- Lipids are heterogenous group of compounds that are relatively *insoluble in water and soluble in nonpolar solvents like ether and chloroform.*
- All major lipids have either **glycerol or sphingosine back bone**, to which *1 or more long chain alkyl groups and a polar head group* are attached. In glycerophospholipid, galacto (sulfo) lipid and triacyl glycerol, the alkyl groups are *fatty acids in ester linkage* whereas, sphingo (both phospho & glyco) lipids contain single fatty acid in amide linkage to sphingosine backbone.

Phospholipids (PL)

- Phospholipids contain **phosphoric acid residue** in addition to *fatty acid and alcohol*
- So PLs are **phosphatidic acid** derivatives in which the *phosphate is esterified with the OH group of suitable alcohol (glycerol or sphingosine).*
- Both types of PLs are found in membranes & play a role in generation of lipid signaling molecules.

Glycolipids (GL)

Glycolipids contain both *carbohydrate* and *lipid*. The carbohydrate portion is antigen determinant and so the glycolipids are antigenic. Two types include

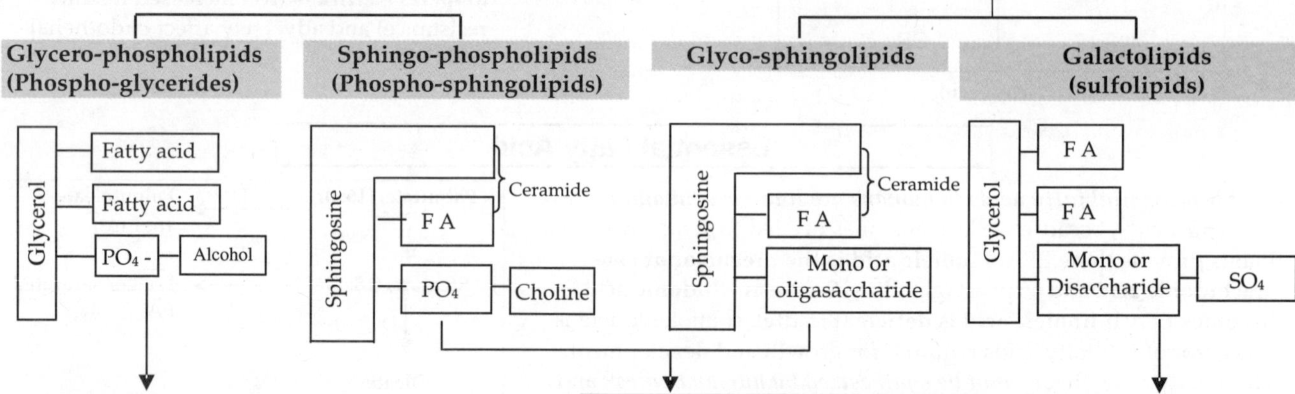

- Phosphoglyceride contain *glycerol backbone linked to 2 fatty acid, a phosphate group and an alcohol* (like serine/ ethanolamine/ choline/ inositol/ glycerol)
- **Phosphatidic acid** is the *simplest (parent)* phosphoglyceride (PG) and is the precursor of other members of this group. All PGs contain (or are derivative of) *phosphatidic acid* (diacyl glycerol with a PO_4 group on 3rd carbon).
- PGs are formed from **phosphatidic acid (PA)** and an alcohol

Glycerophospho-lipid	Components Head group	Common	Net charge (at pH7)
Phosphatidic acid (PA)	(Parent compound)		-1
Phosphotidyl choline (**Lecithin**)	Choline		0
Phosphatidyl ethanolamine (**cephalin**)	Ethanolamine	**PA**	0
Phosphatidyl serine	Serine		-1
Phosphatidyl glycerol	Glycerol		-1
Phosphatidyl inosital 4- 5, biphosphate	Myo Inositol 4, 5-biphosphate		-4
Cardiolipin	Diphosphatidyl glycerol		-2

- All **sphingo-lipids** (ie **sphingosine containing lipids)** are formed from ceramide. **Ceramide** is synthesized from **serine aa in ER** and works as 2nd messenger in cell cycle/differentiation/ senescence and apoptosis. 3 types of sphingolipids are: **phosphosphingolipids (eg sphingomyelin), glycosphingolipids (eg cerebrosides, globosides** and **gangliosides)** and **sulfatides (or sulfo-glyco sphingolipids).**
- Sphingolipids are composed of 1 mol of long chain **amino alcohol sphingosine (4-sphingenine) backbone** linked to 1 mol of **long chain fatty acid** through an amide linkage (at C_2) (i.e. = **ceramide**) and a polar head (PO_4 in phosphospingolipids & mono/oligo-saccharide in glycosphingolipid) group joined by **phosphodiester bond** in phosphosphingolipids and by **O-glycosidic bond** in glycosphingolipids.
- C- 2 bears fatty acid (saturated or monounsaturated with 16, 18, 22 or 24 carbon) in amide linkage.
- **Ceramide** is structurally similar to diacyl glycerol & is parent compound.

- In **galactolipids**, 1 or 2 galactose residues are connected by glycosidic linkage to C-3 of 1, 2 diacyl glycerol
- Galactolipids found predominantly in plants are localized in *internal (thylakoid) membrane of chloroplasts.* They make 70-80% of total membrane lipids of vascular plants and are *most abundant membrane lipid in biosphere.*

Sphingomyelin (sphingophospho-lipid)

Glycosphingolipids

- It consists of **ceramide (sphingosine + fatty acid) and**

- Saturated (C_{16} or C_{18}) fatty acid at C_1 and unsaturated fatty acid (C_{18} or C_{20}) is attached in ester linkage to C_2 (2nd carbon) of glycerol.
- A highly charged or polar head group is attached through a phosphodiester linkage to third carbon. In this head group PO_4^{-3} *bears a negative charge at neutral pH. The polar alcohol may be negatively charged (phosphotidylinositol 4, 5, biphosphate), neutral (phosphotidyl serine) or positively charged (phosphotidyl choline or phosphotidylethanolamine).*
- Phosphoacylglycerol containing choline (i.e. **phosphotidyl choline / Lecithins)** ***are the most abundant phospholipids of cell membrane***[Q] & represent a large proportion of body's *store of choline.* Choline is important in nervous transmission as acetylcholine and as store of labile methyl groups.
- **Dipalmitoyl lecithin** is very active surface active agent and a major constituent of the ***surfactant***[Q].
- **Phosphatidyl ethanolamine (cephalin) & phosphatidylserine** (found in most tissue) differ from phosphatidyl choline only in that *ethanolamine or serine, respectively, replaces choline.*
- **Phosphatidylinosilot** is a ***precursor of second messengers (i.e. help in signal transduction)***[Q].
- **Lysophospholipids** are intermediates in the metabolism of phosphoglycerols.
- In **cardiolipin** 2 phosphatidic acids (PA) share a single glycerol (i.e. 2PA esterified through their PO_4 groups to glycerol) hence the name is **diphosphatidyl glycerol**. It is found exclusively in **inner mitochondrial membrane**, where it maintain ETC. **It is antigenic and is recognized by antibodies raised against *Treponema pallidum (syhillis bacteria)***[Q].
- Some PGs have **ether linked fatty acids (Ether lipids)** like

1. **Plasmalogens** which constitute 10% of PL of brain & heart muscles. These resemble *phosphotidyl ethanolamine (abundant in nerve tissue) &/ or phosphotidylcholine* (abundant in heart muscle) but possess an ether link on Sn -1 instead of ester link (i.e. ester linked fatty acid at carbon 1 is replaced by **ether linked unsaturated alkyl group**).
2. **Platelet activating factor (PAF)**, an unusual ether phosphoglyceride **has saturated alkyl group in ether link** to carbon 1 and an acetyl residue (rather than FA) at carbon 2 of glycerol backbone. PAF is synthesized by variety of cells. It **binds to surface receptors** triggering potent ***acute inflammatory & thrombotic events***[Q]. PAF is one of the most potent bioactive molecule it ***activates inflammatory cells & mediates hypersensitivity, anaphylactic & acute inflammatory reactions***[Q]. It causes ***platelet aggregation & degranulation***[Q] and activate neutrophils & alveolar macrophages ***to generate superoxide radicals***[Q] (killing bacteria).

- It consists of **ceramide** (i.e. **sphingosine amino alcohol** backbone attached at C_2 to **long chain FA** through an amide linkage) and a polar head group. **Phosphoryl choline** or **phosphoethanolamine** (as polar head groups) are attached to carbon 1 of sphingosine through *phosphodiester bond.*
- It is found in as an constituent of **myelin** in nervous tissue.

antigenic carbohydrate (mono/oligosaccharide)
- Like phospholipids, these are essentially present in all membranes but are particularly abundant in **nerve tissue**. They are located in **outer leaflet of plasma membrane**, where they interact with extracellular environment and play role in regulation of cellular inter action, growth and development. So when the cell division/growth is dysregulated, there is dramatic change in glycosphingolipid composition of plasmamembrane
- Glycosphingolipids have been identified as a source of *blood group antigens, embryonic antigens, tumor antigens.*
- They serve as cell surface receptors for *cholera & tetanus toxins* and for certain microbes & viruses.
- Genetic disorder a/w inability to degrade glycosphingolipids l/t lysosomal accumulation of these compounds.
- These can be of two types

- This phosphate free lipid is evolved to conserve PO4, a limiting plant nutrient in soil, for more critical roles
- **Sulfolipids** in plant membrane bear negative charged sulfonate head group
- In this sulfonated lipid, glucose residue is joined to diacylglycerol in glycosidic linkage.

Neutral (Uncharged) glycosphingolipids = Neutral glycolipids	Acidic (Negatively charged) glycosphingolipids
- It consists of **ceramide linked to 1 or more sugar residues** at carbon 1 1. **Cerebroside** (i.e. **ceramide mono saccharide)**/are the simplest neutral glycosphingolipids and they contain either a galactose (**galactocerebroside**) or glucose (**glucocerebroside**). Galactocerebroside are found in plasma membranes of neural tissue and gluco cerebroside, which occur in *plasmamembrane of non neural tissue* serves primarily as an *intermediate in the synthesis & degradation of more complex glycosphingolipids.* ▪ As the name suggest, cerebrosides are found mainly *in brain & peripheral nervous tissue.* Different galacto /gluco-cerebrosides may differ in type	- It consists of **ceramide** l/t **N-acetyl neuraminic acid = NANA/sialic acid (in gangliosides)** or a **sulfate group** on a galactose (in **sulfatides**) - Negative charge at physiological pH is provided by *NANA/sulfate group* 1. **Gangliosides** are derivatives of *ceramide oligosaccharide* (glucosyl ceramide) that contain oligosaccharide as their polar head group & **≥1N acetyl neuraminic acid (Neu 5 Ac = NANA)** a sialic acid at termini. These are found in ganglionic cells of CNS, particularly at the nerve endings. They

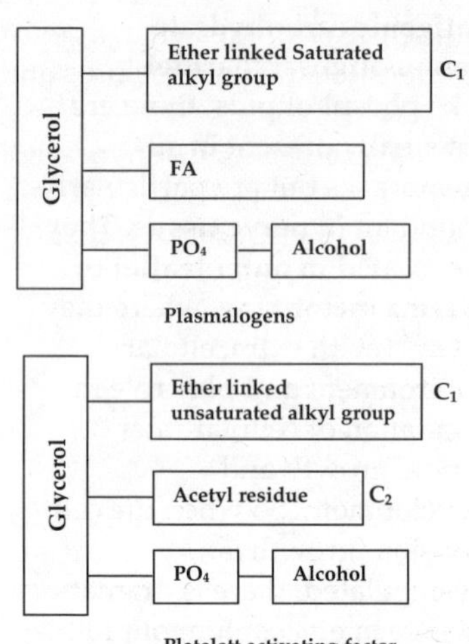

- ★ All cells except mature RBCs can synthesize phospholipids, whereas triacyl glycerol synthesis occurs only in liver, lactating mammary glands, adipose tissue and intestinal mucosal gland.
- ★ Lung maturity of fetus is gauged by determining the **dipalmitoyl lecithin (DPPC) to sphingomyelin (L/S ratio)** in amniotic fluid. A ≥ 2 ratio indicate maturity and major shift from sphingomyelin to DPPC synthesis that occur in pneumocyte at 32 weeks gestation.
- ★ A ceramide (containing 30 carbon FA) is major component of skin & regulates it's *water permeability*.

of FA attached to sphingosine.

2. **Globoside (ceramide oligosaccharide)** are produced by *attaching additional mono saccharide (including N-acetyl galactosamine) to glucocerebrosides.* **Globosides** contain 2 or more sugars, usually D- glucose, D-galactose or N-acetyl D galactosamine

Cerebroside (gluco/galacto) = Ceramide+Glucose/Galactose (Cer – Glc / Gal)
Globoside (Lactosylceramide) = Cer – Glc – Gal
Globoside (Forsman antigen) = Cer – Glc - 2 Gal – 2 Gal Nac

Neutral Storage Lipid (triacyl glycerol)

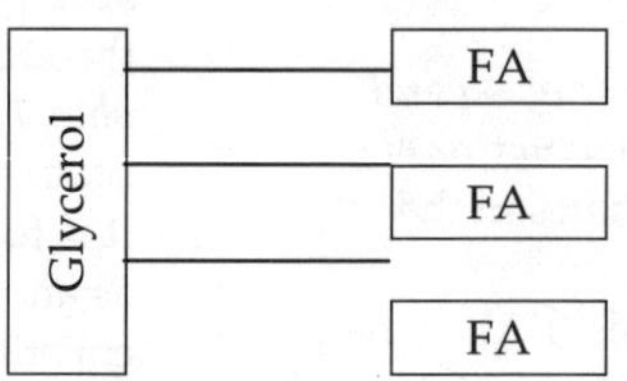

have receptor & other functions. Notation G (for ganglioside). Subscriptio M, D, T, or Q indicate whether there is 1 (mono) 2 (di), 3 (tri) or 4 (quatro) molecules of NANA in ganglioside. Additional number designate monomeric sequence of carbohydrate attached to ceramide. *GM_3* is the simplest ganglioside G represent ganglioside; M is a monosialo containing; & 3 is a number assigned on the basis of chromatographic migration. *Gm_1*,is receptor in intestine for cholera toxin.

2. **Sulfatides** are sulfoglycosphingolipids i.e. cerebrosides that contain **sulfated galactosyl residue.** These sulfogalactosyl ceramide are found predominantly in **nerve tissue (myelin)** & *kidney*.

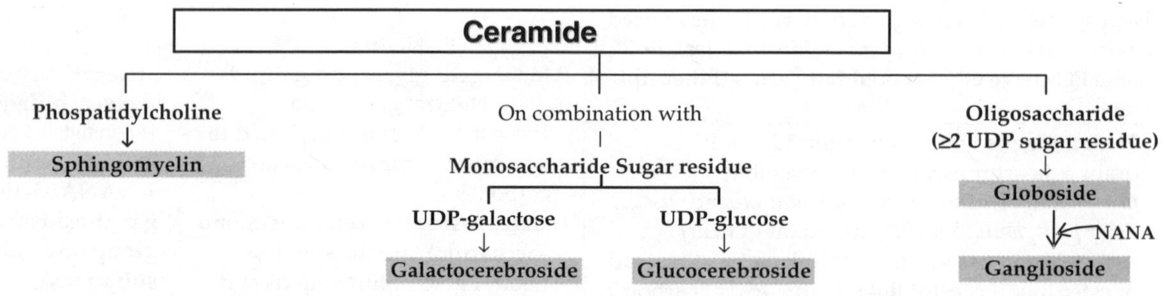

Risk of Atherosclerosis & Coronary Heart Disease (CHD)

- **LDL cholesterol** (especially **oxidized LDL**) uptake by macrophage is responsible for formation **of foam cells** – the hallmark of atherosclerotic plaque. A positive correlation exists b/w plasma LDL cholesterol concentration & atherosclerosis. LDL is degraded in liver (70%) and extrahepatic tissues (30%), both expressing **LDL (apo-B-100, E) receptor**.
- **LDL (apo-B-100, E) receptor** is **defective** in familial hypercholesterolemia, increasing blood LDl cholesterol levels and causing **premature atherosclerosis.**
- **Apoprotein A-I** is a measure of HDL (good) cholesterol & **apo-B** measures LDL (bad) cholesterol. Hence **ratio of Apo B/AI** is the most reliable index of atherosclerosis (cardiovascular disease). Ratio of 0.4 is very good and ratio of 1.4 has highest risk of heart accidents.
- **Lipoprotein (a)**, which inhibits fibrinolysis, consists of 1 mol of LDL attached to 1 mol of apo (a). It increases risk of coronary heart disease (& atherosclerosis) if levels are > 30 mg/dl.

- High plasma **homocysteine** levels (> 15 μmol/L), increased **hs-CRP** (i.e. high sensitivity C-reactive protein), high levels of serum triglyceride & **long chain saturated fatty acids** (e.g. stearic acid), hypertension, diabetes mellitus and smoking are risk factors for atherosclerosis and coronary heart disease.
- **Atherosclerosis & coronary heart disease** occurs in familial **lipoprotein (a)/Lp(a) excess**, familial hypercholesterolemia type II a (**defective LDL receptor apo B-100**), familial type III hyperlipoproteinemia/ broad beta / remnant removal disease/ familial dysbeta lipoproteinemia (**abnormal apo E**). Coronary heart disease also occurs in familial hyper triacylglycerolemia type IV and **hepatic lipase deficiency**.

Sphingolipidoses

- **Sphingolipidoses** (a part of **lysosomal lipid storage diseases)** are a group of **autosomal recessive (except for Fabry disease which is X-linked) inherited** diseases that are caused by a **genetic defect in the degradation (catabolism) of sphingo (or glycosphingo) lipids containing sphingosine.**
- Common features of all sphingolipidoses include
  1. **Rate of synthesis of stored sphingolipid is normal but a specific lysosomal hydrolytic enzyme for degradation is deficient** resulting in accumulation of usually only a single sphingolipid containing ceramide (the substrate for enzyme). It can also result from defects in **lysosomal activator proteins (eg saposins)** that facilitate access of lysosomal hydrolases to short carbohydrate chains as degradation proceeds.
  2. Enzymatic activity is **affected in all tissues similarly.** Accumulation of sphingolipids in neurons cause **neurodegeneration and shortening of lifespan.**
  3. The **incidence is low in most populations except for Gaucher, Tay Sachs and Niemann- Pick disease** (which show high incidence in few ethinic groups). All are **AR except Fabry's disease** which has **x-linked** inheritance.
  4. Can be diagnosed by measuring **enzyme activity** (in cultured fibroblasts or peripheral leukocytes) or by **DNA analysis**. Prenatal diagnosis uses cultured amniocytes or chorionic villi. **Histological examination** can be also useful eg **shell like inclusion bodies in Tay Sachs** and **wrinkled (crumpled) tissue paper appearance of cytoplasm in Gaucher disease.**
  5. Treatment is **not effective** for many diseases. Although **recombinant human enzyme replacement therapy** and **bone marrow transplantation** can successfully treat Fabry's and Gaucher's disease. **Substrate deprivation therapy** (to stop synthesis), **chemical chaperone therapy** and gene therapy (under investigation) are other alternatives.
- Sphingolipidoses include (1) **Neutral glycosphingo lipidoses** (eg **Fabry's, Gaucher's and Niemann Pick disease A and B);** (2) **Generalized GM1 gangliosidoses**; (3) **GM2 gangliosidoses (eg Tay Sachs & Sandhoff's diseases);** (4) **Leukodystrophies (eg Krabbe globoid cell leukodystrophy, metachromatic leukodystrophy** and multiple sulfatase deficiency) (5) **Lactosyl ceramidoses** and; (6) **Farber's disease.**
- **Wolman's disease and cholesteryl ester storage diseases are** not sphingolipidoses as these are a/w **accumulation of triglycerides & cholesterol esters (not sphingolipid/ ceramide).**
- **Multiple sclerosis** is a demyelinating disorder (not sphingolipidoses) in which the lipid composition of white matter resembles that of gray matter because of **loss of both phospholipids** (esp **ethanolamine plasmalogen) and of sphingolipids from white matter.** The CSF shows raised phospholipid levels.

Lysosomal Storage Diseases without

AR inheritance	Neurological involvement	Hepatospleenomegaly
- MPS II – Hunter - Fabry's disease ★ Both are *X-linked*	- MPS IV A, Morquio - MPS VI B, Morquio - MPS VI, Maroteaux- lamy - Cholesterylester storage disease - Gaucher's disease type I	- ***Tay- sach's disease***[Q] - ***Fabry's disease***[Q] - Mucolipidos is III; pseudo- Hurler polydystrophy - ***Krabbe's disease***[Q] - Metachromatic leukodystrophy ★ Cholestery ester storage disease (only hepatomegaly)

Skeletal involvement

- Tay- sach's disease
- Fabry disease
- Niemann- Pick disease, neuropathic type A
- Krabbe's disease
- Metachromatic leukodystrophy
- Wolman's disease
- Cholesteryl ester storage disease
- Farber disease

Opthalmologic involvement

- MPS III (Sanfilippo) A, B, C, D
- Gaucher's disease type I
- Fucosidosis
- β- Mannosidosis
- aspartyl glucosaminuria
- Krabbe's disease
- Wolman disease
- Cholesteryl ester storage disease

Hematological involvement

- GM_2 gangliosidoses (i.e. Tay Sach's & Sandhoff's disease)
- Fabry's disease
- Krabbe's disease
- Metachromatic leukodystrophy
- Disorders of neutral lipids (i.e. Wolman, Faber & cholesteryl ester storage disease)

★ Neurological involvement means mental retardation for all lysosomal storage diseases (LSD) except **Fabry disease** where it is in form of ***painful acroparesthesias (i.e. burning pain in lower extremities)***[Q]. And in *GM_2 gangliosidoses (Tay sach's & Sandhoff's disease), Niemann- Pick disease, β -Mannosidosis* and sialidosis (myoclonus), MR is associated with seizures.

★ In *all MPS and ML* opthalmological involvement, is in form of **corneal clouding** *except in MPS II, Hunter disease,* which causes *retinal degeneration.* And ML III, pseudo- Hurler polydystrophy also show mild retinopathy and hyperopic astigmatism along with corneal clouding. Retinal degeneration is also present in *multiple sulfatase deficiency*; and *macular degeneration* in *Farber disease* & Niemann – Pick disease A & B. Optic atrophy is seen in metachromatic leukodystrophy; corneal dystrophy & vascular lesions in Fabry disease. Cherry red spot is found in ***GM_2 gangliosidoses (Tay sach's & Sandhoff's disease), Sialidoses and, GM1 gangliosidoses***[Q].

Classification and Separation of Lipoproteins (Based on)

Electrophoretic mobility (Frederickson's Method)

- Lipoproteins are separated on their *charge/ size ratio.* Mostly on paper /agarose electrophoretic media.
- **Increasing order of electrophoretic mobility** towards charged (anode) end is

Lipoprotein	Migrate into
Chylomicron	***Do not migrate & remain at origin***[Q]
LDL (β-lipoprotein)	β- globulin region
VLDL (pre-β-lipoprotein)	Pre β-globulin region
HDL (α-lipoprotein)	α_1 globulin region

Density (SP unit) based ultracentrifugation (Gofman-Method)

- Increase in lipid /protein ratio decreases the density of lipoprotein and increase the floatation property of lipoprotein.
- Svedberg units of floatation (SF unit) is the rate at which lipoprotein floats through NaCl and is = 10^{-13} cm/S/dyne/g at 26°c
- In ultracentrifugation separation technique, only *the order of LDL & VLDL* is reversed (as compared to electrophoresis).

Chylomicron	**Floats** d/t lowest density
VLDL	
LDL	
HDL	Settles below d/t highest density

Apolipoproteins (Alaupovic Method)

Lipoprotein Family	Apolipo protein	Density class
A	A-I & AII	HDL
B	Apo B (B_{48} & B_{100})	LDL & VLDL
C	Apo CI, CII, CIII	LDL, VLDL & HDL
D	Apo-D	HDL_3
E	Apo E (arginine rich)	LDL, VLDL & HDL

	Chylomicron	VLDL	LDL	HDL
Triacylglycerol	90%	60%	8%	5%
Protein	2%	5%	20%	40%
Phospholipids	3%	15%	22%	30%
Cholesteral & Cesters	5%	20%	50%	25%

Liporoteins is composed of

Neutral Lipid are (Hydrophobic)	Surrounding shell (Hydrophillic)
- Triacylglycerol - Cholesterol and chlolesterol esters	- Proteins (Apolipoproteins) - Phospholipids - (Unesterified cholesterol)

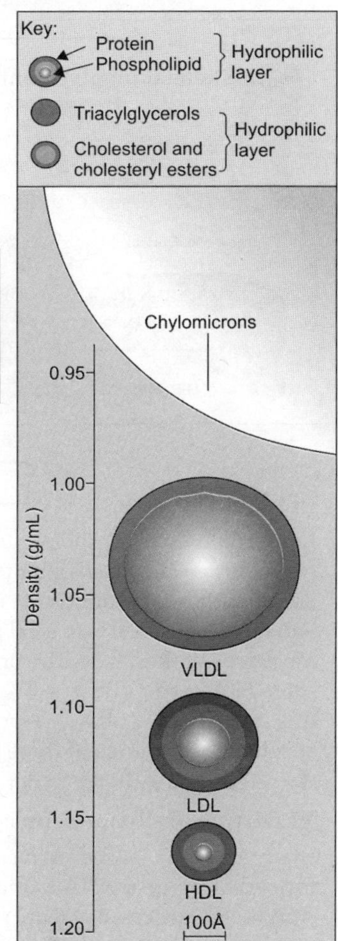

Approximate size and density of serum lipoproteins. Each family of lipoproteins exhibits a range of sizes and densities; this figure shows typical values [Note: The width of the rings approximates the amount of each component]

Chylomicrons & VLDL

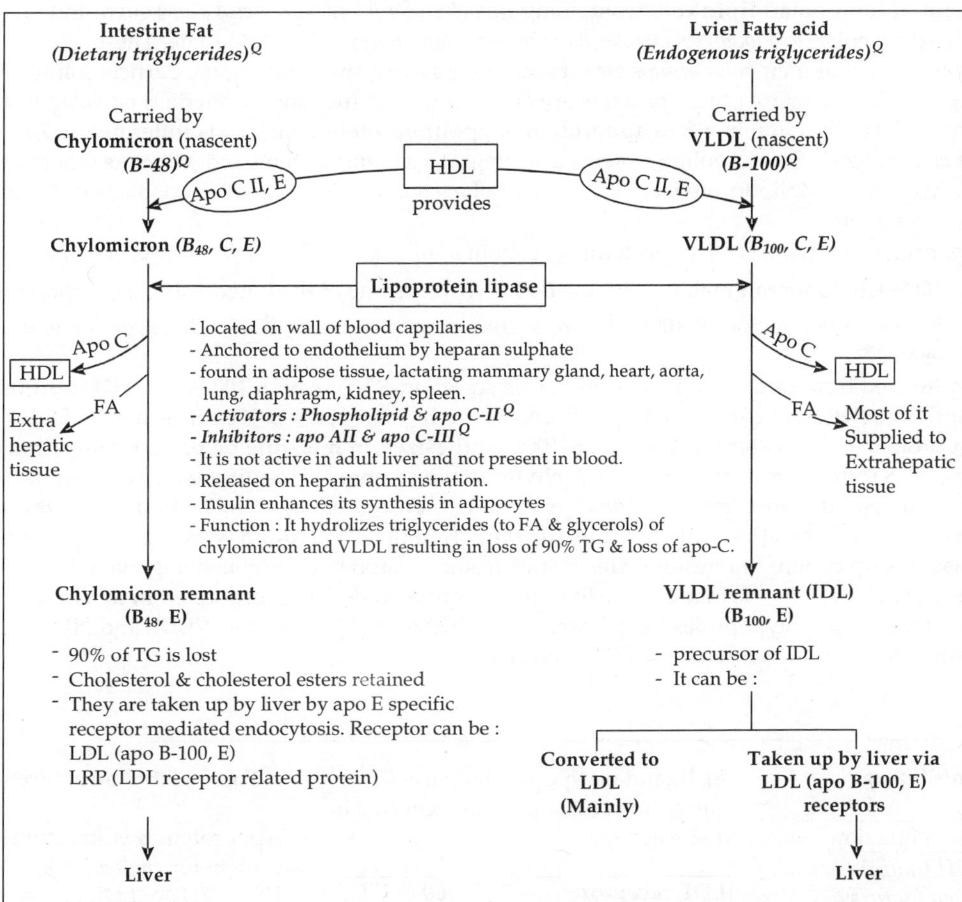

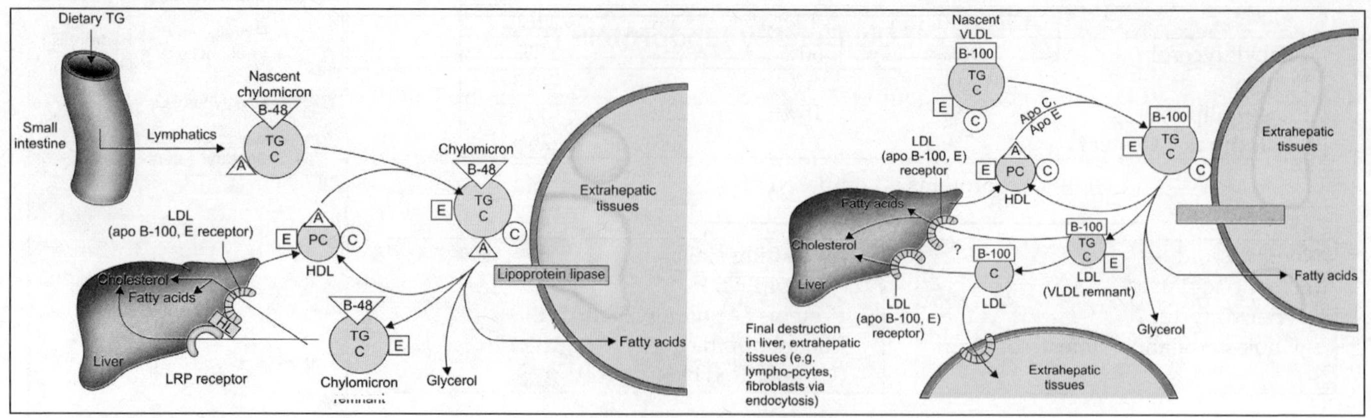

Apolipoprotein

- Lipoproteins are composed of **neutral (non-polar) lipid core** (containing *triacyl glycerol and cholesteryl ester*) surrounded by a *single surface layer shell* of **amphipathic** (polar) *apolipoproteins, phospholipids and nonesterified (free) cholesterol.* These amphipathic compounds are oriented so that their *polar groups are exposed on the surface*, thus making the particle soluble in aqueous solution. The triacyl glycerol & cholesterol of lipo proteins are either *exogenous* (obtained from diet) or *endogenous* (de novo synthesized). The protein part of lipoprotein is k/a **apoprotein** or **apolipoprotein** which constitutes nearly 70% of some HDL and as little as 1% of chylomicron. Some apolipoproteins are integral & cannot be removed, whereas others are free to transfer to other lipoproteins. Actual apolipoprotein & lipid content of each lipoprotein class is variable because of constant interchange of these between them.
- ***Apo AI & apo AII***[Q] are major apoproteins of **HDL (α-lipoprotein)**. The main apoprotein of **LDL (β – lipoprotein)** and **VLDL (pre β-lipoprotein)** is ***B-100***[Q]. **Chylomicron** mainly contains ***B- 48***[Q]. B-100 is one of the longest single polypeptide chain & is synthesized in liver, whereas, B-48 is 48% of B-100 d/t introduction of stop signal by RNA editing enzyme. It is formed by same mRNA but in intestine.
- Apo B-48 and Apo B-100 are synthesized from same Apo B gene and same ApoB- m-RNA. **Apo B 100 is a 100 KDa protein synthesized in liver by full length translation** of corresponding mRNA of Apo B gene. Apo – B-100 forms part of *LDL, IDL and VLDL*. **Apo B-48** is a 48 KDa protein (48% shorter form of Apo B-100) **synthesized in intestine by partial translation of same mRNA of Apo B gene**. Apo B 48 forms part of **chylomicron & chylomicron remnant**. This difference between the sizes of Apo B100 and Apo B48 occurs because **post transcriptional processing (editing)** of Apo B mRNA , **deaminates the cytidine (C) to uracil (U) in intestine** at 2153 position. After **cytidine deamination** the **CAA codon** (which codes **glutamine in liver**) becomes **UAA (nonsense or stop codon)** in intestine. This results in shorter apo B-48 protein being made in intestine (and incorporated into chylomicron) than is made in the liver full length Apo B-100, incorporated in to VLDL.
- **Apoprotein C –I, C- II and C- III** are smaller polypeptides freely transferable between chylomicrons, VLDL and HDL. **Apoprotein E** is found in chylomicron, chylomicron remnant, HDL and IDL.
- Functions of apoproteins are

Enzyme cofactors / inhibitors

Enzyme	Apoprotein function
Lipoprotein lipase	- ***Apo-CII (main) & CI are co factors***[Q] - ***Apo AII & apo C III are inhibitors***[Q]
Lecithin: cholesterol acyl transferase (LCAT)	Apoprotein **AI** is **cofactor**
Cholesteryl ester transfer protein	Apo – **CI** is inhibitor

As ligand on lipoprotein particle for interaction with liprotein receptors in tissue eg.

LDL receptor	***B-100 & E***[Q]
LDL receptor related protein (LRP) or remnant receptor	APo-E
HDL receptor	Apo AI

Form part of structure

- Apoprotein **B** is structural protein for *chylomicron, VLDL, IDL & LDL*
- Apoprotein **AI** is structural protein for *HDL.*

★ LCAT is also a part of HDL

Low Density Lipoprotein (LDL)

- It is derived **from VLDL** (after going through **IDL stage**) by *loss of triacyl glycerol.*
- Each LDL paricle ***contain a single apo B-100 molecule***Q and is derived from single VLDL precursor
- It has ***highest cholesterol and cholesteryl ester content***Q. It transports 70% of total cholesterol
- The *primary function of LDL particle is to provide cholesterol to peripheral tissues* (or return it to liver).
- Cholesterol in LDl is called **bad cholesterol** because it is transported to arteries, where it is oxidized by free radicals and retained in arterial proteoglycans starting the formation of ***atherosclerotic plaques. So it increases risk of coronary artery disease***Q, stroke and peripheral vascular disease.
- While there is growing consensus that ***levels of apolipoprotein (apo) B and the ratio of apo B/apo- AI*** are more accurate predictors of CVD risk but it will take time before apoprotein terminology is recognized by general public & recommended by National cholesterol Education program. Till then it may be more efficacious to continue adhering to already familiar & proven measurements of ***LDL-cholesterol / HDL- cholesterol ratio.***

- It is measured indirectly by using *Friedewald equation* i.e.
  1. LDL cholesterol (in mg/dl) = Total cholesterol – HDL cholesterol – (0.20 x Triglycerides)
  2. LDL cholesterol (in mmol/l) = Total cholesterol – HDL cholesterol – (0.45 x Triglycerides)
- American Heart Association guide lines (2003) for fasting LDL cholesterol levels & risk of CAD

LDL Fasting Level		**CAD Risk**
Mg/dL	Mmol/L	
<100	< 2.6	Optimal LDL, corresponding to reduced but not zero risk
100-129	2.6-3.3	Near optimal LDL
130-159	3.3-4.1	Borderline High LDL
160-189	4.1-4.9	High LDL level
>190	>4.9	Very high LDL, corresponding to highest risk of heart disease

LDL (apo B 100, and apo E) Receptors

- **Liver** and many **extrahepatic tissues** express the ***negatively charged glycoprotein LDL (apo B-100, E) receptors***Q on the *cell membrane in depressed coated pits* that are coated on cytosolic side with a protein called **clathrin** (which stabilizes the shape of pit)
- It is so designated because it is ***specific for apo B-100 but not B-48***Q, which lacks the carboxy terminal domain of B-100 containing the LDL receptor ligand, and it ***also takes up lipoproteins rich in apo E***Q.
- So these receptors can take up LDL, VLDL remnant (i.e IDL), and chylomicron remnant. The LDL is metabolized via LDL receptor. Approximately 30% of LDL is degraded in extrahepatic tissue and 70% in liver.
- The glycoprotein LDL receptor spans the membrane, the B100 binding region being at the exposed amino terminal end. After binding , ***LDL is take up intact with receptor by endocytosis***Q. The vesicle containing LDL loses its clathrin coat & fuses wit similar vesicles, forming larger vesicles called **endosomes**. The pH of endosomes fall d/t proton pumping activity of **endosomal ATPase** which allows separation of LDL from its receptor. The receptor migrates to one side of endosome, whereas LDL stays free within the lumen of vesicle. This structure is called **CURL – Compartment for uncoupling of Receptor & Ligand**. This leads to

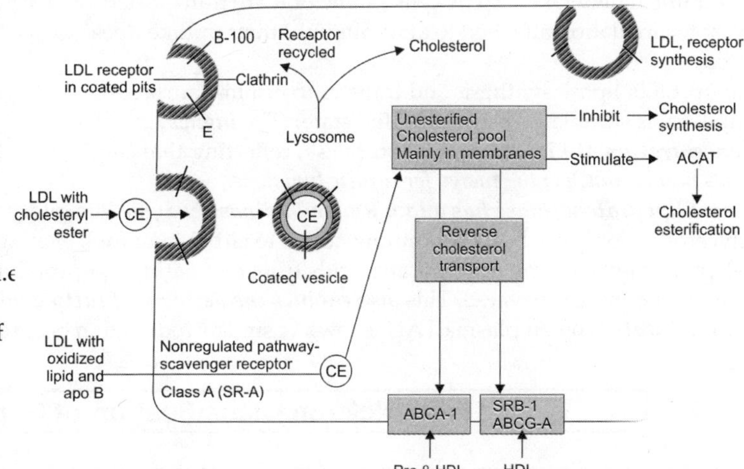

Hydrolysis of apoprotein and cholesteryl esters (present in LDL) **in lysosome** and ***translocation of cholesterol into the cells***Q

LDL receptors are **recycled** back to the cell surface

This influx of cholesterol inhibits cholesterol synthesis and uptake by

- *Inhibiting transcription of genes encoding HMG CoA synthase, HMG CoA reductase* & other enzymes involved in cholesterol synthesis
- ***Inhibiting synthesis (replenishment/recruitment or transcription) of new LDL receptors***Q via SREBP (sterol regulatory element binding protein) pathway, thus decreasing their number in plasma membrane

Because cholesterol is esterified by **ACAT** ***(acetyl CoA-cholesterol acyl transferase), cholesterol influx stimulates ACATactivity promoting cholesterol esterification***Q

- ***LDL receptor is defective***Q in *familial hyper cholesterolemia*, a genetic condition which increases blood LDL cholesterol levels and ***cause premature atherosclerosis and coronary artery disease (CAD)***Q.

Lipoprotein Lipase (LL)

- It is an *extracellular enzyme* that is located on capillary walls, anchored to *endothelium by negatively charged proteioglycan chains of heparan sulfate.*
- It is *not normally found in blood*; however following *heparin injection*, LL is released from its heparan sulfate binding sites into circulation.
- Lipoprotein lipase is found in capillaries of most tissues but ***predominantly in adipose tissue, cardiac & skeletal muscles, lactating mammary glands***Q, and also in spleen, lung, renal medulla, aorta and diaphragm. ***Adult liver does not have this enzyme***Q (Lippincot) / It is not active in liver - *Harper*
- Hepatic lipase , bound to sinusoidal surface of liver cells, does not significantly attack chylomicrons or VLDL triacylglycerol, but rather is involved in chylomicron remnant and HDL metabolism. It is also released by heparin.
- ***Triacyl glycerols (TAG) of chylomicron and VLDL are hydrolyzed by lipoprotein lipase***Q, progressively through diacyl glycerol to mono acyl glycerol and finally to free fatty acids and glycerol. ***Both phospholipids & apo CII are required as cofactors for LL activity, while apo A II and apo CIII act as inhibitors***Q.
- The formed fatty acids are stored (by adipocyte) & used for energy (by cardiac & skeletal muscles, and renal cortex). And if not immediately taken up by cells , some of it are transported back to circulation attached to albumin until their uptake does occur.
- Lipoprotein lipase synthesis and transfer to luminal surface of capillary is stimulated by insulin (fed state). The ***highest concentration of LL is in cardiac muscles***Q, reflecting that *fatty acids provide much of the energy for cardiac functions.* 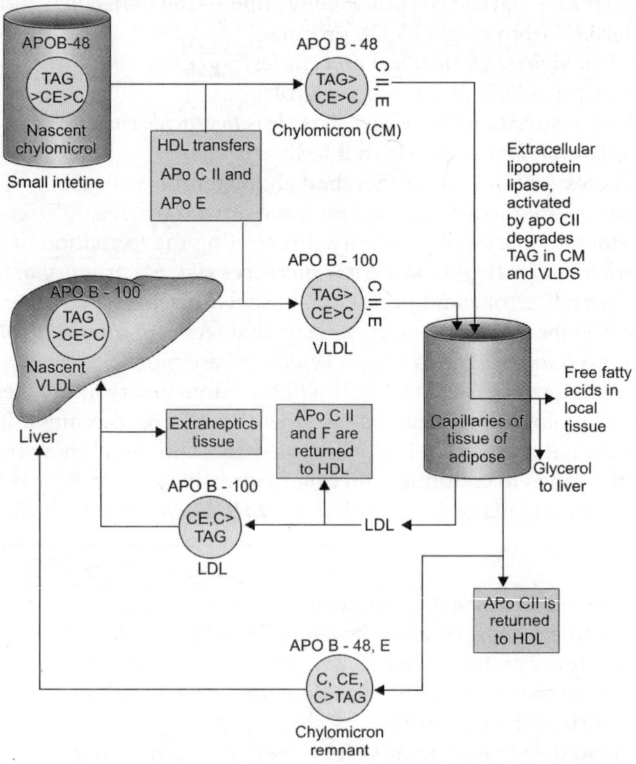
- ***Heart lipoprotein lipase has a low Km and adipose enzyme has a large Km***Q (about 10 times more than heart LL) for triacyl glycerol. This allows heart continuing access to circulating fuel, even when plasma lipoprotein concentrations are low whereas, *adipocytes* can remove fatty acids from circulating lipoproteins and store them as TAG only when lipoprotein concentrations are elevated. This also ***enables the delivery of fatty acids to be redirected from adipose tissue to heart in starved state***Q (when plasma TAG is low). A similar redirection occurs in **lactating mammary glands** for milk synthesis.

Frederickson Classification of Hyperlipoproteinemias

Type	Name	Basic defect	Elevated lipoprotein	Electrophoretic classification	Triglycerides	VLDL (pre β)	LDL (β)	HDL (α)	Cholesterol	Refrigeration test	Clinical feature
I	**Familial lipoprotein lipase deficiency /chylomicronemia syndrome**	- ***LPL deficiency***Q - Abnormal LPL - ***Apo C-II deficiency***Q causing inactive LPL	***Chylomicrons***Q	Hyper chylomicronaemia	↑	↑	↓	↓	Normal	Creamy layer, infranate clear or slightly turbid (Lactescent)	- Erruptive xanthomas - Pancreatitis - Autosomal recessive - ***No atherosclerosis***Q
IIa	**Familial hyper cholesterolemia/defective apo B /sitosterolemia**	- ***Defective LDL receptor***Q - Mutation is apo-B 100, PCSK-9, ABCG8, - ABCG S & ARH	***↑LDL & hypercholesterolemia***Q	Hyper β-lipoproteinemia (heavy βband)	Normal (-) or ↑	↑ (may be)	↑ -	-	↑ -	Clear (yello orange tint)	- Tendon tuberous xanthomas - Coronary & peripheral atherosclerosis - ***Autosomal dominant***Q - No pancreatitis

IIb	**Familial combined hyperlipidemia**	Unknown	*LDL & VLDL*Q	Heavy β and pre β band	N	↑	↑	-	N or ↑	Clear to slightly turbid	- Coronary & peripheral atherosclerosis - No pancreatitis & no xanthoma
III	**Familial dysbetalipoproteinemia/Broad β disease / Remnant removal disease**	- ***Abnormality in apo E***Q	***Chylomicron & VLDL remnants of density <1.019 (*** *(β – VLDL)*Q	**Broad β** lipoproteinaemia **(Broad floating β band)**	↑	↑	↓	-	↑Q	Turbid to opaque with thin clear layer	- Palmar tuberoeruptive Xanthomas - Coronary & peripheral atherosclerosis - Autosomal dominant - No pancreatitis
IV	**Familial hyper triacylglycerolemia**	- Over production of VLDL often with glucose intolerance & hyperinsulinemia - Un known /Apo A-V	*VLDL*Q with cholesterol rise and HDL & LDL tend to be subnormal	Hyper pre β lipoproteinaemia	↑	↑	↓	↓	↑	Turbid to opaque	- Autosomal dominant - Commonly associated with coronary heart disease, type II diabetes mellitus, obesity, alcoholism & administration of progestational hormones - No pancreatitis & no xanthoma
V	**Familial hyper triacylglycerolemia**	- Apo A – V / unknown	*Chylomicron & VlDL*Q	Heavy (hyper) chylomicron & pre β bands	↑	↑	↓	↓	↑	Creamy layer infranate turbid to opaque (Lactescent)	- Autosomal dominant - Eruptive xanthomas - pancreatitis

★ ***Normal TG's in 2 & ↑ed s. cholesterol in 2,3***Q

	Abetalipoproteinemia	**Dysbetalipoproteinemia**
Pathogenesis	Caused by *mutation* in the gene encoding *microsomal triglyceride transfer protein (MTP)*, this prevent loading of apo – B with lipid & there is ***defective synthesis or secretion of Apo- B***Q	Is due to ***defective form of apoprotein E***Q. [Apo- E plays a crucial role in the catabolism of chylomicron and VLDL.]
Lipoprteins level	Absent / ***↓Chylomicron***Q Absent / ***↓VLDL***Q Absent / ***↓LDL***Q	***↑Chylomicron remnant***Q ***↑VLDL remnant***Q LDL normal
Plasma lipid abnormalities	*Low cholesterol*Q (d/t decreased LDL) *Low TG,s*Q (d/t decreased chylomicron & VLDL)	**Increased TG's (mainly)**Q ***Increased VLDL cholesterol***Q
Clinical features	- ***Malabsorption of fat***Q - Early childhood diarrhea & failure to thrive. - ***Neuropathy***Q - ***Spinocerebellar degeneration (Ataxia)***Q - ***Retinitis pigmentosa***Q - ***Acanthocytosis***Q	- ***Tuberous xanthoma***Q - Deposition of cholesterol in palmar creases ***(striae palmaris)***Q - ***Risk for atherosclerosis***Q & its complication is increased
Treatment	- Vitamin E - Low fat, High caloric diet	• Drugs:- HMG COA reductase inhibitor - Febrates, Niacin - Estrogen replacement therapy (In postmeno – pausal women) • Low – cholesterol, low fat diet

Cholesterol: Structure, Esterification & Transport

- **Sterols** are structural lipids present in the membranes of most eukaryotic cells. It has **steroid nucleus**, consisting of 4 fused rings, 3 with 6 carbons and 1 with 5 carbons. The steroid nucleus is almost planar and is relatively rigid; the fused ring do not allow rotation about C-C bonds.
- **Cholesterol**, the **major sterol of animal tissues**, is amphipathic, with a polar head (OH group at C3) and a non polar hydrocarbon body (steroid nucleus & hydrocarbon side chain at C-17) about as long as a 16 carbon fatty acid in its extended form.
- Plants have **stigmasterol** & fungi have **ergosterol.** Bacteria cannot synthesize sterols. The sterols of all eukaryotes are synthesized from 5 carbon **isoprene subunits**, as are **fat soluble vitamins**, **quinones** and **dolichols**
- **Cholesterol** is the *most important steroid (sterol)* and precursor of all other steroids in body eg: - Corticosteroids, Sex hormones, ***Bile acid***[Q], ***Vitamin D***[Q].
- Cholesterol occurs in body as **free form** (that exchanges readily between tissues & liproproteins) and **ester form.** Of the cholesterol absorbed, 80-90% in the lymph is **esterified with long chain fatty acids** (to form cholesterol ester). Esterified form is transported as lipoproteins & is not readily exchangeable and used for storage also. ***Highest proportion of circulating cholesterol is found in LDL (beta lipoproteins) which takes cholesterol to tissue & also in HDL which carry it from tissues to liver for degradation (scavanger)***[Q].
- **Esterfication of cholesterol**: Cholesterol may be combined with long chain FA such as Linoleic acid (50%), Oleic acid (18%), Palmitic acid (11%), Arachidonic acid (5%), and other fatty acid (16%).

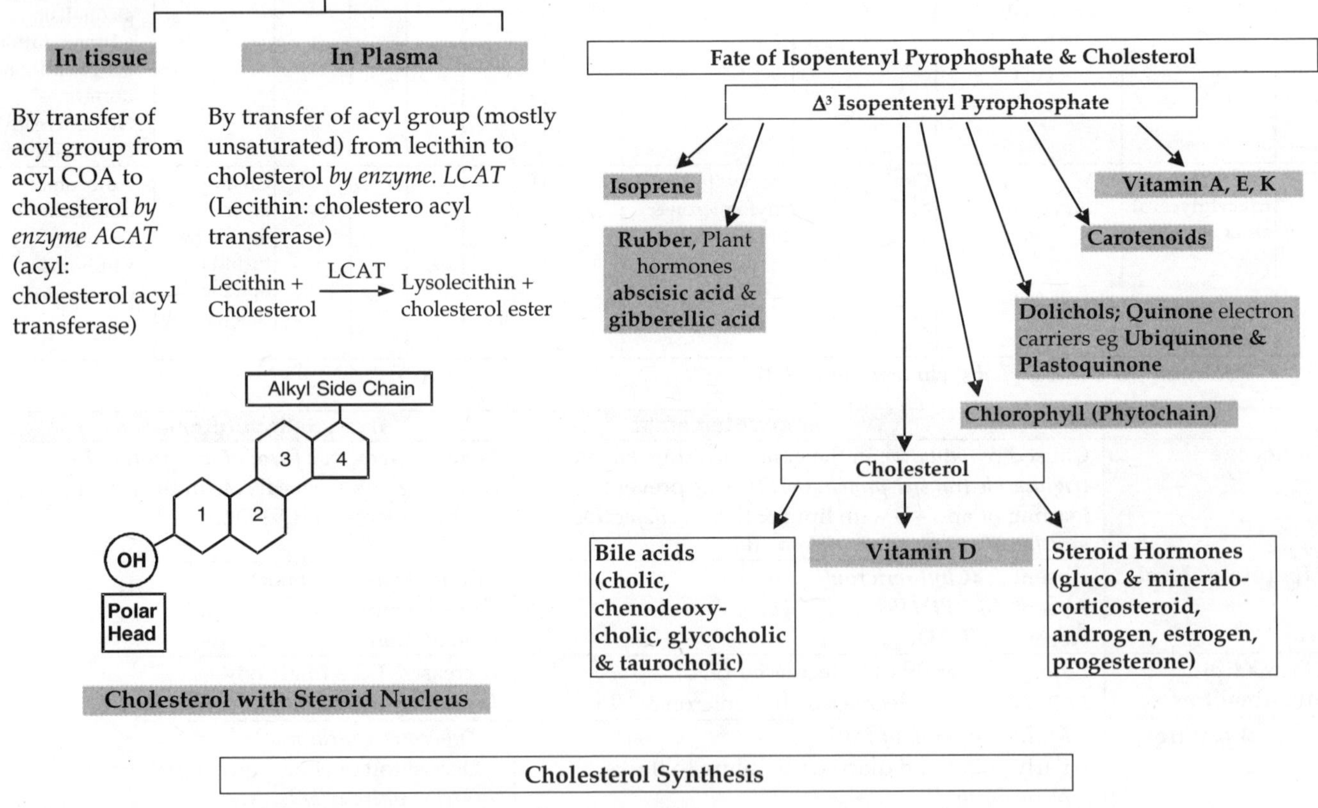

Cholesterol Synthesis

- Sir **John Cornforth** & **Vladimir Prelog** described synthetic pathway and received Nobel Prize (1975).
- Cholesterol is synthesized in **liver, adrenal cortex, testes, ovaries & intestine. Although all nucleated cells** can synthesize cholesterol, including arterial walls. Enzymes for cholesterol synthesis are partly located in **endoplasmic reticulum (ER)** and partly in **cytoplasm**.
- ***Acetyl CoA is the starting material & source of all carbon atoms in cholesterol***[Q]. The synthesis can be divided into 5 steps.

1. Synthesis of Mevalonate

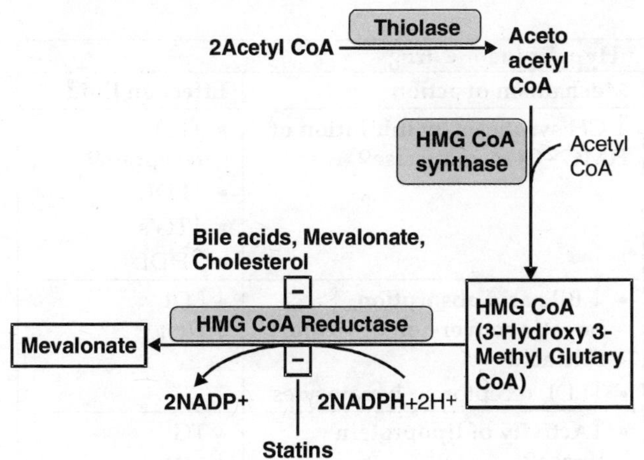

Cholesterol synthesis is controlled by ***regulation of HMG COA reductase, which is a rate limiting enzyme***[Q]**.**

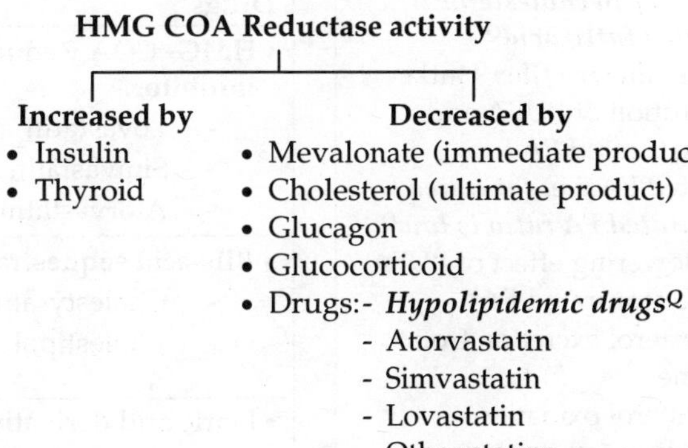

2. Formation of Isoprenoid units by loss of CO_2

Mevalonate is phosphorylated sequentially using ATP by **3 kinases (mevalonate, 5 phospho mevalonate & 5 diphosphomevalonate kinase)** and then decarboxylated by 3, 5 diphospho mevalonate decarboxylase to form **5 carbon atom active isoprenoid unit (ie isopentenyl diphosphate).**

3. Condensation of 6 Isprenoid units form Squaline

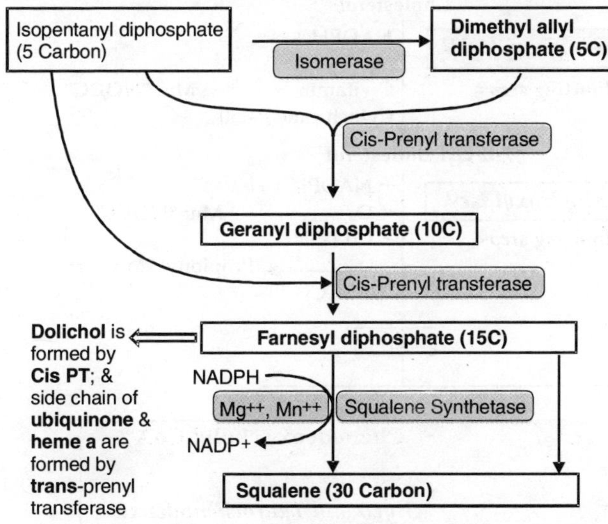

4. Formation of parental steroid, Lanosterol by Cylization of Squalene

Endoplasmic reticulum enzyme, squalene epoxidase converts squalene to squalene 2,3 epoxide by transferring methyl group on C14 to C13 and on C8 to C14. **Ring closure (cyclization)** is catabolize by **oxidosqualene-lanosterol cyclase** to form lanosterol.

5. Formation Cholesterol (in ER membrane)

Methyl groups on C_{14} & C_4 are removed to form **14 desmethyl lanosterol** & then **zymosterol**; The double bond, between C_8-C_9 is remove to C_5-C_6 in 2 steps forming $\Delta^{7,24}$ Cholestadienol and then **desmosterol (24-dehydrocholesterol)**. The double bond of side chain is reduced to finally produce cholesterol by **Δ^{24} reductase** (enzyme inhibited by **triparanol**).

Measures to Lower Blood Cholesterol (CH)

Dietary alteration

- Diet *lower in cholesterol & saturated fatty acid*[Q]
- *Increase dietery fiber*[Q] intke
- Substitution of PUFA and monosaturated FA for saturated FA. i.e. *saturated / unsaturated FA ratio is low*[Q].
- Lipid lowering effect of PUFA (Poly Unsaturated FA):
  - ↑cholesterol excretion from intestine
  - ↑cholesterol oxidation (catabolism to bile acid)
  - LDL receptor upregulation.

Hypolipidemic drugs

Drugs	Mechanism of action	Effect on lipid
• **HMG- COA Reductase inhibitor** - Lovastatin - Simvastatin - Atorvastatin	**↓ CH synthesis by inhibition of HMG –COA reductase**[Q]	• **↑LDL receptors**[Q] • ↓LDL • ↓TG's • ↑HDL
• **Bile acid sequestrant** - Cholestyramine - Cholestipol	• **↓ Bile acid absorption, ↑ hepatic conversion of CH to bile acid**[Q] • ↑LDL receptor on hepatocytes	↓ LDL ↑ HDL
• Fibric acid derivatives - Gemfibrozil	• **↑Activity of lipoprotein lipase**[Q] • ↓ release of FA from adipose tissue	↓ TG ↓ LDL ↑ HDL
• **Nicotinic acid**	• ***↓Lipolysis in adipocytes***[Q] • ↓ Production of VLDL	↓ LDL ↓ TG's ↑ HDL

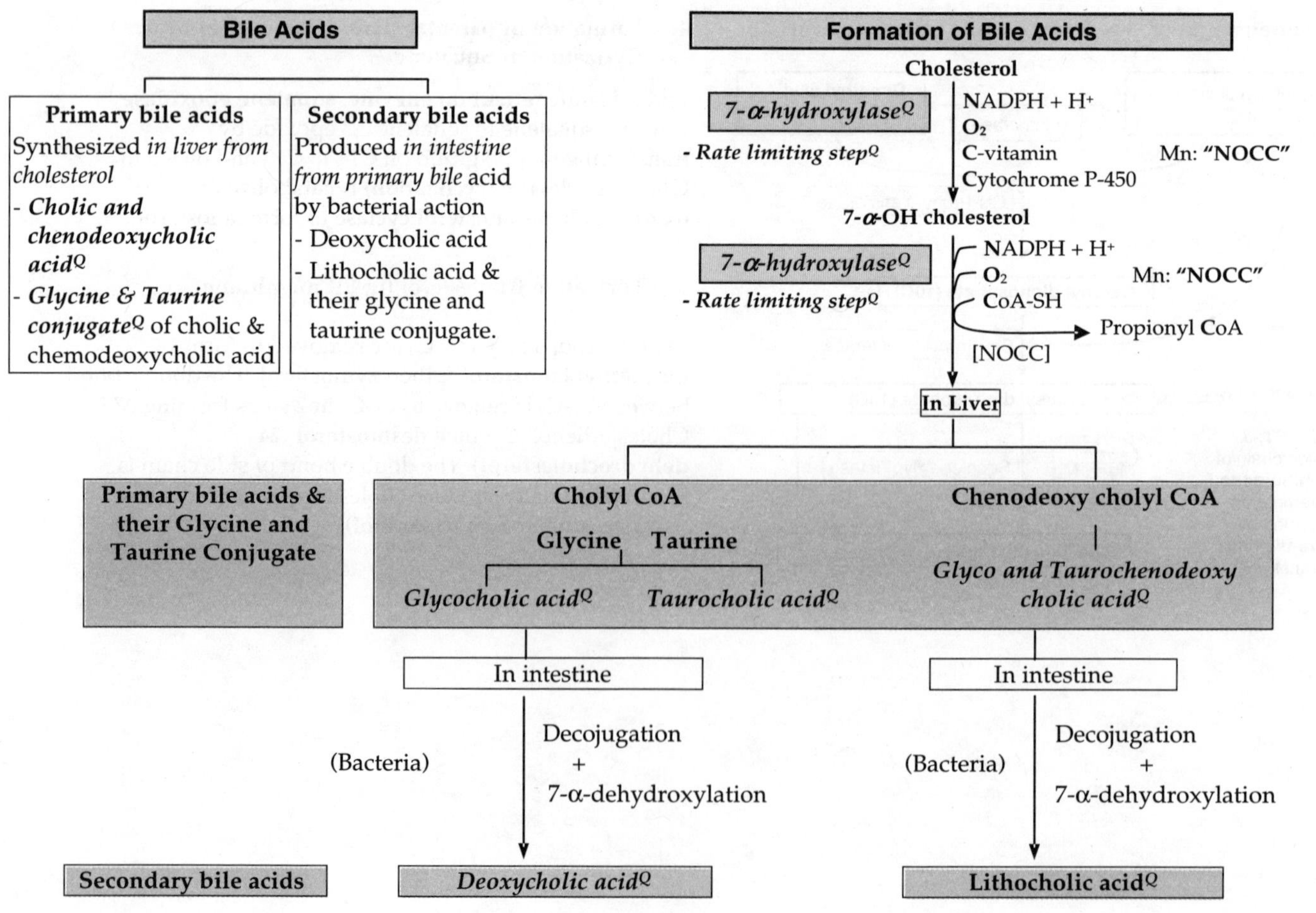

De Novo Fatty Acid Synthesis

- Fatty acid synthesis requires

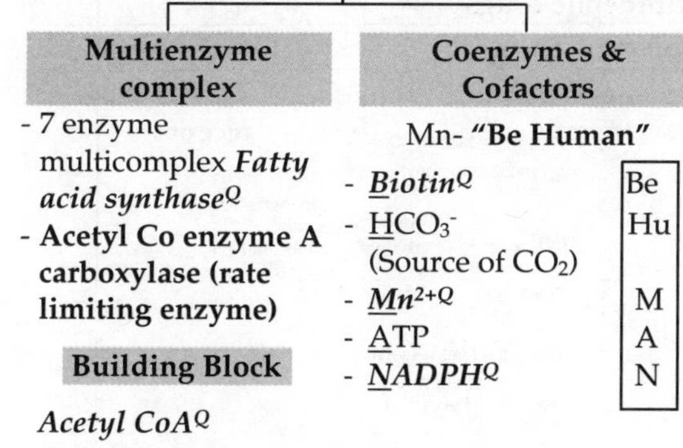

- This takes place in cytosol. ***Acetyl Co enzyme A***Q is *primer (starting material)* for formation of *palmitic acid (palmitate C_{16} fatty acid)*. ***Propionyl CoA*** acts as primer for synthesis of *long chain* fatty acid having an *odd number* of carbon atoms.
- ***Ist** and **rate limiting step** is **formation of malonyl from acetyl CoA***Q in presence of ***acetyl CoA carboxylase***Q by fixation of CO_2 (so called *CO_2 fixation reaction*.)

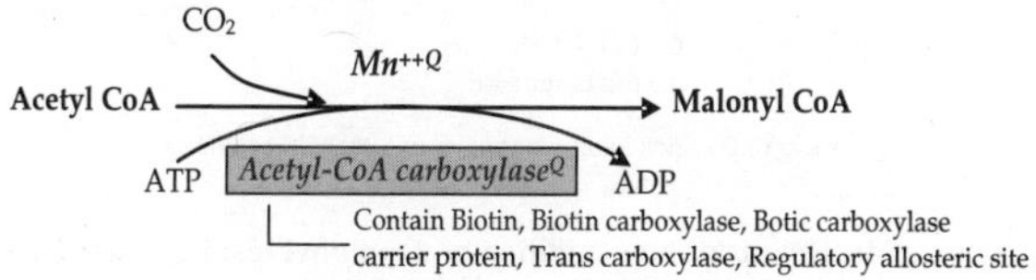

* This is a ***rate limiting irreversible reaction***Q

* **Citrate** is an *activator* and **palmityl CoA** is *inhibitor* of enzyme

Fatty Acid Synthesis

Once malonyl CoA is synthesized rest of fatty acid synthesis reaction takesplace with FA synthase complex. Now *Acetyl CoA binds to cys –SH end of KAS (unit I) and malonyl CoA binds to Pan-SH end of ACP (unit II)* The *coenzyme A is removed* from both of these and *Acetyl (acyl) – malonyl enzyme* is formed This whole reaction is catalyzed by enzyme transacylase.

↓

Now, the acetate attacks malonate (that means acetyl group from Cys-SH site is shifted to malonyl group of Pan-SH site) to form 'aceto – acyl- ACP'. As Aceto acetate is attached to pan – SH of monomer II, Cys – SH of monomer I becomes free. This is a ***condensation reaction*** catalyzed by

Fatty Acid Synthase Complex 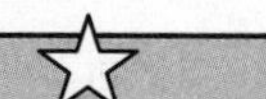

- It is a polypeptide containing 7 *enzyme activities* – Harper
- It is a multienzyme complex, made up of an ellipsoid dimer of identical polypeptide monomeric units arranged in head to tail fashion. Each monomeric unit contains *six enzymes & an ACP molecule (Acyl carrier protein) – Chaterjae.*
- It is functional only when the two monomeric units are in association with each other. Order of enzyme from end to end in each monomeric unit is.

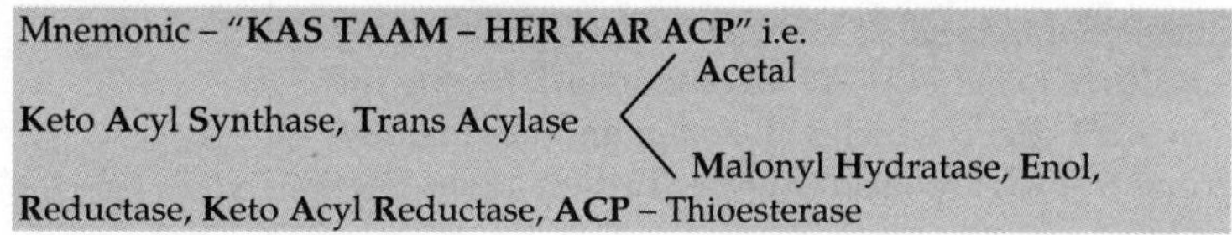

- Active sites of enzyme

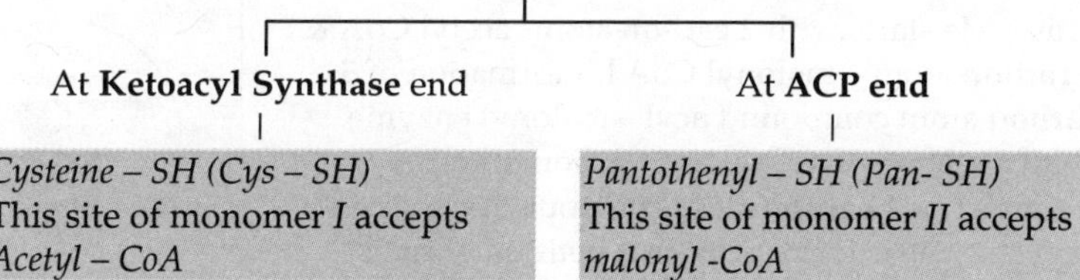

Mnemonic- "**Ist AC of IInd PM**" i.e. Monomer **I** accepts **A**cetyl CoA & has **C**ys – SH active site; Monomer **II** has **P**an-SH active site & accepts **M**alonyl CoA.

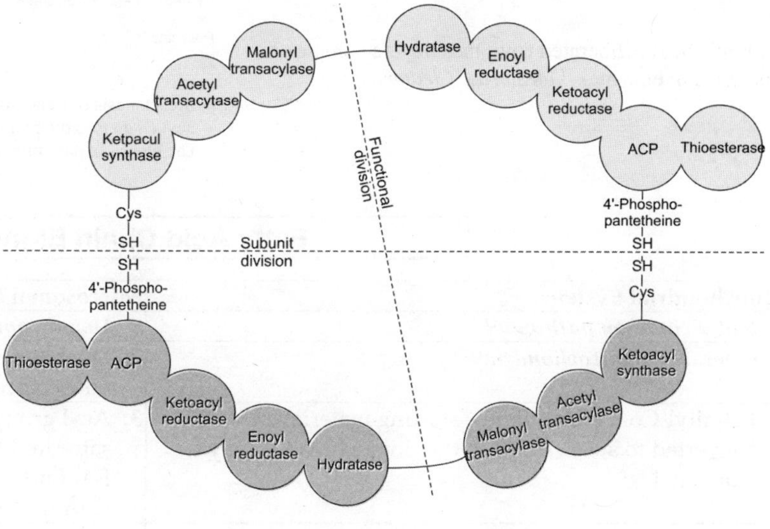

condensing enzyme – ketoacyl synthase. There is ***loss of one molecule of CO_2***

↓

Now aceto- acetate (or 3- ketoacyl group) undergoes ***reduction, dehydration and reduction*** again, catalyzed by ketocyl reductase, Hydratase an enoyl recuctase respectively, to ultimately form *saturated acyl – S- enzyme.* All the above three reactions occur *on Pan-SH of monomer II.*

Once *saturated acyl – S – enzyme* is formed; it is now *transferred to the 'cys –SH'* of monomer I, ***freeing the Pan – SH site***[Q]. (which will accept another malonyl group in each cycle, adding two carbon atoms per cycle)

This cycle starts with **2 carbon** atom- acetyl CoA & **3 carbon** atom – malonyl CoA l/t formation of **5 carbon** atom compound acyl – malonyl enzyme. With a release of CO_2 (i.e. **1 Carbon atom**) ultimately a **4 carbon** atom compound, saturated acyl enzyme is formed. With repetition of each cycle 3 carbon atoms are added (in form of malonyl CoA) and 1 carbon atom is released (in form of CO_2); thus resulting in ***addition of 2 carbon atom in each cycle***[Q]. So after 7 cycles ***(1 first + 6 repetitions = 4+ 6x2 = 16C)***[Q]
Palmitic acid (16 – C compound) is formed.

Palmitic acid is liberated from the enzyme complex by the seventh enzyme- *thioesterase (deacylase)*

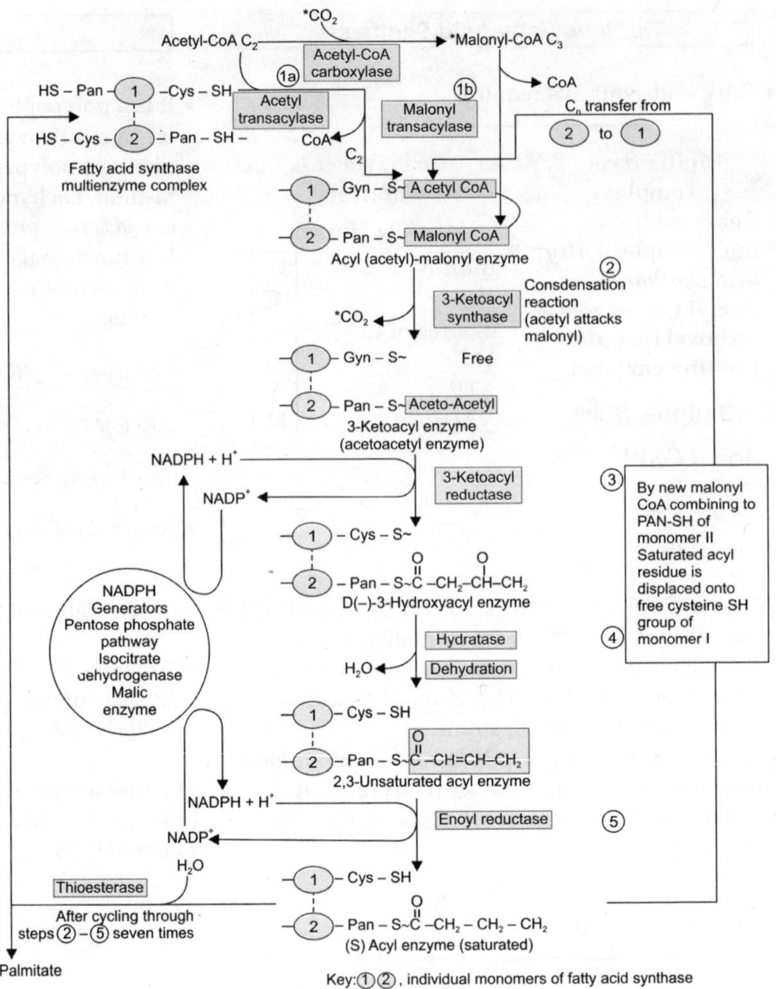

Biosynthesis of long-chain fatty acids. Details of how addition of a malonyl residue causes the acyl chain to grow by two carbon atoms. (Cys, cysteine residue; Pan, 4'-phosphopantetheine). The blocks in dark blue contain initially a C2 unit derived from acetyl-CoA (as illustrated) and subsequently the Co unit formed in reaction 5.

Fatty Acid Chain Elongation

Mitochondrial System	Microsomal System
1. ***Not a common pathway***[Q]	1. ***Usual common pathway for chian elongation***[Q]
2. Operates in ***mitochondria***[Q]	2. Operates in "microsomal" system. Chain elongation of FA takes place in ***endoplasmic reticulum (ER)***[Q]
3. Palmityl-CoA is usually the starting material and converted to stearyl-CoA. Other long-chain FA may be elongated.	3. Acyl group that may acts as "Primer" molecule; May be saturated FA series from C10 to C16 and some unsaturated C18 FA. End-product is next higher homologue of the 'Primer' acyl-CoA molecule.
4. ***Operates under "anaerobic" conditions. It is favoured by a high NADH/NAD⁺ ratio in cells***[Q]. Also in presence of excessive ethanol oxidation in liver.	4. ***Requires presence of O_2***[Q]
5. Acetyl-CoA (two carbon unit) is directly incorporated into the palmityl CoA molecule	5. Acetyl moiety (two carbon) is added through Malonyl CoA and not directly by incorporating C-2 units.
6. NADPH is required which is provided by HMP shunt.	6. NADPH is required as a reductant provided by HMP shunt.
7. ***Pyridoxal-P is required as a coenzyme***[Q] of the "condensing enzyme" in the first reaction to incorporate C-2 unit.	7. ***Pyridoxal-P is not required***[Q]

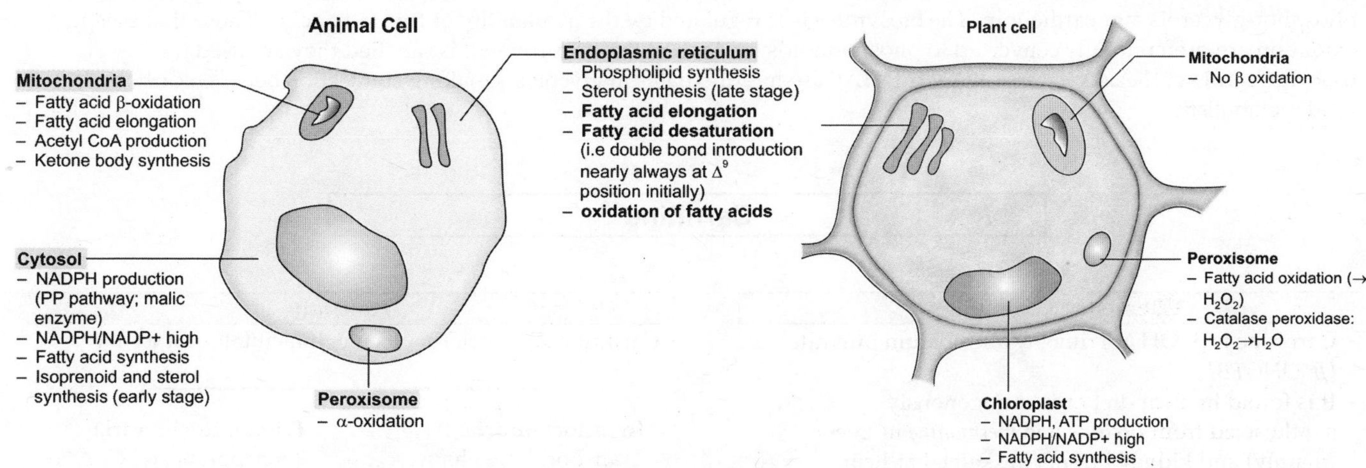

Triacyl Glycerol and Phosphoglycerol Synthesis

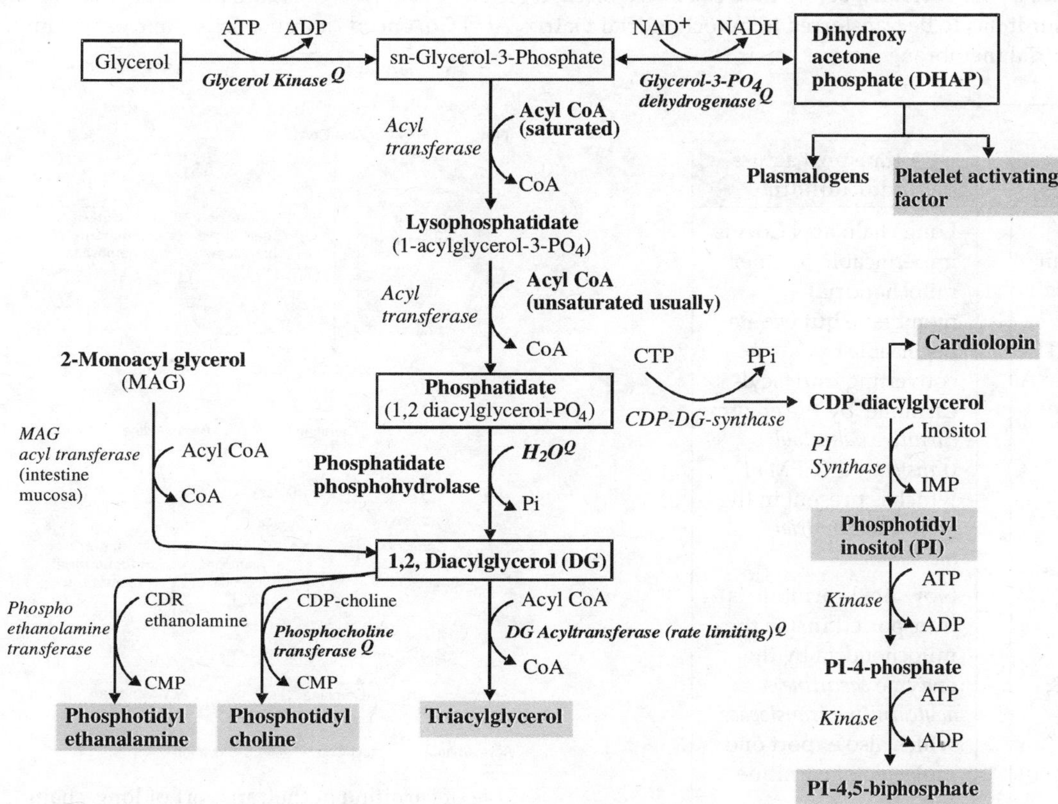

- So **2 molcules of acyl CoA,** combines with **glycerol 3 PO_4** to form phosphatidate in two steps catalyzed by glycerol 3 PO_4 acyltransferase and 1 acylglycerol-3-PO_4 acyl transferase. ***Phosphatidate is hydrolyzed by phosphorylase into 1, 2 diacyl glycerol***Q. **Diacyl glycerol acyl transferase, *rate limiting enzyme,* catalyzes the *only step specific for triacyl glycerol synthesis.***
- Choline & ethanolamine are first activated by *ATP phosphorylation followed by CTP linkage* to form CDP – choline or CDP – ethanolamine which reacts with 1, 2 – diacylglycerol to form either phosphotidyl choline or phosphotidylethanol-amine. Phosphotidyl serine is formed from phosphotidyl ethanolamine by reaction with serine, and decarboxylation reverses the reaction. In liver phosphotidyl ethanolamine gives rise to phosphotidyl choline by methylation.

- These are formed by acylation of triose phosphates; and **phosphatidate** is the common precursor of triacylglycerols, many phosphor-glycerols and cardiolipin. The biosynthesis is regulated by the availability of free fatty acids. Those that escape oxidation are preferentially converted to phospholipids, and when this requirement is satisfied they are used for triacylglycerol synthesis. Glycerol 3 PO_4 & DHAP are intermediates in glycolysis making connection between carbohydrate & lipid metabolism.

Carnitine

Chemistry & Synthesis

- Carnitine is β- OH Y Trimethy ammonium butyrate *[β- OHGTB]*
- It is found in meat diet or is endogenously synthesized from ***lysine***Q and *methionine* in liver (mainly) and kidney but not in skeletal or heat muscles.
- Skeletal muscle contains about *97% of all carnitine* in body.

Functions

Carnitine is a carrier molecule. It facilitates transpost

In mitochondria
Transport long chain acyl – CoA in mitochondria for β-oxidation

From mitochondria
Transport acetyl CoA & acetoacetyl Co from mitochondria to cytosol

Fatty acids must be first activated before they can be oxidizedQ. 'Active' FA (acyl – CoA) are formed in cytosol and for β-oxidation to occur it has to be transferred to mitochondrial matrix. Acyl CoA needs a transport system as it is impermeable to inner mitochondrial membrane.

FA activation	FA transport across mitochondria
- Fatty acid is converted to an *'active fatty acid' or acyl CoA* in presence of ATP and co enzyme A by the enzyme acyl – CoA *synthetase (thiokinase).* - Acy- CoA synthetase is present in endoplasmic reticulum, peroxisomes & mitochondria (inside & on outer membrane) - This is the ***only step in FA degradation where ATP is used & form AMP***Q.	- Long chain acyl CoA is impermeable to inner mitochondrial membrane but bcome permeable by converting into 'acyl-carnitine' by the enzyme *carnitine palmitoyl transferase 1* (CPMT1) which is present in the *outer mtochondrial membrane.* - Now Acyl carnitine is transported inside the mitochondria by the enzyme *carnitine – acylcarnitine translocase* which also export one molecule of carnitine out. - Acyl – carnitine is converted to acyl CoA in mitochondrial matrix by *Carnitine palmtoyl transfase II* (CPMT-2) located on the *inner membrane*

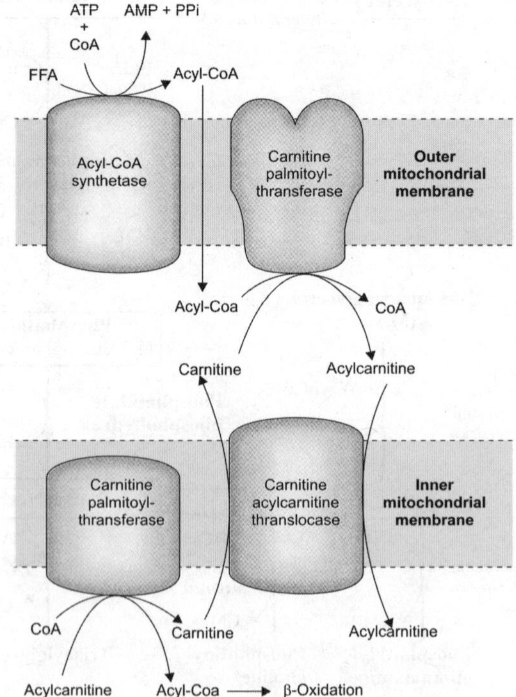

Role of carnitine in thetransport of long-chain faty acids through the inner mitochondrial membrane. Long-chain acyl-CoA cannot pass through the inner mitochondrial membrane, but its metabolic product, acylcarnitine, can.

β - Oxidation of Fatty Acid

It involves successive cleavage of FA chain *between the $\alpha(2)$ and $\beta(3)$ – carbon atom* (hence the name β-oxidation) with release of Acetyl CoA.

Oxidation of acyl CoA to acetyl CoA is catalyzed by *'Fatty acid oxidase complex'* in mitochondrial matrix

The successive steps are:
Dehydrogenation → Hydration → Dehydrogenation. In 1st Dehydrogenation reaction, 2H atoms are removed with the formation of *$FADH_2$ (2ATP)* in presence of acyl –COA dehydrogenase, and E*noyl CoA* (Δ^2 trans enoyl) is formed.

The hydration (addition of $2H_2O$) occurs in presence of enoyl CoA hydratase with the formation of *3-OH (hydro) acyl CoA*

↓

Further dehydrogenation (removal of H_2) catalyzed by 3 –OH- acyl CoA dehydrogenase to form ***keto acyl CoA & NADH (3ATP)***Q.

↓

Dehydrogenation f/b Hydration f/b Dehydrogenation = **Reactions**
Enoyl CoA f/b Hydroacyl CoA f/b ketoacyl CoA = **Products**

↓

Finally 3 – keto acyl CoA is split by *thiolase* and result in formation of:

One Acetyl CoA which enters TCA cycle to form H_2O & CO_2	One Aceyl CoA containing 2 carbon less than original molecules & enters for reoxidation by acyl dehydrogenase.

In this way a long chain fatty acid is degraded completely to acetyl CoA (C-2unit). Thus *palmitoyl – CoA (C_{16}) form 8 acetyl CoA from 7 cycles.*

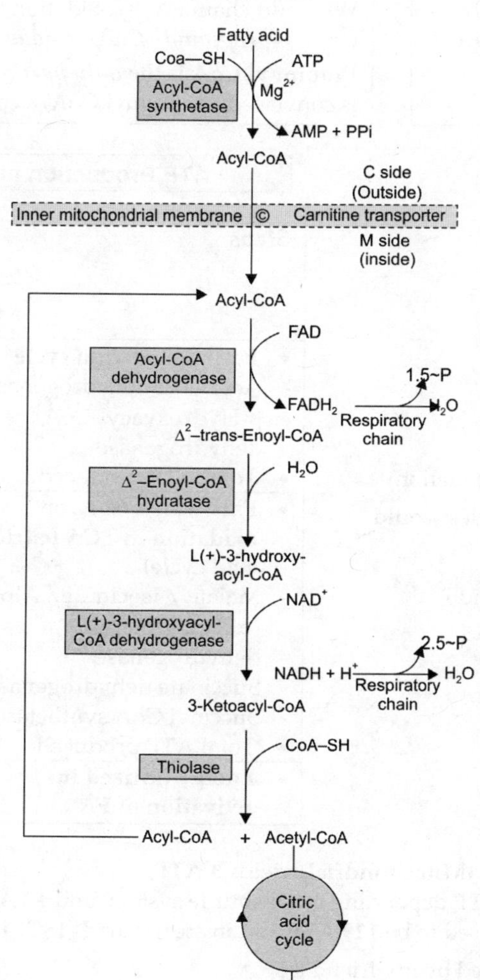

Comparison of long chain, even numbered, saturated FA synthesis & B oxidation (degradation)

Feature	FA synthesis	Degradation
Occurs in	**Fed state** (after carbohydrate rich meal)	**Fasting & starvation**
Favouring hormone	**High insulin/** glucagon ratio	**Low insulin / glucagon ratio**
Primary site Cellular site	**Liver** **Cytosol**	**Muscle, liver** **Mitochondria**
Acyl (acetyl) group carrier	**Citrate** From mitochondria to cytosol	**Carnitine** From cytosol to mitochondria
Phosphopantetheine containing active carriers	Acyl carrier protein, coenzyme A	Coenzyme A
Coenzymers	**NADPH** (reduction)	**NAD+, FAD** (oxidation)
2 Carbon donor / product	**Malonyl CoA** (donor of 1 acetyl group)	**Acetyl CoA** (product of beta oxidation)
Activator	Citrate	
Inhibitor	**Long chain fatty acyl CoA** (inhibits acetyl CoA carboxylase)	***Malonyl CoA (inhibits CPTI)***Q
Product of pathways	Palmitate	Acetyl CoA
Repetitive 4 steps	**Condensation, reduction, dehydration, reduction (CRDR)**	**Dehydrogenation, hydration, dehydrogenation, thiolysis (DHDT)**

β - Oxidation of fatty acid

Even Chain FA
2 carbons at a time are cleaved from acyl – CoA in every cycle to form *Acetyl – CoA (2carbon unit substance)*[Q]

Odd Chain FA
With odd chain FA, β- oxidation produces *acetyl CoA*, until a ***three-carbon (propionyl –CoA) residue remains***[Q]. **Propionyl CoA** is the ***only part of fatty acid that is glucogenic***[Q] [as it is converted to succinyl CoA, a consituent of TCA cycle]

Fatty Acid	Number of C atoms
Acetic	2
Propionic	3
Butyric	4
Valeric	5
Caproic	6
Lauric	12
Myristic	14
Palmitic[Q]	**16**
Stearic[Q]	**18**

★ In any even numbered FA, the no, of β oxidation cycles would be $\frac{n}{2}-1$, and no. of TCA cycles would be n/2

★ So ATP produced by palmitic (no- 16) acid is

$-\frac{16}{2}-1=7\times4=28$ ATP

$-\frac{16}{2}=8\times10=80$ ATP i.e. 108 ATP – 2ATP = 106 *ATP*

ATP Production in β-oxidation of Fatty Acids

Steps	Product	ATP formed Old concept	New concept
• **Each β oxidation cycle**			
- Acyl CoA dehydrogenase	**1 $FADH_2$**	2	1.5
- β-Hydroxyacyl-CoA dehydrogenase	**1 NADH**	3	2.5
• Total ATP produced		5	**4**
• Each **acetyl CoA, on oxidation in TCA (citric acid cycle)**			
- Malate / Isocitrate/ Alpha (α) ketoglutarate dehydrogenase	**3 NADH**	9	7.5
- Succinate dehydrogenase	**1 $FADH_2$**	2	1.5
- Succinyl CoA synthetase	1 GTP	1	1
• Total ATP produced		**12**	**10**
• **Energy utilized in activation of FA**	**-2 ATP**	In all cycles	

- Acording to **older concept 1NADH (Mitochondrial)** yields **3 ATP,**
1 NADH (cytosolic) yields **3 or 2 ATP** depending upon shuttle system, and **1 $FADH_2$** yields **2 ATP**. So net gain of ATPs in **palmitic acid** (16 carbon) used to be **129 ATP** and in **stearic acid** (18C) **146 ATP**.
For calculating this a formula derived by my friend is

$$\text{Net ATP gain} = \frac{17\times no\ of\ carbon\ atoms}{2}-7=\frac{7n}{2}-7$$
(in even number fatty acid)

- But according to **new concept 1 NADH (mitochondrial)** yields **2.5 ATP, 1 NADH (cytosolic) yields 1.5 or 2.5 ATP depending** on the shuttle syste and **1 $FADH_2$** yields **1.5 ATP**. Therefore, net gain in **palmitic acid** would be ***106 ATP***[Q] and in ***stearic acid 120 ATP***[Q]. So now suggested formula is

Net ATP gain (in even number fatty acid) = 7n- 6

★ The formulas are also valid for even numbered unsaturated fatty acids.

- 1 mol. Of palmitate involves net production of **106 mol of ATP** via β oxidation, whereas only **26 mol of ATP** are produced when acetoacetate is the end product and only **21 mol of ATP** when 3 hydroxybutyrate is the end product.

ATP Production (old)

Stearic Acid

Stearic acid (C_{18}) is $C_{17}H_{31}$ COOH. In β- oxidation it will undergo *8 cycle* [2-C removed in each cycle +2 (C2) units remaining in last cycle], producing *9 acetyl CoA*

- Each cycle produces	= 5 ATP.
∴ 8 cycle produces	= 8x 5 = 40 ATP
- Each acetyl CoA produces	= 12 ATP
∴ 9 acetyl CoA produces	= 12x 9 = 108 ATP
- Total ATP produced	= 148 ATP – 2 ATP
Net gain	**= 146 ATP**

Palmitic Acid

Palmitic acid is *16 carbon compounds* Q and it will undergo ***7 cycles & produce 8 acetyl CoA*** Q (for **citric acid cycle**) i.e.

- ATP from NADH & FADH2 in cycle = 7 x 5 = ***35 ATP*** Q
- ATP from acetyl CoA in Citric acid cycle = 12 x 8 = ***96 ATP*** Q
- ATP spend in activation = -2ATP

Net gain = ***129 ATP*** Q

β- Oxidation

In peroxisomes	In Mitochondria
• Facilitates oxidation of *very long chain FA* (C_{20}, C_{22}), do not attack shorter chain FA.	• Oxidation of *both long & short* chain FA.
• β - oxidation sequence *ends at octanoyl – CoA & acetyl CoA*. Both further oxidized in mitochondria.	• End product is acetyl CoA.
• **In 1st oxidation step**: (i.e. Ist dehydrogenation step; FAD linked) Flavoprotein dehydrogenase passes electrons to ***O_2 producing H_2O_2*** Q, which is broken down by catalase into H_2O & O_2. *Energy released dissipates as heat*	• **In 1st oxidation step:** Electron removed from flavoprotein dehydrogenase passes through *respiratory chain to O2 to produce H2O* & this process is accompanied by *ATP synthesis*.
• This system is *not linked directly* to phosphorylation & ATP generation	• This system is directly linked to ATP generation.
• **Other functions:** - *To shorten side chain of cholesterol* in bile acid formation. - Synthesis of ether glycerolipids, cholesterol and dolichol.	

Impaired oxidation of Fatty Acids: l/t disease often associated with hypoglycemia

Carnitine deficiencies

- Secondary deficiency occurs in
- Decreased synthesis of carnitine in patients of *liver disease, malnutrition* or those on *strictly vegetarian* diets
- Increased requirements as result of *pregnancy, trauma, severe burn, infection*
- Increased losses d/t hemodialysis or renal leakage (eg in preterm infants).
- Genetic deficiency may be of 2 types
- **CPT-1 deficiency *affects only liver*** Q, where an inability to use long chain fatty acid for fuel greatly impairs the tissues ability to synthesize glucose during a fast, resulting in reduced fatty acid oxidation and ketogenesis with hypoglycemia, coma and death.
- **CPT II deficiency** affects ***primarily skeletal and cardiac muscles*** Q and, when severe, the liver resulting in *cardiomyopathy, muscle weakness with myoglobinemia* following prolonged exercise

Medium Chain fatty Acyl CoA Dehydrogenase (MCAD) deficiency

- *Autosomal recessive, most common* inborn error of fatty acid oxidation
- *Infants* are particularly affected because they rely on milk (which contains primarily medium chain FA) for their nourishment
- **Dicarboxylic auduria** is characterized by *excretion of C6 – C10*

Zellweger's (Cerebrohepatorenal) syndrome

- Very long chain fatty acids (VLCFA) i.e. >20 carbons, undergo a preliminary β oxidation in peroxidomes. The shortend FA is then transferred to mitochondria for further oxidation
- So **absence of peroxisomes in all tissues (i.e. Zellweger syndrome)** or the inability to transport VLCFA across peroxisomal membrane (i.e. **X-linked adrenoleukodystrophy)** l/t accumulation of *VLCFA (C_{26}-C_{38})*
- In ZS, accumulation of polyenoic

- *Sulfonylurea drugs (glyburide / glybenclamide, and tolbutamide)* used in tt of type 2 diabetes reduce fatty acid oxidation & therefore hyper glycemia by *inhibiting CPT-1*
- ***Malonyl CoA inhibits CPT-1 thus preventing long chain acyl group entery into mitochondrial matrix. The phosphorylation & inhibition of acetyl CoA carboxylase decrease malonyl CoA production, removing the break on fatty acid oxidation***[Q].

★ *Presence of methyl group on β-carbon* (eg in branched chain phytanic acid) *makes β oxidation impossible* and these fatty acids are catabolize in **peroxisomes by α oxidation**.

★ **ω oxidation** (of ω cabon i.e. most distant from carboxyl group) occurs in **endoplasmic reticulum** of liver & kidney, and preffered substrates are fatty acids of 10-12 carbon atoms.

ω- dicarboxylic acids & by non ketotic hypoglycemia, caused by MCAD deficiency.

Jamaican Vomiting Sickness

- Eating of *unripe fruit of akee tree, containing hypoglycin toxin* causes JVS
- Toxin inactivates *medium & short chain acyl CoA dehydrogenase,* inhibiting β-oxidation and causing *hypoglycemia.*

acids in brain causes severe neurological symptoms & death in 1st year of life

Refsum's Disease

- AR disorder caused by ***deficiency of phytanic -α oxidase / α hydroxylase / phytanoyl CoA hydroxylase***[Q] resulting in accumulation of phytanic acid d/t its decreased *α oxidation in peroxisome.*
- Phytanic acid impairs membrane function, protein prenylation and gene expression causing primarily neurological symptoms.
- Phytanic acid is found in *dairy products, & ruminant fat & meat.* It involves dietary restrictions.

Ketogenesis: Synthesis of Ketone Bodies in Liver

- *Acetoacyetyl CoA* is the *starting material &* this can arise in two ways:
- directly from terminal 4- carbon of fatty acid during β- oxidation
- as a result of **condensation of two acetyl CoA molecule** (i.e. 2 C units) formed in β oxidation by ***reversal of thiolase reaction.***
- *Acetoacetate is the Ist ketone body to be formed.* It can be formed from Acetoacyetal in two steps:
- Initially condensation of Acetoacyetyl with another acetyl CoA to form β -OH - β- methyl glutaryl CoA *(HMG CoA)* by enzyme HMG CoA synthesis.
- Then HMG CoA is split into Acetoacetate and Acetyl CoA by the enzyme HMG CoA lyase. This is a commited step.
- Both **enzymes (HMG Co synthase & lyase) of ketogenesis** must be present in **mitochondria** for ketogenesis to take place. This occurs only in **liver** and **rumen epithelium. D(-) – 3 – Hydroxybutyrate** is quantitatively the predominant ketone body *present in blood stream* (ketonemia or hyper ketonemia) and urine (**ketonuria**) in ketosis.

Ketolysis: Use of ketone Bodies in Periphral Tissues as Fuel

- Although *liver constantly produces low levels of ketone bodies,* their production becomes much more significant during **fasting, starvation, type II diabetes mellitus,** twin lamb disease & in lactating cattle. Non pathological form of ketosis occurs under conditions of **high fat feeding & after severe exercise** in post absorptive state.
- Under certain metabolic conditions (depletion of available carbohydrate coupled with increased mobilization/lipolysis of FFF) associated with high rate of fatty acid oxidation, liver produces ketone bodies, which is used as respiratory substrate (fuel) by extrahepatic tissue. ***Ketone bodies is collective name given to 3 compounds***[Q]**: 1. Acetone 2. Acetoacetate 3. Beta hydroxybutyrate. In a well fed state, concentraton of ketone bodies in blood does not exceed *1mg /100ml***[Q]**.**
- Extrahepatic tissues including brain but **excluding cells lacking mitochondria (RBC)** efficiently oxidize acetoacetate & 3(OH) butyrate. In contrast, ***liver actively produces ketone bodies but lacks thiophorase (Succinyl CoA : acetoacetate CoA transferase) and so is unable to use ketone bodies as fuel***[Q]**.**
- Substrate utilized for energy production

Organ	Fed	Fasting	Starvation
Brain	Glucose	Glucose	***Ketone bodies***[Q]
Heart	***Fatty acid***[Q]	Fatty acid	Ketone bodies
Liver	Glucose	Fatty acid	Amino acid
Muscles	Glucose	Fatty acid	Fatty acid

Heart utilizes F.A even in fed state. Resting muscles use FFA as fuel source while exercising muscle initially use glycogen reserve (glucose) and then FFF.

- While **acetoacetate & 3(OH) butyrate** are oxidized by **extrahepatic tissue as fuel, acetone** is difficult to oxidize (in vivo) and is mainly **volatilized in lungs.** Both acetoaectate & 3(OH) butyrate are ***moderately strong acids*** and are buffered depleting alkaline reserve, thus causing **fatal ketoacidosis** (in very severe cases).

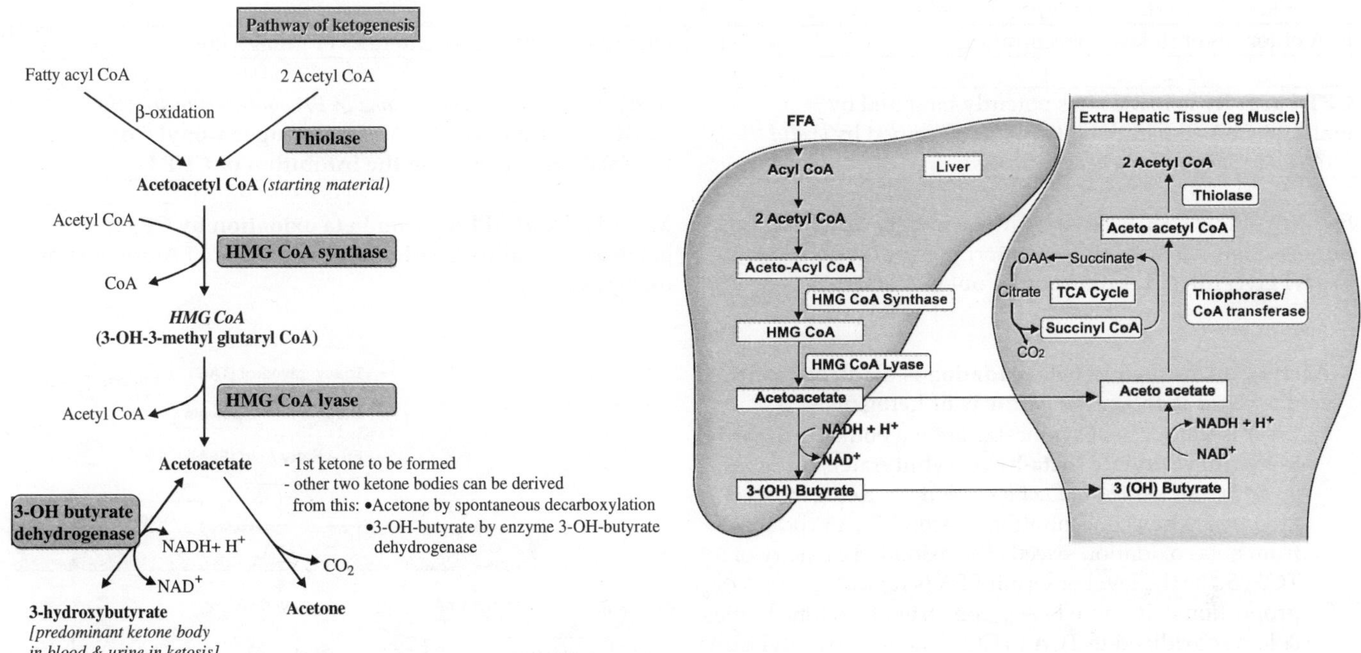

Regulation of Ketogenesis

Ketogenesis is regulated at 3 crucial steps

1. During **mobilization of FFA (free fatty acids) from adipose tissue (lipolysis):** Liver extracts ~ 30% of FFA passing through it both in fed & fasting condition. **FFA are the precursors of ketone bodies in liver**. Therefore factors increasing /decreasing FFA mobilization from adipose tissue increase / decrease ketogenesis. So factors affecting **adipose tissue lipolysis, FFA release and ketogenesis** include

Decreasing Factors	Increasing Factors
- **Insulin, Nicotinic acid, Prostaglandin E_1, Adenosine** & high concentration of **FFA** inhibit lipolysis *by inhibiting synthesis of c-AMP at adenylyl cyclase* site acting through Gi protein. - *Lipolysis is more sensitive to changes in concentration of insulin than are glucose utilization & esterification*. Insulin also stimulates **phosphodiesterase** (removing c-AMP) and **lipase phosphatase** that inactivates hormone sensitive lipase (HSL). FFAs also inhibit HSL. - **Perilipin** protein is involved in formation of lipid droplets in adipocytes and *inhibit lipolysis in basal condition* by preventing access of lipase enzyme to stored triacyl glycerol.	- **Epinephrine, norepinephrine, glucagon, ACTH**, alpha and beta **MSH (melanocyte stimulating hormone), TSH, GH and Vasopressin** increase lipolysis of triacyl glycerol by activating **hormone sensitive lipase** (through adenyl cyclase) - For optimal effect most of these require **glucocorticoids and thyroid hormones as facilitatory or permissive lipolytic endocrinal factors.** - On stimulation with lipolytic hormones, **perilipin** promote TAG degradation; thus regulating balance between TAG storage & lipolysis in adipocytes

2. **During entery of FFAs for B oxidation pathway by CPTI (into mitochondria):** After uptake by liver, FFAs are either **beta-oxidized** (in fasting/ starving) **or esterified** to TAG & phospholipid (in fed state). The ***entery of FFAs into Beta oxidation pathway is regulated by CPTI (carnitine palmitoyl transferase I)***[Q] and the remainder of FA taken up by liver is esterified.

In Fed State	In Fasting / Starvation
↓	↓
FFA enters liver in low concentration	Due to lipolysis FFAs entere liver in high concentration
↓	↓
CPT I activity is low as it is potently inhibited by **malonyl CoA** (the initial intermediate formed by *acetyl CoA carboxylase in fatty acid synthesis*)	*Acetyl CoA carboxylase enzyme in FA synthesis is directly inhibited* by acyl CoA (FFA) **decreasing malonyl CoA levels**; thereby **releasing the inhibition of CPT I**
↓	↓
Because of low CPT I activity, **fatty acid beta oxidation is depressed** and **nearly all FFA** entering liver is esterified to acyl glycerol and is transported out in **VLDL**	**More acyl CoA (FFA) enter beta oxidation by CPTI gateway into mitochondria** and balance of FFA uptake not oxidized is esterified

3. **Acetyl CoA formed in beta oxidation is oxidized in citric acid cycle or it enters the pathway of ketogensis.**
   - Liver is unique as it synthesize ketone bodies, **primarily 3- hydroxybutyrate (beta-hydroxybutyrate)** *for use as fuel by peripheral tissues, but not by liver itself*. Ketogenesis is favoured when concentration of acetyl CoA produced from beta- oxidation, exeeds the oxidative capacity of TCA. So as the level of serum FFA is raised, proportionately more FFA is converted to ketone bodies & less is oxidized in TCA to CO_2. The fate of acetyl CoA between ketogenesis & TCA is regulated *so that the total ATP produced from the oxidation of FFA remains constant* as concentration of FFA in serum changes.
   - 1 mol of **palmitate** produces **106** mol of ATP via beta oxidation & CO_2 production in TCA, whereas only **26 ATP** are produced when **acetoacetate** is end product and only **21 ATP** when **3 hydroxybutyrate** is end product. **So ketogenesis allows liver to oxidize increasing quantities of FAs.** At the same time, ketogenesis releases CoA, ensuring its availability for continued fatty acid oxidation.

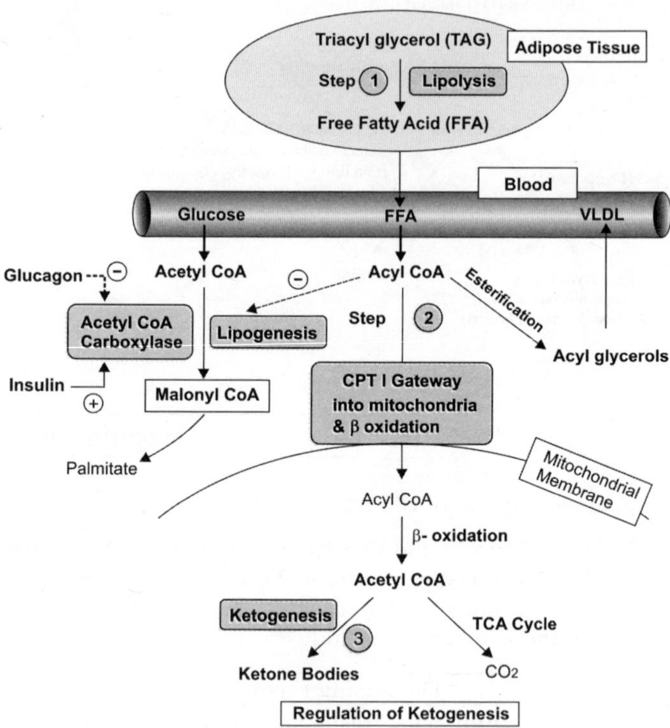

Metabolism In Fed & Fasting

Brain Metabolism

- **Brain tissue** uses *glucose as an exclusive fluel , both during the fed state as well as in fasting state*[Q], except *during starvation* when it can adapt to *use ketonebodies as an energy source*[Q].
- Brian does *not utilize fatty acids as a fuel*[Q]. And brain contains *no fuel reserves*[Q] and so must be continuously supplied with fuel from the blood. *In brain 60% of total energy is utilized during the resting stage*[Q]

Other Organs

- ***Liver is the only source of ketone body production, but it does not utilize ketone bodies***[Q]
- **Liver** utilize *glucose in fed, fatty acid in fasting*, and *aminoacid in starvation*
- **Heart** utilize *fatty acid* as main substrate *in fed & fasting state;* and *ketone bodies* in *starvation.*
- ***Muscles do not utilize ketone bodies***[Q]. They utilize glucose in fed state and fatty acid in fasting and starvation.

Effects of Starvation On Metabolism

I[st] Stage
(first **2 to 3 days** i.e. **48-72 hour**)

- **Glycogenolysis**: *liver glycogen* is first metabolized but d/t its limited storage it cannot last long
- **Gluconeogenesis**: initially from glucogenic amino acids ***(alanine glutamate[Q])*** and then by glycerol & lactate

> **Glucagon secretion** increases during starvation. It reaches a ***peak on 3rd day of fast at the time of maximal gluconeogenesis[Q]***. There after glucagons level declines as the ketones & fatty acids become the major source of energy. Ganong- 350

IInd Stage (last for *longest* period, usually *over 2 weaks*)

- 90% of energy requirement will be derived from fat & remainder 10% from protein
- Since the adipose tissue represents largest amount of stored fat 2nd stage will last for longest period
- Adipose tissue is broken into FFA which is oxidized for energy production and used for ketone body formation.
- The burning of fat is reflected by a lower RQ (~ 0.73) ↓

IIIrd – Stage

- When the fat stores are almost exhausted energy is derived from *breakdown of tissue protein*
- Digestive enzymes. Followed by muscle protein are first to be utilized, as these are least required
- This stage last for *less than one* week & leads to death.

Metabolic Alterations During Fasting / Starvation

Absorptive (fed) state is **2-4 hours period** after ingestion of a normal meal. During this period, *transient increase in plasma glucose, amino acids and triacyl glycerol* (TAG; d/t increased chylomicron synthesis in intestinal mucosa) occur. The elevated insulin to glucagon ratio (in response to increased glucose) make it **anabolic phase** characterized by **increased synthesis of TAG, and glycogen to replenish fuel stores and enhanced synthesis of protein**. During absorptive phase, virtually all tissues use glucose as fuel.

Fasting begins if no food is ingested after absorptive phase. Metabolic changes include

Features	During Brief Fasting	During Prolonged Fasting
Liver	- **Glycogenolysis (glycogen degradation)** maintains blood glucose level initially (a **transient early response**) - **Gluconeogenesis** begins 4-6 hours after last meal and becomes fully active after depletion of liver glycogen stores. *Glucogenic amino acids & lactate from muscles and glycerol from adipose tissue* is utilized. - **Beta-oxidation of fatty acids is increased** for energy production and **ketone body formation.** FAs obtainjm,ed from adipose tissue lipolysis becomes the main fuel. However **RBC and brain continue to use glucose mainly**. Blood levels of ketone bodies (esp 3-hydroxy butyrate) increase gradually.	- Liver glycogen is nearly **exhausted after 10-18 hours of fasting**, therefore glycogenolysis can no longer maintain glucose level. - **Rate of gluconeogenesis is decreased in prolonged fasting** to spare functional proteins and therefore less protein is degraded to provide glucogenic aminoacids - **Beta oxidation of FA and production of ketone bodies** continue to be increased. **Ketone bodies** can **be used for fuel by most tissues (except liver) including brain,** once their level in blood is sufficiently high.
Adipose Tissue	- **Decreased FA & TAG synthesis** d/t decreased glucose transport by insulin sensitive GLUT-4 into adipocytes - **Increased degradation of TAG** (by hormone sensitive lipase) resulting in **increased release of FFAs and glycerol.** - **Decreased uptake of FA** (in adipocytes from circulating TAG of lipoproteins) d/t low lipoprotein lipase activity.	
Skeletal Muscle	- **Rapid breakdown of muscle** protein providing aminoacids for gluconeogenesis - Resting muscle use FFA and ketone bodies for fuel	- Rate of ***muscle proteolysis decreases paralleling a decline in the need for glucose as a fuel for brain which has begun using ketone bodies as a source of energy[Q].*** - FA is mainly used as source of fuel. ***The increased use of ketone bodies by the brain as a result of their increased concentration in blood is correlated with decreased use of ketone bodies by muscle[Q].***
Brain, RBCs	- **Urea production d/t proteolysis increases** - **Brain and RBC use glucose as fuel**	- **Urea production by liver decreases** - Brain use of glucose decrease but **RBCs still need glucose as fuel**

Biochemical Tests for Detection of

Ketone Bodies

- Ketone bodies (such as **acetone, acetoacetic acid/ diacetic acid,** and **betahydroxy butyric acid)** are produced ***exclusively in liver***[Q] as ***products of fat catabolism***[Q] usually in **diabetes mellitus** (ketoacidosis) & **starvation.**
- Ketone bodies serve as an *alternate source of energy especially in brain* (& other parts of CNS) providing **50-70% of brain energy needs** during starvation. This is an adaptation for survival during starvation.
- Ketone bodies in urine are detected by **Rothera's and Gerhardt's test.**

Rothera's test	**Gerhardt's test**
Also called **Nitro prusside test**	Also called **ferric chloride test**
Detects **acetone & acetoacetic acid**	Detects **acetoacetic acid**
Urine (5ml) is saturated with *solid ammonium sulphate.* Adding few drops of *sodium nitroprusside f/b liquor ammonia* 1/t appearance of **purple/pink permanganate ring**	$FeCl_3$ is added drop by drop to 3ml urine. And appearance of **red wine** color indicates presence of ketone bodies

Reducing Sugars

- **Benedict's test** and **Fehling's test** are used to detect reucing sugars like glucose in urine.
- So the patient with **diabetic ketoacidosis** will give ***positive Benedict's test and Rothera's test both***[Q], whereas urine of patient with **starvation** will give a ***negative Benedict's test but a positive Rothera's test***[Q].
- Benedict's reagent contain *copper sulphate, sodium carbonate & sodium citrate.*

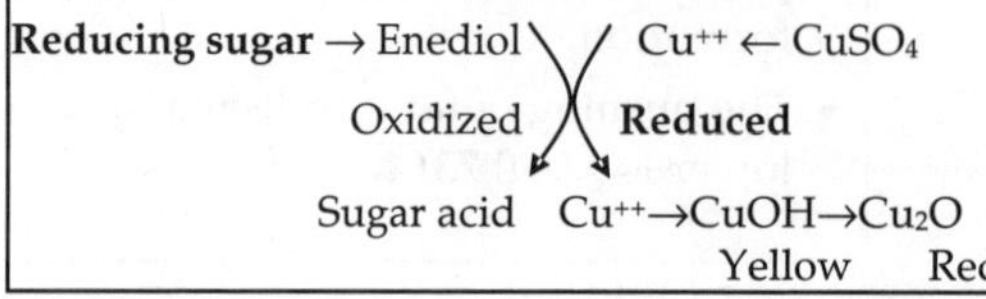

- Benedict's is a semiquantitative test i.e. color roughly indicating concentration of sugar
  - blue (absence), green (0.5%), yellow (1%), orange (1.5%), and red (≥ 2% i.e. ≥ 2 gm/100ml reducing sugar)
- Any reducing sugar (like *glucose, fructose, lactose, galactose and pentose/xylulose*) will give positive Benedict's test. So Benedict's test is positive in
  - **Glucosuria** (diabetes mellitus)
  - **Fructosuria** (fructose intolerance/aldolase B deficiency, fructokinase deficiency)
  - **Lactosuria**
  - **Galactosuria** (galactose – 1-PO_4- uridyl transferase deficiency)
  - **Pentosuria (xylulosuria)**
  - Presence of non carbohydrate reducing substance in urine like *ascorbic acid (vitamin C), homogentisic acid, glucuronides and salicylate.*

★ Presence of **proteins** is detected by ***heat coagulation test, acetic acid test and Haller's nitric acid test***[Q]. Whereas **benzidine test** detects ***presence of blood (hemoglobin > myoglobin)***[Q].

Bile salts

Hay's test detect bile salts *(sodium salts of taurocholic acid & glycocholic acid) in urine.* Positive test indicates obstruction in biliary passage.

Bilirubin

- **Fouchet's** (barium sulphate) test, **Gmelin's** (nitric acid) test and **Vanden Bergh** (diazo/diazotized sulphanilic acid reagent) **tests** detect bilirubin.
- **Conjugated bilirubin** being water soluble gives **direct** Vanden Bergh test (immediate color); whereas **free bilirubin**, being water insoluble give **indirect** reaction (i.e. color after extraction with alcohol)

Bile pigments

- **Uro & steco-bilinogens (UBG & SBG)** give positive **Ehrlich's** (para-amino benzaldehyde reagent) test to form red color.
- **Schlesinger's test** is positive for **Uro & Sterco-bilins** (UB & SB) to give brilliant green fluorescence with zinc ions.
- **Rosenbach's test**

Bile pigments	**Detection – Tests**		
	Fouchet's; Gmelin; Vanden Bergh	**Ehrlich's**	**Schlesingers**
Bilirubin	+	-	-
Bilinogens (UBG, SBG)	-	+	-
Bilins (UB + SB)	-	-	+

Chapter 3. STRUCTURE, FUNCTION AND REPLICATION OF INFORMATIONAL MACROMOLECULES: REVIEW NOTES

Pyrimidine Synthesis & Catabolism

- Unlike purine ring, which is constructed on a preexisting ribosome 5 PO_4, (derived from PRPP) the pyrimidine ring is synthesized from **aspartic acid** (contributing N_1, C_4, C_5, & C_6 atoms), **amine N_2 of glutamine** (source of N_3) and **CO_2** (source of C_2 atom of ring). Although both purine & pyrimidine synthesis require glutamine, aspartic acid & PRPP as essential precursors.

  The steps are Mn- **"GAS CAP AA CAA DHOA OA OMP UMP UDP"** see the rhythm AA, OA, MP, DP
- It uses **2 multifunctional-multicatalytic polypeptides,** which ensures efficient channeling of carbamoyl phosphate to pyrimidine synthesis.

- First 3 enzymes (i.e. CPS II, Aspartate trans carbamoylase and Dihydroorotase) are **three different catalytic domain of single CAD polypeptide chain** (name derived from 1st letter of each domain).
- Next (4th) non multifunctional enzyme **DHOA dehydrogenase** is the ***only mitochondrial enzyme***[Q]
- ***Orotate phosphoribosyl transferase and Orotidylate (OMP) decarboxylase***[Q] are also catalytic domains of a single polypeptide chain of bifunctional enzyme **UMP synthase**. **Orotic aciduria** is caused by defect of single (type II) or both (type I) domains and result in poor growth, megaloblastic anemia & excretion of large amounts of orotate in urine. *Uridine administration* improves condition.

- **Allopurinol & 6-azauridine** drugs may precipitate oritic aciduria & oritidinuria by ***inhibiting OMP decarboxylase (i.e type II orotic aciduria)***[Q]. This enzyme is actually blocked by product of allopurinol & enzyme OPRT and 6-azauridylate.
- Orotic aciduria occurs in **deficiency of liver mitochondrial ornithine transcarbamoylase enzyme of urea cycle** and **Reye syndrome** (in which severly damaged mitochondria is unable to utitize carbamoyl phosphate). ***Excess carbamoyl phosphate exits to cytosol***[Q] and becomes available for cytosolic over production of orotic acid (by stimulating pyrimidine biosynthesis).

	Carbamoyl Phosphate Synthetase	
	I	II
Occur in	Mitochondri	Cytosol
Used in	Urea cycle	Pyrimidine synthesis
Activator	N-acetyl glutamate	PRPP
Nitrogen source	Ammonia	γ-amide group of glutamine

- Unlike purine ring, which is not cleaved in human cells, the pyrimidine ring is opened & degraded by **dihydropyrimidine dehydrogenase** (DHPD) & Beta-ureidopropionase to highly water soluble products *Beta-alanine (from uracil) and Beta-aminoisobutyrate (from thymine)*, with production of NH_3 & CO_2. DHPD deficiency results in *Beta-hydroxybutyric aciduria; a disorder of pyrimidine catabolism (and also of Beta amino acid metabolism* since formation of Beta-alanine & Beta-amine iso butyrate is also impaired) is also k/a **combined uraciluria-thyminuria**. High water solubility of end products results in few clinical features.

Purine Synthesis

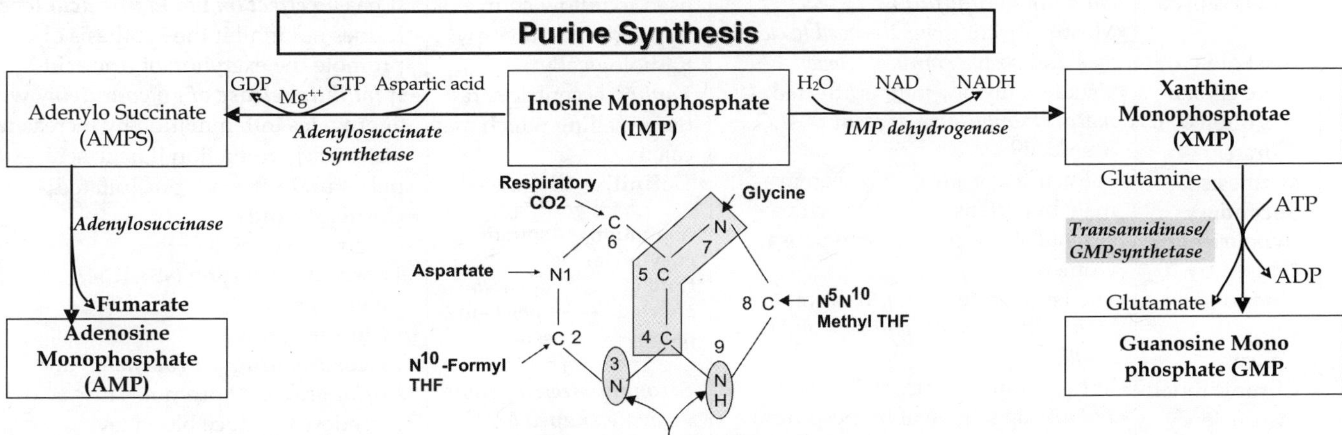

Sources of atoms in purine ring

★ **Mycophenolic acid** is reversible, uncompetitive *inhibitor of IMP dehydrogenase.* It deprives rapidly proliferating T & B cells of nucleic acids and used to prevent *graft rejection.*

Uric Acid Synthesis (Purine Catabolism)

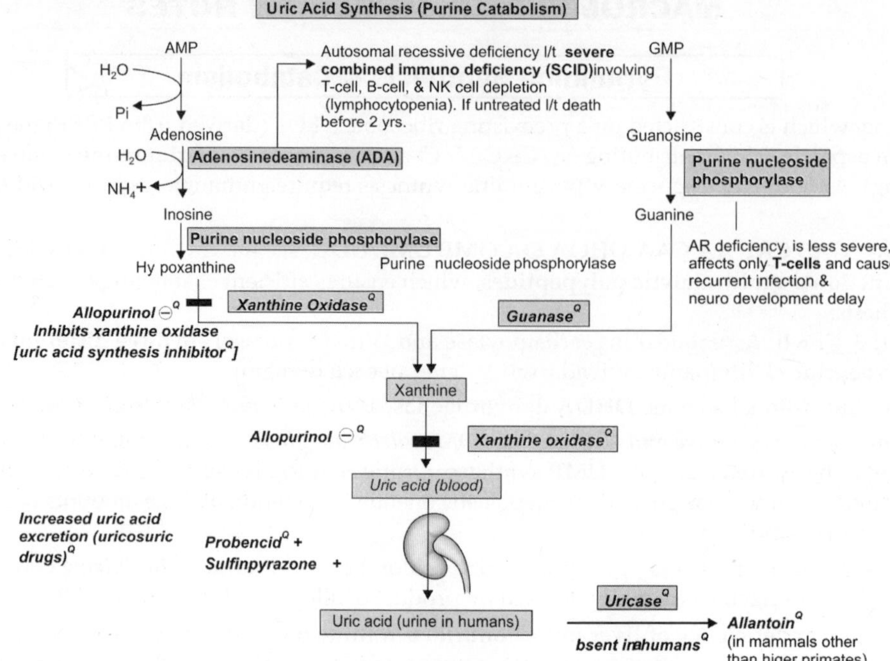

★ Hyperuricemia result in deposition of sodium urate crystals in kidney and joints

★ *Hyperuricemia does not always lead to gout*, but *gout is usually preceded by hyperuricemia.*

Gout

This is characterized by *hyperuricemia* with *recurrent attack of acute arthritic joint inflammation*, caused by *deposition of uric acid crystal.*

Types	Clinical Features	Lab Diagnosis	Treatment
• **Primary gout (hypeuricemia):** Due to inborn error of metabolism and is caused by - most often d/t urate crystal - less often d/t ↑ urate synthesis • **Secondary hypeuricemia:** Caused by other disease eg: - Cancer - Chronic renal insufficiency - Myeloprofiferative disorder - Drugs	• The vast *majority of hyperuricemic patient are asymptomatic.* Any factor that cause ***either an abrupt increase or decrease in the serum urate levels may provoke an acute attack, the best correlations being factors that cause an abrupt fall***Q. • Mostly affecting *middle- aged to elderly men* and *postmenopausal women.* • Usually only one joint is affected, ***1st metatarsophalangeal joint is M.C involved***Q • *Polyarticular acute gout* is seen in – male hypertensive patient with ethanol abuse & postmeno pausal women • The Ist episode *frequently begins at night with dramatic joint pain and swelling* • Joint becomes warm, red & tender • ***Tophi***Q: aggregate of monosodium urate monohydrate (MSU) crystals form in extraarticular & articular structures, cause deformity and destruction of hard and soft tissue.	• *Serum uric acid* level can be ***normal or low at the time of acute attack***Q. • Serum uric acid is ***almost always elevated at some time***Q & can be used to follow cource of hypouricemic therapy. • Radiologically: - ***Tophi***Q: eccentric soft tissue selling which may calcify • **Definitive diagnosis** **Aspiration of synovial fluid of affected joint** / **Aspiration of Tophaceous deposits in tissue** ***Strongly birefringerent needle shaped MSU crystals with negative elongation under polarized light***Q.	<u>**In Acute Gout**</u> • **NSAIDS** : eg. ***Indomethacin***Q **,** Naproxen , Piroxicam - strong anti inflammatory action - ***effective in terminating the attack***Q • **Colchicine** - It has ***no effect on blood uric acid level***Q - It does not inhibit the synthesis or promote the excretion of uric acid. - It ***inhibits release of glycoprotein***Q which aggravates inflammation by increasing lactic acid production [Lactic acid → ↓ pH → urate crystals precipitated] • **Corticosteroids:** - In refractory cases & - Those not tolerating NSAIDs / Colchicine <u>**In Chronic Gout**</u> • **Uricosuric drugs** : ***Probencid***Q and ***sulfinpyrazone***Q promotes uric acid excretion & reduce blood level. • ***Allopurinol***Q inhibits uric acid synthesis by ***inhibiting xamthine oxidase***Q. [an enzyme responsible for uric acid synthesis]

Purine Nucleotide Biosynthesis 

The total- body urate level is the net result between urate production and excretion. Urate production influenced by, dietary intake of purine, pyrimidine, de novo synthesis of purine, nucleic acid turnover and salvage by phosphoribosyl transferase activity.

De novo biosynthesis

- It begins with their metabolic precursors amino acids, ribose 5 phosphate, CO_2 & NH_3.
- Purine ring is contributed by number of compounds
  - A.A [Glycine, Aspartic acid, glutamine]
  - CO_2
  - N^{10} – Formyltatrahydrofolate
  - Ribose –5 PO_4 [Product of HMP shunt]
- Ribose –5- PO_4 is activated by ATP to form phosphoribosyl pyrophosphate (PRPP) by PRPP synthetase.
  - *PRPP concentration is major determinant of purine synthesis*
  - PRPP acts as a substrate in salvage pathway
  - *PRPP synthetase is inhibited by AMP. & GMP* (end product inhibition)

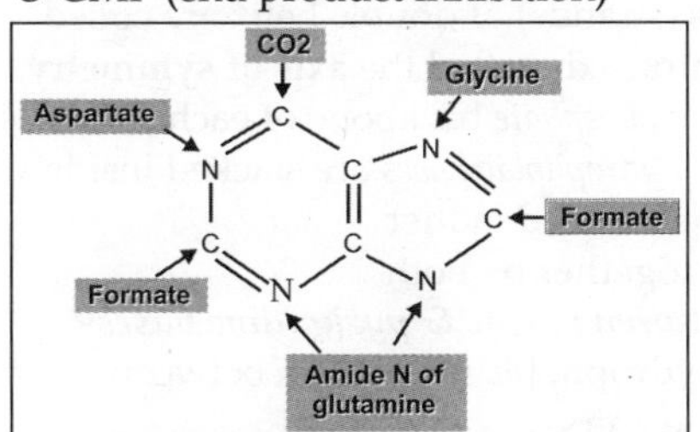

Origin of ring atoms of purine

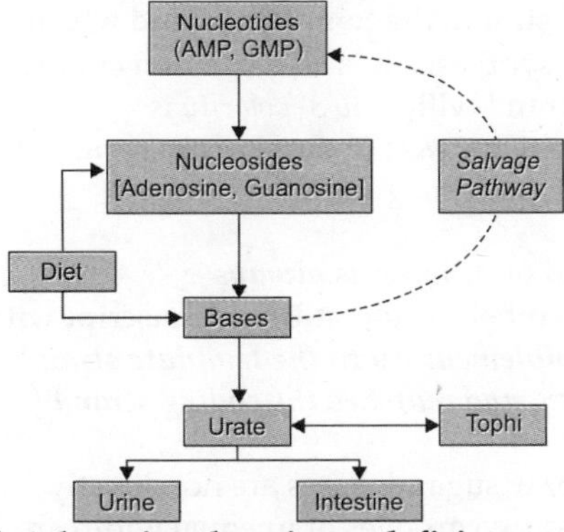

★ **Adenosine deaminase deficiency** l/t immunodeficiency d/t dysfunctional T cells and B cells causing fatal infectios in infants **Purine nucleoside phosphorylase deficiency** is a/w severe deficiency of T cells but apparently normal B cell function.

Salvage Pathway

- It recycles the free bases & nucleotides released from nucleic acid breakdown.
- Purines that result from normal turnover of cellular nucleic acids or obtained from diet and not degraded, can be reconverted into nucleoside triphosphates and used by the body.

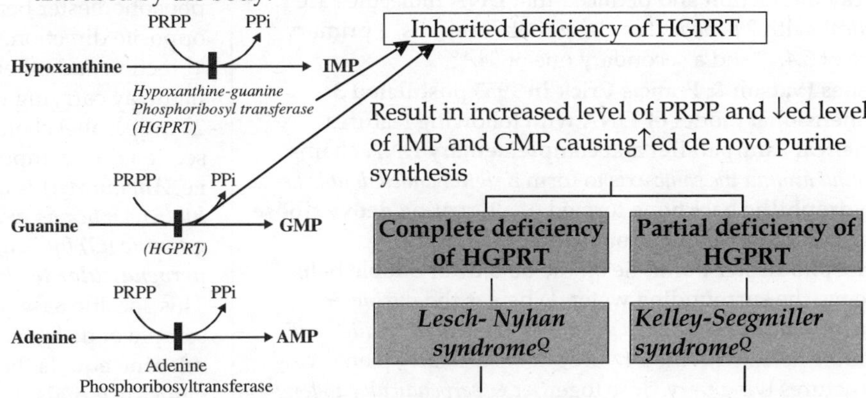

Lesch-Nyhan syndrome

- *X linked recessive disorder* of purine metabolism which becomes manifest by the **age of 2 years** and seen almost exclusively in **male children.**
- Homozygous males are affected & carrier females are asymptomatic
- It demonstrates the importance of salvage pathways. Hypoxanthine & guanine arise constantly d/t breakdown of nucleic acids. In absence of HGPRT-ase, PRPP level rises & purines are produced by denovopathway resulting in high levels of uric acid production and gout like damage to tissue.
- The brain is especially dependent on salvage pathway and this is the reason for central nervous system damage in Lesch-Nyhan syndrome

Kelley-Seegmiller syndrome

- Hyperuricemia
- Gout
- No CNS manifestation

Hyper Uricemic Symptoms	Neurological (CNS) Symptoms
- ***Hyperuricemia, Hyperuricosuria*** - ***Gouty arthritis l/t joint pain***[Q] - Uric acid crystaluria - Nephrolithiasis (urate nephropathy, urinary tract stones) - ***Obstructive uropathy (l/t reduced urinary out put)***[Q]	- ***Mental retardation***[Q] (intellectual disability) - **Poor coordination** (spasticity, choreoathetosis & dystonia) - ***Compulsive aggressiveness (extremely hostile)***[Q] - Show **compulsive self-destructive tendencies** & ***self mutilating behaviour is characteristic feature***[Q] and occurs despite intact sensory (including pain) modalities. Mostly *fingers, mouth & oral mucosa are mutilated.* They mutilate themselves by biting off their fingers, toes & lips.

T/t

Early diagnosis + Allopurinol

- Prevent or eliminate all the problem d/t hyperuricemia
- No effect on neurological abnormalities

Structure of DNA

- **Erwin-Chargaff** in late *1940s* postulated **Charagaff rules** that in a DNA, - Number of adenosine (A) residues is equal to number of thymidine (T) residues **(A=T)** and number of cytidine (C) residues is equal to number of guanosine (G) residues **(C=G)**
- Hence sum of **purine residues (A + G)** = Sum of **pyrimidines residue (T + C)**
- **Rosalind Franklin & Maurice Wilkins** analyzed DNA by **X-ray diffraction** and deduced that DNA molecules are *helical,* with *2 periodicities* along their long axis, a primary one of *3.4A°* and a secondary one of *34A°*.
- **James Watson & Francis Crick in 1953 postulated 3 dimensional model of DNA** with following features
- 2 **helical** , **antiparallel** and **complementary** DNA chains *wound around the same axis* to form a *right handed double helix.*
- **Hydrophillic backbone** formed of alternating **deoxy ribose sugar and phosphate groups** (linked by **3'-5' phosphodiester bond**) lie on the outside of double helix facing, the surrounding water. Whereas the ***purine & pyrimidine bases of both strands are stacked inside***[Q] the double helix, with their hydrophobic & nearly planar ring structures lying very close together & *perpendicular to long axis.*
- Each nucleotide base of one strand is paired with the base of other strand in **same plane**. The *offset pairing* of 2 stands l/t formation of major & minor grooves. Original model had **10 base pairs or 34A° (3.4 nm) per turn of helix** but subsequent measurements revealed **10.5 base pairs or 36 A° (3.6 nm) per turn.**
- **3 hydrogen bonds link C and G (C≡G) and 2 link A and T**. So separation of strands is difficult in DNAs with higher C≡G concentration.)

Primary structure

- Each DNA is a polymer of about 10^{10} *deoxyribo nucleotide* monomers. These deoxynucleotides are of 4 types - deoxy **adenylate** (containing **adenine**), deoxy **guanylate** (containing **guanine**), deoxy **cytidylate** (containing **cytosine**) and deoxy **thymidylate** (containing **thiymine**).
- These monomeric nucleotides are held in polymeric form in each strand by covalent ***3', 5' – phosphodiester linkage***[Q].
- Phosphodiester bond joins 3'- hydroxyl group (OH) of deoxypentose (2'- deoxy D- ribose) sugar of one nucleotide to the 5'-hydroxyl group of deoxy pentose sugar of an adjacent nucleotide through a phosphate group.
- The end of strand which bears 5- hydroxyl or phosphate terminal is called **5 end**. And the opposite end with free 3' OH or 3' phosphate group is k/a **3' end**. ***So the polymer show polarity***[Q]***. The nucleotides are always written and read in 5' → 3' direction***[Q].
- So the primary structure consists of *linear back bone of deoxyribose sugar and phosphate.* While the ***purine or pyrimidine bases project laterally from the backbone at 90° (perpendicular***[Q]***).***

Secondary Structure

- It consists of **2 helical, antiparallel** and **complementary** chains that wound around the same axis to form a double helix. Anti parallel orientation means that the 3'→5' phosphodiester bonds of both chains run in opposite direction.
- The chains are paired in **antiparallel manner** i.e. 5' end of one strand pairs with 3' end of other strand and thus the phosphodiester bonds in two interwoven strands run in opposite direction. In other word one strand run in 5' ti 3' 'direction and other in 3' to 5' direction. (analogous to a highway carrying traffic in opposite directions).
- 2 Antiparallel chains are not identical in either base sequence or composition. Instead they are complementary i.e. ***Adenine (A) is always paired with thymine (T) by 2 hydrogen bonds and cytosine (C) is always paired with guanine (G) by 3 hydrogen bonds***[Q]***. The base pairs are perpendicular to the axis of helix***[Q]. A = T; C ≡G
- This specific base pairing l/t **Chargaff's rule** i.e. in any sample of ds DNA (double stranded DNA) the amount of **adenine equals** the amount of **thymine** and the amount of **cytosine equals** the amount of **guanine**. So the ***total amount of purine equals the total amount of pyrimidine***[Q] $(A+G/T+C\approx 1)$
- Each of the two chains (strands) of double helix are coiled around a common central axis called the **axis of symmetry.**
- *Hydrophillic deoxyribose- phosphate* backbone of each strand is on the *outside* whereas *hydrophobic bases* are stacked inside. The structure resembles twisted ladder.
- **Two strands are held together** by both
  1. ***Hydrogen bonds between purine & pyrimidine bases***[Q]
  2. Vander walls and hydrophobic interaction between stacked adjacent base pairs.
- In ds DNA, **genetic** information resides in the sequence of nucleotides on **3' → 5' strand, the template strand** which is copied during m-RNA synthesis. It is also k/a **non coding strand**. The opposite strand with *5' to 3' polarity* is considered ***coding strand, because it matches the sequence of RNA transcript (but containing uracil in place of thymine)***[Q].
- One polypeptide strand of ds DNA is ***always complementary***[Q] of the other. So the **m-RNA transcript** with a 5' to 3' polarity is ***complementary to the template strand with its 3' to 5' polarity, and matches the coding strand***[Q]. (Harper)
- The glycosidic bonds b/w sugar & bases are not directly opposite each other and two grooves of unequal width are formed. The edge of helix that measures >180° from glycoside bond to glycoside bond is called **major groove**, and if **< 180°**, it is called **minor groove**.
- The hydrogen atoms (proton) in the bases can shift from one ring nitrogen or oxygen atom to another k/a **tautomerisation** – thus interconverting the position that can severe as hydrogen bond donor & acceptor

★ RNA is far less stable than DNA because the **2¹-hydroxyl group** of RNA (absent from DNA) functions as *nucleophile* during hydrolysis of 3′→5′ phosphodiester bonds. However in absence of phosphodiestreases, hydrolysis of phosphodiester bonds of DNA occur only over long periods of time, despite an extremely favourable ΔG. and so DNA even persists in fossils.

DNA Strands

Coding -5′ – TGGAATTGTGAGCGGATAACAATTTCACACAGGAAACAGCTATGACCATG - 3′
Template– 3′- ACCTTAACACTCGCCTATTGTTAAAGTGTGTCCTTTGTCGATACTGGTAC - 5′
RNA transcript 5′- p AUUGUGAGCGGAUAACAAUUUCACACAGGAAACAGCUAUGACCAUG - 3′

Unusual Structures Variations In DNA (Chromosome)

Bending of DNA Helix

DNA helix bends whenever **≥4 adenosine (A) residues** appear sequentially in row in one strand (6 A produce 18° bend).

Triplex DNA & Hoogsteen Pairing

- Nucleotides participating in Watson-Crick base pairing can form additional hydrogen bonds, particularly with functional groups arrayed in the **major groove**. For example protonated cytidine residue (C^+) can pair with guanosine residue of a G ≡ C nucleotide pair; and a thymidine (T) can pair with adenosine of A = T pair.

C ≡ G • C^+ T = A • T

- **Hoogsteen (non Watson-Crick) pairing** at N^7, N^6 and O^6 positions of purines (**Hoogsteen positions**) allow the **formation of triplex DNAs**. The triplexes are formed **most easily within long sequences containing only pyrimidines or only purines in a given strand**; or in **DNAs containing 2 pyrimidine & 1 purine or 2 purine & 1 pyrimidine strands**. The triplexes are most stable at **low pH** because the C ≡ G • C+ triplet requires **protonated cytosine residue** (≡ is WC hydrogen bond & • is Hoogsten hydrogen bond). Normally **pKa** of cytosine is 4.2, which is altered to **> 7.5** in triplex. It is important to understand that Hoogsteen pairing is essential for triplex DNA formation, whereas other factors like long polypyramidine / polypurine only sequences in a strand, 2 + 1 purine / pyramidine strands, **low pH, increased pKa & protonated cytosine** are facilitatory.

Palindromes & Hairpin or Cruciform (Cross shaped) Structures

- Palindrome word / phrase / sentence / sequence is identically read either forward or backward; such as ROTATOR and NURSES RUN.
- Palindromic sequences of DNA have **twofold symmetry over two strands of DNA** and in order to superimpose one repeat on the other, it must be rotated 180° about the horizontal axis then 180° about the vertical axis.

T T A G C A C G T G C T A A
A A T C G T G C A C G A T T

- Palindromic sequences are **self complementary within each strand** and therefor can form **hairpin or cruciform (cross shaped) structures** with **intrastrand** base pairing. When only **one strand** of DNA (or RNA) is involved the structure is called hairpin and when **both strands** of a duplex DNA are involved it is called cruciform.

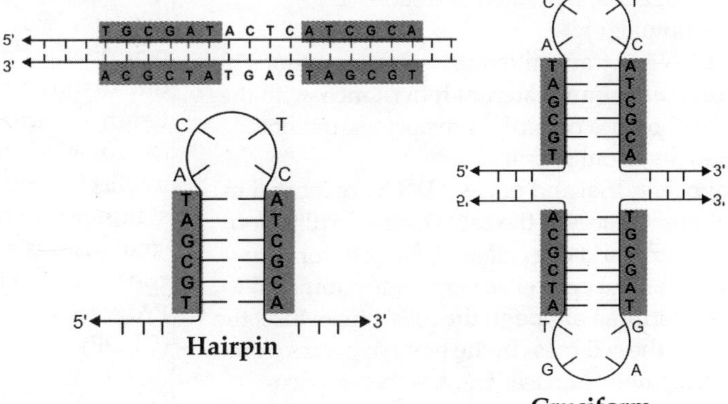

Tetraplex / Quadruplex – DNA & G/Guanosine Tetraplex

- **Four stranded DNA (tetraplex or quadruplex)** occurs only for DNA sequences with **very high proportion of guanosine residue** (or very stable **guanosine /G tetraplex**).
- Guanosine (G) tetraplex is very stable over wide range of conditions

Mirror Repeats

- Mirror repeat has **symmetrical inverted repeat sequence within each strand**. So super imposing one repeat on the other requires only a single 180° rotation about the vertical axis.

T T A G C A C C A C G A T T
A A T C G T G G T G C T A A

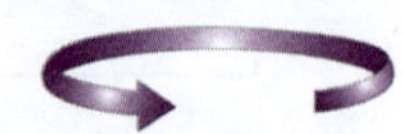

- Mirror repeats **donot have complementary sequences with in the same strand and so cannot form hairpin or cruciform structures.**

Human Mitochondrial DNA (mt DNA)

- Mitochondria contain their own genome which is **a closed circular piece of double stranded DNA**[Q] that is composed of heavy (H) and light (L) strands or chains.
- Mt DNA is double stranded for most of its length except at the replication and transcription control region (the D-loop), It is not packaged in nucleosomes
- Human mt DNA contains 16,569 base pairs (16.599 kb) in length and 37 genes that encode **13 protein complexes of respiratory chain, 2r RNAs and all 22 mt tRNAs required for mitochondrial protein synthesis**[Q]
- However the great majority of mitochondrial proteins – about 900 different types (of which about 54 out of 67/ 66 but of 79 proteins of respiratory chain)- are encoded by nuclear genes, synthesized on cytoplasmic ribosomes, then imported into & assembled in the mitochondria.
- 1% of cellular DNA is in mitochondria as each mitochondria contains 2-10 copies of mt DNA. Each human cell contains variable number of mitochondria depending on the energy requirement of a particular cell. So each cell has large number of mt DNA owing to the fact that mt DNA replication is not limited to one per cell cycle as it is in nuclear genome. This greater abundance, compared with that of nuclear DNA, makes mt DNA attractive for testing applications in which sample DNA is limited (eg crime scene investigation, pathogen detection, & paleontology)
- Mt DNA is transmitted between generations by **non mandalian maternal inheritance**, with the mitochondria coming from oocytes and not (usually) from sperm
- Mitochondrial and nuclear DNA are located in different places in the cell. During fertilization, the sperm and egg cell nuclei fuse to form an embryo. The egg cell is very large compared to the sperm, so although the cells' nuclei fuse, the rest of the cell mass in the embryo comes from the egg only. Nuclear DNA is therefore co-inherited but the mitochondrial DNA, which is

- **Genetic code of mt DNA differs slightly** from standard code: mt RNA reads 4 codons differently

Codon	Normal	Mt DNA
AGA AGG	Arginine	Terminator or stop codon
UGA	Terminator	**Trypthophan**
AUA	Isoleucine	Methionine

- **Proteins & structures encoded by mt DNA**
  - Encodes 2 *mitochondrial ribosomal RNAs large (16s) and small (12S) units*
  - Encodes all 22 *mt tRNA molecules*
  - Encodes **13 protein** subunits of respiratory chain (of a total of about 67-Harper/ 79- Lehninger)

Respiratory chain protein complex	Total no. of subunits	No. of sub units encoded by mt DNA
I NADH dehydrogenase	43	7
II Succinate dehydrogenase	4	0
III Ubiquinone: cytochrome C oxidoreductase (cytochrome b)	11	1
IV Cytochrome oxidase	13	3
V ATP synthase	8	2
Total	79	13

- Disorders due to (*point mutation, large scale rearrangements & some deletions*) defect in mt DNA: (Mn- **"Pearson No Progressive Leigh Deaf Labour Kissed Me Adequtely"**)

Disease & Phenotype	**Mt DNA Mutation & Inheritance (mostly)**
Pearson (PEAR) syndrome i.e. pancreatic & bone marrow failure	Large deletion , Heteroplasmic, Sporadic somatic mutations
NARP syndrome i.e. neurogenic muscle weakess (with sensory or sensory motor neuropathy), ataxia, retinitis pigmentosa due to mutation in MT-ATP 6 gene. **Leigh syndrome** i.e. progressive neurological disease with motor & intellectual developmental delay, signs & symptoms of basal ganglia / or brain stem disease and raised lactate concentration in blood and CSF.	Point mutation in **ATPase subunit 6 gene,** Heteroplasmic; Maternal
Progressive external opthalmoplegia (CEOP)	**Single deletion / duplication**; Heteroplasmic; Sporadic somatic mutations
Deafness: Progressive sensorineural	A 1555 G mutation in **12 s**

located outside of the nucleus, is always maternally inherited because all mitochondria in a foetus and later adult are derived from the mitochondria in the mother's egg. All children from affected mother will inherit the disease but it will not be transmitted from an affected father to his children.

- Mt DNA is **not highly conserved & has high mutation rate** (5-10 times that of nuclear DNA) which accumulate through out the life of organism. It is because
  - Mt DNA suffers greatest exposure to reactive oxygen species produced in respiratory chain
  - It has less effective proof reading system at correcting mistakes made during replication and at repairing DNA damage
  - **It contains no (or very few) introns (or untranslated sequences)**Q
- Rapid accumulation of mutation provides sufficient data, to allow the comparison of closely relatede species or population with in the same species providing **evidence about evolutionary origins** of primates & other species.
- It can be used to study **evolutionary relationship (phylogeny) of organisms** & build evolutionary tree as well as for **genealogical research into person's maternal line** (eg prince Williams has Indian origin maternal line).

deafness induced by amino glycoside antibiotics.	**RNA; Homoplasmic**; Maternal
LHON syndrome i.e. **Leber's** hereditary optic neuropathy (atrophy)	G17778 A, G 3460A, T 14484 C; **Homoplasmic** (±); Maternal
Kearns- Sayre Syndrome (KSS) i.e. opthalmoplegia, pigment degeneration of retina and cardiomyopathy	5Kb **common deletion;** Heteroplasmic; sporadic somatic mutation
MELAS syndrome i.e. mitochondrial myopathy with encephalopathy, lactic acidosis and stroke	Point mutation in **tRNA leu;** Heteroplasmic; Maternal
MERRF syndrome i.e. myoclonic epilepsy and ragged red fibres disease d/t mutation in mitochondrial gene that encodes t RNA specific for lysine (t RNA Lys)	Point mutation in **t RNA lys;** Heteroplasmic; Maternal
MMC syndrome i.e. **M**aternally inherited **m**yopathy and **c**ardiomyopathy	
ADMIMY syndrome i.e. **a**utosomal **d**ominant **mi**tochondrial inherited **my**opathy with mitochondrial deletion.	
Somatic mutations in cytochrome complex III deficiency, muscle pain, ragged red fibers	

★ *Deafness & LHON are homoplasmic* and others are heteroplasmic usually. All have *maternal inheritance* except Pearson syndrome, KKS and chronic progressive external opthalmoplegia (CPEO) which are sporadic somtic mutations mostly.

Types of DNA

Feature	A- DNA	B- DNA	Z- DNA
Prevalence	Not found under physiological conditions. When B DNA crystals are dried, the long thin B- DNA becomes short stubby A- DNA	*Most common*Q	Occurs *in region* that have a sequence of alternating purines & pyrimidines eg poly GC *rich in guanine & cytosine base pairs.*
Helix handedness	Right	*Right*Q	*Left*Q
Sugar pucker conformation	C-3' endo	C-2' endo	**C-2' endo for pyrimidines** and **C-3' endo for purines**
Glycosyl bond confirmation	Anti	Anti	Anti for pyrimidines; Syn for purines
Deoxyribose – phosphate backbone	Linear	Linear	*Zigzag*Q
Major groove	Present	Present	Non existing or convex
Minor groove	Present	Present	Deep cleft
Repeating unit base pairs	1	1	2
Base pairs /turn	11	10.5	12
Inclination of base pair to axis of helix	~ 20° (19°)	~1° (1.2°)	~ 10° (9°)
Base tilt normal to helical axis	20°	6°	7°
Rotation / base pair	~ 33°	~ 35°	30°
Pitch (nm)	2.46	3.40	4.56
Diameter (nm)	2.55	2.37	1.84
Helical Rise / base pair along helix axis (nm)	0.26	0.34	0.37

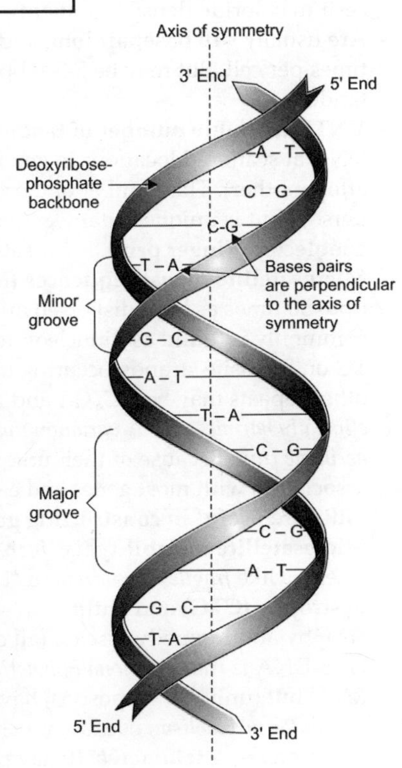

In Human genome

- Haploid genome of each human cell consists of **3×10^9 base pairs (3000 mega bases)** of DNA and about **1.7×10^7 nucleosomes** subdivided into 23 chromosomes (chromatids). Each of these 23 chromatids would contain on the average **1.3×10^8 nucleotides** in one ds DNA molecule.
- Entire haploid genome contains sufficient DNA to have nearly 1.5 million average sized genes but studies suggest that humans have < 1 lakh proteins encoded by ~1% of human genome composed of exonic DNA containing ≤ 25,000 protein coding genes (previously 30-35 thousand). This means most of the DNA is non-protein coding i.e. its information is never translated into an aminoacid sequence of a protein molecule.
- Pathologic effects of genetic diseases are expressed at levels:
  i) DNA ii) RNA iii) Protein iv) Cell & organ consequences.

Eukaryotic DNA: Human Genome

- > 50% of eukaryotic DNA is **unique** or **non repetitive** and at least (i.e. >) 30% consists of **repetitive** sequences, About 30% of genome is genes (for protein) but only 1.5% is **coding sequences (or exons)** carrying information for RNA or protein products.
- **Non coding (non-translated) DNA** segments in genes are called **intervening sequences** or **introns** (28.5%), and the coding segments are called exons. Genes for histones have no introns and genes for muscle protein titin have 178 introns.
- 1% of cellular DNA is in mitochondria. **Repetitive sequence DNA** can be classified as

* Highly Repetitive Sequence (HRS)

- Also called **simple sequence DNA** or **simple sequence repeats (SSR)** and constitute 3% of human genome
- SSR is also called **satellite DNA** because its unsual base composition often causes it to migrate as *satellite bands (separated from the rest of DNA)* when fragmented cellular DNA samples are centrifuged (in cesium chloride density gradient).
- Are usually **<10 basepair long** and sometimes repeated millions of times per cell. But may be 5-500 bp long, repeated many times in tandem
- **VNTR (variable number of tandem repeats)** are short sequences of DNA at scattered locations in genome, repeated in tandem (i.e. one after another). The number of these repeat units varies from person to person, but is unique for any given individual and, therefore, **serves as a molecular finger print**. Microsatellites are a type of VNTR.
- **Microsatellite repeat sequences (MiRS)** consist of 2-6 bp repeated upto 50 times as both dispersed and grouped tandem arrays. It most commonly is found as dinucleotide repeats of AC on ones strand and TG on opposite strands-occuring upto 1 lack times in genome. Several other repeats may be CG, CA and AT. It produces **polymorphism** (i.e. *clinically harmless DNA variation that does not affect phenotype*) & is a *heritable trait*. Because of their unique number (for an indvidual), usual association with most genes and ease of detecting them using PCR, MiRS are **useful in constructing genetic linkage map.**
- **Microsatellite instability** (i.e. *increased tri nucleotide repeats*) can lead to diseases like *fragile X syndrome* d/t unstable p(CGG)n, **myotonic dystrophy (CTG)** and Hutington's chorea, spinobulbar muscular atrophy and Kennedy disease (all d/t unstable CAG).
- HRS-DNA is *transcriptionally inactive (i.e. does not encode proteins or RNA)* but (unlike transposons) have an *identifiable functional importance in cellular metabolism*, because much of it is associated with – **centromeres & telomeres**. It may play a *structural role* also.

Moderately Repititive Sequences

- Defined as being present in numbers of *<10^6 copies per haploid genome, are not clustered but are interspersed* with unique sequences.
- About half (45%) of human genome is made up of MRS which is derived from **transposable elements (transposons) – a kind of molecular parasite,** efficiently *making a home (or trapped) with in the host genome* during evolution.
- These DNA segments range from few *hundred to several thousand bp* long, that can *move from one location to another* in the genome (**transposition**) through an RNA intermediate by action of reverse transcriptase (i.e. **retroposons**).
- Many transposons have genes transcribed by RNA polymerase II encoding m-RNA (containing indistinguishable caps) and proteins that catalyze transposition process.
- Although these do not encode RNA or proteins used in human cells, they have played a major role in human evolution –as movement of transposons can l/t redistribution of other genomic sequences.
- Most transposons are **inactive**, evolutionarily altered by mutations, however, some may be active moving (transcribing) at a low frequency.
- Depending on their length MRS can be

1. Long interspersed repeat sequences (LINEs):

- **6 – 8 Kbp** (1 kbp = 1000bp) long and have 20-50 thousand copies (Harper)/8.5 lack LINEs (Lehninger) in human genome.
- It is species specific families of repeat element.

Centromere

- It is **adenine- thymine-(A-T) rich** region containing repeated DNA sequences from 10^2 – 10^6 bp size (i.e. thousands of tandem copies of short segments in same orientation) which *connects sister chromatids.*
- Metazoan centromere is bound by nucleosome containing CEN P-A (a H3 histone variant protein & other centromere binding proteins, forming **Kinetochore** which *provides the attachment for mitotic spindle.*
- This anchoring is essential for equal & orderly chromosomal segregation (distribution) during mitosis.

Telomere

- Telomeres are **short T-G rich repeats** at the ends of eukaryotic chromosomes that *help stabilize the chromosome.*
- Human telomeres have variable number of **'5' – TTA GGG-3''** repeats which may extend upto several Kb.

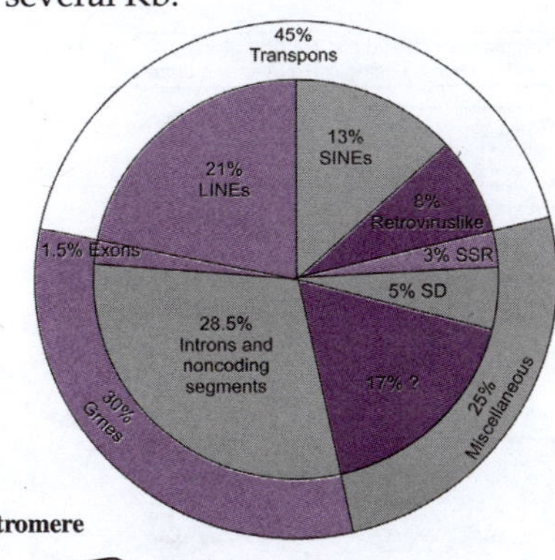

A+T rich centromere

Sister chromatid 1

Sister chromatid 2

TG rich

Telomeres (TTAGGG)n

2. Short interspersed repeat sequences (SINEs)

- Are shorter (70-300 bp long) and have >1 lack copies per genome (Harper)
- Of 1.5 million in human genome >1 million are **Alu family**, so called because they generally have one copy of recognition sequence for AluI, restriction endonuclease (Lehninger).
- Alu elements (family) a/f 5-6% human genome (i.e. 5 lack copies per haploid genome). Harper it is **highly conserved** *within as well as between mammalian species.*
- SINEs are **mobile elements**, capable of jumping from one region to another region of genome and can l/t disastrous events as insertion of Alu sequences may cause *neurofibromatosis.*

3. Retrovirus like transposons

- 1.5 – 11 kbp long, 4.5 lack copies of these are present in human genome.
- Although evolutionarily related to retrovirus they are trapped & cannot move from one cell to another.

4. Transposon remnants that differ greatly in length

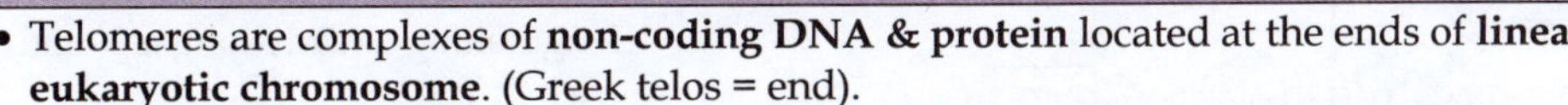

Telomeres

- Telomeres are complexes of **non-coding DNA & protein** located at the ends of **linear eukaryotic chromosome**. (Greek telos = end).
- It consist of **many tandem** (one after another) **repeats** (> 20 to > 1500) **of short DNA sequence /oligo nucleotide** (dimeric to octameric). Telomere usually has **TG rich** *longer strand* and **AC rich** *shorter complementary strand.* The general formula is

5'- $(T_x G_y)n$ 3' – $(A_x C_y)n$

where **x & y** = Between 1 & 4 and number of telomere repeat **n** range from 20 -100 in single cell eukaryotes to >1500 in mammals

5' 3'
3' 5'
Telomere Eukaryotic DNA Telomere

- Telomeres very in length from few dozen bp in protozoa to several thousands bp in mammals (humans). In humans, **non coding hexameric sequence AG_3T_2** base paired to complementary CA sequence forms telomere.

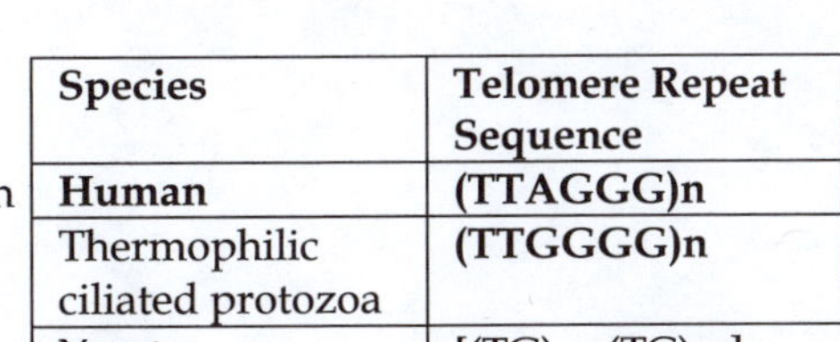

Species	Telomere Repeat Sequence
Human	**(TTAGGG)n**
Thermophilic ciliated protozoa	**(TTGGGG)n**
Yeast	$[(TG)_{1-3}\ (TG)_{2-3}]n$
Plant	(TTTAGGG)n

- The **TG strand is longer** than its AC complement, leving a region of single stranded *(ss) DNA of few hundred nucleotides in length at the 3' end.* Single stranded region (end) is folded back on itself, and paired with its complement in ds portion of telomere, forming a **T-loop structure**. The looped DNA is bound (stabilized) by several **telomere binding proteins**, including

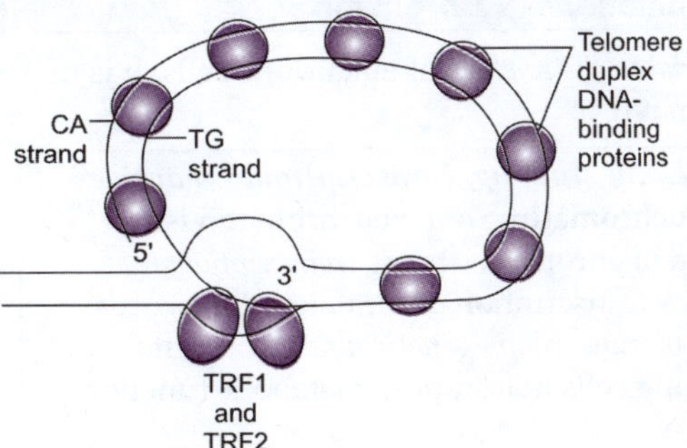

Telomerase Enzyme

- It is a *multisubunit RNA containing-protein complex* with a **RNA dependent DNA polymerase** (i.e. **reverse transcriptase**) activity.
- It is responsible for **telomere synthesis and maintenance of telomere length.**
- Prevention of telomere shortening with every cell division, d/t activity of telomerase enzyme is the cause of **cellular immortality in cancer cells, germline cells and stem cells** as it protects from cellular aging & apoptosis.
- **Somatic cells lack telomerase** and *undergo cellular aging, senescence (i.e. no longer able to divide) and death (apoptosis)*[Q] after 40-60 replications when telomeres become critically short or gone. So cells.

With telomerase activity	Without telomerase activity
- *Germinal (Germline) cells*[Q] - *Cancer (tumor)/ neoplastic cells*[Q] - *Stem cells like hemopoetic cells*[Q]	*Somatic cells*[Q]

TRF-1 & TRF-2 (telomere repeat binding factor) with the latter protein involved in formation of T loop. It maintains the **structural integrity** and **confer stability** to chromosomal ends. T-loops *protect 3′ end,* making them *inaccessible to nucleases and enzymes* that repair double strand breaks, and allow repair system to *distinguish a true end from a break in ds DNA.* So telomeres *protect* chromosomal termini *from fusion & degradation.*

- Because DNA replication (by DNA polymerase) requires a template & primer, and beyond the end (extreme 5′ end) of lagging strand there is *no DNA template available for pairing of an RNA primer.* So **telomeres are not readily replicated by DNA polymerase** and consequently telomeres **shorten with each cell division** in most normal **somatic** human **cells.**
- There is a linear, inverse relationship between telomere length and cell senescence (cessation of cell division) or age. So telomerase is a **mitotic clock** in that their length in most cells is inversely related to the number of times cells have divided.
- Once the telomeres are shortened beyond a certain point, the loss of telomere function leads to activation of p53 dependent cell cycle check points, causing proliferation arrest & apoptosis. Thus *telomere shortening functions as a clock that counts cell divisions.* In germ cells, telomere shortening is prevented by the sustained function of enzyme telomerase, which maintains their ability to self replicate extensively. *Cancer cells show reactivation of telomerase activity* and maintenance of telomere length.

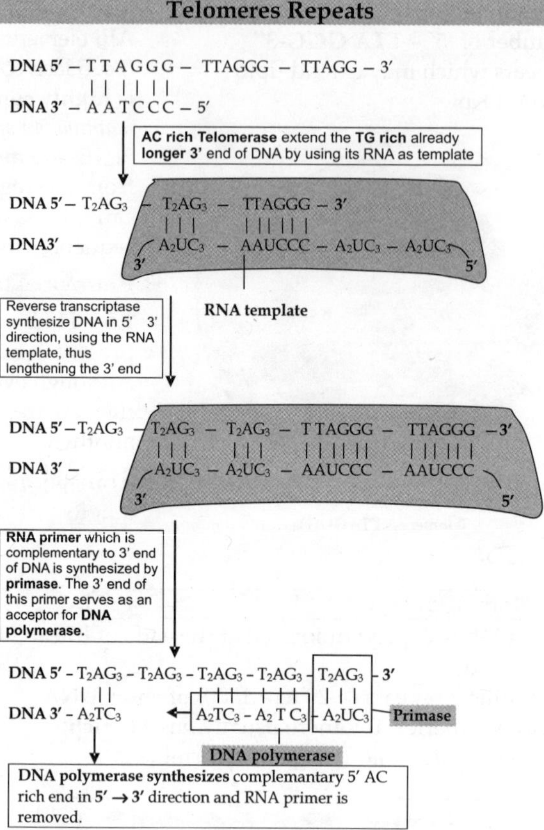

- Telomerase contains a **protein** that acts as **reverse transcriptase and a short piece of (~150 nucleotide long) AC rich RNA** that acts as a **template** for synthesis of already longer TG (3′) strand.
- **CA-rich RNA template** (containing ~ 1.5 copies of Cy Ax telomere repeat) base pairs with *GT rich single stranded 3′ end of telomeric DNA.* The extra overhanging length of this RNA acts as a template for synthesis (lengthening) of already longer Tx Gy strand of telomere. **Reverse transcriptase** uses this RNA template to synthesize DNA in **5′→ 3′ direction**, extending the already longer 3′ (TG) end. However, unlike retroviral reverse transcriptase, telomerase copies only a small segment of RNA that it carries with itself.
- Having synthesized one copy of the repeat, the *telomerase repositions (translocates) to the newly synthesized end and the process is repeated* further lengthening already longer 3′ end (rich in TG).
- Once the GT rich 3′ end (strand) is appropriately lengthened, **primase** can use it as a template to synthesize a complementary **RNA fragment (primer)** opposite to TG strand. The RNA primer is extended by **DNA polymerase** & primer is removed.
- **This means 3′ TG rich end is synthesized by telomerase and complementary 5′ AC rich end is synthesized by DNA polymerase.**

Structure of Chromosome & Chromatin

- Chromatin is the *chromosomal material in the nucleus* of eukaryotic cells. It is of 2 types – euchromatin & heterochromatin.

- ***Less condensed (more open) & weakly staining, transcriptionally active***Q regions of chromatin are called **euchromatin**. So the euchromatin is the **dispersed (uncondensed)** portion of chromatin that is *transcriptionally active during interphase* (when RNA transcription occurs). In other words, *euchromatin contains genes capable of transcribing genetic information into proteins* that are necessary for young cells maturation, metabolic function or DNA repair.

Nucleosomes

- Nucleosomes are *functional or originational units of chromatin* and appear as a **"beads on a string"** arrangement on electron microscopy.
- Flat protein cylinder consisting of **histone octamer** containing **2 molecules each of H3, H4, H2A & H2B** form tine **structural core of** individual **nucleosome beads**
- **(H3-H4)2 tetramer** itself can confer nucleosome like properties on DNA and so

- Whereas, **highly condensed & strongly staining heterochromatin** is defined as a (chromotin) structure that does not alter inits condensation throughout the cell cycle (in contrast to euchromatin that decondense during interphase)

- Chromatin consists of *fibers containing (histone) protein and DNA in nearly equal proportions (by mass)*. Chromatin contains
  - Double stranded (ds) DNA] - Form **nucleosomes**
  - Small **basic proteins** k/a **histones**]
  - Mostly acidic and larger (than histones) **non histone proteins**, that include enzymes involved in DNA replication & repair, and proteins involved in RNA synthesis, processing and transport to cytoplasm in smaller amounts
  - **RNA** (small quantity)
- DNA (in transcriptionally or potentially transcriptionally) active chromatin has larger regions (~ 1 lack bases long) that are relatively *more sensitive to digestion by nuclease* (like **DN ase I**, a *low sequence specific nuclease* that makes *single strand cuts* in nearly any segment of DNA that is not protected , or bound by protein into its component deoxynucleotides). The **sensitivity to DNase I** digestion reflects *only a potential for transcription rather than transcription* itself and can be associated with a relative **lack of 5-methyl deoxycytidine (meC)** in DNA and particular (*phosphorylation, acetylation etc) covalent modification of histones*.
- Shorter (100-300 nucleotides long), **Hypersensitive (10 times more sensitive)** sites to DN ase I exist in larger active chromatin. It is formedby *binding of non-histone regulatory transcriptional factor proteins* and proteins involved in maintaining access to template strand and result in structural conformation that favours access of nuclease to DNA. Hypersensitive regions are often **located immediately upstream from the active gene** that is capable of being transcribed.
- **Inactive chromatin** is *high in meC content in DNA and lower in covalent modifications of histones*. It can be of 2 types
  - **Constitutive hetero chromatin**, found in *centromere and telomeres* (i.e. chromosomal ends), is *always condensed* and thus *essentially inactive*.
  - **Facultative heterochromatin**, is at times condensed but at other times is uncondensed (appears as euchromatin) and is actively transcribed. Like *X chromosome* of females that is active only during gametogenesis.
- Approximately 1 m long DNA of 46 chromosomes is packed in small nucleus of each cell. This becomes possible only b/o multi levels of DNA compaction, condensing it to > 10000 (10^4) folds.

Chromatin form	Packing (Condensation) Ratio	Dia-meter	Features
Nacked double helical DNA	1	2 nm	
10 nm chromatin fibrils of **nucleosomes**	7-10	10 nm	**Beads on string** form of chromatin
30 nm chromatin fiber of superhelical nucleosomes	40-60 (Harper) /100 (Lehninger)	30 nm	10 nm fibril is further supercoiled with *6-7 nucleosomes per turn* to form 30 nm chromatin fiber: H_1 histones stabilize it and faces of nucleosome of successive turns would be nearly parallel to each other.

has a central role in nucleosome formation. Addition of **2 (H2A-H2B) dimmers** stabilize the primary particle & firmly binds two additional half turns of DNA previously bound only loosely to $(H_3\text{-}H_4)_2$.

- **Around the surface of disc shaped histone octamer (i.e. nucleosome protein core), the 1.75 superhelical turns** of DNA are wrapped (wound), forming **left handed solenoidal supercoil** (or **underwound** or **negatively supertwisted helix**), protecting 146 bp of DNA from digestion by a nuclease and forming the **nucleosome core particle.**
- Neighboring nucleosome core particles (beads) are linked by approximately 30 bp (Harper)/50 bp (Lippincot)/**54 bp** (Lehninger) long DNA segment termed as **linker. Histone H1** binds to the linker DNA. The bead plus the connecting DNA that leads to the next bead form the **nucleosome**. So nucleosomes are ***repeating units containing histones & 200 bp DNA (146 bp bound to core & 54 bp linker)***[Q].
- Tight wrapping of DNA around histone core *requires removal of 1 helical turn* in DNA, but because this process does not break the DNA (or change the linking number), the formation of a negative solenoidal supercoil must be accompanied by a compensatory positive super coil in unbound region of DNA. ***Eukaryotic topoisomerase*** *relax the unbound positive supercoil* (leaves the negative supercoil fixed to histone core) and results in an overall decrease in linking number. This is how eukaryotic DNA is underwound even through eukaryotic cells lack enzymes that underwind DNA.
- Majority of *core histone proteins interact with the DNA* on the inside of supercoil without protruding *except their amino terminal tails* which extend outside and are available for covalent modification.
- Nucleosome (histone) core exhibit **non random preferential binding (phasing)** to specific DNA sequence that has a local abundance of **A=T base pairs** in DNA where it is in contact with histones facilitating the compression of minor grooves that is needed for tight wrapping. Nucleosomes bind well to sequences

Loops (Domains)	8000	300 nm	- 20-100 kbp (X 1000 bp) anchored in a **scaffolding (supporting) matrix** with in the nucleus (i.e. **nuclear matrix**) *containing H_1 histone and topoisomerase II, organize to form loops.* - Looped domains contain a set of related genes corresponding to one or more separate genetic functions, containing both coding & non coding regions of cognate gene or genes.
Rosette	6 loops	condense to form 1 rosette	
Coil	30 rosettes	condense to form 1 coil	
Chromatids	10 coils	condense to form each chromatid (of 1400 nm diameter)	

Chromatin Proteins

1. Histone proteins

- Histones are **small, basic proteins**Q, which package the DNA into structural units called **nucleosomes.**
- Carboxy terminal (2/3) of histone molecules are hydrophobic, while amino terminal (1/3) is rich in basic' amino acids.
- Histone proteins are *most abundant chromatin protein.* These are **positively charged** at physiological pH because of their **high content of basic amino acids arginine and lysine** and hence form **ionic bonds** with negatively charge DNA. Histones, along with positively charged ions like Mg^{++} neutralize the negatively charged DNA phosphates.
- There are five classes of histones: *H1, H2A, H2B, H3, H4.* H1 histones are least tightly bound to chromatin and are, therefore, easily removed with salt solution, after which chromatin becomes soluble. The organizational unit of this soluble chromatin is the nucleosome. ***Nucleosome*** contains four type of histones- *H2A, H2B, H3, H4*; collectively called ***core histones.***
- The **histones interact** with each other in a very specific ways. H3 and H4 form a tetramer containing two molecules of each **(H3-H4)$_2$,** while **H2A and H2B form dimmers (H2A-H2B).** Under physiological conditions, these histone oligomers associate to form the **histone octamer (H3-H4)2 – (H2A-H2B)2.**
- **H3** and **H4 histones** are most conserved among eukaryotes f/b other core histones (H2A, H2B). This indicates that function of histones is identical in all eukaryotes and that the entire molecule is involved in carrying out this function.
- H1 histone is most tissue specific & species specific of histones. It facilitates the packing of nucleosoe into more compact structure.
- The four core histones are subjected to at least *six types* of covalent modification. Mn: **"RUPAM"** i.e. **R**ibosylation, **U**biquitin binding, **P**hosphorylation, **A**cetylation, **M**ethylation.

Covalent Modification	DNA Repair
ADP-Ribosylation	- DNA repair
Covalent linkage to Ubiquitin - **Monoubiquitylation** - **Sumoylation** (SUMO; small ubiquitin – related modifier) - **Phosphorylation of H_1**	 - Gene activation, repression, and heterochromatic gene silencing - Transcription repression - Condensation of chromosomes during replication cycle
Acetylation - of core histones - of H3 & H4 histones	 - Chromosomal assembly during DNA-replication - Activation & inactivation of gene transcription
Methylation	- Activation & repression of gene transcription

where **AA** or **AT** or **TT** dinucleotides are staggered at 10 bp intervals. Phasing is d/t physical flexibility of certain sequences that are able to accommodate the regions of kinking within the supercoil.

- Nucleosomes are deposited on DNA in a stepwise manner (during replication or other process that require a transient displacement) mediated by **RCAF** *(replication coupling assembly factor)* which includes acetylated H3 & H4, chromatin assembly factor-1 / **CAF1** and anti silencing factor / **ASF-1**). $(H_3\text{-}H_4)_2$ tetramer binds first f/b (H2A – H2B) dimmer.

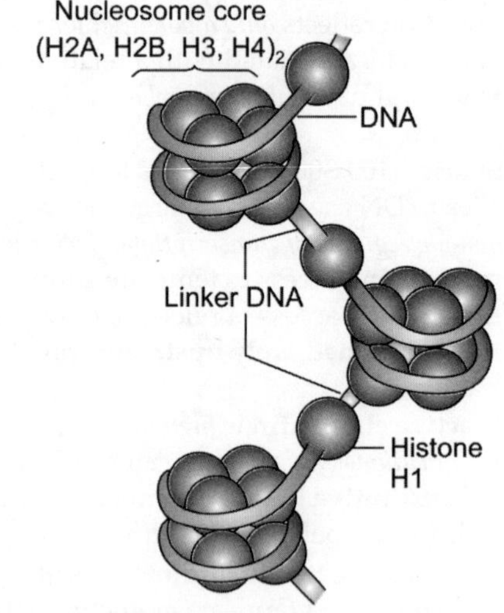

Organization of human DNA illustrating the sequence of nucleosomes

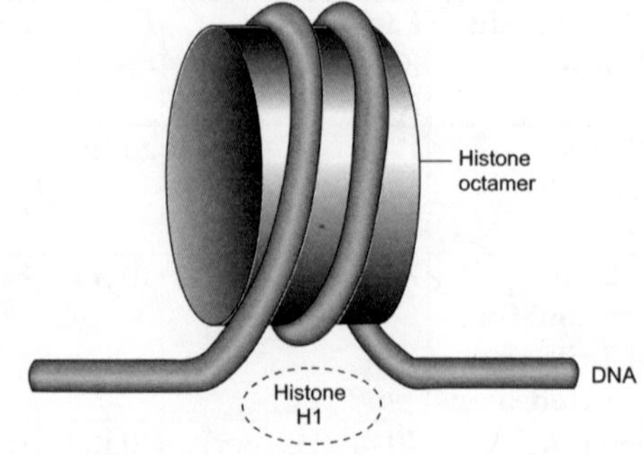

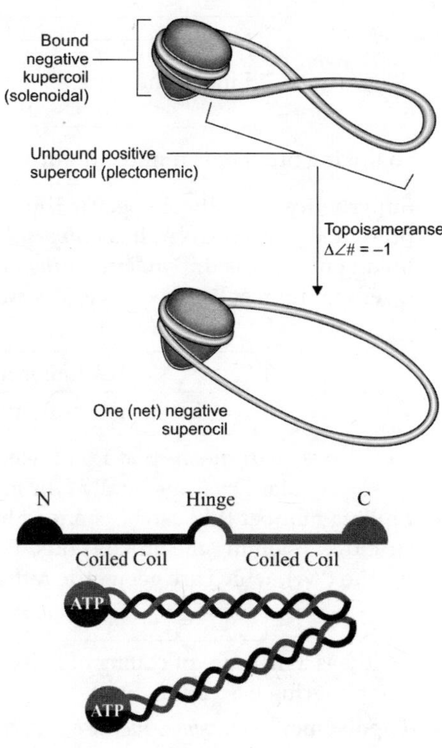

- **Histone acetylation (by histone acetyl transferase = HAT)** causes ***increased (trancriptionally active) relatively uncondensed euchromatin formation***[Q]. Acetylation or phosphorylation of lysine residue at aminoterminal **decreases positive (+) charge of basic histone protein,** there by decreasing their association with negatively (-) charged DNA, thus releasing nucleosomes and allowing access to DNA. **Histone deacetylation (by histone deacetylase = HDAC)** removes acetyl group, restores positive charge and causes **increased formation of transcriptionally inactive hetero chromatin (relatively condensed).**

2. Topoisomerase

It relax *the compensatory positive plectonemic supercoil* in unbound region of DNA produced d/t negative solenoidal supercoiling of DNA around histone core.

3. SMC (Structural maintenance of chromosomes) proteins

- SMC proteins *maintain structures of condensed chromosomes* and consist of 5 domains globular amino (N) & carboxy (C) terminals *with partial ATP hydrolytic site (on each* and becomes complete on joining). These 2 N & C terminals are joined by *2α-helical coiled coil motifs* joined by a hinge domain.
- **Cohesins & Condensins** are 2 SMC proteins. Condensins bind to DNA and *creates positive super coils* (i.e. DNA becomes **over wound** in contrast to underwinding introduced by binding of nucleosomes). So condensins are essential to chromosomal condensation as cell enters mitosis.
- **Cohesins** link sister chromatids together immediately after replication & keep them together as chromosomes condense to metaphase – a process essential for proper segregation of chromosomes at cell division. **Cohesin & Kleisin** form a ring around replicated chromosomes that tie them together (expand & contract in response to ATP hydrolysis) until separation is required at cell division.

Supercoiling & Linking Number

- **Supercoiling** means the coiling of a coil. DNA is coiled in form of a double helix, with both strands of DNA coiling around an axis. The further coiling of that axis upon itself produce DNA super coiling, which is a *manifestation of structural strain.* When there is no net bending of DNA axis upon itself, the DNA is said to be in relaxed state.
- Supercoiling is an *intrinsic property* of DNA *tertiary structure* which is requied for DNA compaction. Replication & transcription of DNA also affect & are affected by supercoiling. It is studied in topology, a branch of mathemetics.
- Closed circular (B form) DNA with **one turn of double helix per 10.5 base pair** is relaxed. Supercoiling is a manifestation of structural strain. And in almost every instance, the strain is a result of **underwinding** of DNA double helix in the closed circle. In other words, *DNA has fewer helical turns than would be expected for the B form* structure. An 84 bp segment of a circular DNA in relaxed state would contain 8 double helical turns, or 1 of every 10.5bp. If one of these turns were removed, there would be (84 bp) / 7= 12 bp / turn rather than 10.5 bp/ turn in B- DNA. This deviation from most stable form would result in a thermodynamically strained DNA

LK = 6

- In principle, the strain could also be accommodated by separating the two DNA strand over a distance of about 10 bp. But in isolated circular DNA the strain introduced by ***under winding is generally accommodated by supercoiling rather than strand seperation***[Q], because coiling the axis of DNA usually requires less energy than breaking the hydrogen bonds that stabilize paired bases. However underwinding represents a *form of stored energy and makes separation of DNA strands easier*
- ***Most cells maintain DNA in under wound state to facilitate its compaction by coiling***[Q].
- **Linking number,** is a topological property of ds DNA, because it does not vary when DNA is bent or deformed, as long as both strands remain intact. Linking number can be defined as the number of times the 2nd strand pierces the surface of 1st strand which is visualized as circle. It is defined **as positive (+ve)** if strands are interwound in *right handed helix and* ***negative (-ve)*** *in left handed helix* (not encountered).

$$\text{Linking number} = \frac{\text{Number of base pairs}}{\text{Number of base pairs per turn (which is 10.5 in relaxed form)}}$$

So linking number is number of turns.

- **Superhelical density** or **specific linking difference (σ)** is a measure of number of turns removed relative to the number present in relaxed DNA. It is *independent of the length of DNA molecule*Q. The **negative** sign indicates that the change in linking number is d/t *underwinding of DNA*Q. So the supercoiling induced by underwinding is called **negative supercoiling**. Over wound results in positive superwinding (which is a mirror image of negative supercoiling).

$$\sigma = \frac{\Delta Lk\ (\text{number of turns removed})}{Lko\ (\text{number of turns present in relaxed DNA})}$$

σ = - 0.01 means that 1% of helical turns present in B form of DNA has been removed. The degree of underwnding in cellular DNAs generally falls in range of 5-7%, that is σ = - 0.05 to - 0.07.

- Linking number (Lk) can be changed by ± 1 by breaking one DNA strand, rotating one of the ends 360° about the unbroken strand, & rejoining the broken ends. This change has no effect on no. of base pairs. Lk can be broken down to **twist (Tw)** and **writhe (Wr)**, which are geometric rather than topological properties, because they may be changed by deformation.

$$Lk = Tw + Wr$$

- Writhe is a measure of coiling of helix axis and twist (Tw) determines the local twisting or spatial relationship of neighbouring base pairs.
- **Topoisomerase** *enzymes increase or decrease the extent of DNA underwinding* and so the linking number
  - **Topoisomerase type I**, act by transiently breaking one of the two strands, passing the unbroken strand through the break & rejoining the broken end; they ***change Lk in increments of 1***Q.
  - **Topoisomerase type II** ***break both DNA strands & change linking number in increments of*** 2Q.

DNA Replication (Initiation, Synthesis, Elongation and Termination) ☆

Initiation of DNA Synthesis

- It ***follows base pair rule and is semiconservative***Q because, although the parental double strands are separated into two halves & therefore is not conserved as entily, each of the individual parental strands remains intact in one of the two daughter chromatids. Each strand of double helix (strand) serves as template for constructing a complementry daughter strand (**semiconservative strand**).
- The site at which the DNA replication is initiated is termed the **origin of replication (Ori)**. In prokaryotes, **Dna A** (a DNA binding protein) binds to **repeated nucleotide consensus (highly conserved) sequences** located within the origin. Binding of 20-30 Dna A molecules to ori induces unwinding, which separates strands in AT rich region adjacent to Dna A- binding sites, that is easy to unwind and is called **DNA unwinding element (DUE)**. The E coli replication origin is called **ori C**. Functionally similar **autonomously replicating sequences (ARS) or replicators** occur in **yeast cells**. The ARS contains degenerate 11 bp sequence, **origin replication element (ORE)** that binds to set of protein analogous to dna A of E.coli and form **origin recognition complex (ORC)**.

Elongation Phase of Replication (Chain Elongation)

- Two strands of double stranded DNA molecules are **antiparallel**. The **DNA replication** in eukaryotes & prokaryotes ***occur on both strands simultaneously by a single asymmetric DNA polymerase III dimer***Q. Because , an enzyme capable of polymerizing DNA in 3′ to 5′ direction does not occur in nature, *so both of newly replicated DNA strands cannot grow in the same direction simultaneously.*
- **Replication exhibits polarity** because DNA polymerases responsible for copying the DNA templates are only able to **read** parental nucleotide sequences **in 3′ → 5′ direction and** they **synthesize** the new DNA strands **only in 5′ → 3′ (antiparallel) direction**
- Because of **unidirectional (5′ → 3′) synthetic activity** of polymerase and the antiparallel nature of two strands, the synthesis of DNA along the two strands is different and in **opposite direction. DNA polymerase** synthesize new DNA strand only in **5′ → 3′**direction, which is *towards (in the direction of advancing) replication fork* in **leading** strand and *away from replication fork* in **lagging** strand. DNA polymerase require **primer** (a short stretch of RNA), synthesized by **DNA primase**. The leading strand only needs one, whereas lagging strand needs *many primers*. The **leading strand** is ***replicated in a continuous fashion***Q. However, for the **lagging strand, *RNA primers are periodically added by DNA primase***Q along the strand. DNA polymerase III elongates these RNA primers to form Okazaki fragments.

- Now the **hexameric protein Dna B** – binds to separated DNA strands. **Dna B has helicase activity** that catelyzes ATP mediated unwinding of DNA helix. DNA gyrase also participates in separation of strands. As this complex continues unwinding DNA strands in both direction from Ori, **SSBP (single stranded DNA- binding protein)** coat the separated strands to ***inhibit their reassociation (i.e. prevent premature reanneiling)***Q. DNA replication ***begins at origin of replication (ori) in S phase. The strands are seperated locally forming*** 2 ***replication forks***Q. Double stranded DNA's replication is **bidirectional. Helicase** *unwinds, seperates the double helix,* which produces *positive supercoil in the region of DNA ahead of replication fork.* **DNA topoisomerase I & II** remove suprecoils.

Proteins Required to Initiate Replication

Protein	No of sub units	Function
Dna A protein	1	- **Recognizes replication origin (ori) sequence** and opens duplex at specific sites in origin. - This member of **AAA + AT pase protein** family has ATP bound active & ADP bound inactive forms. It has higher affinity for **R sites** (5 repeat of 9 base pair consensus sequence = TT (A/T) TNCACC) than I sites in ori. R-sites can bind to both active & inactive Dna A protein whereas, *I sites bind only the active ATP bound Dna A allowing* discrimination. - **8 molecules of ATP bound (active) Dna A proteins form a helical complex and bind at R and I sites in origin (ori)** Tight right handed helical wrapping of DNA around this complex produces a **positive supercoil**. The resultant strain in near by DNA l/t **denaturation in A=T rich DUE (DNA unwinding element) region of ori** (ie tandem array of three 13 bp consensus sequence GATCTNTTNTTTT).
HU, FIS*, IHF	2	- **Histone like bacterial protein (HU) or factor U, factor for**

- So the **leading strand** is produced as a **single, long continuous strand** (in 5'→ 3' direction) **from a single primer** with the same overall forward direction. But the **lagging strand** is synthesized in **small fragments** (1000-5000 bp length) termed **Okazaki fragments** in a **discontinuous manner**, in 5'→ 3' direction, but at the same time it faces towards the back end of the preceding RNA primer rather than toward the unreplicated portion. So overall DNA synthesis is **semi discontinuous (continuous in leading & discontinuous in lagging strand)**.
- Replication proceeds from **single origin (ori) in prokaryotic** bacterial chromosome. In eukaryotic metazoan (mammals etc), the replication is **bidirectional (ie occurs in both directions)** and replication **proceeds from multiple origins** in each chromosome (~ 100 in humans). Thus replication **occurs in both directions and both strands are replicated simultaneously** generating **replication bubbles**.
- Entire protein complex at replication fork k/a **DNA replicase system or replisome** come into action. **Parental DNA is unwound by DNA B helicase** and **resulting topological stress is relieved by topoisomerases (I, II, gyrase)**. Each **separated strand is stabilized by SSB (or RPA)** protein. Dna B helicase and Dna G primase form functional unit within replication complex k/a **primosome. Dna B helicase** bound in front, unwinds the DNA at replication fork as it moves **along the lagging strand template in 5' → 3' direction** and the primer is synthesized by **Dna G primese in 5' → 3' direction** but the direction **opposite to that in which Dna B helicase is moving.** However the first primer laid down serves to prime leading strand DNA synthesis in opposite direction.
- Once the strands are sufficiently unwound (seperated) by helicase, the DnaG primase (of primosome) synthesize RNA oligo nucleotides complementary to each parental DNA strand which serves as primer for DNA synthesis. Once each RNA primer has been laid down, two DNA polymerase III **core subunit** complexes are assembled, one at each of the primed site.
- **Both leading and lagging strands are produced by a single asymmetric DNA polymerase III dimer** tethered to the lagging strand. This is accomplished by **using one set of core subunits (core polymerase)** to synthesize the leading strand, while the other set of core subunits cycles from one Okazaki fragment to the next on the looped lagging strand (ie core subunits are attached to both strands). **Looping of lagging strand** brings together the two points of polymerization.
- Prokaryotic DNA chain elongation is catabolized by **DNA polymerase III** using 5' *deoxyribonucleoside triphosphate as substrate.* It ***proof reads & has 3'→ 5'exonuclease activity. RNA primers are removed by DNA polymerase I using its*** 5' → 3' ***exonuclease activity***Q. *It fills the gap with DNA and proof reads* (during synthesis). So **DNA polymerase I** ***removes the RNA primer, replaces it with DNA and eventually join Okazaki fragments***Q. Finally, ***DNA ligase seals nick and join the lagging strand DNA fragments to form a continuous strand***Q by catalyzing *final phosphodiester linkage.*
- Eukaryotic DNA has 5 types. **Pol** α is a multisubunit enzyme with **primase & 5' → 3'polymerase activity**. It adds a short piece of DNA to RNA, primer. **Pol** δ completes DNA synthesis on leading strand and elongates each lagging strand fragment using 3' → 5'exonuclease

* = Identical sub units		**inversion stimulation (FIS) and Integration host factor (IHF) are DNA binding proteins** which stimulate initiation by *facilitating formation of helical Dna A complex*. - FIS & IHF have specific binding site in ori whereas HUS does not have a specific site. 2 subunits of FIS are identical (not of IHF and HU)
Dna C protein	6*	- An AAA – ATPase protein **required for Dna B (helicase) binding or londing onto separated DNA strands** in the denatured region at origin. **(keystep** in initiation) - Hexamer of Dna C (with ATP bound to each subunit) forms tight complex with hexameric, ring shaped Dna B helicase. This interaction **opens the ring of Dna B and results in loading of 2 ring shaped Dna B hexamers in DUE, one onto each strand**. The ATP bound to Dna C is hydrolyzed, releasing the Dna C and leaving Dna B (helicase) bound to DNA.
DnaB protein (Helicase) & MCM helicase	6*	- Helicase (Dna B) binds to single strand DNA near replication fork (V) and then **move along the SS DNA (that becomes lagging strand) in $5' \to 3'$** direction into the neighboring double stranded region, forcing them apart –in effect **processive unwinding the ds DNA** to provide ss DNA as it travels. It requires energy provided by ATP. Dna B is principal helicase of E.coli. - Thus **both Dna B halicases** loaded on to the two strands of DNA **travel in opposite directions, creating 2 replication V or Y forks**. - All other proteins at replication fork are linked directly or indirectly to Dna B. pol III holoenzyme is linked through τ

activity to *proof read*. **Pol β & pol ε** are involved with *DNA repair*. **Pol** *γ replicates mitochondrial DNA*. Eukaryotes have many more ori and contain a **licencing factor** to insure that excess amount of unfinished replicating DNA do not accumulate.

- When the 3′ end of elongating Okazaki fragment, reaches the 5′ end of previously synthesized, DNA polymerase III release the template & find another primer further back along lagging strand synthesizing another okazaki fragment.
- Proteins of replisome include **Dna B helicase, DnaG primase, DNA gyrase (topoisomerase II), SSB, DNA polymerase III & I and DNA ligase.**

DNA Polymerase	- Polymerize deoxyribonucleotide (DNA) and share 3 comon properties 1. **Chain elongation**: It is d/t **5′ -3′ polymerase activity** accounting for the rate (in nucleotides per second = ntd/s) at which polymerization occurs 2. **Processivity** : It is an expression of number of nucleotides added to nascent (new) chain before the polymerase disengages from the templet. 3. **Proof reading:** It is d/t **3′ – 5′ exonuclease** activity that identifies copying errors & corrects them.
DNA polymerase I	- Gap filling in lagging strand, proof reading & repair - Mostly involved in *host clean up functions* during replication, recombination & repair (d/t $5' \to 3'$ exonuclease activity) - It *locates space (nick) between 3′ end of DNA newly synthesized (by polymerase III) & 5′ end of adjacent RNA primer*. - Next, it removes RNA nucleotides (primer) ahead of itself moving in $5' \to 3'$ direction (by its **(5′ → 3′ exonuclease activity)** and synthesizes DNA/chain elongation (by its **5′ → 3′ polymerase activity)**. During synthesis it also *proofreads* the new chain using **3′ → 5′ exonuclese activity**. - This **removal – synthesis – proofreading** continues one nucleotide at a time, until the RNA is totally degraded & replaced with DNA - The ***5′ → 3′ exonuclease activity is specific to DNA polymerase I and is responsible for Nick translation***[Q] - 5′→ 3′ exonuclease can remove *1 or upto 10, properly base paired or altered*, nucleotides (either ribonucleotides or deoxyribonucleotides) of RNA or DNA at a time. This ability is important in repair of damaged DNA. When 5′ →3′ exouclease domain is removed the remaining large fragment is k/a **Klenow fragment**
DNA polymerase II	- DNA proof reading & repair
DNA polymerse III	- ***Processive leading strand and okazaki fragment synthesis***[Q]. It is a *assembly of 13 protein subunits (of a different types)*

		subunit. - In eukaryotes, a heterohexameric, ring shaped complex of **minichromosome maintenance (MCM) helicase** (MCM 2 to MCM 7) functions like prokaryotic Dna B helicase. MCM is loaded on to DNA by a hexameric protein complex **ORC (origin recognition complex)** = Key step
Stabilizing proteins: Single stranded DNA Binding protein (SSB) & Replication Protein A (RPA)	4*	- Seperation of DNA double helix is promoted by **single stranded DNA binding protein** (SSB) in prokaryotes and **replication protein A (RP-A)** in eukaryotes. - These bind co-operatively & stoichiometrically to SS DNA with out interfering with the abilities of neucleotides to serve as template. So these **stabilizes the single stranded structure as replication fork progresses.** - These proteins (not enzymes) ***keep the two strands of DNA separated by preventing premature reanneiling of ds DNA***[Q]. - *Protect DNA from nuclease that cleaves ss DNA* - Bind to ss DNA created by helicase **cooperatively** – i.e., the binding of one molecule of SSB protein makes it easier for additional molecules of SSB protein to bind tightly.
DNA Grayse	4	- A **DNA topopscmerase II relieves torsional strain / topological stress (positive super coil or suprtwist)** induced ahead of replication fork by the helicase induced unwinding process. - A *type II topoisomerase* that has unusual property of being able to ***introduce negative supercoils into relaxed circular DNA by using energy (ATP)***[Q]. This *facilitates the future replication of DNA* because negative supercoiling neutralize positive supercoils introduced during opening of ds DNA. Also aids *transient strand separation.*

	Subunit	No. per holo-enzyme	Gene	Function
Core polymerase	α ε θ	2 2 2	pol **C** (dna **E**) mut **D** (dna **Q**) hol **E**	**Polymerization activity** **3′ → 5′ Proof reading exonuclease** Stabilization of ε subunit
Clamps	β	4	dna **N**	DNA **donut shaped sliding clamps** required for optimal processivity (one dimer clamp per core subassembly).
Clamp loading (γ) complex	τ	2	dna **X**	Stable template binding; core enzyme dimerization
	γ δ[1] δ	1 1 1	dna **X*** hol **B** hol **A**	Clamp loader Clamp loader Clamp opener — *Clamp loading (γ) complex loads β subunits on lagging strand at each okazaki fragment. It has 5 subunits of 4 different types $\tau^2 \gamma \delta^1 \delta$
	χ (Chi) ψ (Psi)	1 1	hol **C** hol **D**	Interacts with SSB Interacts with γ and χ
DNA ligase	- **Nick sealing enzymes** that **seals (ligates) nick created by removal of DNA polymerase I in lagging strand** (backbone of DNA in form of broken phosphodiester bond) by **using ATP** - Forms final phosphodiester linkage b/w 5′ PO4 group on nascent DNA chain synthesized by DNA polymerase III & 3′ OH group on chain mede by DNA polymerase I			

★ ψ subunit is generated by translational frame shifting (of portion of gene for τ subunit) that l/t premature translational termination

Termination of DNA Synthesis

- 2 replication forks of circular prokaryotic DNA meet at **terminus region containing multiple copies of 20 bp sequences called Ter.** Ter sequences function as **binding sites for protein terminal utilization substance (Tus) and create a trap that a replication fork can enter but cannot leave.**
- Tus – Ter complex can arrest a replication fork **from only one direction**. Only one Tus-Ter complex functions per replication cycle – the complex **first encountered by either** replication fork.
- Because opposing replication forks usually halt when they collide, Ter sequences would not seem essential, but they may **prevent over replication by one fork in the event** that the other is delayed or hated by an encounter with DNA damage or other problem. So, ***when either replication fork first encounters a Tus-Ter complex, it halts; the other replication fork halts when it meets the first arrested fork.***

DnaG (Primase)	1	- DNA primase is a specific **RNA polymerase** that **synthesize** short (~ 10 nucleotide long) stretches of RNA that are complementary and antiparallel to DNA template and are k/e **RNA primer** - As with DNA synthesis the direction of primer synthesis is **5′ → 3′. One primer (& primase) is required for leading strand and many for lagging strand**. - Helicase associates with primase to provide it proper access to the template. This mobile complex of helicase & primase is called **primosome**. - Primer synthesis is important since, DNA polymerase cannot initiate DNA synthesis denovo (without primer).
Hda	-	- **Homologous to Dna A** (or **Hda**) is a AAA + ATPase that *binds to beta subunit of DNA polymerase III* and interacts with Dna A to stimulate hydrolysis of its bound ATP. This ATP hydrolysis **disassembles the Dna A complex at origin**. That is why, *loading of DNA pol III beta subunits on to the DNA signals completion of initiation* phase
Dam Methylase	1	- Methylates N 6 position of adenine within the palindromic sequence (5^1) G ATC at origin (in Ecoli). **Dam stands for DNA adenine methylation** and **it affects timing of replication initiation.** - Immediately after replication, DNA is hemimethylated at ori ie parent strands methylated but newly synthesized strand do not. The DNA **must be fully methylated before** it again binds Dna A and initiates new replication eg cycle.

- Final few hundred bps are replicated by unknown mechanism completing two **topologically interlinked (catenated)** circular chromosomes (k/a **catenanes**). The circles are not covalently linked, but because they are inter wound and each is covalently closed, they cannot be separated. Separation of catenanes requires **topoisomerase IV (a type II topoisomerase)** which transiently breaks both DNA strands of one chromosome and allowing the other chromosome to pass through the break.
- In eukaryotes, telomeres are synthesized.

Topoisomerase	- ***Relieves torsion strain (supercoiling or supertwisting) that result from helicase induced unwinding***[Q] in the region of DNA ahead of replication fork. The swivel function is provided by introducing nicks in strand, thereby allowing unwinding & then resealing the nicks. These are of 2 types
Type I topoisomerase	- Have both **nuclease (strand cutting)** and **ligase (strand / nick sealing)** activity. They *do not require ATP*, but rather appear to *store the energy* for phosphodiester bond they cleave, reusing the energy to reseal the strand. - It *reversibly creates a transient nick (cut) in one strand* of ds DNA. The intact DNA strand is passed through the break before it is resealed, thus relieving (relaxing) accumulated supercoils. - Type I topoisomerase *relax negative supercoils in E. coli, and both negative & positive supercoils in eukaryotes*. (**Positive supercoil** is produced by twisting *in the direction of tightening* of strands so the DNA would contain more turns of helix than relaxed DNA. Whereas, the **negative supercoil** is produced by twisting *in the direction of loosening* the strands; so the negatively super twisted DNA would contain fewer turns of helix than relaxed DNA).
Type II topoisomerase	- Make *transient break in both strands* and *relieve both positive & negative supercoils* by utilizing *ATP* - Required in both prokaryotes & eukaryotes for separation of interlocked molecules of DNA following chromosomal replication.

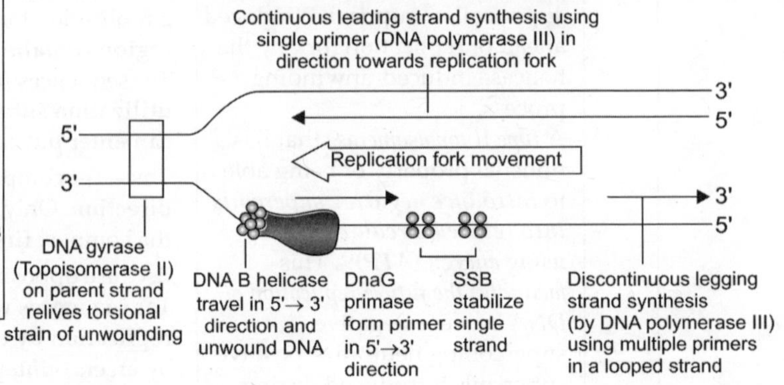

Continuous leading strand synthesis using single primer (DNA polymerase III) in direction towards replication fork

3′ 5′ 5′ 3′ 3′ 5′

Replication fork movement

DNA gyrase (Topoisomerase II) on parent strand relives torsional strain of unwounding

DNA B helicase travel in 5′→ 3′ direction and unwound DNA

DnaG primase form primer in 5′→3′ direction

SSB stabilize single strand

Discontinuous legging strand synthesis (by DNA polymerase III) using multiple primers in a looped strand

Components of Nucleic Acid

Nitrogen -Bases

- Purines & pyrimidines are *nitrogen & carbon containing heterocyclic aromatic compounds with a planar character* (i.e. two or more bases are positioned with the planes of their rings parallel like a stack of coins)- a feature that facilitates their close association or stalking that stabilizes double stranded DNA.
- Larger purine molecules and smaller pyrimidine molecules are numbered in opposite direction for their 6 atom main ring i.e. *clockwise for pyrimidine & anteclockwise for purine.*
- Free purines and pyrimidines with – NH_2 group are **weak bases**. Physiological pH strongly favour **oxo and amino groups** of purine and pyrimidine exhibiting *Keto-enol and amine- imine tautomerism.*

Purine Bases	Pyrmidine Bases	Present in
Adenine = A **Guanine = G**	**Cytosine = C**	Both DNA & RNA
	Thymine = T	**DNA**
	Uracil = U	**RNA**
Hypoxanthine (6 oxopurine) **Xanthine** (2, 6-dioxopurine) **Uric acid** (2, 6, 8-trioxopurine)	-	**Minor bases** formed in catabolism of purines
N6, N6 dimethyl adenine	N4 acetyl cytosine Dihydro uracil	**Unusual Bases**

★ Methylation acetylation, glycosylation or reduction in some viral DNA & tRNA bases forms unusual buses which may aid in its recognition by specific enzymes or protect it from being degraded by nucleases.

★ T and U differ in that only T has a methyl group.

Pentose Sugar : Nucleoside

- Addition of pentose sugar to nitrogenous base produces a **nucleoside**
- Sugar is **D-ribose** in ribonucleoside (of RNA) and **2-deoxy-D-riobse** in deoxy ribionucleotide (of DNA).
- Carbons of pentose sugars are prime numbered 1^1 to 5′ distinguishing them from those of heterocycles. Hence, 5′ carbon of nucleoside (or nucleotide) means a carbon atom in pentose ring rather than atom in base.
- All bases are attached to pentose sugar by a **β-N- glycosidic bond** between 1st carbon of pentose sugar and almost always to the **N-1 of pyrimidine or N-9 of purine.**
- **Nucleosides** are *N-glycosides* formed by addition of **pentose sugar (D-ribose or 2 deoxy D-ribose)** to a **purine (adenine, guanine) or pyrimidine (cytosine, thymine & uracil) bases.** Nucleosides with purine bases (A, G) have – **'sine'** suffix viz – ***adenosine, guanosine***[Q], whereas pyrimidine nucleosides have **'dine'** suppix viz – ***cytidine, thymidine and uridine***[Q].

Phosphate / Phosphoric Acid: Nucleotide

- Nucleotides are **phosphorylated (i.e. phosphate esters of) nucleosides.**

Nuceotide = Nucleoside + Phosphate or Phosphoric acid = Purine / Pyrimidine Base + Pentose (D-ribose / 2 deoxy D-ribose) sugar + Phosphate / Phosphoric acid

- Nucleotides may contain 1, 2 or 3 phosphate groups and are called mono, di or tri phosphate nucleotides (i.e. MP, DP, or TP)
- 1st phosphate (phosphoryl) group is attached (esterified) to hydroxyl (OH) group of pentose sugar by ester linkage on 5' (mostly) or 3' (rarely) position. Since most are 5'-nucleotides or nucleoside 5′ phoshate (i.e. have phosphate at 5' position) the prefix "5'" is usually omitted when naming them.
- Suffix "**– sine/- nylate/- nylic acid**" for purine nucleotides & "**– dine/- dylate/-dylic acid**" for pyrimidine nucleotides are used.

Pentose Sugar	Nitrogenous Base	Nucleoside	Nucleotide (Mono /Di /Tri- phosphate), Mono phosphate (MP)	NDP	NTP
D-ribose sugar forming simple nucleosides & nucleotides in RNA and **2-deoxy ribose** sugar forming **deoxy (or d-) nucleosides & nucleotides** in	**Adenine (A)**	Adeno<u>sine</u>	**Adeno<u>sine</u> /Ade<u>nylate</u> /Ade<u>nylic</u> acid**- mono phosphate (**AMP**)	ADP	ATP
	Guanine (G)	Guano<u>sine</u>	**Guano<u>sine</u> /Gua<u>nylate</u> /Gua<u>nylic</u> <u>acid</u>** – monophosphate (GMP)	GDP	GTP
	Cytosine (C)	Cyti<u>dine</u>	**Cyti<u>dine</u> /Cyti<u>dylate</u> /Cyti<u>dylic</u> acid** mono phosphate (CMP)	CDP	CTP
	Thymine (T)	Thymi<u>dine</u>	Thymi<u>**dine**</u> / Thymi<u>**dylate**</u> / Thymi<u>**dylic**</u> <u>**acid**</u> mono phosphate (TMP)	TDP	TTP
	Uracil (U)	Uri<u>dine</u>	**Uri<u>dine</u> /Uri<u>dylate</u> /Uri<u>dylic</u> <u>acid</u>** mono phosphate (UMP)	UDP	UTP

★ Xanthine base form **Xanthosine** nucleoside and hypoxanthine base forms **inosine** nucleoside of RNA.

Denaturation / Melting of DNA and T_m

- The ds-DNA can be separated into two strands (melted) in solution by *increasing the temperature or decreasing the salt concentration.* Denaturation is also called **a helix to coil transition.**
- Not only do the two stacks of bases pull apart but the bases themselves unstack while still connected in the polymer by the phosphodiester backbone.
- **Concomitant with the denaturation of DNA molecule** is *an increase in the optical absorbance of purines & pyrimidine bases* – a phenomenon referred to as ***hyperchromocity*** of denaturation. DNA loses its viscosity on denaturation .
- The denaturation (melting) is used to analyze the structure of DNA. Denaturation & renaturation of DNA are basis of **nucleic acid hybridization.**
- Separate strands of DNA will renature or reassociate when appropriate physiological temperature & salt conditions are achieved; this **reannealing** process is often referred to as **hybridization.** If melted sample of DNA is slowly cooled the absorbance of solution decreases, which is an indication of complementary strands being pulled again. Annealing can occur at a temperature below Tm of DNA (i.e. 70°c). It is fastest at 20°c below Tm (i.e. 50°c)
- Hybridization when combined with **gel electrophoresis (that separate nucleic acids by size)** & radioactive or fluorescent labeling resulting analytic technique is called **southern (DNA-DNA) & Northern (RNA - DNA) blotting.**

Tm & Factors affecting Tm

- It is the *temperature at which DNA is half denatured.* In other words, the strand of a given DNA molecule separate over a temperature range. The midpoint is called the **melting temperature** or **Tm**. It is calculated by nearest neighbour method.
- At Tm, the absorbance of DNA at **260 nm** is increased by **18.5%** i.e. half of **37%** increased in absorbane when DNA is completely denatured. It is called **hyperchromicity phenomenon or hyperchromic effect**.
- It is in influenced by

- Both *length of DNA molecule & specific nucleotide sequence.* DNA rich in C≡G base pairs with 3 H bonds melts at higher temperature than that rich in **A = T base pairs with 2 hydrogen bonds.**
- **Salt concentration of solution** influence the Tm because negatively charged PO4 in two strands are *shielded by positively charged ion (cation).* Decreased ionic concentration decrease the shielding effect, thus increase the repulsive forces b/w strands and reducing Tm.
- So ***a ten fold increase in movalent cation concentration increase the Tm by 16.6°C***[Q]
- ***Formamide,*** which is commonly used in recombinant DNA experiments and **urea** both of them destabilizes hydrogen bonding between bases, thereby lowering Tm. This allows the strands of DNA or DNA hybrids to be separated at much lower temperatures and minimizes the phosphodiester bond breakage that can occur at higher temperatures.

Applications of Tm

- Estimate amount of G & C content
- In PCR
- To detect sequence differences b/w strands & different DNAs
- As a proxy for equalizing the hybridization strength of molecule eg oligonucleotide probe of DNA microarray.

Ultraviolet Spectrophotometry of Nucleic Acids

- *Electron delocalization* among atoms in aromatic rings of purine & pyrimidine bases give most of the bonds *partial double bond character.* **All nucleotide bases** (d/t conjugated double bond of purine / pyrimidine) ***absorb ultraviolet light***[Q] and nucleic acids (DNA /RNA) are characterized by a strong absorption at near **260 nm** wavelengths.
- *Mutagenic effect* of UV light is d/t its absorption by nucleotides in DNA l/t chemical modification.
- Although spectra is *pH dependent,* all nucleotides of DNA /RNA absorb light at wave length close to 260 nm, at pH 7. So **concentration of nucleotides & nucleic acids** are often expressed in terms of "**absorbance at 260 nm**".
- **DNA purity (quality) measurement** is based on the fact that the *clean/pure DNA has twice (1.8 -2 times more) optical density (OD) at 260 nm then at 280nm.* So if OD-260/OD-280 is lesser, it indicates *contamination,* which decreases OD ratio. Hence purify the DNA again.

Resultant DNA Damages

I. **Single base alteration**
- **Depurination** (rarely depyrimidination)
- **Deamination of cytosine (C) to uracil (U)** and adenine (A) to hypoxanthine
- **Alkylation** of base
- Base-analog incorporation
- Insertion or deletion of nucleotide

II. **2 - Base alteration**
- UV induced **thymine- thymine (pyrimidine)** dimer
- Bifunctional **alkylating cross linkage**

III. **Chain breaks** d/t ionizing radiation, oxidative free radicle formation or radioactive disintegration of backbone element

IV. **Cross linkage** between
- Bases in same & opposite strands
- DNA & protein molecules eg histone

DNA Repair Mechanism

DNA Damaging Agents	DNA lesion produced	DNA Repair Pathway	Fidelity of Repair	Procedure
Replication (copying) errors	**Base** (single or 2-5 base unpaired loops) **mismatch**; Insertions; Deletions	**Mismatch Repair (MMR)**	+++	Corrects a single mismatch base pair (eg C to A rather than T to A) or short region of unpaired DNA. The **defective region in newly synthesized unmethylated strand is recognized by (mut H) endo nuclease** that makes a single strand cut at an adjacent **methylated GATC palindrome sequence** (present in opposite orientation on two strands) . The defective DNA strand is removed through mutation (by **exonuclease**), replicated or replaced (by **DNA helicase II, SSB, DNA polymerase III**) and relegated (by **DNA ligase**). Dam methylase methylates N^6 adenines within (5^1) GATC sequence of parent (template) strand. Replication mismatches in vicinity of hemimethylated GATC sequence are then repaired according to information in methylated template strand. **If both strands are methylated** (in vitro) at GATC, **few mismatches are repaired and if neither strand is methylated repair occurs but does not favor either strand.**
Oxygen radicles ; Hydrolysis; Alkylating agents	Abnormal bases like uracil, hypoxanthine, xanthine, alkylated bases, small pyrimidine dimmers, Abasic sites; single strand breaks; 8 oxoguanine lesions	**Base Excision Repair (BER)**	+ + +	Base removal by N-glycosylase, a basic sugar removal, replacement
UV light, chemicals	Large structural DNA lesions like **pyrimidine dimmers**, Bulky adducts	**Nucleotide Excision Repair (N E R)**	+++	Removal of an approximately 30-nucleotide oligomer and replacement
Ionizing radiation, X-rays, Antitumor drugs	Double / Single strand breaks; intra / inter strand cross links	**Double strand break repair.** - **Homologous recombination (HR)** - **Non Homologous End Joining (NHEJ)**	 ++ +	Synapsis, unwinding, alignment, ligation
Any	**Pyrimidine dimmers** O^6 methyl guanine **Alk B protein**	**Direct Repair** **DNA photolyases** O^6 methyl-guanine -DNA methyl transferase 1 methyl guanine 3 methyl cytosine		

Mismatch Repair (MMR)

- **Mut L protein** forms complex with **Mut S protein** and the complex binds to all mismatched bases (except C-C). **Mut H** binds to Mut L and unmethylated GATC (encountered by Mut L- Mut S complex).
- *DNA on both sides of mismatch is threaded (looped) through Mut L- Mut S complex* and both legs of loop move through complex simultaneously (equivalent to complex moving in both directions along DNA). Mut H attached to complex has site specific **endonuclease activity** which is activated on encountering hemimethylated GATC sequence and cleaves unmethylated strand on 5′ side of G in GATC.
- When mismatch is on **5′ side (right)** of cleavage site the unmethylated strand is unwound (by helicase II) and cleaved in 3′ → 5′ direction from cleavage site by **exonuclease I** or **exonuclease X** (both of which degrade DNA strand in 3′ → 5′ direction).

  Whereas mismatch or **3′ side (left) use** either **exonuclease VII** (which degrade ssDNA in 5′ → 3′ or 3′→ 5′ direction) or **Rec J nuclease** (which degrade ss DNA in 5′→3′ direction).

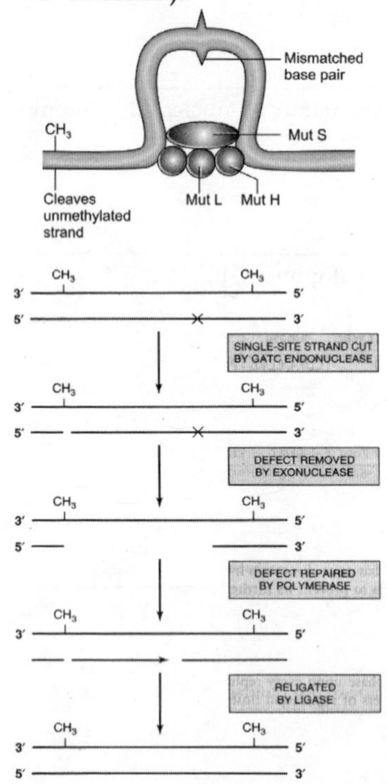

Double Strand Break Repair

The protein Ku and DNA-dependent protein kinase combine to approximate the two strands and unwind them. The aligned fragments form base pairs; the extra

Base Excision Repair (BER)

- **DNA glycosylases** remove purine / pyrimidine created by spontaneous deamination and create **AP (abasic or apurinic) site**. eg uracil DNA glycosylase removes the uracil created by spontaneous deamination of cytosine in DNA (it does not remove T from DNA or U from RNA).
- Humans have **4 types of DNA uracil glycosylase**: most abundant **UNG** is a/w replisome & *removes occasional U* inserted in place of T during replication; **h SMUG1** removes any U residues that occur in ss DNA during replication or transcription; **TDG & MBD 4** ***remove either U or T residues paired with G, generated by deamination of cytosine or* 5 *methyl cytosine respectively***[Q].
- **AP endonuclease** cut DNA strand containing the AP site and a segment of DNA containing AP site is removed.
- **Repair polymerase (DNA polymerase I)** replaces DNA and fills the defect and **DNA ligase** seals the remaining nick (ligates the space created by DNA polymerase I removal)

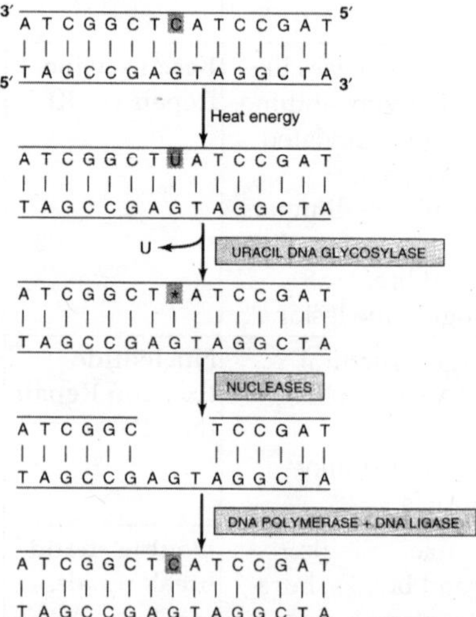

Nucleotid Excision Repair (NER)

- Larger DNA defects that cause large distortion in DNA helix are repaired by NER.
- A multisubunit **excinuclease enzyme** hydrolyze 2 phosphodiester bonds one on either side of distortion. This corresponds in E.coli & bacteria to 5th phosphodiester bond (PDB) on 3′ side & 8th PDB on 5′ side creating 12 to 13 nucleotide fragment; and in humans to 6th PDB on 3′ & 22nd on 5′ side producing a fragment of 27-29 nucleotides.
- **Excinuclease** is a endonuclease with a unique capacity to catalyze 2 specific endonucleolytic cleavages. Following the **dual incision** the excised oligonucleotide are replaced from duplex and resulting gap is filled by **DNA- polymerase I** in E.coli and **DNA polymerase ε/δ** in humans. **DNA ligase** seals nick.
- In E.coli **ABC excinuclease** has 3 subunits **Uvr A, Uvr B** (A_2B complex of both units scans DNA and binds to site of lesion; Uvr A_2 dimer then dissociates leaving a tight Uvr B- DNA complex) and **Uvr C** (binds to B

ends are removed, probably by a DNA-PK-associated endo-or exonuclease, and the gaps are filled in; and continuity is restored by ligation.

subunit and Uvr B makes an incision at 5th PDB on 3′ side whereas Uvr C makes an incision at 8th PDB on 5′ side of lesion).

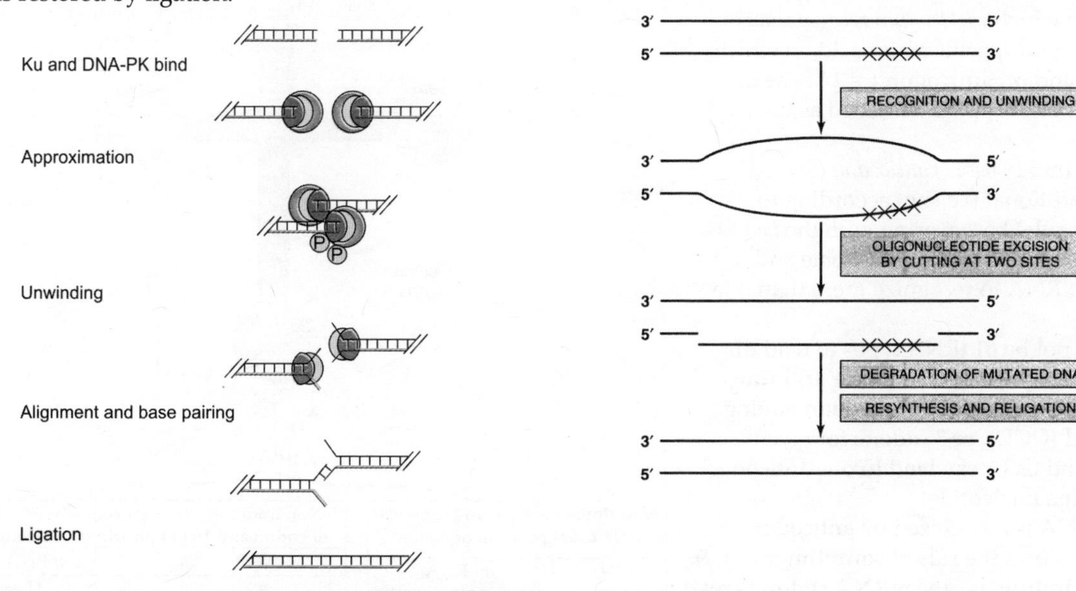

Disease	Defect in DNA repair	Feature
Xeroderma pigmentosa	**Nucleotide excision repair** *pathway* specilly thymine dimmers cannot be incised d/t *deficiency of enzyme nicking endonuclease* (m.c), DNA polymerase I or DNA ligase, helicase (Subunits of transcription factor TFIIH)	- Autosomal recessive (AR) - Marked sensitivity to sunlight (UV rays) l/t multiple skin cancers and premature death
Ataxia telangiectasia		- Autosoml recessive (AR)Q - Cerebellar ataxia, lymphoreticular neoplasms, increased sensitivity to damage by x-ray, oculo cutaneous telangiectasia & IgE deficiency.
Fanconi's anemia	Chromosomal instability & *defective repair of cross linking damage*	- Autosomal recessive (AR) - Anemia & increased frequency of cancer - Defective gene located on chromosome 20q & 9q
Bloom's syndrome	Chromosomal breaks & rearrangements are seen d/t *defective DNA ligase*	- Facial erythema, photosensitivity and telangiectasia
Heriditary non polyposis colon cancer (HNPCC)	**Faulty mismatch repair** due mutation in **hMSH 2** gene (located inchromosome 2) that encodes human analog of E.coli ***Muts protein*** that is involved in mismatch repair.	- Most common inherited cancer - Cells which harbour hMSH2 (50-60% cases) or hMSH-1 mismatch repair enzyme, are unable to remove small loops of unpaired DNA, & the *microsatellite* DNA thus *increase in size.* It affects either expression or function of a protein critical in surveillance of cell cycle in colon cells.

Wobble Hypothesis

- It *explains the degeneracy of genetic code,* a mechanism by which *t RNAs can recognize more than one codon* for a specific aminoacid, in which the **base at 5′ end of anticodon (= 1st base of anticodon)** is not as spatially defined as the two other bases.
- Movement of this *1st base of anticodon (5′ end)* allows non traditional (i.e., not according to watson- Crick rule) base pairing with the *last base of codon (at 3′ end).* This is called wobble and allows single t RNA to recognize more than one codon.
- So there need not be 61 tRNA types to read 61 codons. For example **two codons for arginine, AGA & AGG, bind to same anticodon** having uracil at 5' end (UCU), or 3 codons for glycine – GGU, GGC, and GGA can bind to one anticodon CCI. (I = inosine nucleotide)

★ Codon of mRNA is recognized by anticodon of tRNA and it follows the rule of **complimentary & antiparallel binding**, i.e. the **mRNA codon is read 5′ →3′** by an **anticodon** pairing in the flipped **3′→5′ orientation.** When writing the sequences of both codons & anticodon, the nucleotide sequence must always be listed in the 5′→3′ order.

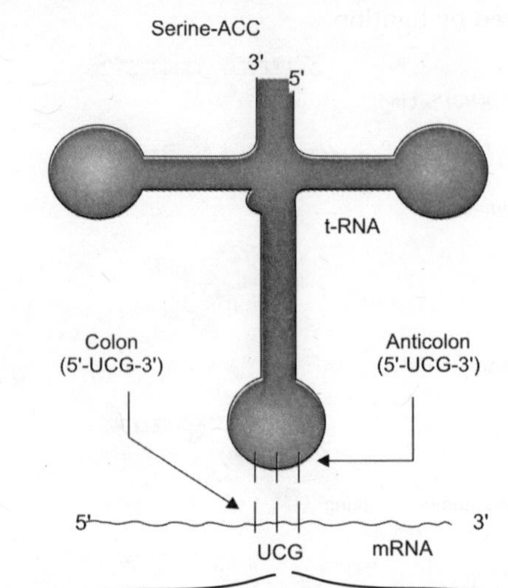

Traditional base pairing observed in **1st & 2nd position of codon:**	
tRNA	m- RNA
A	U
G	C
U	A
C	G

Non traditional base pairing b/w 3rd (3′) position of codon and 1st (5′) positin of anticodon: Wobble	
t- RNA	mRNA
A	U
G	C, U
H	C,U,A
U	A,G

★ H = hypoxanthine (base of inosine)

Characteristics of Motif Containing Proteins

- ***Control of transcription requires high affinity and specificity in binding of regulatory proteins to the correct region of DNA, which is provided by motifs*Q.** Binding must be high affinity to specific sites and low affinity to others. Binding must be *high affinity to specific sites and low affinity to others.* The DNA – protein interactions are maintained by *hydrogen bonds & vander waals forces.* The presence of motifs in unknown protein *suggest that the protein may bind to DNA.*
- *Small regions of motif make direct contact with DNA.* The rest of protein may provide ligand binding sites, trans activation domains, or contact surface for formation of hetero dimers, & interaction with coactivatior or corepressor. It may be involved in dimerization of monomers of binding ***protein. Proteins with helix turn helix & leucine zipper motifs form symmetrical palidromes and their DNA binding sites are symmetrical palindromes*Q.** Whereas, ***in proteins with zinc finger motif, the binding site is repeated 2- 9 times*Q.**

Helix turn helix motif

- Each monomer consist of *three antiparallel β- sheets & three α- helix.*
  - β3 sheets for dimmer.
  - α3 helices form DNA recognition surface.
- Examples of transcription regulatory proteins containing helix turn helix motif

Regulatory protein	Organism
lac repressor, CAP	E. Coli
Cro, λ cl, tryptophan & 434 represor	Phage
Homeo box proteins, pit 1, Oct1, Oct2	Mammals

Zinc- finger motif

- They are series of *repeated domains (2-9)* in which each is centered on a tetrahedral coordination ***with Zn*Q.**
- In TF III A (transcription regulatory protein) *9 zinc* ions present in repeating Co0 ordination complex formed by *pair of cystine (C) separated by 12-13 amino acid from a pair of histidine residue.*
- Transcription regulatory proteins containing Zn-finger motif

Leucine- zipper motif

- Carboxyl terminal of DNA binding protein C/EBP, forms an α- helix in which ***there is periodic repeat of leucine residue at every 7th position*Q.**
- This structure allow two identical monomer or hetero dimer (eg, fos- Jun or Jun- Jun) to 'Zip together' in a coiled coil & form tight dimeric complex.
- This enhance association of separate DNA binding domain with their target

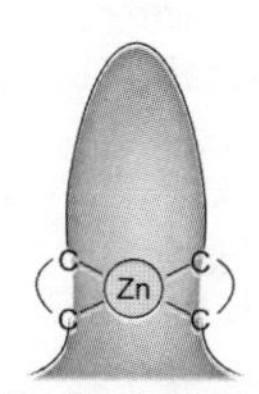

Cys-Cys zinc finger

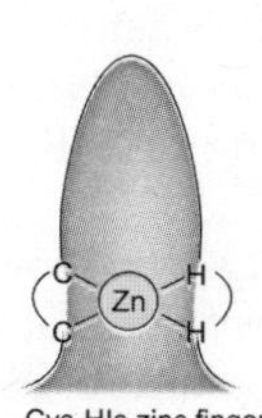

Cys-His zinc finger

Zn finger motif

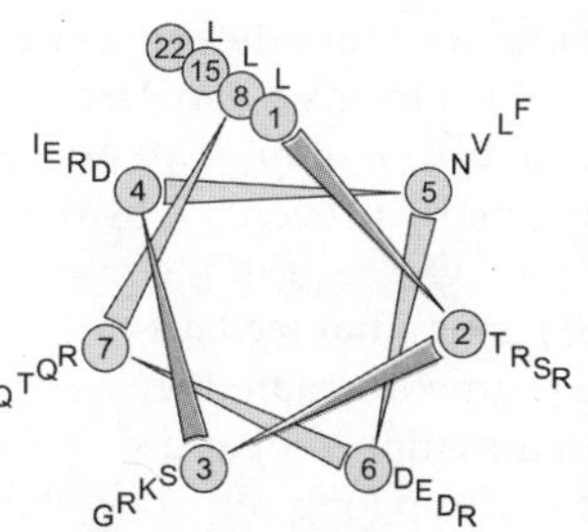

Leucine Zipper motif

Regulatory protien	Orgainsm
Gene 32 protein	E. coli
Gal 4	Yeast
Serendipity, Hunch back	Drosophila
TF III A	Xenopus
Steroid receptor family[Q], Sp1	Mammals

- Transcription regulatory containing leucine zipper motif

Regulatory protein	Organism
GCN-4	Yeast
C- myc, n- myc, l-myc CRE binding protein C/EBP Fra 1, fos Jun	Mammals

★ Gene expression is controlled by **regulatory sequences of DNA** that lie in *non coding regions* of genome *flanking a coding gene*. These are **Cis - acting**, if they influence expression of gene only *on same chromosome* and **transacting** if influences the expression of gene on other chromosome (that is different from its site of origin).

Gene	Cistron
- A *segment of DNA* molecule that *contains the information* required for *synthesis* of a functional biological product, whether *protein or RNA*, is referred to as a *gene* - Edward **Tatum** & George **Beadle** proposed molecular definition of gene in 1940 a/t which a gene is a *segment of genetic material that determines or codes for one enzyme" the **one gene-one enzyme*** **hypothesis**. Later this concept was broadened to **1 gene-1 polypeptide**, because many genes code for a protein that is not an enzyme or for one polypeptide of a multi subunit protein. - A/t modern biochemical definition, a gene is *all the DNA that encodes the primary sequence of some final gene product*, which can either be polypeptide or an RNA with a structural or catalytic function. - **Gene** is a **functional unit** that *encodes a RNA* product which is *mostly (but not always) translated into a protein*, which exerts activity within or outside the cell. (Harrison-385). Gene is regulated by transcription & corresponds to a *unit of inheritance* - **Inducible genes**, with relatively *low basal rates of transcription* are upregulated (i.e. expression increased) in response to an **inducer** or **activator** (a **positive regulator**). By contrast repressible genes, with high basal rate of transcription are often down regulated by **repressor** (negative regulator). - **Housekeeping genes** are **constitutively** expressed meaning that they are expressed at a reasonably constant rate & not known to be subject to regulation. A mutation resulting in constitutive expression of what was formerly a regulated gene is k/a **constitutive mutation.** - **Care taker** (or **stability) genes** encodes proteins that function in *repair of major genetic defect* that result from aberrant DNA replication, environmental carcinogens or ionizing radiation. So mutation in these genes *l/t mutation* (unrepaired damage) in other genes including protoonchogenes & tumor suppressor genes and thus to cancer. Examples include ATM gene, XP gene (l/t Xeroderma pigmentosa), BRCA1 gene (l/t breast cancer), and p53 gene (l/t *Li Fraumeni cancer syndrome.*)	- As we know; some enzymes & proteins are composed of 2 or more *non identical subunits. Thus 1 gene- 1 enzyme concept is not always valid.* - **Cistron** is the ***smallest unit of genetic expression***[Q]. It is the basic genetic unit ***coding for one polypeptide chain / structure of subunit of a protein molecule***[Q]. - So one gene- one enzyme concept might more accurately be regarded as **one cistron-one subunit** concept. - A single mRNA that encodes >.1 sepeatily translated proteins is referred to as **polycistronic m RNA**. Eg polycistronic lac operon m-RNA. - But this concept is also changing as many cistrons could be spliced & rearranged. In other words, **many genes together can produce one peptide chain by** means of **transposition** of genes or **gene rearrangement** or **somatic recombination of DNA or gene shuffling** (described by Susumu Tonegawa for antibodies).

Jacob & Monod's Operon Concept for Prokaryotic Gene 

In prokaryotes, genes involved in a metabolic pathway are often present in a linear array called an **operon**. The **cistron** is the smallest unit of genetic expression coding for subunit of a protein molecule (One cistron – one subunit concept). **Polycistronic mRNA,** predominantly found in prokeryotes is a m-RNA that encodes more than one seperately translated proteins. Operon (transcription unit of prokaryotes) consists of

Structural (coding) genes

- Carries the codon that code for proteins involved in a particular metabolic pathway
- In lac operon of E coli (responsible for lactose metabolism), 3

Regulatory region consisting

Promoter (P) gene

- It is situated on the upstream (5′- side of transcription start site b/w operator & regulator gene.
- It is the site, where ***DNA dependent – RNA polymerase (RNP) binds to form preinitiation complex (PIC)***[Q], and commence transcription.

structural genes **lac Z, lac Y, & lac A** code respectively for *β*-galactosidase, (hydrolyze lactose or *β- galactoside* to galactose & glucose), *permease* (responsible for permeation of galactose into cell), and *thiogalactoside transacetylase.*

Inducible regulated genes	Constitutive (house keeping) genes
- Their expression *increases in response to an* **inducer** or **activator** (a positive regulatory signal) - In general, inducible genes have relatively *low rates of transcription*	- They are expressed at ***a reasonably constant rate and are not subjected to regulation***[Q] - The *product* of these genes are ***required all the time***[Q] in a cell. - A mutation resulting in constitutive expression of what was formerly a regulated gene is called **constitutive mutation**

- **Catabolite gene activator protein (CAP)** in **conjunction with c-AMP** (als k/a c-AMP regulatory protein = **CRP**) is required for efficient formation of PIC. So it is a **positive regulator**. Adenylate cyclase which forms c-AMP from ATP, is activated by *absence of glucose*. So the lac operon ***transcription only occurs in absence of glucose***[Q] **(catabolite repression)**. And presence of glucose prevents it by depleting c-AMP.

Operator (O) genes

- It is a segment of ds DNA (i.e., gene) that *regulates the activity of the structural genes.*
- In lac operon, it is 27 bp long segment situated *between promoter site* (at which RNAP binds) *and lac Z* (transcription initiation site) and show a **twofold rotational symmetry** and **an inverted palindrome** in 21 bp long region as shown below

```
5′- AATTGT →      G -----------  3′
3′ -------------- C -----  TGTTAA 5′
```

When attached to operator (o) gene, the **repressor** (LacI) acts as a **negative regulator** and prevents transcription of operator and structural (lac /Y/A) genes.

Regulator (I) genes

- It is a *constitutive gene, that forms subunits* of lac repressor (MW 38,000), A lac repressor molecule (**Lac I repressor protein**) is formed by union of *4 subunits* and has ***high affinity for operator locus***[Q].
- At any time only *2 subunits* of repressor *binds to operator* , mostly in its *major groove without interrupting the base paired double helical nature of operator DNA.*
- Normally 20-40 repressor tetramers, occupy > 95% of lac operator, thus ensuring a low (but not zero) lac operon transcription in absence of inducer.
- **Presence of lactose or gratuitous inducer** (i.e., lactose analog which induces lac operon but is not a substrate) such as **isopropylthio galactoside (IPTG)** on bacteria growing on poorly utilized carbon source (eg succinate) results induction of lac operon enzymes by **de-repression.** This occurs because lactose / IPTG bind to free & attached repressor & decrease its affinity 10^3 times for operator by inducing coformational change.

★ The first base at transcription start site (of DNA) is assigned a position of **+1**. There is **no** base designated **"O"**. A base is assigned a **negative number**, if it occurs *upstream* (i.e., *prior* to or on *left side* or towards the *5′end* of) the transcription start site. And in the same way **more positivity** indicates *more downstream* (i.e., *after to* or on the *right side* or *towards 3′-end*) distance from +1 position.

★ **Enhancer** and **repressor (silencer)**, can either increase or decrease the rate of transcription initiation of eukaryotic gene respectively. They ***can be located upstream or downstream of transcription start site (+1) and even within transcribed portion of some genes***[Q]. **In contrast to** proximal & upstream **promoters**, these *can exert their effect when located even hundreds or thousand bases away* from transcription unit on same chromosome and function in *orientation independent fashion*. Enhancers are promiscuous, they can stimulate any promoter (homologous or hetrologus). Enhancers work by binding one or more proteins and by facilitating binding of basal transcription complex to promoter.

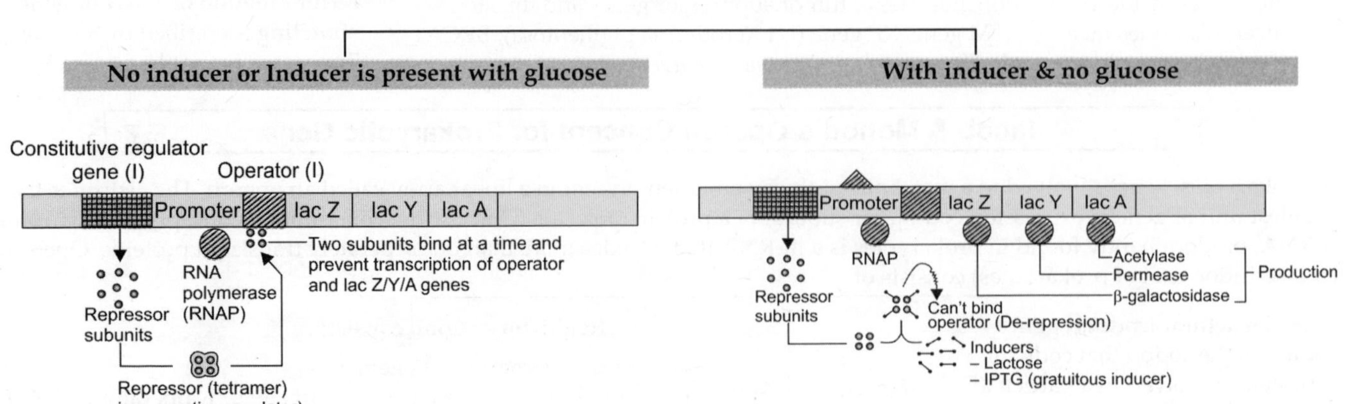

Bacteriophage Lambda (λ) : Gentetic Switch & Lysogenic and Lytic Pathways

- Bacteriophage lambda (λ) is a temperate virus that infects E. coli bacteria and injects its 45, 000 -bp- ds linear – DNA genome into the cell.
- Depending upon the nutritional state of host , the (λ) virus will ***enter either lysogenic or lytic pathways***Q depending on which of 2 sets of viral genes is turned on

Lysogenic Pathway

- *Poor growth conditions* favor lysogeny
- In lysogenic pathway, the viral DNA becomes integrated into bacterial chromosome where it *replicates passively as the bacterial DNA and cell divides.*
- This **dormant genomically integrated** virus is called **prophage** and the cell that horbours it is called a **lysogen**.
- A prophage can be induced by DNA damaging agents such as ultraviolet rays to enter lytic phase by turning on different set of genes (genetic switch)

Lytic Pathway

- *Good growth conditions* promote lytic pathway
- In lytic pathway, *viral DNA replicates* itself and direct synthesis of viral proteins
- About 100 new complete protein packed viral particles are formed. And the proliferating viruses induce the lysis of cell

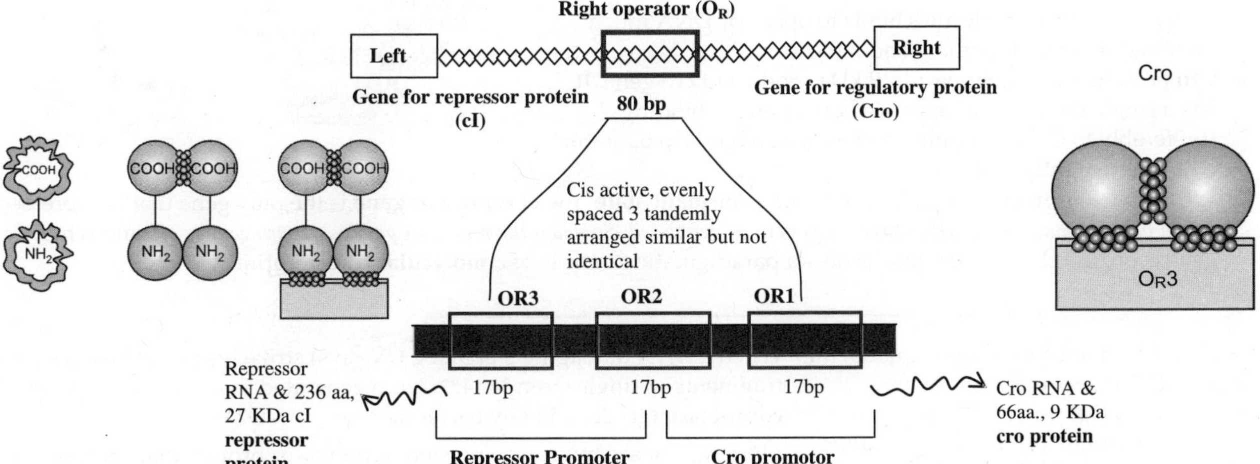

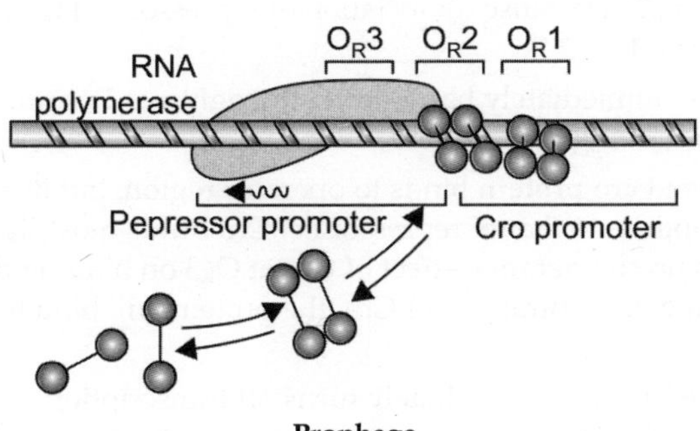

Prophage

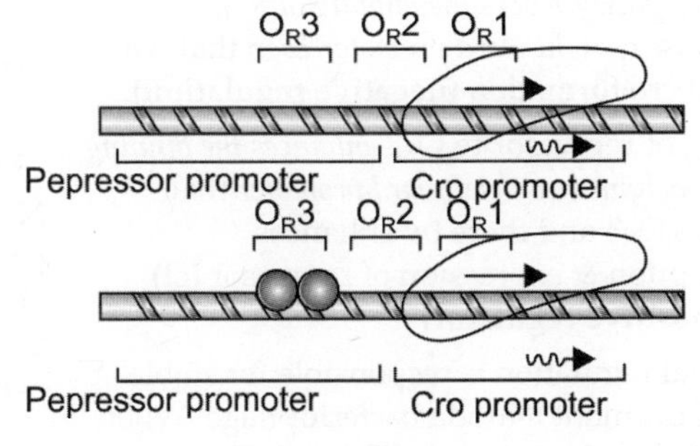

Early lytic phase

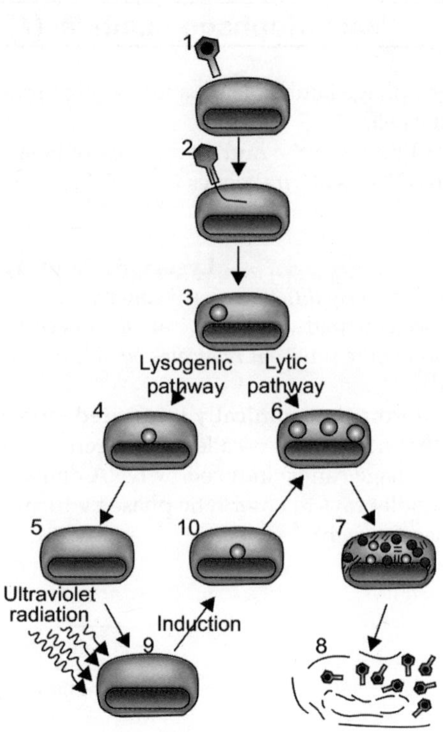

- The lytic – lysogenic genetic switching in (λ) is centered around 80 bp ds DNA **right operator (O_R) genome** which is flanked on its **left side** by **gene for repressor protein (cI)** and on its **right side** by genes encoding regulatory protein **cro** (Mn *"R is not on right side"*)
- O_R can be subdivided into 3 discrete, evenly spaced, tandemly arranged, similar but not identical, 17 bp cis active DNA elements termed **operators O_R1, O_R2, O_R3**. These can be bound by either cI or cro proteins, however *by different binding affinities*, a feature that regulates molecular switch.
- DNA between cro & repressor genes also contain **2 promoter sequences** that over lap the recognition (O_R) sites and direct binding of RNA polymerase in either **right ward** direction (& so transcribing **cro protein**) or **leftward** direction (& so transcribing **cI protein**)
- **Repressor protein (cI)** is a 236 aminoacid, 27 kDa product of repressor gene. It exists as two domain molecule in which the amino terminal domain binds to operator DNA (preferably O_R1) and carboxy terminal domain promotes the association of one repressor protein with another to form a dimer. A dimer of repressor molecules binds to operator DNA much more tightly than does the monomeric form.
- **Cro protein** is a 66 aminoacids, 9 kDa product of cro gene. It has a single domain that operates both operator binding (preferably to O_R3) and dimerization. It also binds to operator DNA more tightly as dimer.
- When the (λ) is in its **lysogenic- prophage – dormant state**- the **cI repressor gene** is the only gene that is expressed. *When bacteriophage is in **lytic state** – **cro gene** is expressed. So when the repressor gene is on, cro gene is off,* and when the cro gene is on, the cI repressor gene is off – a paradigmatic example of a **molecular transcription switch**.

1
2
3
Lysogenic pathway
Lytic pathway
4
6
5
10
7
Ultraviolet radiation
Induction
9
8

- In lysogenic (dormant- prophage) lambda, the **repressor (cI) dimer protein binds preferentially to O_R1** and and enhances binding (by a factor of 10) of another cI dimer to O_R2. The affinity of repressor for O_R3 is least
- O_R1 occupancy *blocks the binding of RNA polymerase to right ward promoter* & in that way prevent cro formation **(negative regulation).**
- Binding of repressor to O_R2 *enhances the binding of RNA polymerase to leftward promoter* that overlaps O_R3 and there by enhances transcription & expression of repressor (cI) gene **(positive regulator)**
- This dual regulation is responsible for stable state of dormant lambda bacteriophage. When intracellular cI protein concentration becomes very high, this *excessive repressor will bind to O_R3 and by doing so diminish transcription of repressor gene* from leftward promoter until the cI concentration drops & repressor dissociates itself from O_R3

When a DNA damaging signal (eg UV rays) strike lysogenic host bacteria, fragments of single stranded DNA are generated that activate a specific **coprotease rec- A** coded by bacterial gene

- Rec A protease hydrolyze portion of repressor protein that connects the amino terminal to carboxy terminal
- Such cleavage of repressor domains causes the repressor dimers to dissociate, which in turn cause dissociation of repressor (cI) from O_R2 & eventually from O_R1
- RNA polymerase immediately has acess to the rightward promoter & commences transcribing the cro gene
- Newly synthesized **cro protein** binds to operator region, but its order of preference is opposite to that of repressor i.e. **Cro binds most lightly to O_R3** but there is no co operative effect of Cro at O_R3 on binding of Cro to O_R2. At increasing concentrations of Cro, the protein will bind to O_R2 and eventually O_R1
- Occupancy of O_R3 by Cro immediately turns off transcription from the left ward cI promoter & so preventing any further expression of repressor gene. Molecular switch is thus completely thrown in lytic direction. The cro is expressed and repressor gene is fully turned off irreversibly
- In very high concentrations Cro occupy O_R1 and reduce expression of its own gene in the final stages of lytic cycle.

DNA Dependent – RNA – Polymerase (RNAP) 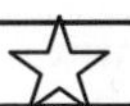

It is the *key enzyme in transcription*Q. In both, prokaryotes & eukaryotes, RNA polymerase *does not require primer & has no proof reading activity*Q.

Prokaryotic RNA polymerase (Bacterial DNA dependent)

RNAP lacks a separate proof reading 3′ → 5′ exonuclease active site (as of DNA polymerase) & so **error rate for transcription is higher than that for DNA replication.** Because many copies of RNA are produced from single gene and eventually all are degraded, so a mistake in RNA is of less significance to cell as compared to DNA which is permanently stored.

Structure & Function

- It *recognizes promoter nucleotide sequence*Q at the begining of length of DNA that is to be transcribed.
- It *makes a complementary RNA copy of DNA templete (antisense) strand, which is identical to coding (sense) strand*Q; with U replacing the T. RNA is synthesized from its 5′ end to its 3′ end, antiparallel to its DNA template strand.
- And then it *recognizes the termination region* (i.e., the end of DNA sequence to be transcribed).
- It is a multisubunit- enzyme, with ~400 kDa **core complex** consisting of *two identical α subunits, similar but not identical β and β′ subunits and a Ω/w subunit* **(αββ′ω). β subunit binds Mg^{++}** and composes **catalytic** subunit.
- It is *multi subunit metalloenzyme* containing 2 *zinc molecules* and

Requirements

RNA polymerase holoenzyme reuires:

1. *Template* of double stranded DNA (or occasionally single stranded DNA)
2. ***Four ribonucleotide triphosphates GTP, UTP, ATP, CTP*Q.**
3. *Mg^{++}* or *Mn^{++}*Q

Type

Only one type of RNAP ***synthetizes all of RNAs (i.e. m-RNA, t-RNA, & r-RNA) except for the short RNA primers needed for DNA replication*Q**. RNA primers are synthesized by **primase** enzyme.

Core- complex (E)

It is ~ 400 kDa complex formed by 5units **($\alpha_2\beta\beta'\omega$)**

Coreenzyme

- Consists of two ***identical α subunits, similar but not identical β and β′ subunits ($\alpha_2\beta\beta'$*Q*, and possess 5′→3′ polymerase activity*Q**
- It *lacks specificity* and *cannot recognize promoter region*

ω/Ω subunit

Function of this 5th subunit is unclear

★ Termination of transcription requires termination factors, such **ρ factor** of E. coli.

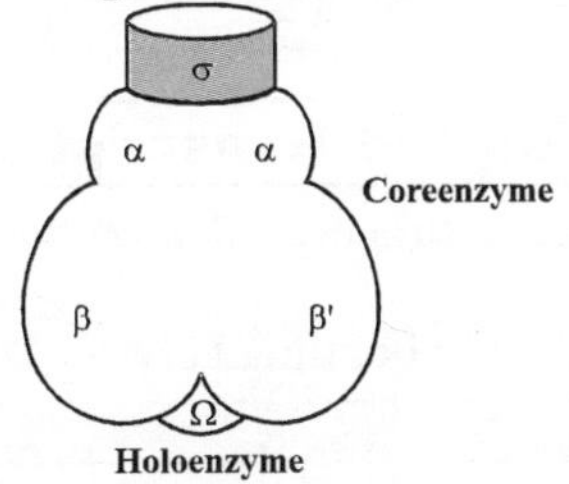

Sigma (σ) subunit

- Sigma factor binds **transiently** to core & directs the enzyme to specific binding sites on DNA. ***It enables RNAP to recognize promoter regions on DNA*Q** and to form the preinitiation complex (PIC).
- It *decreases RNAP's affinity for non promoter regions, while simultaneously increasing holoenzyme affinity for promoter* DNA (dual role)
- It is responsible for **promoter recognization specificity** of RNAP as bacteria has multiple σ factors recognizing different genes. **σ** 70 is the most common type
- Sigma (σ) unit plus the core enzyme makes up the **holoenzyme ($\alpha_2\beta\beta'\omega$+σ)**.

Eukaryotic (Mammation) RNA Polymerase (Nuclear DNA dependent)

- Eukaryotes have **3 types** of RNA polymerases (RNAPs) with size ranging from 5 lack to 6 lack MW and all having **2 larger and multiple** (upto 14 in pol-III) **smaller** subunits. However, these subunits do **exhibit extensive amino acid (& 3 dimensional structure) homologies** with prokaryotic RNA polymerase.
- α- Amantin obtained from **Amanita phalloides (death cap)** is a specific **differential inhibitor** (i.e. differentiates different types) of eukaryotic RNAP. ***It blocks translocation of RNAP during phosphodiester bond formation*Q**. Different forms/types of eukaryotic RNAPs are

RNAP-type	α-Amantin sensitivity	Product	
		Main	**Detailed**
I/ Pol I	**Insensitive**	**r-RNA**	Synthesize only one type of pre-r **RNA (pre ribosomal RNA)** in nucleolus which forms 28S, 18S and 5.8S rRNAs
II (Pol II)	**High**	**m-RNA, mi-RNA, sn RNA**	Synthesize **nuclear precursor of m-RNA** and certain small non coding (nc) RNAs such as **mi-RNA, sn RNA and sno RNA**
III (Pol III)	**Intermediate**	**t-RNA, 5S r RNA**	Forms small RNAs including **t-RNA, 5S rRNA** & some **sn RNA & sno RNA**

- Pol II, responsible for transcription and eukaryotic gene expression consists of **12 subunits**. The two largest subunits **RBP1** (190 KDa) and **RBP 2** (150 kDa) are **structurally similar (homologous)** to prokaryotic **β′** and **β subunits** respectively. *RBP 3 and 11 are homologous to prokaryotic α- subunits.*
- Largest subunit has characteristic **long carboxy tail** consisting of many **repeats of consensus 7 (hepted), aminoacid sequence – Y SPT SPS – (i.e. Tyro – Ser – Pro – Thr – Ser – Pro - Ser). This carboxy terminal repeat domain (CTD)** has 27 repeated units (18 exactly matching the consensus) in yeast and **52 (21 exact)** in mammalian (mouse & human) pol II. The CTD is separated from main enzyme by unstructured linker sequence.
- **Phosphorylation of Ser & Thr** aminoacids of CTD **activates** and **dephosphorylation** of these residues **deactivates** pol II (i.e. increasing & decreasing activity respectively). The phosphorylation & dephosphorylation is essential for *promoter clearance, elongation, termination and even appropriate RNA processing*. So cells with pol II lacking CTD tail are *incapable of activating transcription* and hence are *inviable.*
- CTD is both a *substrate for various kinases (including kinase of TF II H) and binding site for many RNA processing enymes* as well as nuclear transport proteins – thus serves to *couple transcription initiation with m-RNA splicing, 3′ end formation and transport to cytoplasm.*
- Pol II can a/w **Mediator** or **Med** proteins to form **pol II holoenzyme**. Meds are essential for *activating & repressing (i.e. regulating) transcription.* Since mediators (like **TF IID**) are required for actions of activators, they are also called **coactivators /co regulators**. Over 30 meds (Med 1- Med 31) are described in human cells.

★ **Mitochondrial RNA polymerase** more closely resembles bacterial (than eukaryotic) enzyme and is *single* (1 in number).

★ **RNA polymerase leaves its footprints on a promoter**. Foot printing analysis tells the precise location of protein, binding site (like that for RNAP) in a DNA by showing *missing bands (gaps i.e. foot prints)* corresponding to that location. In this 2 identical radioactively labeled DNA (one with and other without RNAP) are cut with DNase and separated by **polyacrylamide gel electrophoresis** (side by side) – the missing bands / gaps in DNA bound to RNA indicate the prescise location of protein binding site.

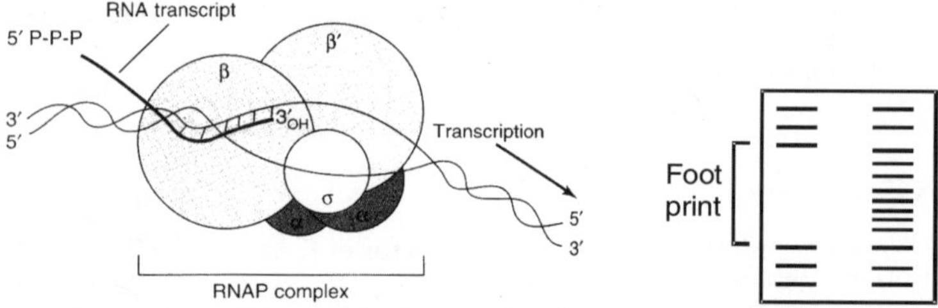

Comparison Between DNA-Replication and Transcription

Similarities: 1) The general steps of initiation, elongation and termination occurs in *5′- 3′ direction*[Q]
2) Both involve large, multi component initiation complex.
3) Adherence to Watson – Crick base pairing rule (i.e. Hydrogen bonding between A= T & between C ≡ G)

DNA Replication	Differences	Transcription
In this process *DNA molecule serves as a template for the formation of daughter DNA molecule*	Definition	In this process *mRNA is synthesized from a DNA template*
Deoxyribonucleotides are used in DNA synthesis	**Nucleotides**	*Ribonucleotides* are used in RNA synthesis
----	**Bases**	'U' replaces 'T' as the complementary base pair for 'A'
Entire genome is copied.	**Copied Genome**	Only a *small portion of genome* is transcribed.
Proof reading occurs.	Proof Reading	No proof reading
Present in DNA polymerase	Endonuclease & Exonuclease activity	***Absent***[Q] in RNA polymerase
Initiation of DNA synthesis ***requires Primer***[Q] [a short length of RNA, about 10-200 nucleotides]	***Primer***[Q]	***Not needed***[Q]

Semiconservative Replication: When the two strands of DNA double helix are separated, each can serve as template for replication of new complementary strand producing two daughter molecule. This process is called semiconservative replication because ***although the parental duplex is separated in two halves (& therefore not conserved as an entity), each of individual parental strands remains intact in one of the two new duplexes***[Q].

Transcription ☆

- DNA constitutes the genetic master plan of an organism, which is however, expressed through RNA – "the working copie of DNA" – This copying process (i.e. synthesis of mRNA from DNA) in which a DNA strand serves as a template is called **transcription**. The 2 complementary DNA strands (of ds DNA) have different roles.

Template Strand	Non-template or Coding Strand
- Template strand of DNA is **transcribed or copied** into an m-RNA molecule. In other words it **is used as a template to make the copy** of that part of DNA (i.e. gene). - The ***information of template strand is readout in 3′ to 5′ direction***[Q]. - So **template strand is complemantary to mRNA transcript** in nucleotide / base sequence.	- The opposite DNA strand (which is complementary to template strand) is called **non template strand**. - Non template DNA strand is also called **coding strand** because **with the exception of T for U changes**, it **corresponds exactly to the sequene of mRNA** primary transcript, which encodes the protein product of that gene. - So **Coding (non-template) strand of DNA is identical to mRNA transcript (except T for U)**

- This means that the information for protein to be produced is encoded in (or is identical to) coding / non template strand of DNA (oriented 5′ to 3′). But the opposite DNA strand acts as template for transcription and is read in 3′ to 5′ direction.
- In ds DNA containing many genes the template strand for each gene will not necessarily be the same strand. So any strand can serve as a *template strand for some genes and coding strand for other genes*. So genes can be transcribed off both strands of DNA.

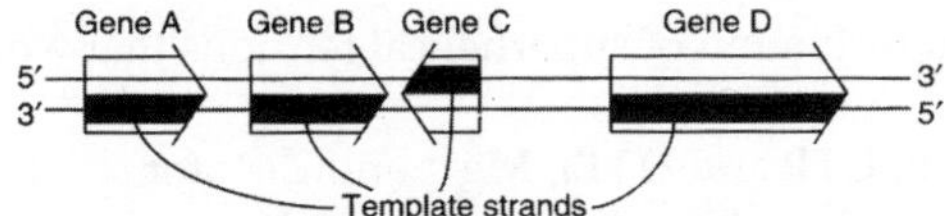

Arrow indicates direction (polarity) of transcription

(5′) CGC TAT AGCG TTT (3′)	DNA **coding strand strand**
(3′) GCGA TAT CGCAAA (5′)	DNA **template strand**
(5′) CGC UAU AGCG UUU (3′)	**mRNA transcript**

- **Regulatory sequences** that control transcription are designated by the sequences in the **coding strand**.

- **Transcription unit** (TU) is the region of DNA that includes signals for all 3 phases of transcription i.e. **initiation, elongation & termination**. TU extends *from promoter to termination region* and the initial RNA product of RNA polymerase (RNAP) which is synthesized in 5′ to 3′direction is called **primary transcript**.
- The **stranting point of transcription in DNA (usually) corresponds** to the 5′ nucleotide of m-RNA. The **base at the transcription start site** is assigned **+1 (first positive) position**. There is **no** base designated **"O"**. By convention, DNA base pairs that corresponds to the beginning of an RNA molecule are given positive numbers & those preceding the RNA start site are given negative numbers. In other words, a base is assigned a **negative number** if it occurs **prior to (towards the 5′ end** or **upstream** of or to the **left** of) transcription start site (+1) and these bases are called **5′ flanking sequences.** Whereas the bases situated **after / down stream / towards 3′ end & right of TSS (+1)** are assigned **positive** numbers in increasing order (i.e. + 10 is more distal to +3). The sequenes down stream of transcription termination site are termed **3′- Flanking sequences**. Although all regulatory sequences function only in ds DNA, by convention, these elements (eg TATA box etc) are **described in 5′ to 3′ direction as being on coding strand**.

1. Initiation

- Transcription begins with the **assembly/binding of RNA polymerase (RNAP) holoenzyme** to (the template strand of) **promoter region** of DNA – forming a **pre-initiation complex (PIC)**. The RNAP can bind with low affinity to many regions of DNA, but instead it scans DNA at a rate of **10^3 bp/s** to find a specific DNA region to which it binds with **higher affinity**. These higher affinity binding, non-transcribing zones are termed **promoters** and it is the binding of RNAP with promoters that **ensures accurate initiation (fidelity)** of transcription.

- Promoter contains characteristic consensus sequences (i.e. ideal sequences in which the base shown at each position is the base most frequently but not necessarily always encountered at that position). Because these sequences are on the same molecule of DNA as the gene being transcribed, they are called **Cis-acting elements**. No one consensus sequence (CS) is found in all core promoters i.e. different bacteria / organism have slightly different CS, but all promoter have 2 common features.

- These tend to be in the *same position relative to transcription start site (+1).*
- *Sequences b/w 2 promoters have no similarity* but still provide **critical spacing functions** that facilitate recognition.

- Promoter regions *can be located upstream & downstream both.* (eg it extends b/w – 70 and +30 in E.coli). **Prokaryotic promoters (-35 sequene, -10/pribnow box)** are recognized by **σ (sigma) subunit** of RNAP holoenzyme. **Eukaryotic** promoters **(TATA box, Inr, DPE** etc) are recognized & assembled to RNAP by **general transcription factors (GTF) like transcription factor II** (i.e. TF required by RNAP II) A to H (except C & G) Because these TFs are encdoded by different genes, synthesized in cytosol, and must transit to their site of action – they are called **trans acting factors**.

2. Elongation

- Beginning of elongation phase is defined when,

- Primary transcript (characteristically starting with purine is **> 10 nucleotides** in length)
- **Sigma (σ)** subunit is **released** and protein **NusA** binds to elongating RNAP competitively
- **Core enzyme** forming elongation complex is able to leave / clear the promoter sequence and move along the template strand in a processive manner (i.e. **promoter clearance**)

- Prokaryotic RNAP has an intrinsic unwindase activity l/t formation of **transcription bubble** (DNA unwinding) of about **20 bp/ RNAP molecule** which remains constant through out transcription (i.e. initiation & elongation). Its size is **determined by RNAP** & is independent of **DNA sequene**.
- Elongation proceeds at a rate of **50-90 nucleotides per second.** Because DNA is a helix, movement of transcription bubble requires considerable strand rotations. So movement of RNAP along DNA tends to generate a **positive superoil (i.e overwound DNA) in front** of transcription bubble and **negative supercoil (underwound DNA) behind** it. This topological problem in cells is relieved by action of **topoisomerases** which rapidly eliminates positive supercoils & regulate the level of negative supercoiling.
- So **topoisomerases both preceeds & follows progressing RNAP** to prevent formation of superhelical tensions that would increase the energy demand to unwind the DNA in front of RNAP.
- RNAP requires, **DNA template**, all 4 nucleotide 5′ triphosphates (**ATP, GTP, CTP and UTP), Mg^{++}** and **Zn^{++}** for synthesis (elongation) of RNA strand – by adding ribonucleotide units to 3′ hydroxyl end, building RNA in **5′→3′ direction**.
- Just like DNA replication, transcription (RNA elongation) is in **5′ to 3′ direction antiparallel to its template strand** (which is read & copied in 3′ to 5′ direction). But unlike it , RNAP **does not require primer** for initiation & has **no proof reading** activity
- Bases are added a/t Watson-Crick base pairing rule and **pyrophosphate (PPi) is released** after each addition (except of 1st initiating purine base, which remains intact throughout transcription). PPi is rapidly degraded to 2 mol of inorganic phosphate (Pi) by ubiquitous pyrophosphatases, making over all reaction irreversible.
- Growing end of newly synthesized RNA strand base pairs temporarily with DNA template strand to form short **8 bp long RNA-DNA double helix** in the transcription bubble.
- RNA hybrid duplex peels off shortly after its formation & DNA duplex reforms.
- In **eukaryotes,** TF IIF remains associated with pol II throughout elongation. **Elongation factors** like Ell; pTEFb, SII (TF IIS) and elongin (S III)- greatly enhance the activity of pol II. pTEFb phosphorylates pol II within CTD and suppress pausing.

3. Termination

- RNAP is **highly processive** (i.e. adds) great number of bases before dissociation)- necessarily so because if it gets detached prematurely, it would have to start from beginning again. So *elongation of SS-RNA continues until termination signal is reached.*
- 2 types of termination are

1. Spontaneous / Intrinsic Rho (ρ) independent termination.

- In mot **prokaryotic genes** a sequence in DNA template strand is spontaneously terminating which produces
- Nascent (newly formed) RNA transcript with self complementary sequences, permitting the RNA to fold back on itself forming a **hair pin structure** centered **15 to 20 nucleotides before** the projected end of RNA strand. This hair pin has **GC rich stem** stabilized by hydrogen bonds and *loop of non complementary bases.*
- Highy conserved string of 3′ ‘A’ in template DNA is transcribed into a **string of ‘U’s at the 3′ end just beyond hair pin**.
- RNAP pauses on reaching termination site with this structure. The bonding of string of Us to complementary As of DNA template is weak. Dissociation of RNA transcription from DNA template in this area is facilitated by formation of hair pin structure and zipping up of DNA double helix behind RNAP.

2. Rho (ρ) dependent termination

- Termination site (in template strand of DNA) **lacks repeated A string** but usually includes **CA-rich** sequence k/a **rut (rho utilization) element**
- This requies addition **ρ protein** that is a **hexameric ATPase** (adenosine triphosphatase) **with helicase activity**.
- Rho binds to **C rich-ρ-recognition site** near the 3′ end of nascent RNA and migrates in **5′ → 3′ direction**, along RNA using its ATPase activity until it reaches the transcription complex (RNAP) that is paused at termination site.
- **ATP dependent RNA-DNA helicase** activity of ρ- protein separates the RNA-DNA hybrid helix-causing the release of RNA. (this enz also promotes translocation along RNA-Lehninger.)

- On completion of transcription NusA dissociates from RNAP, which itself dissociates from DNA. The σ- factor can now bind to RNAP to initiate new transcription – in a cycle called **sigma (σ) cycle**.
- Summary: Transcription initiates with **binding of RNAP to promoter region** of DNA (on **template strand**) to form **PIC** – a process which is guided by **σ- subunit** in prokaryotes & **TFs** in eukaryotes. This l/t formation of **closed (wound DNA) f/b open complex** (with unwound DNA) or **transcription bubble**. Nucleotides are added (i.e. RNA is synthesized) in **5'→ 3' direction antiparalled to temlate strand** a/t base pairing rule. In both prokaryotes & eukaryotes 1st nucleotide is usually purine and its 5′ triphosphate end is maintained (not degraded) in mRNA.

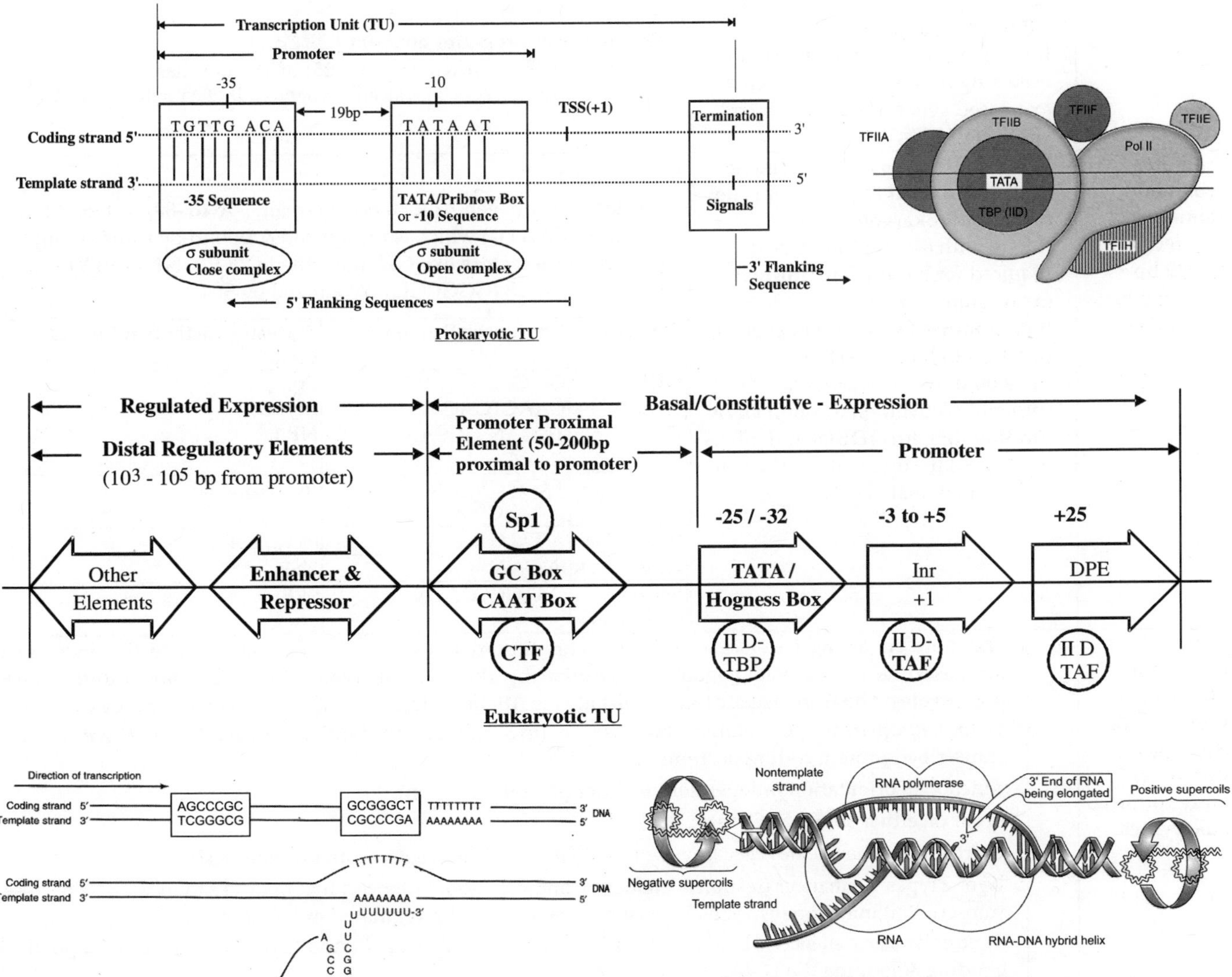

Local unwinding of DNA caused by RNA polymerase

<table>
<tr><th></th><th>Prokaryotes</th><th>Eukaryotes</th></tr>
<tr>
<td>Promoters (Cis-acting element):
Named & positioned a/t location of 5′to3′ base sequence in coding/non-template strand</td>
<td>1. "-35 sequence": It is a consensus sequence of 8 nucleotie pairs (5′-TGTTG-ACA-3′) centered approximately 35 bp upstream (left) of transcription start site (+1). RNA binds & forms closed complex.
2. "-10 sequence" or Pribnow/TATA-box: It is a 6 nucleotide pairs of A+T rich consensus sequence (5′-TATA-AT-3′) centered more proximally about 10 bp upstream (left) to TSS (+1). Closed f/b open complex (k/a transcription bubble) is formed d/t melting /unwinding of short stretch (~14 bases) of DNA-as TATA box lack GC base pairs.
3. UP (Upstream promoter):
It is AT rich recognition element occurring b/w -40 & -60 in highly expressed genes. It is bound by α-subunit of RNAP.</td>
<td>1. Hogness/TATA-box (-25 or -32 sequence):
It is the major assembly point usually located 25 bp upstream from TSS (+1). This region has a sequence of TATAAAG and the consensus sequene is 5′ – TATA-AA-3′, which is recognized by TATA- binding protein (TBP) subunit of TF IID It is functionally similar to prokaryotic TATA box
2. Initiator sequence (Inr): It spans the transcription start site (from-3 to +5) and consist of CS
"Y Y A N T Y Y", where N is any nucleotide and
A Y is pyrimmidine (Lehninger)
T C A_{+1} G T T , where A_{+1} is first transcribed
T C nucleotide. (Harper).
TSS is very near or usually within Inr hence forming open complex with unwound DNA. TBP associated factor (TAFs) subunit of TFIID recognize & help binding it to pol II.
3. Downstream promoter element (DPE):
It is located 25 bp downstream (+25) of TSS and has CS - (5′-A G A CGTG – 3′) which is recognized by TAF subunit of TF IID
G T</td>
</tr>
<tr>
<td>Promoter proximal elements (located b/w 50-200 bp proximal to promoter)</td>
<td>- This cis acting upstream element located proximal to promoter is not found in prokaryotes
- It long with (a/w) promoters is required for basal (Constitutive) expression of gene.
- It determines frequency of even and function in both direction.
- PPEs bind to trans elements (proteins/activators) through DNA binding domains (DBD) and others (eg TF, pol II, coregulators) through activation domain (AD)</td>
<td>1. CAAT box:
It is located between 70 & 80 bp upstream (-70 to -80) of TSS (+1) and has CS (CCAATC) which is recognized & bound by trans acting transcription factors like CTF (als called C/E PB, NF-1, NFY)
2. GC box with CS (GGGCGG) recognized by Sp1
<table>
<tr><th>Element</th><th>Consensus Sequence (CS)</th><th>Activator/Factor that bind to them</th></tr>
<tr><td>GC</td><td>G_3CG_2
CAACTGAC
$TGGAN_5GCCAA$
C C</td><td>Sp1
MyoD
NF-1</td></tr>
<tr><td>AP1</td><td>T G A G T C A
C A</td><td>Jun, Fos, ATF</td></tr>
<tr><td>Ig Octamer</td><td>A T G C A A A T</td><td>Oct 1, 2, 4, 6</td></tr>
<tr><td>Heat Shock</td><td>$(NGAAN)_3$</td><td>HSF</td></tr>
<tr><td>Serum response</td><td>GATGCCCATA</td><td>SRF</td></tr>
</table></td>
</tr>
<tr>
<td>Distal Regulatory Elements – Enhancer & Repressor (Silencer) Only found in eukaryotes</td>
<td colspan="2">- These are cis acting (i.e. located on same chromosome) DNA sequences that regulate (i.e. increase or decrease) the rate of initiation of transcription by Pot IIin eukaryotes. These are not found in these prokaryotes. These are usually located distally (i.e. 10^3 to 10^5 from promoter site. However they can
1. be located upstream (to 5′ end) or down stream (to 3′ end) of transcription start site and even within the transcribed protein coding portions.
2. function in orientation independent manner (in both direction).
3. occur on either strand of DNA.
4. exert effects when located close to or even tens of thousands of bp away from promoter/TU.
5. be of 2 types – enhancer (response elements) and repressor (silencer) that bind TFs to increase & decrese transcription initiation respectively. So these are required for regulated expression.
- These enhancer / silencer – binding TFs can interact with other TFs bound to promoter with RNA pol II by bending & looping the DNA.</td>
</tr>
<tr>
<td>Factors for promoter specific binding</td>
<td>- Sigma (σ) subunit of prokaryotic RNAP is responsible for promoter recognition specificity of enzyme and its binding to promoter l/t formation of PIC</td>
<td>- Various general transcription factors (GTFs) like transcription factor for pol II i.e. TF II from A to H (except C & G) are required for PIC formation as RNAP II alone</td>
</tr>
</table>

- Functions of different sigma subunits are

σ 70	**House keeping**
σ54	Modulations of cellular *nitrogen levels*
σ38	Stationary phase gene
σ32	**Heat shock gene**
σ28	Chemotaxis & flagella genes
σ24	Extracytoplasmic functions like *heat shock functions*
σ18	Extracytoplasmic functions like *ferric citrate transport*

cannot discriminate b/w promoter & other regions of DNA. GTFs in order of binding assembly (i.e. basal components of transcription and their functions) are

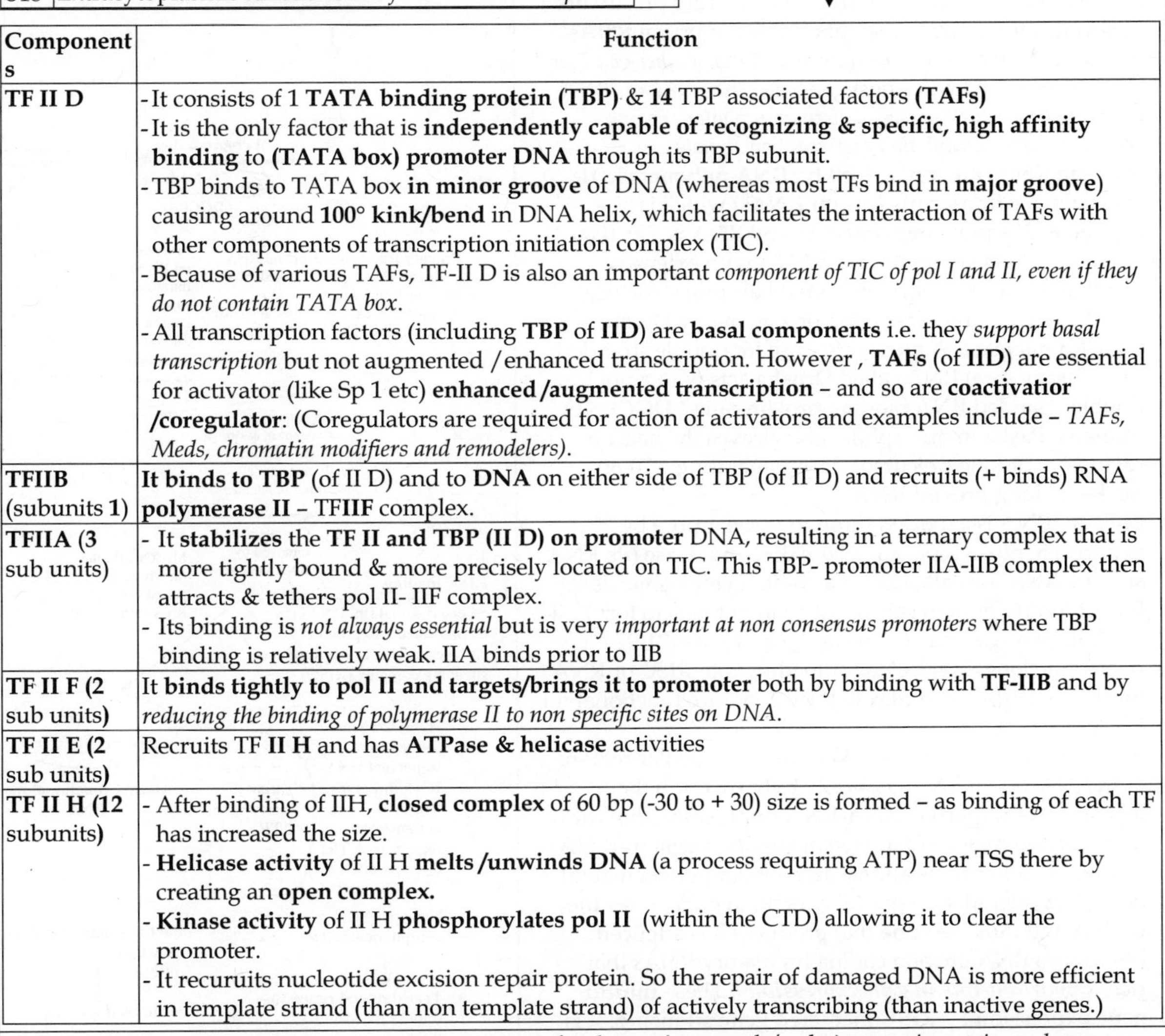

Components	Function
TF II D	-It consists of 1 **TATA binding protein (TBP)** & **14** TBP associated factors **(TAFs)** -It is the only factor that is **independently capable of recognizing & specific, high affinity binding** to **(TATA box) promoter DNA** through its TBP subunit. -TBP binds to TATA box **in minor groove** of DNA (whereas most TFs bind in **major groove**) causing around **100° kink/bend** in DNA helix, which facilitates the interaction of TAFs with other components of transcription initiation complex (TIC). -Because of various TAFs, TF-II D is also an important *component of TIC of pol I and II, even if they do not contain TATA box.* -All transcription factors (including **TBP** of **IID**) are **basal components** i.e. they *support basal transcription* but not augmented /enhanced transcription. However , **TAFs** (of **IID**) are essential for activator (like Sp 1 etc) **enhanced /augmented transcription** – and so are **coactivatior /coregulator**: (Coregulators are required for action of activators and examples include – *TAFs, Meds, chromatin modifiers and remodelers).*
TFIIB (subunits **1**)	**It binds to TBP** (of II D) and to **DNA** on either side of TBP (of II D) and recruits (+ binds) RNA **polymerase II** – TF**IIF** complex.
TFIIA (3 sub units)	- It **stabilizes** the **TF II and TBP (II D) on promoter** DNA, resulting in a ternary complex that is more tightly bound & more precisely located on TIC. This TBP- promoter IIA-IIB complex then attracts & tethers pol II- IIF complex. - Its binding is *not always essential* but is very *important at non consensus promoters* where TBP binding is relatively weak. IIA binds prior to IIB
TF II F (2 sub units**)**	It **binds tightly to pol II and targets/brings it to promoter** both by binding with **TF-IIB** and by *reducing the binding of polymerase II to non specific sites on DNA.*
TF II E (2 sub units**)**	Recruits TF **II H** and has **ATPase & helicase** activities
TF II H (12 subunits**)**	- After binding of IIH, **closed complex** of 60 bp (-30 to + 30) size is formed – as binding of each TF has increased the size. - **Helicase activity** of II H **melts /unwinds DNA** (a process requiring ATP) near TSS there by creating an **open complex.** - **Kinase activity** of II H **phosphorylates pol II** (within the CTD) allowing it to clear the promoter. - It recuruits nucleotide excision repair protein. So the repair of damaged DNA is more efficient in template strand (than non template strand) of actively transcribing (than inactive genes.)

Promoter Acessibility

- Transcription machinery cannot access promoter of **eukaryotic genes** b/o their *wrapping up in nucleosomes.* Binding of TFs to enhancers causes recruitment of **chromatin remodeling & modifying coregulatory factors** (like Swi/Snf, SRC-1, p300 /CBP or P/CAF) – ultimately l/t **nucleosome eviction (removal)** and opening of promoter to become accessible.
- **Interconversion of hetero chromatin** (i.e. highly condensed, most inactive segments of DNA) and **euchromatin** (i.e. relatively relaved, highly transcribing genes) is k/a **chromatin remodeling. Acetylation**, mediated by **HATs (histone acetyl transferases)** *removes positive* charge on **lysine** residues at amino terminal of histone and thus decreases the interaction b/w histones and negatively charged DNA – ultimately converting hetero chromatin to euchromatin and removing nucleosomes. **HDACs (histone deacetylase)** *restores positive charge* building stronger interactions b/w histones & DNA thus forming nucleosomes.
- So this **epigenetic code of histone – protein modifications** can increase or decrease gene transcription. Mutations in **code writers** (proteins that catalyze) or **code readers** (proteins that differentially bind) modified histones l/t diseases.

Micro- RNA (mi-RNA), si RNAs, st RNAs, sRNAs & RNA interference

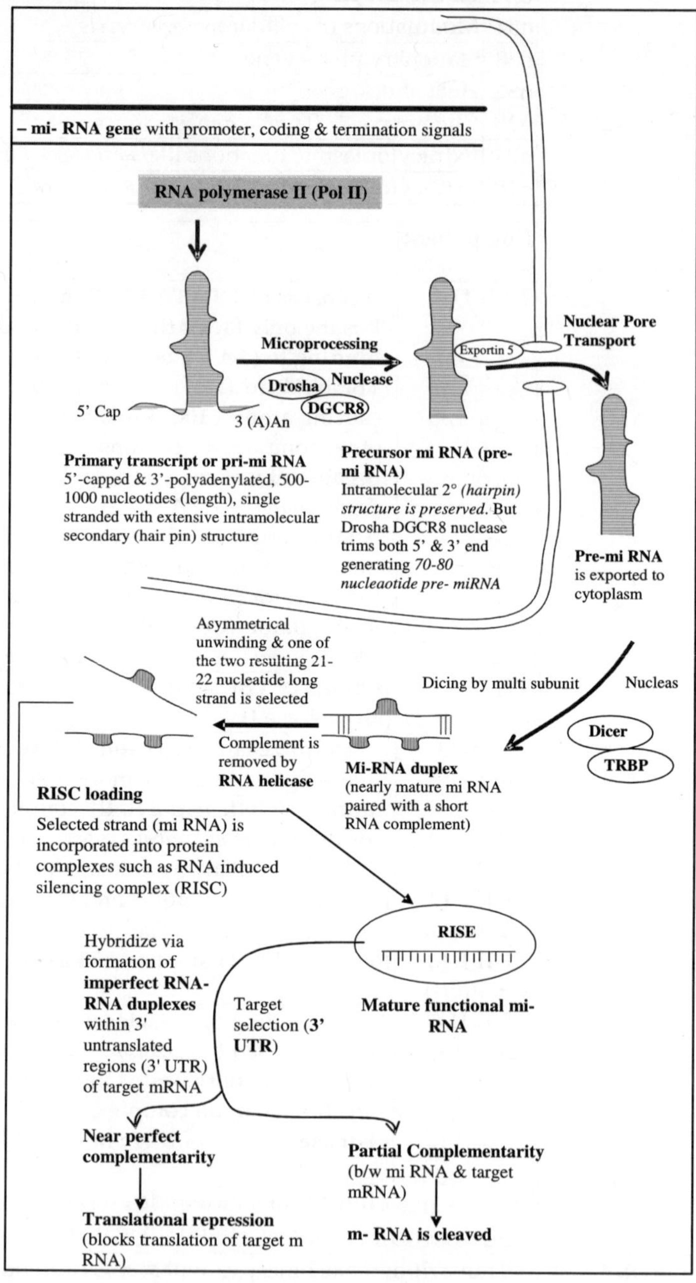

- Micro-RNAs are *non coding (nc RNA* i.e. they do not encode protein) *RNAs about 22 (21-25) nucleotide long*, found in *multicelluar eukaryotes* (eg worms, flies, plants & mammals).
- Upto *1% of human genome* may encode *mi RNAs & mi RNAs may target upto 1/3rd of human m-RNAs*
- mi – RNAs are synthesized from much larger precursors in several steps. The transcription units of pri-mi RNAs are located *either in introns (intronic DNA) of other genes* or (and coexpressed with) host genome. Therefore m*i RNA encoding genes must possess a distinct promotor , coding region, and polyadenylation / termination signals.*
- Most mi RNAs are transcribed by **RNA polymerase II** into **primary transcripts (pri-mi RNAs)** which is **5′ – capped & 3′ – polyadenylated**. pri-mi RNA is 500-1000 nucleotide long single stranded RNA with extensive intramolecular 2° (double stranded hair pin) structure, which is maintained following processing by **Drosha – DGCR8 nuclease.** A nuclear RN ase for double stranded (d/t 2° structure) RNA called **Drosha** acts with a nuclear double stranded RNA binding protein called **DGCR8** in humans (**Pasha** in drosophila) and cleaves the hair pin region out of long precursor RNA generating a 70-80 nucletide long **pre- mi RNA**
- pre – mi RNA is exported through nuclear pore by **exportin 5** into cytoplasm, where **dicer nuclease** (ds RNA specific RNA ase called Dicer act with cytoplasmic ds RNA binding protein called TRBP) in humans to form mi-RNA duplex. Ultimately one of the 2 strands (21-22 nucleotide long) is selected for loading into RISC or RNA induced silencing complex to form a mature functional mi RNA.
- mi RNA is *complementary in sequence* to particular regions of m RNA. So mi RNAs typically hybridize, via the formation of **imperfect RNA-RNA duplexes** within the 3′ untranslated regions (3′ UTRs) of specific target m-R NAs leading to either translational arrest (near perfect match) or mRNA degradation (partal match). In either case, the mRNA and thus the **gene** that produces it is **silenced.**
- Micro (mi) RNA are non coding regulatory RNAs that play ***important role in gene expression***[Q]. These **inhibit gene expression** by **RISC mediated gene silencing.** It is used as a mechanism to protect against invading RNA viruses (esp important in plants which lack an immune system) & to control the activity of transposons & developmental timing.
- Many mi RNAs are present only transiently during development , & are referred to as **small temporal RNAS (st RNAs)**.
- If an investigator introduces into an organism a duplex RNA molecule corresponding in sequence to virtually any mRNA, Dicer nuclease cleaves the duplex into short segments, called **small interfering RNAs (siRNAs).** These short (21-25 nucleotide long) si RNAs usually form **perfect RNA-RNA hybrid** with their targets potentially anywhere within the length of m RNA where the complementary sequence exists. Formation of such RNA-RNA duplexes between si RNAs and mRNA results in reduced specific protein production because the si **RNA – mRNA complexes are degraded,** mostly in specific cytoplasmic organelles termed **P- bodies**. The process is k/a **RNA interference RNAi** for which **Nobel prize** was given to Andrew Fire & Craig Mello in 2006.

- **RNAi** is activated when RNA molecule occurs in double stranded pairs in cell. Ds RNA activates biochemical machinery which degrades those mRNA that carry a genetic code identical to that of ds RNA. When such m RNA molecules disappear, the corresponding gene is silenced and no protein of encoded type is made.
- So **RNA i** is extremely useful research tool as it allows genetic researchers to **knock out specific genes**, observe the consequent disruptions, and so determine exactly what the gene does. It has already revealed genes responsible for diabetes and muscle problems. In lab it has been used to block HIV and polio virus infections.
- **Nearly all mi RNAs and si RNAs cause inhibition of gene expression**. Bacteria also contain small hetrogenous regulatory RNAs called sRNAs. Bacterial sRNAs range in size from 50-500 nucleotides, and like eukaryotic mi RNA / si RNA also control a large array of genes. Similary sRNAS often repress, but some times activate protein synthesis by binding to specific m RNA
- *Mi RNAs are considered to be endogenously expressed counterparts of Si RNAs*

Mechanism &Types of Splicing

There are 4 classes of introns

1 & 2 Self Splicing Introns (SSI)

- It **function as ribozyme,** does *not require protin enzymes and high energy cofactors* (such as ATP) for splicing
- Splicing mechanism involves **two transesterification** reactions in which a new phosphodiester bond *(5′ – 3′ PDB in group I and 5′-2′ PDB in group II) is formed at the expense of old bond* maintaining the balance of energy. These reactions are very similar to DNA breaking and rejoining reactions promoted by topoisomerase and site specific recombinases.
- Self splicing introns may be of 2 types

Group I SSI	Group II SSI
Found in some nuclear, mitochondrial and chloroplast genes that code for r RNAs, mRNAs & t-RNAs; and some introns in bacteria	Found in primary transcript of mitochondrial or chloroplast m RNAs in fungi, algae & plants; and some introns in bacteria
- Nucleophile in first transesterification reaction is **3′-hydroxyl group of guanine nucleoside or nucleotide (guanosine, GMP, GDT, or GTP)** - 3′ → 5′ phosphodiester bond is formed but **lariat (loop) like intermediate is not formed**	- **2′ hydroxyl group of adenosine (A) residue** (known as **branch site**) in intron is nucleophile. - **2′→ 5′ phosphodiester bond and branched lariat (loop) like intermediate structure is formed.** The excised intron is released as a lariat, in which adenosine has 3 phosphodiester bonds. Lariat is degraded.
2 Transeterifications reactions include - **3′ (OH) of G (guanosine, GMP, GDP, GTP cofactors)** is used for nucleophile attack (not energy). It **attacks the phosphate at 5′ splice site (junction of 5′ exon & intron = 5′ end of intron = splice donor site) forming a normal 3′- 5′ phosphodiester bond** with 5[1] end of intron. - 3′(OH) of 5′ exon that is displaced in this step then acts as nuceophile and triggers 2nd transesterification reaction by attacking **5′ phosphate** at **splice acceptor site (3′ end** of **intron** or **3′ splice site**) forming 3′→5′ phosphodiester bond. This results in precise excision of introns & ligation of exons.	2 Transesterification reactions are - **2′ (OH) group of A (adenosine)** in the branch point sequence of intron act as nucleophile, attacking the phosphate at 5′ splice site forming ***unusual 2′ → 5′ phosphodiester bond and creating a lariat (loop) like structure***[Q]. - Newly freed 3′ (OH) of 5′ exon attacks 5′ phosphate at splice acceptor site (3′ end of intron or 3′ splice site) forming 3′ → 5′ phospodiester bond, resulting in excision of introns & ligation of exons.

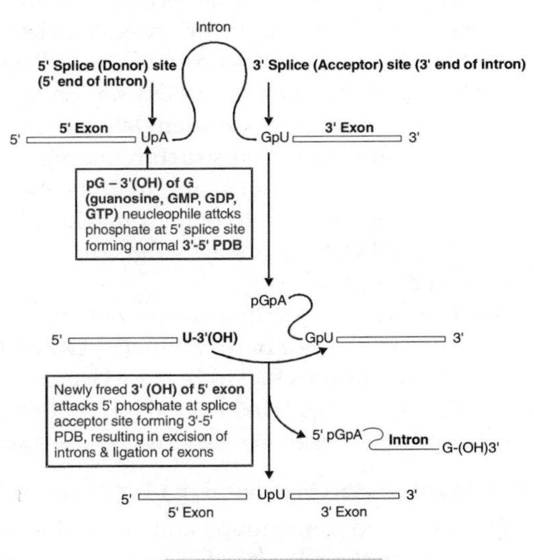

Group I SSI

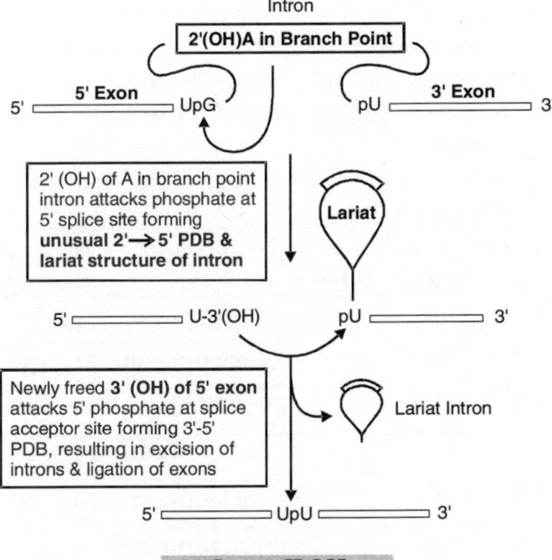

Group II SSI

3. Splicesomal Introns

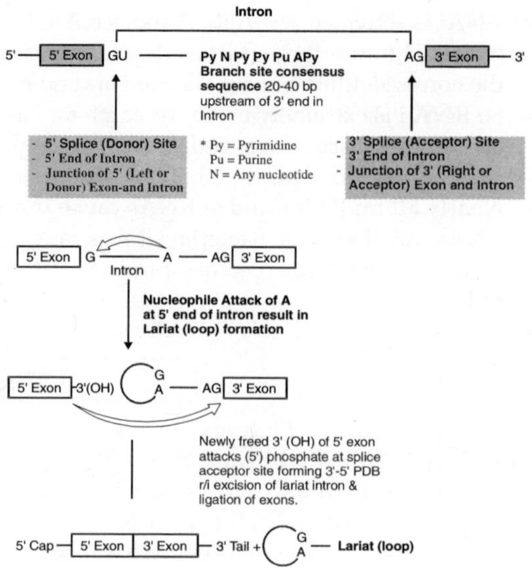

- Most introns are not self **splicing**. This *largest class* of introns includes those *found in nuclear mRNA primary transcripts*
- These are called splicesomal introns, *because their removal occurs within and is catalyzed by large protein complex called **splicesome**. Within the splicesome,* the introns undergo splicing by same ***lariat (loop) forming mechanism as group II introns***[Q].
- Splicesomal introns have **dinucleotide sequence GU at 5′ end and AG at 3′** end and these **mark the site where splicing occurs**. The GU and AG sequences at the beginning and end respectively, of introns are invariant.
- **U1 sn RNA** contains a sequence complementary to sequences near the **5′ splice site of nuclear mRNA introns**; and **U1** binds to this region of primary transcript. **U2** is paired *to intron at a position encompassing the A residue that become nucleophile.* This adenyl residue in branch point sequence is typically located 20-40 nucleotides upstream from 3′ end of intron being removed. *The branch site identifies the 3′ splice site.* Base pairing of U2 causes a bulge that displaces and activate **adenylate (of branch site in intron), whose 2′ (OH) will form the lariat structure through a 2′- 5′ phosphodiester bond.**

Intron

5′ — 5′ Exon GU — Py N Py Py Pu APy — AG 3′ Exon — 3′

Branch site consensus sequence 20-40 bp upstream of 3′ end in Intron

- 5′ Splice (Donor) Site
- 5′ End of Intron
- Junction of 5′ (Left or Donor) Exon-and Intron

* Py = Pyrimidine
Pu = Purine
N = Any nucleotide

- 3′ Splice (Acceptor) Site
- 3′ End of Intron
- Junction of 3′ (Right or Acceptor) Exon and Intron

5′ Exon G — A — AG 3′ Exon
Intron

Nucleophile Attack of A at 5′ end of intron result in Lariat (loop) formation

5′ Exon 3′(OH) G A — AG 3′ Exon

Newly freed 3′ (OH) of 5′ exon attacks (5′) phosphate at splice acceptor site forming 3′-5′ PDB r/i excision of lariat intron & ligation of exons.

5′ Cap — 5′ Exon 3′ Exon — 3′ Tail + G A — Lariat (loop)

- After U_1 and U_2, the remaining sn RNPs (U_4 – U_6 complex and U_5) bind to form an inactive spliceosome. Internal rearrangements activate complex in which U_1 & U_4 have been expelled and U6 is paired with both U2 and 5′ splice site. This is followed by catalytic steps similar to and group II SSI. **ATP is required for the assembly of spliceosome, but not for RNA cleavage - ligation**
- Some less common spliceosomes contain **U_{11} and U_{12} snRNPs** in place of U^1 and U^2. Whereas **U1 and U2** containing spliceosome remove introns with **(5′) GU and AG (3′) terminal sequences**, the U^{11} and U^{12} containing spliceosome remove rare class of introns that have **(5′) AU and AC (3′) terminal sequence** to mark the intrionic splice site.
- Splicing apparatus is tethered to *CTD of RNA polymerase III* coordinating splicing & transcription and providing a mechanism for bringing 2 splice sites together. **After splicing introns (lariat) remains in nucleus and is degraded.**

4. Class 4 Introns are found in t RNAs

- Distinguished from group I and group II introns in that the splicing reaction **requires ATP and endonuclease**
- **Splicing endonuclease (ribonuclease) cleaves the phosphodiester bond** at both ends of introns and two **exons are joined by** a mechanism similar to DNA **ligase** reaction.

Splicing and sn RNAs

- Uracil rich Small nuclear RNAs (sn RNAs) are **non coding RNAs** that play pivotal ***role in RNA processing and splicing***[Q] by forming **small nuclear ribonucleo protein particles (SnRNPs or "snurps")**
- SnRNAs vary in size from *90-300 Nucleotides*. Some example include.

Name	Length (nucleotides)	Localization	Molecules per cell
U1	165	Nucleoplasm	1×10^6
U2	188	Nucleoplasm	5×10^5
U3	216	**Nucleolus**	3×10^5
U4	139	Nucleoplasm	1×10^5
U5	118	Nucleoplasm	2×10^5
U6	106	**Perichromatin granules**	3×10^5
4.55	95	Nucleus & cytoplasm	3×10^5
7 SK	280	Nucleus & cytoplasm	5×10^5

sno RNAs and r RNA modification

- Small nucleolar RNAs (sno RNAs) are nc RNAs that guide nucleoside modification and cleavage reactions in pre- rRNAs.
- In yeast about 70 and in humans > 200 sno RNAs are found
- sno RNAs are *60-300 nucleotides* long and many are encoded with in the *introns of other genes.*
- Each sno RNA includes a *10-21 nucleotide* sequence that is perfectly *complementary to some site in rRNA.* The conserved sequence elements in the remainder of sno RNA fold into structures that are bound by sno RNP proteins.
- The most common nucleoside modification in eukaryotic r RNAs are, again, conversion of uridine to pseudouridine and ado met dependent nucleoside methylation (often at 2′ –OH groups). These reactions rely on **sno-RNA protein complexes** or **sno RNPs**, each consisting of a sno RNA & 4-5 proteins
- There are 2 classes of sno RNPs, both defined by *Key conserved sequence elements referred* to as lettered boxes.

1. **Box C/D** sno RNPs function in *2′ – O – methylations*
2. **Box H/ACA** sno RNPs are involved in *pseudouridylylation*

- Besides its role in splicing, the **sn RNA U1** directly binds to transcription factor TF II H and may regulate TF II H or affect the *coupling between transcription & splicing.*
- **U_1, U_2, U_4, U_5 & U_6** – SnRNAs are involved in intron removal and processing of mRNA precursors into mRNA. **U_7** – snRNA is involved in **production of correct 3′ ends of histone mRNA,** which lacks a poly (A) tail.
- A 331 nucleotide nc RNA called **7SK**, abundant in mammals, binds to *pol II transcription elongation factor P-TEFb* (that modulates mRNA gene transcription elongation by RNA polymerase II) and repress transcriptase elongation.
- In **SLE**, autoantibodies develop against their own nuclear proteins like SnRNPs.

Splice Site Mutation & Alternative Splicing

- Splice site mutation can l/t improper splicing & production of aberrant proteins. 15% of all genetic disease are caused b/o **faculty splicing** and example includes beta thalassemia (with defective beta -globin protein)
- **Alterantive patterns of mRNA splicing** result from *tissue specific developmental & adaptive control mechanism (such as chromatin epigenetic markers). This produces diverse set of proteins from a limited set of genes and example includes multiple isoforms of **tropomyosin protein.***
- Tissue specific regulation of gene expression can be provided by alternative splicing by control elements in promoter or by use of alternative promoters. Example, **insulin & cAMP control glucokinase (GK) gene transcription in liver while glucose controls GK expression in pancreatic beta-cells**.

Splicing of Primary Transcript

- **Primary transcript** contains 2 types of sequences

Introns (Intervening) sequence that do not code the genetic information	**Exon (Expressed) sequence** that contain genetic information & code for various amino acids

- It undergoes extensive processing **(RNA splicing)** to convert into functional RNA which involves **cleaving out of introns** and **splicing together of exons,** facilitated by **Sn RNP or snurp of spliceosome.** This process occurs in nucleus and mature m RNA is then transported to cytoplasm where it is translated into protein.
- *The process of removing introns (RNA sequences which do not code for proteins) and joining exons (RNA sequences that code for proteins) is called 'Splicing'.*
- ***The process of splicing is mediated by Small nuclear ribonucleoprotein particles (sn RNP) or 'Snurps' which are formed from sn RNA***
- *The molecular machinery that accomplishes splicing is called a **spliceosome** which is formed when the primary transcript combines with the Sn RNP.* **Spliceosome** consists of *primary transcript, **five (Sn-RNA) small nuclear RNAs (U1, U2, U4, U5, U6)*** and > 60 proteins collectively these form a **small nuclear ribo nucleoprotein (Sn RNP) complex** or **snurp.**
- *The binding of sn RNP brings the sequences of neighboring exons into correct alignment for splicing.*

U_1	1st binds to 5′ **exon-interon boundary**
U_2	Binds to **branch site** and this **expose the nucleophilic A residue**
$U_5/U_4/U_6$	Mediate an ATP dependent protein mediated **unwinding** that results in disruption of the base paired U4-U6 complex with the release of U4. U6 is then able to interact first with U2, then with U1. This approximate the 5′ splice end, the branch point with its reactive A, and 3′ splice site. This alignment is enhanced by U5. This process also results in formation of **loop or lariat** structure.
U_2-U_6	**Two ends are cleaved**, by U2-U6 with in the SnRNP complex.

U6 is essential since yeast deficient in this are not viable.

Primary Transcript and Post Transcriptional Modification of hn-RNA

- The RNA formed and released from DNA template is known as **primary transcript**. The **primary transcript** of m-RNA is **hn-RNA** (and of mi-RNA is **pri-miRNA**).
- A **primary transcript** is a linear, RNA copy of a trancriptional unit – i.e., segment of DNA between initiation & termination sequence. The primary transcripts of both **prokaryotic & eukaryotic t-RNA and r-RNA** as well as **eukaryotic m-RNA**, 55 RNA, Sn RNAs, RNA processing mechinary are inactive and undergoes modifications for activation. In contrast, ***prokaryotic mRNA is generally identical to its primary transcript***[Q].
- ***Nearly all eukaryotic & prokaryotic RNA (except prokaryotic m-RNA) are extensively processed primariy with in the nucleus (for eukaryotes) before they become functional***[Q]. The processes of transcription, RNA processing & RNA transport from nucleus are highly co-ordinated by – **SAGA** (in yeast) & **P/CAF** (in humans) and **TREX** (transcription export). Transcriptional co-activator (SAGA or P/CAF) link *transcription activation to RNA processing* by recruiting TREX that links *transcription elongation complex, RNA splicing machinery and nuclear export.*

Modification of Eukaryotic mRNA

- All primary transcript synthesized in nucleus by **RNA polymerase II** is k/a **heterogenous nuclear (hn) RNA**. This **pre-mRNA** (primary transcript) the immediate product of gene transcription, is very heterogenous and can be > *10-50 times longer* than mature m-RNA. This hn RNA is very unstable, exists as hn RNP (ribonucleoprotein) and must undego post transcriptional modification (processing) to appear in cytoplasm as m-RNA.
- Addition of **7-methylguanosine cap** at 5′ terminal, **poly (A) tail** at 3′ terminal; secondary **methylation** of **2′ hydroxy** and **N^7 adenyl** residues and **splicing** (introns removed & exons joined) converts hn-RNA to m-RNA.

• Capping

- It is the 1st *processing reaction* for hn-RNA occuring in the ***nucleus***[Q].
- ***Cap structure (7 methyl guanosine) is attached backwards to 5′ end of hn RNA***[Q] forming unusual *5′ → 5′ triphosphate* linkage.
- *Nuclear guanylyl transferease* enzyme is required for creation of GTP (guanosine triphosphate) part of cap.
- **Secondary methylation** of 2′ hydroxy (of 1st & 2nd nucleotide) & N^7 of adenylyl residues of terminal guanine occurs in ***cytosol***[Q], and is catalyzed by *guanine-7 methyl transferase*. S- adenosylmethionine is the source of methyl group.
- ***5′ capping is required for recognization of mRNA by translation machinery, efficient translation initiation and protection of*** 5′ ***end of m-RNA from attack by 5′ → 3′exonuclease***[Q]. Cap ***facilitates binding of m-RNA to 43 S initiation complex***[Q] (Harper) / ***40 S ribosome unit***[Q] (Lippincot).
- The **guanine** of cap is methylated at **N^7** position, and **Ist & 2nd nucleotides** adjacent to cap (of m RNA) are methylated at 2^1 -OH position. So the 7-methyl guanosine triphosphate cap is linked to 5′ end (at 5′- hydroxyl position of 2′ – O – methyl ribonucleoside) through three phosphate *(i.e. triphosphate linkage)*.

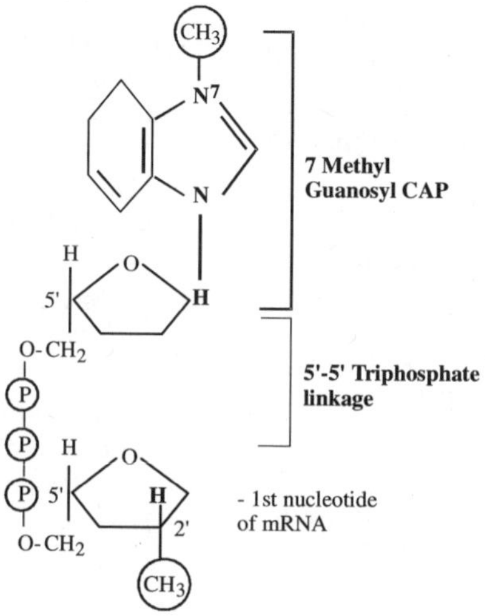

7 Methyl Guanosyl CAP

5'-5' Triphosphate linkage

- 1st nucleotide of mRNA

• Addition of poly (A) tail at 3′ end

- The m-RNA is cleaved ***about 20 nucleotides down stream of a consensus recognition sequence, called the poly adenylation signal sequence (AAUAAA)***[Q] found near 3′ end.
- Poly (A) tail is added to new 3′ end by ***nuclear enzyme polyadenylate polymerase***[Q], using ATP as the substrate. This tail is not transcribed from DNA and contain *40-200 adenine nucleotide*.
- Tail helps stabilize the m-RNA, facilitate their exit from nucleus and protects 3′ end from attack of 3′ → 5′exonuclease[Q].
- The presence of poly (A) tail does not necessarily means that the precurssor mRNA will appear in cytoplasm, ***because all poly (A) taild hnRNA do not contribute to hn-RNA***[Q]. Similarly ***not all cyto plasmic m-RNA have poly A tails (although most have)***[Q]; m-RNA *coding for histones & some interferons* do not have poly (A) tails
- Poly (A) tail is gradually shortened as m-RNA enters cytoplasm.

• Removal of introns & joining of exons (splicing)

- Maturation of m-RNA involves ***removal of non- coding (introns or intervening sequences***[Q]) from primary transcript and ***joining of remaining coding sequenes (or exons)***[Q]

Modification of Transfer (t) RNA

Both eukaryotic & prokaryotic t-RNA precursor molecules are modified by

- *Removal of introns from anticodon loop*
- **Trimming of sequences both at 5′ and 3′ end.** 16 nucleotide sequence at 5′ end is cleaved by RNase P (a ribozyme).
- ***Replacement of uracil residues at 3′ end by CCA sequence***[Q], catalyzed by *nucleotidyl transferase*. 3′ OH of A ribose is point of attachment
- Many bases are converted to modified unusual bases including ***Dihydrouracil (D), pseudo uracil (Ψ) and methylated bases (m)***[Q] by methylation, reduction, deamination, rearranging glycosidic bonds & nucleotide alkylation
- ***Methylation occurs in nucleus whereas cleavage & attachment* of CCA are cytoplasmic functions.**

Modification of Ribosomal (r) RNA

- Both prokaryotic (5S, 16S & 23S) & eukaryotic (5.8S, 18S, & 28S) rRNA are synthesized from long precursor molecule
- All ribosomal (r) RNA molecules except 5S r-RNA, are processed from a single **45 S precursor RNA** molecule in nucleolus
- ***Eukaryotic 5S rRNA is synthesized by RNA polymerase II & modified seperately***[Q].
- The ***r-RNA genes are located in nucleoli (in eukaryotes)***[Q]. Because of *lack of amplification*, large number of genes and high transcription rate is required to synthesize

- The process of removing introns & joining exons is called **splicing** and the molecular machine accomplishing the task is k/a **spliceosome.** The splicing occurs in nucleus &serves to bring the actual aminoacid coding sequences (exons) together.
- Primary tanscript from histone genes contain no interons
- A hn RNA can be spliced in >2 ways to produce multiple variations of m-RNA & therefore proteins.

sufficient copies of rRNA to form the 10^7 *ribosomes* required for each cell replication.

- The precursor (pre ribosome RNA) are cleaved in nucleolus by **ribonucleases** to yield intermediate size pieces of RNA, which are further trimmed to produce required rRNA

- **RNA Editing**

- It *changes the coding information at m-RNA level,* so that coding sequence of mRNA diffes from that of cognate DNA (exception to central dogma)
- **APo B gene** transcribes *100 kDa apo B-100 protein in liver and 48 kDa apo B-48 protein in intestine;* because **cytidine deaminase** converts a *CAA codon* in m-RNA *to UAA* at single specific site. So rather than coding *glutamine* this becomes *termination codon.*
- In **parasitic protozoa (trypanosomes)** large regions of m-RNA are synthesized without uridylate and U residues are inserted later by RNA editing.

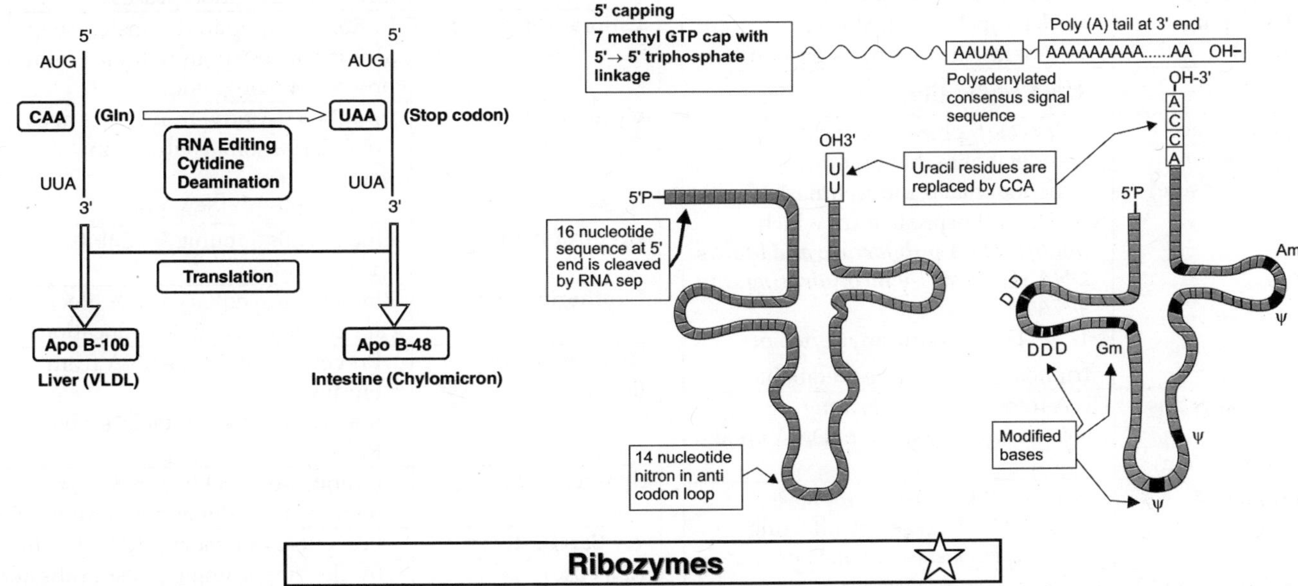

Ribozymes ☆

- Ribozymes are **RNA molecules with enzymatic /catalytic activity**. Examples include **peptidyl transferase**[Q], **self splicing group I introns, RN ase P,** and **hammerhead ribozyme.** Most of the activities of these ribozymes are based on 2 fundamental reactions: **transesterification** and **phosphodiester bond hydrolysis (cleavage)**. The substrate for ribozyme is often an RNA molecule and it may even be part of ribozyme itself; so most ribozyme are concerned with RNA metabolism (**splicing & endoribonuclease**). Recently a r-RNA component has been implicated in *hydrolyzing an aminoacylester & **plays a central role in peptide bond formation (peptidyl transferases)***[Q].
- Ribozymes vary greatly in size (40 nucleotide hammer head to 400 nucleotide SS group I intron). 3-dimensional structure is important for function. Ribozymes are inactivated by melting, or by addition of denaturing agents or complimentary oligonucleotides which disrupt normal base pairing patterns or by changing essential nucleotides.
- Certain virusoids (virus like elements) have small RNA genomes and usually require other virus to assist in their replication and / or packaging. **Hammer head ribozymes** are small segments of virusoidal RNAs, that *promote site specific RNA cleavage reactions associated with replication.* Hammerhead ribozyme is a *metalloenzyme requiring Mg++ ions* for activity and their secondary structures is shaped like a head of hammer.
- **Sidney Altman & Thomas Czech** were awarded Nobel Prize (in 1989, Chemestry) for discovering catalytic property of RNAs. And this discovery changed the central dogma (DNA→RNA→protein) that RNAs are not just the transmitters of genetic information but can also act as enzyme.

Inhibitors of ☆

Transcription

Refamycin, Streptovaricin	Binds with β-*subunit of polymerase to block initiation of transcription*
Actinomycin D	Forms a *complex with double stranded DNA* & prevents movement of core enzyme & thus ***inhibiting process of chain elongation***Q
Streptoglydigin	Binds with β-subunit of prokaryotic polymerase & thus *inhibiting elongation*
Heparin	Binds to β-subunit & inhibits transcription in vitro
α-Amanitin (Death cap, destroying angel)	- ***Blocks m-RNA formation by inhibiting RNA polymerase II***Q - Blocks translocation of RNA polymerase during transcription.

DNA replication

Cytarabine (cytosine arabinoside)	- Cell cycle S phase specific antimetabolite that becomes phosphorylated intracellularly to an active triphosphate form which ***inhibits DNA polymerase and blocks DNA synthesis by incorporating into DNA***Q - 1- β - D-arabinofuranyl cytosine-triphosphate is active metabolite
Anthracyclins (eg daxaorubicin)	DNA inter calaters, *inhibiting topoisomerase II,* leading to DNA breaks
Etopaside	- Arrest cell growth in G_2 phase - Causes DNA breaks by affecting *DNA topoisomerase II function*
Nalidixic acid	Inhibits *bacterial DNA gyrase*
Ciprofloxacin	Inhibits *bacterial DNA gyrase* , which nicks the double stranded DNA, induces negative supercoil and reseals the nicked ends

Translation (protein synthesis)

Streptomycin (highly basic trisaccharide)	- Interferes with binding of f-met t RNA to ribosomes & thus inhibiting initiation process - Leads to misreding of m- RNA
Puromycin	Release nascent polypeptide chains before their synthesis is complete. It binds to A site on ribosome and inhibits the entry of aminocyl t-RNA (both in bactarial & mammalian cells).
Tetracycline	Binds to 30 S subunit & inhibits binding of aminoacyl t-RNA & so inhibiting initiation process.
Chloramphenicol	Inhibits the peptidyl transferase activity of 50s subunit, thus inhibiting process of elongation.
Cycloheximide	- Inhibits peptidyl transferase activity of 60S ribosomal subunit in eukaryotes - Also inhibits elongation.
Erythromycin	Binds to 50s subunit & inhibits translocation
Diptheria toxin	Binds EF-2 in eukaryates & blocks its capacity to carryout translocation
Ricin & abrin (lectins)	- Prevent aminoacyl t-RNA from binding to A site - Inactivates eukaryotic 28 s ribosomal RNA
Sparcomycin	- Inhibits peptidyl transferase & release factor dependent termination
α **- Sarcin** (toxic RNA ase)	- Prevents aminoacyl t- RNA binding by cleaving a single phosphodiester bond in 28 S r- RNA

★ **Paclitaxel** *enhances polymerization of tubulin;* a mechanism opposite to that of vinca alkaloids

★ **Actinomycin D (dactinomycin)** intercalates into the *narrow groove* of DNA double helix, thus ***interfering with DNA and RNA synthesis***Q.

RNA structure

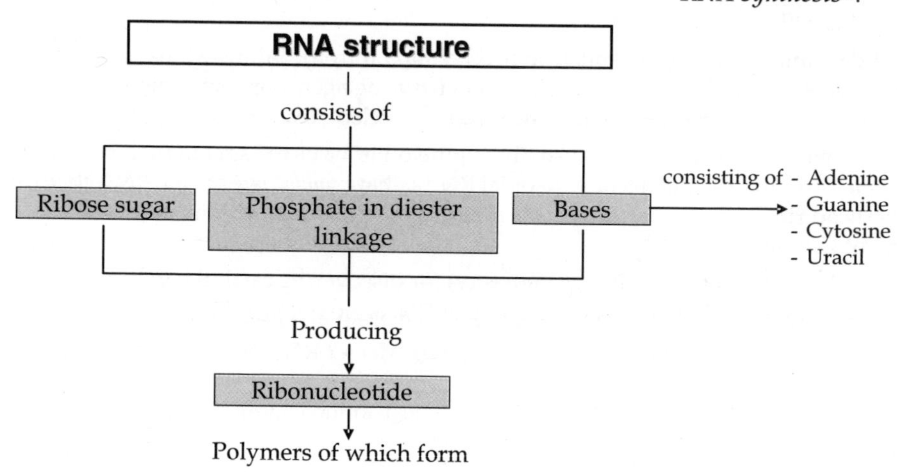

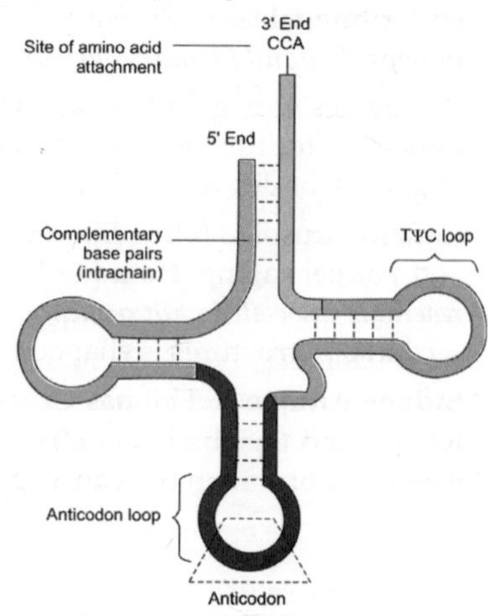

Characteristic tRNA structure

rRNA	tRNA	mRNA
- ***80% of RNA in cell***[Q] - Associates with protein - Four size species in eukaryotes (28S, 18S, 5.8S and 5S) - *Sructural component of ribosomes* - Serve as site ***for protein synthesis***[Q]. ['S' – Svedberg unit, related to molecular wt & shape of compound]	- *15%* of total RNA - *Smallest* of the three species of RNA - ***Contains unusual bases (pseudouridine, thymine)***[Q] - ***Extensive intrachain base pairing***[Q] - ***Clover leaf pattern***[Q] - At least ***one specific type of molecule for each of 20 amino acids found in portein***[Q]. - Serve as adaptor molecule that carries a specific a.a. to ribosome / mRNA complex	- *5%* of total RNA - *Most heterogenous* type - *5' 'Cap'* of 7- methyl guanosine - *3' Poly- A 'tail'* - Used as ***template for protein synthesis***[Q]. It carries genetic information from DNA to cytoplasm.

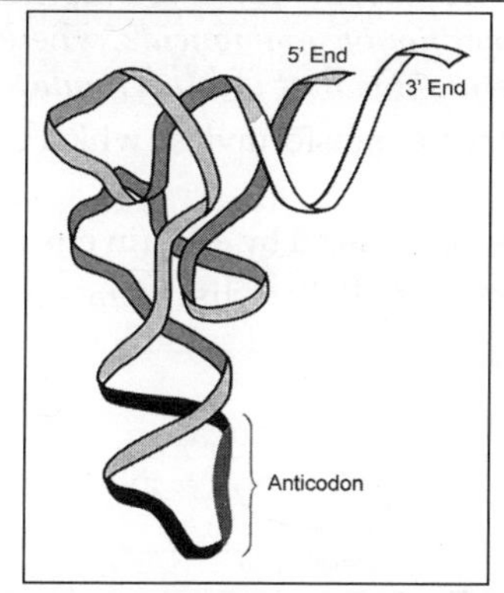

Folder tRNA structure found in cells

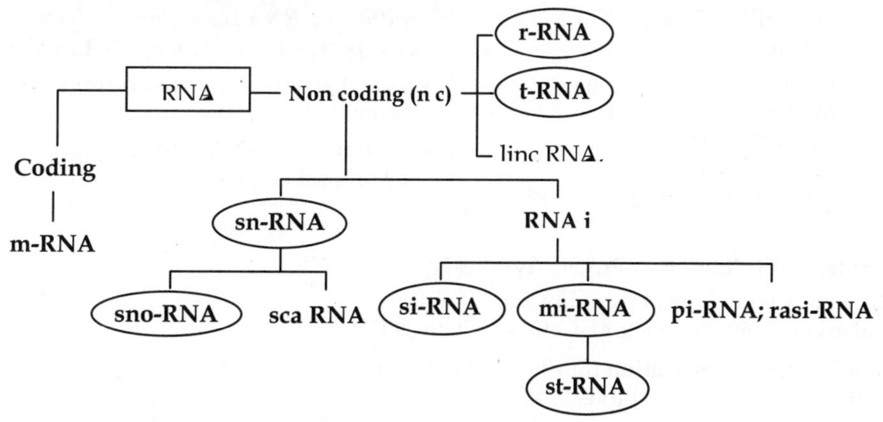

Translation (Protein Synthesis) ☆

The translation of mRNA commences near its 5' terminal. The message is read from 5' to 3', concluding with the formation of carboxyl terminal of the protein[Q]. Occurs in three phases: Initiation, Elongation & Termination

Initiation Sequence

Shine Dalgarno Sequence	Kozak Consensus Sequence
• Present in *prokaryotes.* **Shine Dalgarno sequence** is a ***sequence of nucleotide bases (5' – UAGGAGG-3') located 6- 10 base upstream of AUG codon on mRNA molecule***[Q]. It helps ribosomes in recognizing the nucleotide sequence that is *essential for initiation of translation.* • Sequence of nucleotide base (5'- UAGGAGG-3')	• Present in *eukaryotes* • This sequence *surrounds AUG and determines the initiating codon of mRNA.* • In this sequence *–3 and +4* positions relative to AUG are *occupied by purine* (A&G)

Initiation Codon

- Although amino acid **methionine (Met)** has only one codon **AUG**, all organism have 2 types of t RNA for methionine tRNA ^{fMet} incorporating **N-formyl methionine (f-met)** in response to **initiation codon** AUG and **tRNA^{Met}** incorporating **methionine (Met)** in response to AUG codon in **internal position.**

Codon – **AUG**

In prokaryotes

At-Initiation site	At Internal site
N-formyl methionine (f-Met) is incorporated by **t RNA^{fMet}**	**Methionine (Met)** is incorporated by **t-RNA ^{Met}**

In Eukaryotes

Mitochondria & Chloroplast	Cytosolic Ribosomes
N-formyl methionine (f-Met) is incorporated by **t RNA^{fMet}**	Polypeptide synthesis begin with **Methionine (rather than f-Met)** but again cells use *specialized initiating t-RNA* that is distinct from tRNA^{Met} used at AUG codons at interior positions of m-RNA.

- Initiating amino acid **N-formyl – methionine (f-Met)** arrives with **tRNA $^{f-met}$** at ribosome as **N-formyl methionyl tRNA^{f-Met} (f-Met – t RNA ^{fMet})**, which is formed in 2 steps.

- **Met –tRNA synthetase** aminoacylates (attaches) aminoacid methionine to tRNA ^{fMet} (and also tRNA ^{Met}) with the help of ATP

located 6- 10bp upstream of AUG codon on mRNA at its 5′ end. • The 16 S ribosomal RNA component of 30 S ribosomal subunit has a nucleotide sequence at its 3′ end, that is complementary to all or part of shine Dalgarno sequence • Thus mRNA 5′ end & 3′ end, of 16 S rRNA can form complementary base pair & *facilitating binding of mRNA on 30 S ribosomal subunit.*	GCCA^{-3} / GCC**AUGG**$^{+4}$

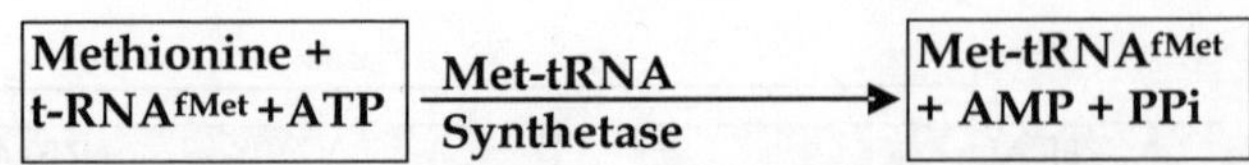

- More selective & specific (for only Met residue attached to tRNA^{fMet}) – **transformylase** transfer a formyl group from N^{10}-formyl tetrahydrofolate to amino group of met residue.

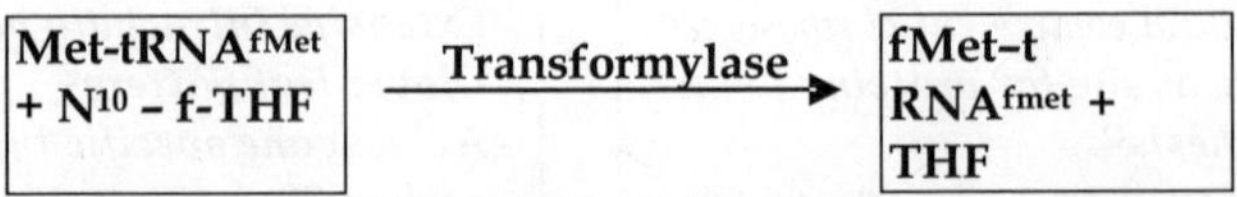

- **Methionine** having anticodon **UAC** is the first amino acid required in binding to the initiation codon AUG on mRNA. In **bacteria (prokaryotes)** & **mitochondria** the *initiator t-RNA carries an N – formylated methionine aminoacid*[Q], whereas in **eukaryotes**, the *initiator tRNA carries a methionine that is not formylated*[Q].
- Formyl group is added to methionine by enzyme transformylase which uses N^{10} formyl THF as carbon donor.
- The initiator t-RNA is the only t – RNA to be recognized by eIF2 (in eukaryotes) / IF2 (in prokaryotes) and the only t RNA to go directly to P site.

I. Steps of Initiation of Protein Synthesis

It can be divided into 4 steps (for ease of writing eukaryotic initiation factor i.e. eIF is written as IF)

1. **Ribosomal dissociation into 40s & 60s subunits.** IF (i.e. e IF) 1A and 3 binds to 40 s subunit which delays its reassociation.
2. **Formation of 40s/43 S preinitiation complex by binding of ternary complex & 40s** subunit

- **GTP** binds to **IF2** to form binary complex & then to **met t RNAi** (a t RNA that binds initiation codon AUG & code methionine) to form **ternary complex**
- Ternary complex binds to 40 s subunit to for 43 s preinitiation complex, which is stabilized by IF 1A & 3
- IF (elf)2 is one of the two **control points** for protein synthesis initiation in eukaryotes and ***consists of α, β & γ subunits***[Q]. **IF2α** is phosphorylated (on serine 51) by at least 4 different protein kinase (HCR, PKR, PERK & GCN2) that are activated when a cell is under stress and energy expenditure required for protein synthesis would be deleterious. Phosphorylated IF-2α binds tightly to and **inactivates the *GTP-GDP recycling protein e IF-2B***. Thus *preventing formation* of 43 s preinitiation complex & blocking protein synthesis.

3. **Formation of 43/48 S initiation complex** by binding of 40/43s preinitiation complex to mRNA.

- ***MGTP (methyguanosyl triphosphate) cap at 5′ terminal of most eukaryotic m RNA facilitate its binding to 43S preinitiation complex***[Q].

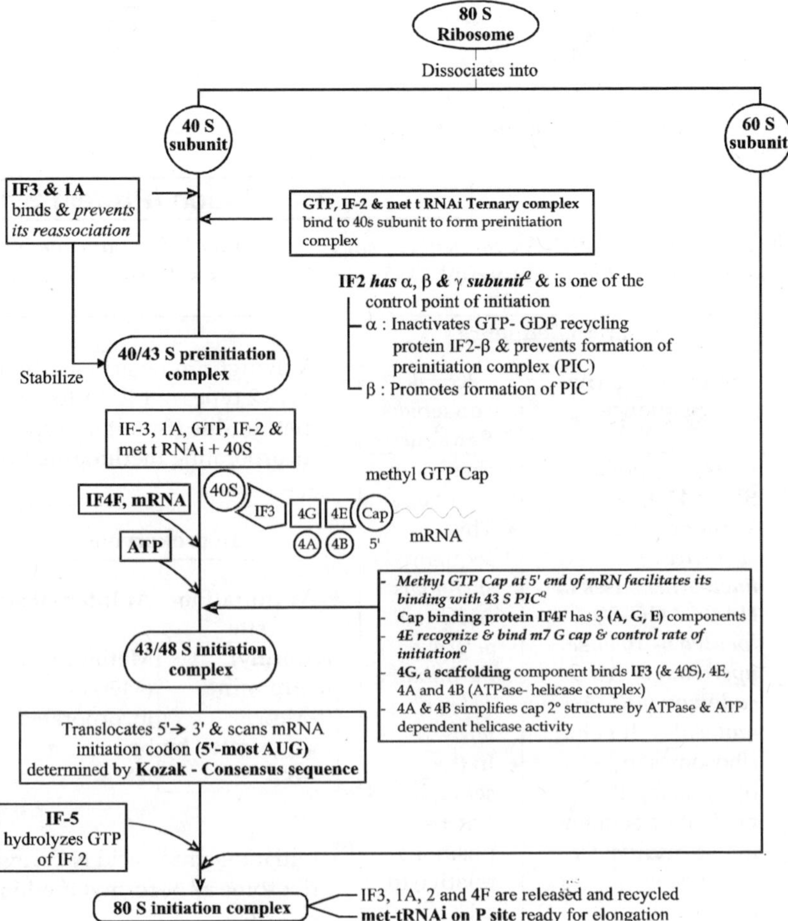

- **Cap binding protein IF 4F** (which consist of 4A, 4G, 4E units) binds to the cap through 4E protein and to 40 S ribosome subunit through 4G component. IF (eIF)3 is a key protein because it binds to 4G component of 4F with high affinity and it links this complex to 40 S ribosomal subunit (in 43 S preinitiation complex)
- **IF 4B (4B)** binds & reduces (melts) the complex 2° structure of 5′ end of mRNA through **ATPase & ATP dependent helicase activity**. Formation of 48 s initiation comlex require ATP hydrolysis
- **4E** is responsible for recognition & binding of m7 G cap structure at 5′ end of m RNA, ***a rate limiting step in translation. So 4E control rate of initiation***[Q]. **4G** is a ***scaffoiding rotein***[Q] which binds to 4E, 4A and 4B (i.e. ATP ase-helicase complex that unwinds RNA) and to eIF3, which links the complex to 40 s ribosomal subunit.

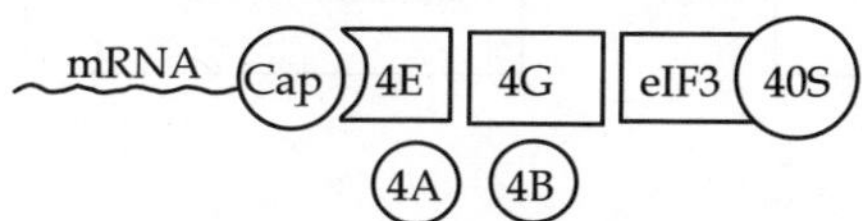

- After binding of 43 S preinitiation complex with m RNA cap, and melting of 2° structure near 5′ end of mRNA through the action of 4B helicase and ATP, the 43/48 S initiation complex translocates 5′ – 3′ & scans mRNA for suitable initiation codon. Generally this is 5′-most AUG, precisely determined by **Kozak-consensus sequence** that surround AUG (i.e. *purine at – 3 and + 4 positions relative to AUG*).

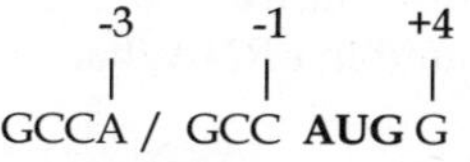

4. **Formation of 80 S initiation complex** by combination of 43 S initiation complex with 60 S ribosomal subunit

- Involves hydrolysis of GTP bound to IF2 by IF5, resulting in release and recycling of initiation factor bound to 48 s initiation complex and rapid association of 40S & 60S subunits to form 80 S ribosome.
- met – t RNAi is on P site ready for elongation.

Difference	Prokaryotes	Eukaryotes
m- RNA	**Polycistronic** i.e. have several coding regions; each with its initiation & termination codon producing a seperate polypeptide	**Monocistronic** with one coding region
Amino acid incorporation rate	**18 aa/sec**	**6 aa/sec**
Initial amino acid	***Formylated methionine*** (f-met)	***Methionine***[Q] (Met)
Initial t-RNA	**t-RNA ^{fMet}**	**tRNA^{Met}**
Transcription & translation	Translation starts before transcription is ended (coupled)	Uncoupled
Initiation factors (IF)	3 i.e. IF1, IF2, IF3	>10 designated eIF
Determination of initiating codon	- ***Shine Dalgarno sequence***[Q] - Facilitated by IF-2 bound to GTP	***Kozak consensus sequence***[Q] Facilitated by eIF-2 bound to GTP (plus additional eIF)
Elongation: Delivery of aminoacyl t-RNA to A site	- Facilitated by EF-Tu & EF-Ts	Facilitated by EF1 α and EF 1 βγ
Nucleotide exchange factors	- EF – Ts (as it exchanges its GTP for GDP on EFTu)	EF 1βγ (as it exchanges its GTP for GDP on EF 1α
Peptidyl transferase activity catalyzing peptide bond formation	*23 S rRNA of 50 S* ribosomal subunit (ribozyme)	*28 S rRNA of 60 S* ribosomal subunit (ribozyme)
Translocation	Requires EF-G & GTP	Requires EF-2 & GTP
Termination	- **Release factor (RF) 1** recognizes UAA & UAG, **RF2** recognizes UAA & UGA - **RF-3** (bound to GTP) causes release of RF-1 or RF-2 as GTP is hydrolysed	- **eRF** recognizes all 3 UAA, UAG and UGA and release nascent polypeptide chain - **eRF-3** (bound to GTP) function like prokaryotic RF-3 & release eRF

II. Elongation

It involves the addition of aminoacids to carboxy end of growing chain and movement of ribosome from 5′ end 3′ end of mRNA that is being translated (translocation)

III. Termination

Termination of protein synthesis occurs when *a stop codon of m-RNA (UAA, UAG, UGA) appears in 'A' site.* These codons are recognized by release factors (RF-1, RF-3). ***RF with GTP & peptidyl transferase promotes hydrolysis of bond between the peptide & t RNA occupying the 'P' site***[Q].

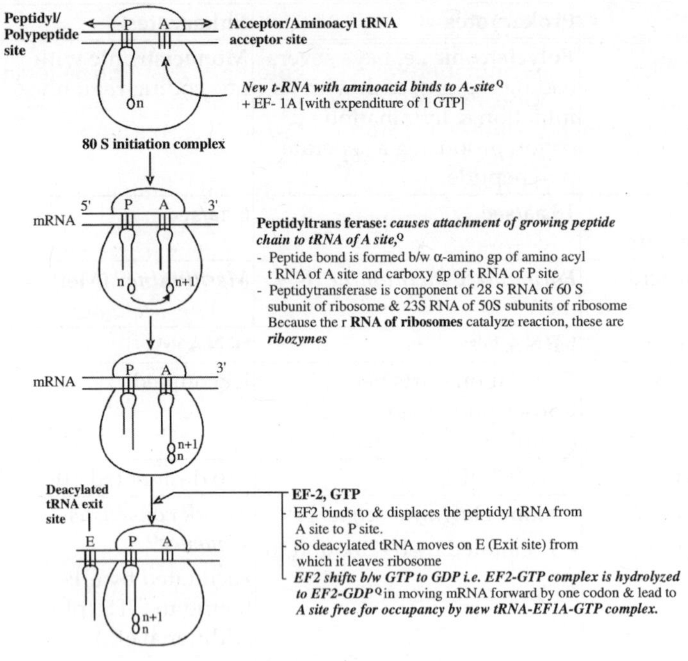

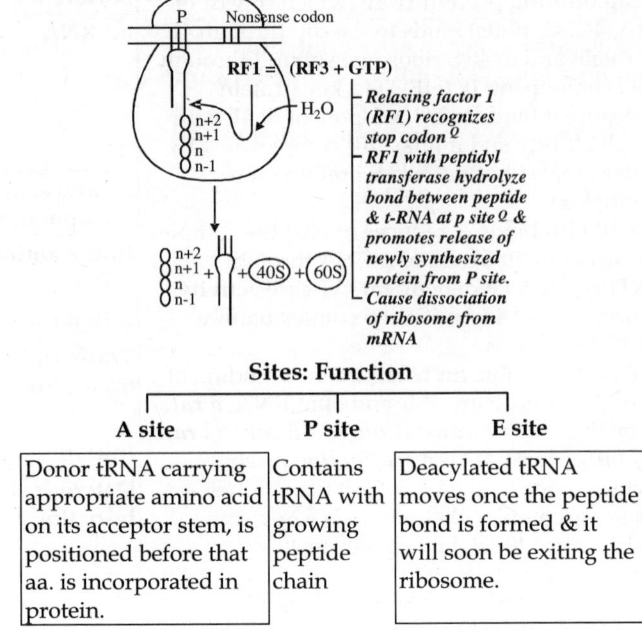

A site	P site	E site
Donor tRNA carrying appropriate amino acid on its acceptor stem, is positioned before that aa. is incorporated in protein.	Contains tRNA with growing peptide chain	Deacylated tRNA moves once the peptide bond is formed & it will soon be exiting the ribosome.

* **Total energy expenditure**: tRNA+A.A= 2ATP
- 2 GTP in elongation } 4ATP

Peptide Bond Formation & Translocation

- **Peptidyl transferase** activity (of ***23S rRNA of 50 s or 28 S rRNA of 60 S ribosome)***[Q] is responsible for peptide bond formation.
- This **ribozyme** catalyzes the reaction between the amino group of aminoacyl t RNA at A site and carboxy carbon of peptidyl tRNA in the P site, forming a peptide bond from an ester bond.
- Because the amino acid on aminoacyl t RNA is already activated *no further energy is required for this reaction*
- The reaction *result in attachment of the growing peptide chain to the t RNA in the A site,* the which makes t RNA of P site to become deacylated.
- The **recently deacylated tRNA** is attached to P site by its anticodon and to an exit (E) site by the open CCA tail.
- **Elongation factor (EF)-2** binds and ***shifts between GTP to GDP (i.e. EF2 GTP is hydrolyzed to EF2 GDP)***[Q] to move the ribosome down one codon on m RNA, so that
  1. A site is vacant & ready to receive next charged t RNA
  2. P site contain peptidyl tRNA that has been translocated (displaced) from A site
  3. Deacylated t RNA is on E site, from which it leaves the ribosome.

Evidence that rRNA is Peptidyl Transferase

- Ribosomes can *form peptide bonds even when proteins are removed* or inactivated
- *Few r RNA sequences are highly conserved* in all species
- These conserved regions are *on the surface of RNA molecule*
- RNA can be catalyst
- Mutations that result in antibiotic resistance at the level of protein synthesis are more often found in r RNA than in protein component of ribosome
- X-ray crystal structure of large subunit bound to tRNA suggest this.

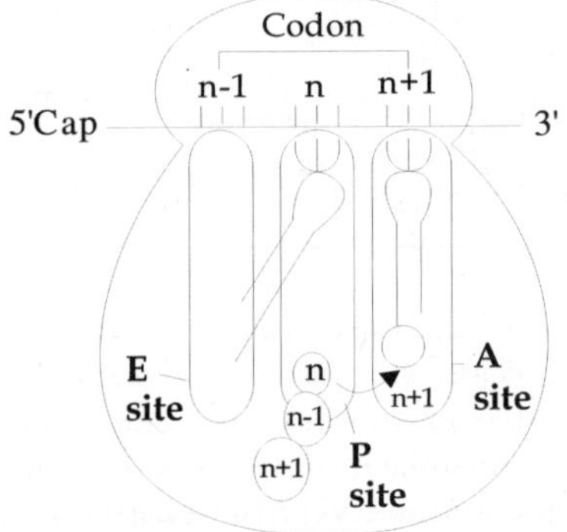

Essential Components Required for 5 Steps of Protein Synthesis (in Prokaryotes)

Activation of amino acids	Initiation	Elongation	Termination & Ribosome recycling	Folding & Post translational modification
- 20 aminoacids - 20 aminoacyl-tRNA synthetase (of 2 classes) - ≥ 32 t RNAs - **ATP** - Mg^{++}	- **mRNA (Shine-Dalgarno** sequence) - **Initiation codon (AUG)** in mRNA - **N-formylmethionyl tRNA** ^{fMet} (i.e. f-Met + tRNA ^{fMet}) - 30S subunit of ribosome - 50 S subunit of ribosome - **Initiation factors (IF-1, IF-2, IF-3)** - **GTP** - Mg^{++}	- Functional 70S ribosome **(initiation complex)** - Aminoacyl tRNAs (as specified by codon) - **Elongation factors** (EF-Tu, EF-Ts, EF-G) - GTP - Mg^{++}	- **Termination /Stop codons (UAA,UAG, UGA** in mRNA - **Release /Termination factors** (RF-1, RF-2, RF-3, RRF) - **EF - G** - **IF - 3**	Enzymes & cofactors required for - Removal of initiating & signal sequences - Addition of acetyl, methyl carboxyl, phosphoryl group etc or oligosaccharide or prosthetic groups to aminoacid residues - Proteolytic cleavage & modification of terminal residues.

Aminoacyl t- RNA Synthetase (AtRS) ☆

- This family of enzyme is *required for attachment of amino acids to their corresponding t RNAs*. ***Each amino acyl tRNA synthetase recognizes one specific amino acid and one or more corresponding t RNAs (isoaccepting t RNAs)***[Q]. **For amino acids with 2 or more corresponding tRNAs**, the same enzyme usually aminoacylates all of them. The *extreme specificity of synthetase* in recognizing both A.A & t-RNA is ***responsible for high fidelity of tranlation of genetic message***[Q]. So, it ***implement genetic code by acting as molecular dictionaries***[Q] that can read both 3 letter code of nucleic acid and 20 letter code of aminoacid.
- Based on substantial differences in primary & tertiary structures and in reaction mechanism AtRS has been divided into **2 classes.**

Class I	Class II
Arg, Cys, Gln, Glu, Ile, Leu, Met, Trp, Tyr, Val – (add tRNA synthetase to each)	Ala, Asn, Asp, Gly, His, Lys, Phe, Pro, Ser, Thr (tRNa synthetase)
In 2nd step, the aminoacyl group is transferred **initially to 2[1](OH) group of 3′ terminal A** residue **then to 3′ (OH) group** by transesterification reaction	In 2nd step, aminoacyl group is **directly transferred to 3[1] hydroxyl group of terminal A adenylate**

- It catalyzes **2 step reaction** that result in ***covalent attachment of carboxyl group of a specific aminoacid to the 3′ end of its corresponding / cognate / isoaccepting tRNA***[Q]. The overall reaction **requires ATP** which is *cleaved to AMP and inorganic pyro phosphate (PPi)*. Thus ***2 high energy phosphate bonds are expended for activation of each aminoacid molecule***[Q], making the over all reaction irreversible. In 1st step the enzyme bound intermediate – aminoacyl adenylate (aminoacyl - AMP) is formed and in 2nd step the aminoacyl group is transferred from **enzyme bound aminoacyl AMP intermediate to 3' (OH) of terminal A (adenylate)** of corresponding tRNA.
- Amino acyl tRNA synthetase, aminoacylates tRNA that accomplishes 2 ends: (1) **it activates an amino acid for peptide bond formation** and (2) **it ensures appropriate placement of aminoacids in growing polypeptide chain**. As the identity of amino acids attached to tRNA is not checked on ribosome, the attachment of correct amino acid to tRNA is ***essential for fidelity of protein synthesis***[Q].

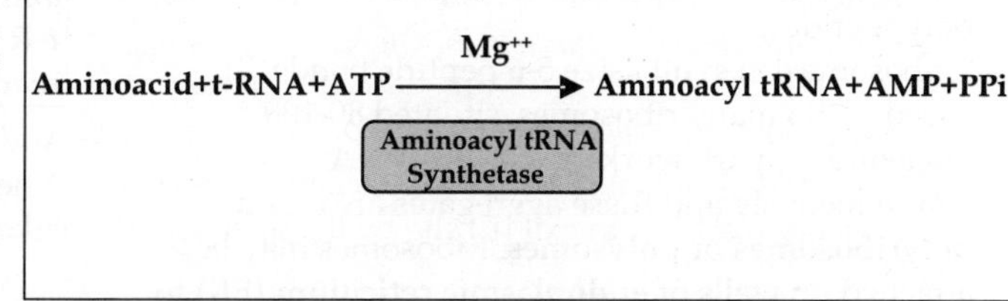

- In addition to extreme specificity & high fidelity it has a ***proof reading or editing activity***[Q] that can remove mischarged aminoacid from the enzyme or tRNA molecule. *The effect of forcing the substrate specific binding through 2 sucessive steps (filters) is multiplicative in proof reading.*
- Incorrect aminoacids bind to **separate hydrolytic (proofreading)** site in few AtRS. The active site of some AtRS that activate aminoacids with no close structural relatives (**eg Cys-tRNA synthetase**) can sufficiently discriminate between the proper substrate and incorrect aminoacids, and demonstrate **little or no proof reading activity**. Overall error rate of protein synthesis (1 mistake in 10^{-4} aa incorporated) is higher than that of DNA relication.
- **Interaction between aminoacyl tRNA synthetase and tRNA is called the second genetic code** b/o its critical role in maintaining accuracy of protein synthesis. Conserved sequences of tRNA cannot be used for discrimination. Discriminatory sequences are mostly concentrated in aminoacid & anticodon arm of tRNA. For example primary determinant of tRNA recognition by Ala-tRNA synthetase is **single G = U base pair in the amino acid arm** of t RNA ^{Ala}. So even a short synthetic RNA minihelix with **critical G=U basepairing** but lacking most of remaining tRNA structure is amino acetylated specifically with alanine almost as efficiently as the complete tRNA^{Ala}.

3' 5' G U 70

Energy Requirements In Protein Synthesis

Energy requirements

Total **4 ATP** and **5GTP** are used in protein synthesis in following steps

- **Activation of aminoacid & formation of aminoacyl t- RNA complex**	**2 high energy PO_4 bonds** (ATP - → AMP)	**Formation of 43 S pre initiation complex** involves binding of *GTP by eIF- 2*. This binary complex binds to *met t RNAi*, (methionine having anticodon *UAC*) specifically involved in binding to initiation codon.	1 GTP
- Formation of 43 S initiation complex when **e IF4A and eIF 4B bind and reduce** the complex secondary structure 5′ end of **m RNA** through ATPase and ATP dependent heticase activity	**1 ATP** (or high energy PO_4 bond)	**Formation of 80 S initiation complex** (i.e. binding of 60 S subunit and 48 S initiation complex) involves hydrolysis of GTP bound to eIF- 2 by eIF- 5	1 GTP
		Binding of aminoacyl t RNA to 'A' site requires elongation factor EF 1A and GTP	1 GTP
- **Formation of 48 S initiation cmplex** by association of m-RNA with 43 S pre initiation complex.	**1 ATP (PO_4 bond)**	For **translocation movment** of m-RNA forward by 1 codon and leaving the A site open for occupancy of another tRNA- EF1A-GTP- aminoacid complex requires EF2 and GTP	1 GPT
		Releasing factor 3 (RF3) with bound GTP is required for **termination** process	1 GTP

Formation of peptide bond

- It is catalyzed by **peptidyl transferase,** a component of **28 S RNA** of **60S** (Harper) /**50 S** (Lippincott) ribosomal subunit. It is an example of ***ribozyme activity (i.e. r-RNA catalyzes the reaction)***Q and a *direct role of RBA in protein synthesis.*
- *α - amino (NH2) group of new aminoacyl t- RNA* in **'A' site** combines with carboxyl (COOH) group of peptidyl t-RNA occupying the ***'P' (peptidyl or polypeptide)*** *side*. At initiation, P site is occupied by ***aminoacyl – t RNA met^{i}. Because the aminoacid on aminoacyl t RNA is already activated, no further energy source is required for this reaction***Q.
- In eukaryotic cell, a single ribosome is capable of synthesizing 400 peptide bonds each minute.
- **Energy required for formation of one peptide bond** include the equivalent of hydrolysis of *2 ATP to ADP and 2GTP to GDP*, or the hydrolysis of **4 high energy phosphate bonds**

Ribosomes

- Ribosome is a *cytoplasmic nucleoprotein* structure that acts as a ***machinery for protein synthesis*** from m RNA templates. Its role is to ***bring m-RNA and t-RNA together***Q to translate the information encoded in m-RNA (and transcribed from genes) into polypeptides.
- 1 ribosome can synthesize 5-6 peptide bonds /second. So many ribosomes, situated 80-100 nucleotides apart, work on same m-RNA simultaneously and these aggregates are called **polyribosomes** or **polysomes**. Ribosomes may be attached on walls of **endoplasmic reticulum (ER)** to form rough ER or may **exist free in cytoplasm.**
- **RER associated ribosomes** synthesize proteins that are exported from cell, are integrated into plasma, ER or golgi membranes or *lysosomes*. Free **cytosolic ribosomes** synthesize protein required in cytosol, nucleus, mitochondria & *peroxisomes*Q. However mitochondria contain its own ribosome
- Ribosomes can be **free (cytoplasmic)** or **membrane (ER) bound**, contain about 65% of r-RNA and 35% of protein, are roughly spherical with a diameter of about 18nm – seen only on electron microscope and accounts for almost 25% of dry weight of cell.
- Ribosomes are large complexes of r-RNA and

Energy Required in Protein Synthesis

- **4 high energy bonds** are required for addition of one aminoacid to growing polypeptide chain

2 from ATP in ***aminoacyl t-RNA synthetase reaction***Q.	**2 from GTP** - ***1 for binding of aminoacyl tRNA to A site***Q - ***1 – for translocation***Q

- Additional ATP & GTP are required for **initiation** *in eukaryotes.* Whereas additional **GTP** is ***required for termination in both eukaryotes & prokaryotes***Q.

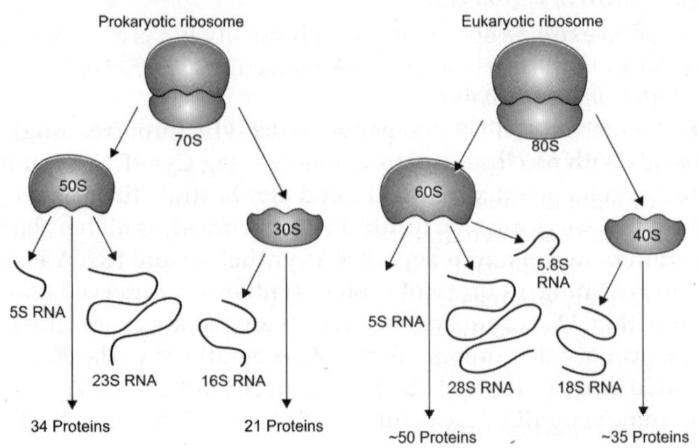

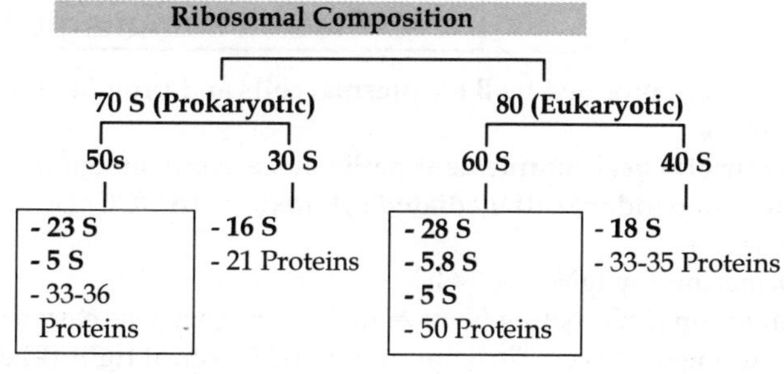

proteins with *one large and one small subunits*. The **small subunit** *binds m-RNA*, thus guiding *interaction b/w m-RNA codon and anticodon of t-RNA* to read the genetic information with exiquisite **fidelity**. Hence small subunit is responsible for accuracy, whereas the **large subunit** catalyzes the **formation of peptide bond.**

- Prokaryotic ribosome with sedimentation coefficient 70S (S=Svedberg units, a parameter sensitive to molecular size & shape) is composed of 2 unequal subunits with sedimentation coefficient of 30 S and 50S. Whereas eukaryotic 80S ribosome has 60S & 40S.
- Each *ribosome has 3 binding sites for t-RNA* – **A** *(for incoming aminoacyl t RNA)*, **P** *(for peptidyl – t RNA)* and **E** (for empty t RNA about to exit), each of which **extend over both subunits**. Together they cover 3 neighbouring codes.
- Both ribosomal subunits *can be broken down into their RNA and protein components, then reconstituted* in vitro nearly identical in structure and activity to native subunit. Ribosomal subunits are *huge r-RNA molecules* that form the structural core. The *proteins are secondary elements* in complex *decorating the surface (forming Worm like structures)*. There is no protein within 18A° of active site for peptide bond formation. The large r-RNA component performs **peptidyl transferase** activity and thus ribosome is a **ribozyme.**
- *Ribosomal RNAs (28S + 16S)* constitute nearly 70% of total eukaryotic cellular RNA. All r-RNA molecules *except 5S r RNA*, which is independently transcribed are processed from a single 45S precursor RNA molecule in nucleolus. The highly methylated r-RNA are packaged in nucleolus with the specific ribosomal proteins. In cytoplasm, ribosomes remain quite stable and capable of *many translational cycles*.
- ***16s r-RNA of 30 subunit of prokaryotic ribosome identifies and binds shine – Dalgarno sequence***[Q].
- The r-RNA residues of large subunit of ribosomes that catalyze peptide bond formation (and have peptidyl tranferase activity) contain highly conserved nucleotide sequence[Q] – the ribonucleotide octet (5′) AUAACAGG (3′) in all cells.
- *Many negatively charged phosphoryl groups* in RNA backbone limit the stability of very large RNA molecules. So incorporation of *divalent cations or positively charged groups* and certain *peptides promote stability*. Ribozyme catalyzed synthesis of peptides could thus initially have evolved for structural maintenance of large RNA molecules but the greater catalytic potential of proteins marked the beginning of new era of protein dominated metabolic system.

Protein Kinase & Protein Phosphorylation

Eukaryotic Protein Kinase (PK)	Phosphorylate
Serine-Threonine PK	Serine (95%); also recognizes threonine (3%)
Tyrosine PK	Tyrosin (< 1%) only
Dual Function PK	Serine (Sr), threonine (Thr), tyrosine (Tyr)

ATP
ADP
Mg^{++}
Protein Kinase
NH_2 - Protein - COOH
NH_2 - Phospho-Protein - O - PO_4^{2-}
Phospho Protein phosphatase
Mg^{++}
PO_4
H_2O

- **Attachment of phosphoryl groups** to specific aminoacid residue of a **protein is catalyzed by protein kinases; removal of phosphoryl groups** is **catalyzed by phospho protein phosphatases.**
- Phosphorylation is the *commonest type of regulatory post translational modification*. **The addition of phosphoryl group to a Ser, Thr**, or **Tyr** residue introduces a bulky charged group into a region that was only moderately polar. The oxygen atoms of a phosphoryl group can hydrogen bond with one or several groups in a protein, commonly the amide groups of peptide backbone at the start of an α-helix or the charged *guanidinium group of an Arg residiue*. The 2 negative charges on a phosphorylated side chain can also repel neighbouring negatively charged (Asp or Glu) residue. The interactions with **arginine, aspartic acid or glutamic acid, histidine & lysine** side chains is usually secondary to and after primary attachment with **serine (Sr) , threonine (Thr) or Tyrosine (Tyr)**
- When modifications caused by phosphorylation occur in a region of an enzyme critical to its three dimensional structure, phosphorylation can have dramatic effects on enzyme conformation and thus on substrate binding and catalysis. (either stimulating or inhibiting). For example phosphorylation **stimulates substrate binding & catalysis in glycogen phosphorylase** of muscle & liver, whereas it **inhibits isocitrate dehydrogenase.**
- Protein kinases catalyze the transfer of negatively charge phosphoryl (phosphate) group of ATP to hydroxyl moiety of only three aminoacids ie **serine (Sr, 95%), threonine (Thr, 3-4%) and tyrosine (Tyr** in < 1%) to form chemically stable phosphate ester **in eukaryotes**. Whereas **in prokaryotic** bacteria, fungi & plants phosphorylate **histidine and aspartate (or glutamate)** by **histidine** and aspartate protein kinases.

Plasma Immunoglobulins (Antibodies)

- Antibodies are produed by **B** (or **plasma**) **cells** and provide **humoral immunity**. It destroyes target cells by following mechanisms.
- **Activating classical complement pathway** i.e. complement fixation (by IgG & IgM)
- **Antibody dependent cell mediated cytotoxicity (ADCC)** i.e. antibody coating will sensitize the target cells for killing by *killer (k) cells* (IgG)
- **Agglutination** (by IgM > A > G)
- **Opsonization** (IgG coating helps & makes phagocytosis easy as its Fc portion can fix with macrophage).
- All immunoglobins contain a minimum of 2 identical **light (L) chains** (23 -kDa) and **2** identical **heavy (H)** chains (53 – 75 kDa) joined together by **disulfide bonds** forming a **Y shaped tetramer ($L_2 H_2$)**. Each chain has 2 ends – **amino (NH_3^+)** and *carboxy (COO^-)* and 2 regions.

Constant (C) region

- It has *constant amino acid sequence*, and located *towards carboxy* (C) terminal.
- **Half (1/2) of light (L) chain** towards carboxy end (k/a C_L) and approximately three quarters **(3/4)** in IgG, A, D or 4/5 in Ig M,E of **heavy chain** towards carboxy terminal (k/a C_H) – constitute the constant region.
- Constant domain have a *characteristic, well conserved structural motif* – the **immunoglobulin fold** in all β-class of proteins. There are **3 to 4** of these constant domains in each heavy and 1 in each light chain.

C_H

- Constant region of heavy chain (C_H) is divided into **3** (in **IgG, IgA, Ig D**) or **4** (in **IgM, IgE**) **parts** – C_{H1}, C_{H2}, C_{H3}, C_{H4}.
- Distinguished by **differences in their CH regions**, humans have **5** different **types of heavy chains – determining 5 classes of immunoglobulin**. These are.

Immuno-globulin	Heavy Chain	CH domains (number)
IgG	Gamma (γ)	3 } C_H1, C_H2, C_H3
IgA	Alpha (α)	3
IgD	Delta (δ)	3
IgM	Mu (μ)	4 } Also C_H**4**
IgE	Epsilon (ε)	4

- **Hinge region between CH_1 and CH_2** domains is the area in which **papain** (proteolytic enzyme obtained from **papaya**) and pepsin cleave the immunoglobulin molecule. Papain cleaves distal disulfide bond to produce **2** antigne binding fragments **(Fab)** and 1 crystallizable fragment **(Fc)** whereas, pepsin digestion cleaves proximal S-S bond to generate 2 Fab fragments joined together by distal S-S bond and 1Fc.
- Hinge region allows both Fab arms to move independently thus confers **flexibility** to bind to antigen sites which may be at variable distance (on bacterial surface).
- **Constant regions** of immunoglobulin ***particularly basal crystalizable fragment (Fc)*** i.e. **CH2, CH3** (and **CH4 in IgM & IgE**) are responsible for **class specific effector functions** (like transplacental passage, complement fixation, opsonization, agglutination, binding to macrophage & mast cells, mediation of allergic response, presence in secretions, antigen receptors on B cells and polymeric forms containing J chains of immunoglobulins.
- 1 molecule of Ig has 2 Fab so it is termed **divalent**.

C_L

- Distinguished by **differences** in their C_L (constant region of light chain), humans have **2** different **types** of light chain – **kappa (κ)** and **lambda (λ)**.
- Any immunoglobulin molecule always contains **either 2λ or 2k** but never a mixture of both.
- In human k chains are more frequent (60%).

Variable (V) region

- It has *variable amio acid sequence* & located towards *amino terminal.*
- First 108 amino acids (out of 214) in light chain i.e. amino terminal half of light chain (V_L) and first 118 aa (out of 440) in heavy chain i.e. approximately **one quarter (1/4)** of **heavy chain** towards amino terminal **(V_H)** constitute the variable region.
- Variable region are quite **heterogenous** and **no two** variable regions **have identical amino acid sequence.**
- Variable regions are comprised of relatively invariable regions and **hypervariable regions.**
- L chains have **3** and H chains have **4 complementarity determining regions (CDRs)** or **hyper variable regions** – which comprise the antigen binding site located on amino tips of Y and dictates amazing **specificity** of antibodies.
- Polypeptide zone b/w 2 hyper variable regions is k/a **frame work regions.**
- About 5 to 10 aminoacis in each hypervariable CD region contribute to antigen binding site, which is formed by CDRs of both V_H & V_L
- **Epitope or antigenic determinant** is the site on antigen to which an antibody binds. Large antigen binds with all of CDRs whereas small antigen interact with only few (or one) CDR i.e. ----- a **mutual complementarity** b/w epitope & CDR surface. Binding involves **non covalent forces** and

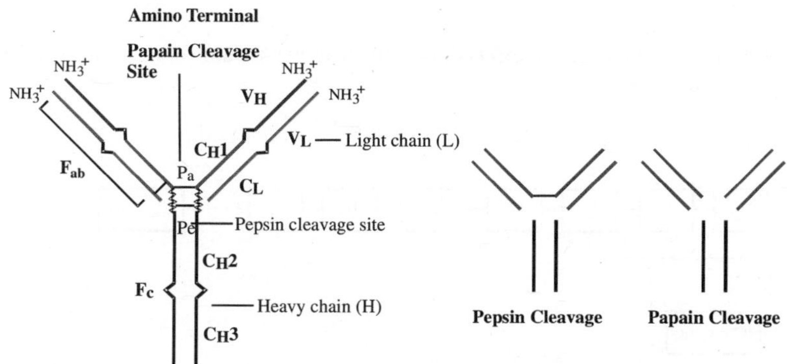

bonds (electrostatic, vander Walls, hydrogen and hydrophobic **bonds)**

- Various combinations of H & L chain CDRs can give rise to tremendous diversity of antibodies (specificity) k/a **combinatorial diversity.**
- **Antigen binding fragment (Fab)** has light chain (V_L & C_L) and V_H & C_{H1} of heavy chain.

- Both light chain and heavy chain products of multiple genes like – variable region **(V)** gene, joining region **(J)** gene, constant region **(C)** gene and diversity region **(D)** genes. **V, J, & C** genes occur for both **L & H** chains – **V_L/V_H, J, $C_{L/H}$** genes whereas diversity region **(D) genes occur only for heavy (H) chains.** *J gene bears no relationship to J chain of IgA or IgM.*
- All normal classes & subclasses of immunoglobins are called **isotopes** if they contin **same light chain** and ***identical variable domains of both their light chains (V_L) and heavy chains (V_H)*** indicating **same antigen specificity**. This means different classes (isotopes) of immunoglobulins are differentiated by their **different C_H regions** which are combined with the *same antigen specific V_H region.*
- Human genome contains only ~ 29,000 coding genes but can produce 10^9- 10^{10} different immunoglobin types b/o **gene rearrangements**, providing the immease diversity needed for recognition of enormous number of antigens. **Immense antibody diversity** depends on a number of factors including – **the existence of multiple gene segments** (30 λV, 300 kapa (κ) V; 1000 heavy chain V, 4J, 15D, 1C segments), ***their recombinations (somatic rearrangement of DNA or transposition of genes)***[Q], the **combinations of different light (L) & heavy (H) chains, junctional diversity** (i.e. addition or deletion of random number of nucleotides in joining certain gene segments l/t inaccuracies in V-J, V-D and D-J recombination), **N-region insertion** (nucleotides inserted b/w D and J by terminal transferase), combinatorial association, multispecificity, and a ***high frequency of somatic mutation***[Q].
- **C- terminal transmembrane domain** is present in membrane bound antibodies

	IgG	IgA	IgM	IgD	IgE
Heavy (H) Chain	γ	A (α)	μ	δ	ε
Heavy chain domains	4	4	5	4	5
Usual Structrue /Units	Monomer (1)	Monomer (1) Dimer (2)	Monomer (1), Pentamer (5) Hexamer (6) Dimmer (2)	Monomer (1)	Monomer (1)
Antibody valence	2	2, 4	10, 12	2	2
Additional Units in polymers	-	**S & J**	**J piece**	-	-
Subclasses (Isotypes)	G1, G2, G3, G4	A1, A2	-	-	-
% of total Ig in serum	75	15	9	0.2	0.004
Serum concentration (mg/dl)	1000	200	120	3	0.05
Serum half life (days)	23	6	5/10	3	2.5
Rate of synthesis (mg/kg/day)	35	65	5	0.4	0.016
Sedimentation coefficient (S)	7	7 or 11★	19	7	8
Molecular weight (X1000)	150	170 or 400★	900	180	190
Complement Fixation-Classical	+ (G_1, G_2, G_3)		+	-	-
Alternative complement activation	+(G_4)	+	-	+	-
Natural antibodies, Primary response antibody Antigen recetors on B cells	-	-	+	-	-
Transplacental passage, Opsonization (produce opsonin C_{3b}), Antibody dependent cell mediated cytolysis (ADCC)	+	-	-	-	-
Fixation to **mast cells Mediation of allergic responses**	-	-	-	-	+
Found in secretions	-	+	-	-	-
Agglutination	+	++	+++		

but absent in secreted (circulating) antibodies. The shift from membrane bound form to secreted form of immunoglobulins ***involves poly A-site choice (i.e. differential RNA processing)***[Q].

★ Form is found in secretions (saliva, milk, tear etc) & fluids of respiratory, genital & intestinal tracts.

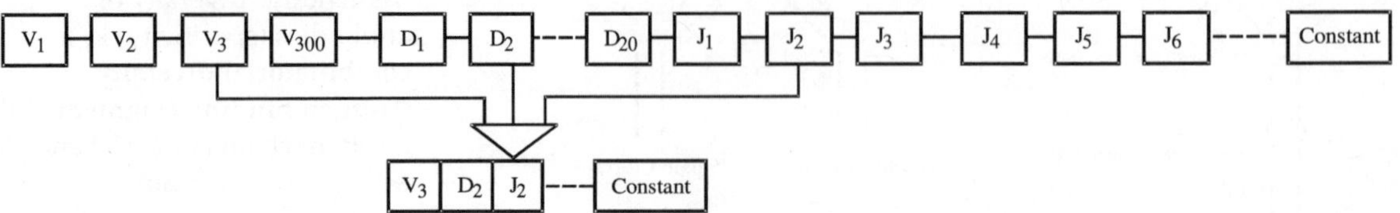

- A gene can give rise to multiple products by **differential RNA processing** i.e. – either by poly A site choice or alternative splicing or both. If there are ≥2 sites for cleavage and polyadenylation, use of one closest to 5′ end will remove more (& use of one closest to 3′ end will remove less) of primary transcript sequence-thus generating diversity in variable domain of Ig heavy chain. The mRNA site where cleavage occurs is marked by 2 sequences.

- Highly conserved (5′) **AAU AAA** (3′) sequences about 10 to 30 bases upstream on the 5′ side of cleavage site
- Less well defined **GU rich** sequence, 20 to 40 nucleotides downstream of the cleavage site.

Cleavage generates free 3′-OH end of mRNA. Poly (80 - 250) A residues are immediately added by polyadenylate polymerase enzyme that does not require template but uses cleaved mRNA as primer. Poly A site choice generates diversity in variable domains and is responsible for *deciding whether an antibody will remain membrane bound or get secreted*[Q]. Alternative spling produce 3 different form of myosin heavy chains whereas, both mechanism come into play to produce 2 different hormones calcium regulating hormone clacitonin in thyroid and calcitonin gene regulated peptide (CGRP) in brain from single transcript.

Protein Sorting (Localization /Targetting)

A major *sorting decision is made early when proteins are synthesized either on membrane bound polyribosomes (of RER) or on free polyribosomes of cytoplasm*. Protein synthesized on

Cytosolic-Free Polyribosomes

- Protein synthesized on free ribosome **lack signal peptide** and are delivered into cytosol.
- They may be further directed to *mitochondria, nuclei,* and *peroxisomes* by specific signals or remain in cytosol if they lack a signal.

★ Proteins that contain targeting sequence that is subsequently removed are called **pre proteins**. Whereas in **pre-pro-proteins** a second peptide also has to be removed.

Membrane bound (RER)- Polyribosomes

- Proteins synthesized in RER contain a **signal peptide** that mediate their attachment to membrane of endoplasmic reticulum.
- Proteins synthesized on RER may be destined to various membranes (eg ER membrane, golgi apparatus membrane and plasma membrane), to lysosome and for secretion.
- Golgi apparatus (all parts) is involved in **O-glycosylation** and *processing of oligosaccharide chains* of membrane & other N-linked glycoproteins and *sorting of various proteins* prior to their delivery to appropriate intracellular destination. (*trans golgi network* performs this role)

Secretory Proteins destined for **regulated secretion** are carried in **secretory vesicles**

Transport proteins for various intracellular (eg lysosome, plasma membrane etc) destinations, and proteins that are **sereted in a constitutive manner** are carried in **transport vesicles.**

Intracellular Traffic & Sorting of Proteins

Signal peptides & protein localization

- Signal peptide is an extension that is found in proteins ***synthesized on membrane bound polyribosomes***[Q]. But proteins whose entire synthesis occurs on free polyribosome lack this signal peptide (Blobel – Sabatini hypothesis)

Chaperone (Folding) Proteins 

- **Chaperone** (literally meaning *older women incharge of young unmarried woman on certain social occasions*) are the proteins that have a role in *assembly and proper folding of newly synthesized proteins* so that they have biological

- Signal peptide is also k/a ***leader or signal sequence, presequence or transient insertion singal.*** And it
  - Contain *12-35 amino acids with a central cluster of hydrophobic amino acids & at least one positively charged aminoacid near amino terminal.* Methionine is usually the amino terminal aminoacid
  - Is usually (not always) located at the amino terminal; and cleaved off at the carboxyl terminal end of an Ala residue by *signal peptidase*
- Signal peptide is *involved in process of protein insertion into ER membrane & lumen* in following manner
  - The m-RNA encodes an *amino terminal* **signal peptide**. It is recognized by **signal recognition particle (SRP)** that ***blocks translation after about 70 amino acids***Q have been polymerized (40 buried in large ribosomal subunit & 30 exposed).
  - SRP causing **elongation arrest** has 6 proteins & 7 S RNA (related to Alu family of highly repeated DNA sequences)
  - **SRP-R** (a receptor for SRP) is an integral **docking protein** on ER membrane, which has α and β subunits. β subunit spans the membrane & α is ***bound to GDP/GTP***Q
  - SRP imposed **elongation block is released** *as* the SRP-signal peptide-polyribosome complex binds to ***SRP-R***Q; thus *SRP guides the signal peptide to SRP-R & prevents premature folding and expulsion of proteins.*
  - **Translocation** consists of 3 membrane bound proteins (**Sec 61 complex**) that form a ***protein conducting channel***Q in ER. The *insertion of signal peptide into conducting channel, while the other end of parent protein is still attached to ribosome* is termed **cotranslational insertion**
  - Protein should be in *unfolded state* prior to entering conducting channel- otherwise it may not be able to gain access to the channel. When the process is complete the ribosome is dissociated into 2 subunits and signal peptide is hydrolysed by signal peptidase, located on luminal side of ER.
  - Amino acid sequence k/a **halt** or **stop transfer signal, retains proteins in membrane** as it prevents passage through membrane of ER, of proteins that are integral ER membrane proteins eg. cytochrome p 450
  - N- glycine chains are added (**cotranslational glycosylation**) occurs as proteins transverse the inner part of ER membrane.
- Some sequences that direct proteins to specific organelle

Targeting sequence (or compound)	**Targeted organelle**
Signal peptide sequence	Membrane of ER
Amino terminal KDEL sequence (Lys- Asp - Glu- Leu) in ER resident proteins in COPI vesicles	Luminal surface of ER
Di-acidic sequences (Asp-X-Glu) in membrane proteins in COP-II vesicles	Golgi membranes
Amino terminal sequence (20 – 80 residues)	Mitochondrial matrix
Nuclear localization signal (NLS) eg Pro_2 – Lys_2 – Arg – Lys- Val	Nucleus
PTS (peroxisomal matrix targeting sequence) eg Ser – Lys – Leu	Peroxisome
Mannose 6 phosphate	***Lysosome***Q

activity. The exit of properly folded protein after synthesis from ER may be a rate limiting step.

- **Present** ***in a wide range*** **of species from bacteria to humans in various cellular compartments such as** ***cytosol, mitochondria, & lumen of endoplasmic reticulum*** **and many are so called** ***heat shock protein (hsp)***Q
- Bind mainly to *hydrophobic regions* of unfolded & aggregated proteins and act as ***a quality control or editing mechanism for detecting misfolded*** **or otherwise defective proteins.**
- Some are *induced by* conditions that cause unfolding of newly synthesized proteins eg. ***any stress to cell like radiation, heavy metals, free radicals, toxins, elevated temperature & chemicals***Q; and hence called **stress proteins. Heat shock proteins** were first identified in response to heat shock.
- Most exhibit **ATP ase activity** & bind ADP & ATP. The chaperon- ADP complex has high affinity for unfolded proteins, when bound ADP is replaced by ATP. Chaperon – ATP complex releases segments of proteins that has folded properly.
- Some **chaperone folding protein & enzyme located in rough endoplasmic reticulum are**

- **Immunoglobin heavy chain binding protein (BiP, prewent in lumen)**
- **Glucose regulated protein (GRP) 94**
- **Calnexin** (calcium binding protein located in ER membrane that also binds to MHC antigen) & variety of other serum proteins, retaining them in ER until glycoprotein has folded properly.
- **Calreticulin** (calcium binding protein)
- **Protein disulfide isomerase (PDI),** an enzyme that promotes ***rapid reshuffling of disulfide bonds***Q until correct set is achieved.
- **Peptidyl prolyl isomerase (PPI)** enzyme ***accelerates folding of proline containing proteins***Q by catalyzing the cis-trans isomerization aminoacid residue (x) – Pro bond

- Misfolded proteins in ER are transported back to **proteasomes** present in cytosol by **retrograde transport** through *translocon* for ERAD. It may be powered by ATP ase present in proteasomes. Before entering proteasomes, most proteins are ubiquitinated.

★ About other options: **Proteases** are ***enzymes that hydrolyze proteins***Q. **Proteosomes** (eg 26 S component) ***help in degrading the proteins marked with ubiquitin***Q. **Template** is involved in the synthesis of nucleic acid.

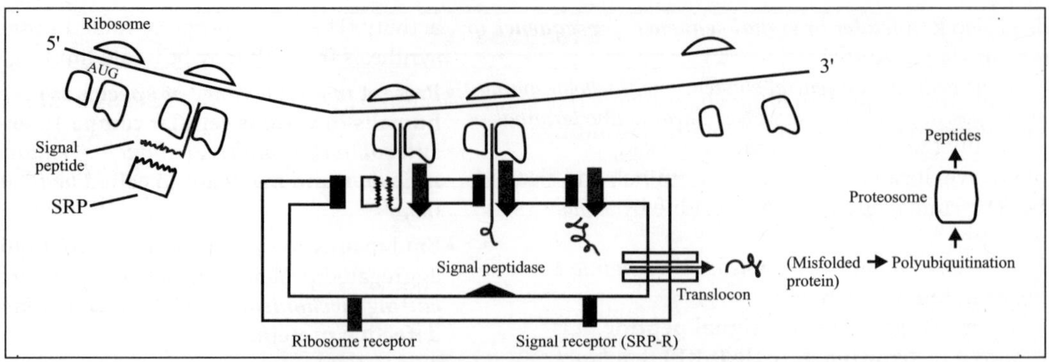

Protein Degradation and Traffic

- Accumulation of misfolded proteins in endoplasmic reticulum (**ER stress**) can induce **unfolded protein response** (**UPR**). This results in increased folding capacity of ER (by increasing chaperones) and prevents a buildup of unproductive & potentially toxic protein products by inhibition of translation of misfolded proteins & induction of protein synthesis involved in degradation of misfolded proteins.
- **Retrotranslocation or dislocation** is the process by which misfolded proteins are transported back across ER to enter ***proteasomes*** in cytoplasm. **Chaperones** (of ER & cytosol) target misfolded proteins and ***polyubiquitin-binding proteins*** *escort* them to proteasomes. Energy for translocation is partly supplied by **p97** an **AAA-ATPase** (i.e. ATP Associated with various cellular Activities).
- **3** enzymes –**activating, conjugating** and **ligase** (latter confers substrate specificity) are involved in attaching ubiquitin to target protein. Minimum of 4 ubiquitin molecules must be attached to commit a target molecules for degradation. Ubiquitin can be **reused** after cleaving by **deubiquitinating** enzymes.
- Proteasome is *a large cylindrical structure composed of 50 subunits*. It has *1-2 regulatory caps containing ATPase* for unfolding target proteins and a *hollow core* for degrading it to small peptides. It has a important role in presenting small peptides (produced by degradation of viruses etc) to major histocompatibility *(MHC) class I molecules*, a key step in *antigen presentation to T-lymphocytes*.
- Vesicles involved in **endocytosis** and / or carrying cargo to *lysosomes* are **coated with clathrin**. Clathrin is involved in transport in post golgi apparatus locations including *endosomes, plasma membrane (PM) and trans golgi network (TGN)*.
- Proteins synthesized on membrane bound polyribosomes (RER) is destined for golgi apparatus (GA) or PM. **COP II (Calthrin free) transport vesides** are involved in *antegrade (ER to GA) transport* and ***COPI (clathrin free) transport vesicles*** are involved in *retrograde (GA to ER) transport. Secretory* & transport **vesicles** carrying cargo from GA to PM are also clathrin free.
- *Key steps* and **molecular switches** in the life cycle of non clathrin coated vesicles are **budding** [*Sar 1* (GTPase); *Sec 12* (guanine nucleotide exchange factor = 'GERF), *coat proteins* (complet bud formation & contribute to curvature)] ; **pinching off** bud, **Uncoating /coat disassembly** (Sar1 has key role in both assembly & uncoating of coat proteins), vesicle **targeting** (*Rab proteins* / Ras related proteins / monomeric GTPases first observed in rabbit brain), **tetering** (or attachment) of vesicles to membrane (*Rab effector proteins*), **docking** (Vesicle or V- *SNAREs* pair with cognate target or t-*SNAREs*, forming 4 helix bundle; *SNAREs* = *SNAP* Receptors), **fusion** (interaction of SNAREs on same membrane forms eis – SNARE complex and on two different membranes forms trans SNARE complex or **SNARE pin**) and **dissociation** (require NSF or NEM sensitive ATPase and *α-SNAP* or soluble NSF attachment protein). ARF (a GTPase or ADP ribosylated factor) is involved in formation of both COP I & clathrin coated vesicles.

There are two major enzyme system responsible for degradation.

Ubiquitin- Proteasome pathway or Endoplasmic reticulum associated degeneration (ERAD)	Lysosomes
• *Energy dependent*, requires ATP • Mainly *degrade endogenous protein* (synthesized within cell) • α- carboxyl glycine of ubiquitine becomes co- valently attached to lysine residue of protein ↓ Protein tagged with ubiquitine is *recognized by proteolytic proteasome* ↓ Protein degraded to Amino acid	• Non energy dependent • Degrade extracellular protein: - Plasma protein - Cell surface membrane protein • Extracellular proteins are taken into cell by endocytosis & then degraded by lysosomal enzyme

Diseases d/t

Conformational abnormalities in *intracellular transport of proteins and enzymes* (d/t mutation) resulting in **ER stress** and **protein misfolding**.

Disease	Affected protein
Alzheimer's disease	***β-amyloid***[Q]
Prion diseases (like kuru, Creutzfeldt Jakob's disease, fatal familia insomnia)	**Pr Psc**
Cystic fibrosis	CFTR
α-Antitrypsin deficiency with liver disease	α1-Antitrypsin
Chediak Higashi syndrome	Lysosomal trafficking regulator
Combined deficiency of factor 5 & 8	Mannose binding lectin (ERGIC 53)
Diabetes mellitus (some)	Insulin receptor (α-subunit)
AD familial hypercholesterolemia	LDL receptor
Gaucher disease	β-glucosidase
Hemophilia A	Factors 8, 9
Hereditary hemochromatosis	HFE
Hermansky-Pudlak syndrome	β-3A subunit of AP-3 adaptor complex
I-cell disease	N- acetyl glucosamie phospho transferase
Lowe oculocerebrorenal syndrome	PIP2- 5- phosphatase
Tay Sach's disease	β-hexosaminidase
Von Willebrand disease	Von Willebrand factor

Peroxisomal abnormalities

1. **Hyper** oxaluria type 1
2. **Hyper** pipecolic academia
3. **Zellweger** and pseudo zell wager syndromes
4. **Adrenoleuko dystrophy** (ALD), neonatal ALD and psoudo neonatal ALD
5. **A**catalasemia
6. **R**izomelic chondrodysplasia punctuata
7. Infantile *Refsum* disease
8. **G**lutaryl CoA oxidase **deficiency**

Mn-"**Hyper ZAR-G deficiency**"

Prion Proteins & Prion Disease

It is a protein that is highly resistant to proteolytic degradation. It exists in two isoforms

Noninfectious normal cellular prion protein (PrP^c^)

- Human prion related protein is a *glycoprotein*, encoded on ***short arm of chromosome 20***[Q]
- It is monomeric, ***rich in α – helix***[Q] and does not cause disease
- It is precursor of PrP^{sc}.

Pathological prion protein (PrPsc)

- It ***rich in β-sheets***[Q] with many hydrophobic aminoacyl side chains exposed to solvents. PrP^{sc} molecules therefore *associates strongly with one another forming insoluble protease resistant aggregates* of fibrils (similar to amyloid)
- One pathological prion or prion related protein can serve as template for conformational transformation of many PrP^{c} molecules. So the prion disease ***can be transmitted by protein alone without involvement of DNA or RNA***[Q].
- It causes transmissible spongiform encephalopathies (TSE) or prion disease. These fatal neurodegenerative diseases are characterized by spongiform changes, astrocytic gliomas & neuronal loss resulting from insoluble aggregates in neural cells. These include ***mad cow disease (bovine spongiform encephalopathy) in cattles, scrapie in sheep, and Creutzfeldt- Jacob disease (most common), Gerstmann- Straussler – Sheinker disease, Kuru, & fatal familial insomnia in humans***[Q].

Protein Misfolding

Any alteration in protein folding causes wide variety of neurodegenerative disease in mammals, perhaps the *most common of which is prions disease.* Prions diseases include:

- ***Fatal familial insomnia***[Q] ┐
- Creutzfeldt – Jakob's disease ├ → Humans
- ***Kuru***[Q] ┘
- Scrapie → Sheep
- Bovine spongiform encephalopathy → Cow

Protein folding is a complex, trial and error process that can sometimes result in improperly folded molecules. Deposits of these misfolded proteins are associated with a number of neurological diseases.

Prions diseases

- Occur because of defect in the secondary – tertiary protein structure ***due to defect of folding of the peptide chain***[Q].
- Prions stands for ***proteinaceous infections particle devoid of nucleic acid***[Q].

Alzheimer's disease

- Occurs due to ***accumulation of misfolded protein called β- amyloid***[Q].
- The *A β amyloid* that is deposited in brain is *derived by proteolytic cleavages from larger amyloid precursor protein*
- A β peptide when aggregated in β-pleated sheet, is neurotoxic.
- **Apolipoprotein E** has been implicated as a potential mediator of this conformational transformation

Gene Duplication

- **Gene duplication** is any duplication or amplification of segment of DNA (chromosome) that contains a gene.
- This **second copy of a whole gene** is introduced into chromosome as a result of *defective replication of the DNA (chromosome)* such as *inhomologus recombination, retrotransposition* or duplication of entire chromosome.
- The *second gene copy is superfluous (extra) and free from selective pressure (the process of natural selection) and mutation in this gene will not be deleterious.* So it becomes a means by which the **cell may evolve, by producing a new gene with a new function (protein/enzyme)** while retaining the original gene & gene function because (organism with) extra gene accumulate mutations faster than (organism with) single function gene.
- Freedom from pressure of natural selection and consequences of mutations in extra copy of gene allow them to acquire new capability (such as metabolism of new substrate) that may increase the fitness of organism for survival in new ecological niche (environment).

Homologs, Paralogs & Orthologs

- When 2 genes share readily detectable sequence similarities (nucleotide sequence in DNA or aminoacid sequence in proteins they encode), their sequences are called **homologous** and proteins they encode are **homologs**.
- 2 homologous genes occurring **in the same species** are called **paralogous** and their protein products are **paralogs.** Paralogous genes are **derived from gene duplication** followed by gradual changes in the sequences of both copies. Paralog proteins are similar in sequence of aminoacid & three dimensional structure both, although they commonly acquire different functions during their evolution
- 2 homologous genes occurring **in different species** are called **orthologous** and their protein products are **orthologs**. Orthologs are commonly have **same functions in both organisms**.
- **Synteny is conserved order of genes on chromosome** over a large segment of genome of closely related species (eg human & mouse). It provides additional evidence for an **orthologous relationship between genes at identical location** within the related segment.
- Genes in segments of **human chromosome 9 & mouse chromosome 2** exhibit very high degree of homology **(orthology)** as well as **synteny (same gene order).**

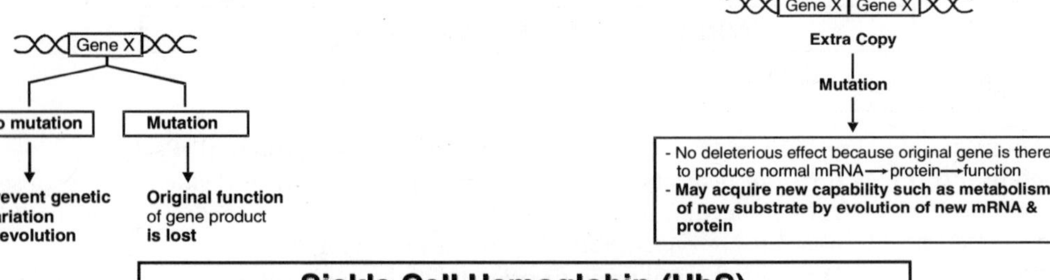

Sickle Cell Hemoglobin (HbS)

- A **point mutation** involving **T- to - A** *DNA substitution* (which inturn results in an **'A - to- U'** change in the *m-RNA*) corresponding to the 6th codon of β globin gene result in sickle cell disease

Partially accecpted missense (Point) mutation involving (T) to (A) substitution in β globulin gene (DNA) at 6th position → (A) to (U) substitution in corresponding positionof m RNA and so codon

Codon	Codes Amino acid	In protein
GAA / GAG	Polar Negatively Charged Glutamate at β6	HbA β chain
becomes GUA / GUG	Non polar hydrophobic Valine at β6	HbS - β chain

- The corresponding single nucleotide change within the codon would be **GAA or GAG of glutamic acid to GUA or GUG of valine**. This is a **partially accepted missense mutation**; partially accepted because HbS does bind & release O_2, albeit abnormally; missense because it hinders normal function & result in sickle cell anemia.
- Restriction fragment length polymorphism (RFLP) is an inherited difference in the pattern of restriction (endonuclease) enzyme digestion d/t presence or absence of an extra restriction site. This single base *change in sickle cell disease result in RFLP*[Q].
- The mutation results in **single amino acid substitution (GLu $^{6(\beta)}$ – Val):** i.e. ***a surface localized charged (polar, hydrophilic) aminoacid glutamate is replaced by hydrophobic (non polar) amino acid valine (without any charge)***[Q] ***at position 6 in two β-chains***. The R group of valine has no electric charge, whereas glutamate has a negative charge at pH 7.4. So HbS has 2 fewer negative charges than HbA (1 for each β-chain)

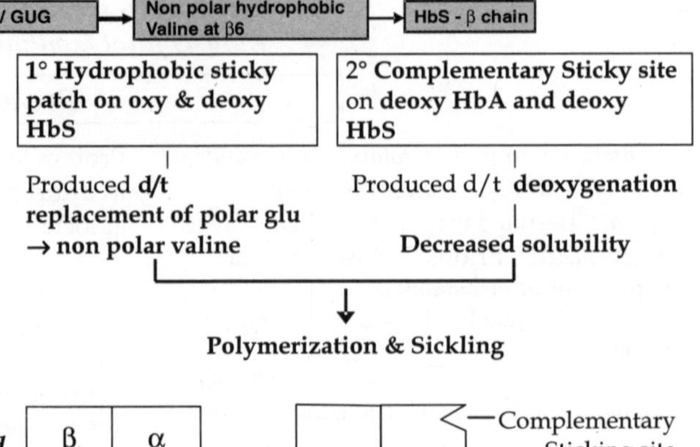

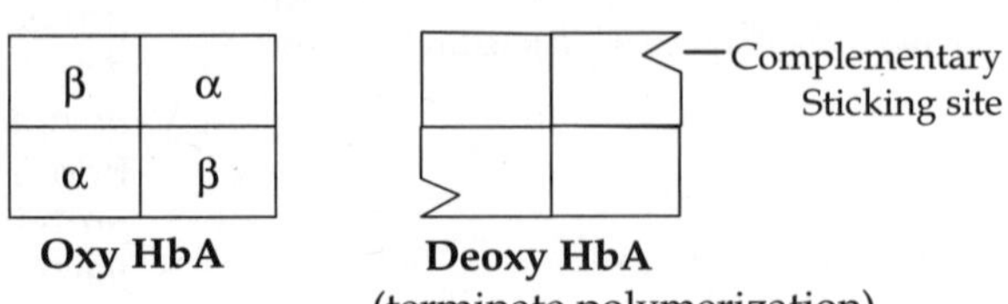

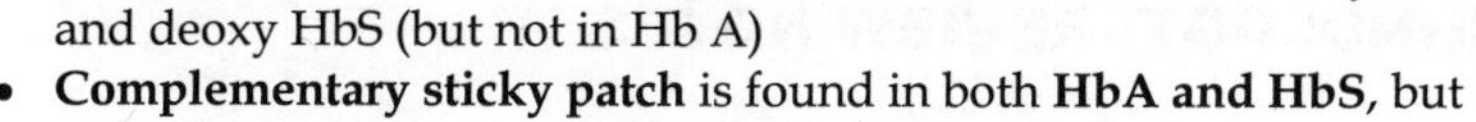

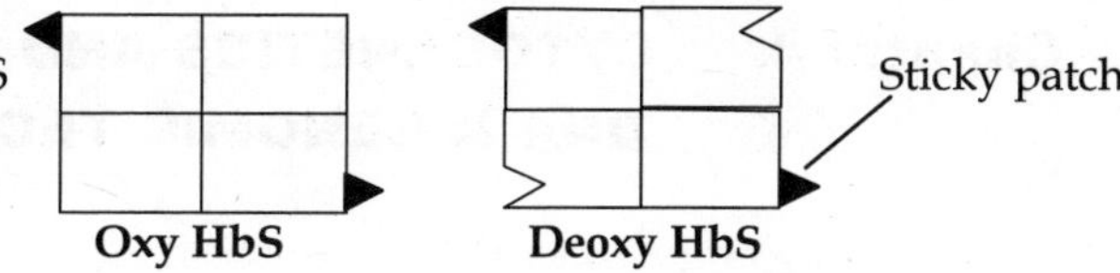

- This replacement creates a **'Sticky hydrophobic patch'** (contact point) on the outer surface at position 6 of β-chain of both oxy HbS and deoxy HbS (but not in Hb A)
- **Complementary sticky patch** is found in both **HbA and HbS**, but is exposed only in their **deoxygenated (T) state.**

- HbA remains a true solute at rather higher concentrations because of polar exterior surface that is compatable and non reactive with nearby Hb molecules. In contrast ***HbS when deoxygenated is less soluble***[Q].
  Thus at low PO_2, deoxy HbS can polymerize to form long, insoluble fibers. These twisted helical fibers ***distort the erythrocyte into characteristic sickle shape***[Q].
- Binding of **deoxy Hb A** *terminates fiber polymerization*, since HbA lacks the second sticky patch necessary to bind another Hb molecule.
- In dilute solutions, HbS has interactions with O_2 (P_{50}, Hill coefficient) that are similar to those for HbA. However *Bohr effect on concentrated HbS is more pronounced* l/t greater release of O_2 in the capillaries & increased propensity for sickling. Sickled RBCs are less deformable less freely mobile through microvasculature & often block blood flow especially in *spleen & joints*. These cells lose water, become fragile, & have a considerable short life span l/t hemolysis & anemia.
- In **heterozygous (Hb A/ HbS, sickle cell trait)** individuals, sickling decreases by at least a factor of 1000, thereby accounting for the *asymptomatic natue except during extreme physical exertion*. For reasons that remain to be elucidated, ***hetrozygosity is associated with an increased resistance to malaria***[Q], specially for lethal forms like *plasmodium falciparum*. HbS trait causes parasites to grow poorly or die at low O_2 concentration b/o *low K^+ levels caused by potassium efflux* from RBC on heboglobin sickling.
- This is the selective advantage that HbA/HbS hetrozygotes exhibit over either normal HbA/HbA or homozygous HbS/ HbS and offer an explanation for persistence of HbS in gene pool d/t natural selection. Emerging t/t include *inducing HbF expression* to inhibit polymerization.

★ 90% of human genome variation occurs d/t **single base change in DNA** and is k/a **single nucleotide polymorphism (SNPs** or pronounced "**snips**"). This results in **disappearance** (of already present) or **creation** of a new **restriction site** by a particular restriction, endonuclease enzyme.
In either case, cleavage with that restriction endonuclease results in fragments of **lengths differing from normal** (i.e. **RFLP**=restriction fragment length polymorphism), which can be detected by *DNA - hybridization (southern bloting).* In Hbs, point mutation abolishes the recognition site of **restriction endonuclease Mst II** that recognizes the nucleotide sequence **C C T N A G G** (N=any nucleotide). A to T mutation in β^s globin gene codon *eliminates a cleavage site*, resulting in generation of **larger 1.35 kg fragments** (in place of *normal 1.15 kb fragments*) on DNA digestion with Mst II restriction endonuclease.

Methods used for Detection of Mutation

Common Techniques	Principle
Cytogenetic analysis	Unique visual appearance of various
Fluorescent in situ hybridization (FISH)	Hybridization to chromosomes with fluorescently labeled probes
Southern blot	Hybridization with genomic probe or cDNA probe after digestion of high molecular DNA
Polymerase chain reaction (PCR)	Amplification of DNA segment
Reverse transcriptase PCR (RT-PCR)	Reverse transcription, amplification of DNA segment - absence or reduction of mRNA transcription
DNA sequencing	Direct sequencing of PCR products Sequencing of DNA segments cloned into plasmid vectors
Restriction fragment polymorphism (RFLP)	Detection of altered restriction pattern of genomic DNA (southern blot) or PCR products

Other Techniques	Principle
Single-strand conformational polymorphism (SSCP)	PCR of DNA segment: Mutations result in conformational change and altered mobility
Denaturing gradient gel electrophoresis (DGGE)	PCR of DNA segment: Mutations result in conformational change and altered mobility
RNAse cleavage	Cleavage of mismatch between mutated and wild type sequence
Oligonucleotide specific hybridization (OSH)	Hybridization of PCR products to wild -type or mutated oligonucleotides immobilized on chips or slides
Microarrays	Hybridization of PCR products to wild-type or mutated oligonucleotides
Protein truncation test (PTT)	Transcription/translation of cDNA isolated from tissue sample
Pyrosequencing	Clonal amplification of single DNA fragments on microparticles followed by massive parallel sequencing
Multiplex ligation-dependent probe amplification (MLPA)	Quantification of PCR-generated amplicons reflecting the number of copies of a specific DNA sequence

Chapter 4. CYTOGENETICS AND MOLECULAR GENETICS, RECOMBINANT DNA & GENOMIC TECHNOLOGY: REVIEW NOTES

Normal Karyotype & Chromosomal Nomenclature

- The study of chromosomes – Karyotyping – is the basic tool of cytogenetics. Chromosome spread is produced by use of mitotic spindle inhibitors (eg. colcemid) to arrest mitosis in dividing cells in metaphase, and then to stain the chromosome. In **metaphase spread** every chromosome takes the form of two chromatids connected at the centromere. A Karyotype is a photograph (image) of stained chromosome pairs arranged in order of decreasing length (in metaphase spread stage). Idiogram is details of banding of chromosome.
- Chromosomes have characteristic banding patterns created by *trypsin and Giemsa stain;* hence called **G banding**. The chromosomes need to be stained in order to see them with a microscope. When stained the chromosomes look like strings with light and dark 'bands'. Each chromosome arm is defined further by numbering the bands, ***the higher the number, the further that area is from the centromere.***

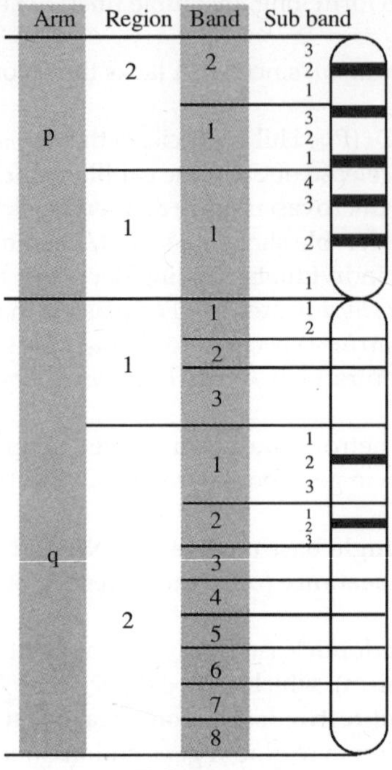

Arm	Region	Band	Sub band
p	2	2	3, 2, 1
		1	3, 2, 1
	1	1	4, 3, 2, 1
q	1	1	1, 2
		2	
		3	
	2	1	1, 2, 3
		2	1, 2, 3
		3	
		4	
		5	
		6	
		7	
		8	

X-Chromosome

- Every cell of the human body has 46 chromosomes occurring in 23 pairs. Chromosomes are laid out in pairs, from largest (#1) to smallest (#22). The last pair are called the sex chromosomes labeled X or Y. Female have two X chromosomes (XX), and males have an X and a Y chromosome (XY).
- Each chromosomes has a p and q arm; ***P (petit) is the short arm and q (next latter in the alphabet) is the long arm***[Q]. When a karyotype is made the q arm is always put on the bottom and the p on the top. The arms are separated by a region known as the centromere. So Xp 21.2 means segment located on short arm of X-chromosome, in region 2, band 1 and subband 2.

p	Short arm
Q	Long arm
+	additional chromosome
-	missing chromosome
T	translocation
del	deletion
dup	duplication
inv	inversion
der	derivative
r	ring chromosome
I	isochromosome

Conventional Cytogenetic Analysis

- Theoritically, chromosomal preparations for analysis can be obtained *from any actively dividing tissue* by causing the cells to arrest **in metaphase** (the stage of cell cycle when chromosomes are maximally condensed). However, in practice only **amniocytes or chorionic villi** (for prenatal testing) and **blood, bone marrow or skin fibroblasts** (for post natal studies) are used.
- Analysis of *blood, bone marrow & chorionic villi* involve **short term culture** technique that yield result in **1-3 days**; whereas other tissues require **long term culture (1-3 weeks of processing)**.
- Cells are isolated at metaphase or prometaphase and treated chemically or enzymatically to reveal chromosome bands. Analysis of number of chromosomes and distribution of bands on individual chromosome allow the identification of numerical or major structural abnormalities.
- Each human chromosome has a ***centromere /primary constriction (that divides chromosome into short (p) and long (q) arms***[Q] and is responsible for segregation during cell division) and **telomeres or chromosomal ends** capping the p & q arms. Each chromosome consists of **single chromatid** copy of double helix DNA *prior to DNA replication* and **2 identical sister chromatids** after DNA replication (until cell division including metaphase)

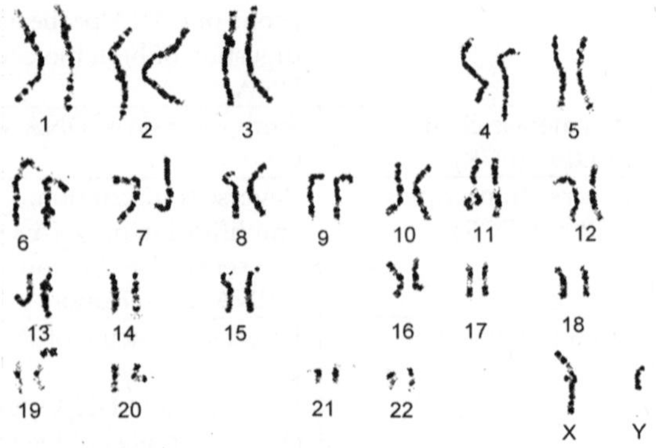

1 2 3 4 5
6 7 8 9 10 11 12
13 14 15 16 17 18
19 20 21 22 X Y

Karyotype

Different Types of Banding

G- Banding

- It is a technique used in cyto genetics to produce visible karyotype by staining *condensed chromosomes* in cells *blocked in mitosis.*
- The metaphase chromosomes are *treated with trypsin* (to partially digest the protein) & stained *with giemsa*. The acid- saline- giemsa protocol utilizes acetic acid fixation, air drying, denaturing chromosomes mildly with proteolytic enzymes, salts, heats, detergents or urea , and finally giemsa stain.
- It yields a series of lightly & darkly stained bands. The **dark regions** tend to be *hetrochromatin, late replicating, AT rich and the light bands are euchromatic, early replicating GC rich.*

FUdR (Fluro- deoxy- uridine Banding)

- FUdR is used to induce fragile sites in chromosomes. Fragile sites on chromosome undergo breakage at an increased frequency under certain culture conditions
- Common or constitutive fragile sites (c- fra) can be induced by low folate levels. Chemicals such as FUdR, aphidicolin and caffeine also enhance c- fra.
- **Rare or heritable fragile sites (h-fra)** are located on autosomes (16), and the 17th is on x- chromosome.

R – Banding

- It is **reverse G banding** i.e. the dark regions are euchromatic, guanine – cytosine rich regions and the bright bands are hetrochromatic adenine – thymine rich regions.

T- Banding

Visualize *telomeres*

C- Banding

Giemsa specifically stain the centromere and other *regions* containing constitutive hetrochromatin i.e. 2° constrictions of human chromosomes 1, 9, 16, & distal segment of Y chromosome long arm.

Q- Banding

- Metaphase chromosomes ae stained with a **fluorescent quinacrine mustard** stain to produce temporary Q bands on chromosome. The pattern of bands is similar to that seen in G banding
- It is useful in identifying *Y chromosome, Y bodies in interphase nuclei and various DNA polymorphisms* involving satellites and centromeres.

Molecular Cytogenetics: Fluorescence in Situ Hybridization (FISH)

Conventional cytogenetic karyotyping *is applicable only to cells that are dividing or can be induced to divide in vitro*. This limitation can be overcome with *DNA probes labelled with fluorescent dyes* that recognizes chromosome specific sequences – a technique k/a FISH. ***The primary advantage of interphase FISH is that it can be performed very rapidly (usually <24 hours) because cell growth is not required***Q.

Method

- In principle, FISH is similar to other **DNA-DNA hybridization method** in which fluorescent labeled DNA probe is hybridized with target DNA to counterstain it & allow its detection under fluorescene microscope
- Sample DNA (**interphase nuclei**, or **metaphase spread chromosome**) is denatured into complimentary strands and *fluorescent labelled DNA probe* is added. *Probe hybridizes with sample DNA* at the target site as the sample DNA reanneals (reforms) back into double

Types of FISH & Array Technology & their Utilty

- FISH can be utilized to **identity specific chromosomes, characterize de novo duplications or deletions and clarify subtle chromosomal rearrangements.** However, its greatest utilization in constitutional analysis is in *detection of microdeletions* and in cancer cytogenetics for analysis of *structural rearrangements.* Though conventional cytogenetic studies can detect some microdeletions, initial detection &/or **confirmation with FISH, is essential.**
- **It can demonstrate *subtle microdeletions, complex translocations, telomere alterations, & specific rearrangements* in metaphase cell that are not readily detectable by routine karyotyping**
- To physically map (localize) a newly isolated gene & to identify extra material of unknown origin.
- It diagnose microdeletion syndromes such as Cri-du-chat / Miller – Dieker / Smith-Magenis/Kallman / Williams / Wolf-Hirschhorn/Prader-Willi-Angelman/Di-George/Velo cardial- facial / CATCH-22 / Shprintzen – syndromes.
- In addition to **metaphase FISH, other types include**

1. Interphase FISH

- It can be used **to make a rapid diagnosis** in instances when metaphase chromosome preparations are not yet available; also *increases number of cells available for examination* , allows for investigation of nuclear organization, and provides results when cell do not progress to metaphase.

helix.

- Then the probe signals are *visualized under fluorescent microscope* & sample *DNA is scored for presence or absence of the signals.*

Types of FISH Probes

1. **Chromosome libraries (chromosome specific paints)** are probes that *hybridize to sequence that span the entirety of chromosome* from which they are derived and as a result they can used to **paint individual chromosomes**
2. **Repetitive probes recognize amplified DNA sequences** present in chromosomes. Eg **alpha-satellite DNA probes** are complementary to DNA sequences found at the **centromeric regions of all human chromosomes.**
3. **Single copy probes,** available d/t human genomic project, can be as small as 1kb (though normally are much larger) and are **packaged into fosmids** (40 kb) or **bacterial artificial chromosomes** (BACs) (100-200kb).

★ The *mobility of ds DNA* in gel electrophoresis depends on strand size & length but *is relatively independent of nucleotide sequence.* However, *mobility of single stranded DNA is highly affected by a small change in nucleotide* sequence because relatively unstable SS DNA forms intrastrand base pairing, loop & folds that give the single strand a unique 3rd structure, regardless of its length. **Single stranded**

- When there is strong clinical indication of any trisomy, the **aneuploid screen test (uncultured amniotic fluid interphase FISH study)** is performed on *amniotic fluid cells, using DNA probes for chromosomes 13, 18, 21 X and Y.* The results are obtained usually within 24 -48 hours and will ascertain ~60% abnormalities detected prenatally.
- *Interphase FISH* is used to *enumerate* one or more *chromosomes in interphase nuclei,* as well as to detect specific chromosomal rearrangements characteristic of certain cancers However, its application is not only limited to interphase nuclei. Many site specific translocations a/w specific types of malignancies (cancer cytogenetics) can be identified. For example, probes for both **Abelson (Abl) onchogene** and **break point cluster region (bcr)** involved in **CML** are labeled in red and green respectively; so the fusion of both genes in CML combines the fluorescence and appears as a yellow hybridization signal.
- **Oncogene activation by DNA sequence amplification** (& overexpression of gene product) leads to increase *in DNA copy number* causing cytogenetically recognizable chromosome alteration k/a **homogenous staining regions (HSRs)** if *integrated within chromosome or* ***double minutes (d mins)*** *if extrachromosomal.* It can be *identified through comparative geneomic hybridization, FISH* which allow visualization of chromosomal aberrations. Microarray based, non cytogenetic approaches identify changes in copy number and short tag based sequencing approaches are used to evaluate amplification. With both microarrays & sequencing technologies, the entire genome can be surveyed for gains and losses of DNA sequences, thus pinpointing chromosomal region likely to contain gene important in development or progression of cancer

- In addition to standard metaphase & interphase FISH, several **enhanced techniques** include.

2. Spectral Karyotyping (SKY) and **multicolor FISH (mFISH)**

- In, **chromosomal painting** whole chromosomes can be labeled with a series of fluorescent DNA probes that binds to a particular chromosome at multiple sites. Chromosomal painting has limited ability *to visualize all 46 human chromosomes simultaneously.* This hurdle has been overcome by **spectral karyotyping (or spectacular Karyotyping = SKY)** which uses a combination of 5 fluorochromes & computer generated signals to visualize entire human genome.
- SKY and m-FISH use combinatorially labeled probes that *create a unique color for individual chromosomes.* It is *useful in identification of unknown chromosome material* (eg accessory marker chromosomes containing additional material) and most commonly *in complex rearrangements* seen in cancer specimen

3. Fiber FISH

- Chromosomes are mechanically stretched which provides a higher **resolution of analysis than conventional FISH**

4. FISH – Comparative Genomic Hybridization (CGH)

- ***Comparative genomic hybridization (FISH-CGH) can be used to detect chromosomal differences between neoplastic cells and their counterparts***[Q]. *It can quickly and efficiently analyse copy number variations (CNVs) in relation to ploidy level* in a test sample DNA compared to another reference sample (which is mostly related). It detects amplification or deletions of smaller DNA region or whole chromosome by comparing DNA of a patient (target) with a normal person.
- It can be used only when DNA in available from a specimen of interest (eg cancer). The entire DNA specimen from the sample of interest is labeled in one color (eg green) and the normal control DNA specimen is labeled by another (eg red) color. These are mixed in equal amounts and hybridized to normal metaphase chromosomes. Computerized analysis of (red to green) color ratio determines where the DNA of interest may have gains or losses of material.

5. Array – CGH (a-CGH, Chromosomal Microarray Analysis / CMA, Virtual Karyotyping)

- Similar to FISH – CGH, except that the test DNA is hybridized to DNAs that are **spread on arrays, rather than hybridized to normal chromosomes.**
- *Comparitive genomic hybridization (CGH) directly compares the DNA, content of differentially labelled normal & tumor cells* by their co- hybridization to normal metaphase chromosome spread or to series of genomic DNA clones aligned on glass slides **(array CGH)**. In this way

conformation polymorphism (SSCP) is electrophoretic seperation of single stranded nucleic acids based on their differences in nucleotide sequence (often a single base pair) that results in a different secondary structure & a measurable difference in its mobility through gel. So the SSCP *can detect point mutations.*

tumor specific alterations in gene copy number can be ascertained.

- It provides a *higher resolution* (upto 50kb). **CGH arrays** utilize either BACs or **oligonucleotides,** whereas **genotyping arrays** utilize *single nucleotide polymorphisms* **(SNP arrays).** It is used in prenatal diagnosis & study of ***cryptic chromosomal imbalances in patients with mental retardation and multiple congenital anomalies.*** It is also used to ***detect microdeletions and micro duplications in cancer and previously unidentified genomic disorder***Q. This technology is still in development, but it will ultimately be the **initial method of study for constitutional abnormalities.**

★ Both **MAPH (multiplex amplification & probe hybridization)** and **MLAP (multiplex ligation dependent probe amplification)** techniques for detection of small scale copy number changes & gene deletions rely on sequence specific probe hybridization to genomic DNA followed by PCR amplification of hybridized probe and semiquantitative analysis of resultant PCR product. The relative peak heights / band intensities indicate initial concentration of each target.

Barr Body

- When two X chromosomes are present in a cell (as in a normal female) one of them becomes inactivated and condensed on the nuclear membrane and is called the **'Barr body'**. This process is termed as X chromosome lyonization (inactivation)
- Presence or absence of Barr bodies helps in *ascertaining the sex of an individuals*
  - ***Absence of Barr body indicates that the patient has only one X chromosome (eg. Normal male XY or Turner's syndrome(XO))***
  - Nuclei of cells in females (XX) contain a darkly staining Barr body that is not present in the nuclei of cells in males.
- Barr bodies are most easily seen in a smear of squamous epithelial cells obtained by **scraping the buccal mucosa** Q
- Barr bodies react differently to histological stains and are best seen as dark staining bodies with in ***the nucleus*** of ***non dividing interphase cells.***

Fluorescence Recovery After Photobleaching (FRAP)

Lateral diffusion can be shown experimentally by attaching **fluorescent probes** to the head groups of lipids/proteins and using the **fluorescence microscopy** to follow the probes over time. Two techniques involve

Fluorescence Tagging of Membrane Surface	Single Particle Tracking
• Lipids (protein etc) on the outer leaflet (layer) of membrane are **labeled by** reaction with a membrane –impermanent **fluorescent probe, so the surface is uniformly labeled when viewed with fluorescence microscope**. A small area ($5\mu m^2$) of a cell surface with fluorescent tagged lipids is **photobleached by intense laser radiation** so that the irradiated patch **no longer fluoresces** (emit fluorescent light) when viewed with less intense (non bleaching) light in the florescence microscope. • However, the photo bleached membrane region **recovers its fluorescence within milliseconds** as unbleached lipid molecules diffused into the bleached patch and bleached lipid molecules diffuse away from it by rapid lateral diffusion. • The **rate of fluorescence recovery after**	• The *motion (movement) of a single fluorescently labeled lipid (protein / etc) molecule* in the cell membrane is *recorded on video by fluorescence microscopy on a much shorter time scale* (eg 50 ms = 2250 frames with time resolution of 25μs=40000 frames/s). • The pattern of movement confirms **rapid lateral diffusion within a confined (small discrete) region with occasional hops** into an adjoining region. It suggests that lipids are corralled by molecular fences that they can occasionally jump by **hop diffusion**. Membrane *proteins (like glycophorin & Cl^- - HCO_3- exchanger in RBC) immobilized by their association with spectrin* (a filamentous cytoskeleton protein)

Fluorescence Resonance Energy Tranfer (FRET)

- **Fluorescent probes** derived from naturally occurring fluorescent protein, the **green fluorescent protein (GFP)** of jelly fish Aequorea victoria or other variants like **BFP (blue), YFP (yellow), CFP (cyan)** along with **fluorescence microscopy** are used to visualize biochemistry of living cells by means of **FRET (fluorescence resonance energy transfer)**. FRET can be used **to measure cAMP and activity of PKA (pyruvate kinase A)**.
- When two molecules are **very close (within 1 to 50A°)**, the energy of excited donor molecule passes directly to near by acceptor molecule without emission of a photon, exciting the acceptor (the efficiency of FRET is **inversely proportional to 6th power of distance between donor & acceptor)**. The acceptor now decays to its ground state by **fluorescence** (which can be located to specific regions of single living cell); ***the emitted photon has lower energy (longer wave length) than both exciting light and the fluorescence emission of donor***Q.

photo bleaching or FRAP is a measure of rate of lateral diffusion of the lipids • FRAP can be used to *assess structure of membranes* (biological & artificial both), *define fluid mosaic model* and investigate ***diffusion (motion) of biological macromolecules including lateral diffusion movements with in the plane of membranes and movements into & out of nucleus***[Q].	form the fences that define the regions of relatively unrestricted lipid motion. 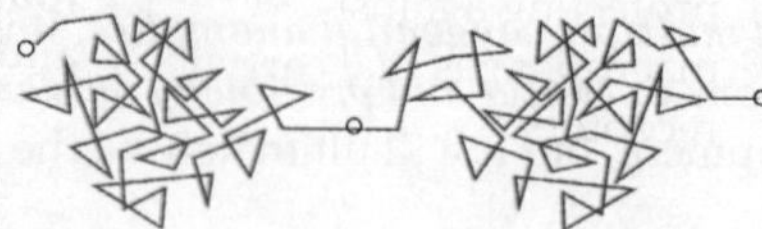 **Hop Diffusion of Single Lipid Molecule**

Photobleaching of small area by intense laser beam

Labeled by Fluorescent probe

Normal cell membrane

Uniformly labeled view on fluorescence microscope (FM)

Non fluorescent irradiated photo bleached patch (on FM)

Recovery of fluorescence d/t lateral diffusion

Atomic Force Microscopy (AFM)

In AFM, the **sharp tip of a microscope probe** attached to a (flexible) cantilever **is moved across an uneven surface eg membrane. Electrostatic & vander Walls interactions** between the tip and sample produce a force that moves the probe or sample up and down (in z dimension) as the probe encounters hills (up) and valleys (downs) in the sample. A laser beam reflected from the cantilever detects motion of 1A°. A series of scans in plane of membrane (x & y dimensions) yields a **three dimensional contour map of the surface** with resolution near the atomic scale – 0.1 nm in vertical and 0.5 to 1 nm in lateral dimensions. When several images of individual units are superimposed with compute, **a high resolution image of protein** is yielded. So AFM is **used to visualize membrane proteins** such as **membrane (microdomains) rafts** (enriched in sphingolipids, cholesterol & GPI linked proteins) or **single membrane protein** such as bacteriorhodopsin, aquaporin & Fo (proton driven rotor of chloroplast ATP synthase) etc.

Movements of Lipid in Membrane Bilayer

Uncatalyzed Lateral Diffusion

Lipid and protein molecules **diffuse laterally (or undergo Brownian movement within the bilayer)** by changing places with neighbouring molecules at very fast rate (1μm/s). This *rapid uncatalyzed lateral diffusion in the plane of membrane bilayer* tends to randomize the position of individual molecules in a few seconds.

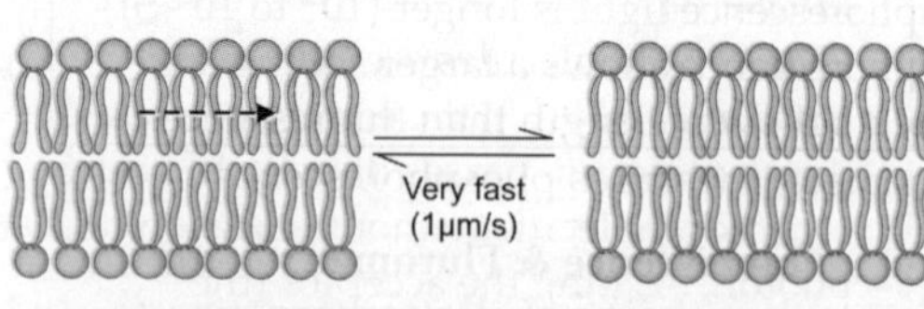

Uncatalyzed Transbilayer (Flip-Flop) Diffusion

Transbilayer (flip-flop) diffusion of a lipid molecule from one leaflet of membrane to other occurs **very slowly** ($t_{1/2}$ in days) because it requires polar (charged) head group to leave its aqueous environment and move into hydrophobic interior of membrane, a process with large, positive free energy

Catalyzed Transbilayer Translocations

- **Use translocaters (flippases, floppases & scramblases)** to facilitate transbilayer movement of lipid by a path that is much **faster and more energetically favourable**.
- The combination of asymmetric biosynthesis of membrane lipids (ie different lipids on different sides), slow flip flop diffusion and presence of selective energy dependent translocaters is responsible for transbilayer asymmetry in lipid composition, *creating a larger surface on one side of membrane and generating curvature essential in budding of vesicles.*
- **3-types of translocater's include**

Flippase	Floppase	Scramblase
- Structurally & functionally related to **P type ATPase** (active transporters); move **PE** (phosphatidylethanolamine) & **PS** (phosphatidyl serine) **from outer (extracellular) to cytosolic (lumenal) leaflet (side) of plasma membrane**. They consume about 1 ATP per molecule of phospholipid translocated	- Are members of **ABC transporter family**; all of which actively *transport hydrophobic substrates outward across the* plasma membrane. - Flippase transport plasma membrane	- Are proteins that move any **membrane phospholipid** across the membrane **down its concentration gradient** (from leaflet where it is i higher concentration to leaflet where it has a lower concentration), ie in **either direction towards equilibrium**. - They **do not require AT** **but are activated by**

change. However, in the *endoplasmic reticulum* this movement is essential for lipids to get from their site of synthesis to their eventual point of deposition as *membrane glycerophospholipids are synthesized on cytosolic surface whereas sphingolipids are synthesized / modified on luminal surface of ER membrane.*

- Keeping PS out of extracellular surface *protects cells from apoptosis (programmed cell death)* by protecting against macrophages that carry PS receptors.

phospholipids **from cytosolic (inner) to extracellular (outer) leaflet and use ATP**

increase in cytosolic calcium (Ca^{++}), which may result from cell *activation, cell injury or apoptosis.*

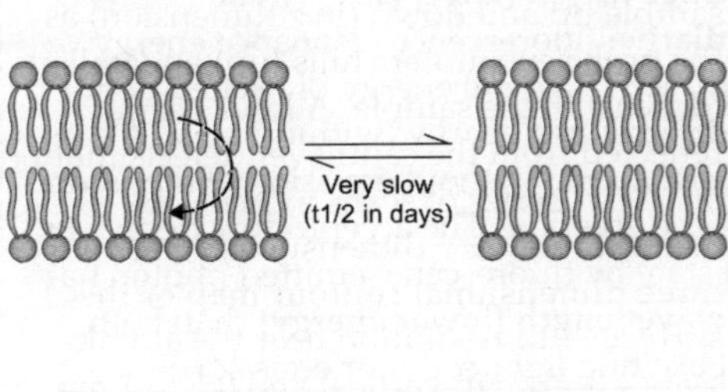

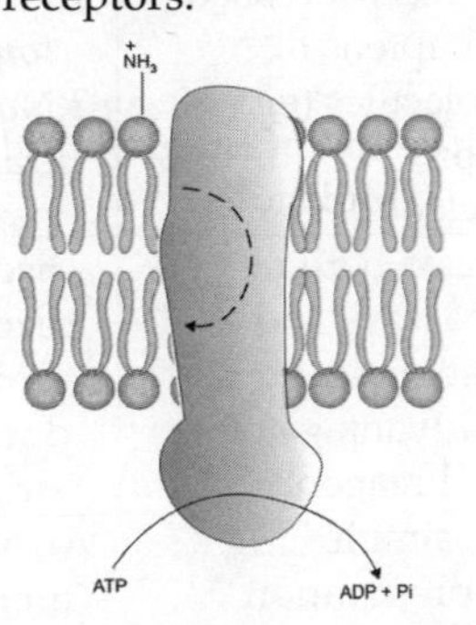

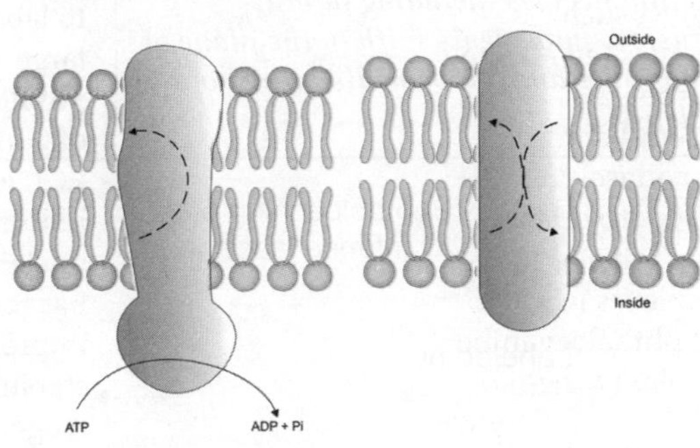

Luminescence

It is the emission of light or radiant energy when an electron returns from an excited or higher energy level to a lower energy level[Q]. It can be **caused by chemical or biochemical reactions, electrochemical reaction, electro magnetic radiation (photons)**, subatomic movements or stress on crystal. It is a **cold body radiation** as the emission of light by a substance is not resulting from heating, which differentiates it from **incandescence** (ie light emitted by a substance after heating). It can be of various types.

Chemi /Bio / Electrochemiluminescence & Luminometry

- These are types of luminescence in which the ***excitation event is caused by a chemical, biochemical or electrochemical reaction and not by photo illumination (or photoluminescence)***[Q] as seen in fluorescence.
- Physical event for light emission in chemi / bio / electro-chemiluminescence is similar to fluorescence in that it occurs from an excited singlet state, & the light is emitted when the electron returns to the ground state
- This type of light emission is measured by **luminometry**

Chemiluminescence

- It is emission of light when *an electron returns from an excited or a higher energy level to a lower energy level*
- Excitation event is caused by **chemical reaction** & involves oxidation of an organic compound such as luminol, isoluminol, acridinum ester, or luciferin by an oxidant such as

Bioluminescence

- It is ***special form of chemiluminescenc e found in biological systems***[Q]
- In it an enzyme or photoprotein or **biological catalyst (eg luciferase & acquorin)** increase the efficiency of luminescence reaction

Electrochemiluminescence (ECL)

- It differs from chemiluminescence in that the reactive species that produce electro chemiluminescent reaction are ***electro chemically generated from stable precursors at the surface of an electrode***[Q]
- Ruthenium (Ru+2), tris (bipyridyl) chelate is the M.C. used ECL label & ECL is generated at an

Photoluminescence

It is a kind of luminescence where energy is supplied by **photons (electromagnetic radiation)**. It can be of 2 types

I. Phosphorescence & Phosphometry

- It is a type of luminescence ***produced by certain substances after absorbing radiant energy or other type of energy***[Q]
- It is distinguished from fluorescence in that

1. It continues even after radiation causing it has ceased
2. The decay time of emission of phosphorescence light is longer (10^{-4} to 10^{-2} S)
3. Phosphorescence shows a larger shift in emitted light wavelength than fluorescence.

- Phosphometry measures phosphorescence

Fluorescence & Flurometry

- Fluorescence is emission of electromagnetic radiation by a substance after the absorption of energy in some form (eg the emission of light of one color / wave length when a substance is excited by irradiation with light of a different wavelength. In other words fluorescence ***occurs when a molecule absorbs light at one wave length and reemits light at a longer wave length (or lower energy)***[Q]
- It is differentiated from phosphorescence in that its life time is < 10 mili seconds after excitation ceases. Eg. fluorescent paint stops glowing as soon as UV

H_2O_2, hypochlorite, or O_2
- Light is emited from the excited product formed in oxidation. These reactions occur in presence catalyst such as enzymes (eg alkaline phosphatase, horseradish peroxidase, & microperoxidase), metal ion and metal complexes (Cu^{++} & Fe^{+3} phthalocyanine complex) & hemin

- The quantum yield is ~ 0.1 – 10% for chemiluminescence and 10-30% for bioluminescence

electrode via oxidation reduction type of reaction with tripropylamine.
- This chelate is relatively small, very stable & has been used to label haptens or large molecules (eg protein or oligonucleotides)
- ECL is used both in immunoassays and nucleic acid assays. It has the advantage of improved reagent stability, simple reagent preparation and enhanced sensitivity.

lamp is turned off but phosphorescent paint keeps glowing for a while.
- An excited fluorescent molecules such as **green fluorescent protein (GFP) or YFP or CFP** etc can dispose of the energy from absorbed photon by either

1. **Fluorescence** ie ***emitting a photon of slightly longer wave length (lower energy)***Q or
2. **Non radiative** fluorescence resonance energy transfer **(FRET)**, where energy of excited donor passes directly to a nearby (within 1 to 50 A°) acceptor molecule without emission of a photon, exciting the acceptor. The acceptor ow decays to ground state by fluorescene; emitted photon has **longer wave length (lower energy)** than both original exciting light & donor emission.

- An atom / molecule that fluoresces is termed **fluorophore**
- **Fluorometry** is measurement of emitted fluorescence light.

Bioluminescence Cycle

- **Bioluminescence** is a ***special form of chemiluminescence found in biological system***Q.
- Bioluminescence requires considerable amount of energy. In firefly, ATP is used in a set of reactions that ***convert chemical energy into light energy***Q
- The light is produced through a chemical reaction involving **luciferin**, (a heat resistant complex carboxylic acid substrate), **luciferase** (enzyme), **ATP** and O_2
- The generation of light flashes requires activation of luciferin by pyrophosphate cleavage of ATP to form **luciferyl adenylate**. In the presence of molecular oxygen (O2) and luciferase, the luciferin (adenylate) undergoes a multistep oxidative decarboxylation to oxyluciferin This process is accompanied by emission of light.
- Colour of flashes differ in different firefly species and seems to be determined by *difference in the structure of luciferase.* Luciferin is regenerated from oxyluciferin in a subsequent series of reactions.
- It has the highest quantum efficiency (Qc= 88%). The quantum yield (total photons emitted per total molecule reacting) is ~ 0.1– 10% for chemiluminescence and 10-30% for bioluminescence

PPi
Luciferyl adenylate
O_2
ATP
Luciferase
Light
Luciferin
CO_2 + AMP
Oxyluciferin

- Since the light producing reaction is **dependent on ATP**. It allows researchers to determine the presence of ATP and hence the **presence of life.**
- In lab, pure firefly luciferin and luciferase are used to measure minute quantities of ATP by the intensity of light flash produced. As little as a few picomoles (10^{-12} mol) of ATP can be measured in this way
- This method is used by NASA **to find life on other planets**. It is also used for **antibiotic susceptibility testing.** If light is produce on mixing above mixture to cultured sample of TB bacteria and antibiotic, it indicates the failure of drug and presence of growing and thriving bacteria.
- In **gene activation therapy**, if light is visible on ultraviolet cameras, this means that genes treated with luciferase are active.

Spectrophotometer : Lambert Beer Law & Absorption of Light by Molecule

- Biomolecules absorb light at characteristic wave lengths, just as **tryptophan, tyrosine** and to a much lesser extent phenylalanine absorb ***ultraviolet light near a wavelength of 280 nm***Q.

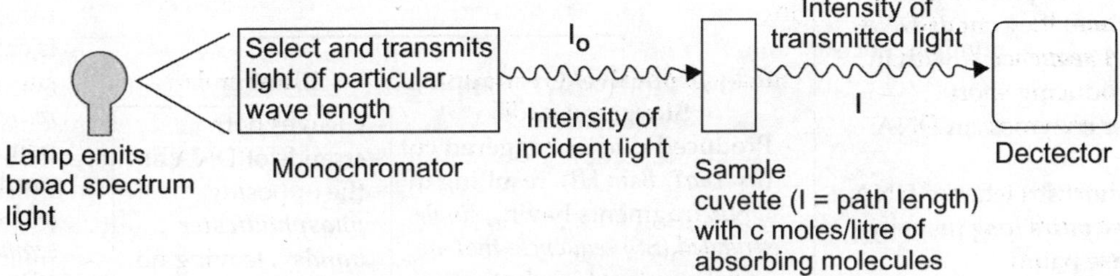

Components of Sphectrophotometer

- The fraction of incident light absorbed by solution at given wavelength depends on thickness of absorbing layer (pathlength) and concentration of the absorbing species. So Lambart Beer Law is **Absorbance** $= \log \frac{I^{\circ}}{I} = \varepsilon Cl$

where ε is molar extinction coefficient and it has been assumed that incident light is parallel, mono chromatic (of single wave length) and solvent & solute are randomaly oriented. So *each successive millimeter path of absorbing solution absorbs not a constant amount but a constant fraction of light*. However, ***with fixed path length absorbing layer, absorbance is directly proportional to the concentration of absorbing solute***Q. ***So it can be used in quatitative estimation of DNA, RNA or aminoacids***Q.

Restriction Enzyme / Restriction Endonucleases (RE) 

- These are originally called **restriction enzymes** because their presence in a given bacteria ***restricted the growth of certain bacterial viruses (i.e. bacteriophages)***Q. This **defensive enzyme** protects the host bacterial DNA from the DNA genome of foreign organisms (particularly infective bacteriophages) by specifically ***inactivating the invading phage DNA by digestion***Q.
- *Werner Arber* discovered that their biological function is to recognize an *cleave foreign DNA* (eg the DNA of infecting virus) and ***such DNA is said to be restricted. RE restrict DNA replication (viral-replication).***Q
- However, REs are found only in cells that also contain **site specific DNA methylase enzyme-*which methylates the host DNA, rendering it an unsuitable substrate for digestion by restriction enzymes (and thus protecting it from RE)***Q. So restriction enzymes and site specific DNA methylase are *companion enzymes* an always exists in pairs in a bacterium – and sometimes called as **restriction modification system.**
- Immense size of DNA was the main obstacle in its molecular analysis, which was over come by a group of bacterial enzyme called restriction endonucleases (restriction enzymes). RE ***cleaves double stranded (d s) DNA into smaller, more manageable & precisely defined DNA segments***Q called **restriction fragments**. RE used as **molecular scissors or chemical knife** is the *key enzyme in recombinant DNA technology or genetic engineering*. There are 3 types of Res
- Restriction endonucleases ***recognize and cleave (cut or splice) double stranded DNA in a predictable manner at specific sequences***Q k/a (**recognition sequences or restriction sites**) that are typically **4-6** (Lehinger) /**4-7** (Harper) bp long, to generate a set of smaller fragments. Restriction enzymes are endonucleases ie they break nucleic acid chains somewhere within the DNA rather than at the ends of molecule.
- To cut DNA, a RE makes ***2 incisions through each sugar – phosphate backbone (i.e. phospho-diester bond of each strand) of double stranded DNA***Q. The **average size of DNA fragments** produced by cleaving genomic DNA with RE depends on the frequency with which a specific restriction site occurs in DNA; which inturn depends on their size. In a DNA in which all 4 nucleotides are equally abundant [i.e. (C=G) = (A = T) =50%] and randomly distributed, a RE tht recognizes a 6 bp sequence cuts once every 4096 (4^6), whereas another RE that recognizes a 4 bp sequence cuts once every 256 bp (4^4) and so produces smaller DNA fragments. The fragment size produced by RE cleavage can be increased by simply terminating the reaction before completion – **partial digest** – or by using special class of endonuclease called **homing endonuclease** (by group I introns) which cleave *14-20 bp DNA sequence*. However, in natural DNA the recognition sequence tend to occur less frequently because neucleotides are neither random nor equally abundant.
- If a piece of DNA from a species is made to react with a specific RE, a characteristic array of cut DNA fragments will be produced, this is k/a **restriction map**. The ends of all fragments have same DNA sequence. These restriction fragments of known size are isolated (enriched) by ***electrophoresis on agarose or polyacrylamide gel***Q or **HPLC**. Restriction map serves as DNA fingerprint because the fragments of DNA from one organism will have a characteristic pattern.

Specificity

- Restriction endonucleases have specific recognition sites with **palindrome arrangement** where they cut ***ds DNA (at specific DNA sequence)***Q with in the molecule producing short fragments (other enzymes cut DNA randomly)
- RE recognizes short stretches of DNA ***about 4 to 7 base pairs long*** (usually having 4 or 6 base pairs)
- These sequences differ for each RE and are **palindromes**, i.e., they show *two fold rotational symmetry.* **Palindrome** (meaning to **run backwards**) are also known as **inverted repeat sequences**. It is similar to a *word that reads backwards or forwards similarly* eg madam. Which means with in a short region of double helix, the nucleotide sequence on one strand, read *5¹ → 3¹, is identical* to that of the 2nd *strand,* also read in *5¹ → 3¹ direction.* So, if rolated 180 degrees around the axis of symmetry – the structure remains same.

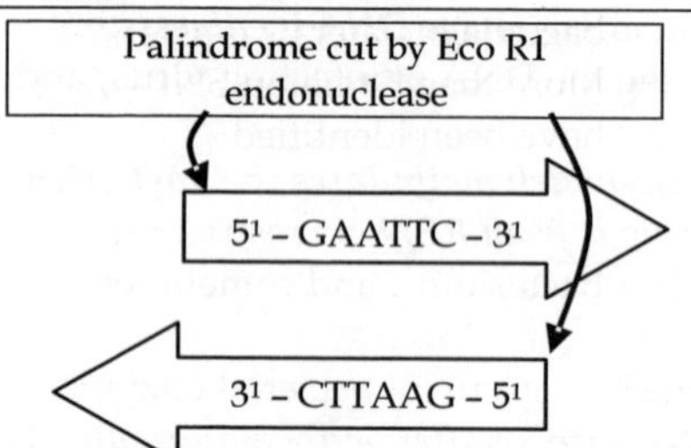

Sticky & Blunt ends

RE cleaves DNA so as to produce a 3′ – OH group on one end & 5¹ – PO_4 group on other end. DNA cut results in

Sticky /Cohesive/ Overlapping/ Staggered ends

- Produced due to **staggered cut** (by *Taq1, Bam HI*), resulting in DNA fragments having *single stranded (SS) sequences that are complementary to each other.*
- This leaves 2-4 nucleotides of one strand unpaired at each resulting end. These unpaired strands are called **sticky-ends** because these can base pair with each other or with complementary sticky ends of other DNA fragments.
- **DNA ligase** joins sticky ends produced by same RE
- **Terminal transferase** enzyme add new ends & change it into blunt end.

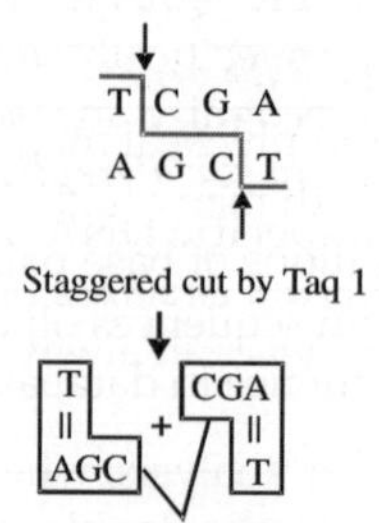

Blunt ends

- Cleaves both strands of DNA at the opposing ***phosphodiester bonds***Q, leaving no unpaired bases on the ends.
- Produced d/t straight cut, (by HpaI, Hae III) that are double stranded & therefore donot form hydrogen bonds with each other.
- **Bacteriophage T_4 ligase** can covalently joint blunt ended fragments.

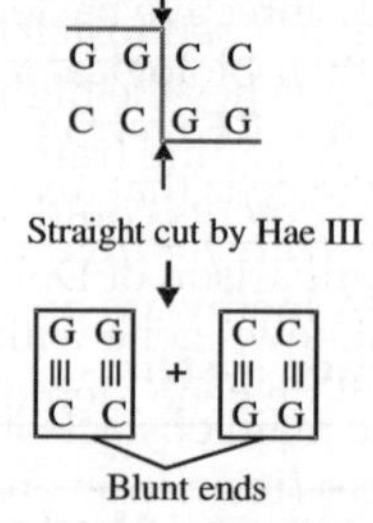

Restriction site & nomenclature

- A DNA sequence recognized by RE is called restriction site. RE that *recognizes 4 base* pair sequences produces *more cuts and shorter segments* than the RE requiring sequence of 6 base pairs.
- The 1st letter of name of RE is from the *genus of bacterium* from which it is isolated (E). Next two letters are from *name of species (Co).* The additional subscript letter indicates the *type or strain (R)* and a *final roman number* indicate the *order in which the enzyme was discovered* in that particular organism (I) eg. ECoRI.

- After isolating target DNA (restriction) fragment, it is joined to similarly digested cloning vector (i.e. vector digested by some RE) by ***DNA ligase***Q (*which catalyzes formation of new phosphodiester bonds by using ATP*). Fragments produced by 2 RE (eg EcoRI & Bam HI) will not link. New DNA sequences can be created by inserting synthetic DNA fragments (**linkers**) b/w the ends that are being ligated. **Poly linkers** are inserted DNA fragments with multiple recognition sequences for RE (often useful later as points for inserting DNA by cleavage & ligation). So it has an *important role in recombinant DNA technology* and preparing *chimeric DNA molecules.*
- Ligating sticky ends is technically easy but is a/w the problems like sticky ends may reconnect with themselves, without net gain of DNA, forming heterogeneous tandom inserts or sticky end sites may not be available in a required (convenient) position. To escape these problems blunt ends can be generated. Blunt ends can be ligated directly (however not directional) by **bacteriophage T_4 ligase** – a technique though less efficient than sticky end ligation, has advantage of ligation of any pairs of ends. 2 alternatives to circumvent problems listed above include

1. **Homopolymer tailing** by **terminal transferase** i.e. if poly d (G) is added to vector and poly d (C) is added to 3′ end of foreign DNA, the two molecules can ony link to each other.
2. Adding synthetic sticky ends (**linkers**)

- Some pro /eu-karyotic **recombinases** (like *CRE recombinase* identifying bacterial lox P sites or *Flp recombinase* identifying yeast FRT sites) are used as an adjunct to RE to catalyze DNA in corporation.

Polymorphism

Any two nonrelated individuals share 99.9% of their DNA sequences. So the remarkable diversity of humans is encoded in only 0.1% of DNA (~ 3 million base pairs). Genomic variations are differences in sequence of DNA among individuals. And genomes of non-related people differ at *about 1 of 1200 to 1,500 DNA bases* (or *0.1% of genome*). These variations are due to.

Polymorphism

- It is **normal, clinically harmless variations of DNA sequence, that does not affect the phenotype**[Q]
- Traditionally defined as **sequence variation at a given locus (allele) in >1% population.**
- It occurs ~ once in every 500 nucleotides or about 10^7 times per genome due to deletion, insertion or single base substitution occuring in non-coding region like introns & intergenic region or at sites that cause no change in function of encoded protein.
- So **polymorphism is single phenotype single locus and multiple normal allele**[Q].

Mutations

- It is **infrequent (<1%) but potentially harmful genome variation that is associated with specific human disease**
- Single mutation may l/t many end effects (**pleiotropism**) or mutations at several genetic loci may produce the several genetic loci may produce the same trait **(genetic heterogeneity).**
- Structural alterations of β-globin

Alteration	Disease	Function affected
Point mutation	Sickel cell disease	Protein folding
	β-Thalassemia	Transcription control, Frame shift & non sense mutation RNA processing.
Deletion	β°- Thalassemia Hemoglobin lepore	MRNA production
Rearragnement	β-Thalassemia type III	MRNA production

Restriction Fragment Length Polymorphism (RFLP)

- Human genome contains **sequence variations at a given locus (allele) that do not affect phenotype in >1% population**. This property of the molecule to exist in >1 form is k/a **polymorphism**. So polymorphism is **presence of single normal phenotype, single locus (site) and multiple allele (sequence variations)** in >1% of population. Polymorphism is a normal variation and is clinically harmless. Whereas mutation is *infrequent, (seen in <1%), abnormal, and potentially deleterious genetic variation that may lead to pleiotropism (one mutation – many effects) or genetic heterogeneity (many mutation – one effect).*
- **Restriction fragment length polymorphism (RFLP)** is a **genetic variation that can be observed by cleaving the DNA into fragments (restriction fragments) with a restriction endonuclease**. The existence of two or more types of restriction fragment patterns is called RFLP. The length of restriction fragment is altered if the genetic variation (polymorphism, mutation etc) alters the DNA so as to create or abolish a site of restriction endonuclease cleavage (a restriction site). Differences in DNA sequence (**polymorphism or mutation**) can *create or abolish a site of restriction endonuclease cleavage* (a **restriction site**) and thus *result in variation in length of restriction fragments.* If DNA of an individual has **gained a restriction site**, then restriction enzyme cleavage *yields at least one additional fragement.* And if mutation cause a **loss of restriction site** *fewer fragments are produced.* Two types of DNA variation that result in RFLP are.

Single nucleotide polymorphism (SNPs, pronounced Snips) or site polymorphism

- It is DNA variation that just *involves single base.* SNPs are *responsible for 90% of human genome* variation.
- Typically the SNPs are *biallelic* (i.e., only two choices exist at a given site) and can occur anywhere in genome – within intron, exon or intergenic regions. However, *<1% of SNPs occur in coding region.*
- Serve both as physical landmark within the genome & as a genetic marker whose transmission can be followed from – parent to child. It *is genetic marker of choice for* study of complex genetic traits.

Length polymorphism / Tandem repeats

- Human DNA contains short repetitive sequence of non coding DNA. This ***variable number of tandem (one after another) repeats* (VNTR), is unique for any individual & therefore serve as a molecular finger print**
- It may be of two types

Microsatellite DNA polymorphism

- ***Short (2-6 base pairs) inherited tandem repeats of usually < 1kb***[Q]
- Occurs ~ 50,000-1 lac times in human

Minisatellite repeats

- Larger *(1-3 kb)*, & repeat motifs is usually *15-70 base pairs.*

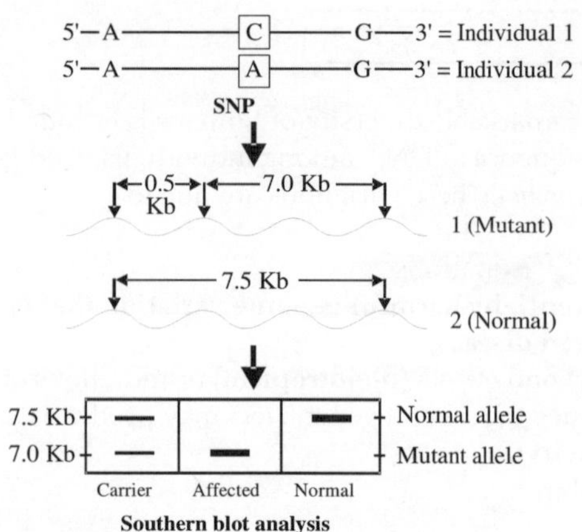

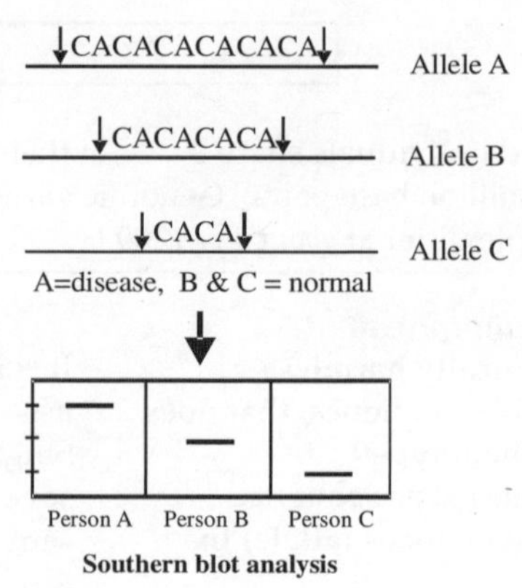

- **Procedure**

DNA sample is treated with **restriction endonuclease enzymes** which cleaves DNA in restriction fragments of defined length. These fragments are **separated by agarose gel electrophoresis on the basis of size. Detection** of RFLP relies **on southern blotting hybridization** procedure. DNA is denatured by soaking agarose get in alkali, and then blotted on to nylon (nitrocellulose) paper

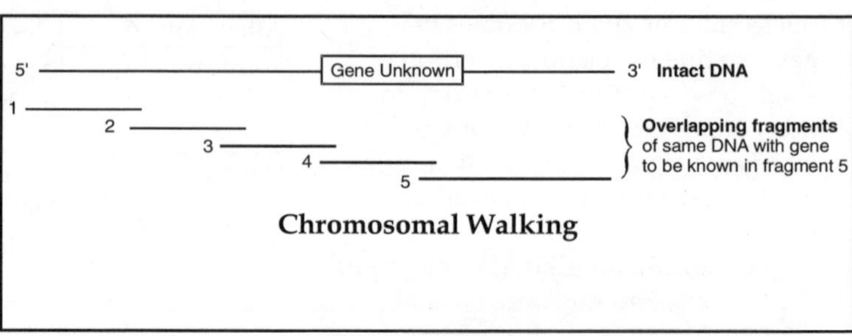

Chromosomal Walking

to reproduce the distribution RFs in gel. This *nitrocellulose membrane is immersed in radioactively labeled DNA probe* (southern-blotting). Autoradiography (x-ray exposure to film) reveals the fragments to which the probe hybridizes. The method is *very accurate*: However, it *requires large samples of undergraded DNA (>25ng)* that is often not available at crime scene.

- **Clinical Applications of RFLP**

- **Tracing chromosome from parent to offspring:** An individual who is heterozygous for a polymorphism has a sequence variation in the DNA of one chromosome and not in the DNA of companion (homolgous) chromosome. In such cases each chromosome can be traced from parent to offspring by determining the absence or presence of polymorphism. This is useful in **disputed parenthood.**
- **Prenatal diagnosis of genetic disease:** Disease will produce alteration in size & distribution of RE fragments of DNA obtained from fetus (blood, amniotic fluid or chorionic villi). Examples include

1. *Sickel cell anemia* can be directly diagnosed by RFLP, as the point ($A \rightarrow T$) mutation *abolishes recognition site of restriction endonuclease mst II* that recognizes nucleotide sequence CCTNAGG (N = any nucleotide). Normal DNA digested with Mst II yields a 1.15 kb fragment whereas a 1.35 kb fragment is generated from β^Sgene.
2. *Phenyl ketonuria* can be indirectly diagnosed using RFLP. Mutation in phenylalanine hydroxylase (PAH) gene do not directly affect any RE site. To establish diagnosis one has *to analyze DNA of affected family member with a goal to identify genetic markers or variants (RFLP) that are tightly linked to the disease.* Once these polymorphism marker that are consistently / closely linked to a disease producing mutation gene – (ie they closely show close linkage and are coinherited) are identified. The RFLP analysis can be carried out for prenatal diagnosis.

- **RFLP results from single base changes /mutation (eg sickle cell disease)** or **from deletions or insertions (copy number variations = CNVs)** of DNA into a restriction fragment (eg thalssemias) and have proved to be **useful diagnostic tools**. Thy have been found at known gene loci and in sequence that have no known function; thus RFLPs may disrupt the function of gene or may have no apperent biological consequence.
- **RFLPs / SNPs are inherited in mendilian fashion**, so these can be used in *definition of inherited disease in which the functional deficit is unknown.* RFLPs / SNPs can be used to **establish linkage** groups, which in turn by the process of **chromosomal walking**, will eventually **define the disease locus**. Chromosomal walking involves *repeated cloning of overlapping DNA segments (of 100-200 kb) to isolate/determine any gene in unknown location of large piece of DNA. In chromosomal walking, a fragment representing one end of long piece of* DNA is used to isolate the next overlapping segment. The direction of extension is determined by restriction mapping and the procedure is repeated sequentially until the desired sequence is obtained. **X chromosome linked disorders** are particularly amenable to chromosomal walking since only a single allele is expressed and a complete **linkage map (& genomic sequence)** of this chromosome have been determined. The gene for X-linked disorder **Duchenne muscular dystrophy** was found using RFLPS (& chromosomal walking). Similarly, defect was localized (linked) to terminal region of short arm of chromosome 4 in **Huntington disease** and to alpha-globin locus on chromosome 16 in **polycystic disease**.

- Comparison of **genetic makeup** of humans & related species **(genetic maping)**
- **For DNA finger printing (DNA typing or DNA profiling):** Alee Jaffreys described this technique in 1985. It is based on **sequence polymorphisms** (slight sequence differences) between individuals. It is a potent weapon of crime detection (forensic medicine).

1. *Some sequence changes affects restriction site and result in RFLPs.* It is very accurate method but requires larg sample of undergraded DNA (>25ng). That amount of DNA is often not available at a crime scene.
2. More sensitive DNA typing method use PCR and focus on **short tandem repeats (STRs)**. An STR locus is a short DNA sequence, repeated many times in tandem at a particular location in a chromosome; mostly & 4bp long. The DNA sequences flanking STR are unique to each type of STR & identical (except for very rare mutations) in all humans. PCR primers are added to this flanking DNA & designed to amplify the DNA across the STR. Since each human inherits one chromosome from each parent, the STR lengths on two chromosomes are often different generating 2 signals from 1 individuals. If multiple STR loci are analyzed, *a profile can be generated that is essentially unique to a particular individual.* PCR amplification allows DNA fingerprints to be obtained from **< 1ng of partially degraded DNA**, an amount that can be obtained from a single hair follicle, a drop of blood, a small semen sample that might be months or years old. Combined DNA Index System **(CODIS)** uses **13 STR loci** for DNA typing in USA. The **amelogenin gene** present on human sex chromosome, has slightly different flanking DNA on X and Y chromosomes. It is used as a marker for sex determination of DNA donor. **Multiplex STR kits** include 13 CODIS loci, amelogenin and 2 additional loci (total 16) . The chances of accidental match between two individuals in human population is < 1 in 10^8 (quintillion).

Microsatellites

- Microsatellites" are defined as loci (or regions within DNA sequences) where short sequences of DNA (nucleotides; adenine- A, thiamine- T, guanine- G, cytosine- C) are repeated in tandem arrays. This means that the sequences are repeated one right after the other. The lengths of sequences used most often are di-, tri-, or tetra-nucleotides.
- They can be used for DNA fingerprinting, in forensic and paternity/parentage work. At the same location within the genomic DNA the number of times the sequence (eg.AC) is repeated often varies between individuals, within population, and/or between species. So one population may commonly have 13 AC's (dinucleotide repeat sequence) repeated in a row while another population has 18 AC's repeated at the same location within the genomic DNA.
- Predicting the progression of disease: Microsatellites are acutely prone to replication errors that result in expansions and contractions of repeat unit (repeat length variability) because of misalignment of the template and daughter strands. Variability of microsatellite repeat lengths leads to genomic instability and, plays a role in the progression of disease, presumably by gene inactivation. DNA mismatch repair (MMR) enzymes maintain genomic stability by removing replication errors from DNA.
- Defective DNA mismatch repair (MMR) enzymes in association with microsatellite instability (MSI) are thus implicated in the progression of several diseases and cancers. Examples includes : Fragile syndrome, Huntington's chorea, Myotonic dystroply, Spinobulbar muscular atrophy, Kennedy's disease, Hereditary non polyposis colon cancer
- Provides clue to genetic bases of disease: The association of a specific polymorphism in affected family members and the lack of this association in unaffected members may be the first clue about genetic bases of a disease.

DNA Fingerprinting (DNA Typing or Profiling)

- *Alec J. Jeffrey*[Q] of Leicester University (U.K), in 1984 serendipitously discovered *fundamentals of genetic finger printing.*
- Because every person's DNA sequence is different, the fragment in DNA specimen from one individual to another are different in number & length. DNA finger printing uses restriction fragment length polymorphism (RFLP) or repeat sequence DNA to establish a unique pattern of DNA fragments for an individual. The DNA markers analyzed for such finger printing are most commonly ***short tandem repeat polymorphisms.*** VNTR (variable number of tandem repeats) are short sequences of DNA at scattered locations in genome, repeated in tandem (one after another) that give rise to polymorphism in chromosome. Short tandem repeats are similar to VNTR but smaller in size.
- **DNA fingerprinting (by PCR)** has revolutinized the analysis of evidence from crime scenes in determining whether the ***sample comes from specific individual and varification of paternity***[Q]. DNA fingerprinting is ***done by nucleated cells***[Q] eg ***blood***[Q] (WBC & RBC), semen, vaginal epithelial cells, tooth pulp, bone marrow, hair roots, muscle, skin, mucous membrane.

Polymerase Chain Reaction (PCR) 

- PCR, invented by **Karry Mullis**, is an **in vitro (test tube) enzymatic method of amplifying** a **selected (target) sequence of DNA**. It is like *Xerox machine for gene copying*. It is **sensitive, selective (specific) and extremely rapid means of amplifying any desired DNA sequence** which can be as short as 50-100 bp and as long as 10kb.
- It is so sensitive that it allows the DNA in a single cell, sperm or hair follicle; from any source – virus, bacteria, plant, animal or, human even when the targetedsequence makes up less than one part in a million of the total initial sample to be amplified. PCR has allowed successful **enzymatic cloning** of DNA from > 40,000 years old sample.
- **Specificity** is based on the use of 2 ***oligonucleotide primers that hybridize to complementary sequences on opposite strands of separated ds (double standed) DNA***[Q]. (So ds DNA is required not SS DNA).
- Each newly synthesized strand can act as a template for the successive cycles thus each cycle of amplification **doubles the amount of DNA** in sample resulting in an **exponential increase** in target DNA, hence the name **polymerase chain reaction**. Typically *20-30 cycles* run during PCR amplify the DNA by a *million to billion folds in a few hours*. 20 cycles provide amplification of 2^{20} (i.e. 10^6) and 30 cycles 2^{30} (i.e. 10^9).
- Major **advantages of PCR over traditional cloning methods** (using recombinant DNA techniques), as a mechanism for amplifying specific DNA sequence are *sensitivity, speed and less technical difficulty*. It is an **in vitro (test tube)** method not requiring living cell. The cycles are generally repeated by automated **Tempcycler**.
- The **double stranded (ds) DNA** is first heated to separate (melt) the 2 strands of template DNA containing the target sequence (**denaturation**); Vast excess of **2 primers** (one for each flanking sequence) is added and allowed to bind DNA (**annealing** or **priming**); each DNA strand is copied by **thermostable DNA (Taq) polymerase enzyme** obtained from Thermus aquaticus, starting from the primer sites **(chain extension)** in presence of **all 4 dXTPs / dNTPs (deoxyribo nucleoside triphosphate**). So it is **enzymatic (non-recombinant) DNA amplification**. The cycles of denaturation, annealing & chain extension are repeated.
- **Clinical applications of PCR** *utilize its ability to amplifly (increase) the minimal (or almost negligable) amount of DNA*, which is then detected by southern blot technique. So it is used in detecting low abundance nucleic acid sequence (DNA). For example.

Detection of infectious disease

- To detect bacterial, viral etc infectious disease agents in early and latent phase (when the agent load is very less). So PCR offers rapid & sensitive method of detecting viruses that have long latency such as HIV.
- Can detect even one virus or bacteria present in sample
- To detect viral load by reality-PCR

★ PCR uses cells obtained from amniocentesis or chorionic villus sampling for prenatal diagnosis; somatic cells for postnatal dignosis and nucleated cells for finger printing.

Detection of variations & mutations in genes

- To ***detect allelic polymorphism, specific aneuploidy***[Q]; to compare normal cloned gene with an uncloned mutant gene and to study evolution using DNA from archeological samples.
- PCR (f/b electrophoresis & southern blot) is used for detection of **direct mutational analysis to prenatally or postnatally diagnose** the presence or absence of inherited disorders like ***Cystic fibrosis, hemophilia, β-thalassemia & sickle cell anemia etc***[Q]. It also detects carriers.
- Detects DNA abnormalities characteristic to cancer and establish precise tissue types for transplantation.
- For quantitative RNA analysis after RNA copying & m-RNA quantitation by RT-PCR (using retroviral reverse transcriptase).
- To score in vivo protein – DNA occupancy using chromatin immunoprecipitation assay.

PCR in Law

- **DNA fingerprinting** by means of PCR has revolutionized *forensic analysis of crime scene and paternity verification*. The DNA markers analyzed for such fingerprinting are most commonly *short tandem repeat polymorphism*.
- Sex determination

Steps of a PCR

- **Each *cycle doubles the amount of DNA*** in the sample, leading to an *exponential (logarithmic) increase in DNA* with repeated cycles. Steps in each cycle are.

1. **Primer construction**:- **Flanking sequence** is nucleotide sequence of short segment on each side of *target DNA*. It brackets the DNA *sequence of interest*. In PCR ***it is not necessary to know the nucleotide sequence of target DNA but it is necessary to know the flanking sequence***[Q].

Types of PCR

1. Conventional DNA based PCR
2. **Reverse transcriptase PCR (RT-PCR)**
   - In this mRNA or rRNA is starting material which is converted to *complementary DNA (c-DNA) by reverse transcriptase*. So it is a normal PCR preceded by reverse transcription
   - **Tth polymerase** (instead of Taq polymerase) from *Thermus thermophilus* is used which has both reverse transcriptase & DNA polymerase activity.
   - In normal PCR, DNA is detected which could be from living or non living organism but in RT-PCR, mRNA is detected indicating its origin from living organism (only living cells chang DNA to mRNA).

- Two *synthetic single stranded oligonucleotides* (usually 20-35 nucleotides long) which are ***complementary to respective flanking sequence***Q are constructed. These serve as primers. ***The 3′- OH end of each primer points towards the target sequence***Q**.** Primer is added in vast excess.

2. **Denaturation of DNA duplex (94-98°C).** The DNA to be amplified is heated to seperated double stranded DNA (ds DNA) into single strands. (SSDNA)
3. **Annealing of primers to SSDNA (37-60°C).** Separated strands are cooled & allowed to ***bind (anneal) to the 2 primers (one for each strand) at flanking sequence***Q. Primer is added in vast excess.
4. **Chain extension of primer (~72°C)**

- ***DNA polymerase & deoxyribo nucleoside triphosphate (d-NTP)***Q are **added in excess** to initiate synthesis of two new chains complementary to original DNA chains, *starting at primer site.* ***DNA polymease adds nucleotides to 3¹- OH end of primer***Q and strand grows across the target DNA making complementary copies of target.
- ***Magnesium concentration is critical***Q as it affects DNA polymerase activity and fidelity, denaturation temperature , primer annealing & dimer formation and PCR specificity. 0.5-5mM is usually used Mg^{++} concentration. Excess results in *accumulation of nonspecific amplification products seen as multiple bands on agarose gel, whereas, insufficient* Mg^{++} *result in reduced* yield of desired PCR products.

• Cycles of heat denaturation (seperation), annealing (binding) of primers to flanking sequence and extension of annealed primer with DNA polymerase are repeated. Initially, *E.coli DNA polymerase* was used in PCR, that was destroyed & so has to be added by each heat denaturation cycle. The advantage of using thermostable DNA polymerase (such as ***Taq polymerase from a thermophilic bacteria Thermus aquaticus***Q***) is that the enzyme itself is not denatured and therefore does not have to be added at each successive cycle***Q.

• The amplified DNA sequences can be analyzed by *gel electrophoresis & ethidium bromide staining, southern hybridization (blotting), direct sequence determination, RFLP / sequencing and incorporation of biotin / digoxigenin labeled dUTP during amplification and detection by colorimetric / luminescent techniques.*

So it is used in *expression mapping* i.e. determining when & where certain genes are expressed.

3. **Asymmetrical PCR** is used to generate single strands by adjusting primer concentrations to favor one strand. After 10-15 cycles the second primer is used up and only one strand complementary to first strand continues to be copied up.
4. **Inverse PCR** amplifies the sequences on either side of known stretch by circularizing a piece of DNA & hybridizing primers in an opposite orientation.
5. **Nested PCR**, improves *sensitivity & specificity by using 2 sets of primers in 2 successive PCR runs.* This means a fragment is amplified by using a set of primers (eg genus specific) and second amplification of some internal sequence is done by using another set of primers in first run product.

- This reduces contamination in products d/t amplification of unexpected primer binding sites but requires more detailed knowledge of sequence and proves hybridization may not be necessary.

6. **Anchored (one sided) PCR or RACE** (rapid amplification of (cDNA ends)

- It is used to amplify the ends of m-RNA transcripts when one end of sequence is known using a specialized *reverse transcription – (RT) PCR*
- To unknown end a segment of *guanine is covalently* attached which serves as template with polycytosine primer. It is used to obtain (amplify) unknown 5′ end (5′ RACE-PCR) or 3′ end (3′ RACE-PCR).

7. **PCR using other DNA polymerases**

- ***DNA ligase in ligation amplification reactions***Q
- **T7 RNA polymerase** in transcription based systems
- **Q β replicase** from bacteriophage

8. **In situ** (paraffin embedded or cytospin coated glass slides) **PCR amplification** (by protease + DNA polymerase) **and product detection** (by hybridization or direct incorporation of biotin / digoxigenin labeled nucleotides)
9. **Real Time PCR (RT- PCR)** has many advantages over conventional RT-PCR

- **RT-PCR or quantitative (q)PCR, combines PCR (DNA) amplification and detection into a single step** by eliminating gel electrophoresis for detection. *It is a software driven automated easy to perform procedure that can be easily standardized. It has higher sensitivity, specificity, reproducibility and sample output (~ 200 samples / day)*
- Allows for *quantitative measurement* and rapidity d/t reduced cycle times & removal of post PCR detection procedure. The amplicon could be visualized as amplification progressed. It is **used to know *how much amplification of DNA has occurred***Q.
- ***All real time PCR rely upon fluorescent reporter (probes) such as SYBER – green, Taq man, and molecular Beacons***Q for detection & quantitation. The signal of which increases in ***direct proportion to the amount of PCR product in reaction*** **[Quantitative Real time PCR (RQ-PCR)].**
- It can detect viral load *(no. of viruses present in sample) so help planning treatment.*

10. **Quantitative (Q-) PCR** (preferably real time) is used to quantify PCR product i.e. determining whether a sequence is present or not and if it is present the number of copies in sample.
11. **Multiplex PCR** uses multiple – unique primer sets within a single PCR targeting multiple genes in a single test run that would otherwise reuire several repeated PCR runs.

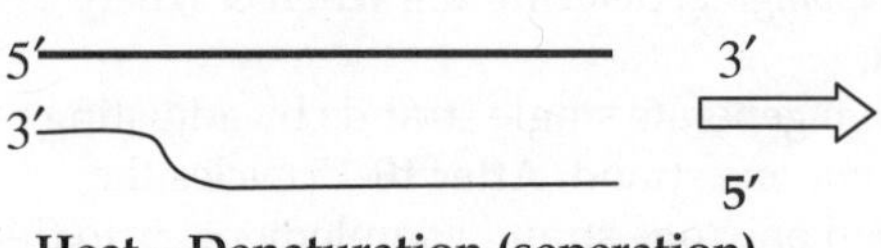

Heat – Denaturation (seperation)

Flanking Sequence Target Sequence Flanking Sequence

5′ 3′

Direction of chain growth ← 3′ 5′ Primer

Primer

5′ 3′ → Direction of Growth

3′ 5′

Annealing & chain extension

5′ 3′

3′ 5′

5′ 3′

3′ 5′

Formation of double copy

Detection of pre or post natal disease with known mutation eg cystic fibrosis, sickle cell anemia, β-thallasemia & hemophila

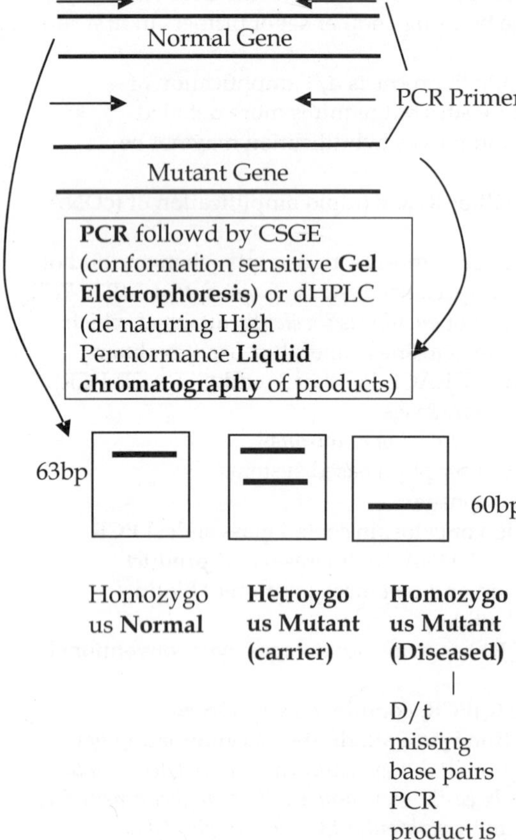

Direct Mutation Analysis (eg by **PCR**)	**Indirect linkage Analysis**
Involves *identification of specific base pair change or mutation responsible for disease*	Involves *segregation of genetic markers known to be linked to a gene* responsible for disease. And it is determined that wheres an individual inherited a chromose present in family that carries the abnormal gene
As it is a direct method, not based on segregation of genetic markers in family members, it does not require DNA analysis of multiple family members.	DNA analysis of multiple family members is required to identify the markers that segregate with abnormal chromosome in each affected pedigree
Involves physical isolation and sequencing of gene	Dose not involve physical isolation & sequencing of gene
Determines unequivocally whether suspect has inherited the disease or not. So has become **gold standard**	Being less specific it's use is restricted to genetic diseases if mutation sequence is not known.

Ligase Chain Reaction (LCR)

- LCR, is amplification of target DNA after multiple rounds of denaturation, annealing & ligation of two pairs of synthetic nucleotide (which hybridize to complementary strands of a target DNA) with a thermostable ligase
- **Gap- LCR** reduces the background generated by target independent blunt end ligation. In this DNA polymerase fills in a gap b/w annealed probes which are sub sequently joined by DNA ligase.

Nucleic Acid Sequence Based Amplification

- NASBA is a *continuous, isothermal, enzyme based* method of nucleic acid *amplification. It amplifies RNA (especially or DNA* from a pool of total nucleic acid.
- It uses a mixture of *reverse transcriptase, RNA polymerase, ribonuclease- H, and 2 transcript specific DNA primers*
- 5[1] extension of *forward primer* contain promoter sequence for bacteriophage T7 DNA dependent RNA polymerase and 5[1] extension of *reverse primer* has complementary binding sequence for an electro chemiluminescent (ECL) tag.

★ **DNA sequencing** is the process of determining the exact order of 3 billion bases (A,T, C & G) that make up the DNA of 24 different human chromosomes.

Gene / DNA / Molecular Cloning

- It is a technique by which large number of identical DNA molecules can be produced. In this technique a DNA fragment to be cloned (amplified) is inserted into the DNA strands of cloning vector eg. plasmid, phages or cosmids to make a new recombinant or chimeric DNA. When the DNA strand of vector multiplies, it also multiplies the inserted DNA fragment. Clones produced is later removed by using restriction enzymes.
- Cloning of DNA fragment involves 4 steps
  - **Fragmentation** by *restriction endonuclease* involves isolation of DNA of intrest (that is to be cloned) and linearization of circular vector DNA that contain same sticky ends
  - **Ligation** is gluing together of DNA of interest with vector DNA to make a new recombinant or chimeric DNA molecules, by DNA ligase enzyme.
  - **Transfection** is inserting newly formed pieces into cells. And finally the cells are cultured. In this way the chimeric DNA (so the DNA of interest) is amplified.
  - **Screening or selection** ***for selecting or identifying the cells that have been successfully transfected with the vector DNA containing the desired insertional DNA sequence in the required orientation***Q. This can be done by.

Antibiotic resistance markers

Allow only cells in which the vector has been transfected, to grow

Colour selection markers which provide blue white screening (α-factor complementation) on X- gal (a colourless galactose sugar) medium

It is based on *lac operon*. The hydrolysis of x-gal by β glactosidase cause blue colour in colonies & indicate that colonies contain unligated vector. Whereas, white colonies indicate insertion of foreign DNA & loss of cells ability to hydrolyse marker.

PCR, restriction fragment analysis & or DNA sequencing

Congirmatory method

Hybridoma Cells and Monoclonal Antibodies

- Generally when an antigen is injected into an animal it results in formation of *polyclonal (not monospecific)* antibodies by mixture of B cells. These antibodies are directed against a number of different sites (epitomes or determinants on antigen).
- By **Kohler- Milstein** method, limitless amounts of **monoclonal – monospecific** (specific for one epitope)antibodies can be obtained, by producing **hybridoma cell**. The method involves **cell fusion** & resulting permanent cell line is called a **hybridoma**.
- **B cells** previously ***treated with an antigen***Q or mixture of antigens & obtained from mouse spleen are mixed with **mouse myeloma** cells in presence of PEG (polyethylene glycol). PEG causes cell fusion and formation of **hybridoma cell**, which when cloned produce **monoclonal monospecific** antibodies.
- Hybridoma cells can be *frozen & stored and subsequently thawed* when more of antibody is required; this ensures its long term supply. It can also be grown in the abdomen of mice, providing relatively large supplies of antibodies. Attempts to produce human monoclonal antibodies are under-way.
- **Monoclonal antibodies** are produced by **hybridoma technology (in vitro)** or by one clone secreting specific type of antibody in **multiple myeloma (in vivo)**. In **monoclonal antibody preparation** all molecules ***are specific against a particular antigen***Q and have **increased avidity** for attaching with antigen. So in a reaction where polyclonal antibodies require 1ml the **monoclonals require very little (only 1 microliter) quantity**. So the initial cost of production may be high but it decreases gradually in long run.
- Monoclonal antibodies are now useful in detection of **1) serum proteins, 2) enzymes, 3) hormones, 4) drugs 5) bacterial & viral antigens, 6) cell surface receptors, 7) HLA antigen, and 8) Cancer cells etc**

Myeloma cell	B Cell
- Do not produce antibody - Immortal - HGPRT-ve rendering salvage path of purine	- Produce specific antibody - Not immortal - HGPRT +ve

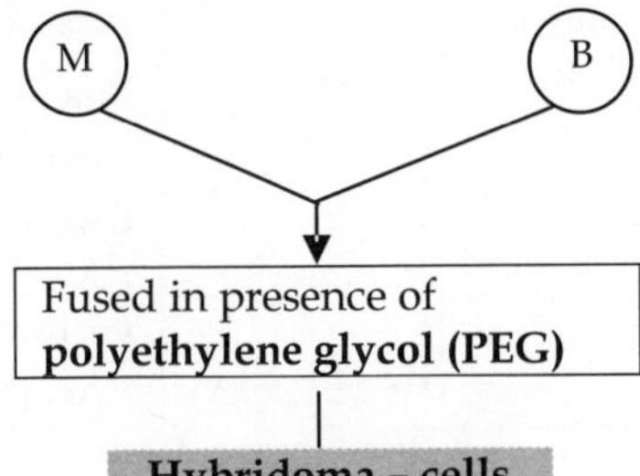

Hybridoma – cells

- Immortalized (like parental myeloma cell)
- Produce antibody & are HGPRT +ve (gained from parental B- cells

Grown in presence of **HAT (Hypoxanthine – aminopterinthymidine)** containing medium

- **Monoclonal monospecific antibodies** are used in
  - To measure the amounts of many individual proteins
  - To determine nature of infectious agent
  - To subclassify both normal (eg lymphocytes) & tumor cells (eg leukemia)
  - To direct therapeutic agents to tumor cells
  - To accelerate removal of drug (eg digoxin) from circulation in toxicities
  - ***Nephelometric assays of blood components** and **blood grouping***[Q]
  - As **immunosuppressants** in clinical conditions like autoimmune disease (Rheumatoid disease)
  - To do ELISA tests
  - Monoclonal antibodies made in mice can be **humanized** (used in humans) by attaching the *complementarity determining regions [CDRs)* (i.e. the sites that binds antigen) onto appropriate sites in a human immunoglobin molecule. This produces an antibody that is very similar to human antibody, thus markedly decreasing immunogenecity & chances of anaphylactic reactions
  - **Quantitative preparation of specific cells and pure antigens**

B Cell will die in medium as they are not immortal

Myeloma cell will also die in presence of HAT, since the aminopterine in HAT suppress purine synthesis by denovo pathway by inhibiting reutilization of tetrahydrofolate

Hybridoma cell will **survive & grow** because they are hypoxanthine – guanine-phosphoribosyl-transferase (HGPRT) +

If cloned produce **monoclonal monospecific antibodies**

Cloning Vectors

Plasmid
- Accept DNA pieces about *6- 10 kb long*
- *Small, circular,* duplex DNA molecules
- Confer *antibiotic resistance to host cell*
- Its complete DNA sequence is known hence precise location of restriction cleavage site for inserting the foreign DNA is available

Phages
- Accept *DNA fragment 10-20 kb long*
- *Linear DNA molecule* into which foreign DNA can be inserted at several restriction enzyme sites.

Cosmids
- ***Accept larger fragment of DNA, 35-50 kb long***[Q]**.**
- Are plasmids that contain DNA sequence, called *cos sites*, required for packaging lambda DNA into phage particle.

Cloning Capacities

Vector	DNA insert size
Plasmid, PBR322	0.01- 10kb (kilobases)
Phage	10- 20kb
Cosmid	***35- 50kb***[Q]
BAC (bacterial artificial chromosome), PAC (E. Coli bacteriophage P1 based) vectors	50- 250kb
YAC (Yeast artificial chromosome)	500- 3000kb

Site Directed Mutagenesis: Alternation in cloned genes produce modified proteins

Cloning can be used not only to overproduce proteins but to produce protein products with *subtle alteration in native* forms. Specific aminoacids may be replaced by **site directed mutagenesis** in two ways

If the appropriate (known) restriction sites flank the sequence to be altered, researchers can simply remove a DNA segment & replace it with a synthetic one that is identical to original except for the desired change

- When known restriction sites are not present, **oligonucleotide - directed mutagenesis** can create a specific DNA sequence change
- A short synthetic DNA strand with a specific base change is annealed to single stranded copy o cloned gene. The mismatch of a single base pair in 15-20 bp does not prevent annealing at appropriate temperatures.
- This annealed strand acts as a primer for synthesis of a duplex DNA (with one mismatch), which is then used to transform cells.
- Cellular DNA repair systems will remove and replace the altered base and restore the gene to its original sequence in 50% cases whereas, ***the other half will remove and replace the normal base , retaining the desired mutation***Q
- Changes can also be introduced that involve more than 1 basepair. Or even the parts of 2 genes can be ligated to create **fused gene** and **fusion protein**.

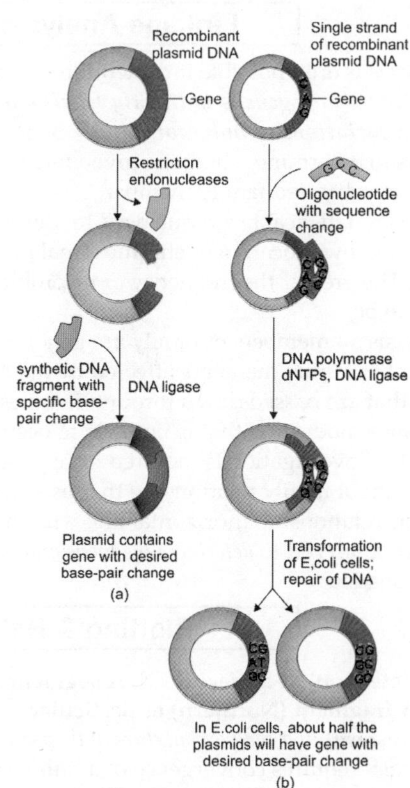

Two approaches to site-directed mutagenesis

Site Specific Recombination (Exchange) / SSR

SSR occurs only at a particular short (20-200 bp), unique DNA sequence - the **recombination site (RS)**, where the recombinase enzyme acts. Recombination sites recognized by site specific recombinase are **non palindromic** ***(partially asymmetrical)***Q and 2 sites align in same orientation during reaction . The outcome depends on location & orientation of recombination sites. If 2 sites are on

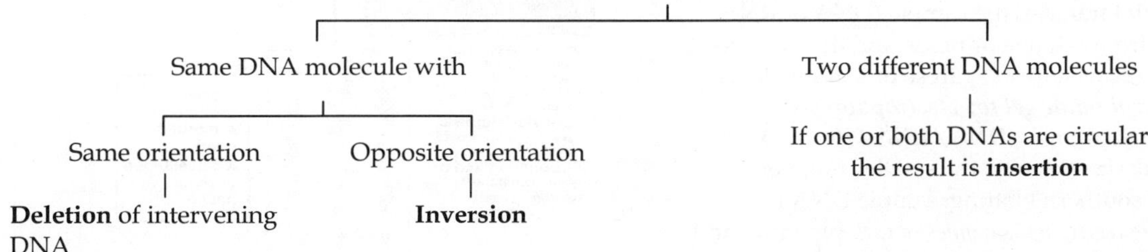

- ***Recombinase is a site specific endonuclease and ligase in one package***Q. Auxillary proteins may regulate timing or outcome of reaction.
- 2 classes of SSR system, with rely on either **Tyr** or **Ser** residues in the active site. A separate recombinase recognize and bind to each RS on same or two different DNA molecules. One DNA strand in each site is cleaved at a specific point & recombinase becomes covalently linked to DNA at cleavage site through phospho tyrosine bond. This transient protein DNA linkage preserves phosphodiester bond that is lost in cleaving the DNA so ATP is unnecessary in subsequent steps. The cleaved DNA strands are rejoined to new parteners to form **Holliday intermediates**, with new phosphodiester bonds created at the expense of protein DNA linkage. The reaction is completed by repeating the process at a 2nd point within each of 2 RS.
- SRS system that employ an **Ser residue active site** , ***both strands of each RS are cut concurrently & rejoined to new partners without the Holliday intemediates***Q. In both systems, ***exchange is precise and reciprocal***Q, regenerating RS when the reaction is complete.

Linkage Analysis : Indirect DNA Diagnosis

- Direct gene diagnosis is only possible if nucleotide sequence of mutant gene is known, which is not the case in most genetic disorders. Therefore ***mutant gene is indirectly tracked on the basis of its linkage to detectable genetic markers such as naturally occuring variations or polymorphism***[Q]; SNPs, RFLP, STRs (short tandem repals or micro satellites)
- In essence, one has to determine whether a given fetus or family member has inherited the same relevent chromosomal region as a previously affected family member.
- **Linkage analysis** is a statistical technique used to identify location on a chromosome of a given gene involved in a trait or disease relative to a known location of chromosomal marker, in terms of recombination frequency rather than as a specific physical distance. The greater the frequency of recombintion (segregation) between two genetic markers, the farther apart they are assumed to be.
- With linkage analysis all members of family are genotyped for polymorphic markers and then compared to determine which markers are present in family members affected by the disorder. So the primary aim is to determine whether there exist pieces of genome that are passed down through families (with multiple patients) in a pattern that is consistent with a particular inheritance model and that is unlikely to occur by chance alone. Since linkage analysis does not detect mutations in gene directly, further investigation is required once genome of interest is identified.
- **Pedigree** is a diagram of family relationship that uses symbols to represent people (square = male, circle = female) and lines to represent genetic relationship (horizontal line = mating, vertical line extending downward from a couple represent their children). It is often analyzed to *determine the mode of inheritance (dominant or recessive)*. All the individuals that possess the trait / disease are shaded.

Blotting & Hybridization Techniques ☆

- **Visualization (or detection) of a specific DNA segment (Southern) or RNA fragment (Northern) or particular antigen/protein (Western)** *in a complex mixture of thousands of containinating molecules* requires convergence of a number of techniques (like *restriction enzymes, Agarose / SDS-PAGE electrophoresis, denaturing, blotting renaturing, fixing, probe hybridization* which are collectively termed **blot transfer**.
- Blot technique was developed by EM Southern in 1975, to detect a specific segment of DNA in the whole genome. Southern blotting is named after its inventor, *Edward Southern* and others (northern, western) began as laboratory jargon.

Procedure

- **Electrophoresis**: For blot transfer, the sample (DNA or RNA or protein) is isolated from cell line or tissue and this complex mixture is pipetted into a well in an agarose or ***sodium dodecyl sulfate (SDS) – polyacrylamide gel for electrophoresis. Electrophoresis seperates sample (DNA / RNA / Protein) according to molecular size (mass)***[Q]; the smaller fragments more most rapidly. In southern blotting, sample DNA is *digested with one or more restriction enzymes* before pipetting and ***exposed to direct electrical current during electrophoresis. DNA being negatively changed move towards anode***[Q].
- **Blotting (Adsorption / Transfer) to Nitrocellulose (Nylon) membrane:** DNA / RNA / Protein within the gel is transferred **(blotted or adsorbed) over to nitrocellulose or nylon paper (membrane)** by covering the gel with paper, resulting in an exact replica of the pattern on the gel. In Southern blotting, *DNA is denatured by exposure to mild alkali (like NaOH) to make it single stranded* before adsorption. During the transfer the SDS is largely removed from some proteins, and there is enough refolding & restoration of conformation so that the antibody probe can react with protein on membrane.

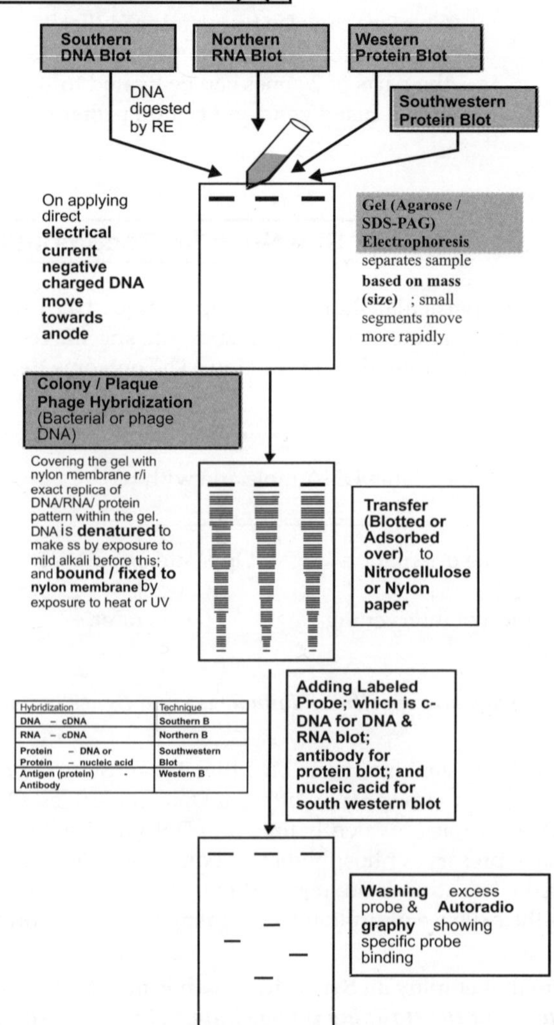

Hybridization	Technique
DNA – cDNA	Southern B
RNA – cDNA	Northern B
Protein – DNA or Protein – nucleic acid	Southwestern Blot
Antigen (protein) - Antibody	Western B

- **Adding Probe & Hybridization:** Before adding probe, DNA is bound (fixed) on the nitrocellulose membrane by exposure to *heat (temp at 80°c) and or UV*. Then paper is **exposed to labeled probe**. The probe is **complementary DNA strand** (c-DNA) labeled with radioisotope or nonradioactive fluorescent label in Southern (DNA) and Northern (RNA) blot tests. *The nucleotide sequence of cDNA is complementary to DNA or RNA*. There will be many DNA/RNA fragments on membrane but only few pieces that contain the target DNA / RNA, hybridize with cDNA probe to make a **DNA-cDNA hybrid in Southern blot or RNA-cDNA hybrid in Northern blot.** Similarly a **labeled antibody probe forms complex with protein (antigen)** in **Western (immuno) blot test** and **labeled nucleic acid probe forms complex with protein in south-Western blot test**.
- **Washing & Autoradiography:** After thorough washing to remove excess probes, the x-ray plate or imaging screen is placed over the nitrocellulose paper in dark for few days. The radiation from fixed probe will produce its *marks in form of several specific bands corresponding to the DNA/RNA/ protein fragment that recognized the probe.*

Variants

- In **Southwestern hybridization blot technique**, proteins are separated by electrophoresis, blotted to a membrane, renatured, and analyzed for an **protein-DNA (nucleic acid) interaction** by incubation with a specific labeled nucleic acid probe.
- **Colony or Plaque or Phage Hybridization** is a method by which **specific clones of bacteria or phage** grown as colonies on agar plate are **identified and purified.** Nitrocellulose paper is overlaid over agar plate sticking clones from each colony which are fixed permanently by heat (UV and denatured or lysed with NaOH so that its DNA is available to hybridize with cDNA probe. It results in a **clonal isolate (bacterial colony) or individual phage plaque** containing a unique DNA insert.

Use

- Blotting procedure are **useful in determining amount of gene (DNA)/RNA/ protein** in a given tissue / sample. If a specific base is changed and a restriction site is altered these procedures **can detect point mutations and gene alterations (deletion, insertion or rearrangements)** because the required electrophoresis step sepeates the molecules on the basis of size. Therefore Southern, Northern & Western blot transfer techniques are used to **size, identify and quantitate specific gene (DNA), RNA and protein – respectively**. Mutant genes like HbS, DMD, PKU & cystic fibrosis as well as presence of viral DNA (HBV, HBC) can be identified by Southern blot method. Similarly ***Western blot method confirms diagnosis of AIDS***[Q] (in ELISA positive or HIV positive patients) by demonstrating presence of antibodies in patients serum to a specific HIV protein.

All hybridization procedures depend on specific base pairing of complementary nucleic acid strands. **Perfect matches hybridize readily & withstand stringent conditions (high temperatures and low salt concentrations).** In the hybridization & washing reactions, less than perfect matches do not tolerate such stringent conditions; thus hybridization either never occur or is disrupted during washing steps. **Gene homology detection and cross species comparison of a gene can be done by varying stringency**.

Probes

DNA probe

- Probe is a *short single stranded piece of DNA*, labelled with a *radioisotope (eg P^{32})* or a *non- radioactive probe (eg. biotin)*, and can pick a specific gene or DNA sequence out of the mixture of thousands or millions of irrelevant DNA fragments cleaved by restriction endonucleases. The nucleotide sequence of a probe is *complementary* to the DNA of interest, called the **target DNA.**
- Utility of probes depends on *phenomenon of hybridization (or annealing)* in which a single stranded sequence of a target DNA binds to a probe containing a complementary nucleotide sequence.

Synthetic oligonucleotide probe

- If sequence of all or part of target DNA is known, single stranded oligonucleotide probes of 20-30 nucleotides can be synthesized that are complementary to gene of interest
- **Allele specific oligonucleotide (ASO)** probe is used to detect the presence of *sickel cell mutation in β-globin gene*

Biotinylated probes

- Disposal of radioactive probes is expansive, so *now vitamin biotin* coupled nucleotide are used to synthesize probes
- Biotin binds to egg white protein avidin. Avidin can be attached to fluorescent dye detectable optically with great sensitivity. Thus a DNA fragment that hybridizes with biotinylated probe can be made visible by immersing the gel in a solution of dye coupled avidin.

Antibodies

- When no information is available to guide the synthesis of a probe for direct detection of DNA of interest.
- In this case ***antibody labeled probe directed against the protein of interest***[Q] is used to identify which bacterial colony produces the protein & therefore contains CDNA of interest.

DNA-Microarray / DNA – Chips

- DNA microarrays *contain thousands* (500-5000) *of immobilized DNA probes /sequences* (few dozen to hundreds of nucleotide long) from known genes organized in an area no longer than a microscope slide. DNA segments (from DNA libraries) are *amplified by PCR* and placed on small wells in a solid polystyrene plates, using robotic devices. Upto million such spots are deposited in a predesigned array on a surface area of just few cm^2. An alternate way is to synthesize DNA directly on the solid surface using *photolithography.*
- C-DNA (obtained directly or from mRNA of patients particular cell type or stage) is added to each well, hybridize and fluorescence is assessed to assess genes being expressed in those cells/stage.
- This is based on principles of nucleic acid hybridization like Southern or Northern blot tests but allows simultaneous study of multiple genes or entire genome rather than single gene. Hybridization means binding of complementary strands of nucleic acid a/t Watson-Crick rules (i.e. A = T and G=C binding). *Southern blot for DNA & Northern blot for RNA allows the study /detection of single gene whereas microarray technique (for DNA & RNA) allows detection of multiple genes or entire genome.* So it can be considered as multiple Southern or Northern blot analysis running in parallel.

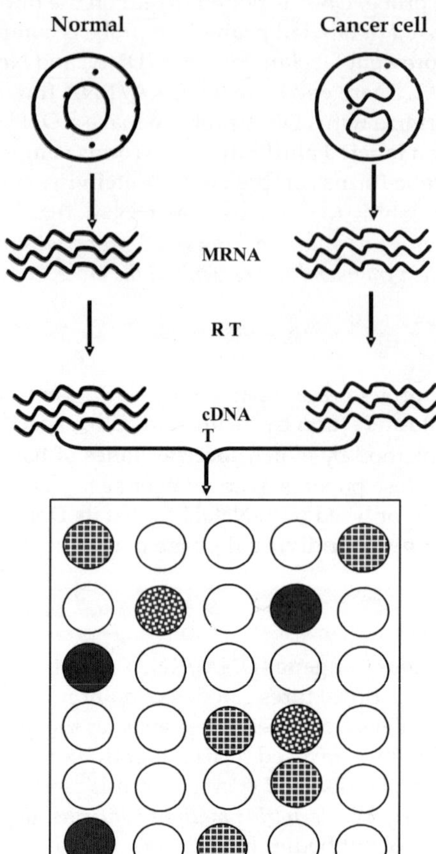

m-RNA is isolated **from 2 types of cells or cells** at 2 **stages of development**; each mRNA represents all genes expressed in that cell or stage.

Convert **mRNA to cDNA** by **reverse transcriptase, using fluorescently labeled deoxy ribonucleotide triphosphates**.

Add cDNAs to microarray; fluorescent cDNAs hybridize to complementary sequences on microarray

Each fluorescent spot represents a gene expressed in that cell or stage. Eg
- Green (crossed) spot for normal cells produce this.
- Red (plain) spot for cancer cells produce this
- Yellow or mixed (dotted spot for both cells produce this

DNA Microarray Analysis of gene expression

- Microarrays are used to analyze a sample for presence of **mutation / gene variation (genotyping)** or to determine the patterns of mRNA production (**gene expression analysis**).

- **For genotyping and mutational analysis**, the cellular sample is genomic DNA. **Microarray based CGH (comparative genomic hybridization)** test can be used as high resolution whole genome scan for the detection or screening of unknown (non specific) abnormalities, mutation or genomic imbalance including deletions, duplication and aneuploidies. Microarray based CGH cannot detect balanced translocations or inversions
- Microarray is the **most powerful tool for screening gene expression profile** of biological samples. It allows researcher to explore, *expression patterns of thousand of genes (or entire genome)* in a single analysis thus permitting **comprehensive analysis of gene expression profile**. For expression analysis the mRNA from a particular cell type (eg normal and cancer cells) or from same cell type in different stags of development is converted to cDNA & labeled with fluorescent tag. This mixture is then exposed to microarray chip. The amount of fluorescence bound to each spot is a measure of the amount of that particular mRNA in the sample. This tells which genes are expressed in which stage of development or in which cells. The spots that fluoresce provide a **snapshot of all genes being expressed** in the cells at the moment they were harvested – gene expression on genome wide scale.
- For a gene of unknown function, the time & circumstances of its expression can provide important *clues about its role in the cells.*
- **Tumor finger print or transcriptional profile** of cancers to tailor treatment regimens.
- *Genetic fingerprint* of different diseases / malignancies – classifying them, understanding genetic pathophysiology and identifying diagnostic or prognostic markers.

Methods for Analysis of Gene (DNA, Mutation) & Products Gene Expression (RNA and Protein)

Methods used for Detection of Mutation (& Analysis of Gene or DNA)

1. Cytogenic analysis
2. Fluorescent in situ hybridization (FISH)
3. ***Southern blot***Q
4. ***Polymerase chain reaction (PCR)***Q
5. ***Reverse transcriptase PCR (RT PCR)***Q
6. ***DNA sequencing and DNA cloning***Q
7. ***Restriction fragment polymorphism (RFLP)***Q
8. ***Single stranded conformational polymorphism (SSCP)***Q.
9. ***Denaturating gradient gel electrophoresis (DGGE)***Q
10. RNAse cleavage
11. Oligonucleotid specific hybridization
12. **Microarrays (c DNA microarrays or DNA chips)**
13. Protein truncation test (PTT).
14. **Pyrosequencing**
15. **Multiplex ligation dependent probe amplification (MLPA)**

Analysis of Gene Expression Product

Determination of mRNA levels

1. ***Northern blot***Q
2. **Microarrays**: In this mRNA from a particular cell is **converted to cDNA** and amplified by **RT-PCR or rererse transcriptase PCR**

Analysis of Proteins

- *Amount of protein in cells donot always directly correspond to amounts of mRNA* as some mRNAs are translated more efficiently & some proteins undergo post translational modifications.
- For detecting **one or limited number of proteins, antigen (protein) labeled antibody binding is used eg in**
  1. **ELISA (Enzyme linked immuo sorbent assay)**
  2. **Western (Immuno) blots**
- When **analyzing abundance & interactions of large number of proteins** (called **proteomics**), automated methods are employed such as.
  1. ***Two dimensional (2D) gel electrophoresis***Q
  2. ***Mass spectroscopy***Q
  3. ***Multidimensional liquid chromatography***Q
  4. **Bioinformatics**

DNA (Gene) Library

DNA or gene library is *collection of cloned restriction fragments of DNA of an organism.* It can be of 2 types

Genomic – DNA library

- It is the *largest type* of DNA library, created when the *complete genome of a particular organism is cleaved into thousands of fragments by restriction endonuclease* and all the fragments are cloned by insertion into a *cloning vector.*
- This (amplified DNA fragments) represent the entire genome of an organism including introns and control regions. It is prepared by RE & cloning in following way
- 1st step **is partial digestion of DNA** (of an organism) by restriction endonucleases (RE) in which either the amount or the time of action of enzyme is limited.
- RE that cut very frequently (recognize 4bp) are generally used. Complete digestion is not done as it would fragment the gene of interest (i.e. it is not contained in any one clone) as most genes contain > 1 restriction sites. Whereas partial digestion provides gene of interet in DNA fragments of range of sizes (~ 20 kb)
- *Too small or too large fragments* (inadequate for cloning) *are removed* by electrophoresis or centrifugation. Clonic vector (BAC or YAC) plasmid is cleaved with the same RE and ligated to partially digested genomic DNA fragments.
- Now each transformed yeast or bacterium cell grows into a colony or clone of identical cells, each bearing the same plasmid containing one of many genes represented in overall library.
- *Hybridization* methods can order individual clones in sequence by identifying clones with overlapping

Complementary (c) DNA library

- It is a *specialized library* designed to *study gene function* – so it includes only those *genes that are expressed i.e. are transcribed into mRNA.* So cDNA libraries lack introns & control regions.
- **It is prepared by *using m-RNA as a template to make a complementary DNA (cDNA) catalyzed by enzyme reverse transcriptase (RNA dependent DNA polymerase)*** Q. (The mRNA is isolated from tRNA and r-RNA by the presence of its poly tail)
- The resulting double stranded c-DNA can be amplified by PCR or cloning (i.e. inserting into a suitable vector and creating a population of clones) resulting in c-DNA libraries.
- To aid mapping of large genomes, cDNAs can be partially sequenced to produce a useful type of STS called **expressed sequence tag (EST)**.
- cDNA libraries are made more specialized by cloning cDNAs into a vector that fuses cDNA sequence with the sequence for **marker** or **reporter gene**-thus forming reporter construct. 2 useful markers include
- **Green fluorescent protein (GFP)** gene which generates fusion protein which is highly fluorescent protein that literally lights up.
- **Epitope tag** protein that bounds mono clonal antibody & precipitates.
- Because cDNA has no intervening (intron & control regions etc) sequences, it can be cloned into an **expression vector**

sequences. **Sequence tagged site (STS)** can provide landmarks for genomic sequencing projects. A set of over lapping clones represents a catalog for a long contiguous segment of a genome, often referred to as a **contig**.

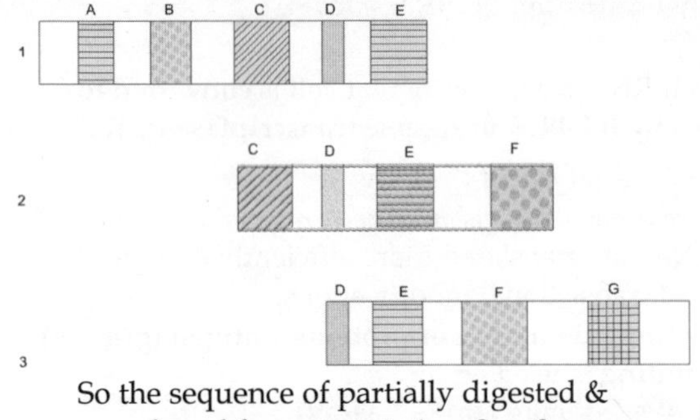

So the sequence of partially digested & cloned fragments is 1 → 2 → 3

for synthesis of eukaryotic proteins (like human insulin) by bacteria. These (plasmid of) expression vector contain bacterial promoter (for transcription) and *Shine Dalgarno sequence* /SDS (to initiate translation).

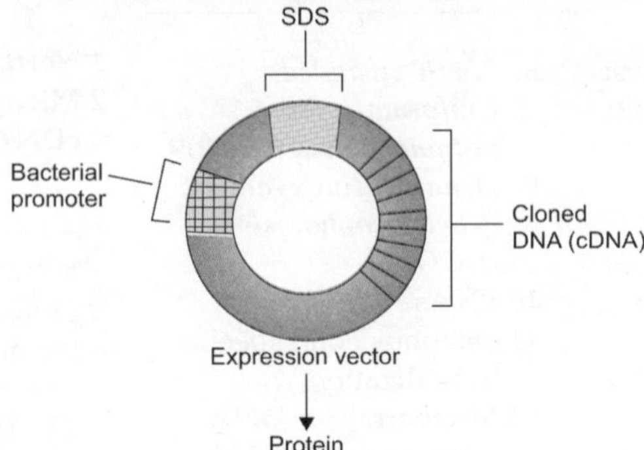

Biotechnology / Recombinant DNA technology / Genetic Engineering

It is a method by which a living organism or its parts (i.e. DNA/genes) are used *to change / incorporate* a particular character to another living organism.

It involves use of *restriction endonuclease* (to cut a particular gene) and PCR or cloning (to amplify it). It can be used for

- **Quantitative production of human biomolecules, genetic products by bacteria eg**
  - Human insulin
  - Erythropoietins, anticoagulants
  - Plasminogen activators
  - Cell growth factos, GF, Colony stimulating factor
  - ***Interferons, interleukins***[Q]
  - *Recombinant vaccines* eg rabies vaccine, hepatitis B vaccine
  - Monoclonal antibodies
  - Superoxide dismutase

  This method produces biological substances without any risk of contamination (like hepatitis B virus)
- **Creation of gene library**

Somatic Gene Therapy

- It is intracellular delivery of desired genes to ***cure a genetic disorder***[Q] by correcting an existing abnormality.
- It is tried in SCID, cystic fibrosis, Duchene MD, familial hyper cholesterolemia etc.

Gene production

New genes can be produced to be incorporated in

- ***Genetic crops***[Q]
- **Transgenic animals**

Production of specific **DNA probes** for diagnosis/ identification of

- Antenatal genetic disease
- Mutation / onchogenesis
- Sex, parent or criminal etc.

Production of Human Insulin by Genetic Engineering

- Because obtaining a human DNA with specific insulin gene is a laborious process, it is easier to ***begin the process by obtaining insulin mRNA from beta cells of pancreas***[Q], where insulin is produced in abundance (and obtaining specific mRNA is easier).
- **Complementary (c) DNA containing the insulin gene** is prepared by using human insulin mRNA (from pancreatic beta cells) as a template and **reverse transcriptase enzyme**.
- This **c-DNA containing insulin gene to be cloned is inserted into plasmid vector**. Bacterial plasmids are small, circular, duplex DNA molecules whose natural function is to confer antibiotic resistance to host cell. They exist as single or multiple copies within bacterium and replicate independtly from the bacterial DNA while using primarily the host replication machinery. The complete DNA sequence of many plasmids are known; so the precise location of RE cleavage sites for inserting foreign DNA (for cloning) is available. Plasmids are easily separated from host chromosome because of smaller size and the desired plasmid – inserted DNA can be easily removed by cutting plasmid with enzyme specific for restriction site into which the original piece of cloned DNA was inserted. **Plasmids produce millions of clones containing same insulin gene.**
- Bacteria (E.coli) containing insulin gene are grown in optimal conditions; insulin produced is isolated, collected & purified.

Insulin mRNA of human pancrease beta cells
↓
c-DNA by reverse transcriptase
↓
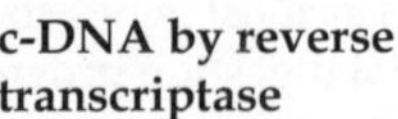
Cloned into plasmid vector to produce many copies of same gene
↓
Bacteria (E.coli) grown in optimal production conditions
↓
Produced insulin is collected isolated & purified

Recombination DNA Technology (Research) & Enzymes Used in it

- It is a *genetic engineering which effects artificial modification* of genetic constitution of a living cell by introduction of foreign DNA experimental techniques. It involves.
  - *Splicing the DNA by restriction endonuclease,*
  - *Preparation of chimeric DNA molecule* followed by
  - *Cloning* for production of large number of target DNA molecules
- The biological tools required are – **enzymes, vector (vehicle) DNA** (i.e. bacterial plasmids, cosmids & bacteriophage), and **passenger (foreign) DNA** (i.e. complementary DNA, synthetic or random DNA to be introduced into the vector). Enzymes used are

Enzymes used in Recombinant DNA Technology / Genetic Engineering

Enzyme	Function	Primary Use
Restriction Endonuclease (Type II)	- Cleave DNAs at a specific base sequences k/a **recognition sequences** or **restriction sites.** - **Cut (splice or cleave)** DNA of any source into short pieces in a **sequence specific manner** in contrast to other methods. eg enzymatic, physical or chemical that break DNA in random fashion.	**Key enzyme** used as **chemical knife,** in recombinant DNA technology Originally called **restriction enzymes** because their presence in a given bacteria restricted the growth of certain viruses (bacterio phages)
Example	**Cleaved Sequence**	**Bacterial Source**
Eco RI	G | AATT C C TTAA | G	E. Coli Ry 13
H Pa I	GTT | AAC CAA | TTG	Haemophilus parainfluenzae
Bam HI	G | GATC C C CTAG | G	Bacillus amylliquifaciens H
Eco RII	| CCTGG GGACC |	E. Coli R 245
Pst I	CTGCA | G G | ACGTC	Providencia stuartii 164
DNA ligase	Catalyzes the formation of new photodiester bonds in a reaction that uses ATP (or similar cofactor) between DNA molecules	***Joining DNA molecules eg after digestion by RE. DNA strands can be joined again by DNA ligase***[Q].
Bacteriophage λ Exonuclease	***Removes nucleotides from 5′ ends of dsDNA to expose single stranded 3′ end***[Q]	DNA sequencing
Exonuclease III	***Removes nucleotides from 3′ ends of DNA***[Q]	DNA sequencing; mapping protein-DNA interactions
BAL 31 Nuclease	Degrades both the 3′ and 5′ ends of DNA	Progressive shortening of DNA molecules
S1 Nuclease	***Degrades single-stranded DNA***[Q]	Removal of "hairpin" in synthesis of cDNA; RNA mapping studies (both 5′ and 3′ ends)
DNase I	Under appropriate conditions, produces single-stranded nicks in DNA	Nick translation; mapping of hypersensitive sites; mapping protein-DNA interactions.
Alkaline phosphatase	- Dephosphorylates 5′ ends of RNA and DNA - Removes terminal phosphate from either 5′ or 3′ ends (or both) - Lehninger	Removal of 5′-PO4 groups prior to kinase labeling to prevent self-ligation.
Thermostable DNA polymerase I (E. coli)	- ***Synthesizes double-stranded DNA from single-stranded DNA***[Q] - ***Fills gap in duplex by stepwise addition of nucleotides to 3′ end***	Synthesis of double-stranded cDNA; nick translation; generation of blunt ends from sticky ends.
Reverse transcriptase *(RNA dependent DNA polymerase)*[Q]	***Synthesizes DNA from RNA template***[Q] (i.e. makes DNA copy of an RNA molecule)	Synthesis of cDNA from mRNA; RNA (5′ end) mapping studies.
Polynucleotide kinase	- Adds a phosphate to 5′-OH end of polynucleotide to label it or permit ligation. - Transfers terminal phosphate (γ position) from ATP to 5′-OH groups of DNA or RNA	^{32}P labeling of DNA or RNA
Terminal transferase	Adds nucleotides (**homopolymer tails**) to 3′-OH ends of DNA (linear duplex).	**Homopolymer tailing**

Genomics

- ***Study of organism's entire genome (i.e. set of genes)***[Q]
- **Genome** is set of all genes expressed by an organism
- *Genome of an organism is constant, so it's less complicated* process and involves study of structure of genome including maping & sequencing and ***enables primary sequence of protein to be identified easily***[Q] from small amounts of sequence data. All that remains is to aquire open reading frame (ORF) that encodes protein.
- Picture provided is both *static & incomplete* and *represents the begining* of the task of undarstanding the dynamics of growth, aging & diseases process.

Glycomics

Deals with the ***structure & function of chains of sugar (oligosaccharides)***[Q]. Glycome refers to the identity of the entirely of carbohydrates in an organism

Bioinformatics

A scientific discipline that combines the tools and techniques of mathematics, computer science and biology with the aim of understanding the biologic significance of variety of data.

Cytogenetics

Branch of genetics concern with structure and function of cell, especially the chromosome.

Pharmacogenomics

The study of genetically determined variations in responses to drugs in human or in laboratory organisms.

Proteomics

- ***Quantitative & qualitative study of entire proteome (all expressed protein)***[Q]. **Preteome** is the set of all proteins expressed by a cell at particularly time. It is *more complicated* as it involves the ***study of all protein expressed by a genome, including their relative abundance, distribution, post translational modifications, functions, & interactions with other macro molecules***[Q].
- It aims to identify the entire complement of proteins expressed by a cell *under diverse condition*. So it provides *more complete, dynamic & advanced picture* of growth, aging & disease. Example includes **identification of proteins whose levels of expression correlate with medically significant events**, like whose appearance or disappearance is associated with a specific physiological condition or disease.
- Basic steps include **sample preparation, protein separation, protein imaging and identification**. It can be done by

1. **Gene Array (DNA Chips)** in which the expression of m RNA that encodes protein is detected. It is more sensitive the 2 D gels, particularly with respect to low abundance proteins. However, changes in expression of mRNA encoding a protein do not necessarily reflect comparable changes in level of corresponding protein.
2. **Multidimensional protein identification technology (Mud PIT)** employs *successive rounds of chromatography* to resolve the peptides produced from digestion of complex biological sample into many simpler fractions that can be analyzed by **mass spectroscopy**.
3. **2-Dimensional electrophoresis: Isoelectric focusing (IEF) is used in conjunction with SDS-PAGE** for 2D (two dimensional) electrophoresis, which *seperates polypeptides based on PI on one dimension and molecular mass (Mr) in second.* 2D electrophoresis is particularly used for separating the components of complex mixtures of proteins. Individual polypeptides are then extracted and analyzed by **Edman sequencing** or **mass spectroscopy**.

★ Proteins & peptides must be **purified** prior to analysis by various **chromatography techniques**. Then protein **purity is assessed by SDS-PAGE** (sodium dodecyl sulfate polyacrylamide gel electrophoresis). **Edman reaction** enables peptide & proteins to be sequenced. **Mass spectroscopy** is more sensitive method for determining sequences of peptides and proteins. MS determines mass of molecules and can be used to *analyze metabolites, carbohydrates and post translational modification* such as phosphorylation or hydroxylation that add *readily identified increaments of mass to a protein.*

Human Genome Project

Principle Methods Used

Procedure	Comments
Detection of specific cytogenic abnormalities	For instance, a small deletion of band Xp21.2 was important in cloning the gene involved in Duchenne muscular dystrophy
Extensive linkage studies	Large families with defined pedigrees are desirable. Dominant genes are easier to recognize than recessives

Major Findings

- More than 90% of the genome has been sequenced; gaps, large and small, remain to be filled in.
- Estimated number of protein –coding genes ranges from

Use of probes to define marker loci	Probes identify STSs, RFLPs, SNPs etc; thousands, covering all the chromosomes, are now available. It is desirable to flank the gene on both sides, clearly delineating it.
Radiation hybrid mapping	Now the *most rapid method of localizing a gene or DNA fragment to a subregion of a human chromosome* and constructing a physical map.
Use of rodent of human somatic cell hybrids	Permits assignment of a gene to one specific chromosome but not to a subregion.
Fluorescence in situ hybridization	Permits localization of a gene to one chromosomal band.
Use of pulsed-field gel electrophoresis (PFGE) to separate large DNA fragments	Permits isolation of a large DNA fragments obtained by use of restriction endonucleases (rare cutters) that result in very limited cutting of DNA.
Chromosome walking	*Involves repeated cloning of overlapping DNA segments*; the procedure is laborious and can usually cover only *100-200 kb.*
Chromosome jumping	By cutting DNA into relatively large fragments and circularizing it, one can *move more quickly and cover greater lengths of DNA than with chromosomal walking.*
Cloning via YACs, BACs, cosmids, phages, plasmids	Permits isolation of fragments of varying lengths
Detection of expression of mRNAs in tissues by Northern blotting using one or more fragments of the gene as a probe	The mRNA should be expressed in affected tissues
PCR	Can be used to *amplify fragments of the gene;*
DNA sequencing	Establishes the highest resolution physical map. Identifies open reading frame. Facilities with many high throughput instruments could sequence millions of base pairs per day.
Databases	Comparison of DNA and protein sequences obtained from unknown gene with known sequence in databases can facilitte gene identification

30,000 to 40,000.
- Only 1.1-1.5% of the genome codes for proteins.
- There are wide variations in feature of individual chromosomes (eg in gene number per Mb, SNP density, GC content, numbers of transposable elements and CpG islands, recombination rate).
- Human genes do more work than those of the roundworm or fruit fly (eg alternative splicing is used more frequently).
- The human proteome is more complex than that found in invertebrates.
- Repeat sequences probably constitute more than 50% of the genome.
- Approximately 100 coding regions have been copied and moved by RNA-based transposons.
- Approximately 200 genes may be derived from bacteria by lateral transfer.
- More than 3 million SNPs have been identified

Nude (Nu) Mouse / Nude Defect

- Nude defect is characterized by **absence of both hair and thymus**. A profound T cell defect can result from faulty thymus development (eg **Di George syndrome** d/t detection in long arm of chromosome 22 and **CHARGE** – coloboma of eye, heart anamoly, choanal atresia, retardation, genital and ear anomalies syndrome d/t CHD 7 deficiency) leading to virtually no T cells. However, expansion of oligo clonal T cells can occur; these cases require thymic graft.
- **Nude mouse** is a laboratory mouse *mutant with disruption of FOX N1 gene* ***(an autosomal recessive mutation on chromosome 11 nu locus), causing lack of body hair and absent/deteriorated thymus (=thymus aplasia)***Q. Because of lack of thymus, nude mice can not produce mature T cell lymphocytes resulting in **deficiency / greatly reduced number of T cells.** Nude mouse **do not generate cytotoxic effector cells, CD 8/4 T cells and are insusceptible to graft versus host disease.** Therefore these **can receive various types of Xenograft and allograft transplants**, in form of tissue and tumor grafts and ***sustain them for weeks***Q (used in research to test new methods of imaging & treating tumors).
- Nude mouse are unable to mount most immune responses such as
  1. **Lack graft rejection** (d/t lack of CD4+ and CD8+ T cells)
  2. Lack **cell mediated immune response** (which requires CD4 + and/or CD8+ Tcells)
  3. Lack **delayed type hypersensitivity response** (requires CD4 + T cells) and some **antibody formation** that require CD4 + helper T cells.
  4. Lack **killing of malignant / virus infected cells** (which requires CD8+ cytotoxic cells)
- Most nude mice are **leaky** (more so on aging) and **have few T cells**. Therefore, now these are less popular in research and **knock out** (eg RAG1 & RAG2 **knock out**) mice with more complete defects in immune system are preferred.

Genetically Modified Animals

Genetically modified animals are produced by *transgenic* pronuclear injection, forward genetics (i.e. mutations created randomly by ENU=N-ethyl-N-nitrourea), *targeted knock in and knock out*, congenic strains (mating of inbred donor, diseased phenotype with inbred recipient strain to identify genome responsible for disorder) and *cloning*.

Transgenic Expression (Animals)

- Transgenic animals are produced by pronuclear injection of transgene (genomic DNA or cDNA construct) into the nuclei of fertilized ovum. There is *no way to control where that gene eventually resides (ie random integration of transgene)*. Transgene has variable copy number and variable expression in each individual founder. Transgenic (animals) expression can be

  1. **Loss of function models** using **antisense** and **dominant negative transgenes**
  2. **Gain of function models** d/t **over expression** using tissue specific promoter
  3. Inducible expression (tetracycline, ecdysone)

- It can be produced by ***microinjecting one or few cloned genes into the nuclei of fertilized egg (ovum) of experimental animal (eg mouse)***[Q]. The successful introduction of recombinant DNA into an animal can be illustrated by an experiment that permanently altered an easily observable inheritable physical trait. Microinjection of DNA into the nuclei of fertilized mouse eggs can produce efficient transformation (chromosomal integration). When the injected eggs are introduced into a female mouse & allowed to develop, the new gene is often expressed in some of new born mice.
- Unlike, somatic cell gene replacement therapy (or gene therapy) which *would not be passed on to offspring, this process of generating transgenic animal would alter germ cell lines and be passed on to offsprings.*
- If gene becomes successfully integrated into a chromosome, it will be present in both somatic cells and germline of resulting animal & is *passed along from generation to generation.*
- So transgenic animals ***have same genome as parents except few (1 or more) genes***[Q] that have been integrated or inactivated. Those in which the germline has been altered can be identified by testing their offspring. By careful breeding of these mice, **transgenic line** in which all the mice are homozygous for new gene or genes can be established.
- Hundreds of transgenic animals are established and these are useful for *analysis of tissue specific effect on gene expression and effects of over production of gene products (eg those from the growth hormone gene or onchogenes)* and in discovering genes involved in development.
- A *giant super mouse* is produced by injecting the gene for rat growth hormone into fertilized mouse egg or transgenic cows or goats can be designed to produce human proteins like *clotting factor in* their *milk.*
- Similarly genetic hypogonadism in mice can be treated (in offsprings) by injecting DNA with coding sequence for GnRH (gonadotropin releasing hormone) precursor.

Targeted (Directed or Conditional) Approaches; Knock out & Knock In

Creation of gene knock in and knock out (targeted) take advantage of the fact that *a segment of DNA (gene) can be substituted by another homologous (identical) or nearly identical DNA segment* by recombination. This allow integration of deletions that disrupt gene function (**targeted knock out**) or integration of selected mutations into **targeted gene** (i.e. targeted knock in).

Targeted Knock In Animals	Targeted Knock Out (Gene Disruption) Animals
• *Introduction of a subtle mutation* (s) into a gene by substitution of a normal endogenous gene with a mutant gene (carrying a specific mutation) by homologous recombination in embryonic stem cell is called **(targeted) knock in**. It occurs d/t substitution of endogenous gene with gene carrying a subtle mutation (i.e. adding few genes). • These are predominantly used in mice and can accurately model human disease • Targeted expression of onchogene is used to study mechanism of neoplasia & to generate immortalized cell lines. Eg expression of simian virus (SV) 40 large T antigen under direction of insulin promoter induces formation of islet cell tumors.	• It is substitution of functional gene with inactive gene by homologous recombination in embryonic stem cell. • It is *selective removal of a gene from genome*. Gene knockout animals are *made by creating a mutation that totally disrupts the function of a gene*. In other words, rather than introducing a functional gene into animal, a non functional version is inserted. • It is a way of *establishing the function of inactivated gene* or to study corresponding human disease. • Both Mi RNAs and DNA recombinases inactivate gene expression. • Techniques disrupting targeted genes take advantage of particular promoter enhancer combinations driving expression of *DNA recombinases or mi RNAs, both of which inactivate gene expression (targeted knock out).* • It is predominantly used in mice. Tissue specific knock out is possible (Cre / lox). ***Absence of phenotype may occur d/t gene redundancy***[Q] or subtle phenotype. For eg **deletion of HPRT gene (Hprt) does not cause characteristic features of Lesch Nyhan syndrome in mice** b/o their reliance on adenine phosphoribosyl transferase (APRT) in purine salvage. **Deletion of retinoblastoma gene (Rb) encoding p 105 does not l/t retinoblastoma** or other human syndromes in mice. However, mice with combinatorial deletion of several Rb related proteins exhibit features similar to human disorder.

This replacement of one gene in embryonic stem cell creates a *heterozygous transgenic animals*. The mating in 2 such animals will

- Transgenic stratigies can be divided into 2 main approches
1) Expression of a gene by random insertion into genome (pronuclear injection of trransgene)
2) Deletion or targeted mutagenesis of a gene by homologous recombination with the native endogenous gene (knock out, knock in).
- Transgenic expression of gene can be useful for studying **disorders that are sensitive to gene dosage**. Eg over expression of PMP 22 gene l/t high level of peripheral myelin protein 22 (type I Charcot-Marie tooth disease); SRY gene in females induce formation of testis. ***Transgenic introduction of CAG trinucleotide repeat causes Hutingtons disease, whereas targeted delition (knock out) of Hutington's disease gene does not induce neurological disorder***Q. (ie gain of function for CAG encoded polyglutamine containing protein)
- Transgenic strategies can be **used as precursors to gene therapy**. Eg expression of dystrophin corrects Duchenne's muscular dystrophy in mouse

result in *25% of homozygous offsprings* (a/t mendelian law). Careful breeding will establish **transgenic (animal) line *in which all animals are homozygous for new gene / genes***Q.

Forward Genetics

- Mutations created randomly by ENU (N-ethyl-N-nitrourea)
- Selection of phenotype followed by genetic characterization
- Useful for identifying novel genes

Congenic strains

- Mating of an inbred donor strain with a disease phenotype with an inbred recipient strain in order to define the genomic region responsible for the disorder
- Useful for mapping disease-causing genes

Cloning

- Introduction of nucleus into enucleated eggs (nuclar transfer)
- Successful in several mammalian species including sheep (Dolly), mice, cows, monkeys
- Cloning of genetically identical individuals
- May effect lifespan
- Ethical concerns

Gene Therapy

- It implies to *correct the basic genetic abnormality*. The principle is to *insert the normal, cloned DNA for defective gene* into somatic cells.
- **Gene therapy** is a procedure involving *inserting (or sometimes deleting portions of gene* in diseased patients for the purpose of cure. In *somatic gene therapy,* the recipient's genome is changed but the change is not passed along the next generation. Whereas, in germ line gene therapy, change is passed to next generation.
- **Antisense gene therapy** or **gene silencing** selectively inactivate (or turn off) a mutated gene by RNA interference using short synthetic double stranded **siRNA (small interfacing RNA)**

- Procedure involves
- ***Replacement***Q: Mutant gene removed & replaced with normal gene.
- **Correction** : Only mutated area of affected gene would be corrected & the remainder will be unchanged.
- ***Augmentation:*** Introduction of foreign genetic material into a cell to compensate for the defective product of mutant gene.
- Gene of interest is usually administered via a **viral** (retro, adeno, adenoassociated, lenti viruses etc) **vector** or **non viral plasmid liposome (cationic lipid) complex**, used as gene transfer vehicle.
- **Gene therapy is used in**
- **SCID (severe combined immunodeficiency disease)** or **bubble bay syndrome,** which occurs d/t mutation in either *adenosine deaminase gene* or a X-linked gene coding for an *interleukin receptor subunit,* is the *first disease that was successfully treated by gene therapy.*
- ***Cystic fibrosis***Q
- Familial hypercholesterolemia
- Duchene muscular dystrophy, Hemophilia, Leber's hereditary optic neuropathy.
- *Lesh – Nyhan syndrome, phenylketonuria (PKU)* are most likely candidates for future gene therapy. Single gene disorders are best candidates for gene therapy. However, unfortunately most prevalent disorders such as heart disease, high BP, Alzheimer's disease, diabetes and arthritis are multigene disorders.

Techniques to transfer genes (foreign material) into cells

- ***Sites directed recombnation***Q
- Soil bacterium Agrobacterium tumefaciens (containing Ti plasmid) and Agrobacterium E. coli are used for plants
- ***Intranuclear microinjection***Q
- **Transduction** using viral vectors like *retrovirus, adenovirus, adeno associated virus, herpes simplex virus and lenti viruses.* Adenovirus lacks a mechanism for integrating DNA into chromosome. Therefore adenoviral vector is expressed for only a short time and then destroyed. This is useful if the objective is **transient expression of gene**. Adenovirus are used for introduction of cystic fibrosis gene in respiratory tract cells. Other possible vectors are- Epstein Barr viruses, herpes, simian virus 40, papilloma, non human lentiviruses, and hepatitis viruses.
- **Transfection** using non-viral methods like plasmid liposome complex using calcium phosphate precipitated DNA. Liposomes (cationic lipids) are small vesicles consisting of lipid bilayer that encloses an aquous compartment.
- **Electroporation :** It employs *pulsed electric field* using small electric current, which *transiently increase the permeability of plasma* membrane thus allowing intake of extracellular macromolecules including DNA.

Mn-"**SITE**"

Inheritance of X-linked Recessive Disease

X linked recessive inheritance is a sex linked disorders i.e. they are transmitted by sex chromosomes. Remember that all sex linked diseases are linked to X chromosome so it is quiet obvious that none of the sex linked disease (whether X-linked recessive or X-linked dominant) will be transmitted from father to son, as **father transmits only 'Y' chromosome to the son.** Other characteristic of this disorder is that it is mostly seen in males. Where as the diseases transmitted through non sex chromosomes (autosomes) have equal male and female incidence.

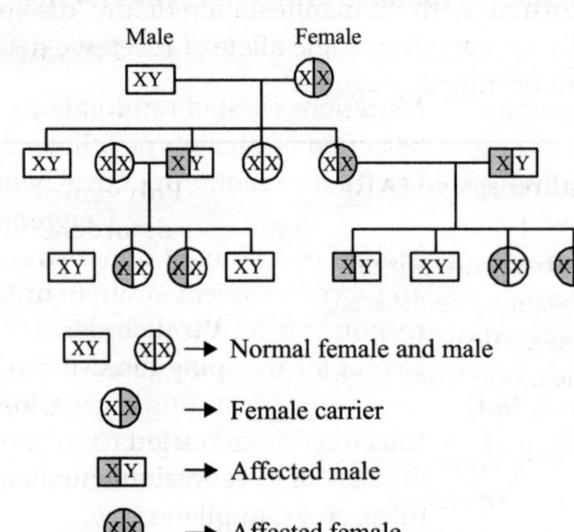

- *An affected male does not transmit the disorder to his sons, but all daughters are carriers*
- *Sons of heterozygous woman have 50% chance of receiving the abnormal gene*
- *It usually affects males because of the presence of Y chromosome which is not homologous to X chromosome and therefore the mutant genes on the X is not paired with alleles on the Y*
- *It is rare in females only possible when mother is carrier and father has overt disease.*

Most of the X linked disorders are X linked recessive. There are only **few X-linked dominant conditions.** These are
- Pseudohypoparathyoidism
- Hypophosphetemic rickets.
- Vit D resistant rickets
- Incontinentia pigmenti

X-linked Recessive Disorders

(1) ***Duchenne & Becker muscular dystrophy***[Q]
(2) ***Hemophilia A and B***[Q]
(3) *Chronic granulomatous disease (70% XLR, 30% AR)*
(4) ***Glucose 6-PO₄ dehydrogenase deficiency***[Q]
(5) *Agammaglobulinemia*
(6) *Wiskott Aldrich syndrome*
(7) *Diabetes insipidus*
(8) *Fragile X syndrome*
(9) *Lesch Nyhan syndrome*
(10) *Fabry disease*
(11) *Hunter's disease*
(12) *Colour blindness*
(13) *Ocular albinism*
(14) *Sideroblastic anemia*

Autosomal Recessive (AR) Disorders

Metabolic

All	Albinism[Q]
Anti	α1 **Antitrypsin deficiency**[Q]
Ha	**Hartnup disease**[Q]
He	**Hemochromatosis**[Q]
Ho	**Homocystinuria**[Q]
Gla	**Galactosemia**[Q]
Gly	**Glycogen storage disease**[Q]
La	**Laurence Moon Biedl** Syndrome[Q]
Ly	**Lysosomal storage disease**[Q]
Will	**Wilson's disease**[Q]
Use	**Usher's syndrome**[Q]
Cystic	**Cystic** Fibrosis[Q]
Urea	Phenylketon**uria**[Q]

Mn – **"All Anti Ha He Ho Gla Gly, La Ly will Use Cystic Urea"**

Hematopoetic

See	**S**ickle cell anemia[Q] Thalasemia - α & β[Q]
And	Leucocyte **adhesion** deficiency
Check	**Che**diak – Higashi syndrome[Q]
My	**My**eloperoxidase deficiency
Fan	**Fan**coni syndrome

Mn – **"See And Check My Fan"**

Endocrine
- Congenital adrenal hyperplasia
- Pendred syndrome

Nervous
- ***Friedrich ataxia***[Q]
- Neurogenic muscular atrophy
- Spinal muscular atrophy

Skeletal

All	**Al**kaptonuria
Pets	Osteo**petr**osis
Fail	Klippel **Feil** syndrome
Don's	**Danlos Ehler syndrome**
Exam	

Urinary
- ***Barter syndrome***[Q]
- ***Gitelman syndrome***[Q]
- Nephronophthisis
- Nephrogenic diabetes insipidus (also XL)
- ***AR polycystic kidney diseasse***[Q]

Gastrointestinal

Familial Mediterranean fever

Other
- Bloom syndrome

Genetically Transmitted Disorders

Normal parents means parents who are 'clinically normal' with no manifestation of any 'disease' during any part of their life time. But these may still be 'abnormal' (1) genetically i.e. carrying single allele of recessive disease that needs 2 recessive alleles to be manifested or (2) non genetically carrying silent or infective agents.

Autosomal dominant (AD)

For a child with an autosomal dominant disorder to be affected at least one parent needs to have the affected allele

Because the allele is dominant it will always express phenotipiclly and hence both parents can not be normal

Genotype of Affected Child with autosomal dominant disorder

Tt (phenotypically abnormal parent 1)	Tt (phenotypically normal parent 2)

T → Tt ← t

Tt (affected offspring in AD disorder)

Autosomal recessive (AR)

For a child with an autosomal recessive disorder to be affected he needs to have atleast two recessive alleles, one from each parent.

Because the allele is recessive, it might not express in either parents and both parents can be phenotypically normal.

Genotype of Affected Child with autosomal recessive disorder

Tt (phenotypically normal parent 1)	Tt (phenotypically normal parent 2)

T → TT ← t

TT (affected offspring in AR disorder)

Polygenic disorder

- A trait is called 'polygenic' if multiple genes on thought to contribute to the phenotype.
- Polygenic disorders include Hypertension Diabetes, Asthma
- ***A male infant with asthma or diabetes may will be born to normal parents***

Vertically transmitted disorder

- Passage of disease causing agent (pathogen) 'vertically' from mother to baby during the perinatal period is called 'vertical transmission'.
- ***A vertically transmitted agent night lie dormant in the mother and not manifest in her clinically (normal mother) but may manifest in the child.***

Types of Defects

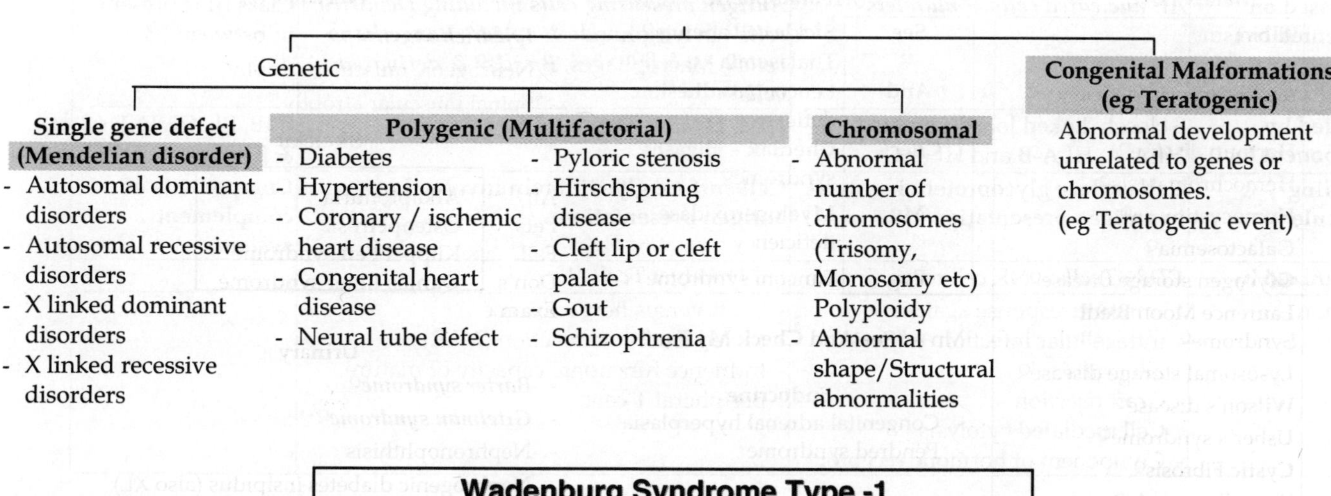

Wadenburg Syndrome Type -1

Waardenburg's Syndrome (WS) is a rare ***autosomal dominant syndrome*** *characterized by pigmentary disturbances (skin,* ***hair****, iris),* ***sensorineural hearing loss****, and other developmental anomalies such as* ***dystopia canthorum (widely spaced eyes)*** *and blepharophimosis.*

Type	I (Waardenburg)
Distinguishing Features	Dystopia canthorum (Widely spaced eyes) Hearing loss (25%)
Inheritance	Autosomal Dominant (AD)
Gene Defect/ Function	P AX3/transactivates promotor for MITF

Facial features

- Broad high nasal root
- Synophrys or medial flaring, or both, of the eyebrows
- Hypoplastic alae nasi
- **Dystopia canthorum (lateral displacement of inner canthi or widely spaced eyes or hypertelorism)**

Hair features

- White forelock (present at birth or developing later; also may disappear later) White body hair, eyebrows, eyelashes
- Dark tufts of hair or black forelock
- Premature graying (i.e. <30 y)

Aural features

- **Sensineural hearing loss (SNHL) (deafness)**

Eye features

- Complete or segmental heterochromia
- Brilliant sapphire blue eyes

Skin features

- Hypopigmentation, possibly on the face, trunk, or limbs with or without an associated white forelock
- Patches ofhyperpigmentation in some families with WS

Less commonly associated findings

- Neural tube defects
- Sprengel shoulder (ie, congenital upward scapular displacement)
- Cleft lip or palate
- Hirschsprung disease (primarily in cases of WS4 but reported in families with WS I and WS2) Contractures and limb muscle hypoplasia (in patients with WS3)

Major Histocompatibility Complex (MHC)/ Human Leukocyte Antigen (HLA) Complex

- In humans the gene encoding MHC or HLA complex are clustered on ***a small segment (4 megabase region) of chromosome 6 short arm***[Q] ***(6p 21.3)***[Q]. HLA class I and class II genes whose products are critical for ***immunological specificity and transplantation histocompatibility***[Q] and they play a major role in **susceptibility to a number of autoimmune diseases.**
- **Function:** Binds peptide fragments of foreign protein for presentation to appropriate *antigen specific T- Cells. Thus involved in:* 1) ***Transplantation reaction***[Q] *2)* Immune response & tolerance 3) Disease susceptibility (***autoimmune ds***[Q], infectious & Inflammatory disease) 4) Complement component.
- They are classified into **3 categories**

Feature	Class I Antigen (MHCI)	Class II Antigen (MHC II)	Class III (MHC III)
Expressed on (presented by)	***All nucleated cells & platelets***[Q]	***Antigen presenting cells including Dendritic cells***[Q] in lymphnode & spleen, ***Langerhans cells***[Q], Macrophages, ***B cells***[Q] ***& activated T cells***[Q]	Class III is present in between I & II
Encoded by (component loci)	3 closely linked loci designated HLA-A, HLA-B and HLA-C	***HLA-D*** (*HLA DP, D*[Q]*, DR*)	C4B, BF, C2 TNF α & β
Encoding molecule	**Cell surface glycoprotein involved in antigen presentation**	**Cell surface glycoprotein involved in antigen presentation**	**Components of complement system**
Recognized by	***CD8+ Tcells***[Q], NK cell recognizition	***CD4+ helper Tcells***[Q]	
Function	- Immune response against intracellular infection, tumors, allografts - Graft rejection - Cell mediated cytolysis - Component of hormone receptor	- Graft versus host response - Mixed leucocyte reaction (MLR) - Influence functional capacity of mature peripheral T cells.	

Chapter 5. STRUCTURE & FUNCTIONS OF PROTEINS AND ENZYMES: REVIEW NOTES

Structural Organization of Protein

Primary Structure

- Primary structure is **linear sequence of aminoacids held together by covalent bonds (mainly peptide and disulfide bonds).** It is **insufficient to perform chemical /physical task.**
- The aminoacids are numbered from N terminal end (free NH_2/amino group of terminal amino acid) as no 1 towards the C (free carboxy) terminal.
- **Peptide bonds form the backbone** and side chains of aminoacid residues project out side the peptide back bone
- α-carbons of adjacent aminoacid residues are separated by three covalent bonds $C_\alpha - C - N - C_\alpha$. **The peptide (C-N) bond has a partial double bond character** that keeps the entire 6 atom peptide group in a **rigid planar configuration.** Peptide C-N bond cannot rotate freely; **rotation is permitted about N-C_α and C_α – C bonds.** So backbone of polypeptide chain can be pictured as a series of rigid planes sharing a **common point of rotation at C_α.**
- Peptide conformation is defined by 3 **dihedral angles** (or **torsion angles**) called **ϕ (phi)** with rotation occurring about **N-C_α bond; ψ(Psi)** with rotation occurring about **C_α–C bond** ; and **ω (omega)** with central peptide (C-N) bond, where rotation is constrained and mostly (99.6% times) peptide bond is in trans configuration (omega = ± 180°) or very rare in cis configuration (ω=0°). Theoritically values of ϕ & ψ can be between – 180° and + 180° but many values (eg both O°) are prohibited d/t steric interferences. Allowed values are obtained by **Ramchandran plot.**

Tertiary Structure

- **Tertiary structure** refers to **over all three dimensional arrangement of all atoms in a protein.** It indicates the **3-D confirmation of a single polypeptide chain** ie in 3D space how secondary structure features helices, sheets, loops and bends assemble to form domains and how these domains relate spatially to one another.
- Tertiary structure refers to ***spatial arrangement of long range aspects of aminoacids***[Q] (in comparison to secondary structure that includes adjacent aminoacids). Proteins with tertiary structure are sufficient to perform a particular task.

Secondary Structure

- **Secondary structure of protein** refers to **description of steric relationship (spatial arrangement) between aminoacids located relatively near each other in a selected segment of main polypeptide chain,** without regard to the conformation of its side chains or its relationship to other segments.
- **A regular secondary structure** occurs when each dihedral angle (ϕ & ψ) remains the same or nearly the same throughout segment. Where a regular pattern is not found, the secondary structure is called **undefined or random coil** (misnomer as polypeptide back bone in any protein is not random).
- The secondary structure of a polypeptide segment can be completely defined if ϕ & ψ angles are known for all aminoacids.
- **Circular dichroism (CD) spectroscopy,** based on principle that structural asymmetry in a molecule gives rise to differences in absorption of left handed versus right handed plane polarized light, is a method for **assessing secondary structure and moniter folding in proteins.** It can determine whether proteins are properly folded, estimate the fraction of protein that is properly folded in either of common secondary structures, an moniter transition b/w folded & unfolded states. For proteins spectra are obtained in **far UV region (190 to 250nm).**
- **Three dimensional secondary structure** is produced by folding or coiling of short (3-30) contiguous segments of polypeptides (peptide chain primary structure) and production of cross linkages or bonds mainly hydrogen bonds. It is *insufficient to perform a particular physical or chemical task.* Organization may result in formation of **geometrically ordered units** such as α helix, β sheets, loops and bends-

α- Helix

- Are *regular- helical coils* of peptide chain
- Formed by ***intra chain hydrogen bonds***[Q] b/w carbonyl O of 1st amino acid and amide N of 4th amino acid residue.
- α- helix may be left handed or right handed
- ***Left handed α helix is less stable***[Q] than right handed α- helix because of steric interference b/w the C=O and the side chains
- Only right handed α- helix has been found in protein structure
- *In one complete turn* of α- helix there are *3.6 amino acid residue.*
- ***Proline is never found in α- helix***[Q].
- Small or uncharged amino acids as *alanine, phenylalanine & leucine* are often found; whereas more polar a.a. such as *arginine, glutamate & serine* may repel & destabilize *α-helix.*

β- Pleated Sheets

- β-pleated structure is formed by ***inter chain hydrogen bonds***[Q].
- They are produced when *hydrogen bonds are formed between carbonyl oxygen and amide hydrogen of two adjacent chains.*
- The adjacent chains may be either parallel or antiparallel.
- Most common a.a to form β- pleated sheet - *Glycine,*

- On the basis of tertiary structure, proteins can be divided into **structural fibrous proteins** (having simple repeating elements of secondary structure) and **globular proteins** (often containing several types of secondary structure in same polypeptide chain).
- Complex structures of globular proteins can be analyzed by examining folding patterns called **motifs (super secondary structures or folds).** A motif is a recognizable folding pattern involving 2 or more elements of secondary structure and the connection (s) between them. It can be very simple as **β -α - β loop** or very elaborate such as **β barrel.** Motif is not a hierarchial structural element falling between secondary & tertiary structure; it is a folding pattern that can describe a small part of protein or an entire polypeptide chain. A motif segment may or may not be independently stable. A **domain** ***is a part of polypeptide chain that can fold stably and independently***Q or could undergo **movements as a** single entity with respect to the entire protein. Multiple domains of large proteins may have different functions and may retain their native 3D structure even when separated. Thousands of known protein structures are assembled from a repertoire of few hundred motifs.

Quaternary Structure

- ***Quarternary structure results from interactions between the subunits of multi subunit (multimeric) proteins***Q. So quaternary structure is **3D arrangement of multiple polypeptide chain proteins**
- Some multimeric proteins have a repeated structural unit, consisting of a single subunit or a group of subunits known as promoter. Promoters are usually related by **rotational or helical symmetry** (ie individual subunit can be super imposed on other). Examples of rotational symmetry include **cyclic symmetry, dihedral symmetry and icosahedral symmetry** (in order of complexity).
- A multimeric protein with few subunits is called **oligomer. Dimer** contains 2 polypeptide chains.

Homodimers	Heterodimers
Contain two copies of same polypeptide chain Represented as X_2	Contain different polypeptide subunits Represented as α β

- Examples: **Creatinine kinase (dimer), lactate dehydrogenase (tetramer), hemoglobulin (tetramer** of 2 alpha + 2 beta chains) and **immunoglobulin (tetramer** of 2 heavy + 2 light chain)

Alpha (α) Helix (Pauley & Corey)

- This *spiral structure* is the *most common and stable* secondary conformation (structure) for a polypeptide chain. The polypeptide bond forms the back bone, side chain of aminoacids extend outward and the structure is **stabilized by hydrogen bond b/w N—H & C= O groups** of main chain
- In α-helix, the polypeptide backbone is *tightly wound (twisted) around an imaginary axis* (drawn longitudinally through the middle of helix) and *side chains (R-groups) protrude outwards* from helical back bone. The polypeptide backbone of α-helix is equally *twisted about each α-carbon atom* with a phi (ϕ) angle = -57° and psi (ψ) angle = -47°. Each complete turn of helix contains ~ **3.6** aminoacyl residues with **translation** (i.e. distance b/w each aminoacid) = 0.15 nm (1.5 A°) and **pitch** (i.e. distance per turn) = 0.54 nm (5.4 A°).
- Structure of α-helix is stabilized primarily by hydrogen bonds formed b/w
  - **Oxygen (O)** of peptide bond carbonyl and **hydrogen (H) atom** of peptide bond nitrogen of **4th** residue down the peptide chain (Harper)
  - Hydrogen (H) atom attached to electronegative nitrogen atom of peptide linkage and the electronegative carbonyl **oxygen (O) atom** of **4th** aminoacid on aminoterminal side of peptide bond (Lehninger).
- Every peptide bond (except those close to end of helix) participate in hydrogen bonding. So each turn is held to adjacent turn by 3-4 **hydrogen bonds** (supplemented by **Van der Walls** interactions), conferring significant stability.
- Experimentally, α-helix can form in polypeptides consisting of *either L or D stereoisomeric* aminoacids, with all residues of one type because *mixing of D & L aminoacids will disrupt the structure.* Theoretically, naturally occurring L aminoacids can form either right or left handed α-helices but extanded left handed α-helices are unstable and not observed.
- **Alanine** show the ***greatest tendency to form α-helix***Q. **Keratins** protein of hair, nail and skin and *hemoglobin / myoglobin* are rich in α-helical structure, whereas chymotrypsin virtually lack it. Not all aminoacids form α-helix, ***proline & glycine have least proclivity to form α-helixes***Q.

Alanine, Serine

- ***Proline occurs although it tends to disrupts β- sheet by producing kinks***Q
- ***Silk fibroins a protein of silk worm is rich in β- pleated sheets***Q.

Triple Helix

- ***Collagen rich in proline and hydroxy proline, can not form α- helix or β- pleated sheet. It forms triple helix***Q.
- Stabilized by interchain hydrogen bonds b/w different polypeptide chains.

Reverse Turns or β- Bends

- β-bends reverse the direction of polypeptide chain, helping it form a compact globular chain.
- Usually occur on the surface of globular protein
- A.A frequently found in β- bends
  - Proline
  - Glycine

Super Secondary Structures

- Greek key
- β-meander: consists of 5 *β- pleated sheets connected by reverse turns.* It contains nearly as many hydrogen bonds as an α-helix.
- β- α- β unit

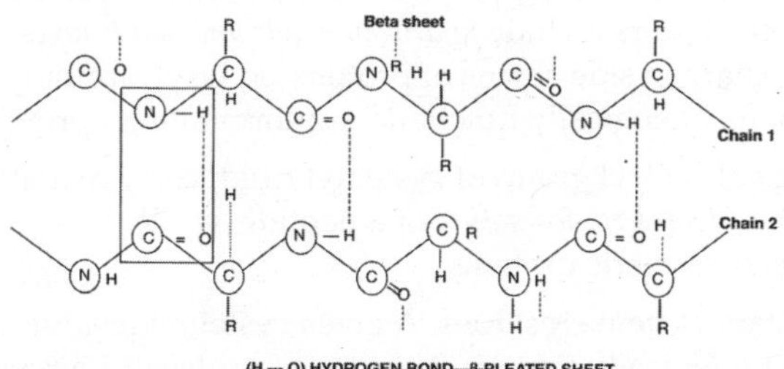

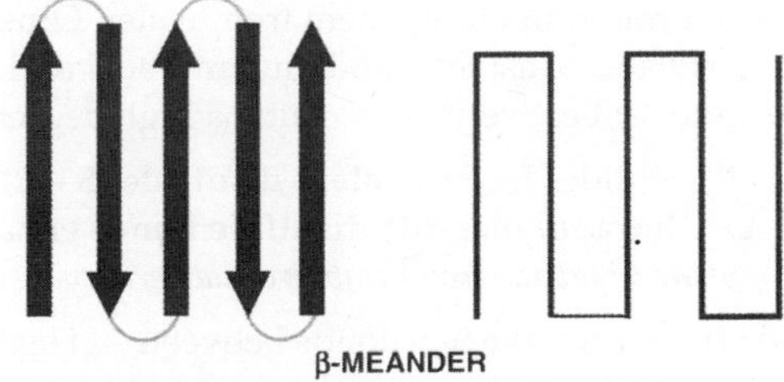

Aminoacids Affecting Stability or Disrupting α-Helices ☆

- Proline
- Hydroxy-proline

- Since peptide bond nitrogen of proline *lacks a hydrogen atom to contribute to a hydrogen bond,* it can only be stably *accommodated within the first turn of α-helix.* When present else where, **proline disrupts α-helix.**
- Nitrogen atom of proline is a part of rigid imino ring & rotation about N-C_α bond is not possible. Hence proline **introduces a destabilizing** kink in α-helix.

Glycine

B/o small size, and more conformational flexibility, it induces bends.

Charged aminoacids

Disrupt α-helix by forming ionic bonds or electro statically repelling each other

+	-
- Arginine - Lysine - Histidine	- ***Aspartate (aspartic acid)***[Q] - Glutamate (glutamic acid)

★ For stability +ve charged aa are found 3 residues away from –ve charge aa.

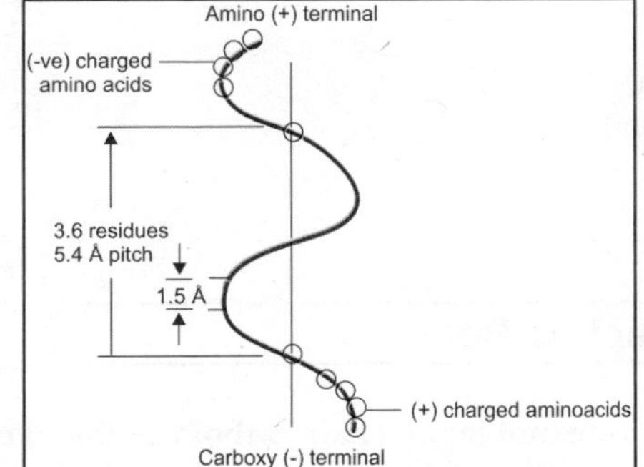

When present in large number or close together

Bulky side chains
- **Tryptopan**

AA that **branch at β carbon** (i.e. **1st C in R group next to α-C)**
- **Valine**
- **Isoleucine**

Bulk & Shape of AA
- Asaparagine
- Serine
- Threonin

Aminoacids at the end of helix

- 4 aminoacids at each end do not fully participate in hydrogen bonding
- Electrical dipole of each peptide bond is aligned through hydrogen bonds of helix, resulting in a net dipole along the helical axis that increases with helix length
- For this reason negatively charged aminoacids are found near amino terminal and positively charged amino acids are found near carboxy terminal of α-helix; where they have stabilizing interaction

Positive (+) charged aminoacid at **amino (+) terminal)** and **negatively (-)** charged aminoacids **at carboxy (-) terminal** of α-helix is destabilizing.

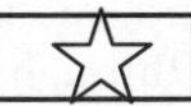

Various Types of Bonds ☆

- **Hydrophobic (weak) interactions** are predominantly important for protein's stabilizing conformation (protein stability)
- Hydrophobic residues are largely buried in the protein interior, away from water and the number of **hydrogen bonds and ionic interactions with in protein is maximized**, thus reducing the number of hydrogen bonding & ionic group that are not paired with suitable partner. Because of favourable free energy change and cooperative bonding (i.e. one bond favours the formation of next bone), the **hydrogen bonds** often ***have an important role in guiding the protein folding process***[Q]. *(Langerhan's 115)*
- After folding into their native conformations, *some protein form interchain or intrachain disulfide bridges between Cys residues.* In eukaryotes, disulfide bonds are common in proteins to be exported from cells. The cross links formed in this way help to *protect the native conformation of protein from denaturation in extracellular environment*, which can differ greatly from intracellular conditions & is generally oxidizing, - *(Lehninger)*

- **Higher order of protein structure (tertiary & quaternary)** are stabilized primarily & often exclusively – by **non covalent** interactions, principle among these are ***hydrophobic interactionns***[Q] that drive most hydrophobic aminoacid side chains into the interior of protein shielding them from water. Other significant contributors include *hydrogen bonds and salt bridges between* carboxylates of aspartic and glutamic acid and the oppositely charged side chains of protonated lysyl, argininyl, and histidyl residue. Collectively these confer a high degree of stability to the biologically functional conformation of protein.
- Some (not all) peptides form **covalent disulfide (S – S) bonds** linking sulfhydryl group of cysteinyl residues by oxidation (requiring O_2). **Intrapolypeptide disulfide bonds** enhance the *stability of folded conformation* of a peptide, while ***interpolypeptide disulfide bond*** *stabilize quarternary structure* of certain oligomeric proteins.
- **Disulphide bonds:** are the S- S bonds between – SH group of two distant cysteine residues. A given cysteinyl residue can form many disulfide bond pairs, only one of which is appropriate for biologically folding. *The enzyme disulphide isomerase* facilitates shuffling of – S-S bonds by accelerating the rate at which disulphide undergo mutual exchange, thereby *accelerating process of protein folding and stabilizing proteins native conformation.*

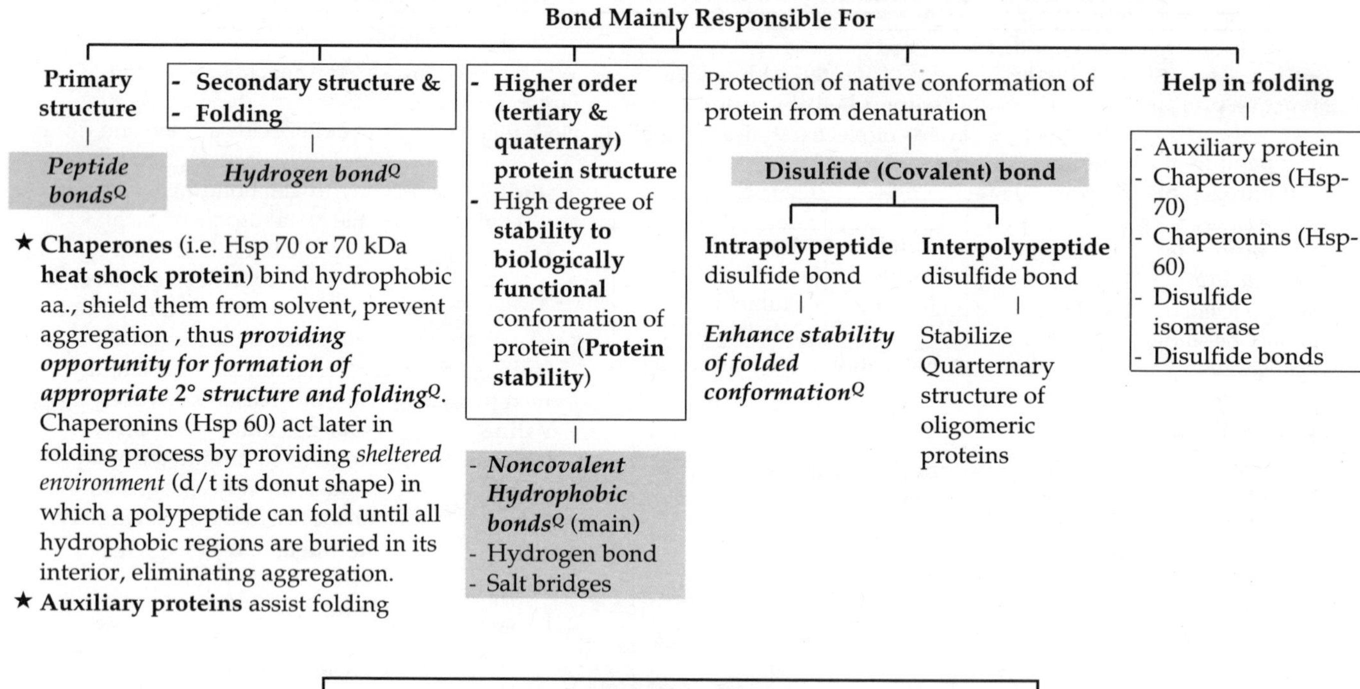

Isopeptide Bond

- **Isopeptide bond** is an amide bond formed **between the side (not main) chain carboxy terminal of one protein** (with either glutamate or aspartate) and **amino group of lysine** residue on side chain of another target protein.
- Bond formation is either **spontaneous** (in gram positive bacterial pilli & HK 97 bacteriophage capsid formation) or **enzyme (transglutaminase) catalyzed** (between lysine & glutamine). **Spontaneous proximity induced isopeptide bond formation** requires presence of glutamic acid, and is used in development of **isopeptag** (a new peptide tag) which can spontaneously & irreversibly react with its target through a covalent isopeptide bond. This molecular tool is used in development of new protein architectures – in vivo protein targeting and fluorescent microscopy imaging.
- Isopeptide bond formation is involved in **post translational modification of proteins**. Interchain isopeptide bonds **make proteins resistant** and produce stably linked protein dimmers, multimers & complexes like blood clots, as only few enzymes can hydrolyze this bond.
- A small peptide **Glutathione**, has isopeptide bond b/w side chain of glutamate & amino group of cysteine. Similary **ubiquitin protein**'s C terminal glycine residue gets attached to lysine side chain of other protein by isopeptide bond.

Keratin: Fibrous – Intermediate Filament (IF) Protein

- **Keratin is a fibrous protein** and like all other fibrous proteins (such as **collagen & silk fibrion**) is adapted for **structural function. Keratins**, like all other **fibrous proteins (eg collagen & silk fibrion) are insoluble in water**, a property conferred by a **high concentration of hydrophobic amino acids both in interior of protein and onits surface**

Right handed Alpha Helix and Left Handed Super Helix with Plenty of Hydrophobic Aminoacids.

- α-keratin (helix) **secondary structure is right handed α helix**. *Two strands of α-keratin (right handed helix), oriented in parallel (with their amino terminals at the same end)*, are wrapped about each other to form a **super twisted coiled coil with its helical axis twisted in a left handed super helix** (forming tertiary structure). The super twisting amplifies the strength of the overall structure, just as strands are twisted to make a strong rope. This super twisting to form a coiled coil is also responsible for discrepancy between the 5.4 A° per turn predicted for α helix by Pauling & Corey and 5.15 to 5.2 A° repeating structures observed in x-ray diffraction (of hair).
- The areas (surfaces) where 2–α helixes touch each other are made up of **hydrophobic aminoacid residues**, their R groups meshed together in a regular interlocking pattern – this **allows a close packing** of polypeptide chains with in left handed supertwist. That's why α keratins are ***rich in hydrophobic aminoacids Ala, Val, Leu, Ile, Met and Phe***[Q].

Disulfide Bonds & Strength of Quaternary Structure

- Intertwinging of 2-α helical polypeptides (coiled coils) forms **quaternary structure** of keratin. It is stabilized by **disulfide cross links** ***between pairs of cysteine (Cyst) residues of adjacent polypeptide chains***[Q] (enhancing the strength of fibrous proteins).
- **Protein α keratin**, formed by all **vertebrates**, is the **chief structural component of hair, nails, horns, hooves, wool, feathers, scales, claws, quills and much of the outer layer of skin**. So α- keratins form tough, insoluble protective structures of varying hardness and flexibility evolved for strength. ***In α-Keratins , the quaternary structure (formed by intertwinging of 2-α-helical polypeptide chains) is stabilized by disulfide bond cross links between pairs of cysteine (cyst) residues of adjacent polypeptide chains***[Q].
- The **extent of hardness, strength and flexibility** of α-keratins depends on the **number of disulfide bonds** (sulfur content / cysteine residues). ***The more the number of disulfide bonds between Cys residues of adjacent polypeptide chains, the more the hardness, toughness & strength and lesser the flexibility of the keratin is***[Q]. So decreasing order of disulfide bonds (or hardness) is
- **Hair can be waved/curled** by moist heat and stretching out α-helix to fully extended β –conformation. **Reducing agent (thiol / or sulfhydryl group)** is applied with moist heat – the reducing agent cleaves disulfide cross link and moist heat breaks hydrogen bonds, thus causing α-helix to uncoil. After some time reducing agent is washed and oxidizing agent is applied to establish new disulfide bond pairs between Cys residues of adjacent polypeptide chains but not the same bond pairs as before the treatment. Similarly straightening of hair can also be done.

IF Proteins

Alpha –keatins are part of a broader family of proteins k/a intermediate filament (IF) proteins. IF is an intracellular fibrous system of filaments with an *axial periodicity of 21 nm and a diameter of 8-10 nm that is intermediate between that of microfilaments (6nm) and microtubules (23nm).*

IF Proteins	Distribution
Keratins **-Type I (Acidic)** **-Type II (Basic)**	**Epithelial cells, hair, nails, horns, hooves, feathers etc**
Lamins A, B and C	**Nuclear lamina**
Neurofilaments **- L (low),** **- M (medium),** **- H (high)**	**Neurons**
Vimentin like **- Peripherin** **- Glial fibrillary acid protein** **- Desmin** **- Vimentin**	 **- Neurons** **- Glial cells** **- Muscle** **- Mesenchymal cells**

They are all elongated, fibrous molecules with a central rod domain, an amino terminal head and a carboxy terminal tail. Mature filaments are composed of tetramers packed together in a helical manner forming a structure like rope. They are structural component of cells, and most are relatively stable components of cytoskeleton, not undergoing rapid assembly and disassembly and not disappearing during mitosis as do actin and microtubular filaments. **Lamins**, which form a *mesh work in apposition to inner nuclear membrane,* is an important exception – lamins subsequent to phosphorylation disassemble at mitosis and **reappear when it ends.**

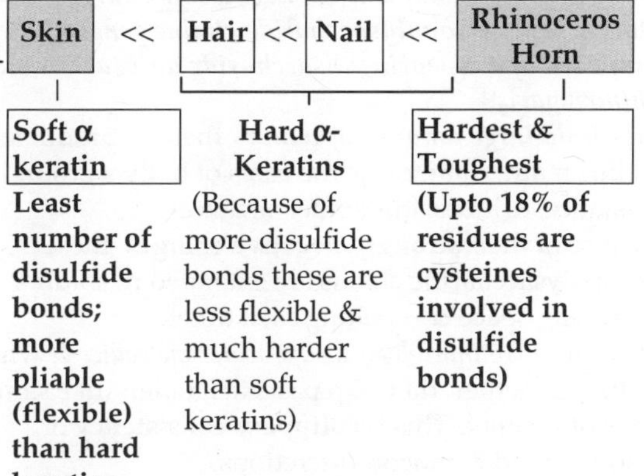

Glycoprotein

- Are ***proteins that contain oligosaccharide (glycan) chains covalently attached to their polypeptide backbones***[Q]
- Carbohydrate chain is usually ***short (2- 10 units), branched & have several repeats***[Q]. Their carbohydrate content ranges from *1- 85%* by weight.
- Once a glycoprotein has been purified, the use of *mass spectrometry* and *high resolution NMR spectroscopy* can often identify the structures of its glycan chains. Analysis of glycoproteins can be complicated by the fact that they often exist as ***glycoforms***; i.e. ***proteins with identical aminoacid sequence but some what different oligosaccharide compositions***[Q].
- *Oligosacchride chains encodes biological information* and this depends upon their constituent sugars, their sequences and their linkages.
- Oligosacchride chain of glycoprotein is responsible for – *physiochemical properties* (eg solubility, viscosity, charge, conformation, denaturation & binding sites), *biological activity, protection against proteolysis, insertion into membranes, intracellular migration, sorting and secretion*. It affects embryonic development & differentiation and site of metastasis.
- Eight sugars predominate in glycoproteins and these are *mannose, fucose* (are GDP linked); *glucose, galactose, xylose, N- Acetyl galactosamine, N- Acetyl glucosamine* (are UDP linked) and *N- Acetyl neuraminic acid* (linked to CMP to form nucleotide sugar)
- *N- Acetyl neuraminic acid (Neu Ac)* is usually found at the *termini* of oligosaccharide chains attached to *subterminal galactose (Gal) or N- acetyl galactosamine (Gal Nac)*. Other sugars are in internal positions. *Neuraminidase* is an *exoglycosidase* (i.e. act externally); endoglycosidase F & H act internally; where as *galactosidase* is both *exo & end glycosidase*
- Based on their linkage between their polypeptide chains & oligosaccharide chains; glycoprotein can be of 3 types:
  i) **O- linked** i.e. containing O- glycosidic linkage, involving hydroxyl chain of serine/ threonine and sugar N- acetyl galactosamine ***(Gal Nac – Ser /Thr)***
  ii) **N- linked** i.e. containing N- glycosidic linkage, involving amide nitrogen of asparagine and N- Acetyl Glucosamine ***(Glc Nac – Asn)***
  iii) **GPI – linked/*Glycophosphatidyl inositol*–linked** i.e. glycan (oligosacchride) is linked to carboxyterminal of a.a. via phosphoryl ethanolamine.

Three inhibitors of enzymes involved in the glycosylation of glycoproteins and their sites of action	
Inhibitor	Site of Action
Tunicamycin	Inhibits GlcNAc-P transferase, the enzyme catalyzing addition of GlcNAc to dolichol-P, the first step in the biosynthesis of oligosaccharide-P-Pdolichol
Deoxynojirimycin	Inhibitor of glucosidases I and II
Swainsonine	Inhibitor of mannosidase II

- ***Glycophorin a RBC glycoprotein contain both O and N linked oligosacchrides***[Q]. Almost all plasma proteins except albumin are glycoproteins. *Selectins* (a glycoprotein) play a key role in *inflammation & lymphocyte homing*. Zona pellucida contain glycoproteins ZP 1- 3, that functions as a *receptor for sperm* (esp *ZP – 3*) & induce *acrosomal reaction*.
- *Asialoglycoprotein receptor* is involved in clearance of glycoprotein from plasma by hepatocytes.
- *Tunicamycin, deoxynojirimycin & swainsonine inhibit N but not O- glycosylation*. The extension of O- linked chains can be prevented by *Gal NAC – benzyl*.

Glycosaminoglycans (GAG)

- GAGs are ***large complexes of negatively charged, long, unbranched, hetropolysaccharide chains generally composed of a repeating disaccharide unit [acidic sugar – aminosugar]$_n$***[Q]
- They ***hold large amount of water***[Q] thereby producing the gel like matrix that forms the basis of body's ground substance, & lubricating other structures
- Because of their **strongly negative charges**, these hetropolysaccharide chains are extended in solution occupying space & repelling each other.
- They are *surrounded by a shell of water molecules* & when brought together, they slip past each other (like same poles of magnet) This l/t **slippery consistency** of synovial fluid & mucous secretions.
- When compressed, the water is squeezed out and GAGs occupy smaller volume. on release of compression the GAGs spring back to their original hydrated volume thus

Proteoglycan

- ***GAGs are generally associated with a small amount of protein forming proteoglycans which contain > 95% carbohydrate***[Q]. Whereas, glycoproteins contain primarily protein & a small amount of carbohydrate
- *All the GAGs, except hyaluronic acid, form proteoglycans*. It is also the only GAG which is *not sulfated* and also found in *bacterias.*
- Proteoglycan monomer resembles a *bottle brush* as it consists of a *core protein to which linear GAG chains* are covalently attached. Each chain may be composed of > *100 monosaccharide chains*, remain separated from each other b/o charge repulsion.

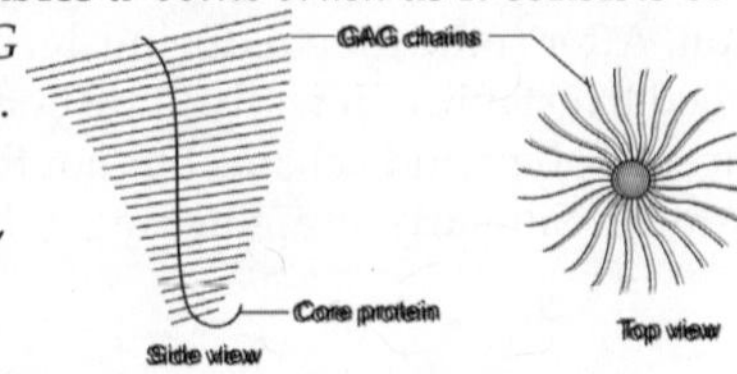

- Linkage b/w core protein & carbohydrate (GAG) chains is most commonly through *a serine residue & a trihexoside (galactose – galactose – xylose)* respectively. An O glycosidic bond is formed b/w hydroxyl group of serine & Xylose.

provides **cushioning**.
- Tend to attract polycations & positive ions such as Na+/K+ which result in their ability to attract water by osmotic pressure.

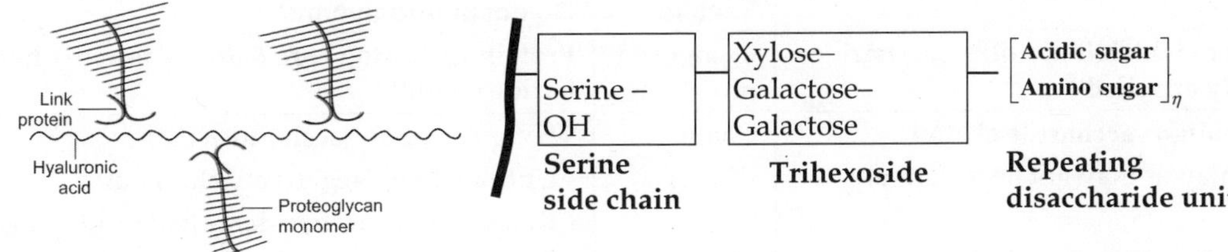

Core protein
- Proteoglycan monomers associate with hyaluronic acid molecule to form proteoglycans aggregates *primarily through ionic interactions*. Association is stabilized by small link proteins.
- PGs can act as **sieves** restricting the passage of large molecules into ECM but allowing free diffusion of small molecules.
- Syndecan (membrane), versican & aggregan (extracellular matrix) and neurocan & cerebrocan (nervous system) are proteoglycans.

★ **So proteoglycan=GAGs+Protein (≤5%) =[Amino & Acidic sugar]$_n$ + proteins**

Glycosylation: Glycosidic Linkages of Glycoproteins

Addition of carbohydrate (sugar or oligosaccharide) side chains to specific aminoacid residues of proteins forming glycoprotein is called **glycosylation**. There are **two types of glycosylation (& glycosides).**

N-Glycosylation and N – Linked Glycosides

- In N-Glycosylation sugar chain is attached to ***amide (NH_2) group of asparagine***[Q] side chain **(Glc Nac – Asn)**
- N-linked oligosaccharide may be of complex or high-mannose variety both containing same **core pentasaccharide**. But additional sugars for complex oligosacchride are NANA (N-acetyl neuraminic acid), Fuc (L-fucose) & Glc NAc (N-acetyl glucosamine), whereas high mannose oligosaccharides contain primarily mannose (Man) only
- **Endo plasmic reticulum (synthesis) & golgi complex (final processing) are involved in N- glycosylation**[Q].

ER
- Protein & **dolichol** (80- 100 carbon ER membrane lipid) linked oligosaccharide are first synthesized.
- Sugars added to dolichol by membrane bound **glycosyl transferase** are first N- acetyl glucosamine f/b mannose & glucose
- Oligosaccharide is transferred from dolichol to asparagine side of protein by **protein – oligosaccharide transferase** present in ER
- **Trimming of carbohydrate chain begins** in ER by removal of mannosyl & glucosyl residues.

Golgicomplex
- **Final trimming & completion** of oligo saccharide chains by addition of variety of sugars (Nac glucosamine, Nac galactosamine, mannose, fucose, NANA) to produce **complex glycoprotein** or
- They are not processed, leaving branched, mannose containing chains in a **high- mannose glycoprotien.**

O- Glycosylation & O-Linked Glycosides

- In O-Glycosylation sugar chain is attached to hydroxy ***(OH) group of either serine or threonine***[Q] R group **(Gal Nac – Ser/Thr)**
- O – glycosylation begins with *transfer of an N-acetyl galactosamine (from UDP-Nac) onto a seryl or threonyl R group.* The **glycosyltransferases** responsible for stepwise synthesis of oligosaccharide are bound to ***membrane of golgi complex***[Q]**.**
- **Tyrosine, hydroxylysine and hydroxyproline** aminoacids may also be involved in O-glycosylation.

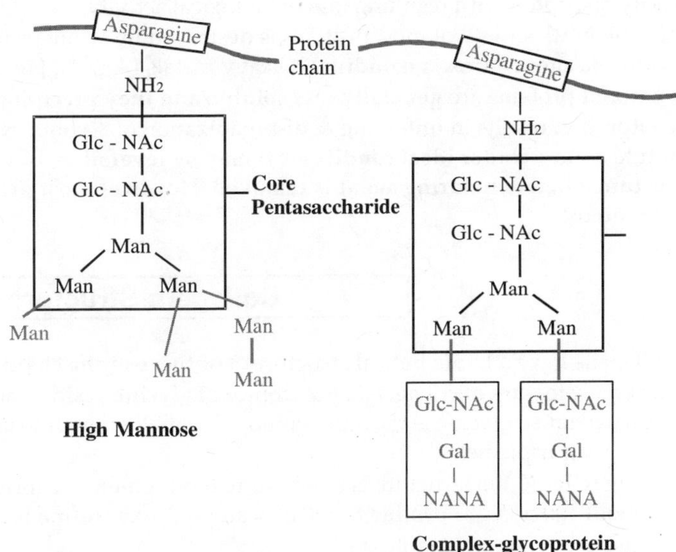

Glycoproteins	Feature	Glycosaminoglycans
Are **proteins to which hetro oligosaccharides are covalently attached**Q	Composed of	**Protein including core & link protein + hetro polysacc haride chain**Q
- **Short hetrooligo saccharide chain**Q - Branched, may or may not be negatively charged. - No repeating disaccharide units	Chain	- Long hetropolysaccharide chain - **Unbranched, Negatively charged**Q. - **Repeating disaccharide units**Q [acidic sugar-amino sugar]$_n$ - Acidic sugar is D- glucronic acid or L- iduronic acid and aminosugar is D-glucosamine or D- galacto-samine
- **Cell surface recognition**Q - Cell surface antigenicity - Components of extracellular matrix & mucin - Globular proteins in plasma	**Function**	- Chondroitin 4 & 6 sulfates, keratan, dermatan & heparan sulfate, heparin & hyaluronic acid are 6 major types - Bind large amounts of water, producing gel like ground substance supporting cellular & fibrous component of tissues - D/t viscosity also k/a mucopolysaccharides - Mediate cell-cell signaling & adhesion
- **N-glycosylation occurs in ER lumen & O-glycosylation in golgi complex**Q - In golgi complex proteins are sorted to their proper destination such as inclusion in cell membrane, lysosome or secretion from cell	Synthesis	- **Glycosaminoglycans are synthesized in golgicomplex**Q - Sulfonation of amino sugar is last step. Source of sulfate is 3′ – phophoadenosyl –5- phosphosulfate. - All except hyaluronic acid form proteoglycan monomer, which consist of a core protein to which linear chains of glycosamino glycans are attached.

Denaturation

- Disruption of native structure is termed denaturation. Physically denaturation may be viewed as **randomizing the conformation of a polypeptide chain**Q with out affecting its primary structure.
- Since no covalent bonds in the back bone of the polypeptide chain are broken during this, the primary structure remains intact
- The comparatively weak forces responsible for maintaining secondary, tertiary and quaternary structure of protein are readily disrupted with resulting loss of biological activity.
- The biological activity of most proteins is destroyed by strong acids or bases, heat, ionic detergents (amphipaths), **chaotropic agents (urea, guanidine)**Q, heavy metals (Ag, Pb, Hg) or organic solvents.
- Denatured proteins are **generally less soluble and they precipitate**Q (not always).
- Denaturation results in unfolding & disorganization of secondary & tertary structure of protein without hydrolysis of peptide bonds. **Under ideal conditions it may be reversible, in which case the protein refolds into original native structure when denaturing agent is removed. However most proteins, once denatured remain permanently disordered**Q.

Collagen: Structure & Formation

- All collagens have a **triple helical** structure. **3 of these alpha chains** are then wound into **right handed superhelix**. A characteristic feature of collagen is occurrence of **glycine residue at every 3rd position** of triple helix of α- chin. This is necessary because glycine is the only amino acid small enough to be accommodated in the limited space available down the central core of triple helix.
- Repeating (Gly- X-Y)n structure is an absolute requirement for formation of triple helix while X & Y can be any other amino acids, about 100 of X are **proline** & 100 of Y are **hydroxyproline** both of which confer rigidity
- Biosynthesis of collagen involves.

Intracellular events in fibroblast, osteoblast or chondroblast

1. **Cleavage of signal or leader peptide to form pro α chains** (from pre-pro α chains)
   Like most secreted proteins produced for export, collagen is synthesized on ribosomes in a precursor form preprocollagen, which contain a leader sequence that facilitates binding of ribosomes to RER & directs the polypeptide chain **into the lumen of endoplasmic reticulum.** The signal sequence is cleaved in ER to yield a precursor of collagen called **pro α chain.**
2. **Hydroxylation of prolyl & some lysyl residues**: proline & lysine residues found at Y position may be *post translationally modified (i.e. hydroxylated) to hydroxy proline & hydroxy lysine residues*, through the action of prolyl hydroxylase & lysyl hydroxylase enzymes. It requires *molecular oxygen (O_2), **reducing agent vitamin C (ascorbic acid)** and α ketoglutarate as cofactors.*
   So in scurvy collagen fibers cannot be cross linked greatly decreasing the tensile strength
3. **Glycosylation of some hydroxyl- lysyl residues** by addition of *galactose or galactosyl- glucose* through an **O-glycosidic linkage** (that is unique to collagen): Like hydroxylation, glycosylation also takes place in ER
4. **Formation of intrachain & interchain disulfide bonds in extension peptides:** Procollagen molecule contains polypeptide extension **(extension peptides)** of 20-35 kDa at both its amino & carboxy terminal. Both extension peptides have cysteine residues. While amino terminal propeptides form only intrachain disulfide (S – S) bonds, the carboxy terminal extension peptide forms both intra & interchain S-S bonds.
5. **Formation o triple helix**:
   Formation of these disulfide bonds assists in formation of triple helix, winding starts from carboxy terminal end. After formation of triple helix, no further hydroxylation or glycosylation can take place. Procollagen molecules are translocated to *golgi apparatus*, where they are packed in *secretory vesicles*. The vesicles fuse the *cell membrane* & release procollagen molecules into extracellular space.

Extracellular events

6. **Cleavage of N and C terminal extension peptides of procollagen molecules.**
   Extracellular enzymes called **procollagen amino proteinase & procollagen carboxy proteinase** remove the extension peptides at amino and carboxy terminal ends, respectively. Cleavage may occur *within crypts or folds in the cell membrane*, releasing triple helical **tropocollagen** molecules which *spontaneously assemble* into collagen fibers.
7. **Self assembly of tropocollagen molecules into quarterly staggered collagen fibrils**
   Tropocollagen molecules spontaneously associate to form collagen fibrils. They form an ordered, parallel, overlapping array, with adjacent collagen molecules arranged in a **quarter staggered pattern** (such that each is displaced longitudinally from its neighbour by slightly less than a quarter of its length)
8. **Oxidtive demination of ε- amino groups of lysyl & hydroxylysyl residues to aldehydes and formation of intra and inter chain cross links**
   Lysyl oxidase, a copper containing enzyme that oxidatively deaminates the ε– amino group of lysine & hydrolysine residues, yielding reactive aldehydes
   The reactive aldehydes (allysine & hydroxy allysine) can condense with ε aminogroup of *unoxidized lysyl or hydroxylysyl residues* in neighbouring collagen molecules to form **collagen crosss links**, & thus, mature collagen fibers
   Histidine may also be involved in certain cross links.

Tropocollagen or Collagen Molecule

It is a subunit of larger collagen aggregates such as fibrils & is approximately **300 nm long and 1.5 nm in diameter**, made up of ***three left-handed alpha* helix *polypeptides strands*** (its name is not to be confused with the commonly occurring alpha helix, a right-handed structure). These three left-handed helices are **twisted together into a *right-handed triple helix or "super helix"***, a quaternary structure stabilized by numerous *hydrogen bonds*. With type I collagen and possibly all fibrillar collagens if not all collagens, each triple-helix associates into *a right-handed super-super-coil* that is referred to as the collagen microfibril. Collagen fibrils are collagen molecules packed into an organized overlapping bundle. Collagen fibers are bundles of fibrils.
A distinctive feature of collagen is the regular arrangement of amino acids in each of the three chains of these collagen subunits - Gly-Pro-Y or Gly-X-Hyp, where X and Y may be any of various other amino acid residues. So ***Proline or hydroxyproline*** constitute about *1/6* &, ***Glycine*** accounting for the *1/3* of the sequence, this means that approximately half of the collagen sequence is not glycine or proline.
In the fibrillar collagens, the tropocollagen molecules are staggered from each other by about ***67nm*** (a **'D' unit** and changes depending upon the hydration state of the aggregate). Each *D-period contains 4 and a fraction collagen molecules*. This is because 300 nm divided by 67 nm does not give an integer (the length of the collagen molecule divided by the stagger distance D).
Collagen fibrils / aggregates are arranged in different combinations and concentrations in various tissues to provide varying tissue properties. **In bone**, entire collagen triple helices lie in a ***parallel, staggered array. 40 nm gaps between the ends of the tropocollagen subunits serve as nucleation sites for the deposition of long, hard, fine crystals of the mineral component, which is (approximately) hydroxyapatite, $Ca_{10}(PO_4)_6(OH)_2$with some phosphate***. It is in this way that certain kinds of cartilage turn into bone. Type I collagen gives bone its tensile strength.

Simple & Conjugated Protein

Proteins can be divided *on the basis of their solubility and their physical properties*

Simple proteins

On complete hydrolysis yield only amino acids

Examples:

- ***Albumin***[Q]
- ***Globulin***[Q]
- Protamines
- Histones

Conjugated protein

Are simple proteins combined with a non- protein group called prosthelic group. Protein part is called **apoprotein** and entire molecule is called holoprotein.

Class	Nucleo-protein	Muco-protein (mucoids)	Lipo protein	Glyco protein	Phospho protein	Chromoprotein			Metallo protein				
						Hemo-protein	Flavo protein	Visual purple					
Prosthetic group	DNA RNA	Hexo-samine	Lipids	Carbo hydrate	Phosphate	Heme (Fe-porphyrin)	Riboflavin (flavin) nucleotide	Caroten-oid	Fe	Zn	Ca	Cu	Mo
Example	Chromatin	Mucin	B_1 lipo-protein	IgG	Casein Ovovitellin	Hb Mb Cytc, P_{450}	Succinate dehydro-genase		Ferritin	Alcohol dehydrogenase, carbonic	Calmodulin	Plastocyanin, ceruloplasmin	Dinitrogenase

Transport or Binding Plasma Proteins

Plasma Proteins	Function (Bind & Transport)
Transthyretin (Prealbumin)	**Thyroxine (T4) and retinol** (forms a complex with retinol binding protein)
Albumin	Osmotic protein binds & transports various ligands like **ions (Ca++), metals (Cu2+, Zn2+), bilirubin , free fatty** acids, metheme, steroids, other hormones & drugs
Retinol binding protein	Binds & transports **retinol**
Ceruloplasmin	Contains & transports **Cu++** (albumin is probably more important in physiological transport of Cu++); has **ferroxidase activity**.
Corticosteroid binding globulin (Transcortin)	Cortisol
Thyroid binding globulin (TBG)	**Thyroxine (T4, T3)**

Plasma Proteins		Function (Bind & Transport)
Haptoglobin		**Extracorpuscular (free) hemoglobin** (phenotype 1-1); **peroxidase activity** (phenotype 2-1)
Sex hormone binding globulin		Testosterone , estradiol
Hemopexin (HPX) = Beta-B-Globulin		**Heme**
Transferrin (Siderophillin)		**Iron (Fe)**
Trans cobalamine I, II, III ($\alpha_2\beta$ mobility)		**Vitamin B_{12}**
Lipoproteins	**α_1 (HDL)**	Transport lipid, fat soluble vitamins, hormones and remove **cholesterol from tissue to liver (scavanger action)**
	β (LDL)	Transport same but **carries cholesterol to tissues.**

★ **Hemoglobin** is a tetrameric protein of RBC that **transport O_2 to tissues and return CO_2 & protons to lungs.**

Storage Proteins

These are **biological reserves of metal ions and aminoacids** such as found in plant seeds, egg whites and milk. Examples includes

1. Plant albumins: **legumelin** in legumes and **leucosin** in cereals.
2. Animal albumins: **ovalbumin** in egg and **lactalbumin & casein** in milk
3. Globulins: ovoglobulin in egg and lactoglobulin in milk
4. **Gliadins (prolamines)** very rich in proline but poor in lysine: gliadin of wheat and **hordein** of barley
5. **Glutelins** (rich in glutamic acid): glutelin in wheat and **oryzenin** of rice
6. **Ferritin and hemosiderin** stores iron
7. **Myoglobin** , a monomeric protein of red muscles stores oxygen as a reserve against oxygen deprivation (Harper 29/48)*

Heat Test for Protein

Take 2/3 of test tube full of urine sample. Hold the test tube from the bottom and heat the top portion of tube. Add a drop of 1% acetic acid. Do not mix.

Normally (when Urine PH is Acidic)	If Urinary pH is Alkaline
White turbidity or precipitates in the heated portion indicating the presence of albumin.	- Proteins may not be precipitated owing to formation of alkaline meta proteins, which are not precipitated on heating - ***Phosphates may however be precipitate and give a false positive test***[Q]. - On acidification with 1% acetic acid, drop by drop, phosphate will disappear and precipitate of albumin will appear on acidification.

Test Methods for Estimation of Substances

Total Serum Protein Estimation

- **Calorimetric Assay (common methods)**

1. ***Biuret***[Q] protein assay
2. ***Lowry's (Folin-Ciocalteu)***[Q] protein assay
3. ***Smith (Bicinchoinic acidd)***[Q] protein assay
4. ***Bradford's (Coomassie G-250 dye) method***[Q]

- Nephelometric, Turbidimetric, Direct photometric, UV visible spectroscopy, Refractometric methods
- Kjeldahl method, Amido black protein assay, O-phthaldehyde & Nano orange methods.

Blood Glucose Concentration

- Aztoor-king, Folin Wu & Nelson-Somogyi chemical methods.
- Glucokinase, Hexokinase & Glucose dehydrogenase enzymatic methods.

Tests of Carbohydrate

- **Molisch's test**
- **Barfoed's, Benedict's and Fehling's tests** for detection of reducing sugar (ie with aldehyde & ketone group). **Seliwanoff's test** differentiate between aldose & ketone sugars.
- **Bial's Resorcinol test** detect presence of pentose (5C sugars)

Tests for Lipids

- Brown paper (grease spot) test
- Sudan red test

Uric Acid

- Phosphotungstic acid (PTA) chemical method
- Uricase enzymatic method

Blood Urea

- Diacetyl monoxime (DAM) chemical method
- Urease & glutamate dehydrogenase enzymatic methods

Clinical Laboratory Based Analytic Systems for Measuring Serum Creatinine to Assess GFR

Alkaline picrate methods

- **Jaffe method** (1886) overestimates serum creatinine by as much as 15-25% d/t presence of interfering substance, particularly *proteins (albumin), acorbate, pyruvate, glucose, bilirubin, fetal hemoglobin & drugs*
- **Kinetic Jaffe assay** have improved specificity & minimized suceptibility to interfering substances.
- **Technicon continuous flow autoanalyzer** (Skeggs) provided the first opportunity to efficiently process increasing workloads & incorporated on line dialysis to remove protein & protein bound interfering substance such as bilirubin, but smaller molecules such as glucose, pyruvate, acetoacetate & cephalosporins were still able to cross the dialysis membrane & cause falsely increased results.

Enzymatic criatinine method

- It uses these enzymes and this reaction

Creatinine —*Creatininase*→ Creatine —*Creatinase*→ Sarcosine —*Sarcosins oxidase*→ Formaldehyde + H_2O_2 + glycine

- The H_2O_2 generated can be measured by spectrophotometrically (Roche creatinine plus assay), using leuco dye (vitros dry chemistry system), or with blood gas analyzer electrodes (Radiometer dual electrode system)
- Bilirubin and creatinine interference is reduced by using more efficient H_2O_2 acceptor (triiodo- hydroxy benzoic acid), potassium ferocyanide& detergents. Ascorbate & dopamine are other interfering substances.

High performance liquid chromatography (HPLC)

Fairly sensitive & specific method and include cation – exchange / normal-phase / reversed-phase and reversed phase ion-pair chromatography. Sample deprotinization improves specificity.

GC- isotope dilution mass spectroscopy

Method of choice

Chromatography

- This is a method of separation of molecules that involves passing (**diffusing**) a solution (the **mobile phase**) through a medium (**immobile or stationary phase**) that shows selective absorption for different solute components based on their size, charge, hydrophobicity & affinity etc. So chromatography separates or purifies proteins on the basis of *charge, size, hydrophobicity or affinity.*
- The stationary /immobile phase or matrix may be a *sheet of filter paper* (**paper chromatography**) or a thin layer of cellulose, silica or alumina (**thin layer chromatography** or **TLC**) or a column (cylinder container of glass, plastic or metal) containing small spherical beads of modified cellulose, acrylamide or silica whose surface has been coated with functional groups)– **Column chromatography**
- Either **ascending** or **descending chromatography** can be done based on the mobile phase being applied *from the bottom or at the top* respectively. Depending on methods of separation types of chromatography include-

Size: Gel Filtration (Size Exclusion) Chromatography

- Separates protein on the basis of ***molecular size*^Q *(stokes radius).***
- A number of gels (sephadex) when hydrated acts as molecular sieves. The pores on the surface of these gel allow smaller molecules to penetrate deeper whereas larger molecules are left outside, hence also called ***exclusion chromatography.***
- The **procedure is *extremely gentle*, permitting seperation of labile substances e.g. protein, nucleic acid like DNA fragments**^Q.
- The procedure is *highly reproducible with minimal losses.*
- Used to *determine molecular weight* of purified protein.

Hydrophobicity: Hydrophobic Interaction Chromatography

- Seperates proteins based on their tendency to associate with a **stationary phase matrix coated with hydrophobic groups** (eg **phenyl Sepharose, octyl Sepharose**)
- *Proteins with exposed hydrophobic surfaces* adhere to the matrix via hydrophobic interactions, that are enhanced by *a mobile phase of high ionic strength*
- Nonadherent proteins are first washed away. The *polarity of mobile phase is then decreased to weaken hydrophobic interactions* by gradually *lowering salt concentration* f/b *adding glycerol or ethanol* (if interactions are very strong).

Solubility: Partition Chromatography

- In this the components of mixture to be separated are partitioned b/w the two phases (eg solid – liquid, liquid-liquid, gas-liquid etc) depending on the **solubility (partition co-efficient)** of the particular substances. Stationary phase may be either solid or liquid over which a liquid or gaseous mobile phase moves
- Purifies proteins based on their relative affinity of different proteins for a given stationary or a mobile phase, which in turn depends on composition of both stationary & mobile phase.
- Proteins that interact more strongly with stationary phase are retained longer and provide a basis of partition (purification)
- Gas liquid chromatography (GLC), TLC or ascending / descending paper chromatography is performed and some **location reagents** (eg ninhydrin for aminoacids & peptides; sulphuric acid for phospholipids; diphenylamine for sugars) is sprayed on paper to identify **RF (relative flow)** value. **RF (ratio of fronts) value** is the *ratio of distance traveled by the substance (solute) to the distance traveled by the solvent* in paper chromatography. The RF is constant for a particular solvent at a given temperature and the substance or aminoacid can be identified by their RF value.

Adsorption coefficients of molecules d/t van der waals interaction with stationary phase: **Absorption Chromatography**

- Protein mixture is applied to a column under conditions where **the protein of interest associates with the stationary phase** so tightly that its partition coefficient is essentially unity
- Non adhering first washed & then stabilizing forces are gradually disrupted by gradient of increasing salt concentration.

Biological Activity: Affinity Chromatography

- Affinity chromatography **separates proteins by their *binding specificities.* The *proteins retained on the column are those that bind specifically to a ligand*^Q** (substance) that has an inherent ability to bind with the target molecule to be purified.
- It exploits the *high selectivity of most proteins for their ligands.* So **enzymes** can be purified by using coenymes or inhibitiors as stationary phase. And so *antigen-antibody, hormone-receptor, enzyme-substrate, inhibitor-cofactor* can be sparated.
- After proteins that do not bind to ligand are washed through Bound proteins are eluted (washed out of column) either by competition with soluble free ligand or by *disrupting protein ligand interactions using urea, guanidine hydrochloride, mildly acidic pH or high salt concentration.*
- Stationary phase matrices available comercialy contain ligands such as *$NADP^+$ or ATP analogs and Ni^{+2}* (that bind protein with an attached polyhistidine tag & a glutathione matrix that binds a recombinant protein linked to glutathione – S- transferase

Charge: Ion- Exchange Chromatography

- Separates proteins depending on the net electric ***charge of protein*^Q.**
- Chromatography ***on carboxymethyl cellulose or diethyl amino methyl cellulose column*^Q** separates protein based on electrostatic attraction b/w charged molecules & oppositely charged groups on ion exchange resins.

Size, affinity & charge; High Performance / Pressure Liquid Chromatograph (HPLC)

- The stationary phase used in classic column chromatography are spongy material whose compressibility limits flow of the mobile phase
- HPLC makes use of **high pressure pumps** that speed the movement of mobile phase (protein molecules) down the column, as well as higher quality chromatographic **incompressible** (sillica or alumina microbeads as) **stationary phase** that can withstand the crushing force of pressurized flow
- Reduced transit time **limits the diffusional spreading** of protein bands & *thus greatly improves resolution.*
- Used for high resolution separation of proteins peptides and aminoacids based on their charge, size & hydrophobicity. The eluates are monitored by *ultraviolet absorption, refractive index or fluorescence.* So it can give **high resolution separation** of mixtures of lipids or peptides whose property differ only slightly.
- **Reversed phase HPCL** uses a *hydrophobic stationary phase of aliphatic polymers* 3-18 carbon atoms in length. And peptide mixtures are eluted (separated) using a gradient of water miscible organic solvent such as *acetonitrile or methanol.*

Ion Exchange Chromatogaphy (IEC) ☆

- It separates (purifies) protein on the basis of differences in the **sign** & **magnitude of net electric** charge at a given pH.
- In IEC, the **stationary phase (column matrix)** is a synthetic polymer (resin) *containing bound (attached) charged groups* – **negatively charged** (carboxylic or sulfonic group) in **cation (+ ion) exchanger;** and **positively charged** (tertiary or quaternary amines) in **anion (- ion) exchanger**. The protein which has to be separated (purified) is percolated through the stationary phase in liquid form and it forms **mobile phase** of IEC. The proteins of mobilephase interact with resin of stationary phase by **charge – charge interaction (electro static attraction)**. Since the *net charge on a protein is determined by the pH,* this separation is also based on *ionic character of proteins & aminoacids* **(isoelectric point)**.
- Proteins, which are *polyvalent compete against monovalent ions* for binding to the stationary phase – thus the term ion exchange

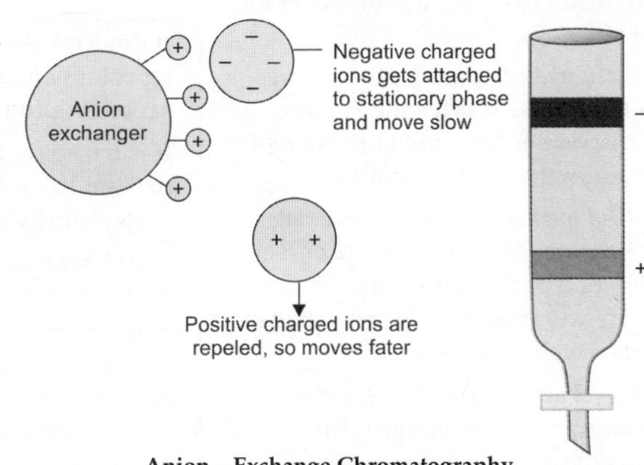

Anion – Exchange Chromatography

- The affinity of each protein for charged group on column (stationary phase) is affected by the pH (which determines the ionization state & net charge of molecule) and **concentration of competing free salt ions**. Separation can be optimized by gradually changing the pH and or salt concentration of the mobile phase so as to create a **pH** or **salt gradient**.

- **On the basis of charge of stationary phase,** It is of 2 types

Cation (Positive ion) Exchanger

When a more positively charged ion (or molecule) is exchanged with another positively charged component bound to **negatively charged stationary phase**, the process is called cation exchanger. Cation exchange resins have **negatively** charged *sulphonic or carboxylic groups*.

Stationary phase (solid matrix) Resin	**Charge**	**Negative**
	Example	- **Carboxymethyl cellulose** ($O\text{-}CH_2\text{-}COO^-$) - Carboxylate (carboxylic) group. - Sulfate (sulphonic) group
Slowest moving amino acids (in mobile phase)		**Positively charged** aa. because they interact with stationary phase
Fastest moving amino acids (in mobile phase)		**Negatively charged**

Anion (Negative ion) Exchanger

When a more negatively charged ion (or molecule) is exchanged with another negatively charged component bound to **positively charged stationary phase** the process is called anion exchanger. Anion exchange resins have positively charged quaternary nitrogen (N^+)

Stationary phase (solid matrix) Resin	**Charge**	**Positive**
	Example	- **Diethyl aminoethyl (DEAE) cellulose** ($\text{- O- } C_2H_4 - NH^+ [C_2H_5]_2$) = Strong anion - Tertiary or quaternary amines (nitrogen) - Dowex – 3 (weak anion) - Amberlite IRC – 50 (weak cation) ?? (Vasudevan)
Slowest moving amino acids		**Negative charged**
Fastest moving amino acids		**Positively charged**

★ At pH 7.5, albumin is negatively charged (pI = 4.8) and immunoglobin is positively charged (pI = ~ 8). So albumin **(anion) will move slowly in an anion exchanger** and immunoglobin **(cation) will move slowly in a cation exchanger.**

Electrophoresis ☆

- **Electrophoresis** is separation of proteins based on ***migration of charged proteins in an electric field***[Q]
- It is ***not geneally used to purify proteins in large amounts because it often adversely affects the structure & function of proteins***[Q] and simpler alternatives are available
- It is an *analytical method that quickly estimates number of different proteins in a mixture or the degree of purity* of a particular prtein preparation. Its advantage is that protein can be visualized as well as separated.
- *Polyacrylamide gel* acts as a molecular sieve slowing the migration of proteine ~ in proportion to **charge – to – mass ratio.** Migration is also affected by **size & shape**[Q].
- The force moving the macromolecule is electrical potential (E)

Isoelectric Focusing

- It determines isoelectric point (pI) of a protein and **separates protein according to their pI.**
- It is based on the fact that each protein has a different pH at which it is electrically neutral (pI)
- A **pH gradient** is generated within polyacrylamide matrix by allowing **ampholytes** or **ionic buffers** (i.e. low molecular weight organic acids & bases) to distribute themselves in an electric field generated across the gel.
- Applied protein migrate until it reaches the region where pH matches its **isoelectric point (pI), the pH at which the molecules net charge is zero.**

Two dimensional Electrophoresis

- It is combining **isoelectric focusing and SDS electrophoresis** sequently
- It is *more sensitive* analytical method than either electrophoretic method alone
- It permits *fractionation of complex mixtures of proteins*
- It separates proteins of identical molecular weight that differ in pI, or protein with similar pI values but different molecular weight

$$\text{Electrophoretic mobility } (\mu) = \frac{\text{Velocity } (V)}{E} = \frac{\text{Net charge } (z)}{\text{Frictional Coffieicnt } (f)}$$

Discrimination / Seperation of Nucleic Acid (DNA & RNA)

- Seperation by size through a gel matrix in presence of an electric field (i.e. gel electrophoresis) is the ***most common technique to discriminate different nucleic acids***[Q]
- Both *DNA & RNA are negatively charged* and will migrate towards a positively charged electrode.
- Seperation is primarily based on **molecular weight** with smaller molecules traveling faster than larger ones. **Physical conformation (or shape)** also affect & form the basis of separation. Because single stranded RNAgenerally hs a high degree of secondary structure. Electrophoresis of RNA is usually performed under denaturating conditions to abolish these structures. Electrophoresis of DNA is performed under non denaturing or denaturing conditions (to abolish hetroduplex, nicked or superhelical circular structures) depending on amplification. Under most gel conditions.

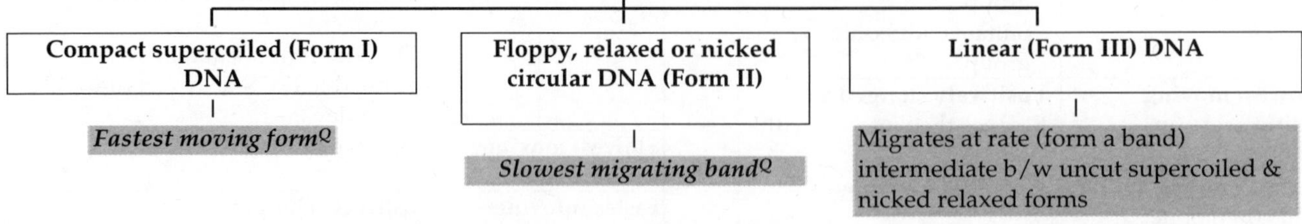

- When very large molecules (> 50kb) have to be separated, **pulsed electrical fields** are employed to help move these molecules through the polymer matrix **(Pulse- field gel electrophoresis, PFGE).** Conventional gel electrophoresis use current applied in single direction. Very large DNA fragments are thought to orient themselves with the voltage field. Once oriented, molecules of different lengths migrate at slow but similar rates. The trick to separating these large fragments is to make them change direction at regular intervals; longer DNAs take longer to orient correctly and so lag behnd shorter fragments. So in PFGE, an alternating current is applied to the gel, changing the direction of electrophoresis at intervals. That's why a normal agarase gel electrophoresis may take 1 – 4 hr, whereas PFEG often require 24 hrs to complete.
- **Polyacrylamide** gel is suited for *high resolution separation* (upto 0.1% size differences) of *short molecules* (upto 2kb), whereas *agarose gel* can separate nucleic acid fragments *from 20 bp to 10 mB (10,000 kb) but with limited resolution* (usually to a size difference 2-5%)

SDS – PAGE

- A *denaturing anionic detergent, sodium dodecyl sulfate (SDS)* [dodecyl denoting 12 carbon chain = $CH_3 (CH_2)_{11}– SO_4 – Na^+$] is used in poly acrylamide gel electrophoresis **(PAGE)** system to separate, resolve & purify protein subunits according to **molecular weight.**
- Acrylamide is polymerized & cross linked to form porous matrix (stationary phase) which acts as a molecular sieve.
- SDS *denatures protein, & disrupts the hydrophobic interactions* of protein so that the protein is *partially unfolded and assumes a similar (rod like) shape.*
- SDS binds to protein at a **ratio of 1 molecule of SDS per 2 peptide bonds (or amino acid residues)** that is roughly *proportional to molecular weight of protein (or length of peptide chain).*
- The large number of bound anionic SDS contribute a **large net negative charge**, rendering the intrinsic charge of protein insignificant and *conferring on each protein a similar charge – to mass ratio.*
- Because SDS treated proteins have similar shape and charge to mass ratio; ***SDS – PAGE separates proteins almost exclusively on the basis of mass (molecular weight)***Q, with smaller polypeptides migrating more rapidly.
- A purified protein preparation can be readily **analyzed for homogeneity (purity)** on SDS-PAGE by staining with sensitive & specific dyes, such as **Coomassie blue**, or with a **silver staining** technique, which *binds to protein but not to gel itself.*
- Thus the researcher can moniter the progress of protein purification as the number of bands decreases after each new fractionation step. When *compared with positions of protein with known molecular weight*, the position of unidentified protein can provide a *good approximation of its molecular weight.*
- SDS- PAGE **separates the component polypeptides of multimeric proteins** when used with **2-merceptoethanol or dithiothreitol** to reduce and break disulfide bonds. **A separate band appears for each component.**

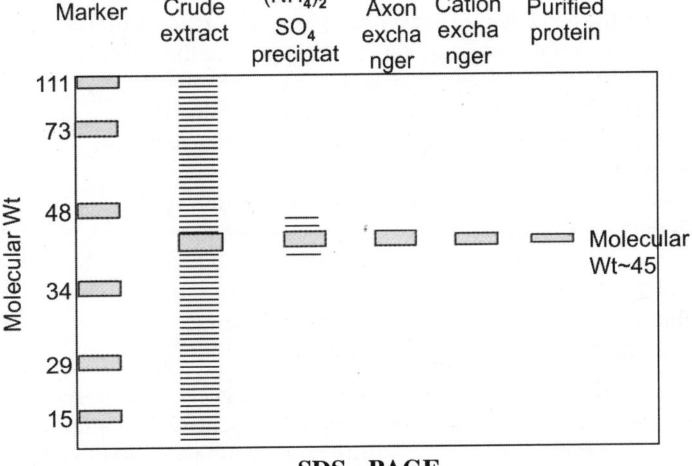

SDS - PAGE

So in above case 100 kD protein has 2 bands of 20 kD & 30 kD.

Hence Protein has 2 components of 20 kD & 30 kD (i.e. 50 kD). Since to be of 100 kD there must be 2 units of 50 kd (50× 2 = 100). So the 100 kD protein is a dimer of 20 kD & 30 kD component.

Detection of Protein Structure

Primary Structure detection

- **Sanger's Reagent Method**
- Fragmenting polypeptide chain by endoproteases & chemical reagents.
- Automated protein sequencer **(sequenator)** using ***Edman's degradation technique***Q and **DNA sequencing.**
- **Mass spectrometry** to ***detect molecular mass, sequence of polypeptides & covalent modifications simultaneously***Q (more commonly used method)
- Protein sequencing, identification and molecular weight determination of intact protein can also be done by **matrix-assisted laser desorption ionization – time of flight (MALDI - TOF) mass spectrometry and Electrospray ionization mass spectrometry (ESI-MS)**
- Once partial aminoacid sequence is obtained, one can determine nucleotide sequence of DNA that encodes this polypeptide segment. Chemically synthesized oligonucleotide primers can be used to identify amplify (by PCR) and isolate gene containing appropriate sequence. **(Indirect hybrid technique)**

Higher three dimensional (Secondary, tertiary and quaternary) structure detection

- ***X ray crystallography (or diffraction)***Q
- **Polychromatic X-ray** crystallography **(Laue diffraction)**
- ***NMR (nuclear magnetic resonance) spectroscopy***Q
- ***Infra-red spectroscopy***Q
- Ultraviolet (UV) light spectroscopy
- Optical rotatory dispersion
- Circular dichromism

Mass Spectrometry

- It determines the ***mass of molecules***Q (< 1000 Da by conventional spectrometers and larger mass by use of **flight spectrometers**)
- Initial difficulty of volatilizing large organic molecules has overcome by ***MALDI (matrix assisted laser desorption and ionization) and electrospray dispersion*** *(eg. Nanospray)* which permit the masses of even large polypeptides (>100000 Da) to be determined with *extraordinary accuracy (±1Da)*
- Peptides inside the mass spectrometer are broken down in smaller units by collisions with *neutral helium atoms (collision induced dissociation)* and the masses of the individual fragments are determined.
- Since peptide bonds are much more labile than the carbon-carbon bonds, the most abundant fragments will differ from one another by units equivalent to one or two amino acids.
- Since with the *exception of leucine and isoleucine*- the molecular mass of each aminoacid is unique, the sequence of the peptide can be reconstructed from the masses of its fragments.
- It *detects covalent modification* i.e. is ideal for detecting the phosphate, hydroxyl and other groups on post translationally modified aminoacids. As each adds a specific and readily identified increment of mass to the modified amino acid
- **Tandem mass spectrometry** can *determine mass by analyzing complex peptide mixture with out prior purification.* It employs the equivalent of 2 mass spectrometers linked in series. It can detect metabolic abnormalities such as PKU, ethyl malonic encephalopathy, & glutaric academia type I.

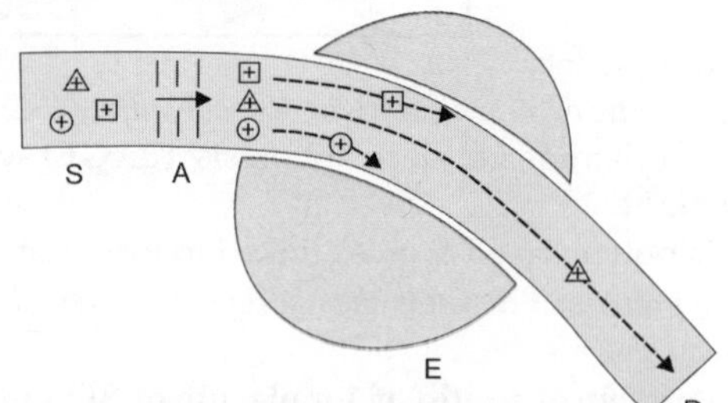

Basic components of a simple mass spectrometer. A mixture of molecules is vaporized in an ionized state in the sample chamber **S.** These molecules are then accelerated down the flight tube by an electrical potential applied to accelerator grid **A.** An adjustable electromagnet, **E,** applies a magnetic field that deflects the flight of the individual ions until they strike the detector, **D.** The greater the mass of the ion, the higher the magnetic field required to focus it onto the detector.

Mass increase resulting from common posttranslational modifications

Modification	Mass Increase (Da)
Phosphorylation	80
Hydroxylation	16
Methylation	14
Acetylation	42
Myristylation	210
Palmitoylation	238
Glycosylation	162

★ **Protein purity** is assessed by ***polyacrylamide gel electrophoresis (PAGE)***Q. The most widely used method is SDS- PAGE i.e. polyacrylamide gel electrophoresis in the presence of the anionic detergent sodium dodecyl sulfate (SDS).

★ **Sanger's reagent (1 fluoro,2, 4- dinitrobenzene)** was used to determine the polypeptide sequence of insulin. It als react with ε- amino group of lysine.

★ **Edman's reagent (phenyl- iso thiocynate)** selectively label the amino terminal residue of a peptide. It enables peptides and proteins to be sequenced.

Enzyme Inhibition ☆

Enzyme/Drug	Competitive Inhibitor	Substrate
Lactate Dehydrogenase	Oxamate	Lactate
Aconitase	Transaconitate	Cis-aconitate
Succinate Dehydrogenase	Malonate	Succinate
HMG-CoA Reductase	HMG	HMG-CoA
Dihydrofolate Reductase	Amethopterin	7,8 Dihydrofolate
Allopurinol	*Xanthine oxidase*, which produce uric acid from hypoxanthine	**Hypoxanthine**
Sulfonamide	Synthesis of folic acid (impermeable to bacterial wall) from PABA	**PABA**
Methotrexate	*Folate reductase* & prevent formation of FH_4	**Folic acid**
MAO Inhibitor eg Ephedrine & amphetamine	*MAO (mono amine oxidase)*	**Cate -cholamines**
Physos-tigmine	Acetyl cholines terase (destroy ACH into choline &acetate)	***Ach***
Dicoumarol	Act as anticoagulant by inhibiting Vit K	***Vit K***
Succinyl Choline	Competitively fixes on post synapti c receptor. As it is not hydrolysed easily by the enzyme acetyl cholinesterase, it produces continued depolarization & muscle relaxation	***Ach***

Regulation of Enzyme Activity

1. Allosteric Inhibition

- Allosteric enzymes are regulated by molecules k/a **effector or modifiers** that bind **noncovalently at a site other than the active site** (k/a allosteric site) on a different region of enzyme molecule. Effector can *alter the affinity &/or the maximal catalytic activity of enzyme.*
- **Positive effectors** increase and **negative effectors** inhibit enzyme activity. When the substrate itself serves as an effector it is called **homotropic effector** but when both are different it is called **heterotropic effector**.
- Does *not follow Michaelis Menten hyperbolic kinetics.* Instead it gives a ***sigmoid curve & show cooperative binding.***Q
- Allosteric ***inhibitors*** shift the substrate saturation curve to the ***right*** & ***activators*** shift it to ***left.***
- Allosteric enzymes may be of *K & M series* according to their kinetics.
- In **K- enzymes** eg *aspartate carbamoylase & phospho fructokinase,* allosteric inhibitor lowers substrate affinity to raise km, but ***Vmax is unchanged***
- In **M-enzymes** eg *acetyl CoA carboxylase,* the allosteric inhibitor reduces the maximum velocity, but ***no change in km or substrate affinity.*** Allosteric activators produce a fall in K enzymes and a rise in Vmax
- When the final product allosterically inhibits the enzyme it is called feed back allosteric inhibition
- ***Asparte transcarbamoylase (AT case)*** which catalyzes first reaction of pyrimidine synthesis is allosterically inhibited by *cytidine triposphate (CTP)*
- *Threonine deaminase* first enz. of isoleucine synthesis is inhibited allosterically by *isoleucine*

Enzyme	*Allosteric activator*	*Allosteric inhibitor*
Glutamate Dehydrogenase	*ADP*	*ATP, NADH*
Hexo kinase ICD	*ADP*	*G-6-P, ATP*
Protein Kinase	*c-AMP*	-
Pyruvate carboxylase	*Acetyl CoA*	*ADP*
Phospho fructo kinase	-	*Citrate*

- A metabolite may cause feed forward allosteric activation eg *F1. 6 Bi PO_4 activates pyruvate kinase*
- Allosteric effector oppositely influences two allosteric enzymes catalyzing reverse reations eg. *AMP activates phospho fructo kinase & inhibits F.D. pase*

2. By covalent modification eg **phosphorylation & dephosphorylation of enzyme.**

Michaelis – Menten model & equation

- According to M-M- model, ***enzyme (E) reversibly combines with its substrate (S) to form enzyme – substrate (ES) complex that subsequently yields product (P), regenerating the free enzyme***Q

$$E + S \underset{K-1}{\overset{K}{\rightleftharpoons}} ES \xrightarrow{K_2} E + P$$

- M- M- equation describes how ***reaction velocity varies with substrate concentration***Q.

$$Initial\ Velocity\ (V_0) = \frac{Maximum\ velocity\ (V_{max})[S]}{Michaelis\ constant\ (K_m) + [S]}$$

Where, [S] is substrate concentration & $K_m = (K-1+K_2)/K_1$. And it is assumed that concentration of substrate is much greater than enzyme, concentration of [ES] does not change with time and [ρ] is very small so rate of back reaction can be ignored. Conclusions extracted are

Catalytic Constant (Kcat) & Efficiency (Kcat/Km)

- Comparision of **relative catalytic activity** of different preparations of same enzyme or different enzymes can be done in
- Impure enzyme preparations by

$$\text{Specific activity} = \frac{V_{max}}{\text{Protein concentration}}$$

- Homogenous enzyme by

$$\text{Turnover number} = \frac{V_{max}}{\text{Moles of enzyme}}$$

- If number of active sites is known

$$\text{Catalytic constant}\ (K_{cat}) = \frac{V_{max}}{\text{Number of active sites}\ (S_t)}$$

Michaelis constant (Km)
- It is characteristic of enzyme & its particular substrate and ***reflects the affinity of enzyme to that substrate***Q
- It is equal to substrate concentration at which ***reaction velocity is equal to 1/2 V_{max}***Q. It ***does not change with enzyme concentration***Q.

Small (low) Km	Large (High) Km
Reflects **high affinity** of enzyme for substrate, as low concentration of S is needed to half saturate E, i.e., to reach 1/2 V_{max}.	Reflects **low affinity** of E for S, because a high concentration of substrate is needed to half saturate enzyme

- **Rate of reaction velocity is *directly proportional to enzyme concentration at all substrate concentrations***Q. Eg. when [E] is halved, V_0 & V_{max} are reduced to half of original
- **Order of reaction**

When [S] << Km	When[S]>> Km
- Velocity of reaction is approximately proportional to substrate concentration i.e., $V\alpha\,[S]$ - **1st order reaction** with respect to substrate.	- Velocity is constant and equal to V_{max} (i.e., V = V_{max}) - **Zero order** reaction, *independent of substrate concentration*

★ **Line weaver – Burk (double – reciprocal) plot** is a straight line obtained by plotting $1/V_0$ versus $1/_{[S]}$. It can be used to calculate Km & V_{max}, as well as to determine the mechanism of action of enzyme inhibitors.

It is best measure and unit is 1/time

- **Catalytic efficiency** is best expressed in terms of **ratio of Kcat/km**

Inhibitory Potency

It is the concentration of inhibitor that produces 50% inhibition (**IC_{50}**)

Calcium – Calmodulin

Calmodulin is calcium dependent (& binding) regulatory protein that is homologus to muscle protein troponin-C in structure & function. It can bind to **4 calcium ions**. Binding of Ca++ with calmodulin activates it (in a similar way of cAMP activates PKA). Enzymes & process activated by Ca^{++} & mediated by calmodulin are

- **Adenylyl *cyclase***Q (brain)
- C-AMP phosphodiesterase
- C-AMP gated olfactory channel
- Cyclic neucleotide **phosphodiesterase**
- ***Guanylate cyclase***Q
- C-GMP gated Na^+ & Ca^{++} channels of rods & cones
- ***Glycogen synthase***Q
- Glycerol-3 phosphate dehydrogenase
- Glutamate decarboxylase

- Ca^{++} dependent protein kinases (CaM kinase I-IV)
- Ca^{++} - Mg^{++} ATPase
- Ca^{++} pump (plasma membrane calcium ATP ase)
- Ca^{++} phospholipid dependent protein kinase
- Ca++ release channels of sarcoplasmic reticulum
- Ca++ dependent Na+ channel (paramecium)
- Calcineurin (phosphoprotein phosphatase 2B)
- L-type calcium channels
- Cytoskeletal protein

- Phosphorylase kinase
- phosphoprotein phosphatase 2B
- Phosphoinositide 3 kinase
- PhospholipaseC
- Phospholipase A2
- Pyruvate carboxylase
- Pyruvate dehydrogenase
- Pyruvate kinase

- RNA helicase
- Myosin light chain kinase
- NAD+ kinase
- Nitric oxide synthase
- NMDA type glutamate receptor

Plasma Enzymes can be of Two Types

Features	Functional Enzymes	Non Functional Enzymes
Function	Has physiological role	No known physiological role
Normal concentration in plasma in comparision to tissue	High	Low
Substrate in blood	Always present	Absent
Site of synthesis	Mostly in liver	In different tissues eg liver, heart, muscle
Cause of origin	Physiological need	Pathological process eg - Cell damage & necrosis in viral hepatitis or MI - Obstruction of normal path (bile duct = alkaline PO_4) - Meastasis
Clinical importance	No	Diagnosis & prognosis of disease
Example	***Lipoprotein lipase***[Q] etc	***Acid & alkaline phosphatase*, *γ glutamyl trnspeptidase***[Q] etc.

Isozymes / Isoenzymes

Isozymes are the physically distinct forms of the same enzyme that catalyze the same reaction, and ***differ from each other structurally, electrophoretically and immunologically***[Q]. Isozymes arise through **gene duplication** in higher organisms. Isoenzymes may differ in their

1. **Quarternary structure** as many **isoenzyme multimeric complexes** contain ***different subunits in different (various) combinations***[Q] such as CPK1 has BB, CPK 2 has MB and CPK 3 has MM compositon.
2. **Physical properties** such as **heat resistance** because of genetically determined ***difference in aminoacid sequence***[Q]
3. **Electrophoretic mobility** (allowing them to be separated from each other by electrophoresis) because of **different electrical charges on the isoenzymes due to difference in contents of charged acidic & basic aminoacids**)
4. Properties such as **sensitivity to particular regulatory factors** or **substrate affinity** (eg glucokinase) **that adapt them to specific tissues or circumstances.**
5. **Tissue distribution**: **Different organs frequently contain characteristic proportions of different isoenzymes.** So pattern of isozyme in plasma may serve as *means of identifying the site of tissue damage.*
6. Although isoenzymes catalyze same reactions they differ in **rate of catalysis, pH optima, Kmax & Vmax** and even **enzyme classification.**

★ Each enzyme has a enzyme code number (EC No) of 4 digits separated by points; first being the main class, second indicating type of group involved in reaction (sub class), third denotes substrate on which group acts (sub sub class) and fourth digit is serial number of a particular enzyme.

Serum **Non functional enzyme**	Diagnostic Use
Amylase,Lipase	Acute Pancreatitis
Lactate dehydrogenase isoenzyme 5	Liver diseases

Isoenzyme of Lactate Dehydrogenase (LDH)

- Lactate dehydrogenase is a tetrameric enzyme & consists of four subunits
- These subunits can occur in two isoform i.e.
  - H isoform (for heart)
  - M isoform (for muscle)
- All these isozymes though different physically they catalyze the same reaction of oxidation of LA to PA
- In normal serum, *LDH2 (H3M) is the most prominent isoenzyme.*

LDH Isoenzymes				
Type	*Polypeptide chains*	*Electrophorectic mobility*	*Tissue rich in isoenzyme type*	
LDH-1	**(H4) H H H H**	**Fastest moving d/t highest negative charge b/o higher Asp & glutamate content**	**found in *myocardium*[Q]**	**Heat resistance**
LDH-2	**(H3M) H H H M**			
LDH-3	**(H2M2) H H M M**			
LDH-4	**(HM3) H M M M**			**Heat labile**
LDH-5	**(M4) M M M M**	**slowest moving**	**found in *liver (Hepatic)*[Q]**	

Isoenzyme of CPK

- **Creatinine phosphokinase exists as three isoenzymes in human tissue:**
  1. CPK- 1 or CPK – BB : Found in *Brain*
  2. CPK- 2 or CPK – MB : Found in *Myocardium and skeletal muscle.*
  3. CPK- 3 or CPK – MM: Found in *skeletal muscle*

Lactate dehydrogenase (isozyme)	Myocardial infarction
Aminotransferase - Aspartae aminotransferase (AST, or SGOT) - Alanine aminotransferase (ALT or SGPT)	 - Myocardial infarction - Vitral Hepatitis
Ceruloplasmin	Hepatolenticular degeneration (Wilson's disease)
γ-Glutamyl transpeptidase	Liver disease
Creatinine kinase (MB)	Muscle disorder, MI
Acid phosphatase	Metastatic Ca of prostate
Alkaline phosphatase	Bone disorders, obstructive liver disease

- Thus creatinine phosphokinase *1* ***is essentially found in brain & would be increased in brain ischaemia***[Q].

Creatine phosphokinase (CPK) -2-CPKMB

Normally	Myocardial infarction
• *CPK –2 (MB isozyme)* occurs in very small quantity accounting for as less as 2% *of total CK activity of plasma.* • CKMB also exists in 2 form: - $CKMB_1$: Extracardiac form - $CKMB_2$: Cardiac form	• *Elevation of CK-MB* isoenzyme occurs within 4 hours, maximum in 24 hrs, then falls rapidly. • A ratio of *$CKMB_1$: $CKMB_2$ above 1.5 is highly sensitive for the diagnosis of acute MI after 4-6 hours of onset of myocardial ischaemia.*

Oxido- Reductase Enzymes

Oxidation involves *removal of electron /hydrogen or hydride* ion from a (reduced) substrate or *incorporation of O_2* into a (reduced) substrate. After which the reduced substrate becomes oxidized. *Oxygen, flavin nucleotides (FMN, FAD) and nicotinamide coenzymes (NAD^+ or $NADP^+$)* are used as hydrogen acceptor. H_2O_2 canbe used as e- acceptor & donor both. Thus *oxidation is always accompanied by reduction* of an electron (hydrogen) acceptor.

Oxidase

- Catalyze removal of hydrogen from substrate using *O_2 as hydrogen acceptor* and forming H_2O or H_2O_2 as product
- ***Cytochrome oxidase (aa_3) contain copper***[Q]
- Flavoprotein containing oxidases are *L amino oxidase (FMN linked), Xanthine oxidase (Mo containing) and aldehyde dehydrogenase* (FAD linked molybdenum & non heme iron containing)

Dehydrogenase

- Dehydrogenaese **cannot use oxygen as hydrogen acceptor**. So these transfer hydrogen from one substrate to another in a coupled oxidation – reduction reaction
- Cytochromes are iron containing hemoproteins in which iron atoms oscillates between Fe+2 & Fe+3 during oxidation & reduction. All cytochromes (except aa3) i.e. *cytochrome b, C_1, c of respiratory chain and cytochrome p-450 & b_5 of endoplasmic reticulum* are regarded dehydrogenase
- They use common coenzyme eg NAD^+ as hydrogen carrier. Because these reactions are reversible, these reducing equivalents (NAD+) are freely transferred in within the cell.

Hydroperoxidase

- These use H_2O_2 or organic peroxide as substrate & protect body from harmful peroxides.
- Are of 2 types: **peroxidases & catalase**
- Catalase is a hemoprotein containing 4 heme group. In addition to possessing peroxidase activity it uses H_2O_2 as electron donor and acceptor

$$2H_2O_2 \xrightarrow[Catalase]{} 2H_2O + O_2$$

- Peroxidases are found in milk & in leukocytes, platelets, & tissues involved in eicosanoid metabolism. It reduces peroxides using electron acceptors such as **ascorbate, quinines, & cytochrome C**

$$H_2O_2 + AH_2 \xrightarrow{Peroxidase} 2H_2O + A$$

Oxygenase

Catalyze direct transfer & incorporation of O_2 into a substrate

Many dehydrogenase employ **(niacin) nicotinamide coenzymes (NAD+ or NADP+)**

- Glucose -6 – phosphate dehydrogenase (NADP+)
- Glutamate dehydrogenase (NADP+ or NAD+)
- Isocitrate dehydrogenase
- α-ketoglutarate dehydrogenase
- Malate dehydrogenase
- Lactate dehydrogenase
- Alcohol dehydrogenase
- Glyceraldehyde-3-PO4 dehydrogenase

(Isocitrate dehydrogenase to Glyceraldehyde-3-PO4 dehydrogenase: NAD^+)

Other depend on **(riboflavin) flavoproteins (FMN or FAD)**

- Glycolate oxidase (FMN)
- NADH dehydrogenase / complex I (FMN)
- Acyl CoA dehydrogenase
- Dihydrolipoyl dehydrogenase
- Succinate dehydrogenase
- Glycerol-3- phosphate dehydrogenase
- Thioredoxin reductase
- Electron transferring Flavoprotein (ETF)

(Acyl CoA dehydrogenase to Electron transferring Flavoprotein: FAD)

Oxygenase

It *oxidizes a substrate* by catalyzing incorporation of oxygen into a substrate. It belongs to *oxido- reductase family* and is called direct oxidase. It is divided into 2 sub groups

Dioxygenase

- ***Cause incorporation of both atoms of O_2 into substate***[Q] i.e.

$$A + O_2 \xrightarrow[\text{Dioxygenase}]{} AO_2$$

- Examples include liver enzymes, iron containing 3- *hydroxy anthranilate* dioxygenase (oxidase), & *homogentisate* dioxygenase (oxidase), and *L- tryptophan 2, 3 dioxygenase (pyrolase)* that utilize heme.

Monooxygenase (Mised function oxidase, Hydroxylase)

- ***Cause incorporation of only one atom of molecular oxygen into substrate***[Q]. The 2nd O_2 atom is reduced to water.
- An electron donor co substrate is necessary. Since main substrate is hydroxylated, it is also c/a **hydroxylase.**

$$A - H \text{ (Main substrate)} + O_2 + ZH_2 \text{ (Cosubstrate)} \xrightarrow[\text{Hydroxylase}]{\text{Monooxygenase}} A - OH \text{ (hydroxylated)} + H_2O + Z$$

- They are also called mixed function oxidase/oxigenase to indicate that they oxidize two different substrate simultaneously. Examples include **cytochrome P-450** and **phenylalanine hydroxylase** (responsible for PKU).
- ***Cytochromes P_{450} are (heme containing) monoxygenases***[Q] which take part in ***hydroxylase cycle***[Q] (NADH, NADPH & $Fe_2 S_2$ required), ***detoxify drugs in liver microsomes***[Q] (with cytochrome b_5, $Fe_2 S_2$ not required).
- **Mitochondrial cytochrome P_{450}** is found in *steroidogenic – adrenal cortex, testis, ovary and placenta* and is concerned with *hydroxylation at C_{22} & C_{20} in side chain* cleavage & at *11B & 18* positions during synthesis of steroid chromones from cholesterol. It catalyzes 1 α & 25 hydroxylation in vit. D metabolism (in kidney) and 7 α hydroxylase & 27 hydroxylase in bile acid synthesis (in liver).

Holoenzyme

It is active enzyme (protein part) with its non protein component

Apoenzyme (protein part)

It is inactive enzyme (protein part) without its non protein component.

Non protein part

Transient association

Coenzyme

- If non-protein part is a **small** thermostable low molecular weight **organic molecule**, it is termed coenzyme
- Coenzyme that only transiently associate with the enzyme are called **cosubstrate** (**second substrate** or **coenzyme – cosubstrate**). Co substrate dissociate from enzyme in an altered state. eg ***NAD^+ & coenzyme A***[Q]
- Coenzyme ***serve as recyclable substrate shuttles –or group transfer agents***[Q] that transport many substrates from their point of generation to their point of utilization. It also *stabilizes unstable substrates* such as hydrogen atoms or hydride ions.
- Components of coenzymes are- ***vitamin B***[Q], adenine, ribose & phosphoryl moieties of AMP or ADP

Cofactor

- If non protein moiety is **metal ion** such as Fe^{++} or Zn^{++}, it is termed cofactor
- Bind reversibly in *transient dissociable manner* either to enzyme or substrate
- Enzymes requiring metal ion as cofactor are k/a **metal activated enzymes.**

Stable & tight incorporation

Prosthetic group

- These are tightly & stability incorporated into protein (enzyme) by covalent or non covalent forces.
- Metals are most common prosthetic groups. Metalloenzymes contain a tightly bound metal ion, that is not dissociated even after several steps of purification.

Vitamin B component	Part of / coenzyme	Function
Pantothenic acid	*Coenzyme A*[Q]	Co ASH is acyl group carrier
Cobalamine (B_{12})	**Cobamide**	***Coenzyme in transfer of 1 carbon fragment & metabolism of folic acid***[Q]
Folic acid	**Tetrahydro folate** (TH_4F)	***Coenzyme in transfer of 1 carbon fragment***[Q]
Niacin (nicotinamide / nicotinic acid)	**NAD & NADP**	Coenzyme in redox (oxidation and reduction) reactions
Riboflavin (B_2)	**FMN & FAD**	
Pyridoxine, pyridoxal, pyridoxamine (B_6)	**Pyridoxal phosphate**	Coenzyme in transmination & decarboxylation of amino acids & glycogen phosphorylase
Thiamine (B_1)	- **Thiamine pyro phosphate (TPP)** - **Thiamine di phosphate (TDP)**	• Coenzyme for **oxidative decarboxylation** by 3 multi enzyme complexes - ***Pyruvate dehydrogenase***[Q] (catalyze pyruvate to acetyl CoA) - ***α -ketoglutarate dehydrogenase***[Q] (in citric acid cycle) - Branched chain ketoacid dehydrogenase for leucine, Isoleucine & valine • Coenzyme for Transketolase (α ketoacid decarboxylation) in pemtose phosphate (PPP)
Biotin	-	***Coenzyme in carboxylation***[Q] reactions in gluco neogenesis & fatty acid synthesis
Vitamin C (ascorbic acid)	***Coenzyme in hydroxylation of proline & lysine in collagen synthesis***[Q]	
Vitamin K (phylloquinoses, menaquinones)	- Coenzyme in **carboxylation** of glutamate residue in proteins of blood clotting (factor 2, 7, 9, 10, protein C, S and Z) and bone matrix (osteocalcin) to form ***γ -carboxy glutamate residue***[Q].	

★ **Coenzyme prosthetic group** are small organic molecules that associate permanently with an enzyme & return to their original form by enzyme. Eg are FMN, FAD, TPP, pyridoxal phosphate, biotin.

Selenium & Selenocysteine

- **Selenium** in form of **selenocysteine** is a component (as a prosthetic groop) of **glutathione peroxidase, thioredoxin**, and **deiodinase** that converts thyroxine to triodothyronine.
- **Selenocysteine**, the **21st aminoacid** is present at the active site of enzymes and participate in catalytic mechanism of these enzymes. So the *replacement of selenocysteine by cysteine can significantly impair catalytic activity*.
- Unlike hydroxy proline & hydroxy lysine, selenocysteine arises by **cotranslational insertion from a previously modified t-RNA (t-RNA^sec). Serine** provides the carbon skeleton of selenocysteine. Biosynthesis of selenocyteine requires **selenate (SeO_4^{2-}), cysteine,** ATP, a specific unusual t RNA^sec and enzymes. The **UGA anticodon of t RNA^sec signals STOP** and this selenocysteine specific UGA stop codon is identified by **selenocysteine insertion element** (ie a stem loop structure in untranslated m RNA).

Enzymes	Cofactors
KG dehydrogenase	***TPP***[Q]
Carbonic anhydrase	***Zn***[Q]
Lactate /Alcohol dehydrogenase	***Zn***[Q]
Xanthine oxidase	Mo
Tyrosinase }	Cu
Cytochrome oxidase }	
Carboxylation	***Biotin***[Q]
Transamination	***Pyridoxine***[Q]
Kinase & peptidase	***Mg***[Q]
Hb & Cytochrome	***Fe***
Hydrolase, decarboxylase & transferase	Manganese

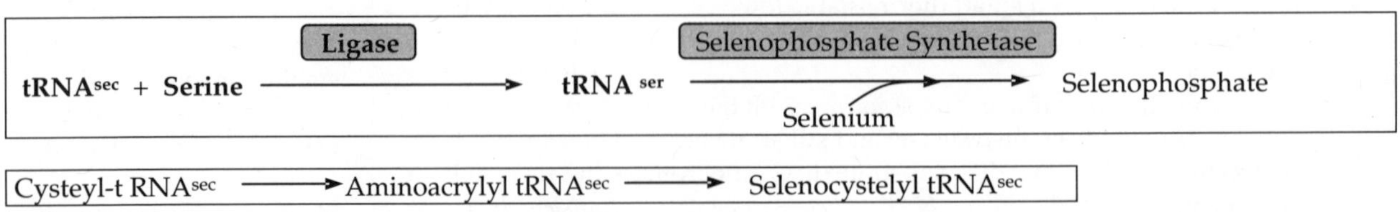

- In presence of specific elongation factors that recognize selenocysteyl – t RNA^sec, selenocysteine is incorporated into protein.
- In erythrocytes pentose phosphate pathway (PPP) is the only source of NADPH for the reduction of oxidized glutathione catalyzed by glutathione reductase (containing FAD). **Reduced glutathione removes H_2O_2** in a reaction catalyzed by **glutathione peroxidase. Glutathione peroxidase *contains selenium analog of cysteine (selenocysteine) as a prosthetic group***[Q]. In erythrocytes and other tissues, it *catalyzes the destruction of H_2O_2 and lipid peroxidases*, protecting membrane lipid

and hemoglobin against oxidation. This reaction is important since accumulation of H_2O_2 decreases life span of RBCs by causing oxidative damage to cell membrane proteins, lipids & nucleic acids l/t hemolysis. In other tissues, NADPH can also be generated by reaction catalyzed by malic enzyme. So **PPP & glutathione peroxidase protect RBCs against hemolysis**.

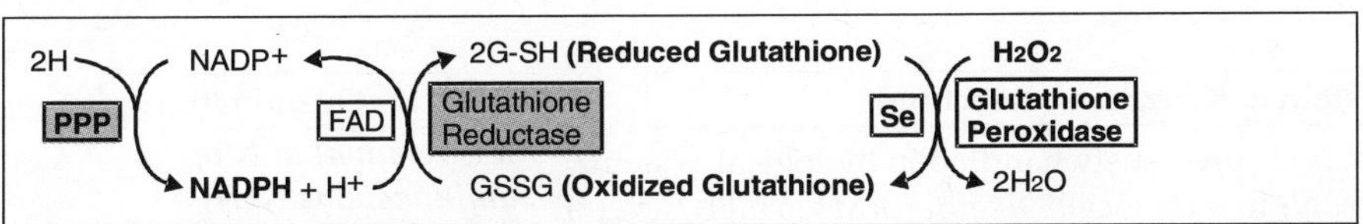

- Selenium has sparing effect on vitamin E reducing its requirements and similarly vitamin E reduces selenium requirement. Selenium & sulphur protect against toxic effects of heavy metals such as cadmium, Hg & Ag (b/o high affinity).
- Seafood, muscle meat & cereals are rich dietary sources of selenium, although the Se content of cereals is determined by soil concentration. Scandinavia, China & New Zealand have low soil Se content. Daily requirement's are 0.1 to 0.2 mg/kg (~ 50-100 Hg in 70 kg adult)

Selenium Deficiency Diseases

1. **Keshan disease**: **Endemic cardiomyopathy** (enlargement, arrhythmia & ECG changes) mainly affecting children & young women with intake < 20μg/d.
2. **Kaschinbeck disease:Endemic degenerative osteoarthritis** (osteopathy) mainly in children between 5 & 13 years with enlarged dysfunctional joints & retarded growth.
3. Liver cell necrosis, exudative diasthesis, pancreatic degeneration, muscular dystrophy, myopathy, infertility, growth failure, and dilatation of heart l/t CCF. (in animals)

Selenium Toxicity

1. **Selenosis** (chronic exposure) presents with **garlicky breath** (d/t dimethyl selenide), chronic **dermatitis**, skin rash, hair & **nail brittleness and loss**, myopathy, irritability & other abnormalities of nervous system (in humans). Animals develop impaired vision, movement disorder (**blind staggers**), alkali disease (anorexia, alopecia, loss of vitality, myocardial atrophy & liver necrosis), paralysis & death.
2. Acute toxicity in animals present with **diarrhea**, raised PR & temperature, tetanic spasm, laboured breathing, respiratory failure & hemorrhagic necrosis of various tissues.

Chapter 6. METABOLISM OF PROTEIN & AMINO ACIDS: REVIEW NOTES

Biosynthesis of Urea

Biosynthesis of urea has 4 stages (1) **transamination, (2) oxidative deamination of glutamate (3) ammonia transport, and (4) urea cycle.**

1. Transamination (Braunstein & Kritzmann Reaction)

- Despite being most abundant in atmosphere, N_2 is preciously handled in biological system, because only few micro organism can convert N_2 to biologically useful form (as NH_3/amino group). Aminoacids derived from dietary protein are the source of amino groups in humans. The presence of this ***α-amino group*** keeps amino acids safely ***locked away from oxidative breakdows***[Q]. So removal of α amino group is essential obligatory step in energy production or catabolism of all aminoacids.
- Transamination is a *reversible* reaction in which α - NH_2 group of one aminoacid is transferred to a α - ketoacid resulting in formation of new amino acid a new keto acid. Once they have reached the **liver, transamination** is the first step in catabolism of most amino acids and involves only intermolecular transfer of amino (NH_2) group without formation (splitting out) of ammonia (NH_3). No net deamination & occurs because α-amino acid is deaminated & α-keto acid (mostly α-keto glutarae) become aminated.

Aminotransferase (Transaminase) Enzyme

- This transfer of α-amino group from L amino acid to α-ketoacid is enzymed by amino transferase or transaminase enzyme
- Enzyme is found in *mitochondria and cytosol of cells through out the body especially those of liver, kidney, intestine, muscle, heart and brain.*
- Each aminotransferase is specific for one pair of substrate but non specific for other pair. Each is specific for 1 or at most few ***amino group donor on which their names are based. Because the acceptor of aminogroup is almost always α-keto (oxo) glutarate***[Q]***. Other rare recipient ketoacids are oxaloacetate or pyruvate.*** Example are

a. Alanine (Alanine-Pyruvate) Aminotransferase (ALT)= Serum Glutamate Pyruvate Transaminase and **Glutamate (Glutamate α-ketoglutarate) Aminotransferase**

Transfer aminogroup of alanine to α-keto (oxo) glutarate, resulting in formation of pyruvate & glutamate (glutamic acid)

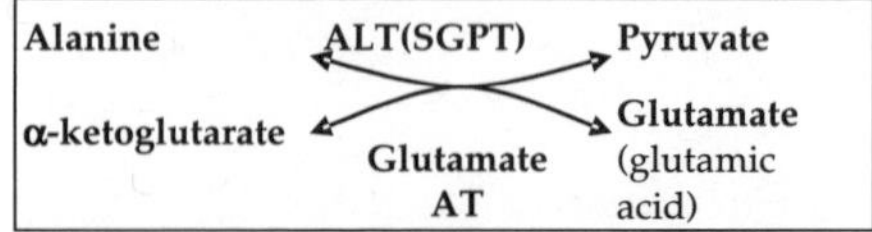

b. Aspartate Aminotransferase (AST)= Serum Glutamate Oxaloacetate, Transaminase (SGOT)

Exception to the rule that aminotransferase enzyme funnel amino groups to form glutamate. Because during aa catabolism, it transfer aminogroup of glutamate to oxaloacetate forming

Salient Features

- **Transamination *interconverts pairs of α-amino acids and α-keto acids, transferring α-amino nitrogen (NH_2 group) without splitting out of ammonia (NH_3) to α-ketoglutarate forming glutamate***[Q].
- Alanine pyruvate (or **alanine) aminotransferase** and glutamate – α-ketoglutarate (**or glutamate) aminotransferase** catalyze the transfer of amino **(NH_2) group to pyruvate (forming alanine) or to α-ketoglutarate (forming glutamate).** Since alanine is also a substrate for glutamate aminotransferase, the α-amino nitrogen from all aminoacids that undergo ***transamination can be concentrated in glutamate. Therefore transamination reaction collects the aminogroup from many different amino acids in form of L-glutamate***[Q]. And then **L-glutamate functions as aminogroup donor for biosynthetic pathways** or **for excretion pathways** that lead to the elimination of nitrogenous waste products.
- **α-ketoglutarate *plays a crucial role by accepting amino (NH_2) groups from most amino acids and thus becoming glutamate***[Q]. So transamination collects amino groups from many different aminoacids in form of **L-glutamate** (i.e. called ***funneling of aminogroups to L-glutamate***). This is important because *L-glutamate is the only amino acid that undergoes oxidative deamination at an appreciable rate* in mammalian tissue. So **formation of ammonia from α-amino group thus occur mainly via α-amino nitrogen of L glutamate**[Q] (by oxidative deamination)

2. Deamination

- It is ***removal of N of aminoacid as NH_3***
- **Oxidative deamination is catalyzed by D & L-aminoacid oxidase.** Despite absence of D aminoacids in tissues, the D-aa-oxidase enzyme is much greater than L-aa-oxidase
- L aminoacid oxidae is *auto oxidizable flavoprotein (FMN)*, which is reoxidized, when reduced, at substrate level directly by O_2 forming H_2O_2 without participation of any electron carrier (like cytochrome or ETS). Toxic H_2O_2 is converted to O_2 & H_2O by catalase.

Feature	L-AA oxidase	D-AA oxidase
Flavoprotein	FMN	FAD
Acts on	L-amino acids	D-amino acids
Extracted with water free form	Not; because bound to tissue	Freely

- **Non oxidative deamination** has a very minor role in NH_3 formation and can occur in

1. **Sulfur containing amino acids** like *cysteine & homocysteine* by **desulfhhydrase** (removing H_2S).
2. **Hydroxy amino acids** like *serine, homoserine & threonine* by **aminoacid dehydrogenases** requiring *pyridoxal (B6)- P as coenzyme.*
3. **Histidine** by **histidase** forming urocanic acid & NH_3.

aspartate (which is used as **source of nitrogen in urea cycle)** & α-ketogluterate.

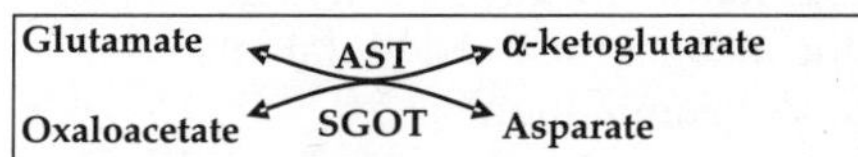

★ However in biosynthesis (when reaction is reversed) the aspartate becomes donor & α-ketoglutarate acceptor.

c. **Formation of alanine by transamination of pyruvate**. Amino donor may be glutamate or aspartate thus forming α-ketoglutarate or oxaloacetate

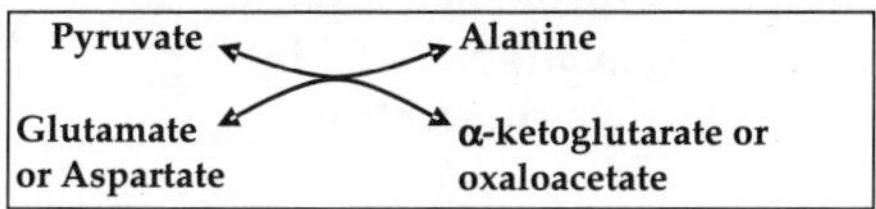

- Transamination occur in almost all amino acids except **threonine, lysine** (loose amino group by deamination), **proline, hydroxyproline**, and *cyclic iminoacids*.
- Transamination is not restricted to α-amino groups. The **δ-amino group** of ornithine (but not ε amino group of lysine) readily undergoes transamination.
- Glutamate produced by transamination can be oxidatively deaminated or used as aminogroup donor in synthesis of non essential amino acids.
- ***Equilibrium constant*** for transamination is **~1** making it readily reversible and *allowing amino acid biosynthesis* (by addition of amino group to keto acid when supply of amino acid in diet is not adequate) **and amino acid degradation** (by removal of amino group when diet is rich in protein) **both.**

Coenzyme Pyridoxal Phosphate (Vitamin B_6 derivative)

- ***Pyridoxal phosphate coenzyme (or prosthetic group) is covalently bound to enzyme's active site by an Schiff base (aldimine) linkage***[Q] to ε amino group of Lys residue and *serves as a carrier of amino group* (and thus generating pyridoxamine phosphate which transfers this amino group to α-keto acid).
- Transamination occurs via **ping pong reaction** which means the 1st substrate reacts & product must leave the active site before 2nd substrate can bind.

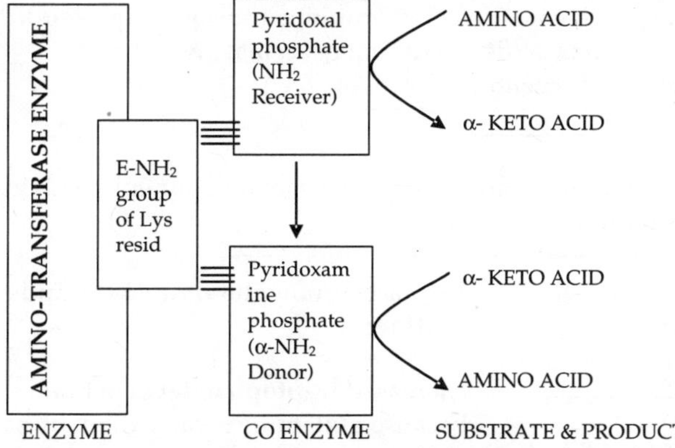

PING-PONG MECHANISM OF TRANSAMINATION

Deamination of L-Glutamate = Transdeamination

- L-Glutamate formed as a main product of transamination is not deaminated by L-amino acid oxidase but by hepatic **L-glutamate dehydrogenase (GDH)**.
- GDH is a tetramer metalloenzyme containing 1 Zn^{++} in each of 4 polypeptide chain. It can use **NAD+ or NADP+ as coenzymes** and release nitrogen as ammonia. It is **allosterically inhibited by ATP, GTP and NADH** and is **activated by ADP**.
- Reaction is freely reversible and equilibrium constant favours glutamate (amino acid) biosynthesis but quick removal of NH_3 to urea cycle & α-ketoglutarate to TCA cycle favours ammonia formation.

L-Glutamate	**L-GDH**	α-ketoglutarate + NH_3
$NAD(P)^+$		$NAD(P)H^+ + H^+$

- Conversion of alpha-amino nitrogen to ammonia by **coupled action of glutamate aminotransferase and GDH** is called **transdeamination**.

Non toxic Transport of Ammonia (& Amino group)

In Brain & Most other tissue

- In most tissues (especially brain) nucleotide degradation produce free ammonia, which being toxic is immediately trapped by glutamate (glutamic acid) to form **nontoxic glutamine**. This reaction is catabolized by **glutamine synthetase** and require ATP.

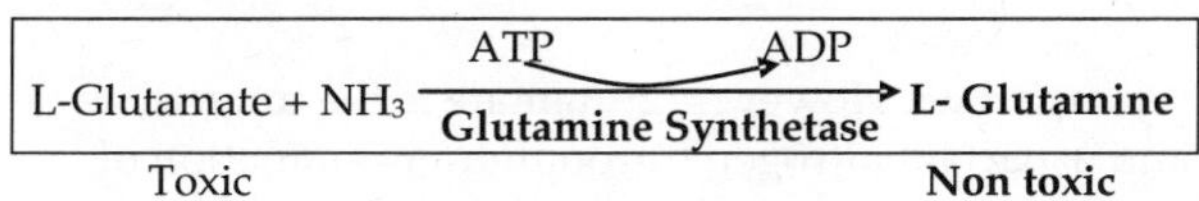

- Aspartic acid may undergo similar reaction to form **asparagine**,

In Skeletal Muscle

- In tissues that degrade aminoacid for fuel (mainly skeletal muscle), amino group is collected in form of L-glutamate (d/t transamination)
- This **glutamate** (containing toxic α-amino group) can be transported to liver by converting it to glutamine or it can transfer its α-amino group to **pyruvate**, a easily available product of muscle glycolysis by the action of **alanine aminotransferase (ALT/SGPT)**. The **alanine** so formed passes into blood to liver.

which traps NH_3 in brain (minor)

- Glutamine is *non toxic transport form of NH_3 and serves as a source of amino group in* biosynthetic reactions. It is normally *present in blood in much higher concentrations* than other amino acids. Excess glutamine (of amount that is required for biosysthesis) is *transported to liver, intestine and kidney*, where enzyme **glutaminase** reverse the reaction and convert glutamine to glutamate (glutamic acid) and NH_3 (NH_4^+). The toxic NH_4^+ from intestine, kidney & other tissues is rapidly removed from blood by liver and converted to urea.
- **In kidney (renal tubular cells)** ***ammonia (NH_4^+) production from intra cellular amino acids mainly glutamine increases in metabolic acidosis and decreases in metabolic alkalosis***[Q]. So in metabolic acidosis not all NH_4^+ produced in kidney is released into blood to form urea in liver; *some is excreted directly into the urine thus facilitating cation (positive ion) conservation and regulating acid base balance.*
- **Glutaminase** and **asparaginase** ***deaminate glutamine & asparagines thus releasing toxic NH_3***[Q]
- In liver cell cytosol **alanine aminotransferase (ALT/SGPT)** transfers amino group from alanine to α-ketoglutarate forming pyruvate (which enters gluconeogenesis) and glutamate (under go oxidative deamination)
- Vigrously contracting muscles operate anerobically producing pyruvate & lactate (from glycolysis) and NH_3 (from aa break down). **Alanine-glucose cycle** in concert with Cori cycle send these products to liver where pyruvate & lactate are incorporated into glucose (by gluconeogenesis and returned back to muscle) and NH_3 is converted to urea for excretion. So the **energetic burden of gluconeogenesis is imposed on liver and all available ATP in muscle is devoted to muscle contraction.**

Hyper-Ammonemia: NH_3 Intoxication

- NH_3 is produced by protein catabolism and is mainly converted to urea (by urea cycle) in liver. Some NH_3 is also used for transamination of α-ketoacid to α-amino acid and in synthesis of glutamine.
- Disorders of urea cycle (i.e. any enzyme of urea cycle) would result in hyper ammonemia, encephalopathy & respiratory alkalosis. Brain is very sensitive to ammonia. Clinical features include mental retardation, lethargy, irritability & vomiting.
- Block in earlier steps of urea cycle results in more symptoms since ammonia itself accumulates, whereas deficiency of later enzymes result in accumulation of less toxic other intermediates and hence symptoms are less. Hyper ammonemia **type I** (d/t **CPS I**- deficiency), hyperammonemia (d/t **OTC** def.), hyperornithinemia (defect in ornithine transporter protein), citrullinemia (def. of argininosuccinate synthetase), argininosuccinicacid uria (def. of argininosuccinate lyase) and *hyperargininemia* (arginase def) are **disorder of urea cycle**. Increase NH_3 concentration causes

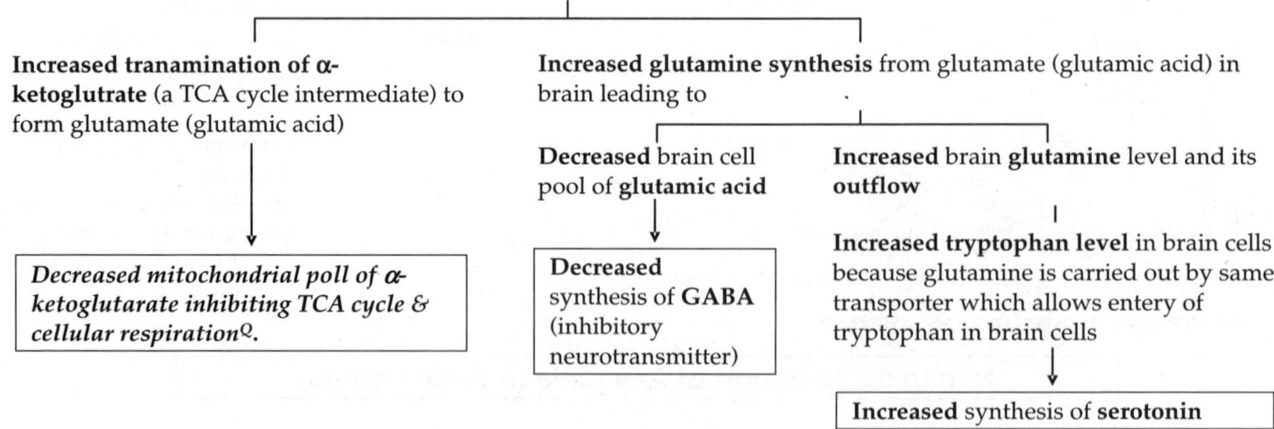

Urea Cycle / Krebs – Henseleit Cycle / Ornithine Cycle 

- ***Urea cycle leading to formation of urea takes place in liver***[Q]. Urea is the most important disposal form of NH_3 or amino group derived from amino acid catabolism. One mol of urea synthesis requires *1 mol each of NH4+ (ammonium ion) & of α-amino* nitrogen of aspartate and **3 mol of ATP (but 4 high energy phosphate bonds** as 1 ATP of these 3 is converted to AMP thus using 2 PO_4 bonds.)
- One nitrogen of urea molecule is supplied by **free ammonia** and other by **aspartate.** However, **glutamate** is the immediate precursor of both ammonia (through oxidative deamination by GDH) and aspartate nitrogen (through trans amination of oxaloacetate by AST). In effect, both nitrogen (N) atoms of urea arise from L-glutamate, which in turn gathers them from aminoacids. The carbon (C) & oxygen (O) atoms of urea are derived from CO_2 (or HCO_3^-)

- It is a cyclic process with 6 participating aminoacids and 5 enzymes. *There is not net loss or gain of ornithine, citrulline, argininosuccinate, or arginine*. However, **ammonium ion (NH4+), CO_2, 3ATP (or 4 high energy phosphate bonds) are consumed and there is net conversion of (oxaloacetate via) aspartate to fumarate.**

Aspartate + NH_3 + CO_2 + H_2O + **3ATP** → **Fumarate + Urea** + 2ADP + 2AMP + 2Pi + PPi

However fumarate formed in urea cycle may be converted to malate, which when oxidized to oxaloacetate produce **1 NADPH** equivalent to **2.5 ATP,** so **net energy expenditure** reduces to only **1.5 high energy phosphates.**

- First two reactions i.e. *formation of carbamoyl phosphate* (catabolized by ***carbamoyl phosphate synthetase I enzyme***) and *formation of citrulline* (catabolized by **ornithine transcarbamoylase**) takes place in **mitochondria**. *Citrulline is transported from mitochondria to cytosol* and remaining steps i.e. formation of argininosuccinate (enz. **argininosuccinate synthetase**), its cleavage to arginine & fumarate (enz. **argininosuccinate lyase**), and cleavage of arginine to ornithine and urea (enz **arginase**) takes place in **cytosol**. Ornithine returns to mitochondria to react with another molecule of carbamoyl PO_4. Ornithine is regenerated with each turn of urea cycle, much in the same way the oxaloacetate is regenerated in citric acid cycle. **Ornithine & citrulline** are basic aminoacids that are not incorporated **into cellular proteins because there are no codons for these amino acids.**
- 2ATP molecules are required to make carbamoyl PO_4 and 1 ATP (2 high energy phosphate bonds) to make argininosuccinate. First step of urea cycle i.e. condensation of CO_2, ammonia and 2 ATP l/t **formation of carbomoyl phosphate by carbamoyl PO_4 synthetase I is the rate limiting step (& enzyme).** This enzyme is only active in presence of **N-acetyl glutamate (NAG)** ***an allosteric activator that enhances the affinity of enzyme for ATP***[Q]. NAG is synthesize by N-acety glutamate synthetase from acetyl CoA and glutamate.
- Because fumarate produced in urea cycle is also an intermediate of citric acid cycle, both cycles are inter connected (k/a **Krebs bicycle**) by **aspartate – argininosuccinate shunt**. However each cycle can operate independently. And fumarase & malate dehydrogenase used in urea cycle are cytosolic (not mitochondrial like TCA cycle).
- *Kidney & Intestine* contribute to most of body arginine because they possess all the urea cycle enzyme except arginase.
- Brain can synthesize urea from citrulline, but lacks enzyme for formation of citrulline from ornithine.
- Thus neither brain nor Kidney can form urea in significant amount.

Serine Proteases

- ***The active site of serine proteases contain three critical amino acids Serine, Histidine and Aspartate. These residues are often referred to as the catalytic triad.*** *Chymotrypsin, Elastase and Trypsin are the three serine proteases that function essentially as enzymes.Each of these enzymes contain the 'catalytic triad' within their active sites but differ with respect to their target cleavage sites.- www.rpc.msue.edu*
- **They are activated by proteolytic activation and not autocatalytic activation.** They are secreted by the pancreas as inactive zymogens into small intestine- and became active through proteolytic cleavage events, either in a subcellular compartment or in an extracellular space where they are required for digestion.
- **Pancreatic trypsin inhibitor** is serine protease inhibitor only for trypsin and not for other serine protease enzymes such as chymotrypsin or elastase. Serine proteases enzymes tightly bind the respective protease inhibitors instead of normal substrates.

Serine protease	Serine protease inhibitor
Trypsin	Pancreatic trypsin inhibitor
Chymotrypsin	Alpha-1 antichymotrypsin
Elastase	Alpha-1 antitrypsin

- **Serine proteases attack the carbonyl group of the peptide bond that is to be cleaved (and not essentially the one adjacent to serine residue)**

Serine protease	Substrate
Chymotrypsin	Peptide bond next to ***aromatic residues (Phenylalanine, Tyrosine Tryptophan)***[Q]
Trypsin	Peptide bond next to ***basic residues (Lysine or Arginine)***[Q]
Elastase	Peptide bonds next to ***Hydrophobic residues (Alanine)***[Q]

Creatinine & Creatinine Biosynthesis ☆

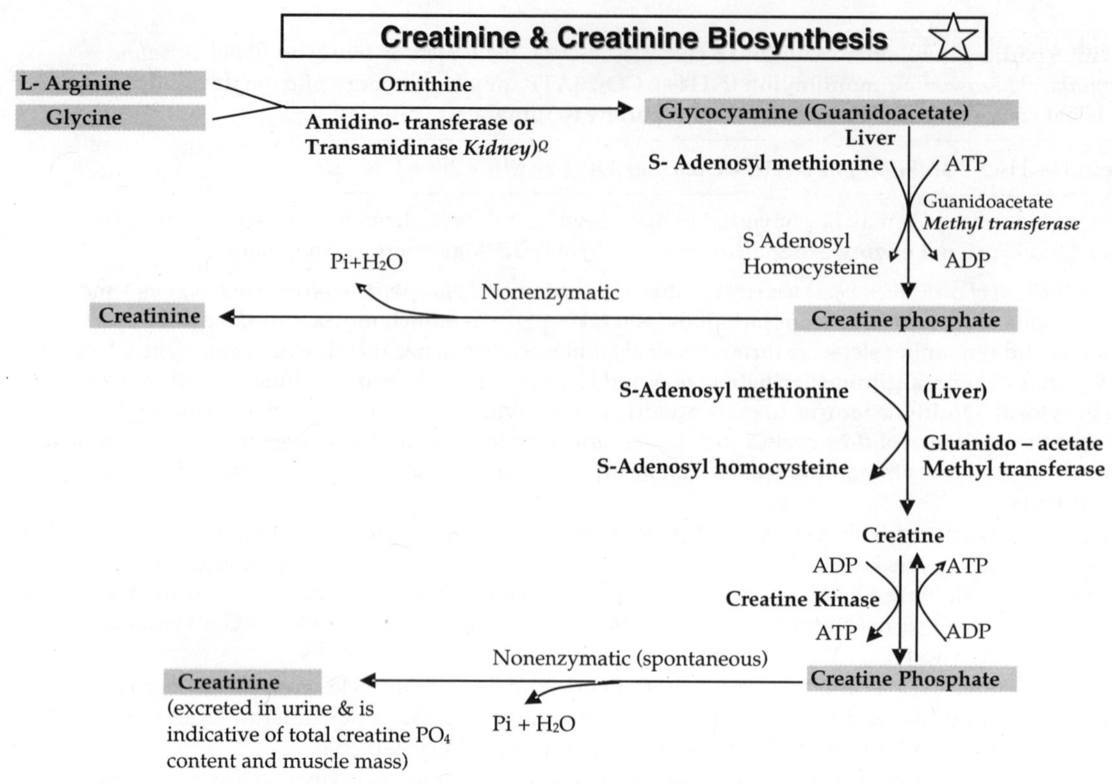

Catabolism of Carbon Skeletons of Aminoacids

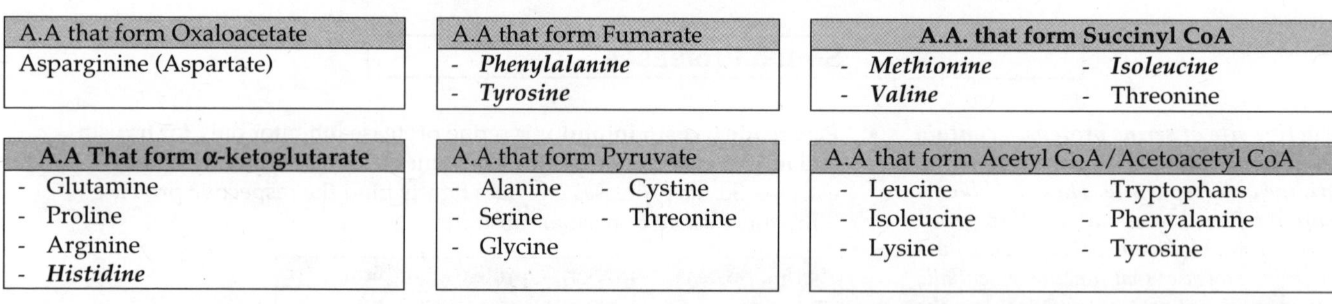

A.A that form Oxaloacetate	A.A that form Fumarate	A.A. that form Succinyl CoA
Asparginine (Aspartate)	- ***Phenylalanine*** - ***Tyrosine***	- ***Methionine*** - ***Isoleucine*** - ***Valine*** - Threonine

A.A That form α-ketoglutarate	A.A.that form Pyruvate	A.A that form Acetyl CoA/Acetoacetyl CoA
- Glutamine - Proline - Arginine - ***Histidine***	- Alanine - Cystine - Serine - Threonine - Glycine	- Leucine - Tryptophans - Isoleucine - Phenyalanine - Lysine - Tyrosine

Classification of Ammino Acids (aa) on the basis of R-Group or Side chains ☆

Nonpolar (Hydrophobic or Water insoluble) side chains

Nonpolar side chains **does not gain or lose protons or participate in hydrogen or ionic bonds**. Oily or *lipid like* side chains promote *hydrophobic interaction*. In proteins found in polar environment or aqueous solutions – the side chains of nonpolar aminoacids tend to cluster together in interior of protein (**hydrophobic effect**) and help give it its three dimensional shape. However in hydrophobic environment such as membranes the nonpolar side chains are found on the outside surface of protein interacting with lipid environment

Aliphatic (Nonpolar / Hydrophobic) Side chain)		Aromatic (Non polar/ relatively Hydrophobic) Side chain
Glycine	***Simplest structure***Q Very small (H) side chain makes no real contribution to hydrophobic interactions	- All can participate in hydrophobic interactions. - ***Tyrosine & tryptophan*** are significantly more polar than **phenyl alanine**, because of tyrosine

Polar (Hydrophillic or Water soluble) side chains

The most hydrophilic (polar) R groups are those that are either positively or negatively charged

Polar, Uncharged (Neutral or Non ionic) side chain

- Have **zero (0) net charge at neutral pH**, although cysteine and tyrosine can lose proton at alkali pH
- They contain functional group that form hydrogen bond with water making them hydrophilic & polar

Serine	Hydroxyl group
Threonine	Hydroxyl group
Cysteine	Sulfhydryl group (weak acid)

Alanine	*Methyl side chain*Q
Valine	C3H7 side chain
Leucine & Isoleucine	C4H9 side chain
Alnine, leucine, Isoleucine & Valine (mn "**ALL Is Well**") tend to cluster together within proteins stabilizing protein structure by means of hydrophobic interactions	
Methionine	**Sulfur containing** amino acid with **thioether side chain**
Proline	Side chain form a distinct **cyclic (ring shaped), rigid 5 membered secondary** (rather than primary **amino group k/a imino group. It reduces structural** flexibility, and contributes in formation of *fibrous structure of collagen* and often **interrupts α-helices** found in globular proteins.

hydroxyl group& nitrogen of tryptophan indole ring

- Tyrosine hydroxyl (OH) group can form hydrogen bonds
- ***Tryptophan & tyrosine, and to much lesser extent phenylalanine absorb ultraviolet light at a wave length of 280nm.***Q **(photochromocity)**
- *Phenylalanine has benzene, tyrosine has phenol and tryptophan has indole groups* respectively.

★**Hydropathy index is negative** (ΔG< O) for polar or charged aminoacids; and positive (ΔG> O) for nonpolar or more hydrophobic aminoacids. All of aliphatic & aromatic aa have (+) value except **glycine** (- 0.4), **tryptophan** (-0.9), **tyrosine** (- 1.3), and **histidine** (-3.2). Hence histidine is not included & tyrosine is relatively included in non polar group

★**Histidine** is a positively charged (basic) aa with **NH_3^+ side chain.** It also has **aromatic imidazole side** chain. As the only aa. having an imidazole side chain with pKa near neutrality, histadine ***may be positively charged (protonated form) or uncharged at pH 7)***Q. It facilitate many reactions by **serving as proton donors / acceptors.**

Asparagine	Amide group
Glutamine	Amide group
Tyrosine	Hydroxyl group

- *Asparagine & glutamine* are the amides of 2 other aa, aspartate & glutamate respectively
- Cysteine is oxidized to form a covalently linked dimeric amino acid called **cystine**, in which 2 cysteine molecules are *joined by disulfide bond making it strongly hydrophobic (non polar)*

★Cysteine & tyrosine may show hydrophobic character when present in interior of protein. Glycine may be included in this group also.

Polar ionic, Positively charged (Basic) side chain /aa

Lysine	Second primary amino at ε position on its aliphatic chain
Arginine	+ve charged guanidinium group
Histidine	Aromatic imidazole group

Polar, Ionic, Negatively charged (Acidic) side chains

- 2 aa. with a net negative charge at pH 7 are **aspartate & glutamate** each of which has 2nd carboxyl (COO-) group.
- **Aspartic acid & glutamic acid** contain β carboxyl and γ carboxyl groups respectively.

★ *α- carbon atom of aminoacid is **optically** or **chirally active** as it is attached to 4 different groups. **Glycine** is the exception and is optically inactive b/o 2 hydrogen atoms attached.

★ Aminoacids with asymmetrical α-carbon center can exist in **two 'D' and 'L'** mirror image forms k/a **optical isomers, stereoisomers or enantiomers**. Only 'L' (levorotatory) alpha aminoacids occur in proteins.

★ **Naturally occurring 'D' – aminoacids are free 'D' serine & 'D'-aspartate in brain; 'D' alanine & 'D' glutamate in cell walls of gram (+) bacteria; D aminoacids in some antibiotics & peptides produced by bacteria, fungi etc.**

Polar –Ionic – Charged – Amino acids

Basic (Positively charged) Monoamino-dicarboxylic acids

- At physiological pH the side chains are *fully ionized (polar) and positively charged* containing an extra positively charged amino group
- These contain one negative charged carboxylic (-COOH / - COO-) group and two positive charged amino (-NH_2) groups. Hence called di amino-mono carboxylic acid
- Basic aminoacids accept protons
- Examples include : **Arginine (most basic)**, lysine, hydroxyl-lysine, and ***histidine (weakly basic /neutral)***Q

Acidic (Negatively charged) Diamino-monocarboxylic acids

- At physiological pH the side chains are fully ionized (polar) and negatively charged *containing an extra negatively charged carboxylic group.*
- Acidic aminoacids contain 1 amino and 2 carboxylic groups. Hence called mono amino dicarboxylic acids
- Acidic aminoacids are *proton donors*
- Examples include **aspartic acid** (or ***aspartate***) and **glutamic acid** (or **glutamate**). These 2 are written in all books but chatterjae also includes ***glutamine & asparagines*** in this group. But these two are included in polar uncharged (neutral) in Lehninger (Go with this)

Functions of Glutathione

NADPH + H^+ → Glutathione Reductase → $NADP^+$; G-S-S-G (oxidized) → 2G-SH (reduced); 2G-SH (reduced) + H_2O_2 → Glutathione Peroxidase → G-S-S-G (oxidized) + $2H_2O$

1. **Antioxidant:**
   - Reduced glutathione (GSH) can ***detoxify H_2O_2 by glutathione peroxidase***[Q] and itself converted into oxidized form (G-S-S-G).
   - Oxidized glutathione contains two glutathione linked by disulphide bond between its cysteine residue, hence its reducing ***property is because of cysteine sulfhydryl group***[Q].
2. It is important *intracellular reductant*, helping to maintain essential SH gp of enzymes in reduced state.
3. **Membrane transport**: It acts as a ***carrier in transport of certain amino acid across membrane in kidney***[Q].
   Amino acid + GSH → γ - Glutamyl amino acid + Cystein glycine
4. ***Helps in conjugation reaction***[Q]***:*** Toxic xenobiotics are conjugated to nucleophilic GSH (glutathione) to convert to more polar, hydroxylated derivatives.

Cystinuria [Mn: "COLA"]

- Is a *disorder of proximal tubule's reabsorption of filtered cystine and dibasic amino acid* (Ornithine, Lysine, Arginine). So there is excretion of – **Cystine, Ornithine, Lysine & Arginine**[Q]
- It is *most common* genetic error of amino acid transport affecting aminoacid carrier in small intestine & proximal tubule of kidney (as both share same transport carrier) for COAL amino acids.
- **Complications**: Cystine is relatively insoluble a.a and therefore precipitates in renal tubules, ureter and bladder to form ***cystine calculi***[Q].
- **Diagnosis**: By ***Cyanide- Nitroprusside test***[Q].

Cysteine

- Cysteine is a ***sulphur containing amino acid***[Q].
- Cystine is formed by two molecules of cysteine, joined together by S- S bond.
- Cysteine can be *synthesized in body from methionine.*
- Prominent a.a in protein of nails, hairs and keratin of skin.

Risk Factors For Altherosclerosis (Hence MI)

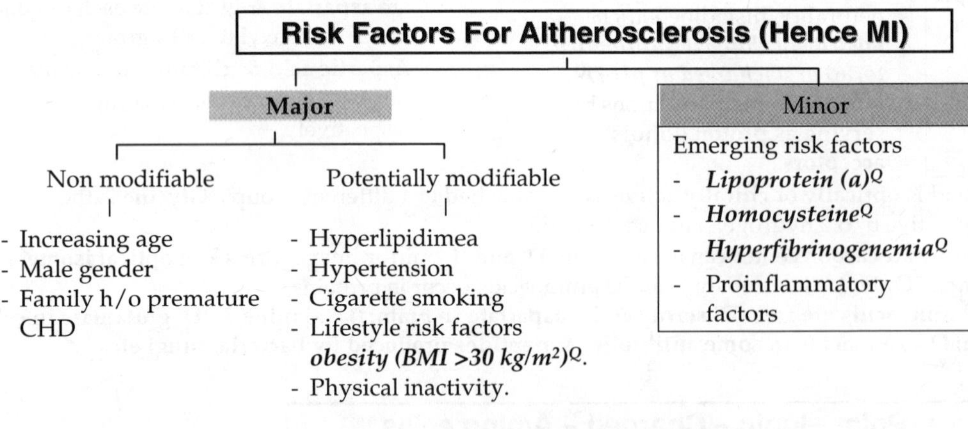

Phenyl Ketonuria (PKU)

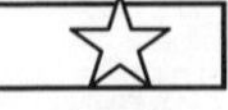

- It is ***most common clinically encountered inborn error of aminoacid metabolism. It is biochemically characterized by accumulation of phenylalanine and a deficiency of tyrosine***[Q].
- In this *autosomal recessive* disorder, due to deficiency of ***phenylalanine*** **hydroxylase (PA- 4 monooxygense**, a mixed function oxidase), *phenylalanine can not be converted to tyrosine*, resulting in elevation of phenylalanine in tissue, plasma & urine. **(Type I , Classic PKU)**
- Phenylalanine hydroxylase requires a **cofactor tetra hydrobiopterin**, which carries e- from NADPH to O_2 & becomes oxidized to dihydrobiopterin. It is subsequently reduced by **enzyme dihydrobiopterin reductase in a reductase** in a rection that requires NADPH. So **hyper phenylataninemia** may also be caused by deficiency of enzymes synthesizing BH_4 or regenerating BH_4 from BH_2 (i.e. dihydrobiopteridine reductase)

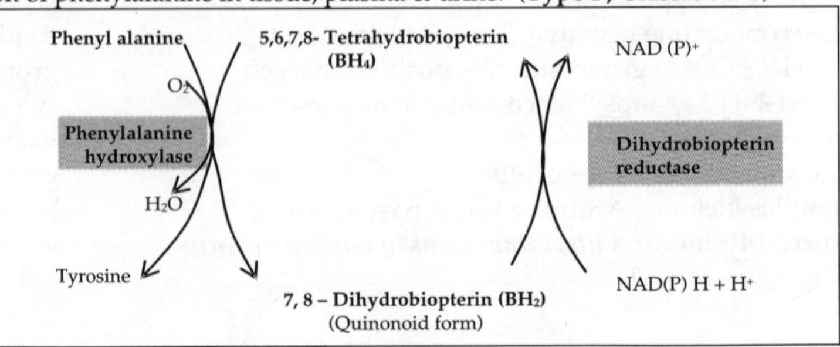

- Hyperphenylalaninemia, d/t **dihydrobiopterine reductase deficiency** (Type II and III), is accompanied with ***BH_4 deficiency. BH4 is also required for tyrosine hydroxylase and tryptophan hydroxylase***[Q] leading to synthesis of *neurotransmitters L-DOPA, catecholamines (from tyrosine) and 5-hydroxy tyrptophan & serotonin (from tryptophan).* So in type II & III PKU simply restricting phenyl alanine and providing tyrosine does not reverse CNS effects d/t deficiencies in neurotransmitters. *Replacement therapy with BH4 or L- DOPA and 5-OH- tryptophan is also needed.* Supplementing the diet with tetrahydro biopterin itself is ineffective as it is unstable and does not cross blood brain barrier.

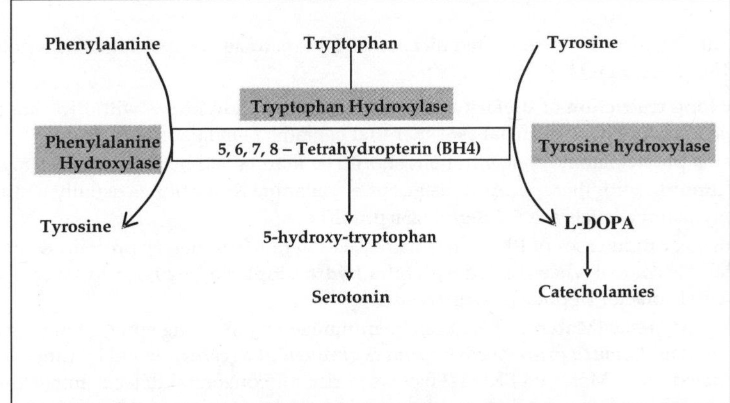

- Elevated phenylalanine undergoes trans amination to form phenyl pyruvate, phenyl lactate and phenyl acetate.

Pathophysiology

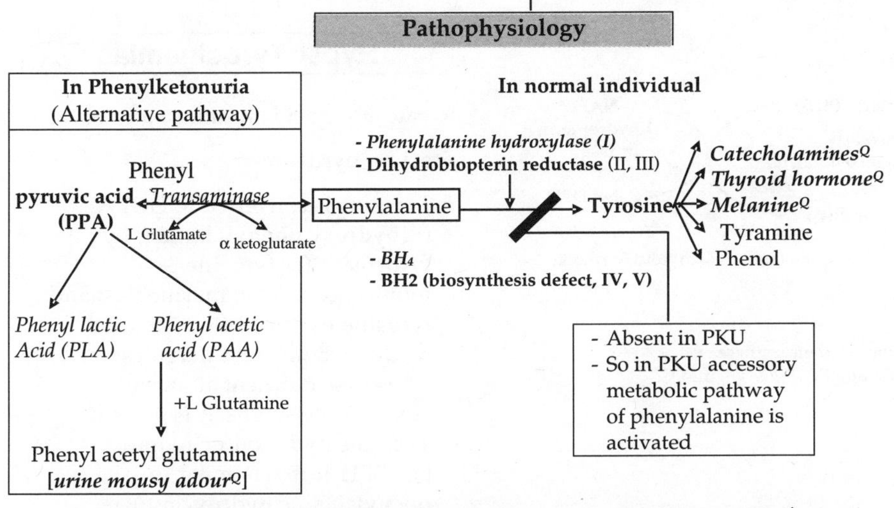

Types of PKU & other PA metabolism defect

I	**Defect in phenylalanine hydroxylase (classic)**[Q]
II III	**Defect in dihydrobiopterin (BH_2) reductase**[Q] 6 Pyruvoyl-tetra hydropterin synthase defect
IV V	Defect in dihydrobiopterin (BH2) biosynthesis
Maternal PKU	When woman with PKU who is not on low phenyl alanine diet become pregnant It causes microcephaly, mental retardation & congenital heart anomalies in fetus)
Transient benign hyper phenylalaninemia	**Pterin-4 carbinolamine dehydratase deficiency**
GTP Cyclohydrolase I deficiency	Defect of PA metabolism

Treatment

- The **main aim for 1st line therapy** is to ***limit the intake of substrate (i.e. phenyl alanine) for deficient enzyme***[Q].
- In PKU, **blood phenyl alanine is maintained close to the normal range by feeding synthetic amino acid preparations low in PA,** supplemented with some natural food (such as fruits, vegetables & some cereals) selected for their low phenylalanine content.
- Because PA is an essential aminoacid, *overzealous treatment that result in blood PA levels below normal should be avoided* because this can l/t poor growth & neurological symptoms
- In PKU, **tyrosine** cannot be synthesized from PA, and therefore it **becomes an essential aminoacid** that must be supplied in diet.
- Treatment must begin during the first **7-10 days** of life to *prevent mental retardation* (as early as better).

■ Clinical features:

- ***Hypopigmentation***[Q] d/t impaired melanin synthesis l/t fair hair, light skin, blue eyes
- **CNS symptoms:** Mental retardation, seizures, hyperactivity, tremors, failure to walk, talk & grow and IQ < 50
- Excretion of phenylalanine & its catabolite in urine: PPA, PAA
- ***Mousy (musty) odour urine***[Q]: PAA conjugates with glutamine and excreted as phenyl acetyl glutamine.

■ Diagnosis

- **Antenatal prenatal diagnosis** is facilitated by ***DNA probes to detect enzyme defect & tandem mass spectrometry*** (most reliable to estimate blood PA levels).
- ***Neonatal screening and diagnosis* of PKU by elevated blood levels of PA**
- It is important because the *disease is treatable by dietary means* and neonates lack symptoms.
- The *infant with PKU has normal blood levels of phenylalanine (PA) at birth* because the mother clears increased blood PA through placenta.
- Normal PA levels may persist until the new born is exposed to **2-4 days** of protein feeding. Thus screening tests are done after this period to avoid false negatives.
- **False positive** in premature infants may reflect delayed maturation of enzymes of PA catabolism.
- The diagnosis is confirmed through **quantitative determination of PA levels**.
- Plasma phenylalanine level: ↑ed to 15- 65mg% (N- 1- 2mg%)

- Discontinuation of PA restricted diet before **8 years of age** is associated with poor performance on IQ test.
- **Life long restriction of dietary PA is recommended.** Individuals with PKU are advised to avoid **aspartame**, an artificial sweetner that contains penylalanine.
- Plasma phenylalanine concentrations should be maintained between **2 and 6 mg/dL (120 and 360 μmol/L)** with therapy. And dietary phenylalanine restriction is usually instituted if blood phenylalanine levels are **> 4 mg/dl (250 μmol/L)**
- Some very mild cases of PKU show increased tolerance to dietary proteins & improved metabolic control when treated with **tetra hydro biopterin** (5-20 mg/kg/day) which is an essential cofactor of phenyl hydroxylase
- Pregnancy risks **(Maternal PKU)** can be minimized by assuring strict phenylalanine restrictions ***2 month prior to conception & through out gestation*** and continuing life long PA restricted diets. Maternal PKU l/t increased risk for congenital defects, microcephaly, congenital heart abnormalities, and severe mental & growth retardation after birth. Phenylalanine is a teratogen.

- **Guthrie** rapid screening **test** uses **Bacillus subtilis** strains which cannot grow in a medium devoid of phenylalanine and the growth is proportional to its content.
- ***$FeCl_3$ test[Q]: (older less reliable test)***
  - Screening test for presence of phenylpyruvate in urine
  - $FeCl_3$ gives ***emerald green with urnie in PKU[Q].***
- Phenylalanine load test (iv) detects PKU carriers.

Phenylalanine

O_2 → H_2O; **Tetrahydrobiopterin (BH_4)** → **Dihydrobiopterin (BH_2)**

Phenylketonuria — **Phenylalanine hydroxylase (4-monoxygenase)**, a mixed function oxidase in liver

NADP⁺ ← **Dihydropterin reductase** ← **NADPH**

Tyrosine ----- Form melanin, catecholamines & thyroid hormone

α - ketoglutarate → Glutamic acid

Richner-Hanhart oculocutaneous Type II tyrosinemia — **Tyrosine** (-α ketoglutarae) **transaminase** (aminotransferase) require **PP (B_6) & vitamin C**

Para Hydroxy phenyl pyruvic acid (pHPPA)

Type III Neonatal tyrosinemia; Hereditary; Hawkinsuria — Cu containing **pHPPA – oxidase / dioxygenase / hydroxylase**, require *vitamin C & B_{12}*

Homogentisic Acid (2, 5-dihydroxy phenyl actic acid)

Alkaptonuria — Fe containing **Homogentisate oxidase** (or **1-2 dioxygenase**), Vitamin C

(4) Maleyl – Acetoacetate (MAA)

MAA **Isomerase,** require *Glutathione*

Fumaryl Acetoacetate

Type I Hepato renal tyrosinemia (Tyrosinosis) — **Fumaryl –acetoacetate hydroxylase**

Fumarate (Glucogenic) | **Aceto-acetate**

Acetate | **Acetyl CoA (Ketogenic)**

Hyper Tyrosinemias

★ - ate & - ic acid are same eg pyruvic acid = pyruvate

★ Tyrosine is converted to DOPA (**dihydroxy phenylalanine**) by **tyrosinase** (or **tyrosine** 3-**monoxygenase**) in melanoblast and **tyrosine hydroxylase** in adrenal medulla. Both are different, so in tyrosinase deficient albinism, epinephrine synthesis is normal. Tyrosine hydroxylase requires NADPH & BH_4 (similar to phenylalanine hydroxylase).

Type / Features	Type I (Tyrosinosis) Hepato renal	Type II (Richner Hanhart syndrome) Oculocutaneous	Neonatal (Type III)	Hereditary	Hawkins-inuria
Enzyme defect	*Fumaryl acetoacetate hydrolase*[Q] Malelyl acetoacetate isomerase (+)	*Tyrosine amino transferase (transaminase)*[Q]	**pHPPA hydroxylase**	**pHPPA- oxidase**	**PHPPA oxidase**
			pHPAA = para Hydroxy phenyl pyruvic acid = p-OH-phenyl pyruvate = 4-OH-phenyl pyruvate		
Inheritance	AR	AR	AR	AR	AD
Clinical Feature	- Manifest in first 6 months of life (acute form) & cause death rapidly d/t liver failure - **Cabbage like odor**, hypoglycemia, vomiting, diarrhea, failure to thrive, rickets. - Major organs affected are *liver, kidney & peripheral nerves* causing cirrhosis, liver failure, ***hepato cellular carcinoma***[Q] (in chronic type when children survve beyond 2-10 years); **renal tubular acidosis** and peripheral neuropathy	- Ocular: *painful corneal erosions with photophobia* - Cutaneous: **palmo-plantar keratosis** - Mental retardation (mild to moderate)	- Transient relative deficiency of enzyme d/t delayed maturation or vitamin C deficiency - Transient hypertyrosine mia with normal liver function - Occasional mental delay	Biochemically similar to type III but differs in that it is - More aggressive & severe - Not suppressed by vitamin C - pHP lactic acid excretion is more - Death occurs before 6 months but those who survive later on develop 1. Renal tubular absorption defects like aminoacid /protein uria, hyper phosphaturia 2. Hypophosphatemic rickets, hypoglycemia 3. Nodular cirrhosis, **hepato cellular carcinoma**	- Transient failure to thrive - Metabolic acidosis in infancy - ***Swimming pool odour***[Q]
Urinarly excretion	- *Fumaryl acetoacetate* & its metabolite succinyl acetone - pHPPA and pHP lactic acid (PHPLA) - Tyrosine	Tyrosine & its metabolites *N-acetyl tyrosine & tyramine*	- pHPPA and its metabolites pHPLA and pHP acetic acid - Tyrosine, N-acetal tyrosine, tyramine	- Same with more pHPLA	Hawkinsin a derivative of pHPPA
Plasma tyrosine	6 -12 mg/dL	4 -5 mg/dL	-	-	-
Treatment	- Dietary restriction of protein especially phenylalanine & tyrosine - Substrate restriction using **nitisinone** in tyrosinemia type I - **Vitamin C** (ascorbic acid) in type III neonatal tyrosinemia				

Alkaptonuria / Alcaptonuria

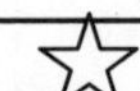

Etio-pathology

- It is *autosomal recessive (AR) inborn error (hereditary defect) in catabolism (degradation) of phenyl alanine & tyrosine* in which *Garrod's* classic ideas concerning heretable metabolic disorder was proposed. Other disorders of Garrod's tetrad are albinism, cystinuria & pentosuria.
- It occurs d/t **deficiency** of Fe containing liver enzyme **homogentisic (homogentisate) oxidase** also k/a **homogentistate 1, 2-dioxygenase** responsible for *cleavage of aromatic benzene ring* of homogentisic acid resulting in formation of 4-maleyl – acetoacetate.
- With lack of this enzyme, levels of *homogentisic acid increase in blood, and spill over into urine* and tissue. It is oxidized by polyphenol oxidase to *benzoquinone acetate,* which polymerizes and binds to connective tissue l/t pigmentation (ochronosis) & arthritis.
- **Vitamin C deficiency** (in premature infants) and experimental

Clinical presentation

- *Mild condition compatible with fairly normal life. Patients are usually asymptomatic* until about ***40 years of age***[Q]. However dark staining of diapers may sometimes indicate the disease in infants but usually no symptoms are present until later in life.
- Most striking clinical feature is ***blackening of urine on standing***[Q]

Management

- **Diets low in protein** especially in **phenylalamine** (< 500 mg/day) & **tyrosine** reduce homogentisic acid levels & pigment deposition (Lippincott)
- **Ascorbic acid (vit.C)** may prevent oxidation of homogentisic acid.
- **Nitisinone** [2-(2-Nitro 4-trifluoromethyl benzyl) 1, 3- Cyclo hexanedione], a drug used in tyrosenemia type I

application of α-α′-dipyridyl-chelating agent of Fe may produce alkaptonuria.

Homogentisic Acid —(Oxidation; Fe containing liver enzyme **Homogentisic** or **Homogentisate oxidase (or 1-2 dioxygenase)**)→ **4- Maleyl Acetoacetate**

Polyphenol oxidase ↓

Benzoquinone acetate

which is also the only sign of disorder in children. As other features develop after 30-40 years age.

- Classical triad in includes–"HOA"

reduces excretion of homogentisic acid in urine and *might prevent long term complications* of alkaptonuria, in conjunction with a low protein diet.

Homogentisic aciduria

- Patient's urinale contain *high levels of homogentisic acid* which is oxidized to dark (black) pigment on standing or exposure to air (sun light and oxygen).
- ***Urine turns black on standing***Q or air exposure when it also *becomes alkaline.* (Alkaptonuria meaning to suck up oxygen greedily in alkali)
- When urine is kept in testube *darkening starts from surface* and involves entire sample with in few hours.
- ***Benedict's test is strongly positive***Q and so is Ferric chloride ($FeCl_3$) test
- *Urine organic acid analysis* or specific *calorimetric test* detect homogentisic acid in urine.

Ochronosis

Deposition & accumulation of oxidized homogentisic acid (benzoquinone acetate) pigment in cartilage and collagenous connective tissue l/t **ochronosis**. This results in **black (gray-blue- brown), pigmentation** and (generalized) **darkening** of

- ***Sclera b/w cornea & canthii***Q
- **Ear cartilage** (concha, anthelix & fnally helix)
- Nose cartilage
- **Tympanic membrane**, larynx, skin, and heart valves.
- Skin (pigmentation) involving ***palmoplantar area***Q, dorsum of hand & feet, face & neck
- ***Intervertebral disc & large joints***Q
- *Pigmented renal and prostatic calculi (stones)* develop occasionally
- D/t pigmentation, valvulitis & calcification (of mitral & aortic) heart valves, the incidence of degenerative heart disease & MI increases.

Arthritis

Ochronosis also involves joint cartilage l/t arthritis which may be severely crippling. It

- Starts with pain, stiffness & limitation of movements of **large joints.**
- It involves **large joints of spine (intervertebral disc) followed by hip, knee & shoulder**.
- It resembles rheumatoid arthritis b/o acute excerbations, but **unlike RA small joints of hands & feet are spared**.
- Black pigment deposition at **intervertebral disc** f/b calcification. Radiological findings resemble osteoarthritis with characteristic ***narrowing of joint spaces & calcification of intervertebral disc***Q.

Maple Syrup Urine Disease (MSUD) or Branched Chain Ketonuria ☆

Biochemical Defect

Reaction	Aminoacids involved	Enzyme
Oxidative decarboxylation	**Leucine** (especially), **isoleucine, valine**	**Branched chain α-ketoacid dehydrogenase**

- *Autosomal recessive (AR) disorder* in which there is deficiency (partial or complete) in **branched chain α-keto acid dehydrogenase (decarboxylase) enzyme complex.** This enzyme is responsible for ***oxidative decarboxylation of branched chain α- keto acids – leucine, isoleucine and valine***Q.
- In MSUD, defect or **deficient decarboxylation of leucine, isoleucine & valine d/t deficiency of branched chain α-ketoacid dehydrogenase** enzyme leads to accumulation of these *aminoacids and their corresponding α-keto acids (α-keto isocaproic acid, α-keto- β-methyl valeric acid, α-ketoisovaleric acid) and α-hydroxy acids (reduced α- ketoacids) in blood (plasma or serum), CSF and urine.* Toxic effects interfere with brain functions.
- Unlike other ketoacidosis, **Rothera's test** is positive even in boiled & cooled urine.

Clinical Features, Types & Management

- Feeding problems, vomiting, dehydration, severe metabolic acidosis and characteristic **sweet maple *syrup or burnt sugar odor of urine***Q, which gives disease its name. If untreated may l/t mental retardation, physical disability & death
- Variants of MSUD are
- **Classic type** is most common & most svere, show symptoms with in first few days of life and lethal in first weeks of life. *Leukocytes or cultured skin fibroblasts of patients show little or no enzyme activity.*
- **Intermediate & intermittent** types have higher (3-15% of normal) enzyme activity. So symptoms are milder & of late onset (from infancy to adulthood)
- **Thiamin dependent MSUD** achieve increased activity of enzyme if given larger doses of thiamin.
- Early prenatal diagnosis (by enzyme analysis in cell), neonatal screening and life long dietary restriction is essential if the child with MSDU is to develop normal. Treatment entails strict control of diet, *restricting the intake of valine, isoleucine and leucine to the minimum required to permit normal growth.*

★ **Hartnup disease** is d/t defect in membrane transport mechanism of monoamino mono carboxylic (neutral) amino acids such as tryptophan by small intestinal mucosa & proximal renal tubule. Indole derivatives of unabsorbed tryptophan formed by intestinal bacteria are excreted. Large losses d/t intestinal malabsorption and failure of renal reabsorption **limits tryptophan availability for niacin biosynthesis** and accounts for pellagia like features.

★ **GM 1 gangliosidosis** is d/t defect in activity of lysosomal enzyme galactosidase resulting in pathological accumulation of GM1 gangliosides in lysosomes.

Catabolism of Branched Chain Aminoacids (BCAA)

- BCAA, leucine, isoleucine & valine are **essential aminoacids**. In contrast to most other aminoacis these are metabolized (oxidized) as fuels primarily by peripheral tissues mainy **muscles, adipose, kidney and brain** rather than by liver. Because these tissues contain aminotransferase, **absent in liver**, that acts on BCAA & produce corresponding α-ketoacids.
- **Branched chain α-ketoacid dehydrogenase** enzyme catalyzes **oxidative decarboxylation** of all three α-ketoacids produce their acyl CoA derivatives & release CO_2. This reaction is analogus to oxidative decarboxylation caused by pyruvate dehydrogenase complex & α-ketoglutarate dehydrogenase as all 3 enzymes are similar in structure, share same mechanism and cofactors – **TPP, NAD, FAD, Lipoate & CoA.** Defect in this step l/t **maple syrup urine disease.**
- **FAD linked dehydrogenation** (analogous to acyl CoA dehydrogenase of β-oxidation yields α-β-unsaturated acy CoA derivatives. Defective **isovaleryl CoA dehydrogenase** is a/w **seaty feet odor in body fluids**)
- **Methyl malonyl CoA mutase (isomerase)** enzyme and coenzyme **vitamin B_{12} (adenosyl cobalamine)** rearrang MMCoA to succinyl CoA. Deficiency of MMCoA mutase or B_{12} result in **methyl malonic academia & aciduria**, in which both propionate & methyl malonate are excreted in urine. Patient presents with metabolic acidosis, developmental retardation, symptoms resembling **ethylene glycol poisoning and death.**
- Leucine is ketogenic (yields acetyl CoA & acetoacetate); isoleucine is both ketogenic & glucogenic (yields acetyl CoA & succinyl CoA) and valine is glucogenic (yield succinyl CoA).

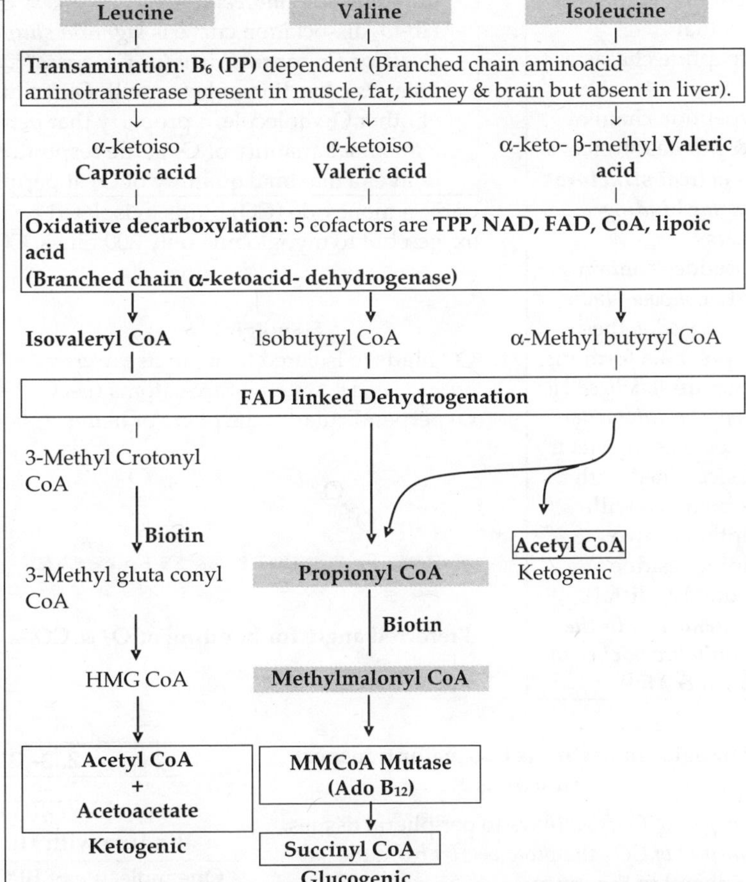

BCAA Disease	Defective Enzyme
MSUD (BC Ketonuria)	BCKA Dehydrogenase
Intermittent branched chain ketonuria	BCKAD (less severe)
Isovaleric acidemia	Isovaleryl CoA dehydrogenase
Hypervalinemia	Valine transaminase

Amphibolic Intermediates formed from the Carbon Skeletons of Amio Acid

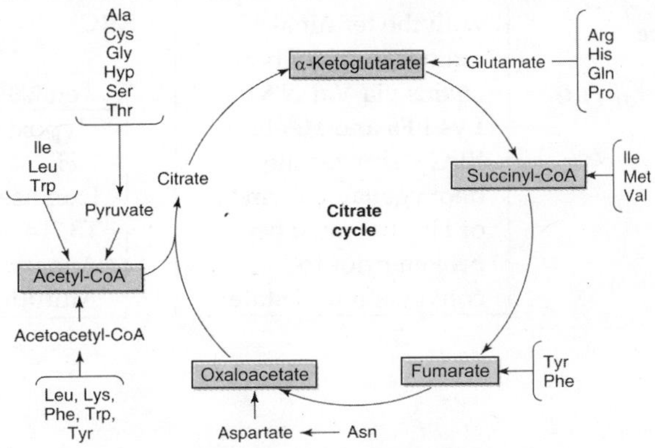

Comparison between Hb & Myoglobin

Similarities

- Single polypeptide chain of myoglobin is structurally similar to individual polypeptide chains of Hb.
- Polypeptide chain of Hb & Mb has stretches of ***α- helical structure* & *a heme binding pockets***[Q].
- Polypetides contain mostly *nonpolar amino acids internally*, these non- polar a.a forming a structure *stabilized by hydrophobic interaction*
- The heme group sits in a cervice, lined with non- polar a.a with exception of two histidine residue (Proximal & distal). Thus ***heme lies in the hydrophobic pocket in both Hb & Mb***[Q].

Differences

Hemoglobin	Myoglobin
- ***Tetrameric structure***[Q], consists of *4 polypeptide chains* - Can ***bind 4 O_2 molecule***[Q] - Hb-O_2 dissociation curve is ***sigmoid shaped***[Q]. - ***Positive Co- operativity (or Co-operative binding kinetics***[Q]: binding of heme with O_2 facilitates binding of other O_2 molecule, a property that permits it to bind a maximal quantity of O_2 at the respiratory organ & to deliver a maximal quantity of O_2 at peripheral tissue.	- Monomeric structure with *one polypeptide chain* - Combines with ***one mole of O_2.*** [Q] - Myoglobin –O_2 dissociation curve is → ***Rectangular hyperbola.*** [Q]

Carbon monoxide (CO) binds to isolated heme about 25000 times more strongly than does oxygen but to myoglobine only 200 times. CO binds to

Hemoglobin

CO binds to isolated heme in its *preferred orientation*, i.e, with all three atoms (Fe, C, O) perpendicular to the plane of heme

Preferred angle for bonding of O_2 & CO

Myoglobin

Presence of ***distal E-7 histidine***[Q]. Hinders binding or CO at 180° angle (Preferred angle) & forces it to bind in a less favoured configuration and reduce the strength of heme – CO bond.

Angles for bonding of O_2 & CO to heme iron of myoglobin

Hemoglobin performs two major transport functions

1. *Transport of O_2 from lungs* to peripheral tissues.
2. *Transport of CO_2 and protons (H^+)* from the peripheral to the lungs.

In Lungs

Binding of O_2 to deoxyhemoglobin cause release of protons (H^+). & this is responsible for the *Bohr effect*

Released H^+ combine with HCO_3^-, forming carbonic acid. Which is broken down into CO_2 & H_2O and CO_2 is exhaled out.

In Tissues

Binding of protons to Hb causes release of O_2.

In tissue ***increase in H^+ conc (i.e. ↓pH), decreases the affinity of hemoglobin for O_2***[Q].

2, 3- Di/Bi-Phosphoglycerate (2, 3- DPG)

Binding with Hb

- One molecule of BPG is bound per Hb tetramer in the central cavity formed by all four subunits. This cavity is sufficient for BPG, *only when the Hb is in the T form* (deoxy genated form)
- BPG forms salt bridges with the terminal aminogroups of both β-chains via **Val NA1** and **Lys EF6 and His H21**.
- BPG stabilizes the deoxygenated form (T) of Hb that must be broken prior to conversion to R state.

Feature

- ***One mole of deoxyhemoglobin binds one mole of 2, 3 DPG***[Q].
- 2,3- DPG binds to deoxygenated (T) form of Hb & binding of O_2 to Hb decreases the binding of 2,3- DPG
- 2,3- DPG decreases the affinity of Hb molecule for O_2 thus increase in DPG conc. *shifts O_2- Hb dissociation curve to right*.
- **Factors that affects conc. of 2,3 DPG in RBC**

↑ed 2,3- DPG	↓ed 2,3- DPG
- Hypoxia - GH - Exercise - T3, T4 - Anemia - Altitude high	- *Fetal Hb*[Q] - In bank blood that is stored→ less O_2 is released to the tissues.

Porphyria

Porophyrias: Are group of disorders *due to abnormalities in the pathway of biosynthesis of heme*, resulting in accumulation & increased excretion of porphyrins or its precursors. Depending on whether enzyme deficiency occurs in Liver or bone marrow.

1. Hepatic Porphyria

Acute Intermittent Porphyria

- D/t deficiency of ***uroporphyrinogen I synthase (Hydroxymethyl bilane synthase)***[Q]
- Porphobilinogen & ALA accumulates in urine.
- Urine darkens on exposure to light and air
- Patient are ***not photosensitive*** [Q]
- Abdominal pain & neuropsychiatric symptoms

Varigate Porphyria

- An acute disease caused by deficiency in ***proto porphyrinogen oxidase*** [Q]
- Protoporphyrinogen III & other intermediates prior to the block accumulate in the urine
- Patients are photosensitive

Hereditary Coproporphyria

- An acute disease caused by deficiency in ***coproporphyrinogen oxidase*** [Q]
- Coproporphyrinogen III accumulate in the urine
- Patients are photosensitive

2. Erythropoietic porphyria

Erythropoietic Protoporphyria

- D/t deficiency in *ferrochelatase*[Q]
- Protoporphyrins accumulates in erythrocytes, bone marrow and plasma
- Patients are photosensitive

Congenital Erythropoietic Porphyria

- D/t deficiency of ***uroporphyrinogen III synthase***[Q]
- Uroporphyrinogen I & coproporphyrinogen I accumulates in urine
- Patients are photosensitive

3. Both

Porphyrea Cutanea Tarda

- *Affects both liver and erythropoietic cells.*
- ***Most common type***[Q].
- *Chronic* disease caused by deficiency in ***uroporphyrinogen decarboxylase.*** [Q]
- Uroporphyrin accumulates in urine
- Patients are photosensitive

Treatment

- Medical support for pain & vomiting during acute attack
- *I.V hemin*: decreases synthesis of ALA synthase
- Avoidance of sunlight

Ingestion of β- carotene (free radical scavanger)

★ *All porphyries are AD* disorder *except* congenital erythropoietic porphyria which is AR

★ **Photosensitivity:** patients skin itches & burns (pruritis) when exposed to visible light (result of porphyrin mediated formation of superoxide radicles from O_2)

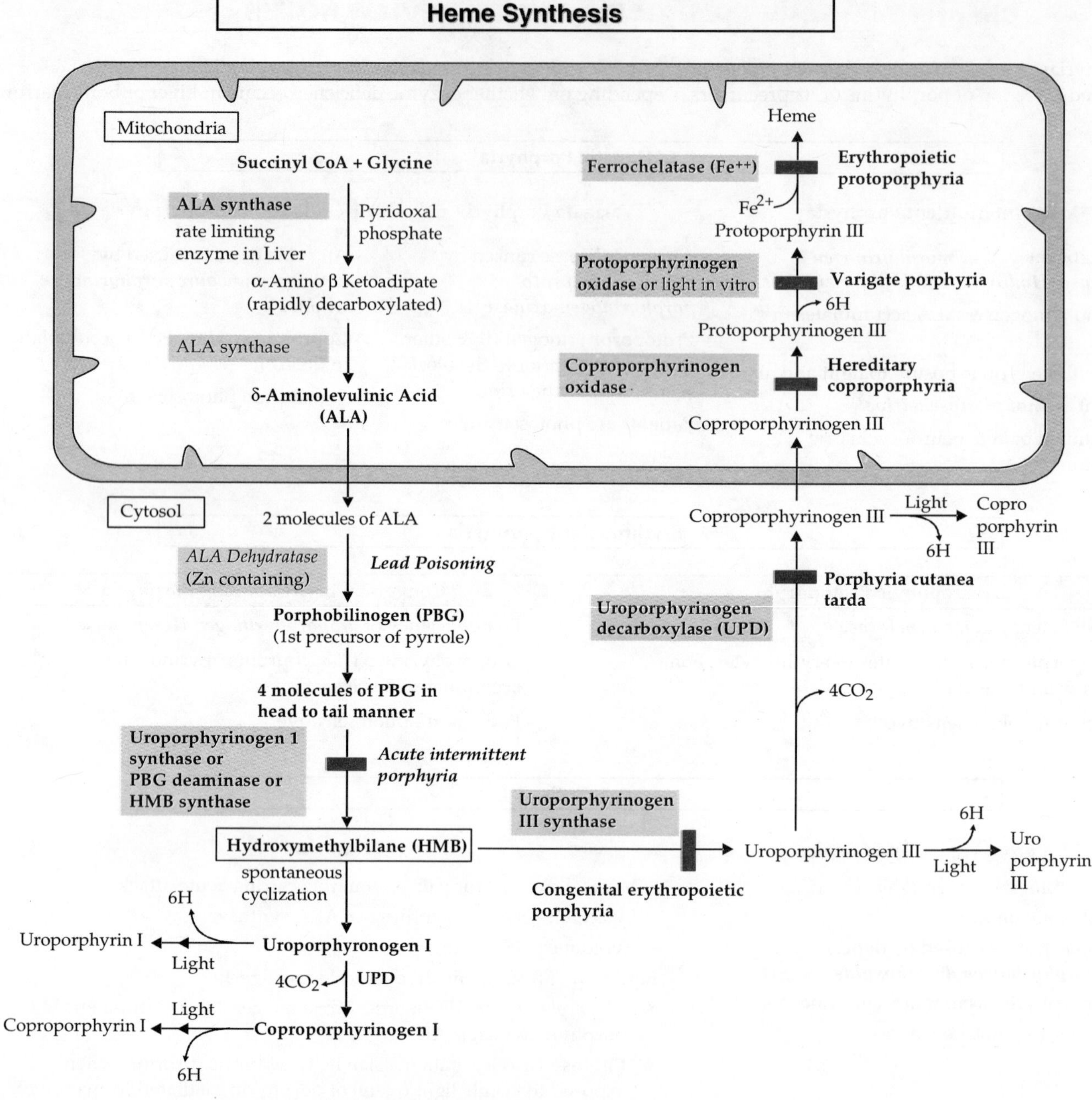

Site of heme biosynthesis are ***Liver & Bone marrow (erythropoietic cells)***[Q]

Chapter 7. GENERAL BIOCHEMISTRY: REVIEW NOTES

Acids

Monoprotic Acids (HA)

These donate *1 proton (H^+) per molecule*

Example include

- Mineral acids – ***HCl (hydrochloric acid) & HNO_3 (Nitric acid)***[Q]
- Monocarboxylic organic acids like ***formic acid (HCOOH), acetic acid (CH_3COOH) and benzoic acid***[Q].

Monoprotic Acids		
Formic	pK	3.75
Lactic	pK	3.86
Acetic	pK	4.76
Ammonium ion	pK	9.25

Polyprotic Acids

Diprotic Acids (H_2A)

- Can donate upto **2 protons** per molecule during process of ionization
- Can undero 2 dissociations (ionizations) & have 2 dissociation constants, first typically greater than second **(K1 > K2)**
- Examples include
  - Sulfuric acid (H_2SO_4)
  - ***Carbonic acid***[Q] (H_2CO_3)

Diprotic Acids		
Carbonic	pK_1	6.37
	pK_2	10.25
Succinic	pK_1	4.21
	pK_2	5.64
Glutaric	pK_1	4.34
	pK_2	5.41

Triprotic Acids (H_3A)

- Can donate upto **3 protons** per molecule during process of ionization
- Can undergo 3 ionization & have 3 dissociation constants (K1>K2>K3)
- Examples include
  - Phosphoric acid (H_3PO_4)
  - ***Citric acid***[Q]

Triprotic Acids		
Phosphoric	pK_1	2.15
	pK_2	6.82
	pK_3	12.38
Citric	pK_1	3.08
	pK_2	4.74
	pK_3	5.40

Different Types of Bonds

Covalent Bond

- *Strongest force* that holds molecules together
- ***Electron have opposite spin***[Q]
- *Each individual DNA strand is held together* by covalent bonds; but the two strands of helix are held together by noncovalent interactions (eg. Hydrogen bonds between nucleotide bases (Watson-Crick base pairing) & vandarwall forces.

Non covalent Interactions

While of lesser magnitude make significant contribution to the structure, stability and functional competence of macro molecules of living cells.

Electrostatic Bonds / Salt Bridges

- Occurs between oppositely charged groups with in or between molecules
- Comparable in strength to hydrogen bond but *act over larger distances*
- Facilitate the binding of charged molecules & ions to proteins and nucleic acids.

Hydrogen Bond

- It is the electrostatic interaction between the hydrogen nucleus of one water molecule and unshared electron pair of another
- Compared to covalent bonds, these are quite weak & requires ~ *4.5 k cal / mole* energy to break it (about *4% of energy)* required to rupture the O-H bond (110 k cal/mol)
- *Influences the physical properties of water and accounts for its exceptionally high viscosity, surface tension and boiling point.*
- In *solid state* each water molecule is associated with *4 other water molecules* and *~ 3.5 in liquid state*
- Responsible for *ice formation*
- Show phenomenon of *co-operativity*

Hydrophobic Interactions

- A tendency of nonpolar compounds to self associate in an aqueous environment. This self association is neither attraction nor bond (so hydrophobic bond is misnomer).
- It arises from the need to minimize energetically unfavourable interactions between nonpolar groups and water
- Contribute stability to the interiors of proteins.

Vandar Wall Forces

- Arise from attraction between transient dipoles *generated by rapid movements of electron* on all neutral atoms
- Significantly weaker than hydrogen bonds but potentially extremely numerous.
- Act over a very short distances (2-4Å)

Glutathione

- Reduced glutathione is **tripeptide thiol (γ- gluatamyl cystein glycine) consisting of 3 amino acids – glutamic acid, cysteine and glycine**Q. The glutamate is linked to cysteine through γ – carboxyl linkage. And **sulfhydryl (SH) or thiol group of cysteine, which accounts for its strong electron donating (nucleophilic) character of glutathione**Q, is the business part of molecule.
- Reduced glutathione is important reducing agent in the tissue, and can chemically detoxify hydrogen peroxide. The reaction is **catabolized by selenium (Se) requiring glutathione peroxidase**Q enzyme and form oxidized glutathione (glutathione di sulfide GSSG) which no longer has protective properties. The cell **regenerates reduced glutathione (GSH) in a reaction catabolized by glutathione reductase, which contains FAD as prosthetic group and uses NADPH as a source of reducing electron**Q.

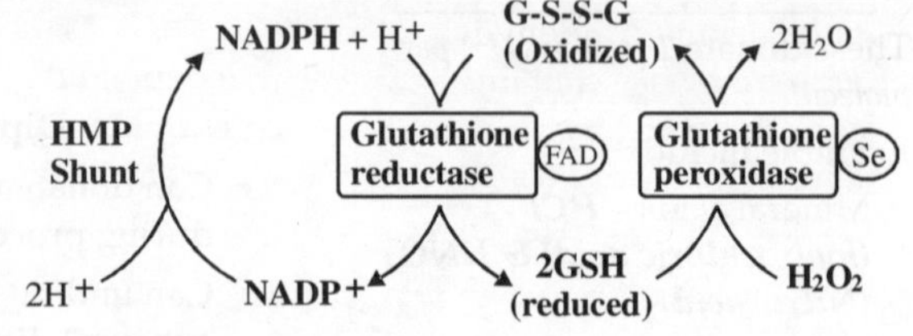

- Liver is the largest GSH reservoir and because of its reducing property it has potent **antioxidant action, protects from oxidative stress conjugates Xenobiotics, acts as carrier and coenzymes & cofactor**Q.

Xenobiotic metabolic conjugation

- Nucleophilic GSH conjugate with toxic electrophilic xenobiotics such as *carcinogens*
- **Glutathione S transferase** present in liver cytosol catalyze the reaction.
- These conjugates are ultimately excreted in urine as mercpturic acid which is formed by removing glutamyl & glycinyl group and addind acetyl group.

Antioxidant: protect from oxidative stress

- Accumulation of H_2O_2 may decrease life span of RBC by causing oxidative damage of cell membrane l/t hemolysis.
- ***Reduced glutathione removes H_2O_2 in a reaction catalyzed by glutathione peroxidase***Q an enzyme that contains the ***selenium analogue of cysteine (selenocysteine)***Q
- *In RBC, HMP shunt is the only pathway that produces NADPH for reduction of oxidized glutathion* (catalyzed by glutathione reductase)
- ***So G6PD deficiency impairs generation of NADPH, and l/t hemolytic anemia*** Q when subjected to antimalarial ***primaquin, aspirin, sulfonamides or fava beans (vicia fava – favism)*** Q

As a carrier: γ-glutamyl cycle

- It transport certain *amino acids* across membranes in kidney

Aminoacid + GSH → γ- Glutamyl amino acid+ cyteinyl- glycine

- The above reaction I catalyzed by **γ- glutamyl tranferase (GGT)** present in plasma membrane of renal tubular & bile ductular cells and in ER of hepatocytes.

As intracellular reductant

- Prevents oxidation of SH group containing enzymes eg glyceraldehyde-3-P-dehydrogenase
- GSH & glutathione trans hydrogenase cause reductive cleavage of S-S linkage of thyroglobulin glycoprotein

Acts as coenzyme / co factor

GSH acts as coenzyme with glutathione transhydrogenase, formaldehyde dehydrogenase, glyoxylase, maleyl acetoacetate isomerase, cyclo- oxygenase (PG synthatase system) and for liver enzyme for activation of methionine to form SAM.

★ ***Measurement*** of erythrocyte transketolase and its activation by thiamine diphosphate is used to ***assess thiamine nutritional status***Q.

Oxido-Redutase

In biological systems, oxidation (loss of electron) is always accompanied by reduction of electron acceptor. Enzymes involved in oxidation & reduction are called **Oxidoredutase** and are classified into four groups.

Oxidase

- Catalyze the removal of hydrogen from a substrate *using oxygen as a hydrogen acceptor*, forming H_2O_2 or H_2O
- Some oxidase contain Cu and others are flavoproteins

Dehydrogenase

- *Cannot use oxygen as a hydrogen acceptor*. They transfer H+ from one substrate to another, thus causing one substrate to be oxidized at the expense of another

Hydroperoxidase

Hydroperoxidase ***protect the body against harmful peroxidases***Q (which can generate free radicals). These are of 2 types

1. Catalase

- *use H_2O_2 as electron donor &*

Oxygenase

Catalyze the direct transfer & incorporation of O2 into a substrate molecule

- Dioxygenase incorporate both

- **Cytochrome oxidase/aa3** is a hemoprotein containing 2 atoms of *Fe atom* (that oscillates between *Fe^{2+} and Fe^{3+})* and 2 *atoms of Cu*.
- **Xanthine oxidase** contain ***molybdenum***Q; aldehyde dehydrogenase contain FAD, molebdenum & non heme iron; L-amino acid oxidase contain FMN
- Poisoned by ***CO cyanides and H_2S***Q.

- Useful in enabling *oxidative process* to occur in the *absence of O_2* such as during anaerobic phase of glycolysis and *as components of respiratory chain*
- These depend on nicotinamide coenzyme (NAD+ or NADP+) or riboflavin (FMN) or FAD
- Except for cytochrome oxidase, other cytochromes are classified as dehydrogenase.

electron acceptorQ & its function is assumed to be the destruction of ***H_2O_2***Q formed by the action of oxidase

- It is found in *blood, bone marrow, mucous membrane, kidney & liver.*

2. Peroxidase

- reduces H_2O_2 using various electron acceptors such as ascorbate, quinones & cytochrome C
- found in milk, leucocytes, platelets and other tissues involved in eicosanoid metabolism
- In erythrocytes ***glutathione peroxidase containing selenium***Q destroy H_2O_2.

atoms of molecular O_2 into the substrate

- Monooxygenases (mixed function oxidase hydroxylase) incorporates only one atom of molecular O_2 into substrate
- Cytochrome p450 are monooxygenase important for detoxification of many drugs & for hydroxylation of steroids.

★ ***Superoxide dismutase protects aerobic organisms against oxygen toxicity (superoxide anion free radicals O_2^-)***Q

$$O_2^{\bar{}} + O_2^{\bar{}} + 2H^+ \xrightarrow[\text{dismutase}]{\text{Superoxide}} H_2O_2 + O_2$$

Oxidative Stress

It is *accumulation of oxygen derived free radicals* due to inappropriate prooxidant – antioxidant balance.

Pro-oxidant

- These are chemical compounds or reactions capable of generating potentially toxic **reactive oxygen species (ROS)** or **free radicals,** which contain single unpaired electron in an outer orbit. These are produced by/in
- Absorption of radiant energy (UV ray, X-ray, ionizing radiation)
- ***Ischemic – reperfusion injury***Q induced by restoration of blood flow in ischemic tissue.
- *Microbial killing by phagocytes* and cellular aging.
- Enzymatic *metabolism of exogenous chemicals* or drugs (eg. CCl_4 generate CCl_3)
- *Reduction – oxidation reactions* of normal metabolism.
- Transition metals such as **iron (Fe) and copper (Cu)** donate or accept free electrons during intracellular reaction and catalyze free radical formation as in *Fenton reaction* (ferrous form is used)
- **Nitric oxide (NO),** can act as free radical and can be converted to highly reactive **peroxynitrite anion ($ONOO^-$)** as well as **NO_2** and **NO_3^-**.

Antioxidants (AO)

These are compound and reactions that *either block free radical formation or inactivate (scavenge) their action*. These include antioxidants

Naturally occurring AO

- Vitamins : **Beta carotene** (a type of vitamin A), **C** (ascorbic acid), **E *(alpha tocopherol)***Q.
- Zinc (trace element), ***selenium***Q
- Caffeine, epigallocatectin gallate = ECGg (in green tea leaves); *clorogenic & melanic acids* (coffee beans); curcuminoids (turmeric);

According to action

- **Preventive AO**: They inhibit chain initiation and initial production of free radicals

- Catalases
- Glutathione peroxidase
- Chelators of metal ions like

1. ***Transferrin, ferritin, lectoferrin and ceruloplasmin*** are storage and transport proteins that minimize levels of reactive Fe and Cu by binding them (and so OH- formation)
2. EDTA (ethylene diamine tetra acetate)
3. DTPA (diethylene triamine penta acetate)

- Used commercially (in vitro) as **food preservatives** to prevent lipid peroxidation (esp PUFA) & increase shelf life

- Propyl gallate (PG)
- Butylated hydroxy anisole

proanthocyanidines (grape seeds); polyphenols (apple); flavonoid querectin (apple & onions); ***lycopene (red tomato)*** Q; α-lipoic acid (yeast & liver); and lutein & zeaxanthin (egg yolk)

Synzyme (M-40403)

A *synthetic enzyme* that works like body's own scavenger anti oxidants (ex SOD) to mop up free radicals. This *manganese based* experimental product (for *treating stroke*) is *more powerful* than traditional antioxidants like vitamin E & C.

- **Chain Breaking AO**: They interfere with chain propogation
  - Superoxide dismutase both cytosolic & mitochondrial
  - ***Vitamin E (alpha tocopherol)***Q is most effective
  - ***Beta carotene***Q (a type of vitamin A)
  - Uric acid (urate)
  - ***Selenium containing glutathione peroxidase***Q
  - Phenols or aromatic amines
- **Scavanger** of free radicals
  - **Superoxide dismutase** (SOD), scavange superoxide anion ($O_2^{\bullet}$) and produce H_2O_2.
  - **Catalase** scavange H_2O_2
  - **Glutathione peroxidase** ***and reduced glutathione (GSH)***Q (Se dependent scavenge H_2O_2)
  - NADPH dependent Glutathione reductase
  - **Vitamin C, uric acid** and **polyphenols** obtained form plant food act as water soluble free radical trapping AO.
  - **Ubiquinone** & **Beta-carotenes** are lipid soluble radical trapping antioxidants in membranes & plasma lipoproteins.

(BHA)
- Butylated hydroxy toluene (BHT)
- Vitamin E

- Used as **therapeutic agents**

Dimethyl thio urea
Dimethyl sulfoxide
Allopurinol
Vitamin C
Vitamin E

Free Radicals or Reactive Oxygen Species (ROS) ☆

Free radicals or **reactive oxygen species (ROS)** are atoms or groups of atoms that have an unpaired electron and are powerful oxidants. These include **superoxide anion ($O_2^{\cdot-}$), hydrogen peroxide (H_2O_2), peroxyl radicals ($ROO^{\cdot}$), hypochlorite (HOCl) and very reactive hydroxyl radicals ($OH^{\cdot}$)** that react with proteins, nucleic acid, lipid etc.

Reaction & enzyme generating free radicals (and causing damage)

- ***NADPH oxidase (produce superoxide anion)***Q
- ***Myeloperoxidase (produce hypohalous acids)*** Q
- ***Fenton and Haber – Weiss reaction (produce hydroxyl radicals)*** Q
- Xanthine oxidase

- **Fenton reaction**:

$Fe^{2+} + H_2O_2 \rightarrow OH^{\circ} + OH^- + Fe^{3+}$

- **Heber – weiss reaction (iron catalysed)**:

$O_2^{\cdot-} + H_2O_2 \rightarrow OH^{\circ} + OH^- + O_2$

Reactions & enaymes scavenging free radicals (protective)

- **Superoxide dismutase** (SOD), scavange superoxide anion ($O_2^{\bullet}$) and produce H_2O_2.
- **Catalase** scavange H_2O_2
- **Glutathione peroxidase** (Se dependent scavenge H_2O_2)
- NADPH dependent Glutathione reductase

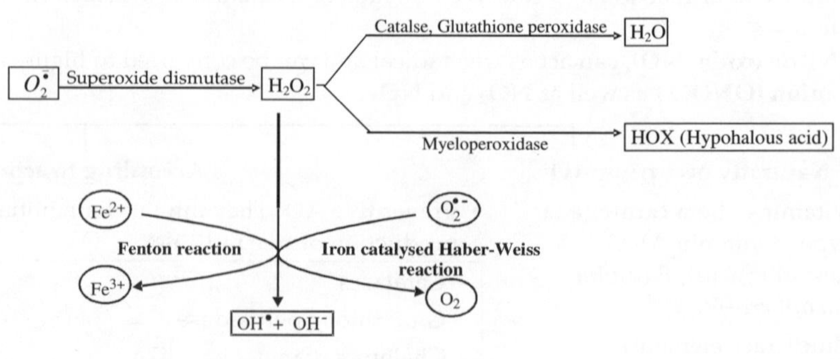

H_2O_2 – Myeloperoxidase (MPO) – Halide System

H_2O_2 – Myeloperoxidase (MPO) – Halide System is the ***most efficienct bactericidal system in neutrophils***Q. It has 3 components.

NADPH – oxidase

- Its activation (when phagocytic cell, engulf bacteria) is associated with *a rapid increase in O_2 consumption and metabolism* (the ***respiratoryu burst***) and *generation of superoxide ($O_2^{\cdot-}$) anion* by following reaction.

$$NADPH + 2O_2 \rightarrow NADP + H^+ + O_2^{\cdot-}$$

- There is only a lag of 15-60 seconds in phenomenon of respiratory burst. NADPH is mainly generated by **pentose phosphate pathway**, whose activity increases markedly during phagocytosis. Electron transport chain system – NADPH oxidase is composed of a hetrodimer polypeptide (of 91 KDa + 22KDa) **cytochrome b558**, located in plasma membrane along with two cytoplasmic polypeptides of 47 and 67 KDa
- Two molecules of superoxide anion spontaneously produce hydrogen peroxide (H_2O_2) by a process of spontaneous dismutation.

$$\bar{O_2^{\bullet}} + \bar{O_2^{\bullet}} + 2H^+ \rightarrow H_2O_2 + O_2$$

Halide & Myeloperoxidase (MPO)

- H_2O_2 generated by NADPH oxidase system (after spontaneous dismutation) is not able to efficiently kill microbes by itself. This is compensated by *enzyme myeloperoxidase present in azurophilic granules of meutriophils.*
- MPO is responsible for *green colour of pus* and act on H_2O_2 in presence of halide to produce **hypophaloius acids**.
- Cl- is the halide usually employed as it is present in high concentration in plasma & body fluids. And hypochlorite (HOCl or bleech) which is a powerful oxidant and is highly microbicidal is usually produced.

$$H_2O_2 + H^+ + X^- \xrightarrow{\text{Myeloperoxidase}} HOX + H_2O$$

(X- = Cl-, Br-, I- or SCN-; HOX = HOCl etc.)

- In normal tissue, HOCl combines with amine and form *chloramines*, which are less powerful oxidants and act as *microbicidal agents without causing tissue damage.*

- **Superoxide dismutases** tremenduously speed up the above reaction. This group includes both **copper-zinc superoxide dismutase** found in cytosol and **manganese superoxide dismutase** localized in *mitochindria.*

★ **Superoxide dismutase=SOD** (present in cytosol & mitochondria), **catalse** (present in peroxisome) and **glutathione peroxidase** (present in cytosol & mitochondria) protects cells from oxidative stress and damage in following way.

$$2 \text{ Superoxide anion } (O_2^{\cdot-}) + 2H^+ \xrightarrow{SOD} H_2O_2 + O_2$$

$$2H_2O + O_2 \xleftarrow{\text{Catalase}} H_2O_2$$

$$H_2O_2 + 2GSH \xrightarrow{\text{Glutathione peroxidase (GPO)}} GSSG + H_2O$$

or

$$2OH + 2GSH \xrightarrow{(GPO)} GSSG + H_2O$$

So intracellular **ratio of oxidized glutathione (GSSG) to reduced glutathione (GSH)** is a reflection of oxidative state of cell & its ability to detoxify reactive oxygen species.

Element /Mineral Requirement

Group 1: Components of **organic macro molecules** (carbohydrate, lipid, protein) which form 90% of solid matter

- Carbon (C)
- Hydrogen (H)
- Oxygen (O)
- Nitrogen (N)

Group 2: Major (Principal or Macro) Elements / Minerals

Are nutrilionally important and requirement **> 100 mg/day** The deficiency can prove fatal. The 7 macrominerals constitute **60-80% of body's inorganic** matter.

- Calcium (Ca)
- Magnesium (Mg)
- Phosphorus (P)
- ***Sodium (Na)***Q
- Potassium (K)
- Chloride (Cl)
- Sulfur (S)

Group 3: Trace or (Minor or Micro) Elements / Minerals

These are essential and required in **<100 mg/day** amount. Dificiency can l/t serious disorders

- ***Iron (Fe)***Q
- Iodine (I)
- Copper (Cu)
- Cobalt (Co)
- Chromium (Cr)
- ***Manganese (Mn)***Q
- Molybdenum(Mo)
- Fluoride (F)
- Selenium (Se)
- Zinc (Zn)

★ Cr & Cd are included in different groups in different books.

Group 4: Additional Trace Elements

Are possibly essential (necessary) but exact function is unknown

- Barium (Ba)
- Bromine (B)
- Cadmium (Cd)
- Nickel (Ni)
- Lithium (Li)
- Silicon (Si)
- Sn
- Vanadium (Vn)
- Chromium (Cr)

Group 5: Non-essential or Toxic Element

No known role and enter body through pollution or contaminants.

Non-essential elements

- Silver (Ag)
- Gold (Au)
- Bismuth (Bi)
- Rubidium (Ru)

Toxic Elements

- ***Lead (Pb)***Q
- Mercury (Hg)
- Aluminium (Al)
- Cyanide (CN^-)
- Arsenic (As)
- Boron (Bo)
- Cadmium (Cd)

Vitamin

Water- Soluble Vitamins

Differs from fat soluble vitamins in following ways
- Readily excreted once their concentration surpasses the threshold, so toxicities are rare
- Deficiency is quick on an inadequate diet as their metabolic stores are labile & depletion occurs in few weeks or months
- Are coenzymes so status can be assayed by measuring enzyme activities

Vitamin B complex[Q]

Energy releasing
- Vitamin B_1 (thiamine)
- Vitamin B_2 (riboflavin)
- Vitamin B_3 (niacin)
- Biotin
- Pantothenic acid

Haemopoietic
- ***Folic acid***[Q]
- Vitamin B_{12} (Cobalamine)

Other
- Vitamin B_6 (pyridoxine)
- Pyridoxal
- Pyridoxamine

Vitamin C (ascorbic acid[Q]**)**

Fat –Soluble Vitamins

- Vitamin **A** (retinol, β carotenes)
- Vitamin **D** (cholecalciferol)
- Vitamin K i.e.
  - **K_1 = Phylloquinone** (in green vegetables)
  - **K_2 = Menaquinone** (synthesized by intestinal bacteria)
  - **K_3 = Menodione** (synthetic compounds that can be metabolized to phylloquinones)
- **Vitamin E** (tocopherols)

Vitamin B_3 (Niacin)

NADP⁺ - Cofactor

- **Glu**cose-6-phosphate dehydrogenase (G-6-PD (glucose-6-PO_4 to 6-phosphogluconate)
- **Glu**tathione **reductase**

Either NADP⁺ or NAD⁺ - Cofactor

- **Glu**tamate dehydrogenase (glutamate → α-ketoglutarate + NH_3)
- **Is**ocitrate dehydrogenase (isocitrate → oxalosuccinate)

Mn- **"Glu³ Is MAL Gly Kit/Pit-PDC"**

All are **dehydrogenase** except glutathione reductase sounds like *"Glue in small gly pit/Kit"*

NAD⁺ - Cofactor

- **Mal**ate dehydrogenase (malate → oxaloacetate)
- **Al**cohol dehydrogenase (ethanol → acetaldehyde
- **La**ctate dehydrogenase (pyruvic acid → lactic acid)
- **Gly**ceraldehyde-3-phosphate dehydrogenase (glyceraldehyde 3P → 1, 3 diphosphoglycerate)
- α-**Gly**cero-P-dehydrogenase
- α-**Keto**glutarate dehydrogenase (α-**keto**glutarate → succinyl CoA)
- Pyruvate dehydrogenase complex (**PDC**) (pyruvate → acetyl CoA)

Vitamin B_1 (Thiamin) or Aneurine (i.e. relieves neuritis)

Chemistry and Mechanism

- Thiamin is a *basic substance* that has a *thiazole ring, pyrimidine & sulphur (S).*
- **Thiamin pyrophosphate (TPP)** also k/a **thiamin diphosphate (TDP)** is **biologically active & storage form** of vitamin B1 and is formed by transfer of pyrophosphate group from ATP

$$\text{Thiamin} \xrightarrow[\textit{TPP Transferase}]{\textit{ATP} \rightarrow \textit{AMP}} \textbf{TPP (TDP)}$$

- **Thiazolium ring**, the functional part of TPP, has a relatively *acidic proton at C-2*. Loss of this acidic (C_2) proton produces a **carbanion**, which is the active species in TPP dependent reactions. In other words, *C_2 in thiazolium ring of TPP ionizes rapidly, thus producing active species carbanion.* Carbanion readily adds to carbonyl groups (eg pyruvate) and thiazolium ring of TPP stabilizes carbanion intermediate by providing an electron deficient (electrophilic) structure into which the carbanion electrons can be delocalized by **resonance**. This **"electron-sink"** action of thiazolium ring facilitate *carbon-carbon bond cleavage adjacent to carbonyl group in reactions like decarboxylation of α-ketoacids (eliminating CO_2) and in chemical rearrangements in which an activated acetaldehyde group is transferred* from one carbon atom to another.

Deficiency

- Thiamin deficiency can l/t 3 distinct syndromes

1. **Chronic peripheral neuritis**
2. **Beriberi** (Singhalese word meaning weakness) occurs in areas where polished rice (lacking aleurone layer) is major diet. It is characterized by dry skin, irritability, disordered thinking, progressive paralysis d/t peripheral neuritis in adults
   - **Acute pernicious (fulminating) beri beri (or shoshin beri beri)** is c/b *high out put cardiac failure, edema and metabolic abnormalities without peripheral neuritis.* (**Wet beri beri**)
   - **Dry beri beri :** Peripheral neuritis & CNS manifestations predominate
   - **Infantile beriberi** occurs in infants born to thiamin deficient mothers and show tachycardia, vomiting, convulsions, death.
3. **Wernicke encephalopathy with Korsakoff psychosis** (W-K syndrome) is a/w thiamin

Physiological Role

- Thiamin has a **central role in energy yielding metabolism** and especially of carbohydrates. ***So thiamin requirements increase in excess intake of carbohydrates and its deficiency leads to decreased energy production***Q
- TDP (TPP) is coenzyme for **oxidative decarboxylation and transketolation reactions** such as

I. Oxidative Decarboxylation of α-Ketoacids

3 Multienzyme complexes that catalyze oxidative decarboxylation are **pyruvate dehydrogenase/PDH** (in carbohydrate metabolism synthesizing Acetyl CoA from pyruvate); **α-ketoglutarate dehydrogenase** (forming succinyl CoA from α-KG, in citric acid cycle); and ***branched chain ketoacid dehydrogenase*** **/BCKD** (in metabolism of **leucine, isoleucine & valine**).

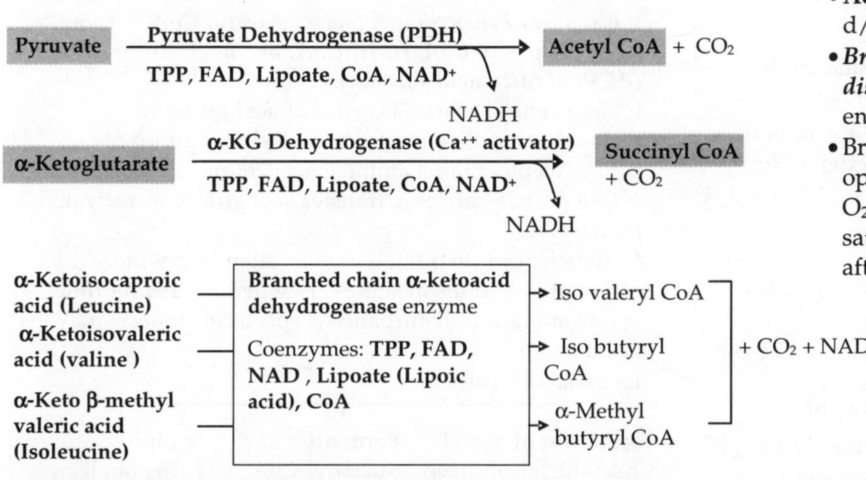

II. Formation and degradation of α-ketols by transketolase (transferring 2 carbons in PPP/HMP shunt)

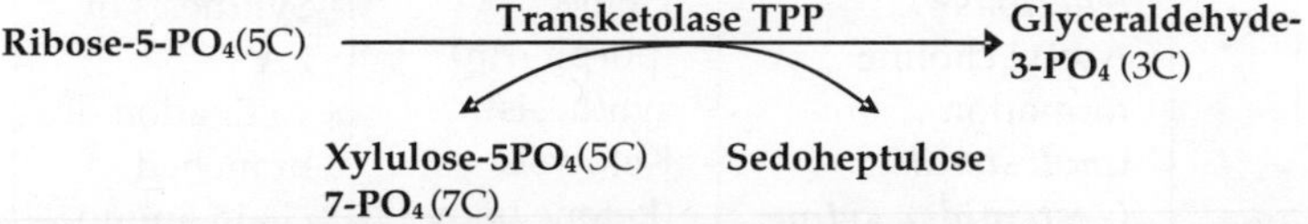

III. Reduction of pyruvate to ethanol (in yeast but not in humans): Fermentation /Non oxidative decarboxylation

Pyruvate —(**Pyruvate decarboxylase**, **TPP**)→ **Ethanol (alcohol)** + CO_2

deficiency in ***chronic alcoholism***Q & narcotic abuse. It is c/b ***apathy, ataxia, ammesia, nystagmus & opthalmoplegia***Q

- **Lactic and pyruvic acidosis**
  High carbohydrate diet in thiamin deficient subjects result in increased level of pyruvic acid **or pyruvate** (d/t **PDH dysfunction**) which is then converted to lactic acid thus causing life threatening **lactic acidosis.** Abnormal blood LA/PA ratio is a specific indicator
- **Decreased energy production** because acetyl CoA is not formed (d/t **PDH dysfunction**) and citric acid cycle is hampered (d/t **α-KGD dysfunction**)
- **Accumulation of pentose (5C) sugar in RBC** d/t retardation of transketolase
- ***Branched chain ketonuria (Maple syrup urine disease)***Q variant (d/t retardation of BCKD enzyme)
- Bracken disease, chastek paralysis, opisthotonus, **catatorulin effect** (i.e. decreased O_2 uptake by B1 deficient brain) and saturation effect (i.e. low urinary excretion after test dose in thiamin deficient) in animals.

Diagnosis

Thiamin (B1) deficiency is **best diagnosed by** observing an **increase in RBC *transketolase activity***Q on ***addition of thiamin pyrophosphate (TPP)***Q

Biotin (Vitamin B_7)

- *Biotin, carboxybiotin & biocytin (ε-aminobiotinyllysine* which require proteolysis to release biotin) is widely distributed in many foods and *synthesized by intestinal flora in excess of requirement. So dietary deficiency is unknown* except among people
  - Maintained on *total parenteral nutrition* for many months
  - Eat abnormally large amount of (>20) raw eggs per day. Uncooked egg white contains

Coenzyme in Carboxylation reaction (by Carboxylase enzyme)

- Coenzyme biotin serves as a *carrier of activated carbon dioxide in biotin dependent carboxylation* reactions. Biotin *covalently binds to ε-amino groups of lysine residues* of biotin dependent carboxylase (apo) enzymes to form *biocytin residue of holoenzyme.* This conversion is catalyzed by *holocarboxylase synthetase.* **1-N-carboxybiocytin** formed from CO_2 in ATP dependent reaction is the *reactive enzyme-biotin-CO_2 intermediate*, which transfers carboxy group to substrate.

glycoprotein **avidin** that tightly binds biotin and prevents its absorption from intestine.
- *Multiple carboxylase deficiency,* results from *defect in ability to link or remove biotin from* carboxylases
- *Congenital holocarboxylase synthetase* deficiency
- Deficiency of biotin l/t anorexia, nausea, glossitis, dermatitis, **spectacle eyed appearance** (d/t circumocular alopecia), and **Leiner's disease** (i.e. exfoliative dermatitis or erythroderma desquamativum in young infants)

- **Biotin dependent 4 carboxylase enzymes are**
  - ***Acetyl CoA carboxylase***Q : catalyzes Acetyl CoA → Malonyl CoA
  - ***Pyruvate carboxylase***Q : Pyruvic acid → Oxaloaceticacid.
  - ***Propionyl CoA Carboxylase***Q : Propionyl CoA → Methyl malonyl CoA
  - **3 Methyl-crotonyl CoA carboxylase:** 3 methyl crotonyl CoA → 3 Methyl glutaconyl CoA
- *Carbamoyl phosphate synthetase* (of urea & pyrimidine synthesis), *malic enzyme* (converting pyruvate to malate) and addition of CO_2 to form C_6 in purine ring are some biotin independent carboxylation reactions.

Pantothenic Acid (Vitamin B$_5$)

Biochemistry

- Pantothenic acid consist of peptide linked β-alanine & pantoic acid (dihydroxy-dimethyl butyric acid).
- Peptide linkage of *pantothenic acid to* ***β-merceptoethanol amine*** (which is obtained from **aminoacid cysteine**) forms **(4-phospho)-pantetheine**. This process requires 2 ATP (or 1 A TP & 1 CTP)
- Terminal **thiol** or **sulfhydryl (-SH)** group of *betamercaptoethanolamine in pantetheine functional moiety is the* **active site** where ***acyl groups are carried***Q.
- Coenzyme (Co) A is formed when pantoic acid moiety (of pantetheine) is linked to *adenosine 3′ phosphate* by pyrophosphate bridge (a process requiring *2ATP*)
- So CoA is a nucleotide and requires expenditure of 4 high energy bonds (ATP) in synthesis. It can be denoted as *CoA-SH to denote the active thiol site.*

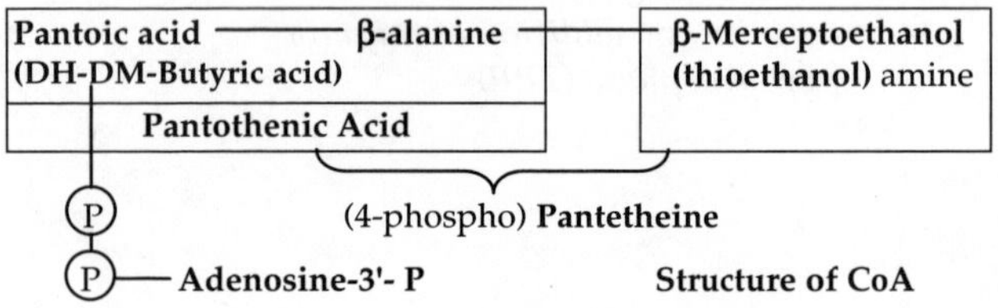

Pantoic acid — **β-alanine** —	**β-Merceptoethanol (thioethanol)** amine
(DH-DM-Butyric acid)	
Pantothenic Acid	

(4-phospho) **Pantetheine**

(P)
(P)— **Adenosine-3'- P**

Structure of CoA

- It is a ***part of coenzyme A (such as acetyl CoA, succinyl CoA, fatty acyl CoA, HMG CoA) and acyl carrier protein (ACP) of fatty acid synthase***Q
- It has a central role as a **carrier of acyl group** in metabolism. Active thiol (sulfhydryl-SH) group of betamerceptoethanol amine in *pantetheine functional moiety of CoA or ACP* carries & transfer acyl groups as activated thiol esters.
- Its deficiency is extremely rare as vitamin is widely distributed (Pantos means every where). **Burning foot syndrome**, sleep disturbance & spectacle alopecia may (±) occur
- Its metabolic roles are

Formation of acetyl CoA which is utilized in	**Formation of Succinyl CoA** which is utilized in	• Lipid metabolism
- ***Acetylation reactions***Q - Acetyl choline formation - ***Cholesterol (→steroids), ketone body & fatty acid synthesis***Q - Elongation of FA - Synthesis of ether lipids eg plasmalogen & PAF - TCA cycle, Detoxification	- Heme (porphyrin) synthesis - Ketolysis (ketone body degradation) by extrahepatic tissue - TCA cycle, detoxification - Gluconeogenesis, activation of acetoacetate	- β oxidation of FA - Synthesis of FA • Activation of branched chain amino acid such as valine & leucine involve CoA • Formation of adreno cortical hormones.

Vitamin B6 / Pyridoxine

- *Six derivatives of pyridine* have vitamin B_6 activity: pyridoxine (occurs primarily in plants); *pyridoxal, pyridoxamine* (in animal foods mainly) and their 5′ phosphates.
- ***Biologically active coenzyme is pyridoxal 5′-phosphate***[Q] which can be obtained for from all 3 precursors i.e. pyridoxine (alcohol), pyridoxal (aldehyde) & pyridoxamine (amine).
- *80% of body's total vitamin B_6 is pyridoxal (5′) phosphate* (PP) in **muscles** mostly a/w **glycogen phosphorylase**. *This is not available in deficiency, but is released* to become available in starvation, when glycogen reserves become depleted. Then it is mainly available in liver & kidney, to meet increased requirements for gluconeogenesis from aminoacids
- PP *terminates the action of steroid hormone* by removing the hormone receptor complex from DNA binding. So there ***is increased sensitivity to actions of low concentrations of cortisol, androgen, estrogen and vitamin D, which may l/t development of hormone dependent cancers of breast, uterus, & prostate and vitamin B_6 status may affect the prognosis***[Q]
- *Isoniazid, OCP, cycloserine and alcohol* may induce B6 deficiency.
- Vit B6 status is assessed by assaying
  - **Activation coefficient** i.e. *activation of RBC transaminase by pyridoxal phosphate added* in vitro.
  - **Xanthurenic acid index (tryptophan loading test)** i.e. *excretion of Xanthurenate (or Xandhurenic acid) in urine after a feeding test dose of tryptophan* is diagnostic of B_6 deficiency
- B_6 is the only water soluble vitamin with significant toxicity. **Sensory neuropathy** occur at > 200 mg / day doses (used to treat *premenstrual syndrome). Substantial improvement with some residual damage (i.e. recovery is not complete) occurs on discontinuation of vitamin.*

Physiological role

- B_6 is important in ***aminoacid metabolism for transamination, deamination, decarboxylation and condensation***[Q].

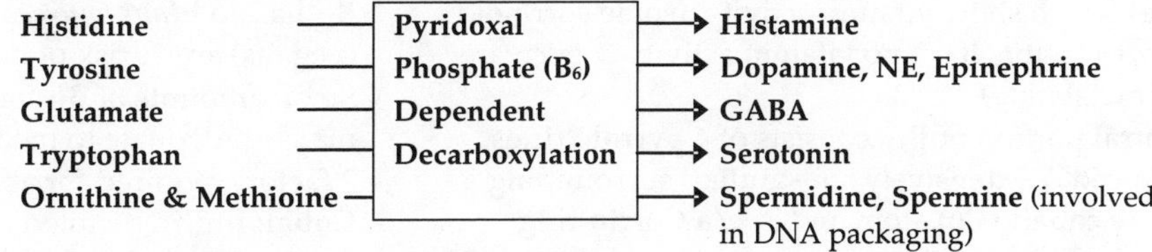

- So defective allergic response & gastric acid secretion (d/t histamine); deterioration of **parkinson's disease** (d/t dopamine); epileptic seizures (d/t GABA, an inhibitory neurotransmitter) can result from B_6 deficiency.

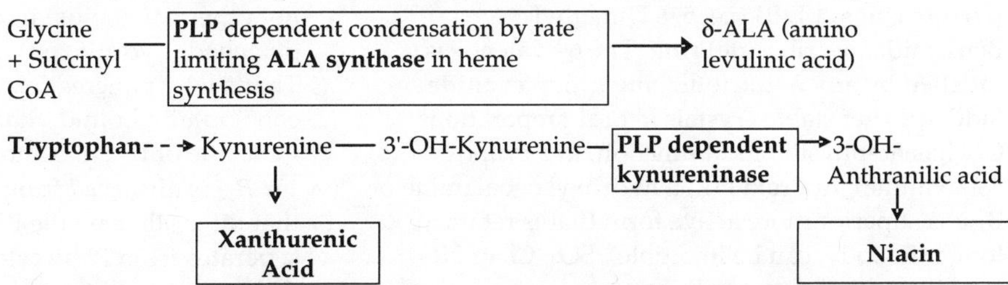

- B_6 deficiency results in (**sideroblastic** / **sidero achrestic** i.e. microcytic hypochromic) **anemia** (d/t defective ALA synthase in heme /porphyrin synthesis), **xanthurenicaciduria** and **pellagra** (d/t defective kynureninase). One vitamin (B_6) is necessary for synthesis of other vitamin (niacin). So niacin is not strictly a vitamin as it can be synthesized from tryptophan (essential aa) in body.

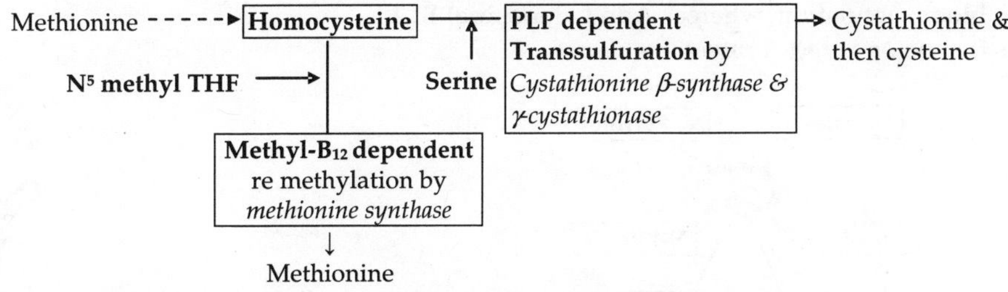

- B_6 deficiency cases **hyperhomomo cystinemia & homocystinuria** l/t cardiovascular diseases and **oxaluria** l/t **kidney stones**.
- B_6 is required in glycogen metabolism as *a cofactor (& constituent of) glycogen phosphorylase* (4 molecule of PLP per enzyme molecule)
- B_6 is required in *CoA synthesis, sphingomyelin synthesis (so def.causes peripheral neuritis d/t defective myelination), arachidonic acid* synthesis (from linoleic acid), intramitochondrial FA synthesis and K^+ transport (from out to inside).

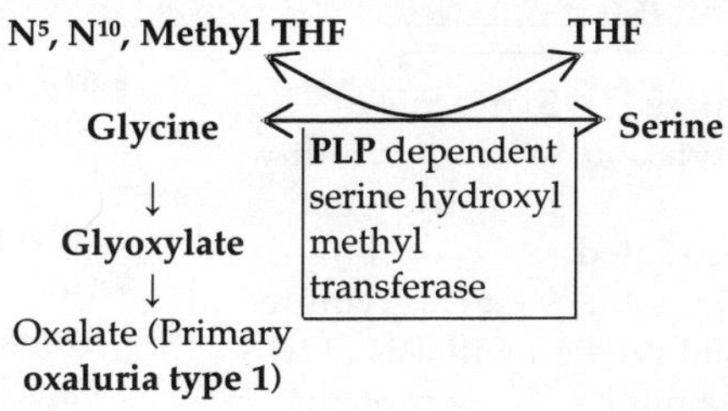

Vitamin B_{12} (Cobalamine, Extrinsic Factor of Castle, Animal protein/Anti Pernicious Anemia-Factor)

Structure

- Vitamin B_{12} or **cobalamins** are *those* **corrinoids** (i.e. **cobalt containing** compounds possessing **corrin ring**) which show vitamin activity. (some corrinoid growth factors have no vitamin activity & even are antimetabolite)
- Central portion of B_{12}, consists of **4 pyrrole rings** (reduced & extensively substituted) surrounding a **single cobalt (Co)** atom and is k/a **Corrin ring system**. This differs from porphyrins only in that 2 of pyrrole rings *(i.e. ring 1 & 4) are linked directly* rather than through a methene bond.
- **1 cobalt (Co) atom** (with 6 valency) is joined to **4 pyrrole rings, 1 DBI** (i.e. 5, 6 Dimethyl Benzimidazole riboside) **ring**. The 6th valency is satisfied by any of the following group **cyanide** (added to get stable crystals in oral preparations CN has no physiological function, k/a cyano-cobalamine); **hydroxyl** (k/a hydroxyl cobalamine or $B_{12}a$ is superior more active form that is retained longer in body; can be injectible), SO_4, Cl^- or NO_2 (i.e. nitro-cobalamine or $B_{12}c$)
- **Coenzyme forms of cobalamine** are methyl and adenosyl cobalamine. These are formed in body when 6th valency (like CN-) is replaced by methyl or 5[1] – deoxyadenosine group respectively. **Methyl-cobalamine** is major form seen in cytoplasm of cells & blood circulation, whereas **Ado (adenosine) B12** is the major *storage form seen in liver*

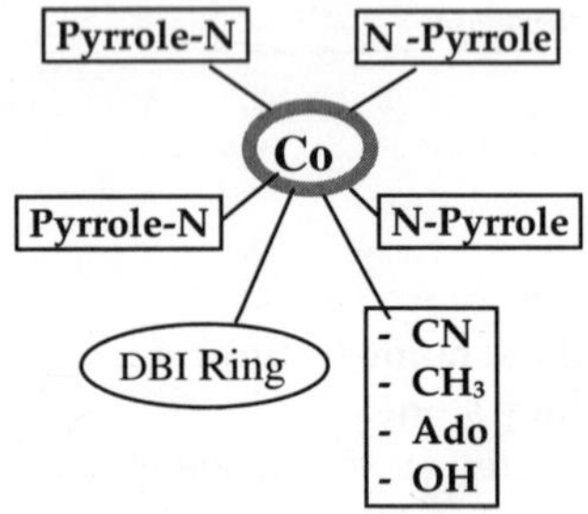

Source & Absorption

- It is synthesized exclusively by **microorganisms** & (for all practical purposes) ***found only in foods of animal origin***[Q]. Vit B_{12} has ***no plant sources***[Q] which means that strict vegetarians (vegans) are at risk of developing B_{12} deficiency.
- Small amounts of B_{12} formed by bacteria on surface of fruits may be adequate to meet the requirements
- 2 factors required for absorption of B_{12} are
  - **Cobalophilin** secreted in *saliva* bind to B_{12} when *gastric acid & pepsin* release the vitamin from protein in food.
  - ***Intrinsic factor (IF) of castle***[Q], a small ***glycoprotein secreted by parietal cells of gastric mucosa***[Q] (in cardiac end & fundus but not in pylorus) **binds only to active vitamin B_{12} vitamers** (and not other corrinoids) **in duodenum**, where cardiophilin is detached (hydrolyzed) from B_{12} by trypsin of pancreatic juice. That's why pancreatic insufficiency result in excretion of cobalophilin bound vitamin B_{12} causing its deficiency. 1 molecule of IF can combine with 2 molecules of B_{12}
- ***Vit B_{12} is absorbed from distal third of ileium***[Q] by receptors that internalize whole IF-B_{12} complex but not free IF or B_{12}. B_{12} seperates from IF by **releasing factor (RF)** secreted by duodenum, and Ca^{++}
- Vitamin B_{12} is transported in blood as methyl B_{12} with *trans cobalamin glycoprotein;* and stored in liver as ado-B_{12} with transcorrin in amounts sufficient for 2-3 years (an exception as B complex is not stored in body)

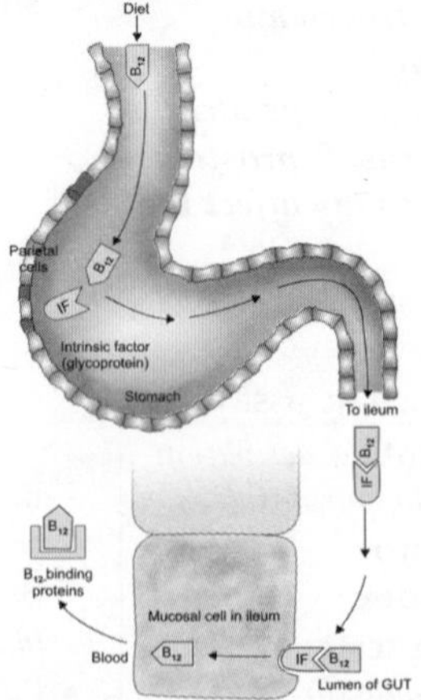

Absorption of Vitamin B_{12}

Functions of Vit K

Synthesis & activation of clotting factors

- Vitamin K is required in **hepatic synthesis** and **post translational modification** (by **γ carboxylation of glutamate residues**) of

Oxidative phosphorylation

- Being associated with mitochondiral lipid, vitamin K is a necessary cofactor in oxiative

Synthesis of calcium binding bone proteins

- Vit K is required in synthesis of two bone proteins. ***Osteocalcin and bone matrix Gla protein***[Q] that

Functions of Vit C (Acorbic acid)

- Main function of ascorbate is as **reducing agent** in different reactions because it can reversibly chang b/w ascorbic acid & dehydro ascorbic acid (reversible oxidation & reduction)
- Co-enzyme for **copper containing hydroxylases** eg
  - **Dopamine β hydroxylase** involved in synthesis of catecholamines (epinephrine & norepinephrine) from tyrosine in CNS and adrenal medulla.
  - Peptidylglycine hydroxylase, hydroxylating terminal glycine residue

calcium binding clotting factors (proteins) **prothrombin,** ***2, 7, 9, 10***[Q], ***protein C & protein S*** [Q].

- Vitamin K dependent clotting factors are **2, 7, 9,** ***10 and protein C & protein S***[Q]
- Carboxylation is inhibited by ***dicumarol (natural analog of vitamin K) and warfarin***[Q] (synthetic analog of vitamin K)
- Vitamin K ***deficiency l/t hemorrhagic disease of newborn (HDN)***[Q]

★ In presence of warfarin, *Vitamin K epoxide* can not be reduced to quinone (by warfarin sensitive reductase), but accumulates & excreted. ***A high dose of vitamin K is an antidote to warfarin overdose***[Q], which is reduced to active hydroquinone by warfarin insensitive enzyme.

phosphorylation.

- ***Dicumarol (vitamin K antagonist)***[Q] is uncoupler of oxidative phosphorylation

contain γ- carboxy glutamate.

- **Osteocalcin** also contains **hydroxyproline,** so its synthesis is also dependent *on both vitamin K and C;* and also its synthesis is induced by *vitamin D.* The release of osteocalcin into circulation *provides an index of vitamin D status.*
- Warfarin treatment in pregnancy 1/t fetal bone abnormalities (fetal Warfarin syndrome) d/t defective synthesis of bone calcium binding proteins caused by vit K deficiency.

- Co enzyme for **α-ketoglutarate linked iron containing hydroxylases,** in which hydroxylation of substrate is linked to decarboxylation of α-ketoglutarate examples are
  - **Proline & lysine hydroxylases** are required for hydroxylation of ***prolyl (proline) & lysyl (lysine) residues of collagen, in postsynthetic modification of procollagen to colagen***[Q].
  - Proline hydroxylase is also required in synthesis of **osteocalcin & C1q** component of **complement.**
  - **Trimethyllysine & γ-butyrobetaine hydroxylases** are required for **carnitine** synthesis.
  - **Aspartate β-hydroxylase** is required for post translational modification of precursor of protein C (a vitamin K dependent protease that hydrolyse activated factor V in blood clotting cascade)
  - *Vitamin C* is **antioxidant** (just like *vitamin E & β carotene*) and can decrease incidence of common cold; and some chronic diseases like cataract, *coronary heart disease & cancer.* Its deficiency 1/t **scurvy,** Barlow's disease (infantile scurvy), hemorrhagic tendency & poor wound healing
  - Help in deposition of collagen in bone
  - Maintenance of Capillary integrity
  - Help in Absorption of Fe
  - Prevent formation of *Atheromatous plaque*
  - Involved in Electron Transport chain: contribute to *microsomal hydroxylation reaction.* **[Mn : "C A T"]**

Vitamin A

Structure

- Active form
  - ***Retinol***[Q]
  - ***Retinal*** [Q]
  - ***Retinoic acid***[Q]
- Retinal is a ***component of visual pigment rhodopsin***[Q].
- **β Carotenes** are found in certain plants, cleaved to yield 2 mol. Of retinal

Transport & Storage

- Dietary retinal is transported as retinyl esters *in chylomicrons*
- Stored form is ***retinyl esters***[Q] mainly in liver & adipose tissue

↓ Zn

Mobilized form

Functions

- ***Vision***[Q]
- Maintenance of reproduction
- ***Antinfective***[Q]
- ***Antioxidant***[Q]
- ***Anticarcinogenic***[Q]

Deficiency

- Night blindness
- Xeropthelmia
- Impotence
- Growth retardation

Visual cycle in Retina

All trans retinol
↓
All trans retinal
↓
11- Cis retinal[Q]
↓ ← Opsin
Rhodopsin
Light ↓ → Opsin
All trans retinal

Prevalence criteria for determining the xeroplathalamia problem

Criteria	**Prevalence in population at risk (6 month –6yr)**
Bitol's spot	>0.5%
Cormeal ulcer	>0.05%
Serum retinal	>5%
Corneal xerosis	>0.01%
Nightblind-ness	>1%

Vitamin A Intoxication

Acute

- Seen after administration of >100 mg in children or > 150 mg in adult
- 1st noticed in arctic explores who ate polar bear liver.
- P manifests as ***increased intracranial pressure, bulging fontanels (in children), seizure, vertigo, diplopia, exfoliative dermatitis***Q *and death.*

Chronic

- Seen after chronic ingestion (for several months) of > *6mg/day in children or >15 mg/day in adults.*
- It manifests as
  - ***Pseudotumor cerebri***Q with increased TCP & papilledema
  - Vomiting
  - Alopecia
  - Dryskin
  - Cheliosis
  - Glossitis
  - Bone demineralization
  - Bone pain
  - Hypercalcemia
  - Hyperlipidemia
  - Lymphadenopathy
  - Liver fibrosis
  - Portal hypertension
  - Hyper lipidemia
  - **Teratogenic effects**
    - Amenorrhea
    - Spontaneous abortion
    - Craniofacial abnormality
    - Valvular heart disease

Vitamin D

D_2D_3 (Diet) + 7-OH-cholecalciferol (Skin) ← UV light
→ Vit D_3
↓ *25(OH)* *Liver*Q
25(OH) Vit D_3
↓ *1 ∝ (OH)* *Kidney*Q
1.25 $(OH)_2$ Vit D_3 [Active form]
→ ↑absorption of Ca^{2+} from gut
→ ↑mineralization of bone

- It behaves like a *steroid hormone*, binding to a nuclear receptor protein.
- **Deficiency:**
  - Rickets (In children)
  - Osteomalacia (In adults)
- **Toxicity:** Vitamin D is most toxic of all vitamins
  - ↑ serum Ca^{2+} → ↑BP; Vaso constriction; Calcinosis [soft tissue calcification]
  - Nausea
  - Stupor